Pharmacy

Drugs

Focus on Pirbuterol and Guanadrel
Patient Compliance
NSAID Interactions
Drug Photosensitivity
Vitamins in Psychiatry
Leukotrienes in Disease
Primary Oesophageal Motility Disorders

July 1985
Vol. 30, No. 1 (pp. 1-84)
DRUGAY 30 (1) 1-84
ISSN: 0012-6667

USA • UNITED KINGDOM • HONG KONG • AUSTRALIA • NEW ZEALAND

Drugs

Cumulated Contents Vol. 30, 1985

Leading Articles

1-5 *Higgs, G.A.* and *Moncada, S.* (Beckenham)
Leukotrienes in Disease: Implications for Drug Development

175-181 *Noble, J.T.* and *Barza, M.* (Boston)
Pharmacokinetic Properties of the Newer Cephalosporins: A Valid Basis for Drug Selection?

377-381 *Brandon, M.L.* (San Diego)
Newer Non-Sedating Antihistamines: Will They Replace Older Agents?

469-474 *Freis, E.D.* and *Papademetriou, V.* (Washington)
How Dangerous are Diuretics?

475-481 *Galko, B.M.* and *Rebuck, A.S.* (Toronto)
Therapeutic Use of Respiratory Stimulants: An Overview of Newer Developments

Drug Evaluations

6-21 *Richards, D.M.* and *Brogden, R.N.* (Auckland)
Pirbuterol: A Preliminary Review of its Pharmacological Properties and Therapeutic Efficacy in Reversible Bronchospastic Disease

22-31 *Finnerty Jr, F.A.* and *Brogden, R.N.* (Arlington and Auckland)
Guanadrel: A Review of its Pharmacodynamic and Pharmacokinetic Properties and Therapeutic Efficacy in Hypertension

85-126 *Carmine, A.A.* and *Brogden, R.N.* (Auckland)
Pirenzepine: A Review of its Pharmacodynamic and Pharmacokinetic Properties and Therapeutic Efficacy in Peptic Ulcer Disease and Other Allied Diseases

127-144 *Ward, A.* and *Holmes, B.* (Auckland)
Nabilone: A Preliminary Review of its Pharmacological Properties and Therapeutic Use

182-274 *Sorkin, E.M.; Clissold, S.P.* and *Brogden, R.N.* (Auckland)
Nifedipine: A Review of Its Pharmacodynamic and Pharmacokinetic Properties, and Therapeutic Efficacy, in Ischaemic Heart Disease, Hypertension and Related Cardiovascular Disorders

285-312 *Holmes, B.* and *Ward, A.* (Auckland)
Meptazinol: A Review of its Pharmacodynamic and Pharmacokinetic Properties and Therapeutic Efficacy

313-332 *Prichard, B.N.C.* and *Brogden, R.N.* (Auckland)
Xipamide: A Review of its Pharmacodynamic and Pharmacokinetic Properties and Therapeutic Efficacy

382-426 *Ward, A.* and *Richards, D.M.* (Auckland)
Cefotetan: A Review of its Antibacterial Activity, Pharmacokinetic Properties and Therapeutic Use

482-513 *Holmes, B.; Brogden, R.N.* and *Richards, D.M.* (Auckland)
Norfloxacin: A Review of Its Antibacterial Activity, Pharmacokinetic Properties and Therapeutic Use

514-538 *Todd, P.A.* and *Heel, R.C.* (Auckland)
Suprofen: A Review of Its Pharmacodynamic and Pharmacokinetic Properties, and Analgesic Efficacy

Review Articles

32-41 *Webster, J.* (Aberdeen)
Interactions of NSAIDs with Diuretics and β-Blockers: Mechanisms and Clinical Implications
42-57 *Epstein, J.H.* and *Wintroub, B.U.* (San Francisco)
Photosensitivity Due to Drugs
58-65 *Petrie, W.M.* and *Ban, T.A.* (Nashville)
Vitamins in Psychiatry: Do They Have a Role?
145-155 *Lambie, D.G.* and *Johnson, R.H.* (Wellington)
Drugs and Folate Metabolism
156-173 *Hosking, D.J.* (Nottingham)
Paget's Disease of Bone: An Update on Management
333-354 *Williams, K.* and *Lee, E.* (Sydney)
Importance of Drug Enantiomers in Clinical Pharmacology
355-367 *Behrens, B.C.; Young, R.C.* and *DeVita Jr, V.T.* (Bethesda)
Current Management of Hodgkin's Disease
427-443 *Brater, D.C.* (Dallas)
Resistance to Loop Diuretics: Why it Happens and What to Do About It
539-551 *Slattery, P.J.* and *Boas, R.A.* (Auckland)
Newer Methods of Delivery of Opiates for Relief of Pain

Research Review

444-460 *Levine, M.N.; Raskob, G.* and *Hirsh, J.* (Hamilton, Ontario)
Risk of Haemorrhage Associated with Long Term Anticoagulant Therapy

Practical Therapeutics

66-77 *Traube, M.* and *McCallum, R.W.* (New Haven)
Primary Oesophageal Motility Disorders: Current Therapeutic Concepts
78-84 *Peck, C.L.* and *King, N.J.* (Bundoora)
Compliance and the Doctor-Patient Relationship
275-283 *Oosterveld, W.J.* (Amsterdam)
Vertigo: Current Concepts in Management
368-375 *Anderson, F.E.* (Tamworth)
Warts: Facts and Fiction
461-468 *Ryan, T.J.* (Oxford)
Current Management of Leg Ulcers
552-560 *Mathews, K.P.* (Ann Arbor)
The Urticarias: Current Concepts in Pathogenesis and Treatment

Leading Article

Drugs 30: 1-5 (1985)
0012-6667/85/0700-0001/$02.50/0

Leukotrienes in Disease
Implications for Drug Development

G.A. Higgs and *S. Moncada*
Department of Prostaglandin Research, Wellcome Research Laboratories, Beckenham

In common with the prostaglandins, interest in the leukotrienes began with the discovery of a biologically active material which contracted smooth muscle. Both groups of substances are present in many pathological conditions but it was not until 1979 that it became apparent that they were derived from the same precursor. Feldberg and Kellaway (1938) observed that after challenging perfused lungs *in vitro* with snake venom, there was a release of a biologically active principal which induced a slow, long-lasting contraction of smooth muscle. Because of this they called it slow-reacting substance, or SRS. Production of SRS by other tissues following different stimuli indicated that there was a group of substances with this property and the SRS produced following immunological or anaphylactic challenge became known as SRS-A (slow-reacting substance of anaphylaxis). Interest focused on SRS-A as it was thought to be an important mediator of human asthma. By the early 1960s, major advances in the structural elucidation of the prostaglandins had been made but the identification of SRS-A remained elusive.

In 1969, Piper and Vane demonstrated the concomitant release of prostaglandins, SRS-A and a labile substance (now known as thromboxane A_2) during the anaphylactic challenge of isolated perfused lungs. Using a preparation of immunologically stimulated human lung tissue, Walker (1973) showed that SRS-A release was enhanced in the presence of inhibitors of prostaglandin synthesis. These experiments led to the suggestion that prostaglandins and SRS-A may be formed from a common precursor.

1. Synthesis of Prostaglandins and Leukotrienes

Prostaglandins are derived from arachidonic acid and other 20-carbon polyunsaturated fatty acids. The study of arachidonic acid metabolism in platelets and leucocytes led Samuelsson and his colleagues to the discovery of a number of oxygenated products which were produced independently of the prostaglandin pathway (Borgeat et al., 1976; Hamberg and Samuelsson, 1974). The formation of these products was catalysed by lipoxygenase enzymes resulting in the synthesis of hydroxy-eicosatetraenoic acids (HETEs). A major product of leucocyte lipoxygenase was found to be a dihydroxy acid with a conjugated triene structure (Borgeat and Samuelsson, 1979) and this led to the term 'leukotriene'. The 5,6-epoxide of arachidonic acid (leukotriene A_4; LTA_4), is an unstable intermediate in the formation of 5,12-dihydroxy arachidonic acid (LTB_4). Alternatively, the addition of glutathione to the epoxide by glutathione-S-transferase results in the formation of a leukotriene with slow-reacting properties on smooth muscle (LTC_4) [Murphy et al., 1979]. Removal of glutamate from LTC_4 by

γ-glutamyl transpeptidase gives LTD_4 which is further metabolised to LTE_4 with the loss of glycine (for review see Samuelsson, 1983). The major component of SRS-A is thought to be LTD_4 (Morris et al., 1980).

2. Leukotrienes in Diseases of the Airways

The release of SRSs in immediate hypersensitivity reactions has been studied for many years and the bronchoconstrictor properties of SRS-A are well documented (Austen, 1978). It is now believed that LTC_4, LTD_4 and LTE_4 account for the biological activity attributed to SRS. The peptide-substituted leukotrienes are 2 to 3 orders of magnitude more potent than histamine as bronchoconstrictors and contractors of isolated airway smooth muscle, although LTC_4 and LTD_4 are more potent than LTE_4. There is considerable species variation in response to the leukotrienes, with human and guinea-pig respiratory smooth muscle being more sensitive than rat, cat or dog airways. LTE_4 is generally less potent but has a longer duration of action than LTC_4 or LTD_4 (Piper, 1984). As well as a bronchoconstrictor action, there is some evidence that leukotrienes also stimulate the secretion of mucus and therefore might impair airway clearance (Ahmed et al., 1981).

Leukotrienes contract isolated preparations of tracheal, bronchial and parenchymal smooth muscle but experiments *in vivo* indicate that they have a selective action on the small airways. LTC_4 and LTD_4 induce a preferential reduction in compliance and are relatively less effective in reducing specific airway conductance (Drazen et al., 1980). When administered to normal volunteers, LTC_4 and LTD_4 caused coughing, bronchoconstriction, wheezing, tightness of the chest and a reduction in expiratory maximum air flow rate (Holroyde et al., 1981; Weiss et al., 1982).

It is clear, therefore, that leukotrienes can cause some of the symptoms of respiratory distress associated with bronchial asthma, and this, coupled with the observation that sputum collected from asthmatics contains leukotrienes (Kay, 1983; Zakrzewski et al., 1985), strengthens the argument that leukotrienes are important mediators of respiratory pathology. Furthermore, leukotrienes C, D and E have been detected in nasal washes of allergic patients following antigen challenge (Creticos et al., 1984). There is preliminary evidence that the leukotriene antagonist FPL 55712 substantially inhibits LTC_4-induced bronchoconstriction and cough (Holroyde et al., 1981), although when administered to chronic asthmatics, FPL 55712 was only weakly active (Lee et al., 1981).

3. Leukotrienes in Inflammation

The long search for the structure of SRS has led to the identification of a group of compounds with a variety of potent biological activities. It is ironic that LTB_4, one of the most interesting members of this group, has no slow-reacting properties. Furthermore, the activities of LTB_4 may well have implications in a wider spectrum of pathology than the respiratory diseases in which it was first thought that SRS played an important role. Turner et al. (1975) originally demonstrated that lipoxygenase products are chemotactic for leucocytes, and this led to the proposal that lipoxygenase activity in damaged tissues could represent a local control mechanism for the accumulation of inflammatory leucocytes. Since then it has been shown that a lipoxygenase inhibitor reduces leucocyte accumulation in inflammation (Higgs et al., 1979), and that LTB_4 is one of the most potent chemotactic factors known (Ford-Hutchinson et al., 1980).

There is increasing evidence that LTB_4 contributes to leucocyte activation in immediate hypersensitivity and inflammatory responses. In common with other chemotactic mediators (such as the complement fraction C5a), LTB_4 induces chemokinesis and lysozomal enzyme secretion from leucocytes (Goetzl and Pickett, 1980). *In vivo*, LTB_4 induces leucocyte accumulation in rabbit and human skin (Brain et al., 1984b; Higgs et al., 1981) and causes leucocyte margination in the microcirculation (Dahlen et al., 1981). The leukotrienes with slow-reacting properties do not induce these effects.

As well as being an important mediator of leucocyte activation, LTB_4 could also contribute to vascular changes in the microcirculation. Vascular permeability in rabbit skin is increased by LTB_4 and this effect is enhanced in the presence of other inflammatory mediators such as bradykinin and prostaglandin E_2 (Higgs et al., 1981). Wedmore and Williams (1981) demonstrated that permeability increases induced by LTB_4 and other chemotactic factors were dependent on circulating neutrophils. It is possible, therefore, that when neutrophils marginate in inflamed blood vessels in response to chemotactic stimuli they generate a factor which increases the permeability of the vessel. This could explain why circulating neutrophils are necessary for the formation of acute oedema (Higgs, 1984). LTC_4 and LTD_4 cause plasma leakage in the microcirculation of rats, guinea-pigs and hamsters but are relatively less active in rabbits (Dahlen et al., 1981; Ueno et al., 1981). In human skin LTB_4, LTC_4 and LTD_4 cause transient wheal and flare responses (Lewis et al., 1982), either by a direct action or through release of other endogenous mediators.

The synthesis of a number of lipoxygenase products has been demonstrated in human inflammatory diseases. Initially, high concentrations of 12-HETE were detected in psoriasis (Hammarstrom, 1975) and now LTB_4 has been found in rheumatoid arthritis (Davidson et al., 1982; Klickstein et al., 1980), gout (Rae et al., 1982) and psoriasis (Brain et al., 1984a). It now remains to be seen whether inhibitors of leukotriene synthesis or antagonists of their actions have any therapeutic value in these diseases.

4. Leukotrienes in Cardiovascular Disease

The release of leukotrienes, prostaglandins and other anaphylactic mediators from the lung could result in effects on the heart and cardiovascular system. LTC_4 and LTD_4 exert vasoconstrictor effects in the coronary circulation and it has been proposed that they may contribute to myocardial ischaemia and angina (Piper, 1984). There is also evidence that leukotrienes produced by blood vessels are involved in the local control of vascular tone. These ideas will certainly be the subject of future research.

5. Leukotrienes and Drug Development

In 1973, Augstein et al. produced a selective SRS antagonist, FPL 55712. With the discovery of the structure of leukotrienes, it has subsequently been shown that FPL 55712 antagonises the actions of synthetic LTC_4, LTD_4 and LTE_4 as well as a number of leukotriene analogues (Sheard et al., 1984). FPL 55712 does not, however, antagonise the chemokinetic effect of LTB_4 on human neutrophils or its contractile activity in guinea-pig lung parenchymal strips (see Sheard et al., 1984). The limited clinical studies performed so far with FPL 55712 have been disappointing, but this is believed to be due to a pharmacokinetic problem associated with this prototype drug.

We have proposed that inhibition of the synthesis of chemotactic lipoxygenase products could represent a new approach to the development of anti-inflammatory drugs. This suggestion was based on the findings that an experimental compound, BW755C, which inhibits both prostaglandin and leukotriene production, is also equiactive in reducing prostaglandin synthesis and leucocyte migration in experimental inflammation (Higgs et al., 1979). The inhibition of prostaglandin synthesis alone, by non-steroidal aspirin-like anti-inflammatory drugs, leads to a reduction in such symptoms as pain, fever and oedema. These drugs do not, however, suppress leucocyte accumulation in human arthritis and they do not modify the course of arthritic diseases. There is a possibility that a dual inhibitor of prostaglandin and leukotriene synthesis, such as BW755C, could extend the therapeutic action of aspirin-like drugs by limiting leucocyte mobilisation.

The pathogenesis of chronic inflammatory conditions is closely associated with the accumulation of phagocytic leucocytes. The release of lysozomal enzymes from these cells, after specific stimuli or cell death, contributes to tissue damage and necrosis (Davis and Allison, 1978). In some types of chronic degenerative disease, such as rheumatoid arthritis, the control of leucocyte accumulation could be an important factor in limiting tissue damage. BW755C reduced tissue damage in inflammation (Higgs et al., 1984) and myocardial infarction (Mullane and Moncada, 1982) and this effect was accompanied by a reduction in leucocyte numbers in the affected tissues.

Anti-inflammatory steroids do not inhibit the enzymes which synthesise prostaglandins or leukotrienes, but they do inhibit the release of arachidonic acid from phospholipids and thereby prevent arachidonic acid metabolism by both pathways (Blackwell et al., 1980; Hirata et al., 1980). This suppression of leukotriene as well as prostaglandin synthesis may explain why steroids provide a more comprehensive anti-inflammatory activity with non-steroidal aspirin-like drugs and also why steroids are useful in the treatment of allergic bronchoconstriction, whereas aspirin-like drugs are not. Thus, compounds like BW755C may provide a steroid-like profile of therapeutic activity without the toxicity normally associated with steroids.

The novel non-steroidal anti-inflammatory drug benoxaprofen (now withdrawn) inhibits leukotriene synthesis *in vitro* (Harvey et al., 1983) and it was thought that this activity contributed to its therapeutic activity, particularly in psoriasis (Allen and Littlewood, 1982). *In vivo,* however, benoxaprofen is a potent inhibitor of prostaglandin synthesis without affecting LTB_4 production (Salmon et al., 1984) and in this respect it is indistinguishable from conventional aspirin-like drugs. There are many reports of different compounds inhibiting arachidonate lipoxygenases *in vitro* but there are relatively few examples of lipoxygenase inhibitors with *in vivo* activity. In fact, only BW755C and dexamethasone have been shown to inhibit leukotriene production *in vivo* (Salmon et al., 1983).

The evaluation of the true clinical importance of the leukotrienes, therefore, awaits the development of drugs which inhibit their synthesis or antagonise their actions.

References

Ahmed, T.; Greenblatt, D.W.; Birch, S.; Marchette, B. and Wanner, A.: Abnormal mucociliary transport in allergic patients with antigen-induced bronchospasm: Role of slow reacting substance of anaphylaxis. American Review of Respiratory Disease 124: 110-114 (1981).

Allen, B.R. and Littlewood, S.M.: Benoxaprofen: Effect on cutaneous lesions in psoriasis. Brit. Med. J. 285: 1241 (1982).

Augstein, J.; Farmer, J.B.; Lee, T.B.; Sheard, P. and Tattersall, M.L.: Selective inhibitor of slow reacting substance of anaphylaxis. Nature – New Biology 245: 215-217 (1973).

Austen, K.: Homeostasis of effector systems which can also be recruited for immunologic reactions. Journal of Immunology 121: 798-805 (1978).

Blackwell, G.J.; Carnuccio, R.; Di Rosa, M.; Flower, R.J.; Parente, L. and Persico, P.: Macrocortin: A polypeptide causing the antiphospholipase effect of glucocorticoids. Nature 287: 147-149 (1980).

Borgeat, P.; Hamberg, M. and Samuelsson, B.: Transformation of arachidonic acid and dihomo-γ-linolenic acid by polymorphonuclear leukocytes. Journal of Biological Chemistry 251: 7816-7820 (1976).

Borgeat, P. and Samuelsson, B.: Arachidonic acid metabolism in polymorphonuclear leukocytes. Effects of ionophore A23187. Proceedings of the National Academy of Sciences, USA 76: 2148-2152 (1979).

Brain, S.D.; Camp, R.D.R.; Cunningham, F.M.; Dowd, P.M.; Greaves, M.W. and Black, A.K.: Leukotriene B_4-like material in scale of psoriatic skin lesions. British Journal of Pharmacology 83: 313-317 (1984a).

Brain, S.D.; Camp, R.D.; Greaves, M.W.; Russell Jones, R. and Woollard, P.M.: The inflammatory responses of human skin to topical application of leukotriene B_4. British Journal of Clinical Pharmacology 17: 610P-611P (1984b).

Creticos, P.S.; Peters, S.P.; Adkinson Jr, N.F.; Naclerio, R.M.; Hayes, E.C.; Norman, P.S. and Lichtenstein, L.M.: Peptide leukotriene release after antigen challenge in patients sensitive to ragweed. New England Journal of Medicine 310: 1626-1630 (1984).

Dahlen, S.E.; Bjork, J.; Hedqvist, P.; Arfors, K-E.; Hammarstrom, S.; Lindgren, J.A. and Samuelsson, B.: Leukotrienes promote plasma leakage and leukocyte adhesion in postcapillary venules: *In vivo* effects with relevance to the acute inflammatory response. Proceedings of the National Academy of Sciences, USA 78: 3887-3891 (1981).

Davidson, E.M.; Rae, S.A. and Smith, M.J.H.: Leukotriene B_4 in synovial fluid. Journal of Pharmacy and Pharmacology 34: 410 (1982).

Davis, P. and Allison, A.C.: The release of hydrolytic enzymes from phagocytic and other cells participating in acute and chronic inflammation; in Vane and Ferreira (Eds) Inflammation, Handbook of Experimental Pharmacology, 50/I, pp. 267-294 (Springer, New York 1978).

Drazen, J.M.; Austen, K.F.; Lewis, R.A.; Clark, D.A.; Goto, G.; Marfat, A. and Corey, E.J.: Comparative airway and vascular activities of leukotrienes C-1 and D *in vivo* and *in vitro.* Proceedings of the National Academy of Sciences, USA 77: 4354-4358 (1980).

Feldberg, W. and Kellaway, C.H.: Liberation of histamine and formation of lysocithin-like substances by cobra venom. Journal of Physiology 94: 187-226 (1938).

Ford-Hutchinson, A.W.; Bray, M.A.; Doig, M.V.; Shipley, M.E. and Smith, M.J.H.: Leukotriene B, a potent chemokinetic and aggregating substance released from polymorphonuclear leukocytes. Nature 286: 264-265 (1980).

Goetzl, E.J. and Pickett, W.C.: The human PMN leukocyte chemotactic activity of complex hydroxy-eicosatetraenoic acids (HETEs). Journal of Immunology, 125: 1789-1791 (1980).

Hamberg, M. and Samuelsson, B.: Prostaglandin endoperoxides. Novel transformations of arachidonic acid in human platelets. Proceedings of the National Academy of Sciences, USA 71: 3400-3404 (1974).

Hammarstrom, S.; Hamberg, M.; Samuelsson, B.; Duell, E.A.; Stawiski, M. and Voorhees, J.: Increased concentrations of free arachidonic acid, prostaglandins E_2 and $F_{2\alpha}$ and of 12L hydroxy-5,8,10,14-eicosatetraenoic acid (HETE) in epidermis of psoriasis: Evidence for perturbed regulation of arachidonic acid levels in psoriasis. Proceedings of the National Academy of Sciences, USA 72: 5130-5134 (1975).

Harvey, J.; Parish, H.; Ho, P.P.K.; Boot, J.R. and Dawson, W.: The preferential inhibition of 5′-lipoxygenase product formation by benoxaprofen. Journal of Pharmacy and Pharmacology 35: 44-45 (1983).

Higgs, G.A.: Acute oedema formation in neutropaenic rats. Proceedings of the 9th International Congress of Pharmacology, London, Abstract 445 (1984).

Higgs, G.A.; Flower, R.J. and Vane, J.R.: A new approach to anti-inflammatory drugs. Biochemical Pharmacology 28: 1959-1961 (1979).

Higgs, G.A.; Mugridge, K.G.; Moncada, S. and Vane, J.R.: Inhibition of tissue damage by the arachidonate lipoxygenase inhibitor BW 755C. Proceedings of the National Academy of Sciences, USA 81: 2890-2892 (1984).

Higgs, G.A.; Salmon, J.A. and Spayne, J.A.: The inflammatory effects of hydroperoxy and hydroxy acid products of arachidonate lipoxygenase in rabbit skin. British Journal of Pharmacology 74: 429-433 (1981).

Hirata, F.; Schiffmann, E.; Venkatasubramanian, K.; Salomon, D. and Axelrod, J.: A phospholipase A_2 inhibitory protein in rabbit neutrophils induced by glucocorticoids. Proceedings of the National Academy of Sciences, USA 77: 2533-2536 (1980).

Holroyde, M.C.; Altounyan, R.E.C.; Cole, M.; Dixon, M. and Elliott, E.V.: Bronchoconstriction produced in man by leukotrienes C and D. Lancet 2: 17-18 (1981).

Kay, A.B.: The sputum in bronchial asthma; in Clark and Godfrey (Eds) Asthma pp. 99-110 (Chapman and Hall, London 1983).

Klickstein, L.B.; Shapleigh, C. and Goetzl, E.J.: Lipoxygenation of arachidonic acid as a source of polymorphonuclear leukocyte chemotactic factors in synovial fluid and tissue in rheumatoid arthritis and spondyloarthritis. Journal of Clinical Investigation 66: 1166-1170 (1980).

Lee, T.H.; Walport, M.J.; Wilkinson, A.H.; Turner-Warick, M. and Kay, A.B.: Slow reacting substance of anaphylaxis antagonist. FPL 55712 in chronic asthma. Lancet 2: 304-305 (1981).

Lewis, R.A.; Austen, K.F.; Drazen, J.M.; Soter, N.A.; Figueiredo, J.C. and Corey, E.J.; Structure, function and metabolism of leukotriene constituents of SRS-A; in Samuelsson and Paoletti (Eds) Advances in Prostaglandin, Thromboxane and Leukotriene Research, pp. 137-151 (Raven Press, New York 1982).

Morris, H.R.; Taylor, G.W.; Piper, P.J. and Tippins, J.R.: Slow reacting substance of anaphylaxis from guinea-pig lung. Nature 285: 104-106 (1980).

Mullane, K.M. and Moncada, S.: The salvage of ischaemic myocardium by BW 755C in anaesthetised dogs. Prostaglandins 24: 255-266 (1982).

Murphy, R.C.; Hammarstrom, S. and Samuelsson, B.: Leukotriene C.: A slow reacting substance from murine mastocytoma cells. Proceedings of the National Academy of Sciences, USA 76: 4275-4279 (1979).

Piper, P.J.: Leukotrienes; in Buckle and Smith (Eds) Development of Anti-Asthmatic Drugs, pp. 55-72 (Butterworths, London 1984).

Piper, P.J. and Vane, J.R.: The release of additional factors in anaphylaxis and its antagonism by anti-inflammatory drugs. Nature 223: 29-35 (1969).

Rae, S.A.; Davidson, E.M. and Smith, M.J.H.: Leukotriene B_4, an inflammatory mediator in gout. Lancet 2: 1122-1124 (1982).

Salmon, J.A.; Higgs, G.A.; Tilling, L.; Moncada, S. and Vane, J.R.: Mode of action of benoxaprofen. Lancet 1: 848 (1984).

Salmon, J.A.; Simmons, P.M. and Moncada, S.: The effects of BW 755C and other anti-inflammatory drugs on eicosanoid concentrations and leukocyte accumulation in experimentally-induced acute inflammation. Journal of Pharmacy and Pharmacology 35: 808-813 (1983).

Samuelsson, B.: Leukotrienes: Mediators of immediate hypersensitivity reactions and inflammation. Science 220: 568-575 (1983).

Sheard, P.; Holroyde, M.C.; Bantinck, J.R. and Lee, J.B.: SRS-A antagonists; in Buckle and Smith (Eds) Development of Anti-Asthmatic Drugs, pp. 133-158 (Butterworths, London 1984).

Turner, S.R.; Tainer, J.A. and Lynn, W.S.: Biogenesis of chemotactic molecules by the arachidonate lipoxygenase system in platelets. Nature 257: 680-681 (1975).

Ueno, A.; Tanaka, K.; Katori, M.; Hayashi, M. and Arai, Y.: Species difference in increased vascular permeability by synthetic leukotrienes C_4 and D_4. Prostaglandins 21: 637-648 (1981).

Walker, J.L.: The regulatory function of prostaglandins in the release of histamine and SRS-A from passively sensitized human lung tissue; in Bergstrom and Bernhard (Eds) Advances in the Biosciences 9, 235-240 (Pergamon, Vieweg 1973).

Wedmore, C.V. and Williams, T.J.: Control of vascular permeability by polymorphonuclear leukocytes in inflammation. Nature 289: 646-650 (1981).

Weiss, J.W.; Drazen, J.M.; Coles, N.; McFadden, E.R.; Weller, P.W.; Corey, E.J.; Lewis, R.A. and Austen, K.F.: Bronchoconstrictor effects of leukotriene C in humans. Science 216: 196-198 (1982).

Zakrzewski, J.T.; Barnes, N.C.; Piper, P.J. and Costello, J.F.: Quantitation of leukotrienes in asthmatic sputum. British Journal of Pharmacology 19: 574P (1985).

Address for correspondence and reprints: Dr *G.A. Higgs*, Department of Prostaglandin Research, Wellcome Research Laboratories, Langley Court, Beckenham, Kent BR3 3BS (England).

Drugs 30: 6-21 (1985)
0012-6667/85/0700-0006/$08.00/0

Pirbuterol
A Preliminary Review of its Pharmacological Properties and Therapeutic Efficacy in Reversible Bronchospastic Disease

D.M. Richards and *R.N. Brogden*

ADIS Drug Information Services, Auckland

Various sections of the manuscript reviewed by: ***W.S. Colucci,*** Department of Medicine, Brigham and Women's Hospital, Boston, Massachusetts, USA; ***R.T. Jackson,*** Section of Otolaryngology, The Emory Clinic, Emory University School of Medicine, Atlanta, Georgia, USA; ***J.W. Jenne,*** Pulmonary Section, Veterans Administration Hospital, Hines, Illinois, USA; ***A.D. Mackay,*** Department of Respiratory Physiology, City General Hospital, Stoke-on-Trent, UK; ***H.S. Nelson,*** Allergy-Immunology Service, Fitzsimons Army Medical Center, Aurora, Colorado, USA; ***N. Weiner,*** Department of Pharmacology, University of Colorado School of Medicine, Denver, Colorado, USA.

Contents

Summary 7
1. Pharmacodynamic Studies 8
   1.1 β-Adrenoceptor Selectivity 8
      1.1.1 *In vitro* Selectivity Studies 8
      1.1.2 Animal Studies 9
   1.2 Bronchial Effects 9
      1.2.1 Studies in Asthmatic Volunteers 9
      1.2.2 Animal Studies 9
   1.3 Cardiovascular Effects 10
      1.3.1 Studies in Healthy Volunteers 10
      1.3.2 Studies in Patients with Pulmonary Diseases 10
      1.3.3 Studies in Patients with Congestive Heart Failure 11
   1.4 Carcinogenicity Studies 12
2. Pharmacokinetic Studies 12
   2.1 Absorption 12
   2.2 Metabolism and Excretion 13
3. Therapeutic Trials in Reversible Airflow Obstruction 13
   3.1 Single-Dose Studies 13
      3.1.1 Aerosol Pirbuterol 13
      3.1.2 Oral Pirbuterol 15
      3.1.3 Aerosol *versus* Oral Pirbuterol 16
   3.2 Long Term Studies 16
      3.2.1 Non-Comparative Studies 16
      3.2.2 Comparative Studies 18
4. Side Effects 18
5. Dosage and Administration 19
6. Place of Pirbuterol in Therapy 19

Summary

Synopsis: *Pirbuterol*[1] *is a β-adrenoceptor agonist which differs structurally from salbutamol in the substitution of a pyridine ring for the benzene ring. In common with salbutamol, pirbuterol demonstrates both bronchodilatory and cardiovascular effects. Generally, improvements of up to 25% are noted in forced expiratory volume in 1 second* (FEV_1)[versus *baseline or placebo*] *in asthmatic patients treated with pirbuterol for several months. In individual 12-week double-blind comparative studies, pirbuterol aerosol appeared similar to orciprenaline (metaproterenol) aerosol, and orally administered pirbuterol appeared similar to orally administered salbutamol in bronchodilator efficacy. However, well-designed long term comparative studies are needed to more clearly define the comparative efficacy of pirbuterol and alternative β-adrenoceptor agonists.*

Pharmacodynamic Studies: Pirbuterol is a relatively β_2-selective adrenoceptor agonist. In guinea-pigs, inhaled, oral or intravenous pirbuterol effectively inhibits inhaled histamine- and inhaled allergen-induced bronchoconstriction, and acetylcholine-induced bronchoconstriction, but it is less potent on a weight basis than salbutamol. In common with other β-adrenoceptor agonists, pirbuterol demonstrates significant vasodilatory and inotropic effects in healthy volunteers (intravenous administration) and in patients with severe irreversible airflow obstruction or congestive heart failure (oral administration). However, the cardiovascular effects of the drug in congestive heart failure patients are attenuated during long term exposure. Adrenoceptor 'down regulation', a decrease in the density of myocardial or vascular (or both) β-adrenoceptors, may be the mechanism of cardiovascular tachyphylaxis. The cardiovascular effects of pirbuterol in asthmatic patients include small decreases in mean blood pressure and increases in mean heart rate, and in a few patients abnormalities of the electrocardiogram. The frequency and/or magnitude of these cardiovascular effects in asthmatics is similar to those seen with other β-adrenoceptor agonist bronchodilators.

Pharmacokinetics: No detailed pirbuterol pharmacokinetic studies exist, but in asthmatic patients single 10 and 15mg oral doses result in mean peak plasma concentrations of 6.2 and 9.8 μg/L, respectively. Pirbuterol has a plasma half-life of 2 to 3 hours and 50% of a 10mg oral dose is excreted in the urine as pirbuterol sulphate; 10% of a 10mg oral dose is excreted in the urine unchanged. Plasma concentrations are undetectable at the maximum aerosol dose of 0.8mg.

Therapeutic Trials: In several double-blind randomised crossover studies in asthmatic patients, single doses of pirbuterol were significantly superior to placebo in bronchodilator efficacy. The onset of pirbuterol activity occurs 5 minutes after aerosol administration and within 1 hour after oral administration. The time to peak activity (30 minutes and within 2 hours, respectively), and magnitude of activity for the duration of testing (3 to 4 hours and 5 to 6 hours after administration, respectively) are similar to those of equipotent doses of salbutamol. However, the duration of activity of pirbuterol 15mg orally is at least 1 to 2 hours longer than that of orciprenaline 20mg orally. Pirbuterol is a less potent bronchodilator than salbutamol on a weight basis: pirbuterol 0.4mg aerosol and 15mg oral are the lowest doses which produce apparently maximum bronchodilation (mean peak improvements of 20 to 60% have been reported).

In unblinded or single-blinded non-comparative studies, long term (up to 6 months) pirbuterol therapy (30 to 60mg daily orally as 3 or 4 divided doses, or 0.2 to 2mg by aerosol 3 or 4 times daily) was generally associated with improvements in FEV_1 of up to 25% *versus* baseline or placebo. However, there were no statistically significant improvements in subjective assessments of bronchodilator efficacy.

In individual double-blind, randomised trials, pirbuterol 0.4mg aerosol was not significantly different from orciprenaline 1.3mg aerosol (3 or 4 doses daily for 12 weeks), and pirbuterol 10mg orally was not significantly different from salbutamol 4mg orally (3

1 'Exirel' (Pfizer).

or 4 doses daily for 10 weeks) in improving daily peak expiratory flow rates or subjective assessments of bronchodilator efficacy. Also, there was no statistically significant difference between the drugs in the degree of improvement of any spirometric parameter. However, in the comparative study of oral dosage forms only salbutamol significantly improved spirometric parameters (FEV_1 and forced vital capacity) compared with placebo, and neither drug appreciably diminished usage of the supplemental salbutamol inhaler. Additionally, in the study comparing pirbuterol and orciprenaline aerosols, one-third of the pirbuterol group (*vs* none of the orciprenaline group) received daily corticosteroid therapy.

Well-designed, long term studies are needed to more clearly define the comparative bronchodilator efficacy of pirbuterol and alternative β-adrenoceptor agonists.

Side Effects: The side effects most frequently associated with oral pirbuterol therapy are tremors (9.4%), nervousness (7.0%), headache (4.5%), tachycardia (2.9%), dry mouth (2%) and palpitations (1.9%). Nervousness and headache appear to be dose related.

Dosage and Administration: The recommended oral dosage of pirbuterol is 10 or 15mg administered 3 or 4 times daily up to a maximum daily dosage of 60mg. 5ml of pirbuterol syrup (7.5 mg/5ml) is recommended 4 times daily in children between the ages of 6 and 12 years. One or 2 inhalations (0.2 or 0.4mg) of pirbuterol aerosol, no more frequently than 4-hourly, and not to exceed 12 inhalations daily, is recommended.

1. *Pharmacodynamic Studies*

Pirbuterol is a relatively selective β_2-adrenoceptor agonist which differs structurally from salbutamol only in the presence of a pyridine as opposed to a benzene ring (fig. 1), and which, in common with salbutamol, has demonstrated both bronchodilatory and cardiovascular effects.

1.1 β-Adrenoceptor Selectivity

The β-adrenoceptor stimulant drugs are agonists of both β_1- and β_2-adrenoceptors, and selectivity arises from, among other differences, varying affinity for the 2 types of β-receptor (Offermeier et al., 1972). Affinity for β_2-adrenoceptors, stimulation of which results in relaxation of bronchial, uterine and vascular smooth muscle, appears to increase with the size of the nitrogen-attached moiety on a catechol or resorcinol base (Brittain et al., 1976; Leiffer and Wittig, 1975).

1.1.1 In vitro *Selectivity Studies*

Moore et al. (1978) assessed the intrinsic relative β-adrenoceptor selectivity of pirbuterol, salbutamol and isoprenaline (isoproterenol) in guinea-pig tissue by comparing the relaxation of tracheal muscle (β_2) to the chronotropic activity in atrial muscle (β_1). Similar concentrations of all 3 drugs relaxed isolated tracheal muscle, but pirbuterol was 9-fold more selective for pulmonary tissue than was salbutamol, and 1520 times more selective than isoprenaline. Similarly, Kenakin and Ferris (1983) reported that pirbuterol produced a maximal chronotropic response in rat atrial muscle that was 75% of the maximal response with isoprenaline, but a pirbuterol concentration 1000-fold higher than the isoprenaline concentration was required to produce 50% of this maximal response. Pirbuterol was a partial agonist in rat atrial tissue, but in tissue samples in which long term exposure to isoprenaline had caused receptor 'down-regulation' (a decrease in the number of β-adrenoceptors but no alteration in the binding affinity) pirbuterol functioned as a β-adrenoceptor antagonist, blocking responses to isoprenaline (Kenakin and Ferris, 1983). Estimates of the equilibrium dissociation constants of pirbuterol (2 μmol/L) and prenalterol (0.9 μmol/L) in these tissues were used to calculate the relative efficacy (relative receptor occupancies required for equal responses). Pirbuterol was shown to have 2.3 times the efficacy of prenalterol on β_1-adrenoceptors (Kenakin and Beek, 1984). These results suggest a mechanism for the tachyphylaxis which has developed to the cardiovascular effects of pirbuterol during long term administration to patients with congestive heart failure: dominance of β-adrenoceptor antagonist activity in tissues having 'down-regulated' receptors due to long term β-adrenoceptor agonist exposure (section 1.3.3).

1.1.2 Animal Studies

β-Adrenoceptor blockade with propranolol almost completely abolished the cardiovascular effects of pirbuterol in conscious dogs, thus pirbuterol demonstrated no apparent α-adrenoceptor agonist effect (Gold and Horowitz, 1981). In both this study and in a second cardiovascular study in conscious dogs (Vatner et al., 1982) pirbuterol caused significant chronotropic and inotropic changes, qualitatively similar to but of a lesser magnitude than those seen with isoprenaline. The changes in pirbuterol haemodynamics noted during selective β_1-adrenoceptor blockade with atenolol or practolol included an abolishment of the increases in left ventricular maximum rate of pressure rise (LV dp/dt) and an attenuation of the increases in heart rate.

1.2 Bronchial Effects

1.2.1 Studies in Asthmatic Volunteers

Exercise-induced bronchoconstriction was produced in 12 asthmatic patients after a 6-minute run on a 10% steep treadmill ergometer. Forced expiratory volume in 1 second (FEV_1) decreased by 12 to 73% (average 27%) of the control value measured before the run and remained constant for 10 to 20 minutes. 21 minutes after the run pirbuterol 0.2mg or salbutamol 0.2mg were inhaled in an open randomised crossover fashion (1 to 3 days separated the crossover challenge and testing). There were no significant differences between pirbuterol and salbutamol in the bronchodilating effect (FEV_1 returned to the control value within 5 minutes) or the effect on pulse rate (Aebischer et al., 1984).

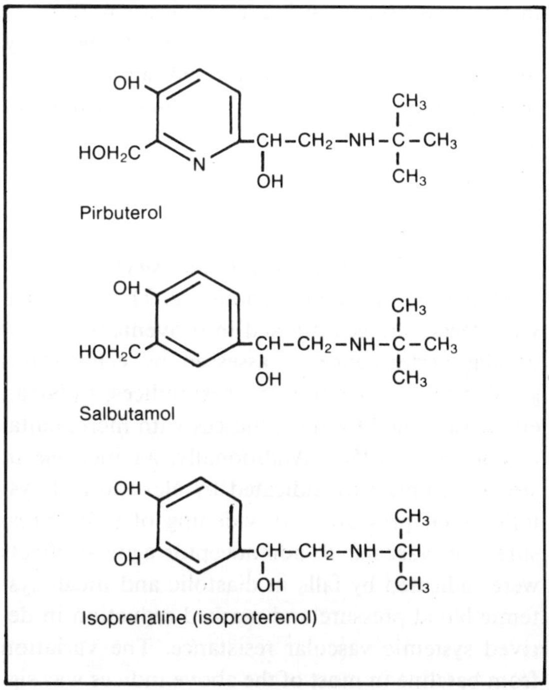

Fig. 1. Formulae of pirbuterol and other β-adrenoceptor agonists.

1.2.2 Animal Studies

Aerosol histamine-induced bronchoconstriction in guinea-pigs was inhibited by isoprenaline, salbutamol and pirbuterol, in order of decreasing potency. The maximum administered aerosol dose of pirbuterol (0.1 g/L) inhibited bronchoconstriction by 75% when given immediately prior to challenge and 33% when given 16 minutes prior to challenge. Percentage inhibition following maximum oral doses was 65% and 32% when the drug was given 5 and 80 minutes prior to challenge, respectively. Additionally, the combination of pirbuterol plus subeffective theophylline doses demonstrated additive inhibitory effects (Moore et al., 1978).

Intravenous pirbuterol 30 μg/kg given 2 minutes before challenge, and aerosol pirbuterol 0.1 g/L given just before challenge, inhibited bronchoconstriction due to inhaled albumin by 56% and 54%, respectively, in passively sensitised guinea-pigs. Results obtained for salbutamol 30 μg/kg intravenous and 0.1 g/L aerosol doses were 63%. Aerosol pirbuterol 0.1 g/L given immediately prior to challenge also inhibited acetylcholine-induced bronchoconstriction by 58% (Moore et al., 1978).

1.3 Cardiovascular Effects

1.3.1 Studies in Healthy Volunteers

Pirbuterol, given intravenously to 9 healthy male volunteers, induced marked improvement in ventricular performance as assessed by echocardiographic and systolic time interval indices; a plateau effect was noted for most indices with incremental dosing above 125μg. Additionally, an increase in stroke volume was indicated by elevation of systolic blood pressure and widening of pulse pressure, and vascular β_2-adrenoceptor agonist effects were indicated by falls in diastolic and mean systemic blood pressure and marked reduction in derived systemic vascular resistance. The variation from baseline in most of the above indices was significant ($p < 0.05$) even at the lowest dose administered (62.5μg) [Leier et al., 1982].

1.3.2 Studies in Patients with Pulmonary Diseases

Patients with Reversible Airway Obstruction

In many single-dose studies (section 3.1) oral or aerosol administration of pirbuterol did not cause statistically significant changes in the mean blood pressure or mean heart rate of patients with reversible airway obstruction. However, heart rate was significantly increased (*vs* baseline) at 15 to 120 minutes (supine) and 15 to 30 minutes (standing) following a dose of 0.8mg (the largest tested aerosol dose of the drug) [Littner et al., 1982]. Also, in 1 study, heart rate was significantly increased 2 hours after 10 or 15mg oral doses, but had returned to baseline 1 hour later (Willey and Grant, 1976). In another study, standing diastolic blood pressure 2 and 4 hours after 10 or 15mg oral doses was significantly decreased (6% decrease from baseline) [Ence et al., 1979]. In a double-blind comparison, there was no significant difference in the mean increase in heart rate caused by pirbuterol 15mg or salbutamol 4mg (Willey and Grant, 1976).

Most of these single-dose studies reported no abnormalities, other than previously diagnosed ones, in the electrocardiograms (ECG) of patients treated with pirbuterol. However, new ECG abnormalities were reported in a few patients following long term administration of the drug, and included premature atrial, supraventricular and/or ventricular contractions, ventricular ectopic beats, right atrial hypertrophy, sinus tachycardia, and sinus bradycardia (Beumer, 1983a,b; Dyson and Mackay, 1980; Steen et al., 1983). In 12-week double-blind crossover studies, no significant differences were reported in the incidences of ECG abnormalities between patients treated with pirbuterol or orciprenaline (metaproterenol) aerosol (Beumer, 1983b), or between patients treated with pirbuterol or salbutamol orally (Dyson and Mackay, 1980).

Patients with Severe Irreversible Airflow Obstruction

The cardiovascular effects of pirbuterol have been assessed in patients with severe irreversible airflow obstruction and moderate or severe hypoxaemia (table I). Single oral doses of pirbuterol or 6 weeks' administration of the drug significantly decreased pulmonary vascular resistance, but apparently at the cost of decreases in arterial oxygen tension. However, the decrease in tissue oxygen perfusion that this decrease in tension represents may be compensated for by the increased right ventricular ejection fraction, stroke volume, heart rate and cardiac output.

In an open comparative study, sodium nitroprusside (1 to 5 mg/kg intravenously) reduced mean pulmonary arterial pressure and total pulmonary vascular resistance significantly, without change in cardiac output or right ventricular ejection fraction. However, pirbuterol 22.5mg produced a greater reduction in total pulmonary vascular resistance than nitroprusside, largely as a result of increasing cardiac output (MacNee et al., 1983).

In a randomised double-blind crossover comparison, single equipotent bronchodilator doses of

Table I. Changes in some cardiovascular variables in patients with severe irreversible airflow obstruction following administration of oral pirbuterol or salbutamol, or intravenous infusion of sodium nitroprusside

References	Study design	No. of pts	AOT (baseline)	Drug, dosage	PVR[a]	PAP_{syst} (mm Hg)	HR (beats/min)	CO (L/min)	SV (ml)	RVEF	AOT (pK_a)
MacNee et al. (1983)	Open	12	7.28 kPa (55mm Hg)	Pirbuterol 15mg × 1	↓ 23%***	↑ 4%	↑ 13%*	↑ 30%***	↑ 12%*	↑ 12%*	↓ 13%
				Nitroprusside 1-5 mg/kg × 1	↓ 26%	↓ 20%***	↑ 13%	↑ 6%	↓ 6%	↑ 17%	
				Pirbuterol 22.5mg × 1	↓ 27%***	↓ 17%*	↑ 7%*	↑ 21%***	↑ 17%***	↑ 20%***	↓ 6%
				Nitroprusside 1-5 mg/kg × 1	↓ 21%***	↓ 27%***	↑ 7%	↓ 2%	↓ 8%	↑ 7%	
				Pirbuterol 15mg tid × 6 wks		↓ 19%*	↑ 7%			↑ 15%*	↓ 4%
Peacock et al. (1983)	Open	9	8.4 kPa (63mm Hg)	Pirbuterol 15mg × 1	↓ 19%**	↓ 8%		↑ 24%**			↓ 7%**
Winter et al. (1984)	Double-blind, randomised, crossover	12	8.2 kPa (62mm Hg)	Pirbuterol 15mg × 1						↑ 19%***	
				Salbutamol 4mg × 1						↑ 22%***	

a kPa · sec · cm^{-5} (MacNee et al., 1983) and dyne · sec · cm^{-5} (Peacock et al., 1983).

Abbreviations: AOT = arterial oxygen tension; PVR = pulmonary vascular resistance; PAP = pulmonary artery pressure; HR = heart rate; CO = cardiac output; SV = stroke volume; RVEF = right ventricular ejection fraction; * = $p < 0.05$; ** = $p < 0.02$; *** = $p < 0.01$; ↑ = increase; ↓ = decrease; tid = thrice daily.

pirbuterol and salbutamol (15 and 4mg, respectively) did not differ significantly in their effect (increases) on right and left ventricular ejection fractions (Winter et al., 1984). The effect of pirbuterol on systolic pulmonary artery pressure varied with dose (table I). However, a statistically significant decrease followed administration of single 22.5mg doses or 6 weeks' administration of 15mg thrice daily (MacNee et al., 1983).

1.3.3 Studies in Patients with Congestive Heart Failure

In small numbers of patients with severe congestive heart failure [New York Heart Association (NYHA) classes III or IV] due to various aetiologies, who were stabilised on digoxin and diuretics, single oral doses of pirbuterol (usual dose 20mg) were generally reported to significantly increase indices of cardiac function at rest (cardiac index, left ventricular ejection fraction and stroke volume index) and to significantly decrease left ventricular filling pressure and total systemic vascular resistance. The slight increases in heart rate and decreases in mean arterial pressure and pulmonary capillary wedge pressure only occasionally attained statistical significance (Awan et al., 1981; Bayliss et al., 1983; Colucci et al., 1981a,b; Kunze et al., 1983; Pamelia et al., 1983; Rude et al., 1981a,b; Sharma et al., 1981; Weber et al., 1982). Peak increases in cardiac output occurred 2 to 3 hours after 20 and 30mg doses and were sustained for 6 hours (Weber et al., 1982).

During exercise, Kunze et al. (1983) found no significant difference (*vs* baseline exercise values) in measurements of cardiovascular function in 12 patients pretreated with single oral doses of pirbuterol 20mg. However, Nelson et al. (1982) reported that pulmonary arterial pressure ($p < 0.01$), pulmonary vascular resistance ($p < 0.01$), and both diastolic and mean arterial pressure ($p < 0.01$), but not systolic arterial pressure, were decreased when pirbuterol 10 or 20mg preceded exercise by 1 hour.

Importantly, the effects of oral pirbuterol on haemodynamics were achieved without maldistribution of skeletal or organ blood flow (Canepa-Anson et al., 1982; Hoback et al., 1980) and without significant metabolic increases as assessed by myocardial oxygen consumption at rest (Awan et al., 1981; Rude et al., 1981a,b; Timmis et al., 1981), total oxygen uptake at rest or during exercise (Nelson et al., 1982; Weber et al., 1982), or the myocardial lactate, glucose or free fatty acid extraction ratios at rest (Rude et al., 1981b; Timmis et al., 1981). However, Fowler et al. (1982) reported that among 6 patients with left ventricular failure complicating coronary artery disease, intravenous infusion of pirbuterol 5 to 20 μg/min was associated with increased myocardial oxygen uptake and a decreased lactate extraction ratio. One patient developed angina.

Canepa-Anson et al. (1983) reported that acute administration of oral pirbuterol 10 to 20mg to patients with congestive heart failure resulted in decreases in plasma potassium, hydrocortisone (cortisol) and free fatty acid concentrations, and increases in glucose, insulin and lactate concentrations. Long term treatment (20mg thrice daily for 3 months) resulted in sustained effects on glucose and insulin, but loss of all other metabolic and endocrine effects.

In several uncontrolled, non-blinded studies, long term administration of oral pirbuterol (usual dosage 10 to 20mg thrice daily for up to 6 weeks) was associated with significant improvements in exercise duration and subjective assessments of New York Heart Association functional class (Awan et al., 1981; Colucci et al., 1981a,b; Dawson et al., 1982; Pamelia et al., 1983). However, in a well-designed double-blind randomised study, neither placebo nor pirbuterol (10mg thrice daily for 2 weeks then 20mg thrice daily for 5 weeks) significantly improved exercise tolerance (Weber et al., 1982). Additionally, the resting haemodynamic effects seen with acute administration of oral pirbuterol were generally not significantly sustained during long term administration of the drug (Colucci et al., 1981a,b; Kunze et al., 1983) except in the 2 studies which only retested the patients who responded to treatment (29 of 63 and 14 of 20 patients, respectively) [Dawson et al., 1982; Pamelia et al., 1983]. In 7 patients with ischaemic heart failure, vasodilator effects (mean and diastolic arterial pressure, pulmonary arterial pressure and pulmonary vascular resistance) during exercise were maintained during an entire month of pirbuterol therapy, but no significant positive inotropic effects were demonstrated (Nelson et al., 1982).

Colucci et al. (1981b) demonstrated a decrease in the density of β-adrenoceptor receptors on lymphocytes from patients treated with pirbuterol compared with untreated patients – a finding also reported with other selective β-agonists (Conolly et al., 1982). It was proposed by Colucci et al. (1981b) that the tolerance to the haemodynamic and clinical effects of pirbuterol which appears to develop during long term administration may be related to a decrease in the density of myocardial or vascular (or both) β-adrenoceptors.

1.4 Carcinogenicity Studies

Tumourigenesis in the form of mesovarial leiomyomas and pituitary adenomata have been found in rats following administration of β_2-adrenoceptor agonists (soterenol hydrochloride and mesuprine hydrochloride) [Nelson and Kelly, 1971; Nelson et al., 1972; Poynter et al., 1978]. However, there was no evidence of carcinogenicity following pirbuterol treatment of rats and mice for 24 and 18 months, respectively, at doses representing 8 times the recommended human dose (Pitts et al., 1983; Weber and Nelson, 1984).

2. Pharmacokinetic Studies

High performance liquid chromatography and a selected ion monitoring assay have been developed to measure plasma concentrations of pirbuterol (Falkner and McIlhenny, 1976). However, as no detailed bioavailability studies exist, the pharmacokinetics of pirbuterol in man have been poorly defined.

2.1 Absorption

Pirbuterol plasma concentrations in asthmatic patients were undetectable at the maximum aerosol dose of 0.8mg (limit of assay sensitivity 5 μg/L) [Littner et al., 1982].

Following administration of single oral doses to asthmatics, the mean peak plasma concentrations were 6.2 μg/L (10mg dose), and 9.8 μg/L (15mg dose). Peak plasma concentrations were seen within 3 hours (Pitts et al., 1983).

More detailed plasma concentration data were available on patients with congestive heart failure. These data revealed a rapid rise in plasma concentrations following oral administration, with peak concentrations at 2 hours and sustained plasma concentrations for a further 4 hours (Canepa-Anson et al., 1981; Dawson et al., 1982). Following long term administration of 20mg oral doses thrice daily to patients with congestive heart failure, mean plasma pirbuterol concentrations had increased 33% after 4 weeks of therapy (Colucci et al., 1981a) and 72% after 12 weeks' therapy (Nelson et al., 1982) *versus* concentrations following the initial doses. However, an increase in mean plasma concentrations *versus* that following the first dose was not noted following long term administration of 10mg thrice daily (Nelson et al., 1982). These results are perplexing in light of the reported pirbuterol half-life of 2 to 3 hours (see below).

2.2 Metabolism and Excretion

Pirbuterol has a plasma half-life of 2 to 3 hours. 50% of a 10mg oral dose was excreted in the urine as pirbuterol sulphate, indicating that sulphate conjugation is the major pathway of metabolism. 10% of the dose was excreted in the urine unchanged (McIlhenny and Ghaly, 1979).

3. *Therapeutic Trials in Reversible Airflow Obstruction*

The clinical efficacy of pirbuterol in patients with reversible airflow obstruction (intrinsic or extrinsic asthma, or chronic asthmatic bronchitis) has been assessed in several small single-dose crossover studies, a few long term unblinded or single-blind non-comparative studies, and in 2 long term double-blind, randomised comparative studies. Additionally, in a multicentre open trial, pirbuterol aerosol was assessed in over 2000 patients in the UK for periods of 4 weeks or greater (unpublished data on file, Pfizer).

In the clinical trials, history and an increase of at least 15 to 25% in FEV_1 following a test dose of aerosol isoprenaline or salbutamol were generally used to confirm the diagnosis. Most of these studies reported that patients were taken off other oral bronchodilators (aerosol pirbuterol studies) at least 12 hours, and supplemental inhaled bronchodilators (oral pirbuterol studies) at least 4 to 6 hours, before testing respiratory function. Measurement of specific airway resistance by whole body plethysmography is the preferred method of evaluating bronchodilators, since it is independent of patient cooperation and can be measured during normal breathing. However, spirometric assessment of airway function is easier to perform and has been utilised in most of the studies of pirbuterol.

3.1 Single-Dose Studies

Several small double-blind crossover studies have compared the bronchodilator efficacy of single aerosol or oral doses of pirbuterol with that of a placebo and alternative bronchodilators (Verstraeten, 1978; table II). Intervals of 1 to 14 days separated treatments. Additionally, 1 small study compared the combined efficacy of aerosol and oral pirbuterol (administered 2 hours apart) with the efficacy of the 2 formulations administered separately. Three of the studies failed to comment on the concurrent administration of other bronchodilator drugs (Stam, 1984; Vialatte et al., 1982; Willey and Grant, 1976). Baseline pulmonary function tests were performed at least once before administration of a treatment, and efficacy as percentage improvement of baseline values was compared between treatments.

3.1.1 Aerosol Pirbuterol

Among a series of 23 patients, pirbuterol aerosol doses as low as 0.1mg improved FEV_1 and forced vital capacity (FVC) significantly more so *versus* baseline than did placebo, but 0.4mg was the

Table II. Double-blind randomised crossover studies comparing the effect of single doses of pirbuterol (PB), salbutamol (S), orciprenaline (O), a combination product (theophylline 130mg, ephedrine 24mg and phenobarbitone 8mg) [T] and placebo (P) on respiratory function tests in patients with reversible airflow obstruction

References	No. of pts	Route	Parameters assessed	Improvement in mean parameter from baseline [time]
Comparisons with placebo				
Brandon (1980)	12	Oral	FEV_1	PB 10 or 15mg > P [0-∞][a]
			MMF	PB 10 or 15mg ≥ P [0-∞]
			SA	PB 10 or 15mg > P
Littner et al. (1982)	23	Aerosol	FEV_1	PB 0.1-0.8mg > P [5 min to 3-4h]
			FVC	PB 0.1-0.8mg > P [5 min to 3-4h]
			SA	PB 0.3-0.8mg > P [5 min to 4h][b]
Vialatte et al. (1982)	15[c]	Oral	FEV_1	PB 2.5-7.5mg ≥ P [0-∞]
			R	PB 2.5-7.5mg > P [0-∞]
Comparisons with other bronchodilators and placebo				
Beumer (1980)	12	Aerosol	FEV_1	(PB 0.2, 0.4 or 0.6mg = S 0.2mg) > P [0-∞]
			FVC, MEFR, MBC	(PB 0.4 or 0.6mg = S 0.2mg) > PB 0.2mg > P [0-6h]
Ence et al. (1979)	24	Oral	8 different spirometric and plethysmographic parameters	(PB 10 or 15mg = O 20mg) > P [0-≈ 3h][d] PB 15mg > O 20mg (4-6h)[e]
Votteri and Melcher (1979)	10	Oral	FEV_1, MMF	(PB 10 or 15mg = T or 2 T) ≥ P
Willey and Grant (1976)	10	Oral	FEV_1	(PB 10, 15 or 20mg = S 4, 6 or 8mg) > (PB 5 or 7.5mg = S 2mg = P) [5h][f]
Comparison of oral pirbuterol and aerosol pirbuterol				
Stam (1984)	10[c]	Oral *vs* aerosol	FEV_1, VC	PB 15mg (oral) + PB 0.2mg (aerosol) > [PB 15mg (oral) = PB 0.2mg (aerosol)][g]

a Mean area under the treatment/response curve.
b PB 0.2mg > placebo (15 min to 4h).
c Children.
d For most parameters assessed.
e For 4 of 8 parameters.
f Intertreatment significance of results at other times was not reported, but overall results for most doses are given in fig. 3.
g Oral and aerosol dosage forms were administered 2 hours apart. Combined efficacy was compared to individual efficacies.
Abbreviations: FEV_1 = forced expiratory volume in 1 second; FVC = forced vital capacity; VC = vital capacity; SA = self assessment; R = specific airway resistance; MEFR = maximum expiratory flow rate; MBC = maximum breathing capacity; MMF = maximum mid-expiratory flow rate; > = statistically significant difference; ≥ = non-significant trend.

lowest dose consistently producing an apparently maximum increase in both FEV_1 and FVC during the first 2 hours after administration (Littner et al., 1982). A mean peak improvement in FEV_1 of approximately 50% was reported following a single 0.4mg dose (Beumer, 1980).

During the 4 hours following administration, pirbuterol 0.4 and 0.6mg were not significantly different in efficacy from salbutamol 0.2mg, but all 3 treatments were more effective than pirbuterol

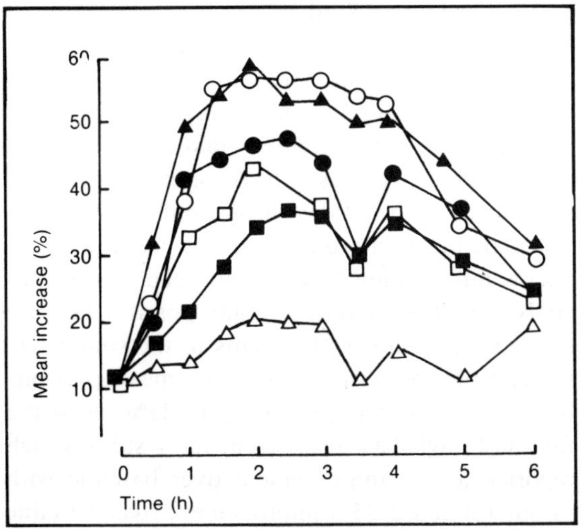

Fig. 2. Mean percentage increase of forced expiratory volume in 1 second from baseline values in 10 patients with reversible bronchospastic disease after oral administration of placebo (△), pirbuterol 7.5mg (■), pirbuterol 10mg (●), pirbuterol 20mg (▲), salbutamol 2mg (□) and salbutamol 8mg (○) [after Willey and Grant, 1976].

0.2mg [FEV_1, FVC, maximum expiratory flow rate (MEFR) and maximum breathing capacity (MBC) were assessed; Beumer, 1980]. The onset of activity of pirbuterol aerosol was within approximately 5 minutes, peak activity occurred at from 30 minutes (0.4mg dose) to 60 minutes (0.6mg dose), and a single dose of pirbuterol 0.1 to 0.8mg maintained statistically significant bronchodilation for 3 to 4 hours (Beumer, 1980; Littner et al., 1982). However, in a review of published and unpublished double-blind comparisons of pirbuterol and placebo, Pitts et al. (1983) concluded that the duration of action of pirbuterol aerosol may be longer: of the patients 'responding' (defined as 15% improvement in FEV_1 on 3 successive occasions) 66.7% still responded to the final (5-hour) evaluation – this persisting effect averaged 77.7% of the original peak response.

3.1.2 Oral Pirbuterol

The usual oral dose of pirbuterol was 10 or 15mg, which generally improved mean FEV_1 20 to 30% *versus* baseline (Ence et al., 1979; Vialatte et al., 1982; Votteri and Melcher, 1979), mean FVC 12 to 18% *versus* baseline (Ence et al., 1979), mean maximum mid-expiratory flow rate (MMEF) 45 to 50% *versus* baseline (Votteri and Melcher, 1979) and mean specific airways conductance 30 to 50% *versus* baseline (Ence et al., 1979). These doses were generally not significantly different in bronchodilator efficacy from salbutamol 4, 6 or 8mg, orciprenaline 20mg, or 1 to 2 tablets of a theophylline combination product, but were significantly more effective than placebo or lower doses of pirbuterol (figs 2 to 4). Pirbuterol 15mg was the lowest dose to produce apparently near maximum bronchodilation (Willey and Grant, 1976). Pirbuterol 10 and 15mg did not differ significantly from the tested doses of salbutamol and the theophylline combination product in time to onset of activity (within 1 hour), peak activity (within 2 hours) and magnitude of activity remaining at the end of testing (5 to 6 hours) [Brandon, 1980; Votteri and Melcher, 1979; Willey and Grant, 1976]. However, the duration of activity of pirbuterol 15mg was longer than that of orciprenaline 20mg, and thus the former demonstrated a significantly greater bronchodilator effect during the period 4 to 6 hours after administration (Ence et al., 1979).

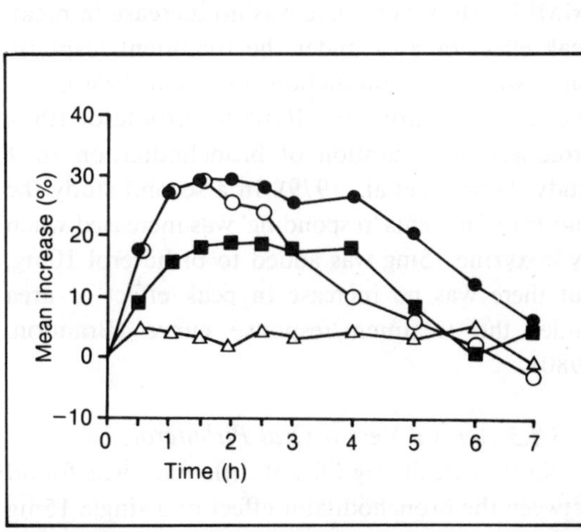

Fig. 3. Mean percentage increase of forced expiratory volume in 1 second from baseline values in 24 patients with reversible bronchospastic disease after oral administration of placebo (△), pirbuterol 10mg (■), pirbuterol 15mg (●) and orciprenaline (metaproterenol) 20mg (○) [after Ence et al., 1979].

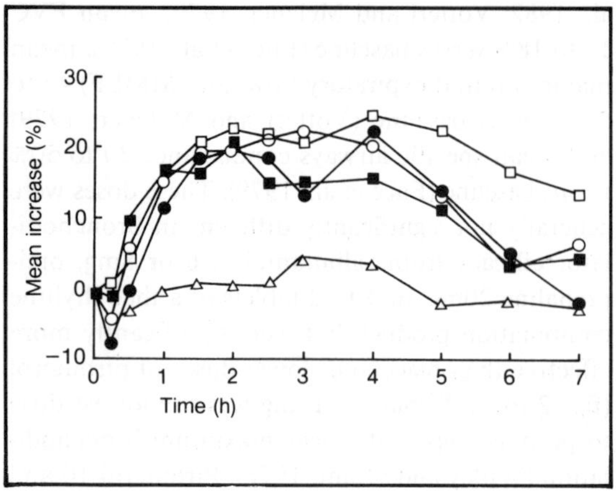

Fig. 4. Mean percentage increase of forced expiratory volume in 1 second from baseline values in 10 patients with reversible bronchospastic disease after oral administration of placebo (△), pirbuterol 10mg (■), pirbuterol 15mg (●), 'Tedral' (theophylline 130mg, ephedrine 24mg and phenobarbitone 8mg) 1 tab (○) and 'Tedral' 2 tabs (□) [after Votteri and Melcher, 1979].

The addition of theophylline 130mg to pirbuterol 10mg resulted in an increase in the number of patients 'responding', defined as 3 or more consecutive assessments that were improved 15% above baseline (FEV_1) or 20% above baseline (MMEF). However, there was no increase in mean peak effect or area under the treatment/response curve with this combination (Brandon, 1980). The addition of hydroxyzine 10mg to pirbuterol 10mg prolonged the duration of bronchodilation in 1 study (Poppius et al., 1979). In a second study the number of patients 'responding' was increased when hydroxyzine 15mg was added to pirbuterol 10mg, but there was no increase in peak effect or area under the treatment/response curve (Brandon, 1980).

3.1.3 Aerosol Versus *Oral Pirbuterol*

No statistically significant difference was found between the bronchodilator effect of a single 15mg oral and single 0.2mg aerosol dose of pirbuterol. Lung function was significantly better ($p < 0.05$) in patients receiving both formulations (2 hours apart) than in patients receiving either formulation alone (Stam, 1984).

3.2 Long Term Studies

3.2.1 Non-Comparative Studies

In the unblinded or single-blinded non-comparative long term studies (table III) baseline measurements were taken before administration of the drug on each test day throughout the study period. The mean improvement from baseline FEV_1 after administration of the pirbuterol dose was generally not statistically significant, possibly because of the small number of patients in the studies. At the end of long term therapy, the mean post-pirbuterol FEV_1 was improved up to 25% *versus* the final test day's baseline, except for 1 study which reported a 58% improvement over baseline with pirbuterol and a 35% improvement over baseline with placebo (table III).

Viallat et al. (1984) reported that the gradual improvement in baseline FEV_1, FVC and MMEF over the 13-week study period masked the corresponding increase in peak post-administration values when percentage increase from baseline was used as the assessment criterion. In this study on all test days both baseline and peak FEV_1 and FVC were significantly ($p < 0.01$) superior to those recorded during the placebo run-in period. Stam (1981) also reported superior responses in lung function following pirbuterol administration than following placebo administration; statistical significance was not reported. However, neither Stam (1981) nor the other studies in table III confirm the continuing improvement in lung function with time reported by Viallat et al. (1984); baseline and peak respiratory function fluctuated during the duration of the pirbuterol treatment period with no apparent trends.

Paterson et al. (1977) reported that the improvement in FEV_1 following administration of the pirbuterol 10mg (oral) dose reached statistical significance ($p < 0.05$) on only 1 of 4 test days throughout the 16-week study. However, subsequent administration of salbutamol 0.5% for 3 minutes (intermittent positive pressure ventilation) resulted in a 29 to 38% further increase in FEV_1 over that seen with pirbuterol alone ($p < 0.01$ on all 4 test days).

Table III. Uncontrolled studies assessing the improvement in respiratory function values (*vs* baseline for the same test day) following long term administration of pirbuterol to patients with reversible airflow obstruction

References	No. of patients	Drug, dosage, duration	Baseline FEV_1/peak FEV_1 (ml)		% imp. in FEV_1 from baseline	
			after initial dose	after final dose	after initial dose	after final dose
Beumer (1979)	21	Pirbuterol 15mg tid (oral) × 4-11 mo. (mean 7 mo.)	1664/2005	1704/1946	20*	14*
Beumer (1983a)	25	Pirbuterol 0.4mg tid-qid (aerosol)[a] × 6 mo.			30[b]	25[b]
Burki and Diamond (1978)	12	Pirbuterol 30-60mg daily as 3-4 divided doses (oral) × 6 mo.	1650/2100[b]	1810/1820[b]	27[b]	1[b]
Paterson et al. (1977)	16	Placebo × 4 wk Pirbuterol 10mg qid (oral) × 12 wk	1359/1528	1175/1413	12	20
Stam (1981)	16	Placebo × 2 wk Pirbuterol 0.2-2mg daily (aerosol)[a] × 4 wk			76[b]	35[b] 58[b]
Viallat et al. (1984)	31[c]	Pirbuterol 7.5mg qid (oral) × 1 mo.	1230/1560	1470/1670	27	14
	33[c]	Pirbuterol 7.5mg qid (oral) × 3 mo.	1230/1560	1530/1750	27	14

a Patients were allowed to adjust their dosage within an allowable range.
b Results derived from a graph.
c Paediatric patients.
Abbreviations: FEV_1 = forced expiratory volume in 1 second; tid = thrice daily; qid = 4 times daily; * = $p < 0.05$.

Subjective assessments were disappointing. Beumer (1979) noted that all 21 patients reported 'no change' in their asthma with long term pirbuterol therapy. The investigators' assessments in this study were more favourable but can be questioned, given the unblinded design. Beumer (1983a) reported no significant improvement in the number of asthmatic attacks (day or night), cough or malaise during a 6-month treatment period, and Paterson et al. (1977) reported only small (approximately 6%) and non-significant decreases in mean daily symptom scores and mean daily supplemental inhaled bronchodilator use during 12 weeks of pirbuterol administration (*vs* placebo).

The development of subsensitivity to the bronchodilatory effects of β-adrenoceptor agonists is seldom clinically significant in asthmatics (Tattersfield, 1983). In a review of studies which reported the development of subsensitivity to various β-adrenoceptor agonists, Nelson (1982) found that the decreases seen in peak FEV_1 ranged from 14 to 58% and usually occurred after 1 to 2 weeks, with no further loss of bronchodilator effect during continuous observation for up to 12 months. In 2 of the studies in table III, a placebo washout period was employed which allowed the magnitude of any potential subsensitivity to be assessed. Viallat et al. (1984) reported no development of subsensitivity during 13 weeks of pirbuterol therapy. However, the 5-day washout period may have been too short to allow complete β-adrenoceptor recovery. Stam (1981) reported that between weeks 2 and 4 of pirbuterol therapy, a decrease of approximately 25% [vital capacity (VC)] and 15% (FEV_1) occurred in the mean percentage change from baseline values. However, as absolute values were not provided for VC and FEV_1 it is difficult to assess whether subsensitivity actually occurred. In a follow-up study involving 8 of the patients in this study, there was no further decline in VC or FEV_1 during 2 more years of therapy (Stam, 1984).

3.2.2 Comparative Studies

Pirbuterol has only been compared with alternative bronchodilators in two 12-week double-blind randomised trials, and so definitive statements on comparative efficacy would be premature. Both studies included only patients with reversible airways obstruction (≥ 15% or ≥20% improvements in FEV_1 after aerosol isoprenaline inhalation), and used a 1-week placebo run-in period to establish placebo response, but neither study stated whether assessments were performed at the same time on each test days.

38 male outpatients were randomly assigned to therapy with pirbuterol aerosol 0.4mg 3 to 4 times daily or orciprenaline aerosol 1.3mg 3 or 4 times daily. There were no statistically significant differences between the pirbuterol group (18 patients assessed) and the orciprenaline group (15 patients assessed) in the improvement in any spirometric parameter on any test day, the improvement in daily PEFR, or in scores for daytime and night-time assessment of cough and malaise, number of daytime asthmatic attacks or number of times awakened by asthma at night. However, while the patient groups appeared similar regarding age, weight, primary diagnosis (including severity and duration of illness), and response to previous therapy, 6 of the 19 pirbuterol patients (*vs* none of the orciprenaline patients) received daily corticosteroids (betamethasone 0.5 to 1.5mg or dexamethasone 0.5mg). It was not reported whether ancillary therapy was kept stable and constant during the trial (Beumer, 1983b).

72 patients received pirbuterol 10mg or salbutamol 4mg orally, 3 to 4 times daily for 10 weeks, before crossing over to the alternative therapy for 2 weeks. Treatment groups were reported to be comparable in terms of percentage predicted FEV_1, age, sex, and initial steroid usage. 10 salbutamol patients and 6 pirbuterol patients were given a short course of oral corticosteroids for exacerbations of asthma, and were excluded from the analysis. Thus, the remaining patients probably had only mild disease. Both treatments significantly improved PEFR scores ($p < 0.005$ and $p < 0.01$ for pirbuterol and salbutamol, respectively, *vs* placebo), and there was no significant difference between the drugs. Also, both treatments significantly improved subjective assessments of breathing, wellbeing and nocturnal symptoms. However, only salbutamol produced a statistically significant increase in FEV_1 ($p < 0.005$) and FVC ($p < 0.02$) compared with placebo, and neither drug appreciably diminished usage of the supplemental salbutamol inhaler from the usage during the placebo run-in period (mean number of weekly puffs was 23 on placebo, 19 on pirbuterol and 20 on salbutamol) [Dyson and Mackay, 1980].

4. Side Effects

The side effect profile of orally administered pirbuterol was summarised by Pitts et al. (1983) from results obtained in open studies and comparative trials. The discussion below is based on this report.

The most frequently reported side effects were tremors, nervousness, headache, tachycardia, dry mouth and palpitations (table IV). In a double-blind crossover comparison of 95 patients, 1 patient receiving salbutamol (4mg thrice daily) withdrew due to tremor and 4 patients receiving pirbuterol (30 to 40mg daily as 3 divided doses) withdrew due to tremor. Two of the patients who withdrew from pirbuterol therapy also experienced palpitations (Dyson and Mackay, 1980).

Laboratory values from 292 patients in single-dose studies and 646 patients in multiple-dose studies (mean duration of therapy, 7.3 months; maximum duration, 3.7 years) revealed no evidence of significant organ toxicity. However, Dyson and Mackay (1980) found creatine phosphokinase (CPK) elevations in 6 of 93 patients receiving oral pirbuterol and 6 of 93 receiving oral salbutamol in a 12-week crossover study. Seven other

Table IV. A summary of the side effects of oral pirbuterol. 30 patients (7.4%) discontinued therapy due to the severity of side effects (after Pitts et al., 1983)

Side effect	No. of side effects (%)				Totals (%)
	10mg tid [27 days][a] (255 pts)	10mg qid [56 days] (418 pts)	15mg tid [123 days] (247 pts)	15mg qid [177 days] (113 pts)	(1033pts)
Central nervous system					
nervousness	11 (4.3)	28 (6.7)	24 (9.7)	10 (8.8)	73 (7.0)
headache	8 (3.1)	20 (4.8)	18 (7.3)	1 (0.9)	47 (4.5)
dizziness	5 (2.0)	4 (1.0)	5 (2.0)	0	14 (1.3)
other	4 (1.6)	13 (3.1)	4 (1.6)	0	21 (2.0)
Tremor	22 (8.6)	48 (11.5)	23 (9.3)	4 (3.5)	97 (9.4)
Cardiovascular					
palpitations	5 (2.0)	9 (2.2)	5 (2.0)	1 (0.9)	20 (1.9)
tachycardia	8 (3.1)	8 (1.9)	13 (5.3)	1 (0.9)	30 (2.9)
Gastrointestinal					
dry mouth	6 (2.3)	10 (2.4)	5 (2.0)	1 (0.9)	22 (2.1)
nausea	4 (1.6)	6 (1.4)	3 (1.2)	1 (0.9)	14 (1.4)
other	3 (1.2)	15 (3.6)	1 (0.4)	2 (1.8)	21 (2.0)

a Mean duration of therapy

patients had elevated CPK concentrations while receiving either drug.

Pirbuterol was associated with small decreases in mean blood pressure and increases in mean heart rate, and in a few patients with abnormalities of the ECG (section 1.3.2). The frequency and/or magnitude of these cardiovascular effects was similar to those seen with other β-adrenoceptor agonist bronchodilators.

5. Dosage and Administration

Pirbuterol is contraindicated in patients sensitive to sympathomimetic drugs, and in those receiving non-selective β-adrenoceptor blocking agents. The drug should be used with caution in patients with thyrotoxicosis, coronary artery disease or cardiac dysrhythmias.

Patients should be warned of the possible danger of overuse. If the usual dose does not provide the usual relief, a non-responsive state may be developing. Other therapy is then indicated as there is probably a severe form of asthma present.

Oral administration: The recommended oral dose of pirbuterol is 10 or 15mg administered 3 or 4 times daily, with a maximum recommended daily dosage of 60mg. For children between the ages of 6 and 12 years the syrup formulation in a dosage of 7.5mg (5ml) is recommended 4 times daily.

Aerosol administration: One or 2 inhalations (0.2 or 0.4mg) 3 or 4 times daily, not repeated more frequently than 4-hourly, and not to exceed 12 inhalations daily, is recommended for adults. Patients should actuate the valve shortly after beginning a slow inhalation which should be followed by at least 10 seconds of breath holding.

6. Place of Pirbuterol in Therapy

Oral and aerosol pirbuterol in single doses of 10 to 15mg and 0.4mg, respectively, effected significant bronchodilation *versus* baseline values in asthmatic patients. With long term therapy the mean improvement in FEV_1 *versus* baseline or placebo was generally up to 25%. Single 12-week double-blind studies found pirbuterol aerosol to appear similar to orciprenaline aerosol, and orally administered pirbuterol to appear similar to orally administered salbutamol in bronchodilator efficacy. However, well-designed long term trials are needed to more clearly define the comparative efficacy of pirbuterol and alternative β-adrenoceptor agonists.

References

Aebischer, J.C.; Benoit, R.C. and Scherrer, M.: Pirbuterol- und salbutamol-aerosol gegen die anstengung-iduzierte bronchokonstriktion. Schweizerische Medizinische Wochenschrift 114: 1660-1664 (1984).

Awan, N.A.; Needham, K.; Evenson, M.K.; Hermanovich, J.; Joye, J.A. et al.: Therapeutic efficacy of oral pirbuterol in severe congestive heart failure: Acute hemodynamic and long-term ambulatory evaluation. American Heart Journal 102: 555-563 (1981).

Bayliss, J.; Norell, M.; Canepa-Anson, R.; Reuben, S.R.; Poole-Wilson, P.A. and Sutton, G.C.: Acute haemodynamic comparison of amrinone and pirbuterol in chronic heart failure. British Heart Journal 49: 214-221 (1983).

Beumer, H.M.: Pirbuterol in the treatment of bronchial asthma. International Journal of Clinical Pharmacology and Biopharmacy 17: 18-25 (1979).

Beumer, H.M.: Pirbuterol aerosol *versus* salbutamol and placebo aerosols in bronchial asthma. Drugs Under Experimental and Clinical Research 2: 77-83 (1980).

Beumer, H.M.: Long-term treatment of bronchial asthma with pirbuterol aerosol. International Journal of Clinical Pharmacology, Therapy and Toxicology 21: 172-175 (1983a).

Beumer, H.M.: Pirbuterol *versus* orciprenaline aerosols in the treatment of bronchial asthma. International Journal of Clinical Pharmacology, Therapy and Toxicology 21: 147-166 (1983b).

Brandon, M.L.: Pirbuterol *vs* hydroxyzine *vs* theophylline in the treatment of bronchial asthma. Annals of Allergy 45: 8-12 (1980).

Brittain, R.T.; Dean, C.M. and Jack, D.: Sympathomimetic bronchodilator drugs. Pharmacology and Therapeutics, Part B 2: 423-462 (1976).

Burki, N.K. and Diamond, L.: Long-term oral bronchodilator therapy of asthma with pirbuterol. Clinical Pharmacology and Therapeutics 24: 84-89 (1978).

Canepa-Anson, R.; Dawson, R.; Kuan, P.; Poole-Wilson, P.; Sutton, G. et al.: Differences between acute and long term metabolic and endocrine effects of oral beta adrenergic agonist therapy for cardiac failure. (Abstract 98.) European Heart Journal 4 (Suppl. E): 109 (1983).

Canepa-Anson, R.; Dawson, J.R.; Kuan, P.; Warnes, C.A.; Poole-Wilson, P.A. et al.: Single-dose and dose-response studies with oral pirbuterol, a new beta agonist in chronic heart failure. American Heart Journal 102: 578-583 (1981).

Canepa-Anson, R.; Ilsley, C.; Bayliss, J.; Reuben, S.; Sutton, G. and Poole-Wilson, P.: Effects of oral pirbuterol on haemodynamics, distribution of blood flow and lactate production during treadmill exercise in patients with chronic heart failure. (Abstract.) American Journal of Cardiology 49: 1001 (1982).

Colucci, W.S.; Alexander, R.W.; Mudge, G.H.; Rude, R.E.; Holman, B.L. et al.: Acute and chronic effects of pirbuterol on left ventricular ejection fraction and clinical status in severe congestive heart failure. American Heart Journal 102: 564-568 (1981a).

Colucci, W.S.; Alexander, R.W.; Williams, G.H.; Rude, R.E.; Holman, B.L. et al.: Decreased lymphocyte beta-adrenergic-receptor density in patients with heart failure and tolerance to the beta-adrenergic agonist pirbuterol. New England Journal of Medicine 305: 185-190 (1981b).

Conolly, M.E.; Tashkin, D.P.; Hui, K.K.P.; Lither, M.R. and Wolfe, R.N.: Selective subsensitization of β-adrenergic receptors in central airways of asthmatics and normal subjects during long-term therapy with inhaled salbutamol. Journal of Allergy and Clinical Immunology 70: 423-431 (1982).

Ence, T.J.; Tashkin, D.P.; Ho, D. and Child, J.S.: Acute bronchial and cardiovascular effects of oral pirbuterol and metaproterenol. Annals of Allergy 43: 229-236 (1979).

Dawson, J.R.; Bayliss, J.; Norell, M.S.; Canepa-Anson, R.; Kuan, P. et al.: Clinical studies with $beta_2$ adrenoceptor agonists in heart failure. European Heart Journal 3 (Suppl. D): 135-141 (1982).

Dyson, A.J. and Mackay, A.D.: Two oral beta-adrenergic stimulant drugs, pirbuterol and salbutamol, in reversible airway obstruction. British Journal of Diseases of the Chest 74: 70-74 (1980).

Falkner, F.C. and McIlhenny, H.M.: Selected ion monitoring assay for the bronchodilator pirbuterol. Biomedical Mass Spectrometry 3: 207-211 (1976).

Fowler, M.B.; Bergman, G.; Timmis, A.D.; Atkinson, L.; Howell, L. and Jewitt, D.E.: Is pirbuterol therapy in left ventricular failure associated with a positive inotropic action and what is its metabolic cost? (Abstract 547.) Circulation 66 (Suppl. II): 137 (1982).

Gold, F.L. and Horowitz, L.D.: Hemodynamic effects of pirbuterol in conscious dogs. American Heart Journal 102: 591-596 (1981).

Hoback, J.; Sharma, P.; Maxim, D. and Erllen, D.: Pirbuterol in congestive heart failure: Regional flow-response. (Abstract 1148.) Circulation 62 (Suppl. III): 299 (1980).

Kenakin, T.P. and Beek, D.: Relative efficacy of prenalterol and pirbuterol for beta-1 adrenoceptors: Measurement of agonist affinity by alteration of receptor number. Journal of Pharmacology and Experimental Therapeutics 229: 340-345 (1984).

Kenakin, T.P. and Ferris, R.M.: Effect of *in vivo* β-adrenoceptor down-regulation on cardiac responses to prenalterol and pirbuterol. Journal of Cardiovascular Pharmacology 5: 90-97 (1983).

Kunze, K.P.; Kluck, H.; Costard, A. and Bleifeld, W.: Acute and long-term effects of oral pirbuterol in patients with chronic congestive heart failure. (Abstract 1497.) Circulation 68 (Suppl. III): 374 (1983).

Leier, C.V.; Nelson, S.; Huss, P.; Bianchine, J.R.; Olukotun, A.Y. et al.: Intravenous pirbuterol. Clinical Pharmacology and Therapeutics 31: 89-94 (1982).

Leiffer, K.N. and Wittig, H.S.: Beta-2 sympathomimetic aerosols in the treatment of asthma. Annals of Allergy 35: 69-80 (1975).

Littner, M.R.; Tashkin, D.P.; Calvarese, B. and Bautista, M.: Acute bronchial and cardiovascular effects of increasing doses of pirbuterol acetate aerosol in asthma. Annals of Allergy 48: 14-20 (1982).

MacNee, W.; Wathen, C.G.; Hannan, W.J.; Flenley, D.C. and Muir, A.L.: Effects of pirbuterol and sodium nitroprusside on pulmonary haemodynamics in hypoxic cor pulmonale. British Medical Journal 287: 1169-1172 (1983).

McIlhenny, H.M. and Ghaly, M.S.D.: Biotransformation of pirbuterol by the rat, dog and human. (Abstract 1130.) Federation Proceedings 38: 442 (1979).

Moore, P.F.; Constantine, J.W. and Barth, W.E.: Pirbuterol, a selective $beta_2$ adrenergic bronchodilator. Journal of Pharmacology and Experimental Therapeutics 207: 410-418 (1978).

Nelson, G.I.C.; Silke, B.; Barker, M.C.J.; Saxton, C.A.P.D. and

Taylor, S.H.: New beta-2 adrenoceptor agonist (pirbuterol) in the treatment of ischaemic heart failure. European Heart Journal 3: 238-245 (1982).

Nelson, H.S.: Beta adrenergic agonists. Chest 82 (Suppl.): 33-38 (1982).

Nelson, L.W. and Kelly, W.A.: Mesovarial leiomyomas in rats in a chronic toxicity study of soterenol hydrochloride. Veterinary Pathology 8: 452-457 (1971).

Nelson, L.W.; Kelly, W.A. and Weikel Jr, J.H.: Mesovarial leiomyomas in rats in a chronic toxicity study of mesuprine hydrochloride. Toxicity and Applied Pharmacology 23: 731-737 (1972).

Offermeier, J.; Dreyer, A.C.; Brandt, H.D. and Steinberg, S.: The β_2-selectivity of various β-adrenergic drugs. Medical Proceedings 18: 5-8 (1972).

Pamelia, F.X.; Georghiade, M.; Beller, G.A.; Bishop, H.L.; Olukotun, A.Y. et al.: Acute and long-term hemodynamic effects of oral pirbuterol in patients with chronic severe congestive heart failure: Randomized double-blind trial. American Heart Journal 106: 1369-1376 (1983).

Paterson, I.C.; Willey, R.F. and Grant, I.W.B.: Effects of prolonged administration of pirbuterol by mouth in chronic asthma. British Journal of Clinical Pharmacology 4: 376-377 (1977).

Peacock, A.; Busst, C.; Dawkins, K. and Denison, D.M.: Response of pulmonary circulation to oral pirbuterol in chronic airflow obstruction. British Medical Journal 287: 1178-1180 (1983).

Pitts, N.E.; Borger, A.P.; Ghaly, M.S.; Salsburg, D.S. and Gans, D.J.: Pirbuterol – a new selective beta-agonist; in Richardson, R.G. (Ed.) Pulmonary and Circulatory Abnormalities in Chronic Obstructive Airways Disease: An Evaluation of Pirbuterol, pp. 1-31 (Academic Press and the Royal Society of Medicine, London 1983).

Poppius, H.; Lehti, H. and Stenius-Aarniala, B.: Comparison of pirbuterol and pirbuterol and hydroxyzine in patients with reversible airway obstruction. European Journal of Clinical Pharmacology 15: 389-393 (1979).

Poynter, D.; Harris, D.M. and Jack, D.: Salbutamol: Lack of evidence of tumour induction in man. British Medical Journal 1: 46-47 (1978).

Rude, R.E.; Grossman, W.; Colucci, W.S.; Benotti, J.R.; Carabello, B.A. et al.: Problems in assessment of new pharmacologic agents for the heart failure patient. American Heart Journal 102: 584-590 (1981a).

Rude, R.E.; Turi, Z.; Brown, E.J.; Lorell, B.H.; Colucci, W.S. et al.: Acute effects of oral pirbuterol on myocardial oxygen metabolism and systemic hemodynamics in chronic congestive heart failure. Circulation 64: 139-145 (1981b).

Sharma, B.; Hoback, J.; Francis, G.S.; Hodges, M.; Asinger, R.W. et al.: Pirbuterol: A new oral sympathomimetic amine for the treatment of congestive heart failure. American Heart Journal 102: 533-541 (1981).

Stam, J.: Open study of the bronchodilator efficacy and safety of multiple doses of pirbuterol aerosol. European Journal of Respiratory Diseases 62 (Suppl. 113): 181-182 (1981).

Stam, J.: Comparison of oral, inhalation and combined routes of administration of pirbuterol on lung function in patients with bronchospastic disease. (Abstract.) Respiration 46 (Suppl. 1): 57-58 (1984).

Steen, S.N.; Smith, R.L. and Thomas, J.S.: Pirbuterol as long-term bronchodilator therapy. (Abstract 339.) 2nd World Conference on Clinical Pharmacology and Therapeutics, Washington D.C. (Jul-Aug 1983).

Tattersfield, A.E.: Autonomic bronchodilators; in Godfrey and Clark (Eds) Asthma, 2nd ed., pp. 323-325 (Chapman and Hall, London (1983).

Timmis, A.D.; Bergman, G.; Atkinson, L.; Monaghan, M. and Jewitt, D.E.: Potential value of oral β_2 adrenoceptor agonists in left ventricular failure. (Abstract.) American Journal of Cardiology 47: 427 (1981).

Vatner, S.F.; Hintze, T.H. and Macho, P.: Regulation of large coronary arteries by β-adrenergic mechanisms in the conscious dog. Circulation Research 51: 56-66 (1982).

Verstraeten, J.M.: Vergelijkende studie met pirbuterol, salbutamol en een placebo toegediend onder vorm van gedoseerde aerosols bij asmatische patienten. Revue de l'Institut d'Hygiène des Mines 33: 200-203 (1978).

Viallat, J.R.; Boutin, C. and Razzouk, H.: Pirbuterol syrup – treatment of asthma in children in a residential asthma clinic. British Journal of Clinical Practice 38: 362-367 (1984).

Vialatte, J.; Rufin, P. and Paupe, J.: Action bronchodilatatrice du pirbutérol chez l'enfant asthmatique. Revue Française d'Allergologie et d'Immunologie Clinique 22: 141-145 (1982).

Votteri, B.A. and Melcher, L.: Comparative trial of pirbuterol and tedral in patients with reversible airway obstruction. Annals of Allergy 43: 348-351 (1979).

Weber, K.T.; Andrews, V.; Janicki, J.S.; Likoff, M. and Reichek, N.: Pirbuterol, an oral beta-adrenergic receptor agonist in the treatment of chronic cardiac failure. Circulation 66: 1262-1267 (1982).

Weber, R.W. and Nelson, H.S.: Pirbuterol hydrochloride: evaluation of beta adrenergic agonist activity in reversible obstructive pulmonary disease and congestive heart failure. Pharmacotherapy 4: 1-10 (1984).

Willey, R.F. and Grant, I.W.B.: Effects of oral salbutamol and pirbuterol on FEV_1, heart rate and blood pressure in asthmatics. British Journal of Clinical Pharmacology 3: 595-600 (1976).

Winter, R.J.D.; Langford, J.A. and Rudd, R.M.: Effects of oral and inhaled salbutamol and oral pirbuterol on right and left ventricular function in chronic bronchitis. British Medical Journal 288: 824-825 (1984).

Authors' address: *Deborah Richards*, ADIS Drug Information Services, P.O. Box 34-030, Birkenhead, Auckland 10 (New Zealand).

Drugs 30: 22-31 (1985)
0012-6667/85/0700-0022/$05.00/0

Guanadrel
A Review of its Pharmacodynamic and Pharmacokinetic Properties and Therapeutic Use in Hypertension

F.A. Finnerty Jr and *R.N. Brogden*

George Washington University, Arlington, and ADIS Drug Information Services, Auckland

Manuscript reviewed by: ***J.F. Burris,*** Cardiovascular Center of Northern Virginia, Alexandria, Virginia, USA; ***J.L. Cangiano,*** Veterans Administration, San Juan, Puerto Rico; ***D. Hansson,*** Department of Medicine, Östra Hospital, Göteborg, Sweden; ***D.C. Harrison,*** Falk Cardiovascular Research Center, Stanford University School of Medicine, Stanford, California, USA; ***N.M. Kaplan,*** Department of Internal Medicine, The University of Texas, Dallas, Texas, USA; ***F.G. McMahon,*** Clinical Research Center, New Orleans, Louisiana, USA; ***F.O. Simpson,*** Department of Medicine, University of Otago, Dunedin, New Zealand; ***D. Sloman,*** Department of Cardiology, Epworth Medical Centre, Richmond, Victoria, Australia; ***P. Turner,*** Department of Clinical Pharmacology, St Bartholomew's Hospital Medical College, London, England; ***N. Weiner,*** Department of Pharmacology, University of Colorado Health Sciences Center, Denver, Colorado, USA.

Contents

Summary 23
1. Pharmacodynamic Properties 24
   1.1 Haemodynamic Effects 24
   1.2 Effect on Peripheral Sympathetic Neurons 24
   1.3 Effect on the Central Nervous System 25
   1.4 Miscellaneous Effects 25
2. Pharmacokinetic Studies 25
   2.1 Guanadrel Compared with Guanethidine 26
3. Therapeutic Trials 26
   3.1 Open Studies 26
   3.2 Comparisons with Guanethidine 26
   3.3 Comparisons with Methyldopa 27
   3.4 Studies in Patients who had Failed to Respond to Other Treatment 28
4. Side Effects 29
5. Drug Interactions 29
6. Dosage and Administration 30
7. Overdosage 30
8. The Place of Guanadrel in Therapy 30

Summary

Synopsis: *Guanadrel[1] sulphate is an orally active peripheral sympathetic inhibitor (adrenergic neuron-blocking drug). In comparative studies, guanadrel was comparable in efficacy with guanethidine or methyldopa in mild to moderately severe hypertension, although generally it caused fewer central nervous system side effects than methyldopa and less orthostatic dizziness and diarrhoea than guanethidine. However, its efficacy in patients whose blood pressure remains inadequately controlled by other drugs (except diuretics alone) has yet to be adequately demonstrated. Guanadrel has a rapid onset of action and a half-life of about 10 hours, thus dose titration can be achieved more rapidly than with guanethidine, and twice daily administration is appropriate. Generally, guanadrel has been well tolerated, withdrawal of treatment due to adverse effects seldom being necessary. Thus, guanadrel appears to be a suitable alternative to methyldopa for the treatment of mild to moderately severe hypertension not controlled adequately by diuretics alone.*

Pharmacodynamic Properties: Blockade of noradrenaline (norepinephrine) release and depletion of noradrenaline stores by guanadrel have been demonstrated in a wide range of animal and human studies. The mechanism by which guanadrel is taken up in the nerve endings appears to be sensitive to blockade by tricyclic antidepressants, but no inhibition of monoamine oxidase metabolism has been reported. Guanadrel reduces both standing and supine blood pressures. Since it is a peripherally acting agent, a significantly greater reduction in standing blood pressure over supine pressure has been noted. Blood pressure reduction in humans is accompanied by only modest decreases in heart rate and by no significant change in cardiac output, the primary antihypertensive action being through a reduction in peripheral resistance.

Pharmacokinetic Properties: Because the antihypertensive action of guanadrel starts and dissipates quickly, and since drug accumulation is limited, rapid titration and drug withdrawal are easily accomplished compared with guanethidine. Peak plasma concentrations in humans are generally reached within 1.5 to 2 hours after oral administration, and urinary excretion is approximately 85% complete within 24 hours. The elimination half-life of guanadrel is about 10 hours. Studies in animals and man have shown that less than 20% of guanadrel binds to plasma protein.

Therapeutic Trials: In published studies to date, guanadrel 20 to 400mg daily has been found similar in efficacy to methyldopa 500 to 3000mg daily when either drug was given with a diuretic. Comparisons with guanethidine have also shown a comparable antihypertensive effect at equipotent dosages in small groups of patients with mild to moderately severe hypertension not adequately controlled with diuretics alone. In these studies, drowsiness was more common with methyldopa than with guanadrel and orthostatic dizziness and diarrhoea appeared to be more of a problem with guanethidine than with guanadrel.

Side Effects: The side effect profile of guanadrel is similar to that of the other peripheral sympathetic inhibitors, but in published comparative studies there appears to be a lower incidence of orthostatic dizziness with guanadrel than with guanethidine. Sexual dysfunction in men occurred with similar frequency during treatment with either peripheral sympathetic inhibitor. Early morning orthostatic hypotension has not been reported to be a problem with guanadrel.

Dosage and Administration: Guanadrel (available as 10 and 25mg tablets) should be employed as an adjunct to diuretic therapy. A starting dose of 10 mg/day is recom-

1 'Hylorel' (Pennwalt Corporation).

mended, with weekly upward titration at 10mg increments. In most patients, control of blood pressure is achieved with dosages of 20 to 75 mg/day. The maximum daily dose is 400mg. The daily dosage should be divided and taken in the morning and the evening.

1. Pharmacodynamic Properties

Guanadrel sulphate is an orally active postganglionic sympathetic inhibitor (adrenergic neuron-blocking drug). The antihypertensive effect of guanadrel, like that of guanethidine, derives from its ability to block the release of noradrenaline (norepinephrine) at sympathetic nerve terminals. In addition, guanadrel depletes neuronal stores of noradrenaline at these sites. This peripheral sympathetic blockade results in relaxation of vascular smooth muscle, with a consequent decrease in total peripheral resistance and in blood pressure.

1.1 Haemodynamic Effects

In dogs, administration of guanadrel 5 mg/kg via catheter into the femoral vein inhibited the reflex increase in mean arterial and femoral perfusion blood pressures induced by bilateral carotid occlusion. The same inhibition was seen to occur with oral guanadrel administration (Pruss and Hidalgo, 1972) and is indicative of postganglionic sympathetic blockade.

In 6 humans with essential hypertension, who were studied before and after treatment with 75 to 400 mg/day of oral guanadrel, a reduction of 13% was observed in mean supine arterial pressure, while total peripheral resistance in the supine position decreased by 21%. Supine heart rate, cardiac output, stroke volume, renal blood flow, glomerular filtration rate, and renal vascular resistance were not significantly affected (table I). The effects of oral guanadrel were somewhat more pronounced in the erect position. Mean arterial pressure was decreased 29% and total peripheral resistance by 37%. Heart rate, cardiac output and stroke volume were not affected. However, in the erect position, renal blood flow and glomerular filtration were noticeably lower and renal vascular resistance was somewhat higher than when the patients were supine. Only the change in renal blood flow, however, was significantly different from control values (Cangiano and Bloomfield, 1969).

A recent small study compared the antihypertensive and cardiac effects of guanadrel and propranolol. Ultrasound measurements of cardiac output revealed no changes with guanadrel. The concurrent use of guanadrel and hydrochlorothiazide produced a significant decrease in peripheral vascular resistance, whereas this was increased by propranolol. Measurements in the same study also showed that guanadrel had no negative effects on cardiac contractility (DeQuattro and Allen, 1984).

These results have formed the basis for concluding that the blood pressure-lowering effect of guanadrel is achieved principally through a lessening of total peripheral resistance and that the drug does not significantly alter cardiac output.

1.2 Effect on Peripheral Sympathetic Neurons

The blockade of noradrenaline release from sympathetic nerve endings by guanadrel is evidenced by: inhibition of nictitating membrane contraction induced by electrical stimulation of pre- or post-ganglionic innervation; suppression of the overall increase in cardiac rate induced by electrical stimulation of the sympathetic nerves to the heart; and the counteraction of arterial blood pressure elevation in response to direct stimulation (data on file, Pennwalt Pharmaceutical Div.).

Noradrenaline depletion after guanadrel administration has been demonstrated by the inhibition of the pressor response associated with tyramine and by the disappearance of the initial transient pressor response to intravenous administration of guanadrel upon repeated injections of the drug (data on file, Pennwalt Pharmaceutical Div.). Direct tissue radioassays have also documented the deple-

Table I. Mean haemodynamic response in 6 patients treated with guanadrel, expressed as percentage of control value (adapted from Cangiano and Bloomfield, 1969, with permission)

	MAP	HR	CO	SV	TPR	RBF	RVR	GFR
Supine position	87*	95	112	122	79**	83	95	90
Standing position	71*	96	108	119	63**	58*	220	70

* $p < 0.05$, ** $p < 0.01$, significant difference from control values.
Abbreviations: SV = stroke volume (ml/min); MAP = mean arterial pressure (mm Hg); HR = heart rate (beats/min); CO = cardiac output (L/min); TPR = total peripheral resistance (units); RBF = renal blood flow (ml/min); GFR = glomerular filtration rate (ml/min) RVR = renal vascular resistance (units).

tion by guanadrel of noradrenaline from synaptic storage vesicles (Rhet et al., 1976).

The uptake of guanadrel appears to be sensitive to blockade by tricyclic antidepressants which may therefore interfere with the antihypertensive effect of guanadrel (see section 5). Pretreatment of rats with desmethylimipramine effectively blocks the depletion of myocardial noradrenaline induced by guanadrel (data on file, Pennwalt Pharmaceutical Div.).

1.3 Effect on the Central Nervous System

Guanadrel does not enter the central nervous system (CNS) of experimental animals in significant amounts and was devoid of CNS activity in a variety of tests. Thus, overt behaviour in mice was normal and no effect on coordination or muscle strength was observed following administration of guanadrel. The drug exhibited no anticonvulsant or analgesic activity and did not potentiate hexobarbitone hypnosis (data on file, Pennwalt Pharmaceutical Div.). The low incidence of clinical CNS side effects during treatment of hypertension with guanadrel is logically related to these findings (section 4).

1.4 Miscellaneous Effects

In vitro, guanadrel did not significantly inhibit monoamine oxidase, although a related compound, debrisoquine, did inhibit the enzyme. The concentrations of serotonin (5-hydroxytryptamine) in the brain and intestine of guinea-pigs were not influenced by guanadrel. The drug did not affect plasma concentrations of cholesterol in normal rats or Grollman hypertensive dogs, nor platelet aggregation in rats or rabbits. A moderate increase in the weight of the accessory reproductive organs in male rats was the only indication of any endocrine activity (data on file, Pennwalt Pharmaceutical Div.).

2. *Pharmacokinetic Studies*

Following oral administration, peak plasma concentrations of guanadrel are attained within 1.5 to 2 hours and are proportional to the dose after ingestion of 25 or 50mg. There is little accumulation after repeated doses (data on file, Pennwalt Pharmaceutical Division).

Guanadrel is extensively distributed throughout the body but concentrations are low in the brain and eye and in the fetus of the mouse. Protein binding is 20%; it is thus unlikely that guanadrel will be involved in drug-protein displacement reactions. However, few clinically significant drug interactions are due solely to displacement from protein binding.

In man, approximately 85% of guanadrel is excreted in the urine as intact drug (about half the dose) and metabolites within 24 hours. The latter are equally divided between an as yet unidentified metabolite and polar materials (primarily 2,3-dihydroxypropylguanidine). The elimination half-life of guanadrel in healthy subjects is approximately

Table II. Comparison of some of the pharmacokinetic properties of guanadrel and guanethidine following oral administration

Variable	Guanethidine	Guanadrel	References
Absorption	Variable (3-50%)	More complete	3, 5
Onset of effect	2-3 days	1-2 hours	4, 6
Urinary excretion (24h)	≈ 13-20%	85%	2, 5
Elimination half-life	≈ 120-240 hours	10 hours	1, 5
Duration of effect after drug withdrawal	Up to 14 days	4-14 hours	2, 5

Key to references: 1 Avery (1980); 2 Goodman and Gilman (1975); 3 McMartin and Simpson (1971); 4 Martindale (1972); 5 Data on file (Pennwalt Pharmaceutical Division); 6 Pascual and Julius (1972).

10 hours (data on file, Pennwalt Pharmaceutical Division).

2.1 Guanadrel Compared with Guanethidine

The onset of action of guanadrel is much quicker and the duration of action shorter than that of guanethidine (table II). Therefore, the dosage of guanadrel can be quickly titrated to individual requirements (unlike the gradual adjustment of dosage necessary with guanethidine), any troublesome side effects disappear more quickly after guanadrel withdrawal, and there is a shorter withdrawal period prior to surgery in patients receiving guanadrel than in those receiving guanethidine.

3. Therapeutic Trials

Guanadrel has been studied in trials of mostly single-blind or non-blind design in patients with mild to moderately severe hypertension not adequately controlled by diuretics alone. Guanadrel was comparable in efficacy with guanethidine and methyldopa in such patients, but its efficacy in patients unresponsive to other antihypertensive drugs has yet to be adequately demonstrated.

3.1 Open Studies

In an open multicentre trial in 199 outpatients with supine diastolic blood pressures from 95 to 120mm Hg, Dunn and Dunlap (1981) reported good control (140/85mm Hg) of standing blood pressure in 75% of patients receiving a wide range of doses of guanadrel (5 to 600mg daily) plus hydrochlorothiazide. A good to excellent response (reduction of 11 to 20mm Hg in mean blood pressure) in the erect position in 75% of 20 Black patients was also reported by Bloomfield and Cangiano (1969). Chlorthalidone was administered concurrently with guanadrel in 8 of these patients.

3.2 Comparisons with Guanethidine

Guanadrel has been compared with guanethidine in a small number of trials, each involving small groups of patients (table III). Patients with uncomplicated essential hypertension ranging in severity from mild to severe had in all but one trial failed to achieve satisfactory control of blood pressure with diuretic treatment which was continued unchanged during subsequent treatment with a peripheral sympathetic inhibitor. None of the trials was truly double-blind, although a modified double-blind design was employed by Bloomfield and Cangiano (1970) in which the investigator dispensing the medication took no part in the evaluation of the patients. All studies have defined their criteria of efficacy, but reported results in some have not been related to these criteria. A flexible dosage regimen was used in all studies and the antihypertensive efficacy of the two drugs was generally similar, except in the study of Malinow (1983) where the rate of response to guanadrel was about twice that of guanethidine (table III). The wide range of dosages used in some studies indicated the need for individualised dosage adjustment with both drugs.

A tendency for more even control of blood pressure with guanadrel administered 3 or 4 times daily (rather than twice daily as presently recommended) than with guanethidine was noted by Hansson et al. (1973) and Pascual and Julius (1972). Guanethidine was administered once daily by Hansson and his colleagues, but the frequency of administration was not stated in either the study of Pascual and Julius (1972), or in those of Bloomfield and Cangiano (1970) and Malinow (1983).

Side effects, which were elicited by a checklist in 3 studies (Chrysant and Frohlich, 1976; Hansson et al., 1973; Malinow, 1983), occurred about twice as often with guanethidine as with guanadrel. However, the high initial incidence of symptoms and the probable influence of a checklist in hypertensive patients was evident in the study of Hansson et al. (1973), where the frequency of side effects during placebo was also high (see also section 4).

3.3 Comparisons with Methyldopa

Guanadrel has been compared with methyldopa in 2 studies involving large numbers of patients (331 and 547) with hypertension (Mroczek, 1984; Nugent et al., 1982) and in one smaller trial in 40 patients (McMahon et al., 1977). These studies were conducted over periods of 6 months to 2 years.

In two multicentre non-blinded comparisons, the addition of either guanadrel or methyldopa to ex-

Table III. Results of controlled trials comparing guanadrel (Gl) and guanethidine (Get) in patients with essential hypertension. All drugs were used in combination with a thiazide diuretic except for the majority of patients in study of Bloomfield and Cangiano (1970)

References	No. of patients	Dosage (mg/day)	Design	Duration (weeks)	Efficacy criteria	Response rate (%) supine	Response rate (%) erect	Side effects incidence[a]
Bloomfield and Cangiano (1970)	40 moderate to severe	Gl 30-400 Get 10-200	mdb, p	15.5 mean	MBP decreased 20mm Hg = ex; decreased 10-20mm Hg = g	GL 60 Get 55	75 70	Get > Gl
Chrysant and Frohlich (1976)	12 moderate to severe	Gl 72 mean Get 90 mean	nb, p	24	BP ≤ 150/95	Gl 60 Get 71	60 71	Get > Gl
Hansson et al. (1973)	13 moderately severe	Gl 70 average Get 57 average	sb, co	6[b]	Best practical control	Both drugs better than placebo		Get > Gl; Gl = placebo
Malinow (1983)	18	Gl 10-75 Get 10-200	nb, r, p	24	BP ≤ 150/90 40 yr or less BP ≤ 155/95 over 40 years	GL 70 Get 25	73 38	Get > Gl
Pascual and Julius (1972)	8	Gl 82.8 mean Get 62 mean	nb, co	GL 5-17 Get 5-30	Lowest with acceptable side effects	Equivalent		Get > Gl

a Get > Gl indicates about twice as many side effects overall with guanethidine.
b Duration on each drug.
Abbreviations: mdb = modified double-blind; p = parallel groups; nb = non-blind; sb = single-blind; co = crossover; r = randomised; MBP = mean blood pressure; ex = excellent; g = good.

Table IV. Criteria of antihypertensive efficacy used in 2 large trials that compared guanadrel and methyldopa

Goal of treatment	Decrease supine diastolic blood pressure to ⩽ 90-95mm Hg[a]
Good control	A reduction of supine diastolic blood pressure of ⩾ 75% toward ideal goal
Fair control	A reduction of supine diastolic blood pressure of 25-74% toward ideal goal
Poor control	A reduction of supine diastolic blood pressure of < 25% toward ideal goal

a Goal was ⩽ 90mm Hg in Nugent et al. (1982) study. The same goal was set for patients under 40 years in the study of Mroczek et al. (1984), this being increased to ⩽ 95mm Hg in patients over 40 years of age.

isting diuretic therapy resulted in a similar decrease in blood pressure with both drugs (Mroczek et al., 1984; Nugent et al., 1982). Both of these studies used almost the same criteria of efficacy (table IV) and both used a checklist to elicit side effects. Good control with either drug was achieved in about 70% of patients treated by Nugent et al. (1982) [fig. 1]. The proportion of patients in whom this degree of control was achieved was not reported by Mroczek et al. (1984), although supine diastolic pressure was decreased by about 12% with either drug. Throughout the study of Nugent et al. (1982) the mean daily dosages needed to control blood pressure were 61mg guanadrel and 1210mg methyldopa, although the required dosage varied directly with pretrial diastolic blood pressure (< 100mm Hg: 58mg guanadrel, 997mg methyldopa; 110 to 119mm Hg: 130mg guanadrel, 1540mg methyldopa). However, the mean daily guanadrel dosage rose 20% from the end of the first year to the end of the second year, which suggested development of some tolerance. A similar phenomenon was noted by Pascual and Julius (1972), although too few patients were involved in this study to permit valid conclusions.

Side effects (table V) occurred with similar frequency with each drug in both studies, although methyldopa consistently caused more complaints of drowsiness than did guanadrel (see section 4).

3.4 Studies in Patients who had Failed to Respond to Other Treatment

In a study of guanadrel in 50 patients who had failed to respond optimally to methyldopa therapy, guanadrel was started at 10mg daily after patients were stabilised on 50 or 100mg of hydrochlorothiazide daily (data on file, Pennwalt Pharmaceutical Division). The highest dosages of guanadrel in this study were higher in general than those used in the comparative studies (section 3.3), due to the fact that the patients had failed to respond to methyldopa therapy. Nevertheless, a satisfactory response to guanadrel was achieved in more than half of this resistant group, who had started with relatively high blood pressures.

DeQuattro and Allen (1984) compared the antihypertensive and cardiac effects of guanadrel and propranolol (both in combination with hydrochlorothiazide) in 20 patients, 13 of whom had not responded satisfactorily to treatment with β-

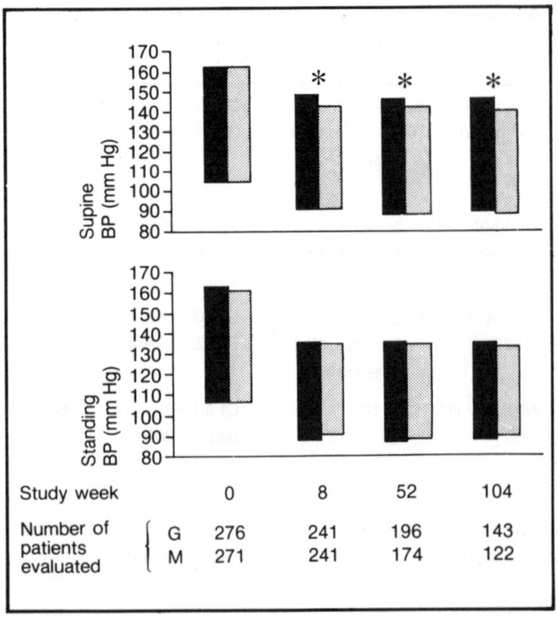

Fig. 1. Mean systolic and diastolic blood pressure responses relative to baseline to guanadrel (■) or methyldopa (□) therapy. The top of each bar represents the mean systolic pressure; the bottom represents mean diastolic pressure; * $p < 0.01$ (after Nugent et al., 1982).

adrenoceptor blocking drugs or methyldopa, each combined with a diuretic. After randomisation according to age, sex, race, and duration of hypertension, dosages of diuretic and either guanadrel or propranolol were titrated for each patient. Following the dose-titration phase, patients were continued on therapy for a 6-week, dose-maintenance period. Both guanadrel and propranolol significantly lowered blood pressure and were well tolerated in combination with diuretic therapy. Guanadrel was slightly more effective in lowering standing pressures and marginally less effective than propranolol for reducing supine pressures.

Thus, preliminary studies suggest that guanadrel may be a useful antihypertensive drug in patients who fail to respond to other second-line therapy, but further well designed trials are needed to demonstrate its value relative to other widely used drugs.

4. *Side Effects*

At dosages of 20 to 400mg daily guanadrel has been well tolerated by most patients with uncomplicated essential hypertension. The rather high incidence of side effects in some studies (e.g. Chrysant and Frohlich, 1976; Malinow, 1983) probably reflects the use of a standardised checklist to evaluate side effects. This is also supported by the high number of side effects reported during placebo administration in the study of Hansson et al. (1973), in which 21 patients noted 70, 67 and 93 effects during 6 weeks' treatment with guanadrel, placebo and guanethidine, respectively. Under these circumstances, guanethidine has usually caused more complaints of dizziness and weakness and of diarrhoea than therapeutically equivalent dosages of guanadrel, but these differences have not been subjected to statistical analysis. In comparative studies, ejaculation disturbances in males have occurred with similar frequency with guanadrel and guanethidine, and in the study of Hansson et al. (1973) with placebo as well.

In comparisons with methyldopa, guanadrel caused significantly less drowsiness and tended to cause less impotence in men. Other side effects, including orthostatic faintness (morning and during the day) and diarrhoea, occurred with similar frequency in patients receiving either drug in the study of Nugent et al. (1982), although in the study of Mroczek et al. (1984), orthostatic faintness, diarrhoea, and sexual dysfunction in men were more frequently reported with guanadrel. The magnitude of the side effect scores was usually directly related to the size of the dose (table V).

Table V. Side effect scores after 2 years of treatment in 265 patients continuing to receive low or high dosages of guanadrel (G) or methyldopa (M) (from Nugent et al., 1982)

Side effect	Side effect scores[a]		
	dose (mg)	G ≤ 50 M ≤ 1000	G > 50 M > 1000
Drowsiness	G	5.6	16.9
	M	17.9[b]	32.7[b]
Orthostatic faintness			
morning	G	4.2	9.1
	M	6.0	10.9
during day	G	5.6	9.9
	M	9.0	12.7
Diarrhoea	G	1.4	12.7
	M	3.0	3.6
Ejaculation disturbances in males	G	6.5	16.1
	M	34.8	16.1

a Side effect score defined as frequency (0-100) × severity (0 to 4) adjusted for pretreatment symptoms.
b Significantly higher with methyldopa.

Data from the manufacturer (table VI), which were derived from a large number of studies, indicate that the rate of withdrawal of treatment because of orthostatic dizziness was significantly higher with guanethidine than with guanadrel and that drowsiness and fatigue necessitated discontinuation of methyldopa significantly more frequently than guanadrel (table VI). Withdrawal of guanadrel because of side effects has been necessary in only 1.2% of patients being treated for hypertension.

5. *Drug Interactions*

Although there are no published data concern-

Table VI. Comparative percentage discontinuation rates of patients taking antihypertensive medication as revealed by combined clinical data (data on file, Pennwalt Corp.)

	Guanadrel	Methyldopa	Guanethidine
Orthostatic faintness, syncope and other faintness	2.2	1.0	8.0
Incresed bowel movements	0.8	0.7	1.4
Drowsiness	0.0	1.9[a]	0.0
Fatigue	0.2	2.6[a]	0.0
Ejaculation disturbances	0.4	0. 0	0.0

a Significantly greater than with guanadrel ($p < 0.0003$).

ing drug interactions with guanadrel, it is to be expected that drug interactions associated with other peripheral sympathetic inhibitors (guanethidine, bethanidine and debrisoquine) will also occur with guanadrel, since, like the others, it decreases adrenergic neuronal activity by inhibiting noradrenaline release (section 1.2). Thus, the antihypertensive effects of guanadrel may be reduced by the addition of sympathomimetic amines such as amphetamines, ephedrine, phenylephrine, phenylpropanolamine and phentermine.

Tricyclic antidepressants prevent the uptake of peripheral sympathetic inhibitors into the nerve endings by inhibiting the noradrenaline pump and thus may markedly decrease the antihypertensive effects of peripheral sympathetic inhibitors if given concurrently. Amitriptyline, imipramine and particularly desipramine have a considerable inhibitory effect on the noradrenaline pump mechanism and are more likely to antagonise the action of peripheral sympathetic inhibitors than doxepin, which has a less marked effect on the noradrenaline pump. Thus, if any of these drugs are given concomitantly with guanadrel and then abruptly discontinued, there may be an excessive lowering of blood pressure.

The antihypertensive effect of the peripheral sympathetic inhibitors may also be antagonised by mazindol (a tricyclic anorectic), pizotifen (a tricyclic drug used in prophylaxis of migraine) and chlorpromazine (Avery and Heel, 1980).

6. *Dosage and Administration*

Guanadrel may be added to diuretic therapy when the diuretic alone fails to control blood pressure adequately. As with other sympathetic suppressant drugs, the dose response to guanadrel varies widely and must be adjusted for each patient until the therapeutic goal is achieved.

The usual starting dosage is 10 mg/day added to a thiazide-type diuretic. The dosage may be increased weekly or monthly until blood pressure is controlled. Most patients require a daily dosage in the range of 20 to 75mg. Maximum recommended dose is 400mg daily. The daily total dosage should be divided and taken in the morning and evening.

Since many 'cold cures' and cough mixtures contain vasoconstrictors, patients should be warned to avoid such substances.

7. *Overdosage*

Symptoms of guanadrel overdose usually include marked dizziness and blurred vision related to postural hypotension and may progress to syncope on standing. If excessive hypotension occurs the patient should be placed in the supine or head-down position. A vasoconstrictor such as phenylephrine may be required to ameliorate the effect of guanadrel. A single dose of vasoconstrictor given intravenously or orally should be sufficient, since guanadrel is rapidly excreted in the urine.

8. *The Place of Guanadrel in Therapy*

The antihypertensive efficacy of guanadrel has been demonstrated in long term multicentre and short term comparative trials involving patients with hypertension not adequately controlled by diuretics alone. In such patients it was similar in efficacy to methyldopa and to guanethidine. The efficacy of guanadrel in treating patients whose blood pressure remains uncontrolled with other antihypertensive drugs remains to be fully evaluated. Generally, guanadrel causes fewer CNS side effects than methyldopa and appears to cause less orthostatic dizziness or diarrhoea than guanethidine. In published studies to date, mild sexual dysfunction in the male (primarily retrograde ejaculation) has occurred with similar frequency during administration of either guanadrel or guanethidine. As guanadrel has a rapid onset of action and is rapidly eliminated compared with guanethidine, it is suited to twice daily administration, and dosage titration can be achieved more rapidly than with guanethidine.

Guanadrel appears to be a useful alternative to other antihypertensive therapy in patients with unacceptable CNS side effects and those patients in whom other widely used antihypertensive drugs are unsuitable. Guanadrel will probably be used most often as a second- or third-line drug to treat patients with moderately severe to severe hypertension rather than the milder forms of the disease. There is a possibility of tolerance developing to the antihypertensive effects of guanadrel, as occurs with other peripherally acting adrenergic drugs, particularly when it is used alone. It is desirable that guanadrel be administered with a diuretic. Nevertheless, further long term studies of this combination are required to determine whether tolerance or pseudotolerance will be a problem.

References

Avery, G.S.: Drug data digest; in Avery (Ed.) Drug Treatment, 2nd ed., p. 1218 (ADIS Press 1980).
Avery, G.S. and Heel, R.C.: Guide to the clinically more important drug interactions; in Avery (Ed.) Drug Treatment, 2nd ed., pp. 1252-1272 (ADIS Press 1980).
Bloomfield, D.K. and Cangiano, J.L.: Clinical experience with a new antihypertensive agent, guanadrel sulfate. Current Therapeutic Research 11: 727 (1969).
Bloomfield, D.K. and Cangiano, J.L.: Guanadrel and guanethidine in hypertension. Clinical Pharmacology and Therapeutics 11: 200 (1970).
Cangiano, J.L. and Bloomfield, D.K.: Haemodynamic effects of a new antihypertensive agent, guanadrel sulfate. Current Therapeutic Research 11: 736 (1969).
Chrysant, S.G. and Frohlich, E.D.: Comparison of the antihypertensive effectiveness of guanadrel and guanethidine. Current Therapeutic Research 19: 379 (1976).
DeQuattro, V. and Allen, J.W.: The comparative antihypertensive and cardiac effects of guanadrel and propranolol. Health Science Review 1 (2): 17 (1984).
Dunn, M.I. and Dunlap, J.L.: Guanadrel – a new antihypertensive drug. Journal of the American Medical Association 245: 1639 (1981).
Goodman, L.S. and Gilman, A.: The Pharmacological Basis of Therapeutics, pp. 553-556 (Macmillan Publishing 1975).
Hansson, L.; Pascual, A. and Julius, S.: Comparison of guanadrel and guanethidine. Clinical Pharmacology and Therapeutics 14: 204 (1973).
Leishman, A.W.; Matthews, H.L. and Smith, A.J.: Guanethidine: Hypotensive drug with prolonged action. Lancet 2: 1044 (1959).
Malinow, S.H.: Comparison of guanadrel and guanethidine efficacy and side effects. Clinical Therapeutics 5: 284 (1983).
Martindale, The extra Pharmacopoeia, 26th ed., p. 786 (Pharmaceutical Press 1972).
McMahon, F.G.; Sosnow, P.; Onel, A.; Ryan, J.R. and Vargas, R.: Comparison of guanadrel sulfate and methyldopa in a two-year study with 40 hypertensive patients, abstracted. Clinical Pharmacology and Therapeutics 21: 110 (1977).
McMartin, C.; Rondel, R.K.; Vinter, J.; Allan, B.R.; Humberstone, P.M. et al.: The fate of guanethidine in two hypertensive patients. Clinical Pharmacology and Therapeutics 11: 423 (1970).
McMartin, C. and Simpson, P.: The absorption and metabolism of guanethidine in hypertensive patients requiring different doses of the drug. Clinical Pharmacology and Therapeutics 12: 73 (1971).
Mroczek, W.J.: A multicenter evaluation of guanadrel sulfate and methyldopa in hypertensive patients. (Abstract.) Clinical Pharmacology and Therapeutics 27 (2): 272 (1980).
Mroczek, W.J.; Burris, J.F. and DeQuattro, V.: A multicenter evaluation of guanadrel sulfate and methyldopa in hypertensive patients receiving a diuretic. Current Therapeutic Research 36: 1004 (1984).
Nugent, C.A.; Palmer, J.D. and Ursprung, J.J.: Guanadrel sulfate compared with methyldopa for mild and moderate hypertension. Pharmacotherapy 2: 378 (1982).
Pascual, A.V. and Julius, S.: Short term effectiveness and hemodynamic actions of guanadrel, a new sympatholytic drug. Current Therapeutic Research 14: 333 (1972).
Pruss, T.P. and Hidalgo, J.: Cardiovascular profile of the antihypertensive agent, guanadrel (36195). Proceedings of the Society for Experimental Biology and Medicine 139: 600 (1972).
Rhet, S.N.; Alexander, N. and Maronde, R.F.: Guanadrel depletion of norepinephrine from storage vesicles of rat vas deferens and atria. Pharmacology 18: 134 (1976).

Address for correspondence and reprints: Dr *F.A. Finnerty Jr*, George Washington University, Washington, D.C. 20052 (USA).

Review Article

Drugs 30: 32-41 (1985)
0012-6667/85/0700-0032/$05.00/0

Interactions of NSAIDs with Diuretics and β-Blockers
Mechanisms and Clinical Implications

J. Webster

Department of Therapeutics and Clinical Pharmacology, University of Aberdeen, Aberdeen

Summary

Indomethacin attenuates the antihypertensive effect of both thiazide diuretics and β-adrenoceptor blocking drugs. The mechanisms of these interactions are poorly understood but sodium and water retention, suppression of plasma renin activity, alterations in adrenoceptor sensitivity and impaired synthesis of vasodilator prostaglandins may all contribute to this effect. Other non-steroidal anti-inflammatory drugs (NSAIDs) may share this property of indomethacin but sulindac, which is a selective inhibitor of extrarenal prostaglandin synthesis, appears not to. This may have important clinical and theoretical implications. Clinicians must beware of this potential interaction in any patient receiving treatment for hypertension.

NSAIDs may also inhibit the natriuretic response to diuretics with resultant adverse effects in patients with heart failure and other forms of oedema. NSAIDs may also have adverse nephrotoxic effects which may be exacerbated by diuretic therapy.

The non-steroidal anti-inflammatory drugs (NSAIDs) are widely prescribed and are commonly implicated in adverse drug reactions. These range from mild, nonspecific symptoms such as dizziness and indigestion to fatal complications such as thrombocytopenia and gastrointestinal haemorrhage. Increasing awareness of such adverse reactions and the identification of new and unpredictable toxicity have contributed in recent years to the imposition of restrictions by various regulatory authorities on the use of NSAIDs such as benoxaprofen, sustained-release indomethacin, indoprofen, zomepirac, phenylbutazone and oxyphenbutazone. In contrast, ibuprofen is now available without prescription in both the United Kingdom and the United States, having been considered by both the Committee for Safety of Medicines (CSM) and the Food and Drug Administration (FDA) to have shown acceptable toxicity over many years of clinical use.

In spite of the recent publicity over the adverse effects of NSAIDs, their propensity to interact adversely with other drugs is not fully appreciated. Such interactions may not be as dramatic or life-threatening as the jaundice produced by benoxaprofen or the aplastic anaemias produced by phenylbutazone, but may be much more common than is generally recognised, reflecting the vast numbers of patients exposed to NSAIDs and other drugs. Another factor contributing to such interactions is that many patients requiring NSAIDs are elderly and require concomitant therapy for other diseases.

Many of these interactions are overlooked because they result in loss of effect of existing therapy rather than augmented toxicity.

1. Interactions of NSAIDs with Diuretics

1.1 Attenuation of Diuretic Action

The first observation that NSAIDs may interact with diuretics was made in 1962 when aspirin was shown to antagonise the action of spironolactone (Elliott, 1962). Since then, a number of reports have indicated that NSAIDs may antagonise the actions of 'loop' diuretics, thiazides and potassium-sparing diuretics.

1.1.1 Mechanisms

The interaction between NSAIDs and diuretics is influenced by patient factors such as age, renal disease and cardiac failure, and by drug factors such as dose, duration of administration and pharmacological profile. As a result, it can be difficult to attribute the interaction to one particular mechanism. Many NSAIDs cause sodium and water retention, especially phenylbutazone and indomethacin, and this tends to negate the action of diuretics in a global fashion. Possible mechanisms include pharmacokinetic interactions, effects on renal tubular handling of salt and water, and alterations in prostaglandin-mediated renal haemodynamics. These may coexist or may vary according to the type of diuretic used.

The interference by NSAIDs, especially indomethacin, with the natriuretic effects of frusemide (furosemide) has been confirmed in several studies (Data et al., 1978; Patak et al., 1975), although the dose and duration of drug administration may be critical (Brater, 1979; Scherer and Weber, 1979). In an elegant study by Chennavasin et al. (1980) it was shown that indomethacin altered the disposition of frusemide in man. Renal clearance of frusemide was reduced, but so also was non-renal clearance. The delivery of frusemide into the urine and to the tubular sites of action was not altered and the pharmacokinetic changes were not sufficient to explain the impaired natriuretic response to frusemide. Indomethacin shifted the serum concentration-response curve of frusemide to the right, while the urinary frusemide excretion-response curve was not altered. The maximum responses in both cases were decreased, indicating a non-competitive pharmacodynamic inhibition of frusemide effects.

Several investigations have shown that activation of renal prostaglandin synthesis accompanies the natriuresis induced by loop diuretics and it seems likely that prostaglandins such as PGE_2 and PGI_2 (prostacyclin) mediate both the natriuresis and the increase in renal blood flow produced by such drugs (Attallah, 1979; Ciabattoni et al., 1979). Nonspecific inhibitors of cyclo-oxygenase, such as indomethacin, block the activation of renal prostaglandins and attenuate the response to diuretics such as frusemide (Mackay et al., 1984). Sulindac is a selective inhibitor of extrarenal cyclo-oxygenase (Ciabattoni et al., 1980) and does not inhibit the natriuretic response to frusemide. This supports the hypothesis of a pharmacodynamic interaction based on inhibition of renal prostaglandin synthesis.

Degree of Inhibition in Relation to Site of Action

Diuretics acting at different sites along the renal tubule may differ in the degree to which their actions may be attenuated by NSAIDs (Favre et al., 1983). The original observation that aspirin blocks the natriuresis induced by spironolactone (Elliott, 1962) has been confirmed by Tweeddale and Ogilvie (1973) who showed that a single 600mg dose of aspirin produced a profound inhibition of the natriuretic response to spironolactone in subjects receiving fludrocortisone. Both indomethacin and diflunisal have been shown to inhibit the natriuretic response to spironolactone in normal volunteers (Favre et al., 1983). In a study designed to elucidate the mechanisms of these interactions, Ramsay et al., (1976) showed that aspirin reduced the fractional urinary excretion of canrenone, the principal unconjugated metabolite of spironolactone. These authors proposed that the most likely explanation for this pharmacokinetic interaction was competition between aspirin and canrenone for active secretion in the proximal renal tubule. Thus it is possible that both pharmacokinetic and pharmacodynamic factors may contribute to this interaction.

NSAIDs undoubtedly antagonise the natriuretic effects of 'loop' diuretics (Brater, 1979; Patak et al., 1975). It has been suggested that prostaglandins also mediate the diuretic action of thiazides (Kramer et al., 1980), but another study found that inhibition of prostaglandin synthesis by either indomethacin or diflunisal did not alter the natriuretic effect of hydrochlorothiazide (Favre et al., 1983).

There is no doubt that prostaglandins are important mediators of renin release (Frolich et al., 1976; Glasson et al., 1979), and inhibition of renal prostaglandin synthesis appears to inhibit activation of the renin-angiotensin-aldosterone system by all types of diuretic.

1.1.2 Clinical Implications

The principal adverse clinical effect of the attenuated natriuretic response to diuretics by NSAIDs is worsening of cardiac failure. Phenylbutazone has long been recognised as a cause of cardiac decompensation, and both oedema and cardiac failure are contraindications to its use. It is likely that many other NSAIDs interact adversely with diuretics in this way, such as ibuprofen (Yeung Laiwah and Mactier, 1981) and piroxicam (Fowler and Arnold, 1983), but such interactions may be overlooked or dealt with by increasing the medication used to treat the heart failure. Patients at greatest risk would appear to be the elderly and those with renal insufficiency.

A recent study has thrown some further light on both the underlying mechanisms and clinical significance of this interaction (Dzau et al., 1984). These authors found that urinary metabolites of PGE_2 and prostacyclin were increased in patients with severe congestive heart failure and that such changes occurred principally in patients with associated hyponatraemia. They postulated that in such patients there is concomitant activation of the renin-angiotensin-aldosterone system – which is predominantly vasoconstrictor – and of the renal prostaglandin system – which is predominantly vasodilator. Activation of these systems serves to maintain circulatory and renal homeostasis. Disturbance of this homeostatic mechanism by inhibition of prostaglandin synthesis resulted in haemodynamic deterioration. When indomethacin was given orally either as a single 75mg dose or as four 50mg doses at intervals of 6 hours, patients with cardiac failure and a serum sodium concentration under 135 mmol/L showed a significant decrease in cardiac index, and increases in capillary wedge pressure, mean arterial pressure and systemic vascular resistance (fig. 1).

Thus, in patients with cardiac failure, NSAIDs may cause deleterious effects by a number of mechanisms, including inhibition of synthesis of vasodilator prostaglandins, interference with natriuretic mechanisms in the renal medulla (Oliw et al., 1976), and attenuation of the natriuretic action

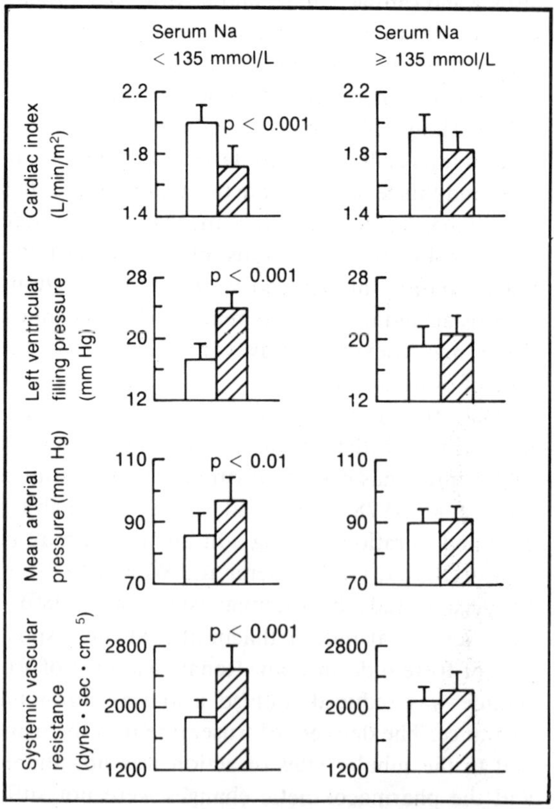

Fig. 1. Changes in mean (± SEM) values of cardiac index, left ventricular filling pressure, mean arterial pressure and systemic vascular resistance before (□) and after (▨) administration of indomethacin in 23 patients with heart failure who underwent haemodynamic evaluation and who were grouped according to their serum sodium concentration (reproduced with permission from Dzau et al., 1984).

of diuretics. It is also possible that some NSAIDs may have deleterious effects on coronary perfusion (Friedman et al., 1981).

In patients with cardiac failure due to ischaemic heart disease, this may adversely affect ventricular function and indirectly reduce the benefit of drugs used to treat the heart failure.

Clinicians should be aware of this important interaction and should exercise great care in the use of NSAIDs in patients with cardiac failure, especially if the failure is severe and associated with hyponatraemia, or if the patient is elderly and has renal impairment.

1.2 Attenuation of Antihypertensive Effect

In spite of the widespread use of thiazide diuretics as antihypertensive therapy for over 20 years, their mode of action is incompletely understood. Extracellular volume depletion and reduced cardiac output occur in the initial phase of treatment, whereas after several weeks of treatment cardiac output returns to normal and total peripheral resistance falls (Conway and Lauwers, 1960). It had appeared that the ability of the kidneys to excrete sodium was essential to the antihypertensive effect of diuretics (Bennett et al., 1977) but a study in patients with chronic renal failure has raised the possibility of a mechanism independent of sodium loss (Jones and Nanra, 1979).

Direct evidence is lacking of a specific vasodilator effect of thiazide diuretics but there is considerable evidence in animals that these drugs reduce vascular reactivity to both angiotensin II (Weinberger et al., 1972) and noradrenaline (norepinephrine) [Eckstein et al., 1962, 1966]. In man, chlorothiazide reduces both local (Jackson and Duff, 1963) and systemic (Fries et al., 1960) vascular reactivity to noradrenaline, the latter being at least partly reversible by volume replacement.

Indomethacin pretreatment has been noted to attenuate the antihypertensive effects of thiazides (Lopez-Ovejero et al., 1978; Watkins et al., 1980) [fig. 2]. Some doubt has recently been raised about the clinical importance of this interaction (Koopmans et al., 1984) but even this report demonstrates a transient adverse interaction of indomethacin with hydrochlorothiazide. Several mechanisms for this interaction have been proposed.

1.2.1 Mechanisms

The first possible mechanism is that NSAIDs may themselves exhibit a pressor effect, negating the relatively mild antihypertensive action of thia-

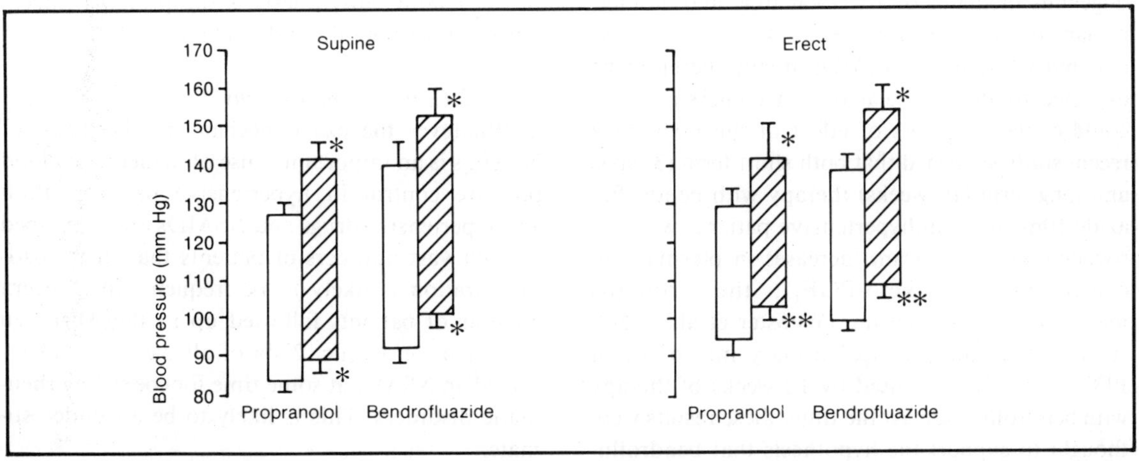

Fig. 2. Effects on supine and erect blood pressures of adding either indomethacin (▨), 100mg daily for 3 weeks, or placebo (□) to hypertensive patients receiving treatment with bendrofluazide (n = 5) or propranolol (n = 8); * $p < 0.05$; ** $p < 0.01$ [reproduced with permission from Watkins et al., 1980].

zides. Intravenous indomethacin administration may cause a short-lived rise in blood pressure (Dzau et al., 1984; Nowak and Wennmalm, 1978). In patients with Parkinsonism and postural hypotension, indomethacin reduced forearm blood flow, significantly reduced the fall in blood pressure on standing, and lessened orthostatic symptoms (Abate et al., 1979). However, there is little evidence to suggest that long term oral therapy has a significant pressor effect in normal or hypertensive subjects.

NSAIDs may cause sufficient fluid retention to reverse the volume depletion caused by diuretics. This might more readily explain the reversal of the short term antihypertensive effect of diuretics than the long term effect, when volume depletion is less evident. Nevertheless, this must be considered as a partial explanation, at least, for this interaction.

Another hypothesis is that thiazides may exhibit their antihypertensive effect directly on arteriolar tone. This would be compatible with the principal net haemodynamic effect of long term thiazide therapy in hypertension, namely a reduction in total peripheral resistance. The possible mediator of such an effect has aroused speculation but no mechanism has yet been established. Prostacyclin is synthesised in blood vessel walls and is a potent vasodilator (Armstrong et al., 1978). It is possible that prostacyclin may be an important endogenous mediator of arteriolar tone and a determinant of blood pressure. Inhibition of prostacyclin biosynthesis by NSAIDs might therefore be expected to alter vascular responsiveness and this could explain the loss of effect of thiazides. One recent study suggested that both short term (3 days) and long term (10 weeks) therapy with bendrofluazide 10mg daily in hypertensive patients were associated with significant increases in plasma concentrations of 6-keto-$PGF_{1\alpha}$, the principal metabolite of prostacyclin, (Webster et al., 1980). In this study the principal urinary metabolite of $PFG_{2\alpha}$ was also increased by 10 weeks of therapy with bendrofluazide. At the time, these results were thought to support the hypothesis that bendrofluazide may have stimulated the biosynthesis of a vasodilator prostaglandin such as prostacyclin. Since then, however, some doubts have emerged about the validity of the assay used in that study for 6-keto-$PGF_{1\alpha}$ in plasma and it now seems certain that prostacyclin does not circulate as a systemically active hormone (Blair et al., 1982; Fitzgerald et al., 1981). Analytical problems continue to plague the assessment of prostaglandin synthesis *in vivo*, and the question of whether thiazides stimulate the systemic biosynthesis of vasodilator prostaglandins remains unanswered.

A recent and important development in the understanding of this interaction has been the demonstration that sulindac, unlike indomethacin, may enhance rather than attenuate the antihypertensive effects of thiazide diuretics (Steiness and Waldorff, 1982). As already mentioned, sulindac differs from indomethacin in being a selective inhibitor of extrarenal prostaglandin biosynthesis (Ciabattoni et al., 1980). This suggests that inhibition of renal prostaglandin synthesis may be the key to the interaction between NSAIDs and thiazides in hypertension.

A series of clinical studies has suggested that indomethacin attenuates the effect of most antihypertensive drugs in a nonspecific way and furthermore that other NSAIDs such as aspirin and naproxen do not share this interaction (Chalmers et al., 1983). These results are a little difficult to reconcile with the hypothesis that inhibition of prostaglandin biosynthesis is the principal mechanism underlying the indomethacin effect.

1.2.2 Clinical Implications

Whatever the exact mechanism, the effect of NSAIDs is an important cause of inadequate blood pressure control in hypertensive patients. Both antihypertensive drugs and NSAIDs are prescribed to such vast numbers of patients that their coadministration is likely to be frequent. In a recent analysis of patients followed up in the Aberdeen Hypertension Clinic, 2.5% of all patients had received an NSAID at some time for coexisting rheumatic disorders. This is likely to be an underestimate.

Patients in whom NSAIDs contribute to severe or refractory hypertension may be uncommon but are relatively easy to identify provided clinicians are aware of the possible interaction. More difficult to identify are the many patients whose blood pressure control is marginally suboptimal but who may escape rigorous clinical audit. Evidence is emerging that the level of blood pressure achieved during follow-up is an important predictor of adverse cardiovascular events (Australian Therapeutic Trial in Mild Hypertension, 1980). Even a partial attenuation of antihypertensive drug action may adversely affect prognosis, and the problem will be overlooked unless clinicians aim to achieve strict 'target pressures'.

All hypertensive patients receiving NSAIDs should have their blood pressure monitored more frequently than usual. If blood pressure control is unsatisfactory, the NSAID should be stopped. If there is a continuing need for NSAID therapy, then a trial of an alternative drug such as sulindac should be undertaken.

1.3 Nephrotoxicity

It is increasingly recognised that NSAIDs produce a variety of toxic effects on the kidney. The various syndromes of NSAID-associated nephrotoxicity have recently been reviewed by Clive and Stoff (1984).

1.3.1 Mechanisms

Water and electrolyte balance may be disturbed by NSAIDs. Sodium retention and oedema are common, affecting over 10% of patients receiving NSAIDs and contributing to the loss of efficacy of diuretics. Occasionally, severe hyponatraemia may result from inhibition of free water excretion (Walker et al., 1981). This may occur if there is pre-existing renal impairment (Blum and Aviram, 1980) and may be exacerbated if diuretics are coadministered. Hyperkalaemia may also occur (Goldszer et al., 1981). This might not in itself be a serious disadvantage in patients receiving either a 'loop' diuretic or a thiazide but might be hazardous in patients receiving potassium-sparing diuretics.

A more serious problem is the precipitation of acute renal failure by NSAIDs. It is generally accepted that NSAIDs do not impair renal function in normal subjects but that inhibition of prostaglandin synthesis may have serious adverse effects on renal function when superimposed on hypovolaemia, salt depletion, cardiac failure or cirrhosis. This supports the hypothesis that prostaglandins may act to maintain renal homeostasis under adverse conditions.

A recent study has provided further persuasive evidence in support of this hypothesis (Ciabattoni et al., 1984). In patients with chronic glomerular disease, urinary excretion of 6-keto-PGF$_{1\alpha}$, the stable hydrolysis product of prostacyclin, appeared to be reduced. In these patients ibuprofen, a non-selective inhibitor of cyclo-oxygenase, increased serum creatinine and reduced the renal clearance of creatinine and para-aminohippurate. In contrast, sulindac did not impair renal function, despite inhibiting extrarenal cyclo-oxygenase.

1.3.2 Clinical Implications

Patients receiving diuretic therapy may be at increased risk of NSAID-induced renal failure. Reversible acute renal failure occurred in 2 healthy medical students receiving indomethacin and triamterene as part of a research study (Favre et al., 1982). A similar interaction has not been observed with other diuretics but may be more difficult to detect and attribute to drugs in patients with coexisting renal disease.

Great care should be taken to avoid the combination of NSAIDs and diuretics in patients with renal disease, cirrhosis or cardiac failure as well as in elderly patients who usually have reduced renal reserve.

2. Interaction of NSAIDs with β-Blockers

2.1 Attenuation of Antihypertensive Action

Indomethacin has been reported to attenuate the antihypertensive effect of propranolol in man (Durao et al., 1977; Watkins et al., 1980). A similar interaction has also been observed between indomethacin and pindolol (Durao et al., 1977), oxprenolol (Salvetti et al., 1982a) and atenolol (Salvetti et al., 1982b). Flurbiprofen attenuates the antihypertensive response to single doses of propranolol (Webster et al., 1983). In contrast, other NSAIDs such as sulindac (Salvetti et al., 1984), naproxen and aspirin (Chalmers et al., 1983) appear not to exhibit this interaction.

This interaction is not only of clinical importance but also may contribute to an understanding of the mode of action of β-blockers in hypertension.

2.1.1 Mechanisms

The mechanism by which β-blockers lower blood pressure remains uncertain. Several explanations have been proposed, including negative cardiac inotropic (Donoso et al., 1967) and chronotropic effects (Dollery et al., 1969), inhibition of renin release (Birkenhager et al., 1977; Buhler et al., 1972; Hollifield et al., 1976), central nervous system effects (Lewis, 1976) and presynaptic inhibition of neurotransmitter release (Langer, 1976).

Initially, systemic vascular resistance rises after β-blockade (Frolich et al., 1968). During long term β-blockade cardiac output remains suppressed (Tarazi and Dunstan, 1972) but the initial effects on peripheral resistance are reversed (Cohn, 1983). The autoregulatory mechanisms underlying this apparent delayed vasodilator response to long term β-blockade remain unclear (Guyton et al., 1974). Largely because of these uncertainties, the mechanism underlying the interaction between NSAIDs and β-blockers is also poorly understood.

The possibility exists that long term use of β-blockers may stimulate the synthesis of vasodilator prostaglandins, such as PGE_2 and prostacyclin, that these may mediate some of the haemodynamic effects of long term β-blockade, and that inhibitors of prostaglandin synthesis may negate these effects. Such an hypothesis is superificially attractive but fails to explain a number of observations.

Webster et al. (1984) have recently reported that flurbiprofen attenuated the hypotensive effect of single doses of propranolol. This effect was observed within 2 hours of oral ingestion of propranolol. At this stage of treatment the predominant haemodynamic effect is a reduction in cardiac output, and total peripheral resistance may be increased; furthermore, it was found that the hypotensive response to single doses of atenolol was not altered by flurbiprofen. This raised the possibility that atenolol and propranolol might differ at least in their short term antihypertensive mode of action.

In this study (Webster et al., 1984) flurbiprofen had no effect on the suppression of post-exercise heart rate by either propranolol or atenolol. Similarly, indomethacin did not interfere with the inhibition of exercise-induced tachycardia by metoprolol (Rolf Smith et al., 1983). These results suggest that NSAIDs do not interfere with cardiac β_1-adrenoceptors.

It has been suggested that inhibition of prostaglandin synthesis might result in increased sensitivity of α-adrenoceptors (Bartter et al., 1976; Rubin et al., 1980). This may be clinically more apparent in the presence of a non-selective β-blocker such as propranolol than in the presence of a cardioselective drug such as atenolol, and might be sufficient to offset the delayed vasodilator response to long term propranolol. However, this explanation would not account for the observation of Salvetti et al. (1982b) that indomethacin attenuates the hypotensive effect of atenolol, and the hypothesis remains speculative.

Another possible mechanism for the interaction between NSAIDs and propranolol may lie in the suppression of plasma renin activity that accompanies administration of NSAIDs. Suppression of plasma renin activity is almost certainly an important, though not exclusive, factor in the antihypertensive action of propranolol and certain other β-blockers (Harms et al., 1978). Prior suppression of plasma renin activity might therefore attenuate the antihypertensive response. This hypothesis is certainly plausible, and may explain the interaction in some subjects.

In other studies, sulindac did not attenuate the antihypertensive action of atenolol (Salvetti et al., 1982c). However, this study also showed that sulindac suppressed plasma renin activity, which is rather surprising in view of its proposed action as a selective inhibitor of extrarenal prostaglandin synthesis. A series of studies by Chalmers and colleagues (1983) tends to confirm this dissociation of changes in plasma renin activity induced by NSAIDs from their attenuation of the antihypertensive effects of β-blockers. These authors also proposed that the interaction of indomethacin with antihypertensive drugs is a general effect and is independent of the specific antihypertensive drug used. Other studies have confirmed that indomethacin attenuates the antihypertensive effect of prazosin in some patients (Rubin et al., 1980) and of captopril (Salvetti et al., 1982c), in addition to its effects on thiazide diuretics as discussed above.

The possibility of a pharmacokinetic interaction between NSAIDs and β-blockers was studied by Webster et al. (1983). They showed that flurbiprofen had no effect on the disposition of either atenolol, a hydrophilic, non-metabolised drug cleared by the kidney, or propranolol, a lipophilic drug that undergoes extensive hepatic extraction. Thus, although NSAIDs may alter hepatic microsomal enzyme activity (Chalmers et al., 1973), apparent hepatic blood flow (Feely and Wood, 1983) and renal elimination of some drugs (Chennavasin et al., 1980), these factors would not appear to explain the attenuation of the effects of β-blockers on blood pressure.

It is distinctly possible that several mechanisms may apply simultaneously, and that many confounding factors (such as sodium balance, renin status, drug dosage, presence of other drugs and severity of hypertension) may influence the resultant effect on blood pressure on combining NSAIDs with β-blockers.

2.1.2 Clinical Importance

The main clinical problem arising from interaction of NSAIDs with β-blockers is loss of blood pressure control. As with the diuretics, this interaction is often overlooked and underestimated. Indomethacin may be more likely to exhibit this interaction than other NSAIDs but there is a need for more reliable comparative data. Sulindac may offer an alternative choice of NSAID if blood pressure control remains unsatisfactory.

Since heart rate response to β-blockade seems to be unaffected by NSAIDs, it is unlikely that these drugs will adversely affect the treatment of angina by β-blockers. However, it should be borne in mind that indomethacin may adversely affect coronary blood flow in some patients (Friedman et al., 1981). Furthermore, it might be predicted that cardiac failure might be more common or more severe as a consequence of combined NSAID/β-blocker therapy than as a consequence of either drug alone.

3. Conclusions

Clinical investigators are faced with several important restrictions on further research into the nature of these interactions, the drugs so affected and their dose-effect relationships.

In the past, many studies have been carried out in patients with mild uncomplicated hypertension. These are not necessarily the patients to suffer most from any potential NSAID interaction. Studies in more severe hypertension carry added risks and may be difficult to justify. Such studies may require patients to take NSAIDs although there may be no clinical indication for the use of such drugs. Awareness of the serious unpredictable adverse effects of NSAIDs makes it increasingly difficult to expose such patients or volunteers to such drugs unless there is a coexisting clinical indication for their use.

Patients with conditions requiring therapy with NSAIDs such as osteoarthritis, rheumatoid arthritis and ankylosing spondylitis may be considered for interaction studies with a reasonable prospect of some personal benefit. However, in these patients it may be difficult to justify withdrawal of NSAIDs and substitution by placebo for other than short term studies. Furthermore, the presence of joint pain, stiffness and disability may confound the interpretation of results. A recent study in patients with arthritis and coexisting hypertension treated with a variety of antihypertensive drugs has confirmed the adverse effect on blood pressure of indomethacin as compared with sulindac and paracetamol (Lewis et al., 1985).

Practical and ethical constraints imply that the collection of further reliable clinical information in this field is likely to be difficult. There will be a continuing need for careful observational studies in individual patients, but randomised studies are indispensible. The importance of patient selection, dose and duration of drug treatments, 'blind' observers and accurate methods of measurement cannot be overemphasised.

References

Abate, G.; Polimeni, R.M.; Cuccurullo, F.; Puddu, P. and Lenzi, S.: Effects indomethacin on postural hypotension in Parkinsonism. British Medical Journal 2: 1466-1468 (1979).

Armstrong, J.M.; Dusting, G.J.; Moncada, S. and Vane, J.R.: Cardiovascular actions of prostacyclin (PGI_2) a metabolite of arachidonic acid which is synthesized by blood vessels. Circulation Research 43 (Suppl. 1): 112-119 (1978).

Attallah, A.A.: Interaction of prostaglandins with diuretics. Prostaglandins 18: 369-375 (1979).

Bartter, F.C.; Gill, J.R.; Frolich, J.C.; Bowden, R.E.; Hollifield, J.W. et al.: Prostaglandins are over produced by the kidneys and mediate hyperreninemia in Bartter's syndrome. Transactions of the Association of American Physicians 89: 77-91 (1976).

Bennett, W.M.; McDonald, W.J.; Kuehnel, E.; Hartnett, M.N. and Porter, G.A.: Do diuretics have antihypertensive properties independent of natriuresis? Clinical Pharmacology and Therapeutics 22: 499-504 (1977).

Birkenhager, W.H.; De Leeuw, P.W.; Wester, A.; Kho, L.T.; Vandongen, R. and Falke, H.E.: Therapeutic effects of β-adrenoceptor blocking agents. Advances in Internal Medicine and Paediatrics 39: 117-134 (1977).

Blair, I.A.; Barrow, S.E.; Waddel, K.A.; Lewis, P.J. and Dollery, C.T.: Prostacyclin is not a circulatory hormone in man. Prostaglandins 23: 579-589 (1982).

Blum, M. and Aviram, A.: Ibuprofen induced hyponatraemia. Rheumatology and Rehabilitation 19: 258-259 (1980).

Brater, D.C.: Analysis of the effect of indomethacin on the response to furosemide in man: Effect of dose of furosemide. Journal of Pharmacology and Experimental Therapeutics 210: 386-390 (1979).

Buhler, F.R.; Laragh, J.H.; Baer, L.; Vaughan, E.D. and Brunner, H.R.: Propranolol inhibition of renin secretion: A specific approach to diagnosis and treatment of renin-dependent hypertensive diseases. New England Journal of Medicine 287: 1209-1214 (1972).

Chalmers, I.M.; Bell, M.A. and Buchanan, W.W.: Effect of flurbiprofen on the metabolism of antypyrine in man. Annals of Rheumatic Disease 32: 58-61 (1973).

Chalmers, J.; Ayres, B.; Bune, A.; Graham, J.; West, M. and Wing, L.: Effects of indomethacin, sulindac, naproxen, aspirin and paracetamol in treated hypertensive patients. (Abstract No. 234.) 2nd World Conference on Clinical Pharmacology and Therapeutics (1983).

Chennavasin, P.; Seiwell, R. and Brater, D.C.: Pharmacokinetic-dynamic analysis of the indomethacin-furosemide interaction in man. Journal of Pharmacology and Experimental Therapeutics 215: 77-81 (1980).

Ciabattoni, G.; Cinotti, G.A.; Pieruccu, A.; Simonetti, B.M.; Manzi, M. et al.: Effects of sulindac and ibuprofen in patients with chronic glomerular disease. New England Journal of Medicine 310: 279-283 (1984).

Ciabattoni, G.; Pugliese, F.; Cinotti, G.A.; Stirati, G.; Ronci, R. et al.: Characterization of furosemide-induced activation of the renal prostaglandin system. European Journal of Pharmacology 60: 181-187 (1979).

Ciabottoni, G.; Pugliese, F.; Cinotti, G.A. and Patrono, C.: Renal effects of anti-inflammatory drugs. European Journal of Rheumatology and Inflammation 3: 210-221 (1980).

Clive, D.M. and Stoff, J.S.: Renal syndromes associated with nonsteroidal anti-inflammatory drugs. New England Journal of Medicine 31: 563-572 (1984).

Cohn, J.N.: Haemodynamic effects of β-blockers. Drugs 25 (Suppl. 2): 100-102 (1983).

Conway, J. and Lauwers, P.: Haemodynamic and hypotensive effects of long-term therapy with chlorothiazide. Circulation 21: 21-27 (1960).

Data, J.L.; Rane, A.; Gierkens, J.; Wilkinson, G.R.; Nies, A.S. and Branch, R.A.: The influence of indomethacin on the pharmacokinetics, diuretic response and haemodynamics of furosemide in the dog. Journal of Pharmacology and Experimental Therapeutics 206: 431-438 (1978).

Dollery, C.T.; Patterson, J.W. and Connelly, M.E.: Clinical pharmacology of beta receptor blocking drugs. Clinical Pharmacology and Therapeutics 10: 765-799 (1969).

Donoso, E.; Cohn, L.J.; Newman, B.J.; Broome, H.S.; Stein, W.G. and Friedberg, C.K.: Effects of propranolol on patients with complete heart block and implanted pacemaker. Circulation 36: 534-538 (1967).

Durao, V.; Martins-Prata, M. and Pires Gonçalves, L.M.: Modification of antihypertensive effect of β-adrenoceptor blocking agents by inhibition of endogenous prostaglandin synthesis. Lancet 2: 1005-1007 (1977).

Dzau, V.J.; Packer, M.; Lilly, L.S.; Swartz, S.L.; Hollenberg, N.K. and Williams, G.H.: Prostaglandins in severe congestive heart failure in relation to activation of the renin-angiotensin system and hyponatremia. New England Journal of Medicine 310: 347-352 (1984).

Eckstein, J.W.; Abboud, F.M. and Pereda, S.A.: Effects of noradrenaline on cardiac output, blood pressure and heart rate in dogs treated with chlorothiazide. Journal of Clinical Investigation 41: 1578-1583 (1962).

Eckstein, J.W.; Wendling, M.G. and Abboud, F.M.: Circulatory responses to noradrenaline after prolonged treatment with chlorothiazide. Circulation Research 28 (Suppl. 1): 48-53 (1966).

Elliott, H.C.: Reduced adrenocortical steroid excretion rates in man following aspirin administration. Metabolism 11: 1015-1018 (1962).

Favre, L.; Glasson, P. and Vallotton, M.B.: Reversible acute renal failure with combined triamterene and indomethacin. A study in healthy subjects. Annals of Internal Medicine 96: 317-320 (1982).

Favre, L.; Glasson, P.H.; Riondel, A. and Vallotton, M.B.: Interaction of diuretics and non-steroidal anti-inflammatory drugs in man. Clinical Science 64: 407-415 (1983).

Fitzgerald, G.A.; Brash, A.R.; Falardeau, P. and Oates, J.A.: Estimated rate of prostacyclin secretion into the circulation of normal man. Journal of Clinical Investigation 68: 1272-1276 (1981).

Feely, J. and Wood, A.J.J.: Effect of inhibition of prostaglandin synthesis on hepatic drug clearance. British Journal of Clinical Pharmacology 15: 109-111 (1983).

Fowler, R.W. and Arnold, K.G.: Non-steroidal analgesic and anti-inflammatory agents. British Medical Journal 287: 835 (1983).

Friedman, P.L.; Brown, E.J.; Gunther, S.; Alexander, R.W.; Barry, W.H.; Mudge, G.H. and Grossman, W.: Coronary vasoconstrictor effect of indomethacin in patients with coronary-artery disease. New England Journal of Medicine 305: 1171-1175 (1981).

Fries, E.D.; Wanko, A.; Schnaper, H.W. and Frolich, E.D.: Mechanism of altered blood pressure responsiveness produced by chlorothiazide. Journal of Clinical Investigation 39: 1277-1281 (1960).

Frolich, E.D.; Tarazi, R.C.; Dunstan, H.C. and Page, I.H.: The

paradox of beta adrenergic blockade in hypertension. Circulation 37: 417-423 (1968).
Frolich, J.C.; Hollifield, J.W.; Dormois, J.C.; Frolich, B.L.; Seyberth, H.; Michelakis, A.M. and Oates, J.A.: Suppression of plasma renin activity by indomethacin in man. Circulation Research 39: 447-452 (1976).
Glasson, P.; Gaillard, R.; Riondel, A. and Vallotton, M.B.: Role of renal prostaglandins and relationships to renin aldosterone and antidiuretic hormone during salt depletion in man. J. Clin. Endocrin. Metab. 49: 176-181 (1979).
Goldszer, R.C.; Goodley, E.L.; Rosner, M.J.; Simons, W.M. and Schwartz, A.B.: Hyperkalemia associated with indomethacin. Archives of Internal Medicine 141: 802-804 (1981).
Guyton, A.C.; Coleman, T.G.; Cowley, A.W.; Manning, R.O.; Norman, R.A. and Ferguson, J.D.: A system analysis approach to understanding long-range arterial blood pressure control. Circulation Research 35: 159-176 (1974).
Harms, H.H.; Gooren, L.; Spoelstra, A.J.G.; Hesse, C. and Verschoor, L.: Blockade of isoprenaline-induced changes in plasma free fatty acids, immunoreactive insulin levels and plasma renin activity in healthy subjects, by propranolol, pindolol, practolol, atenolol, metoprolol and acebutolol. British Journal of Clinical Pharmacology 5: 19-26 (1978).
Hollifield, J.W.; Sherman, K.; van der Zwagg, R. and Shand, D.G.: Proposed mechanism of propranolol's antihypertensive effect in essential hypertension. N. Eng. J. Med. 295: 68-73 (1976).
Jackson, E. and Duff, R.S.: Effect of chlorothiazide on noradrenaline vasoconstriction in man. Clinical Science 24: 24-27 (1963).
Jones, B. and Nanra, R.S.: Double-blind trial of antihypertensive effects of chlorothiazide in severe renal failure. Lancet 2: 1258-1260 (1979).
Koopmans, P.P.; Thien, Th. and Gribnau, F.W.J.: Influence of non-steroidal anti-inflammatory drugs on diuretic treatment of mild to moderate essential hypertension. British Medical Journal 289: 1492-1494 (1984).
Kramer, H.G.; Dusing, R.; Stinnesbeck, B.; Prior, W.; Backer, A. et al.: Interactions of conventional and antikaliuretic diuretics with the renal prostaglandin system. Clinical Science 59: 67-70 (1980).
Langer, S.Z.: The role of α and β presynaptic receptors in the regulation of noradrenaline release elicited by nerve stimulation. Clinical Science 51 (Suppl. 3): 421-426 (1976).
Lewis, P.J.: Propranolol – an antihypertensive drug with a central action; in Davies and Reid (Eds) Central Actions of Drugs in Blood Pressure Regulation, pp. 206-213 (Pitman Medical, Tunbridge Wells 1975).
Lewis, R.V.; Toner, J.M.; Jackson, P.R. and Ramsey, L.E.: Effects of sulindac and indomethacin on the blood pressure of hypertensive patients. (Abstract C44.) Proceedings of the British Pharmacological Society (1985).
Lopez-Ovejero, J.A.; Weber, M.A.; Drayer, J.I.M.; Sealey, J.E. and Laragh, J.H.: Effects of indomethacin alone and during diuretic or β-adrenoceptor-blockade therapy on blood pressure and the renin system in essential hypertension. Clinical Science and Molecular Medicine 55 (Suppl. 4): 203S-205S (1978).
Mackay, G.; Muir, A.L. and Watson, M.L.: Contribution of prostaglandins to the systemic and renal vascular responses to frusemide in normal man. British Journal of Clinical Pharmacology 17: 513-519 (1984).
Nowak, J. and Wennmalm, A.: Influence of indomethacin and of prostaglandin E, on total and regional blood flow in man. Acta Physiologica Scandinavica 102: 484-491 (1978).
Oliw, E.; Kover, G.; Larsson, C. and Anggard, E.: Reduction by indomethacin of furosemide effects in the rabbit. European Journal of Pharmacology 38: 95-100 (1976).
Patak, R.V.; Mookerjee, B.K.; Bentzel, C.J.; Hysert, P.E.; Babej, M. and Lee, J.B.: Antagonism of the effects of furosemide by indomethacin in normal and hypertensive man. Prostaglandins 10: 649-658 (1975).
Ramsay, L.E.; Harrison, I.R.; Shelton, J.R. and Vose, C.W.: Influence of acetylsalicylic acid on the renal handling of a spironolactoine metabolite in healthy subjects. European Journal of Clinical Pharmacology 10: 43-48 (1976).
Rolf Smith, S.; Gibson, R.; Bradley, D. and Kendall, M.J.: Failure of indomethacin to modify adrenoceptor blockade. British Journal of Clinical Pharmacology 15: 267-268 (1983).
Rubin, P.; Jackson, G.; and Blaschke, T.: Studies on the clinical pharmacology of prazosin II: The influence of indomethacin and of prazoson on the action and disposition of prazosin. British Journal of Clinical Pharmacology 10: 33-39 (1980).
Salvetti, A.; Arzilli, F.; Pedrinelli, R.; Beggi, P. and Motolese, M.: Interaction between oxprenolol and indomethacin on blood pressure in essential hypertension patients. European Journal of Clinical Pharmacology 22: 197-201 (1982a).
Salvetti, A.; Pedrinelli, R.; Magagna, A. and Abdel-Haq, B.: The influence of indomethacin on some pharmacological actions of atenolol; in Dunn et al. (Eds). Prostaglandins and the Kidney, pp. 287-295, (Plenum, New York, 1982b).
Salvetti, A.; Pedrinelli, R.; Magagna, A. and Ugenti, P.: Differential effects of selective and non-selective prostaglandin synthesis inhibition on the pharmacological responses to captopril in patients with essential hypertension. Clinical Science 63: 261S-263S (1982c).
Salvetti, A.; Pedrinelli, R.; Alberici, P.; Magagna, A. and Abdel-Haq, B.: The influence of indomethacin and sulindac on some pharmacological actions of atenolol in hypertensive patients. Brit. J. Clin. Pharmacol. 17 (Suppl. 1): 108S-111S (1984).
Scherer, B. and Weber, P.C.: Time dependent changes in prostaglandin excretion in response to frusemide in man. Clinical Science 56: 77-81 (1979).
Steiness, E. and Waldorff, S.: Different interactions of indomethacin and sulindac with thiazides in hypertension. British Medical Journal 285: 1702-1703 (1982).
Tarazi, R.C. and Dunstan, H.P.: Beta adrenergic blockade in hypertension. Practical and theoretical implications of long term haemodynamic variations. American Journal of Cardiology 29: 633-640 (1972).
Tweeddale, M.G. and Ogilvie, R.I.: Antagonism of spironolactone-induced natriuresis by aspirin in man. New England Journal of Medicine 289: 198-200 (1973).
Yeung, Laiwah, A.C. and Mactier, R.A.: Antagonistic effect of non-steroidal anti-inflammatory drugs on frusemide-induced diuresis in cardiac failure. Brit. Med. J. 283: 714A (1981).
Walker, R.M.; Brown, R.S. and Stoff, J.S.: Role of renal prostaglandins during antidiuresis and water diuresis in man. Kidney International 21: 365-370 (1981).
Watkins, J.; Carl Abbott, E.; Hensby, C.N.; Webster, J. and Dollery, C.T.: Attenuation of hypotensive effect of propranolol and thiazide diuretics by indomethacin. British Medical Journal 281: 702-705 (1980).
Webster, J.; Hawksworth, G.M.; McLean, I. and Petrie, J.C.: Flurbiprofen interaction with single doses of atenolol and propranolol. Brit. J. Clin. Pharmacol. 18: 861-866 (1984).
Webster, J.; Hensby, C.N.; Dollery, C.T. and Friedman, L.A.: The antihypertensive action of bendroflumethiazide-increased prostacyclin production. Clinical Pharmacology and Therapeutics 28: 751-758 (1980).
Weinberger, M.H.; Ramsdell, J.W.; Rosner, D.R. and Geddes, J.J.L.: Effect of chlorothiazide and sodium on vascular responsiveness to angiotensin II. American Journal of Physiology 223: 1049-1052 (1972).

Address for correspondence and reprints: Dr *J. Webster*, University of Aberdeen, Department of Therapeutics and Clinical Pharmacology, Aberdeen Royal Infirmary, Foresterhill, Aberdeen AB9 2ZB (Scotland).

Review Article

Drugs 30: 42-57 (1985)
0012-6667/85/0700-0042/$08.00/0

Photosensitivity Due to Drugs

John H. Epstein and *Bruce U. Wintroub*

Department of Dermatology, University of California, and Dermatology Service, Veterans Administration Medical Center, San Francisco

Summary

Photosensitivity reactions induced by drugs may be phototoxic or photoallergic in nature. Acute phototoxic reactions are by far the more common, and are generally characterised by erythema and oedema followed by hyperpigmentation and desquamation. Chronic repeated injury of this type may result in fragility, blistering and milia formation or even actinic keratoses and skin cancers. The photochemical mechanisms involved differ with the chemical photosensitiser involved. They include photoaddition of the chemical to biological targets such as DNA, the formation of toxic products due to absorption of the action spectrum by the photosensitising molecule, or the activation of toxic oxygen species or free radicals. Subsequent activation of the complement pathways may participate in the photoresponse to certain agents.

Photoallergic reactions are uncommon. They represent an acquired altered reactivity dependent on a circulating antibody or a cell-mediated hypersensitivity process. Clinically, they are characterised by an immediate wheal and flare or a delayed papular to eczematous process. Some of the same drugs which cause phototoxic responses occasionally produce photoallergic reactions.

Sun-induced cutaneous reactions have become increasingly common over the past several decades, due not only to social causes centred on desires for a golden suntan, but also to the ever-expanding numbers and amounts of photosensitising chemicals entering our environment – primarily from cosmetic, pharmaceutical and industrial sources. This article is concerned primarily with the photosensitising effects of chemicals that are used as medications therapeutically or as cosmetics.

Two types of photosensitivity reactions may be induced by such chemicals; i.e. they may be *phototoxic* or *photoallergic* in nature. Phototoxic reactions may be oxygen dependent (photodynamic) or oxygen independent (non-photodynamic) [Blum, 1941a; Epstein, 1971]. Photoallergic reactions may be due to immediate antibody-mediated or delayed cell-mediated (CMI) responses (Epstein, 1972; Morison et al., 1979).

Whichever type of response occurs, it must follow the basic law of photochemical absorption which states that non-ionising radiation must be absorbed to produce a photochemical and subsequently a photobiological reaction. This law then stipulates that the photosensitising molecule must be present at the time of the irradiation for the reaction to occur. In addition, the action spectrum for any specific photoreaction must be included in the absorption spectrum of the photosensitiser.

1. Phototoxicity

Phototoxic reactions may be drug-induced or may accompany certain metabolic disorders in which an appropriate photosensitising chemical is available in target tissue. In each case, the phototoxic reaction occurs when enough chromophore (drug or metabolic product) absorbs sufficient radiation in reactive tissue. Drug-induced phototoxic reactions, whether from systemic administration or topical application, can occur in 100% of people on first exposure, and using appropriate experimental conditions a dose-response curve can be demonstrated with the incidence of phototoxicity being related to the concentration of sensitisers and amount of light. This section focuses on the clinical expression and mechanism of phototoxicity due to topically or systemically administered drugs. It only briefly considers phototoxicity which accompanies certain metabolic disorders, such as the porphyrias, in which a phototoxic metabolic product accumulates in skin as the result of an inborn metabolic error.

1.1 Clinical Expressions

1.1.1 Acute Reactions

In general, acute phototoxic reactions are characterised by erythema, oedema, and at times blister formation, followed by hyperpigmentation and desquamation (Epstein, 1983). These reactions are confined to sun-exposed skin. Immediate burning, stinging sensations are characteristic of photosensitisation by certain chemicals such as coal tar, demeclocycline (demethylchlortetracycline), and protoporphyrin (in erythropoietic protoporphyria). The clinical reaction may begin from a few minutes to several hours after the irradiation and reach a peak from several hours to several days later. Acute erythema is usually associated with stimulation of melanin formation, leading to subsequent hyperpigmentation.

Since phototoxic injury results in cell death, sloughing of the dead epidermal cells presents as desquamation or peeling. 'Sunburn' reaction induced by ultraviolet B (UVB; 290 to 320nm) radiation is the classic example of an acute phototoxic reaction.

Host effects may influence the natural history of drug-induced phototoxic reactions. Several factors, including hair, pigment, and thickness of the stratum corneum, influence radiation penetration. Topical photosensitisers are dependent on percutaneous absorption and metabolism in the skin (Anderson and Parrish, 1981). Systemic chromophores are influenced by gastrointestinal absorption, distribution and metabolism of the chemicals. In addition, increased humidity, temperature and wind also enhance phototoxic responses (Levine and Harber, 1969; Owens and Knox, 1978).

Histologically, epidermal cell degeneration may be prominent when the photosensitiser or chromophore is in the epidermis (Epstein, 1971). This is most notable when a potent photosensitiser, such as a psoralen compound, is applied to the skin. In contrast, if the chromophore reaches the skin through the vasculature, the primary site of injury may be in the dermis, with little or no visible epidermal change (Epstein, 1974). In both instances, there is generally little inflammatory cell response in the dermis in human skin. When tissue is examined at a submicroscopic level, vascular injury is associated with protoporphyrin photosensitisation (Hönigsman et al., 1976; Schnait et al., 1975).

1.1.2 Chronic Reactions

Lifelong exposure to the sun (most notably UVB rays) causes clinical cutaneous alterations which include wrinkling, atrophy, hyper- and hypopigmented macules, telangiectasia, yellow papules and plaques, keratotic growths (actinic keratoses), and at times skin cancer formation. A distinctive, furrowed, leathery appearance may be seen on the nuchal area of fair-complexioned individuals. The chronically damaged skin is usually quite fragile, rupturing following mild trauma. In addition, the cutaneous blood vessels rupture easily, leading to areas of purpura; these are due to a loss of structural support by the dermal connective tissue.

Histologically, effacement as well as projections of the rete ridges, a possible thinning of the epidermis, and the presence of many abnormal keratinocytes in disorderly arrangement may be seen. In the dermis, there is a progressive degeneration in the papillary and subpapillary zones. Specific changes include the development of vascular ectasia, the accumulation of acid mucopolysaccharides and abnormal-appearing fibrocytes, the loss of collagen (but an increase in the soluble component), and the marked increase and degeneration of elastic tissue, referred to as actinic elastosis. Although there is still some question as to the origin of the fibres which stain like elastic tissue, biochemical and electron microscopic studies have confirmed that actinic elastosis is due to the accumulation of elastic tissue.

In general, most drug-induced phototoxic reactions are acute and phototoxicity may necessitate discontinuation of the drug. However, chronic actinic changes have been associated with a form of dermatological psoriasis therapy in which photochemotherapy is employed. In a large series of psoriatic patients treated with psoralens and ultraviolet A (UVA; 320 to 400nm) radiation (PUVA), a definite increase in cutaneous cancer formation was noted (Stern et al., 1979). In addition, there is histological evidence of focal dystrophy of epidermal cells, atypical changes in melanocytes, and deposition of colloid bodies and amyloid at the dermoepidermal junction (Abel and Farber, 1980).

More recently, an increased cancer incidence in psoriatic patients who had received very extensive treatment with coal tar and UVB exposures has been reported (Stern et al., 1980). This may represent an additive carcinogenic effect between tar and UVB energy since the action spectrum for coal tar photosensitisation is the UVA range.

A limited form of chronic phototoxic injury occurs in porphyria cutanea tarda, variegate porphyria, hereditary coproporphyria, and low-grade photosensitisation by certain medications such as nalidixic acid, tetracycline hydrochloride, and the sulphones. Clinically, this injury is characterised by fragility, blistering, milia formation, and at times sclerodermoid changes involving the sun-exposed skin. In erythropoietic protoporphyria, the skin frequently becomes quite thick.

1.2 Mechanisms

The interactions of light, phototoxic chemicals and their biological targets may result from several types of photochemical reactions. In each case, damage to biological substrates is initiated by the absorption of light energy by a phototoxic compound. As already noted, phototoxic reactions have been divided into 2 categories: oxygen-dependent (photodynamic) and oxygen-independent (non-photodynamic) [Blum, 1941a; Epstein, 1971]. In the case of drug-induced phototoxicity, recent studies have resulted in a more detailed understanding of the various mechanisms of phototoxicity.

At least 3 distinct photochemical mechanisms have been described in *in vitro* systems (Kochevar, 1981). *Firstly,* the direct reaction between the excited state of a phototoxic molecule and a biological target may result in the formation of a covalent photoaddition product which is comprised of the compound itself and the biological target. Examples include photoaddition of chlorpromazine to protein or DNA, or the light-induced formation of a photoadduct of methoxsalen (8-methoxypsoralen; 8-MOP) and a pyrimidine base in the DNA molecule (Song and Tapley, 1979). *Secondly,* the phototoxic molecule absorbs protons to form stable photoproducts which are toxic to biological substrates. Such photoproducts are usually detected by irradiation of the phototoxic molecule prior to exposure to a potential substrate. Examples include erythrocytolysis caused by formation of a stable photoproduct from chlorpromazine or protriptyline (Kochevar and Lamola, 1979). *Thirdly,* irradiation of a phototoxic molecule may result in the tranfer of energy to oxygen molecules with resultant formation of toxic active oxygen species, such as a singlet oxygen, a superoxide anion, or an hydroxyl radical. Interaction of these species with biological targets produces photo-oxidised molecules. Examples include toxic oxygen species produced by irradiation of protoporphyrin (Lamola and Doleideu, 1980), xanthene dyes (Ito and Kobayashi, 1977), and thiazine dyes (Stratigos and Magnus, 1968).

Each of the above photochemical reactions occurs *in vitro* in a serum-free environment. Recent studies have uncovered a critical role for serum protein-dependent systems in acute, *in vivo,* phototoxic tissue damage due to exogenous agents (Lim et al., 1983). Evidence suggests that complement may participate in the development of phototoxic lesions. Irradiation of normal human serum containing added uroporphyrin or protoporphyrin, or demeclocycline resulted in complement activation and generation of chemotactic activity (Lim et al., 1981, 1983). *In vivo* activation of the complement system was noted after irradiation of patients with erythropoietic protoporphyria or porphyria cutanea tarda (Lim et al., 1982). In addition, normal numbers of polymorphonuclear cells and an intact complement system are required for the full development of demeclocycline-induced phototoxic lesions in an *in vivo* guinea-pig model system (Lim et al., 1983). Therefore, both serum protein-dependent pathways and circulating, mobile effector cells appear to be necessary for certain forms of phototoxic tissue injury.

With the exception of the examples outlined above, the erythrogenic mediators of phototoxic reactions are not well understood. Unlike UVB phototoxicity, prostaglandins do not appear to be involved in methoxsalen and UVA photoreactions. Anthracene phototoxic-induced hyperaemia in mouse skin appears to be mediated by histamine (Argenbright et al., 1980). How this relates to erythematous responses to other molecules and in other animals remains to be seen. In general, much more information is needed to clarify the mechanisms which lead to the changes we see in and during phototoxic cutaneous responses.

1.3 Phototoxic Agents of Special Interest

Certain frequently used orally and topically administered agents are known to cause phototoxicity (table I). In certain cases, phototoxicity is employed for therapeutic benefit, as in the case of psoralens and tar, while in other cases phototoxicity is a distinctly adverse event. In this section, those drugs which are commonly used are reviewed with respect to clinical problems and mechanisms of phototoxicity.

1.3.1 Psoralen Phototoxicity

Furocoumarins are a class of compounds to which the psoralens belong; these compounds consist of a double-ringed coumarin moiety with a furan ring attached. At least 28 different furocoumarins have been isolated from natural sources, but only 4 are used clinically: psoralen, methoxsalen (8-methoxypsoralen), 5-methoxypsoralen, and trioxsalen (4,5,8-trimethylpsoralen). The absorption maxima of psoralens range between 210 and 330nm, but the erythema action spectrum is in the UVA range from 320 to 370nm, with a probable peak at 360nm.

Psoralen combined with sun exposure has been used to treat vitiligo for centuries. The availability of high intensity artificial UVA light sources in the past decade has permitted the use of psoralens in combination with controlled doses of UVA light (Parrish et al., 1974). The acronym PUVA (psoralen and UVA photochemotherapy) is used to indicate this form of dermatological therapy. Three major dermatological diseases are frequently treated with PUVA; vitiligo, psoriasis and mycosis fungoides.

Mechanism of Phototoxicity

The mechanism of psoralen photosensitisation has been intensively studied. Non-photodynamic reactions have been described for psoralen photosensitisation (Pathak et al., 1974). In this instance certain psoralen compounds intercalate into the DNA helix (Song and Tapley, 1979). On photoactivation with UVA radiation, mono- and bifunctional adducts may be formed in the DNA, depending on the structure of the psoralen molecule and the wavelengths utilised for irradiation (Parsons, 1980; Pathak et al., 1974; Song and Tapley, 1979). Photoreactions with proteins may also occur.

It should be noted that psoralens can also produce photodynamic responses (Parsons, 1980). Psoralen photoinduced singlet oxygen formation has been correlated with erythema production by

Table I. Some commonly used drug photosensitisers

Drug	Clinical manifestations	Action spectrum (nm)
Amiodarone	Delayed erythema, slate grey pigmentation	
Benoxaprofen	Pruritus, delayed erythema, photo-onycholysis	310-340
Coal tar derivatives: anthralene methylanthracene acridine phenanthrene benzo(a)pyrene	'Tar smarts', pricking sensation, erythema, melanosis	320-430
Furocoumarins: psoralen 5-methoxypsoralen 8-methoxypsoralen (methoxasalen) 4,5,8-trimethylpsoralen (trioxsalen)	Delayed erythema, phytophotodermatitis	320-380
Halogenated salicylanilides	Photoallergic contact dermatitis	320-400
Musk ambrette	Eczematous reaction	310-380
Nalidixic acid	Bullae, fragility, milia	320-360
Phenothiazines: chlorpromazine thioridazine promethazine trimeprazine	Delayed erythema, eczematous reaction, slate grey pigmentation	320-400
Piroxicam	Bullae, delayed erythema	
Quinidine	Delayed erythema	320-380
Sulphonamides	Delayed erythema, eczematous reaction	315-400
Sulphonylureas	Delayed erythema, eczematous reaction	315-400
Tetracyclines	Delayed erythema; photo-onycholysis, bullae, fragility, milia	350-420
Thiazides	Delayed erythema, eczematous reaction, lichenoid eruption, bullae	300-400
Quindoxin (quinoxaline 1,4-dioxide)	Eczematous reaction	
6-Methylcoumarin	Eczematous reaction	320-380

several psoralens, suggesting that these photodynamic responses may be responsible for some of the effects of psoralen photosensitisation in human skin (Parsons, 1980).

1.3.2 Chlorpromazine Phototoxicity

Chlorpromazine is an antipsychotic drug frequently utilised in psychiatric patients. Clinical photosensitivity to chlorpromazine was first reported in the 1950s (J.H. Epstein et al., 1957) and the drug is now known to be phototoxic in a variety of *in vitro* systems, including red blood cells, bacteria, mammalian cells, bacteriophages and viruses (Kochevar, 1981). Clorpromazine is known to cause several photodermatoses when taken systemically. An exagerated sunburn reaction (phototoxicity) and a hyperpigmentation of purple or slate-grey tone in light exposed skin have been described. The wavelength range required to elicit a clinical reaction has been a topic of controversy. Chlorpromazine has an absorption maximum at 305nm in aqueous solution, but the action spectrum for phototoxicity has been reported to be both below (J.H. Epstein et al., 1957) and above (S. Epstein, 1968) 320nm in man. For phototoxicity in mice, the action spectrum has been reported to be 320 to 340nm with a maximum of 330nm (Hunter et al., 1970).

Mechanisms of Phototoxicity

The mechanisms of chlorpromazine phototoxicity have been extensively studied and at least two possible mechanisms have been demonstrated *in vitro*. Photoaddition of chlorpromazine to protein, DNA, and cell membranes has been reported (Rosenthal et al., 1978). In addition, it appears that stable photoproducts of chlorpromazine elicit cutaneous toxicity in animals and haemolyse red blood cells (Kochevar and Lamola, 1979). In both systems, toxicity was detected induced by pre-irradiated chlorpromazine. In the case of red cell haemolysis, the stable lysis-producing product did not require oxygen for activity nor cause lipid oxidation in the presence of oxygen. Thus, chlorpromazine has been shown to be phototoxic in many systems, but the route of translation of these *in vitro* effects to human phototoxicity is unclear.

1.3.3 Tetracycline Phototoxicity

Of the tetracyclines, demeclocycline (demethylchlortetracycline), is the most potent phototoxic agent. It causes both immediate and delayed reactions in most individuals, according to dose (Kligman, 1962; Maibach et al., 1967). Human studies indicate that the action spectrum for demeclocycline phototoxicity is above 320nm, and studies in mice demonstrate an effective radiation range of 350 to 450nm, with the greatest response at 400nm.

Recent experiments have clearly demonstrated a requirement for complement and polymorphonuclear leucocytes as amplifiers or effectors of demeclocycline phototoxicity (Lim et al., 1983).

1.3.4 Nalidixic Acid Phototoxicity

Nalidixic acid is a bacteriostatic agent commonly used to treat urinary tract infections. In association with extensive sun exposure, nalidixic acid has caused characteristic bullous eruptions, fragility, scarring and milum formation in light-exposed areas, particularly the lower legs and feet (Ramsay and Obreshkova, 1974). Similar reactions have been noted for tetracycline hydrochloride and sulphones (Epstein et al., 1976).

While the mechanisms of nalidixic acid phototoxicity are not known, the clinical and histopathological changes are identical to those found in a number of porphyrias (Epstein et al., 1973).

1.3.5 Phototoxicity Due to Non-Steroidal Anti-Inflammatory Agents

In the past 10 years many new non-steroidal anti-inflammatory drugs have been introduced and are widely used to treat a variety of inflammatory and symptomatic musculoskeletal disorders. Two of these agents, benoxaprofen (now withdrawn) and piroxicam, are known to cause clinically important phototoxicity.

Benoxaprofen is a proprionic acid derivative which was introduced into the European and United States markets for treatment of rheumatoid arthritis, osteoarthritis, ankylosing spondylitis and psoriasis. The drug was suspended because it caused instances of fatal cholestatic hepatitis, especially in the elderly. Unlike other non-steroidal anti-inflammatory drugs which act principally by inhibiting prostaglandin synthetase, benoxaprofen is primarily a 5-lipoxygenase inhibitor. Benoxaprofen caused side effects in up to 65% of patients, and cutaneous reactions were the most common, accounting for 70% of all side effects (Halsey, 1982). The commonest cutaneous side effect was photosensitivity, which occured in up to 29% of patients on the drug, the incidence depending on skin type and amount of UV exposure. The action spectrum of the phototoxic reaction is 310 to 340nm. The reaction is manifested as immediate itching, burning and erythema (Ferguson, 1982). The mechanism of this phototoxicity is unknown.

Piroxicam is an oxicam which inhibits prostaglandin synthetase and is used for treatment of rheumatoid arthritis, osteoarthritis, gout and ankylosing spondylitis. While the incidence of cutaneous side effects is around 2.4%, a unique photosensitivity due to piroxicam has been reported in several patients (Stern and Bigby, 1984). The photosensitivity reaction is usually vesiculobullous and is often pruritic. The spectrum and mechanisms of photosensitivity are unknown.

1.4 Testing for Phototoxicity

Agents capable of producing phototoxic effects have been identified by use of a variety of *in vitro* and *in vivo* systems. However, the ultimate issue concerns the effect these compounds have on human tissue *in vivo* (Emmet, 1979; Kligman and Kaidbey, 1982). In general, the following 4 techniques have been utilised: systemic administration, topical application with occlusion, topical application after the stratum corneum is stripped off, and intradermal injection. Each of the techniques has disadvantages, among which are lack of distribution to the skin of the active photosensitising molecule, metabolism of the chemical to a non-photosensitising structure, lack of metabolism to an active photosensitising structure, lack of penetration to the appropriate target tissue, lack of irradiation with the appropriate wavelengths, and lack of irradiation at the appropriate time.

2. Photoallergy

2.1 Definition

Photoallergic reactions are uncommon. As with allergic responses in general, they are acquired altered reactivities presumably dependent on an antigen antibody or cell-mediated hypersensitivity phenomenon. Clinically, they present as an *immediate* wheal and flare or a *delayed* papular to eczematous dermatitis (J.H. Epstein, 1971, 1972; S. Epstein, 1962; Morison et al., 1979; Storck, 1965). Microscopically, these delayed reactions are characterised by a dense dermal perivascular round cell infiltrate similar to that seen in allergic contact dermatitis. Though vasodilitation and oedema are present in the immediate reaction, these are difficult to discern histologically.

2.2 Photoallergic Reactions to Exogenous Chemicals

Photoallergic reactions to drugs and other exogenous chemicals are almost always of a delayed hypersensitivity or cell-mediated type. An exception was reported by Horio (1975) who studied a patient with clinical expressions of both immediate and delayed reactions induced by chlorpromazine. He was able to reproduce both responses with photopatch and intradermal tests and UVA radiation. In addition, he passively transferred the immediate wheal reaction with the patient's serum. Masuda et al. (1971) noted an immediate wheal response with photopatch tests in 2 of 44 patients who were contact-photosensitive to biothionol. They were also able to passively transfer the reaction. However, the patients did not demonstrate solar urticarial responses clinically.

The skin is the site of photoallergic reactions to exogenous chemicals which may be applied topically or administered systemically. As with phototoxicity, in the photoallergic reactions to these chemicals the action spectrum usually falls in the UVA range. The immunological basis for these reactions is supported primarily by studies on contact photoallergy.

2.2.1 Photoallergic Contact Dermatitis

Clinical Expression

Photoallergic contact reactions are clinically identical to any other type of allergic contact dermatitis. Thus the spectrum of the possible responses may range from a simple erythema to a severe vesiculobullous eruption. The most common picture is eczematous in nature. When the process is chronic, lichenification results from repeated mechanical trauma (rubbing and scratching). The sun-exposed areas of the skin are involved primarily, as would be expected. However, the eruption may extend to unexposed parts of the body and even become generalised due to conditioned irritability and autoeczematisation reactions. Even when this occurs the dermatitis is most notable in the exposed sites.

Histologically, there is generally some intercellular oedema in the epidermis with or without vesicle formation, depending on the clinical pattern. However, the characteristic finding is present in the dermis and consists of a dense perivascular round cell infiltrate, which is identical to that found in any allergic contact dermatitis response.

Adults are much more commonly affected than children. Obviously the reactions will occur in populations that are exposed to sunlight and the photocontactants. Thus, reactions to the optical brighteners are more likely to be seen in occupations where they are used: those to chlorpromazine would more likely occur in people who work in mental institutions, and so on. Perhaps the most extensive statistical data have been compiled on the eruptions induced by the halogenated salicylanilides and related antibacterial compounds because of the large number of people photosensitised by these agents between 1960 and 1970 (Herman and Sams, 1972). The reactions occurred predominantly in men past the age of 40 years. The reason for this age and sex distribution is unknown. Skin colour and race apparently have little influence on the problem, since the reaction occurs readily in Blacks and Orientals as well as Caucasians.

In general, removal of the offending photosensitiser and related compounds will eliminate the problem once the eruption has subsided. A small percentage of patients who have developed this process will become persistent light reactors (Jillson and Baughman, 1963). These are people who continue to develop the dermatitis on sun-exposed areas without apparent further contact with the offending agent or related structures. These patients tend to be exquisitely sensitive to the sun and usually have very low UVB minimal erythema doses. The incidence of this most disturbing problem is unknown, but it probably represents only a small percentage of those who become contact photosensitive. However, up to 25% of patients with photocontact reactions to the halogenated salicylanilides severe enough to necessitate consultation at medical centres have been persistent light reactors. In our studies with antibacterial halogenated salicylanilides we found two types of persistent light reactors: a mild variety that loses its reactivity within 1.5 years and a severe type that appears to persist indefinitely (Epstein et al., 1968).

Chemicals other than the antibacterial halogenated salicylanilides have induced persistent light reactions, including the related antifungal compound buclosamide (Burry, 1970; Burry and Hunter, 1970), chlorpromazine (Amblard et al., 1982; Burdick, 1969; Wiskemann and Wulf, 1959), promethazine (Sidi et al., 1955), musk ambrette (Giovinazzo et al., 1980) and epoxy resins (Allen and Kaidbey, 1979). Persistent light reactions induced in guinea-pigs with sulphonamides have also been noted (Schwarz and Speck, 1957), and one of us has observed a phototoxic persistent light reaction induced by systemic demeclocycline that has persisted 3 years (Epstein, unpublished data). The mechanism or mechanisms of this persistent light reactivity are not clear. Cross-reactions to unknown photocontactants have been considered. Willis and Kligman (1968a) presented evidence suggesting that the reactions could result from the retention of small amounts of the photosensitiser in the dermis. These authors also reported that the lowered minimal erythema dose in persistent light reactors was a photoallergic reaction, which resembled a sunburn.

Photoinduced covalent binding of tetrachlorosalicylanilide to the albumin molecule has been demonstrated by Kochevar (1979). Other possibilities include: (a) the persistence of a sensitised mononuclear infiltrate in the dermis, which will react on minimal antigenic exposure; (b) hypersensitivity to the protein component of the complete antigen, which then becomes an independent photoallergen; or (c) the development of clones of cells that are persistently sensitive to a number of photoallergens (Herman and Sams, 1972). Also, a possible relationship to the chronic eczematous type of polymorphous light eruption has been reported (Epstein et al., 1968).

Diagnosis

The differential diagnosis includes essentially any eruption that may involve the sun-exposed skin. However, for practical purposes, allergic contact dermatitis, the eczematous type of polymorphous light eruption, and phototoxic reactions are by far the most important.

Airborne allergens will primarily contact exposed skin. Unlike photocontactant reactions, the airborne contact eruption will be accentuated in fold areas such as the upper eyelids, antecubital fossae, and the flexural areas of the wrists, etc., because of concentration of the airborne material in these areas. Differentiation from allergic contact reactions to sunscreens, 'suntanning' lotions and creams, and medications used to relieve the discomfort of a sunburn is more difficult since they are confined to the sun-exposed areas and are indistinguishable clinically and histologically. The same is true for the eczematous type of polymorphous light eruption.

Phototoxic reactions induced by topical or systemic exogenous photosensitisers will have the same distribution as the photoallergic reactions. The clinical picture and lack of the dermal round cell infiltrate histologically will usually serve to make this differentiation. However, the most useful diagnostic tools available are the patch, photopatch, and phototesting procedures.

The diagnosis of photocontact dermatitis is suspected by the clinical picture, including the character and distribution of the eruption and the histology. Confirmation and identification of the offending chemical depends on photopatch testing. This is accomplished by the application in duplicate of non-irritating concentrations of the potential photosensitisers in appropriate vehicles (i.e. a 1% concentration of halogenated salicylanilides in petrolatum). The use of an extra layer of black paper over the patches will help prevent a 'masked' positive reaction to the photopatch test (Epstein, 1963); this is unnecessary with the use of aluminium patches. 24 hours later one set of patches is irradiated with the UVA rays. Any light source that emits sufficient amounts of these rays can be utilised, including the sun, hot quartz lamps, fluorescent tubes, zenon arcs, carbon arcs, and monochromatic sources (Harber et al., 1974). Window glass filtration is necessary if there is a significant amount of UVB emitted by the lamp, as in the case of the hot quartz source. 24 hours after the irradiation the closed and exposed sites are compared. The reading techniques are identical to those used in evaluation of ordinary patch tests. A positive reaction to the photopatch tests reproduces the clinical lesions morphologically and histologically. Certain difficulties with patch testing may occur. If the patient is contact allergic to a chemical it may be difficult to determine if he or she is photocontact allergic as well. However, in general, the photopatch test site will be much more reactive than the patch test area in a patient with dual sensitivity.

Another significant problem concerns identifying the potential photoallergen. The history may be helpful in this determination. Unfortunately patients often do not know what they contacted (except for suntan oils or the like). This is especially true of preservatives and ingredients in soaps. We use the following series of compounds routinely and add whatever can be determined from the history: 5% para-aminobenzoic acid (PABA); amyl dimethyl PABA; glyceryl PABA; 5% musk ambrette; octyl dimethyl PABA; oxybenzone; dioxybenzone; 0.25% tetrachlorosalicylanilide: and 1% tribromosalicylanilide.

We also routinely patch test with the screening materials suggested by the North American Contact Dermatitis Groups (NACDG, 1974) to evaluate other potential contactants and phototest to examine for polymorphous light eruption (Epstein, 1966).

Photocontactants

Photoallergic reactions to a number of topically contacted chemicals have been reported. These include: sulphonamides (Epstein, 1962; Schwarz and Speck, 1957; Storck, 1965); phenothiazines (Amblard et al., 1982; Burdick, 1969; Epstein, 1960a, 1968; Epstein and Rowe, 1957; Ertle, 1982; Horio, 1975; Polano, 1964; Sidi et al., 1955; Storck, 1965; Torinuki et al., 1982); sulphonylcarbamides

(Burckhardt and Schwarz-Speck, 1957); men's colognes and after-shave lotions (Epstein, 1969; Starke, 1967); blankophores (optical brighteners) [Burckhardt, 1957]; Persian lime rind (Epstein, 1956); ragweed (Epstein, 1960b); sunscreens (Davies et al., 1982; Fagerlund et al., 1983; Fitzpatrick et al., 1963; Goldman and Epstein, 1969; Hözle and Plewig, 1982; Kaidbey and Allen, 1981; Mathias et al., 1978; Sams, 1956; Satulsky, 1950); diphenhydramine (Emmett, 1974); psoralens (Fulton and Willis, 1968; Sidi and Bourgeois-Cavardin, 1953); epoxy resins (Allen and Kaidbey, 1979); and quindoxin (Scott and Dawson, 1974; Zanoun et al., 1976). However, the halogenated salicylanilides and related antibacterial and antifungal compounds represented the most important group of allergic contact photosensitisers. In the 1960s these chemicals were responsible for almost an epidemic of photoallergic reactions. Tetrachlorosalicylanilide was perhaps the most potent photosensitiser of this type. Between 1960 and 1961 it was responsible for an estimated 10,000 cases in England (Wilkinson, 1961) before it was removed from general use. Subsequently, a number of related phenolic compounds were incorporated into soaps and other vehicles to combat infection, reduce body odour, act as preservatives, and destroy fungi. Photocontact reactions were induced by many of these agents, including bithionol, the brominated salicylanilides, hexachlorophane, dichlorophen, the carbanilides, fenticlor [*bis* (2-hydroxy-5-chlorophenyl) sulphide], bromochlorosalicylanilide, 'Jadit' (a mixture of buclosamide and salicylic acid) [Epstein, 1972; Herman and Sams, 1972], and chloro-2-phenylphenol (Adams, 1972).

Since 1968, there has been a rapid decline in the induction of photocontact dermatitis by the halogenated salicylanilides and related compounds (Smith and Epstein, 1977). This is most likely due to the removal of the more potent of these photosensitisers from general use. However, within the past 5 years, 2 new contactants appear to produce most, if not all, photoallergic responses. These are the two widely used fragrance compounds 6-methylcoumarin (Jackson et al., 1980; Kaidbey and Kligman, 1978) and musk ambrette (Galosi and Plewig, 1982; Giovinazzo et al., 1980; Raugi et al., 1979). In addition, musk ambrette has been reported to be responsible for the induction of a persistent light reactor state similar to that noted with the halogenated salicylanilides (Giovinazzo et al., 1980). The action spectrum for the photoallergic reactions to these fragrances appears to fall in the UVA range (Giovinazzo et al., 1981; Jackson et al., 1980; Kaidbey and Kligman, 1978).

Mechanisms Involved in Development of Photocontact Reactions

The clinical appearance, histology and photopatch test responses strongly suggest that the photoreactions described in this discussion are dependent on a cell-mediated immunity process. A number of experimental studies utilising animal and human models have supported this concept.

Herman and Sams (1972), using micro-ouchterlony immune diffusion techniques, could not demonstrate antibodies to 3,5-dibromosalicylanilide (3,5-DBS) protein complexes in the serum of patients photocontact-sensitive to this chemical. No binding of fluorescein-tagged goat antihuman IgG, IgA, IgM and complement or fibrin was noted in positive photopatch test sites with the direct immunofluorescence methods. In addition, immunoglobulins in serum from patients photosensitive to tetrachlorosalicylanilide and 3,5-DBS did not bind to cutaneous tissues bathed in these chemicals. Thus, no evidence of antibody-mediated hypersensitivity was discovered in patients with photocontact reactions to the halogenated salicylanilides.

Photoallergic reactions in human skin characteristic of cell-mediated immunity responses have been induced by a number of agents including the sulphonamides (Epstein, 1939), phenothiazines (Burdick, 1969), and the halogenated salicylanilides (Willis and Kligman, 1968b). Perhaps the most extensive studies have been performed with the halogenated salicylanilides. Willis and Kligman utilised UVB as well as UVA exposures plus the chemicals to induce photosensitivity, but only UVA and the halogenated salicylanilides were used to elicit the photocontact allergy.

As noted, animal and human studies have confirmed the cell-mediated immunity mechanism for the photocontact allergy reactions, which appears to be identical to the mechanism of contact allergy itself. However, the nature of the antigen has not been settled. The studies of Burckhardt and Schwarz-Speck (1957), Jung and Schwarz (1965) and Schwarz and Speck (1957) with sulphonamide and related compounds, those of Epstein and Enta (1965), Jung and Schültz (1968) and Willis and Kligman (1968b, 1969) with the halogenated salicylanilides, and those of Fulton and Willis (1968) with methoxypsoralens suggested that the haptens were stable photoproducts of these chemicals. *In vitro* binding studies have also supported this concept.

An alternative concept was proposed by Jenkins et al. (1964). They concluded that the photoproducts might well be shortlived free radicals, which would attach to the protein carrier within microseconds to form the complete antigen. Support for this theory has developed from clinical observations (Epstein, 1972; Herman and Sams, 1972; Osmundsen, 1969). In addition, Jung's studies of postirradiation free radical formation and subsequent binding to albumin and β-globulin of chlorpramazine (Jung, 1970) and triplet state induction by radiation of triacetyldiphenylisatin with deactivation by binding to albumin, γ-globulin, and skin protein (Jung, 1967) present further evidence in favour of this concept. The studies of Jung et al. (1968a,b) with 'Jadit' (buclosamide/salicylic acid) were even more supportive of this second theory immunologically. They were able to demonstrate protein binding *in vitro* after irradiation. This *in vitro* protein complex then acted as a full antigen on plain patch testing of 'Jadit'-photosensitive patients.

As can be seen, there is a significant discrepancy between the theories concerning the origin of the antigen in photocontact reactions. Most probably both theories are correct under different circumstances; i.e. it is likely that at least some of the subjects experimentally photosensitised by Willis and Kligman (1968b) were actually contact sensitised by stable photoproducts of the chemicals. In contrast, the available evidence suggests that the haptens in clinically acquired disease are unstable photoproducts, perhaps free radicals, which must be in close proximity to the protein carrier at the time of irradiation.

Experimental Predictive Testing Models

Determination of the potential for a chemical to induce allergic contact sensitisation has depended on demonstration of such reactions in patients who have clinically developed photocontact allergies to the chemical. Though animal models are readily available for phototoxicity studies, their use in evaluation of photoallergic reactions has presented a more complicated problem.

Schwarz and Speck (1957) first reported the induction of photoallergic contact dermatitis to sulphanilamide in guinea-pigs. Subsequently, photoallergic contact reactions in guinea-pigs have been induced by tetrachlorosalicylanilide and related compounds, chlorpromazine, musk ambrette and 6-methylcoumarin (Harber, 1981; Jordan, 1982). *In vitro* and in animals, immunological studies have supported the cell-mediated nature of the hypersensitivity (Harber et al., 1959, 1967; Herman and Sams, 1972; Jung et al., 1968a,b). More recently, mouse models have been shown to be most efficient for experimentally examining this problem (Maguire and Kaidbey, 1982; Miyachi and Takigawa, 1983). Using such animals, demonstration of the necessity of Langerhans cells apparently to process the photoallergen appropriately, the need for genetically dependent T cells for the development of the reactivity, and the inhibiting influence of UVB-induced suppressor T cells, have been established under experimental conditions (Granstein et al., 1983; Miyachi and Takigawa, 1982; Takigawa and Miyachi, 1982). However, to date, no animal models have proved to be predictive for screening the potential for chemicals which had not previously been identified to produce photoallergic contact reactions.

Human Predictive Testing Models

Predictive testing in human skin is even less definitive. In the 1960s, identification of tetrachlorosalicylanilide and related phenolic compounds was accomplished by photopatch testing clinically involved patients. Subsequently, Willis and Kligman (1968b) induced contact photoallergy to certain of these agents in normal human subjects using a modification of the maximisation test developed for evaluating the potential for chemicals to produce contact dermatitis (Kligman, 1966).

Recently, Kaidbey and Kligman (Kaidbey, 1983; Kaidbey and Kligman, 1980) modified the photomaximisation procedure. With the new test they were able to photoallergically contact sensitise normal human volunteers relatively readily to certain methylated coumarin derivatives, tetrachlorosalicylanilide, 3,5-DBS, chlorpromazine, and sodium pyrithione. A lesser number of positive induction responses were noted with tribromosalicylanilide contaminated with 47% dibromosalicylanilide, 4, 5-DBS, buclosamide, and bithionol. However, negative results were noted with para-aminobenzoic acid and musk ambrette which have produced photoallergic contact reactions clinically. The authors considered them weak photosensitisers.

Thus, to date there is no proven effective predictive testing model for photoallergic contact dermatitis.

2.2.2 Systemic Drug Photoallergy

Photoallergic reactions to systemic photosensitisers are less common than those induced by contactants and they are less well understood. However, a few apparent photoallergic reactions have been reported to a number of agents, including the antibacterial sulphonamides (Blum, 1941b; Burckhardt, 1941; Epstein, 1939; Schwarz and Speck, 1957; Stevanovic, 1961), sulphonylurea antidiabetic agents (Hitselberger and Foxnaugh, 1962), the thiazide diuretics (Harber et al., 1959) and quinethazone (Miller and Beltrani, 1966), phenothiazines (Calnan et al., 1962; Schultz et al., 1956), oral contraceptive hormones (Erickson and Peterka, 1968), griseofulvin (Chang, 1965), chlordiazepoxide hydrochloride (Luton and Finchum, 1965), several antihistamines (Schreiber and Naylor, 1962), triacetyldiphenylisatin (Kasuistik and Jung, 1967), the artificial sweetener calcium cyclamate (Kobori and Araki, 1966; Lamberg, 1967; Tatsuji and Toshie, 1963), chloroquine (van Weelden et al., 1982), quinidine (Lang, 1983; Marx et al., 1983), carprofen (Merot et al., 1983) and 5-fluorocytosine (Beardmore, 1979; Shelley and Sica, 1983).

Clinical Expression

The reaction times for these responses appear to be delayed in nature and the clinical eruptions range from lichenoid papules to eczematous changes. Though the problems are generally short term in nature, occasionally persistent light reactivity may be induced by these systemic photosensitisers (S. Epstein, 1962).

Histologically, the lichenoid eruptions resemble lichen planus with a subepidermal band of round cells. In addition, they have a perivascular round cell infiltrate deeper in the dermis. The eczematous eruptions show epidermal oedema and a dermal round cell infiltrate.

Diagnosis

The diagnosis of photoallergy is usually made on morphological, histological, and historical grounds. In some instances reproduction of the photoallergic response has been accomplished by exposure to the appropriate action spectrum. However, the use of injections or topical applications with occlusion or after stripping may be useful if the agent itself, and not a metabolite, is responsible for the photosensitivity.

There is little information concerning the mechanisms involved in the development of these reactions induced by systemic medications. However, they do appear to be delayed hypersensitivity responses. Thus the principles noted in section 2.2.1 on photoallergic contact dermatitis should apply.

3. *Therapy of Drug-Induced Photosensitivity*

Therapy of acute photoallergic or phototoxic responses is identical to that used for any such inflammatory reactions. This includes the use of topical cool wet dressings, soothing shake lotions, topical corticosteroids and systemic antipruritic agents.

If the process is severe enough, systemic corticosteroids may be indicated. As with any topical or systemic drug-induced eruption, removal of the offending agent is essential to the cure of the allergic process. In the case of photoallergy or phototoxicity, either the sun or the chemical could be removed. The radiant energy is more difficult to control; therefore removal of the chemical is usually the most appropriate approach since the patient frequently is made exquisitely sensitive by the drugs. At times, the medication may be indispensable and avoidance of the sun is essential.

As noted previously, some patients may develop persistent light eruptions which persist after discontinuing use of the offending agent. When this occurs, the patient usually becomes markedly photosensitive. Long term anti-inflammatory therapy and avoidance of any sun exposure may be necessary to control such a process.

References

Abel, E.A. and Farber, E.M.: Photochemotherapy; in Rook and Savin (Eds) Recent Advances in Dermatology, pp. 259-283 (Churchill Livingstone, Edinburgh 1980).

Adams, R.M.: Photoallergic contact dermatitis to chloro-2-phenylphenol. Archives of Dermatology 106: 711-714 (1972).

Allen, H. and Kaidbey, K.H.: Persistent photosensitivity following occupational exposure to epoxy resin. Archives of Dermatology 115: 1307-1310 (1979).

Amblard, P.; Beani, J.C. and Reymond, J.L.: Persistent light reaction due to phenothiazines in atopic disease. Annals of Dermatology and Venereology 109: 225-228 (1982).

Anderson, R.R. and Parrish, J.A.: Optics of human skin. Journal of Investigative Dermatology 77: 13-19 (1981).

Argenbright, L.W.; Forbes, P.D. and Stewart, G.J.: Quantitation of phototoxic hyperemia and permeability. II. Inhibition of histamine (H_1 and H_2) receptor antagonists in mouse skin. Journal of Investigative Dermatology 75: 417-420 (1980).

Beardmore, G.L.: Recalcitrant sporotrichosis: A report of a patient treated with various therapies, including oral miconozole and 5-fluorocytosine. Australasian Journal of Dermatology 20: 10-13 (1979).

Blum, H.F.: Photodynamic Action and Diseases Caused by Light (Rhinehold, New York 1941a).

Blum, H.F.: Studies of photosensivity due to sulfanilamide. Journal of Investigative Dermatology 4: 159-173 (1941b).

Burckhardt, W.: Photoallergy eczema due to blankophores (optic brightening agents). Hautarzt 8: 486-488 (1957).

Burckhardt, W.: Untersuchungen über die Photoaktivität einiger Sulfanilamide. Dermatologica 83: 63-83 (1941).

Burckhardt, W. and Schwarz-Speck, M.: Photoallergische Ekzeme durch Nadisan. Schweizerische Medizinische Wochenschrift 87: 954-956 (1957).

Burdick, K.H.: Prolonged sensitivity to intradermal chlorpromazine. Cutis 5: 1113-1114 (1969).

Burry, J.N.: Persistent light reactions from buclosamide. Archives of Dermatology 101: 95-97 (1970).

Burry, J.N. and Hunter, G.A.: Photocontact dermatitis from Jadit. British Journal of Dermatology 82: 244-249 (1970).

Calnan, C.D.; Frain-Bell, W. and Cuthbert, W.I.: Occupational dermatitis from chlorpromazine. Transactions of the St John Hospital Dermatological Society 48: 49-72 (1962).

Chang, T.W.: Cold urticaria and photosensitivity due to griseofulvin. Journal of the American Medical Association 193: 848-850 (1965).

Davies, M.G.; Hawk, J.L. and Rycroft, R.J.: Acute photosensitivity from the sunscreen 2-ethoxyethyl-P-methoxycinnamate. Contact Dermatitis 8: 190-200 (1982).

Emmet, E.A.: Diphenhydramine photoallergy. Archives of Dermatology 110: 249-251 (1974).

Emmet, E.A.: Phototoxicity from exogenous agents. Photochemical Photobiology 38: 429-436 (1979).

Epstein, E.: Persome dermatitis in men. Journal of the American Medical Association 209: 911-913 (1969).

Epstein, J.H.: Polymorphous light eruption. Annals of Allergy 24: 397-405 (1966).

Epstein, J.H.: Adverse cutaneous reactions to the sun; in Malkinson and Pearson (Eds) Yearbook of Dermatology, pp. 5-43 (Yearbook Medical Publishers, Chicago 1971).

Epstein, J.H.: Photoallergy: A review. Archives of Dermatology 106: 741-748 (1972).

Epstein, J.H.: Phototoxicity and photoallergy; in Pathak et al. (Eds) Sunlight and Man, pp. 459-477 (University of Tokyo Press, Tokyo 1974).

Epstein, J.H.: Phototoxicity and photoallergy in man. Journal of the American Academy of Dermatology 8: 141-147 (1983).

Epstein, J.H.; Brunsting, L.A.; Petersen, M.C. et al.: A study of photosensitivity occurring with chlorpromazine therapy. Journal of Investigative Dermatology 28: 329-338 (1957).

Epstein, J.H.; Tuffanelli, D.L. and Epstein, W.L.: Cutaneous changes in the porphyrias: A microscopic study. Archives of Dermatology 107: 689-698 (1973).

Epstein, J.H.; Tuffanelli, D.L.; Seibert, J.S. and Epstein, W.L.: Porphyria-like cutaneous changes induced by tetracycline hydrochloride photosensitization. Archives of Dermatology 112: 661-666 (1976).

Epstein, J.H.; Wuepper, K.D. and Maibach, H.I.: Photocontact dermatitis to halogenated compounds and related compounds. Archives of Dermatology 97: 236-244 (1968).

Epstein, S.: Photoallergy and primary phototoxicity to sulfanilamide. Journal of Investigative Dermatology 2: 43-51 (1939).

Epstein, S.: Discussion of paper by Sams, W.M. Archives of Dermatology 73: 142-148 (1956).

Epstein, S.: Allergic photocontact dermatitis from promethazine (Phenergan). Archives of Dermatology 81: 175-180 (1960a).

Epstein, S.: Role of dermal sensitivity in ragweed contact dermatitis. Archives of Dermatology 82: 48-55 (1960b).

Epstein, S.: Photoallergy versus phototoxicity; in Rees (Ed.) Dermatoses Due to Environmental and Physical Factors, pp. 119-135 (Thomas, Springfield 1962).

Epstein, S.: 'Masked' photopatch tests. Journal of Investigative Dermatology 41: 369-370 (1963).

Epstein, S.: Chlorpromazine photosensitivity: Phototoxic and photoallergic reactions. Archives of Dermatology 98: 354-363 (1968).

Epstein, S. and Enta, T.: Photoallergic contact dermatitis. Journal of the American Medical Association 194: 1016-1017 (1965).

Epstein, S. and Rowe, R.J.: Photoallergy and photocross-sensitivity to Phenergan. Journal of Investigative Dermatology 29: 319-326 (1957).

Erickson, L.R. and Peterka, E.S.: Sunlight sensitivity from oral

contraceptives. Journal of the American Medical Association 203: 980-981 (1968).
Ertle, T.: Work-related contact and photocontact allergy in a farmer caused by chlorpromazine. Dermatosen in Beruf und Umwelt 30: 120-122 (1982).
Fagerlund, V.L.; Kalimo, K. and Jansen, C.: Photocontact allergy from sunscreens. Duodecim 99: 146-150 (1983).
Ferguson, J.: A study of benoxaprofen-induced photosensitivity. British Journal of Dermatology 107: 429-442 (1982).
Fitzpatrick, T.B.; Pathak, M.A.; Magnus, I.A. et al.: Abnormal reactions of man to light. Annual Reviews of Medicine 14: 195-214 (1963).
Fulton Jr, J.E. and Willis, I.: Photoallergy to methoxsalen. Archives of Dermatology 98: 445-450 (1968).
Galosi, A. and Plewig, G.: Photoallergic eczema caused by musk ambrette. Hautarzt 33: 589-594 (1982).
Giovinazzo, V.J.; Harber, L.C.; Bickers, D.R.; Armstrong, R.B. and Silvers, D.N.: Photoallergic contact dermatitis to musk ambrette. Journal of the American Academy of Dermatology 3: 384-393 (1980).
Giovinazzo, V.J.; Ichikawa, H.; Kochevar, I.E.; Armstrong, R.B. and Harber, L.C.: Photoallergic contact dermatitis to musk ambrette: Action spectrum in guinea pigs and man. Photochemical Photobiology 33: 773-777 (1981).
Goldman, G.C. and Epstein Jr, E.: Contact photosensitivity dermatitis from a sun-protective agent. Archives of Dermatology 100: 447-449 (1969).
Granstein, R.D.; Morison, W.L. and Kripke, M.L.: The role of suppressor cells in the induction of murine photoallergic contact dermatitis and in its suppression by prior UVB irradiation. Journal of Immunology 130: 2099-2103 (1983).
Halsey, J.: Benoxaprofen: Side-effect profile in 300 patients. British Medical Journal 284: 1365 (1982).
Harber, L.C.: Current status of mammalian and human models for predicting drug photosensitivity. Journal of Investigative Dermatology 77: 65-70 (1981).
Harber, L.C.; Bickers, D.R.; Epstein, J.H.; Pathak, M.A. and Urbach, F.: Report on ultraviolet light sources. Archives of Dermatology 109: 833-839 (1974).
Harber, L.C.; Lashinsky, A.M. and Baer, R.L.: Photosensitivity due to chlorothiazide and hydrochlorothiazide. New England Journal of Medicine 261: 1378-1381 (1959).
Harber, L.C.; Targovnik, S.E. and Baer, R.L.: Contact photosensitivity patterns to halogenated salicylanilides in man and guinea pigs. Archives of Dermatology 96: 646-656 (1967).
Herman, P.S. and Sams Jr, W.M.: Soap photodermatitis. (Thomas, Springfield 1972).
Hitselberger, J.F. and Foxnaugh, R.P.: Photosensitivity due to chlorpropamide. Journal of the American Medical Association 180: 142-143 (1962).
Hözle, E. and Plewig, G.: Photoallergic contact dermatitis by benzophenone containing sunscreening preparations. Hautarzt 33: 391-393 (1982).
Hönigsman, H.; Scnait, G.S.; Konrad, R.A.; Stingl, G. and Wolff, K.: Mouse model for protoporphyria. Journal of Investigative Dermatology 66: 188-195 (1976).
Horio, T.: Chlorpromazine photoallergy. Archives of Dermatology 11: 1469-1471 (1975).
Hunter, J.A.; Bhutani, L.K. and Magnus, I.A.: Chlorpromazine photosensitivity in mice; Its action spectrum and effect of anti-inflammatory agents. British Journal of Dermatology 82: 157-168 (1970).
Ito, T. and Kobayashi, K.: A survey of *in vivo* photodynamic activity of xanthenes, thiazines and acridines in yeast cells. Photochemical Photobiology 26: 581-587 (1977).
Jackson, R.T.; Nesbit, L.T. and DeLeo, V.A.: 6-Methyl coumarin photocontact dermatitis. Journal of the American Academy of Dermatology 2: 124-127 (1980).
Jenkins, F.P.; Welti, D. and Baines, D.: Photochemicals reactions of tetrachlorosalicylanilide. Nature 201: 827-828 (1964).
Jillson, V.F. and Baughman, R.D.: Contact dermatitis from bithionol. Archives of Dermatology 88: 409-418 (1963).
Jordan Jr, W.P.: The guinea pig model for predicting photoallergic contact dermatitis. Contact Dermatitis 8: 109-116 (1982).
Jung, E.G.: Photoallergie durch Triacetyldiphenolisatin (TDI). II. Photochemische Untersuchungen zur Pathogenese. Archiv für Klinische und Experimentelle Dermatologie 231: 39-49 (1967).
Jung, E.G.: In vitro-Untersuchungen zur Chlorpromazine (CPZ) Photoallergie. Archiv für Klinische und Experimentelle Dermatologie 237: 501-506 (1970).
Jung, E.G.; Dummler, U. and Immich, H.: Photoallergie durch 4-Chlor-2-hydroxy-benzoesäure-n-butylamid. I. Lichtbiologische Untersuchungen zur Antigenbildung. Archiv für Klinische und Experimentelle Dermatologie 232: 403-412 (1968a).
Jung, E.G.; Hornke, J. and Hajde, P.: Photoallergie durch 4-Chlor-2-hydroxy-benzoesäure-n-butylmid. II. Photochemische Untersuchungen. Archiv für Klinische und Experimentelle Deratologie 233: 287-295 (1968b).
Jung, E.G. and Schültz, R.: Kontakt und Photoallergien durch Desinfizienzen. Dermatologica 137: 216-226 (1968).
Jung, E.G. and Schwarz, K.: Photoallergy to 'Jadit' with photo cross-reactions to derivatives of sulfanilamide. International Archives of Allergy and Applied Immunology 27: 313-317 (1965).
Kaidbey, K.H.: The evaluation of photoallergic contact sensitizers in humans; in Marzulli and Maibach (Eds) Dermatotoxicology, 2nd ed., pp. 405-414 (Hemisphere Publishers, Washington 1983).
Kaidbey, K.H. and Allen, H.: Photocontact allergy to benzocaine. Archives of Dermatology 117: 77-79 (1981).
Kaidbey, K.H. and Kligman, A.M.: Contact photoallergy to 6-methyl coumarin in proprietary sunscreens. Archives of Dermatology 114: 1709-1710 (1978).
Kaidbey, K.H. and Kligman, A.M.: Photo-maximization test for identifying photoallergic contact sensitizers. Contact Dermatitis 6: 161-169 (1980).
Kasuistik, I. and Jung, E.G.: Photoallergie durch Triacetyldiphenolisatin (TDI) Archiv für Klinische und Experimentelle Dermatologie 229: 170-173 (1967).
Kligman, A.M.: Identification of contact allergens by human assay. III. The maximization test. A procedure for screening and rating contact sensitizers. Journal of Investigative Dermatology 47: 393-409 (1966).
Kligman, A.M.: Declomycin compendium. (Lederle Laboratories, Pearl River, New York 1962).
Kligman, A.M. and Kaidbey, K.H.: Human models for identification of photosensitizing chemicals. Journal of the National Cancer Institute 69: 264-272 (1982).
Kobori, T. and Araki, H.: Photoallergy in dermatology. Journal of Asthma Research 3: 213-215 (1966).
Kochevar, I.E.: Photoallergic responses to chemicals. Photochemistry and Photobiology 30: 437-442 (1979).
Kochevar, I.E.: Phototoxicity mechanisms: Chlorpromazine photosensitized damage to DNA and cell membranes. Journal of Investigative Dermatology 77: 59-64 (1981).
Kochevar, I.E. and Lamola, A.A.: Chlorpromazine and protriptyline phototoxicity: Photosensitized oxygen-independent red cell hemolysis. Photochemistry and Photobiology 29: 1177-1197 (1979).
Lamberg, S.I.: A new photosensitizer: The artificial cyclamate. J.A.M.A. 201: 121-124 (1967).
Lamola, A.A. and Doleideu, F.H.: Cross-linking of membrane proteins and protoporphyrin-sensitized photohemolysis. Photochemistry and Photobiology 31: 597-601 (1980).
Lang Jr, P.G.: Quinidine-induced photodermatitis confirmed by photopatch testing. Journal of the American Academy of Dermatology 91: 124-128 (1983).
Levine, G.M. and Harber, L.C.: The effect of humidity on the

phototoxic response to 8-methoxypsoralen in guinea pigs. Acta Dermatologica Venereologica 49: 82-86 (1969).

Lim, H.W.; Novotny, H. and Gigli, I.: Role of complement and polymorphonuclear cells in demethylchlortetracycline-induced phototoxicity in guinea pigs. Journal of Clinical Investigation 71: 1326-1335 (1983).

Lim, H.W.; Perez, H.D.; Goldstein, I.M. and Gigli, I.: Complement-derived chemotactic activity is generated in human serum containing uroporphyrin after irradiation with 405 nm light. Journal of Clinical Investigation 67: 1072-1077 (1981).

Lim, H.W.; Poh-Fitzpatrick, M.B. and Gigli, I.: Activation of the complement system and generation of hemotactic activity in vivo in patients with porphyrias. (Abstract). Clinical Research 30: 488a (1982).

Luton E.F. and Finchum, R.N.: Photosensitivity reaction to chlordiazepoxide. Archives of Dermatology 91: 362-363 (1965).

Maguire Jr, H.C. and Kaidbey, K.H.: Experimental photoallergic contact dermatitis: A mouse model. Journal of Investigational Dermatology 79: 147-152 (1982).

Maibach, H.I.; Sams Jr, N.M. and Epstein, J.H.: Screening for drug toxicity by wave lengths greater than 3,100Å. Archives of Dermatology 95: 12-15 (1967).

Mathias, C.G.T.; Maibach, H.I. and Epstein, J.H.: Allergic contact photodermatitis to para-aminobenzoic acid. Archives of Dermatology 114: 1665-1666 (1978).

Marx, J.L.; Eisenstat, B.A. and Gladstein, A.H.: Quinidine photosensitivity. Archives of Dermatology 119: 39-43 (1983).

Masuda, T.; Honda, S.; Nakauchi, Y. et al.: Photocontact dermatitis to bithionol, TBS, diaphene, and hexachlorophene. Japanese Journal of Dermatology, Series B 81: 238-244 (1971).

Merot, Y.; Harms, M. and Saurat, J.H.: Photosensitivity associated with carprofen (Imadyl) a new non-steroidal anti-inflammatory drug. Dermatologica 116: 301-307 (1983).

Miller, R.C. and Beltrani, V.S.: Quinethazone photosensitivity dermatitis. Archives of Dermatology 93: 346-347 (1966).

Miyachi, Y. and Takigawa, M.: Mechanisms of contact photosensitivity in mice. III. Predictive testing of chemicals with photoallergic potential in mice. Archives of Dermatology 119: 736-739 (1983).

Miyachi, Y. and Takigawa, M.: Mechanisms of contact photosensitivity in mice. II. Langerhan cells are required for successful induction of contact photosensitivity to TCSA. Journal of Investigative Dermatology 78: 363-365 (1982).

Morison, W.L.; Parrish, J.A. and Epstein, J.H.: Photoimmunology. Archives of Dermatology 115: 350-354 (1979).

NACDG (North American Contact Dermatitis Group) of the National Program for Dermatology: The Role of Patch Testing in Allergic Contact Dermatitis (Johson and Johson, New Brunswick 1974).

Osmundsen, P.E.: Contact photoallergy to tribromsalicylanilide. British Journal of Dermatology 81: 429-434 (1969).

Owens, D.W. and Knox, J.M.: Influence of heat, wind, and humidity on ultraviolet radiation injury; Kripke and Sass (Eds) ultraviolet Carcinogenesis. National Cancer Institute Monographs 50: 161-167 (1978).

Parrish, J.A.; Fitzpatrick, T.B.; Tannenbaum, L. and Pathak, M.A.: Photochemistry of psoriasis with oral methoxsalen and longwave ultraviolet light. N. Eng. J. Med. 291: 1207-1211 (1974).

Parsons, B.J.: Psoralen photochemistry. Photochemistry and Photobiology 32: 813-821 (1980).

Pathak, M.A.; Krämer, D.M. and Fitzpatrick, T.B.: Photochemistry and photobiology of furocoumarins (psoralens); in Pathak et al. (Eds) Sunlight and Man pp. 335-368 (University of Tokyo Press, Tokyo 1974).

Polano, J.K.: Photosensitivity due to drugs. Exerpta Med. Int. Congr. Ser. 85: 102-107 (1964).

Raugi, G.J.; Storrs, F.J. and Larsen, W.G.: Photoallergic contact dermatitis to men's perfume. Contact Dermatitis 5: 251-260 (1979).

Ramsay, C.A. and Obreshkova, E.: Photosensitivity from nalidixic acid. British Journal of Dermatology 91: 523-528 (1974).

Rosenthal, I.; Ben-Hur, E.; Prager, A. and Riklis, E.: Photochemical reactions of chlorpromazine: Chemical and biochemical implications. Photochemical Photobiology 28: 591-594 (1978).

Sams, W.M.: Contact photodermatitis. Archives of Dermatology 73: 142-148 (1956).

Satulsky, E.M.: Photosensitization induced by monoglycerol paraminobenzoate. Archives of Dermatology 62: 711-713 (1950).

Scott, K.W. and Dawson, T.A.J.: Photocontact dermatitis arising from the presence of quindoxin in animals seeding stuffs. British Journal of Dermatology 90: 543-546 (1974).

Schnait, F.G.; Wolff, K. and Konrad, K.: Erythropoietic protoporphyria-submicroscopic events during the acute photosensitivity flare. British Journal of Dermatology 92: 545-557 (1975).

Schreiber, M.M. and Naylor, L.Z.: Antihistamine photosensitivity. Archives of Dermatology 86: 58-62 (1962).

Schultz, K.H.; Wickemann, A. and Wulf, K.: Klinische and experimentelle untersuchungen über die photodynamische Wirksamkeit von Phenothiazin Derivaten, insbesondere von Magaphen. Archiv für Klinische und Experimentelle Dermatologie 202: 285-298 (1956).

Schwarz, K. and Speck, M.: Experimentelle Untersuchungen zur Frage der Photoallergie der Sulfonamide. Dermatologica 114: 232-243 (1957).

Shelley, W.B. and Sica, P.A.: Disseminate sporotrichosis of skin and bone cured with 5-flurocytosine: Photosensitivity as a complication. Journal of the American Academy of Dermatology 8: 229-235 (1983).

Sidi, E. and Bourgeois-Cavardin, J.: Mise au point du traitement du vitiligo par l'Ammi Majus. Presse Médicale 61L436-440 (1953).

Sidi, E.; Hincky, M. and Gervais, A.: Allergic sensitization and photosensitization to Phenergan cream. Journal of Investigative Dermatology 24: 345-352 (1955).

Smith, S.Z. and Epstein, J.H.: Photocontact dermatitis to halogenated salicylanilides and related compounds. Archives of Dermatology 113: 1372-1374 (1977).

Song, P. and Tapley Jr, K.J.: Photochemistry and photobiology of psoralens. Photochemistry and Photobiology 29: 1177-1197 (1979).

Stern, R.S. and Bigby, M.: An expanded profile of cutaneous reactions to nonsteroidal anti-inflammatory drugs. Journal of American Medical Association 252: 1433-1437 (1984).

Stern, R.S.; Thibodeau, L.A.; Kleinerman, R.A.; Parrish, J.A.; Fitzpatrick, T.B. et al.: Risk of cutaneous carcinoma in patients treated with oral methoxsalen photochemotherapy for psoriasis. New England Journal of Medicine 300: 809-813 (1979).

Stern, R.B.; Ziebler, S. and Parrish, J.A.: Skin carcinoma in patients treated with topical tar and artificial ultraviolet radiation. Lancet 1: 732-735 (1980).

Stevanovic, D.V.: Photosensitivity due to certain drugs. British Journal of Dermatology 73: 233-237 (1961).

Storck, H.: Photoallergy and photosensitivity: Due to systemically administered drugs. Archives of Dermatology 91: 469-482 (1965).

Stratigos, J.D. and Magnus, I.A.: Photosensitivity by demethylchlortetracycline and sulphanilamide. British Journal of Dermatology 80: 391-405 (1968).

Takigawa, M. and Miyachi, Y.: Mechanisms of contact photosensitivity in mice: I. T cell regulation of contact photosensitivity to tetrachlorosalicylanilide under genetic restrictions of the major histocompatibility complex. Journal of Investigative Dermatology 79: 108-115 (1982).

Tatsuji, K. and Toshie, A.: Photoallergic dermatitis probably due to artificial sweetening agents. Med. Culture 5: 795-800 (1963).

Torinuki, W.; Kumai, N. and Miura, T.: Chronic photosensitive dermatitis due to phenothiazines. Tohoku Journal of Experimental Medicine 138: 223-226 (1982).

van Weelden, H.; Bolling, H.H.; Baart de la Faille, H. and van der Leun, J.C.: Photosensitivity caused by chloroquine. (Abstract) Archives of Dermatology 118: 290 (1982).
Wilkinson, D.S.: Photodermatitis due to tetrachlorosalicylanilide. British Journal of Dermatology 73: 213-219 (1961).
Willis, I. and Kligman, A.M.: The mechanism of the persistent light reactor. Journal of Investigative Dermatology 51: 385-394 (1968a).
Willis, I. and Kligman, A.M.: The mechanism of photoallergic contact dermatitis. Journal of Investigative Dermatology 51: 378-384 (1968b).
Willis, I. and Kligman, A.M.: Photocontact allergic reactions: Elicitation by low doses ultraviolet rays. Archives of Dermatology 110: 535-539 (1969).
Wiskemann, A. and Wulf, K.: Untersuchungen über den auslösenden Spektralbereich und die direkte Lichtpigmentierung bei chronischen und akuten Lichtauschlägen. Archiv für Klinische und Experimentelle Dermatologie 209: 443-453 (1959).
Zanoun, S.; Johnson, B.E. and Frain-Bell, W.: The investigation of quindoxin photosensitivity. Contact Dermatitis 2: 342-352 (1976).

Address for correspondence and reprints: Dr *John H. Epstein*, Department of Dermatology A-432, University of California, San Francisco, CA 94143 (USA).

Drugs 30: 58-65 (1985)
0012-6667/85/0700-0058/$04.00/0

Vitamins in Psychiatry
Do They Have a Role?

William M. Petrie and *Thomas A. Ban*

Department of Psychiatry, Vanderbilt University, Nashville

Summary

Deficiencies of specific vitamins produce consistent symptoms of psychiatric disorder. Thiamine deficiency, which is common in alcoholism, can produce confusion and psychotic symptoms, in addition to neurological signs. Vitamin B_{12} and folate deficiency may contribute symptoms of disorientation, depression or psychosis; their measurement is a part of routine dementia work-ups. Pyridoxine deficiency results in seizures, although the effects of exogenously administered pyridoxine are not clearly understood in depression and anxiety – the disorders in which it is most frequently used clinically.

The use of vitamins has been most prominent in psychiatry in the treatment of schizophrenia, where large doses of nicotinic acid were initially given alone and later combined with other vitamins and minerals. Several theoretical models were described to support the use of vitamins in schizophrenia. These included: the parallels of schizophrenia to the psychiatric symptoms of pellagra; hypotheses of a defect in adrenaline metabolism; and the accumulation of psychotoxic substances which produce psychotic symptoms. Initially, positive results were reported over 30 years ago, but have not been replicated by thorough investigations. An extensive series of comprehensive placebo-controlled trials failed to show efficacy for any of the vitamin therapies tested.

Although clearly less effective than antipsychotic drug treatment, vitamin therapy is not without risks – adverse effects have been reported with nicotinic acid, pyridoxine and vitamin C. Although the possible role of vitamins has played an important part in the development of biological psychiatry, vitamin therapy is no longer extensively practised, and claims for its efficacy have not been supported by objective scientific evidence.

The fact that vitamin administration reverses the psychiatric symptoms of specific vitamin deficiencies was a key discovery in biological psychiatry. Deficiencies of vitamin B_1 (thiamine), B_3 (nicotinic acid), B_{12} (cyanocabalamin), C (ascorbic acid) and others produce reliable behavioural symptoms, usually in combination with associated physical signs.

1. Psychiatric Symptoms and Vitamin Deficiency States

1.1 Thiamine Deficiency

Thiamine plays a basic role in the metabolism of carbohydrates. Thiamine deficiency, seen commonly in alcoholism, leads to an accumulation of pyruvate in the blood and might cause neuropathy and encephalopathy (Wernicke's syndrome). It has also been hypothesised that thiamine produces a 'diphosphate effect' and increases transketolase activity in thiamine-deficient individuals (Waldenlind et al., 1981). The clinical symptoms of Wernicke's encephalopathy (global confusional state, ophthalmoplegia, nystagmus and ataxia) are generally attenuated with immediate thiamine treatment.

The symptoms of Korsakoff's psychosis (memory loss, learning deficits and confabulation) may be seen either in short or long term care settings and is felt to be on the continuum of the same pathological process as Wernicke's encephalopathy (Feinberg, 1980). It has been noted that thiamine must be administered early in the course of the illness to produce improvement in the psychiatric symptoms of the Wernicke-Korsakoff syndrome (Leigh et al., 1981).

As well as thiamine, folic acid has also been noted to be deficient in alcoholics, and during the stage of detoxification, reduction of folic acid levels predict cognitive impairment (Albert et al., 1982). In addition, pellagra (nicotinic acid deficiency) has been noted in some chronic alcoholics. Ishii and Nishihara (1981) found characteristic neuropathological changes at autopsy, even when characteristic pellagra skin lesions were not present.

Thiamine has also been used to treat nutritionally deficient, non-alcoholic patients who presented with apparently neurotic symptoms. These patients had abnormally low red cell transketolase activity, which could be gradually corrected by exogenous thiamine administration (Lonsdale and Shamberger, 1980). Carney et al. (1982) assessed levels of thiamine, riboflavine, and pyridoxine in general psychiatric patients. Of the 172 patients in this study, 53% were deficient in at least one vitamin, and 12% were deficient in more than one. Thiamine deficiency was found to be the most common and was seen both in alcoholics and schizophrenics. Patients with affective disorders were noted to have lower levels of riboflavine and pyridoxine.

1.2 Vitamin B_{12} and Folate Deficiency

Vitamin B_{12} deficiency produces the classic symptoms of subacute combined degeneration in addition to psychiatric symptoms of irritability, confusion, disorientation, depression and frank psychosis. At times, the organic psychosis may be present without haematological or spinal column abnormalities (Zucker et al., 1981).

Folate deficiency may also be present with psychiatric and haematological symptoms. Affective symptoms have been specifically related to folate deficiency (Shorvon et al., 1980), and dementia symptoms have been reversed by folate administration (Enk et al., 1980). The relationship of folate to depression has been linked to changes in serotonin metabolism effected by folate (Botez et al., 1982).

1.3 Pyridoxine Deficiency

The vitamin B_6 group (pyridoxine, pyridoxal and pyridoxamine) are important in coenzyme function in the conversion of tryptophan to both nicotinic acid and serotonin, and in the conversion of glutamic acid to γ-aminobutyric acid (GABA). In conditions of pyridoxine deficiency, GABA levels are reduced and the resultant convulsive activity may be controlled by administration of GABA (Tower, 1958). Whereas psychiatric symptoms have not been classically described in pyridoxine deficiency (except in alcoholics), the changes in serotonin and GABA metabolism are of theoretical interest to psychiatry. Disturbances in serotonin metabolism are accepted as a viable hypothesis in the pathogenesis of affective illness, and GABA has been related to anxiety disorders.

Thus, pyridoxine has been administered to depressed patients, both alone and in combination with antidepressant agents. Although anecdotal reports indicate potential efficacy, no conclusive clinical trial has been undertaken. Data are also lacking on pyridoxine's use in anxiety disorders.

In Western countries, inadequate food intake is now rarely seen as a cause of vitamin deficiency. But the refining of current foods, food selection patterns, and pure corn diets may deplete B vitamins, and ω-3 essential fatty acid, a substrate upon which nicotinic acid and other B vitamin coenzymes act to form the prostaglandin-3 series, which may regulate neurohormones (Rudin, 1981). Other investigators (Lonsdale and Shamberger, 1980) have linked overrefined or 'junk' foods to nutritional deficiency in psychiatric patients, but such an hypothesis would require further substantiation.

2. *Vitamins and Schizophrenia*

The use of vitamins to treat schizophrenia was based on the theoretical assumption that the illness was related to a biological imbalance which could be corrected by the addition of vitamins. Initially 'megavitamin therapy' of schizophrenia was carried out with the use of large doses of vitamin B_3 (nicotinic acid or nicotinamide), although later it included the use of the coenzyme nicotinamide adenine dinucleotide (NAD), pyridoxine, ascorbic acid, folic acid, vitamin B_{12}, and other vitamins and minerals.

2.1 Hypotheses Regarding the Possible Mode of Action of Vitamins

Hoffer initially offered 9 separate speculations as to the mode of action of nicotinic acid in the treatment of schizophrenia. He suggested that the psychiatric symptoms of pellagra (nicotinic acid deficiency) resembled elements of schizophrenia (Hoffer et al., 1957). Nicotinic acid had been established as effective treatment for pellagra as late as 1938. It was demonstrated that psychiatric symptoms such as dementia, confusion, neurasthenia and depression could develop on the basis of acute and/or chronic nicotinic acid deficiency (Medlicott, 1945). However, even in patients who have pellagra, less than 10% will have mental symptoms (Henderson and Gillespie, 1946).

Osmond and Smythies (1952) hypothesised that schizophrenia resulted from stress-induced anxiety and an error in adrenaline (epinephrine) metabolism, whereby toxic-hallucinatory, mescaline-like byproducts are formed. The idea that an endogenous, psychotomimetic compound produced many of the clinical symptoms of schizophrenia was further developed by Harley-Mason who postulated that certain such compounds (e.g. 3,4,dimethoxyphenylethylamine; DMPEA) were the result of transmethylation. In such cases, N-methylation of noradrenaline (norepinephrine) is replaced by O-methylation of the phenol ring of dopamine (Harley-Mason, 1952). Alternatively, it was proposed by Hoffer et al. (1954) that another psychotoxic metabolic product, adrenochrome, resulted from increased phenolase activity in the schizophrenic brain (Hoffer, 1962). Thus, nicotinic acid might prevent adrenaline accumulation, thereby preventing the toxic buildup of adrenochrome. Nicotinic acid was thought to compete with noradrenaline for available methyl groups, supplied in the diet by methionine. Large amounts of nicotinic acid, up to 2000 mg/day, would be necessary to counteract this theorised methyl donor accumulation.

Subsequently, Pauling (1968) coined the phrase 'orthomolecular' psychiatry, hypothesising that schizophrenic patients and others were lacking in optimum molecular concentrations of vitamins and other nutrients, resulting in 'abnormal reaction rates', and ultimately psychopathological symptoms. These abnormal reaction rates were supposedly related to genetically idiosyncratic needs for large amounts of vitamins. Pauling reported differences between schizophrenics and normal subjects in their response to oral doses of ascorbic acid, nicotinic acid and pyridoxine, with schizophrenic patients excreting lower amounts. This lower excretion rate was considered as support for megavitamin therapy in the treatment of schizophrenia (Pauling et al., 1973).

Concentrations of trace elements have been reported to be altered in some schizophrenics. Copper levels were reported by Pfeiffer et al. (1973) to be elevated in many schizophrenics, with an accompanying reduced urinary excretion of copper. Copper as well as elevated iron levels in some patients were felt to act as 'tissue enzyme poisons', which could be reduced by the administration of zinc and zinc sulphate plus manganese chloride.

Blood histamine levels have also been reported to be lowered in up to 50% of schizophrenic patients; Pfeiffer et al. (1973) believed these patients have lowered basophil counts with predominantly paranoid symptomatology. Vitamin B_{12} and folic acid were considered to be specifically therapeutic in this group, while patients with high blood histamine concentrations were believed to respond to methionine (which releases histamine), zinc and manganese.

Thus, what began as a theory of a specific vitamin treatment (B_3), became generalised to include a larger number of vitamins and nutrients. This theory was in opposition to a psychogenic aetiology of schizophrenia and other major psychiatric disorders, widely accepted at the time, and was also applied by some to learning disabilities, and depression (Cott, 1971; Hoffer, 1967, 1971). However, megavitamin and orthomolecular therapy has been most widely used in schizophrenia.

2.2 Clinical Trials with Vitamin B_3

Positive findings with megavitamin therapy began in 1952, when nicotinic acid or nicotinamide (in doses of 1 to 5 g/day) were reportedly beneficial in a number of seriously ill schizophrenic patients. The vitamin therapy produced a rapid response in these patients, whereas conventional treatments at that time (antipsychotics had not yet been introduced) had been unable to stop their deterioration. Hoffer (1962) conducted a double-blind study of 30 days' treatment of nicotinic acid and nicotinamide *versus* other treatments, including electroconvulsive therapy (ECT). Although the vitamin-treated patients improved only slightly more than the control group, the relapse rate of the experimental group was significantly lower over the next 4 years. Later studies led Hoffer to believe that acute schizophrenics benefitted more from vitamin treatment than did chronic patients (Hoffer, 1962; Osmond and Hoffer, 1962).

Other positive findings were reported on the basis of open trials (Cott, 1969, 1970; Denson, 1962; Ward, 1967). Hoffer and Osmond's report (1966) on the effectiveness of nicotinamide adenine dinucleotide (NAD) created the greatest interest. They reported dramatic reduction in schizophrenic symptoms in 11 of 18 chronic schizophrenics, with a rapid return of psychopathology when the experimental agent was withdrawn.

However, attempts to replicate this work by other investigators failed (Gallant et al., 1966; Kline et al., 1967; Meltzer et al., 1969). It should also be noted that the methodology of clinical trials at the time of the introduction of megavitamin therapy did not emphasise random selection of patients, precise diagnosis, clearcut criteria for improvement or remission, nor careful follow-up. Electroconvulsive therapy was also used frequently in early megavitamin trials, usually as a concomitant therapy to megavitamins.

Careful attempts at replication were made by Ashby et al. (1960) who studied 39 patients over a 26-week study period. He found no difference between nicotinic acid, nicotinamide, and placebo. Greenbaum (1970) reported a similar lack of efficacy in 57 schizophrenic children given nicotinamide or placebo for 6 months.

It is important to note that as antipsychotic agents were introduced, vitamin therapy was used in addition to these drugs. However, it was felt by megavitamin proponents that vitamin therapy reduced the need for antipsychotics. Nevertheless, Meltzer et al. (1969) was unable to detect any change in phenothiazine efficacy when nicotinic acid was used concomitantly. Studying 265 consecutive admissions, McGrath et al. (1972), in addition to phenothiazine and rehabilitative treatment, gave either 3g of nicotinamide or placebo for a 1-year period. A majority of these patients had been ill for at least a year. No additional improvement was noticeable in the vitamin-treated patients, either after 30 days or after 1 year of treatment.

Wittenborn et al. (1973) examined the effects of 3g of nicotinic acid and placebo in 86 patients over a period of 18 months. 90% of patients completed 2 years of treatment. Careful follow-up was done at monthly intervals. No shortening of hospital stays on nicotinic acid, no difference in rehospitalisation, and no difference in psychological tests or home or community adjustment were noted.

2.2.1 Collaborative Studies

Not only were initial claims of vitamin therapy positive, but with the multiple regimens used, it was difficult to scientifically replicate these findings in any single trial. The Canadian Mental Health Association (CMHA) set up a thorough, systematic trial of the testable hypotheses from megavitamin therapy. These trials were executed over 2 years in a double-blind, placebo-controlled manner.

The first study assessed the effect of nicotinic acid *versus* placebo in acute schizophrenia, with the addition of chlorpromazine as the patient's condition warranted. This study indicated that nicotinic acid was, in fact, not superior to placebo as the sole medication in these newly admitted patients, even with doses as high as 9 g/day. Patients on nicotinic acid and nicotinamide required longer hospital stays than those on placebo, although all 3 patient groups showed significant improvement (Ban, 1974).

A second study measured the effectiveness of nicotinic acid as an adjuvant therapy in addition to phenothiazine drugs. Nicotinic acid or placebo was added to various antipsychotic agents in a double-blind regimen lasting 6 months utilising newly admitted schizophrenic patients. Again, nicotinic acid was not superior to placebo, and with doses of 3 g/day both hospital duration and amount of antipsychotic required were both increased in the experimental group compared with control patients (Ramsey et al., 1970).

In another study, long term hospitalised patients fared no better on nicotinic acid in addition to an antipsychotic agent than on placebo. Interestingly, with these 30 patients the active treatment group fared worse than the placebo group on a variety of assessment measures, including the amount of antipsychotic drug required to control their symptoms (Ban and Lehmann, 1970).

2.2.2 Clinical Trials with Nicotinic Acid in Combination with Pyridoxine and Other Vitamins

As a part of megavitamin, or orthomolecular, therapy, nicotinic acid is almost never given alone (table I). In part using Pauling's rationale, a large number of other vitamins and substances are used. Antipsychotic drugs, special diets and prescribed periods of exercise and diet are also used (Hawkins, 1973). Typically, vitamin therapy consists of at least 1g nicotinamide, 1g ascorbic acid, 50mg pyridoxine, and 40IU of vitamin E, 4 times daily (Hawkins, 1973). Improvement is expected within the first 6 months. Parenteral (intramuscular injection) treatment, with reduced amounts of vitamins injected at weekly intervals or less, has been utilised in an attempt to accelerate the response.

Table I. Vitamin regimens tested in schizophrenia

Nicotinic acid
Nicotinic acid + antipsychotic drugs
Nicotinic acid + pyridoxine[a]
Nicotinic acid + pyridoxine + ascorbic acid[a]
Nicotinic acid + pyridoxine + ascorbic acid + thiamine
Nicotinic acid + pyridoxine + ascorbic acid + hydroxocobalamin[a]

a Generally includes antipsychotic drug treatment.

To address the issue of the efficacy of nicotinic acid in combination with pyridoxine, these two vitamins were compared with either nicotinic acid or pyridoxine given alone. In this placebo-controlled trial, the combination was no more effective than either of its components. Antipsychotic agents were also given to patients throughout the trial. On the Brief Psychiatric Rating Scale (BPRS), the nicotinic acid patients improved by 8.4%, the pyridoxine patients by 8.1% and the combined treatment group by 5.5%. These figures were not significantly different (Ban and Lehmann, 1973).

In another 1-year, 30-patient study, the question of whether nicotinic acid combined with ascorbic acid was more effective than either agent alone was tested. Up to 3g nicotinic acid and 1.5g ascorbic acid was used. Again, these agents were combined with antipsychotic agents. The combination proved of no advantage when compared with either agent alone, there being no significant difference between the 3 groups (Ban, 1981). However, all 3 groups did show significant improvement in total BPRS scores. On individual factor scores, patients on nicotinic acid became slightly worse on anxiety, conceptual disorganisation and uncooperativeness, while patients on ascorbic acid and ascorbic acid plus nicotinic acid improved slightly more on these scores. Patients receiving ascorbic acid alone scored higher on manifest psychosis than did patients in the nicotinic acid plus ascorbic acid group. Therefore, it was concluded that the combination of vitamins was not superior to either (i.e. nicotinic acid or ascorbic acid) given separately (Ban, 1981).

Furthermore, to specifically test the transmethylation hypothesis of nicotinic acid therapy (see section 2.1), a 14-week, double-blind crossover study was performed in 20 hospitalised schizophrenics. Patients were first given a methyldonor (methionine) and a monoamine oxidase inhibitor (tranylcypromine), and nicotinic acid or placebo was then administered. If the theory of nicotinic acid's action was correct, the emergence of increased psychotic symptoms in the nicotinic acid group should be prevented. With the addition of tranylcypromine and methionine, most of the patients showed intensification of their psychotic symptoms, as well as confusional and sexual symptoms. Nicotinic acid had no effect on these changes; thus the hypothesis that nicotinic acid could prevent transmethylation-related symptoms was not supported (Lehmann et al., 1973).

Finally, in a 24-week placebo-controlled study, 20 hospitalised chronic schizophrenics were treated with the entire orthomolecular armamentarium, with daily doses of nicotinic acid (1 to 9g), thiamine (300mg), pyridoxine (150mg), ascorbic acid (1 to 3g) and hydroxocobalamin (0.5mg). Both vitamin and placebo patients also received chlorpromazine. No difference was found between the 2 groups (Ban et al., 1977).

In summary, the findings of the CMHA studies, as well as the most carefully controlled studies by others, point to the unequivocal conclusion that megavitamin therapy has no reliable effect on either acute or chronic schizophrenia. Given the systematic, painstaking method of the CMHA study, it is likely that if such a therapeutic effect – even a subtle one – were present, it would have been discovered in one of the studies.

3. Adverse Effects of Vitamin Therapy

While the therapeutic effects of high dose vitamins are questionable, at best, it is well-known that these agents may produce occasional adverse effects of consequence. High doses of nicotinic acid may produce flushing and itching of the skin, dermatological lesions, nausea, vomiting and activation of peptic ulcer disease. In addition, hypotension, tachycardia and hyperglycaemia have been noted in addition to hypoalbuminaemia, jaundice and elevation of liver enzyme (transaminase) levels.

Megadoses of pyridoxine may produce neurological symptoms such as weakness, impairment of balance, and damage to motor and sensory neurons. Some patients have lost sensation in their arms and legs and 1 patient was reported unable to walk (Schaumberg et al., 1983).

High doses of vitamin C may irritate the gastrointestinal tract and may also lower serum uric acid levels. Vitamin E has produced fatigue and weakness in patients on high dose regimens.

4. Conclusions

Although antipsychotic agents control the symptoms of schizophrenia, the illness remains devastating to its victims, even with the most modern treatment methods. Megavitamin therapy hypothesised a biochemical defect in schizophrenic patients at a time when psychotherapy and long term institutionalisation were the most frequent therapies. Good has no doubt resulted from the treatment, at least through focusing critical attention toward the area. There have been countless anecdotal reports of improvement of patients given vitamin therapies, and if these are reliable, then patients have indeed benefited.

The theoretical basis of orthomolecular and megavitamin therapies, which were attractive 30 years ago, have not been supported by time. The adrenochrome theory of schizophrenia has now been abandoned. The presence of adrenochrome in the plasma of schizophrenic patients could not be confirmed, although adrenochrome itself does have psychotomimetic properties. It is also clear now that nicotinic acid is not a clinically effective methyl acceptor substance. In addition, consistent alterations in vitamins or trace elements have not been found in schizophrenic patients. More importantly, serious attempts to replicate the claims of megavitamin and orthomolecular therapy have clearly failed, as noted in this review.

While these studies are not exhaustive, we advise caution in the assumption that selected schizophrenic patients may benefit from vitamin therapy. Similar claims have been made (unsuccessfully) for insulin coma, psychoanalysis, and other treatments of schizophrenia which have now been largely abandoned. Vitamin therapy of schizophrenia will no doubt continue. However, it should be viewed by clinician and patient alike as unproven.

References

Albert, M.; Butters, N.; Rogers, S.; Pressman, J. and Geller, A.: A preliminary report: Nutritional levels and cognitive performance in chronic alcohol abusers. Drug and Alcohol Dependence 9: 131-142 (1982).

Ashby, W.R.; Collins, G.H. and Bassett, M.: The effects of nicotinamide and placebo on the chronic schizophrenic. Journal of Mental Science 106: 155-159 (1960).

Ban, T.A.: Negative findings with nicotinic acid in the treatment of schizophrenias. International Pharmacopsychiatry 9: 174-187 (1974).

Ban, T.A.: Megavitamin therapy in schizophrenia; in Miller (Ed.) Nutrition and Behavior, pp. 247-253 (Franklin Institute Press, Philadelphia 1981).

Ban, T.A. and Lehmann, H.E.: Nicotinic acid in the treatment of schizophrenias. Canadian Mental Health Association Collaborative Study (Canadian Mental Health Association, Toronto, 1970).

Ban, T.A. and Lehmann, H.E.: Niacin in the treatment of schizophrenias: Alone and in combination; in Ban et al. (Eds) Psychopharmacology, Sexual Disorders and Drug Abuse, pp. 293-299 (North Holland Publishing, Amsterdam 1973).

Ban, T.A.; Lehmann, H.E. and Deutsch, M.: Negative findings with megavitamins in schizophrenic patients: preliminary report. Communications in Psychopharmacology 1: 119-122 (1977).

Botez, M.I.; Young, S.N.; Bachevalier, J. and Gauthier, S.: Effect of folic acid and vitamin B_{12} deficiencies on 5-hydroxyindolacetic acid in human cerebrospinal fluid. Annals of Neurology 12: 479-484 (1982).

Carney, M.W.; Ravindran, A.; Rinsler, M.G. and Williams, D.G.: Thiamine, riboflavin and pyridoxine deficiency in psychiatric patients. British Journal of Psychiatry 141: 271-272 (1982).

Cott, A.: Treating schizophrenic children. Schizophrenia 1: 44-49 (1969).

Cott, A.: The parenteral use of vitamins in the treatment of schizophrenia. Schizophrenia 2: 177-179 (1970).

Cott, A.: Orthomolecular approach to the treatment of learning disabilities. Schizophrenia 3: 95-105 (1971).

Denson, R.: Nicotinamide in the treatment of schizophrenia. Disorders of the Nervous System 23: 167-172 (1962).

Enk, C.; Hougaard, K. and Hippe, E.: Reversible dementia and neuropathy associated with folate deficiency 16 years after partial gastrectomy. Scandinavian Journal of Haematology 25: 63-66 (1980).

Feinberg, J.F.: The Wernicke-Korsakoff syndrome. American Family Physician 22: 129-133 (1980).

Gallant, D.M.; Bishop, M. and Steeler, C.A.: DPN (NAD-oxidized form): A preliminary evaluation in chronic schizophrenic patients. Current Therapeutic Research 8: 542-548 (1966).

Greenbaum, G.H.C.: An evaluation of niacinamide in the treatment of childhood schizophrenia. American Journal of Psychiatry 127: 129-132 (1970).

Harley-Mason, J.: in Osmond and Smythies (Eds) Schizophrenia: A new approach. Journal of Mental Science 98: 309-315 (1952).

Hawkins, D.: in Hawkins and Pauling (Eds) Orthomolecular Psychiatry: Treatment of Schizophrenia, pp. 631-673 (W.H. Freeman, San Francisco 1973).

Henderson, D.K. and Gillespie, R.D.: A Textbook of Psychiatry for Students and Practitioners (Oxford University Press, London, New York 1946).

Hoffer, A.: Niacin Therapy in Psychiatry (C.C. Thomas, Springfield 1962).

Hoffer, A.: A Program for Treating Schizophrenia and Other Conditions Using Megavitamin Therapy (Modern Press, Saskatoon 1967).

Hoffer, A.: Megavitamin B-3 therapy for schizophrenia. Canadian Psychiatric Association Journal 16: 499-504 (1971).

Hoffer, A. and Osmond, H.: Nicotinamide adenine dinucleotide (NAD) as a treatment for schizophrenia. Journal of Psychopharmacology 1: 79-95 (1966).

Hoffer, A.; Osmond, H. and Callbeck, M.: Treatment of schizophrenia with nicotinic acid and nicotinamide. Journal of Clinical Experimental Psychopathology 18: 131-158 (1957).

Hoffer, A.; Osmond, H. and Smythies, J.: Schizophrenia: A new approach. II. Result of a year's research. Journal of Mental Science 100: 29-54 (1954).

Ishii, N. and Nishihara, Y.: Pellagra among chronic alcoholics: Clinical and pathological study of 20 necropsy cases. Journal of Neurology, Neurosurgery and Psychiatry 44: 209-215 (1981).

Kline, N.S.; Barclay, G.L.; Cole, J.O.; Esser, A.H.; Lehman, H. and Wittenborn, J.R.: Controlled evaluation of nicotinamide adenine dinucleotide in the treatment of chronic schizophrenic patients. British Journal of Psychiatry 113: 731-742 (1967).

Lehmann, H.E.; Ban, T.A. and Ananth, J.V.: Nicotinic acid and the transmethylation hypothesis of schizophrenia; in Cole et al. (Eds) Psychopathology and Psychopharmacology, pp. 219-230 (Johns Hopkins University Press, Baltimore 1973).

Leigh, D.; McBurney, A. and McIlwain, H.: Erythrocyte transketolase activity in the Wernicke-Korsakoff syndrome. British Journal of Psychiatry 139: 153-156 (1981).

Lonsdale, D. and Shamberger, R.J.: Red cell transketolase as an indicator of nutritional deficiency. American Journal of Clinical Nutrition 33: 205-211 (1980).

McGrath, S.D.; O'Brien, P.F.; Power, P.J. and Shea, J.R.: Nicotinamide treatment of schizophrenia. Schizophrenia Bulletin 5: 74-76 (1972).

Medlicott, R.W.: Nicotinic acid in treatment of some psychiatric

syndromes. New Zealand Medical Journal 44: 28-33 (1945).
Meltzer, H.; Shader, R. and Grinspoon, L.: The behavioral effects of nicotinamide adenine dinucleotide in chronic schizophrenia. Psychopharmacologia (Berlin) 15: 144-152 (1969).
Osmond, H. and Hoffer, A.: Massive niacin treatment in schizophrenia: Review of a nine-year study. Lancet 1: 316-319 (1962).
Osmond, H. and Smythies, J.: Schizophrenia: A new approach. Journal of Mental Science 98: 309 (1952).
Pauling, L.: Orthomolecular psychiatry. Science 160: 265-271 (1968).
Pauling, L.; Robinson, A.B.; Oxley, S.S.; Bergeson, M.; Harris, A.; Cary, P.; Blethen, J. and Keaveny, I.T.: Results of loading test of ascorbic acid, niacinamide, and pyridoxine in schizophrenic subjects and controls; in Hawkins and Pauling (Eds), Orthomolecular Psychiatry (W.H. Freeman, San Francisco 1973).
Pfeiffer, C.C.; Iliev, V. and Goldstein, L.: Blood histamine basophil counts, and trace elements in the schizophrenias; in Hawkins and Pauling (Eds) Orthomolecular Psychiatry: Treatment of Schizophrenia, pp. 463-512 (W.H. Freeman and Co, San Francisco 1973).
Ramsey, R.A.; Ban, T.A.; Lehmann, H.E.; Saxena, B.M. and Bennett, J.: Nicotinic acid as adjuvant therapy in newly admitted schizophrenic patients. Canadian Medical Association Journal 102: 939-942 (1970).
Rudin, D.O.: The major psychoses and neuroses as omega-3 essential fatty acid deficiency syndrome: Substrate pellagra. Biological Psychiatry 16: 837-850 (1981).
Schaumberg, H.; Kaplan, J.; Windebank, A.; Vick, N.; Rasmus, S.; Pleasure, D. and Brown, M.J.: Sensory neuropathy from pyridoxine abuse. A new megavitamin syndrome. New England Journal of Medicine 309: 445-448 (1983).
Shorvon, S.D.; Carney, M.W.; Chanarin, I. and Reynolds, E.H.: The neuropsychiatry of megaloblastic anaemia. British Medical Journal 281: 1036-1038 (1980).
Tower, D.B.: Pyridoxine and cerebral activity. Nutritional Reviews 16: 161-164 (1958).
Waldenlind, L.; Borg, S. and Vikander, B.: Effect of peroral thiamine treatment on thiamine contents and transketolase activity of red blood cells in alcoholic patients. Acta Medica Scandinavica 209: 209-212 (1981).
Ward, J.L.: Treatment of neurotics and schizophrenics using clinical and HOD criteria. Journal of Schizophrenia 1: 140 (1967).
Wittenborn, J.R.; Weber, E.S.P. and Brown, M.: Niacin in the long-term treatment of schizophrenia. Archives of General Psychiatry 28: 308-315 (1973).
Zucker, D.K.; Livingston, R.L.; Nakra, R. and Clayton, P.L.: B_{12} deficiency and psychiatric disorders: Case report and literature review. Biological Psychiatry 16: 197-205 (1981).

Address for correspondence and reprints: Associate Professor *William M. Petrie*, Department of Psychiatry, Vanderbilt University, Nashville, TN 37232 (USA).

Drugs 30: 66-77 (1985)
0012-6667/85/0700-0066/$06.00/0

Primary Oesophageal Motility Disorders
Current Therapeutic Concepts

Morris Traube and *Richard W. McCallum*
Gastroenterology Unit, Yale University School of Medicine, New Haven

Summary

Various oesophageal manometric disorders have been associated with chest pain or dysphagia. The classic motility disorders are achalasia and diffuse oesophageal spasm. In achalasia, a disorder of aperistalsis in the oesophageal body and incomplete relaxation of the lower oesophageal sphincter, either surgical myotomy or pneumatic dilatation is an effective approach, although some investigators have suggested a role for pharmacological therapy. For the treatment of diffuse oesophageal spasm, a disorder of non-peristaltic motor activity in the oesophagus, various pharmacological approaches with nitrates, anticholinergics, and calcium antagonists have been used. In the presence of associated lower oesophageal sphincter dysfunction, bouginage or pneumatic dilatation may be indicated. Long oesophagomyotomy should be considered for those patients who fail to respond to these measures.

Recent manometric techniques have led to the identification of patients with chest pain or dysphagia who have abnormalities of increased contractile amplitude ('nutcracker' oesophagus) or duration. An association with gastro-oesophageal reflux or with psychiatric disturbance has been suggested. Treatment directed towards these factors is indicated and may be supplemented by pharmacological intervention, e.g. by calcium antagonists or anticholinergics.

The recent flourishing of laboratories performing oesophageal manometry makes a review of the oesophageal 'spastic' disorders timely. This article emphasises our current therapeutic approach to patients with the classic motility disorders, namely achalasia and diffuse oesophageal spasm, as well as those with more recently recognised primary disturbances of motility in the distal oesophagus which also present as chest pain and/or dysphagia.

1. Normal Physiology and Pharmacology of the Oesophagus

Propulsion of a bolus of food down the oesophagus occurs via an orderly propagated contraction (fig. 1). This primary peristalsis is initiated by pharyngeal reflexes and requires cholinergic input. Thus, both parenteral (Dodds et al., 1981) and oral (Hongo et al., 1984b) anticholinergic agents decrease the amplitude of contraction, but only relatively high doses of parenteral atropine inhibit completeness of peristalsis (Richardson and Welch, 1981).

The lower oesophageal sphincter (LOS) separates the oesophagus from the stomach. An anatomic equivalent of the LOS has been identified in cadaveric studies (Liebermann-Meffert et al., 1979), but the physiological aspect is of greater importance. The LOS separates the negative intraoesophageal pressure from the positive intragastric

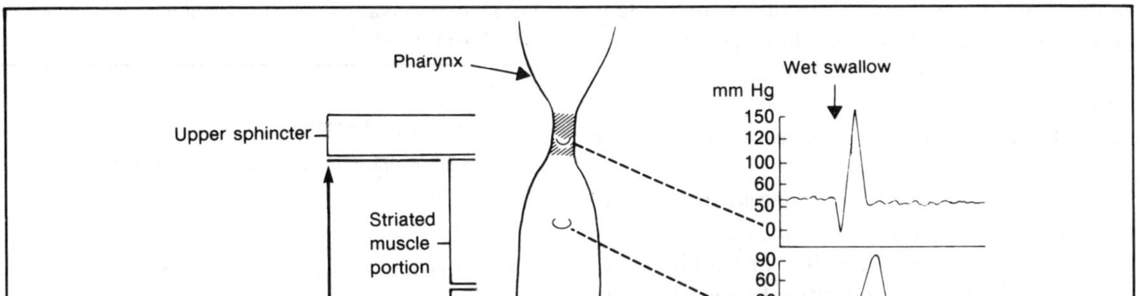

Fig. 1. Schematic representation of oesophageal motor function. The lower oesophageal sphincter relaxes at the onset of swallowing. A propagated contraction is shown from the proximal oesophagus through the lower oesophageal sphincter.

pressure and helps to prevent reflux of gastric material into the oesophagus. Upon swallowing, LOS tone falls, or relaxes, toward intragastric pressure, thus allowing the bolus upon reaching the LOS to traverse the stomach (fig. 1). As the peristaltic contraction from the oesophageal body reaches the sphincter, the latter contracts, following which LOS tone returns to its basal state.

Basal LOS tone is generated by both neural and intrinsic myogenic activity (Dodds et al., 1981). Thus, both parenteral (Dodds et al., 1981) and oral (Hongo et al., 1984b) anticholinergic agents decrease LOS pressure in normal subjects.

Calcium is required for both contraction of muscle in the oesophageal body and for the maintenance of LOS tone (Cohen and Green, 1973; DeCarle et al., 1977). In normal subjects nifedipine, a calcium-antagonist, decreases in a dose-dependent manner both LOS pressure and amplitude of contraction in the oesophageal body (Hongo et al., 1984a). The latter effect, however, is less marked than that seen on the LOS.

2. Classification of Primary Manometric Disorders

The classic disorders of oesophageal motility in the smooth muscle portion of the oesophagus are achalasia and diffuse oesophageal spasm (Vantrappen et al., 1979). In achalasia, two major abnormalities are present: (a) failure of, or incomplete, relaxation of the LOS with swallowing; and (b) absence of peristalsis in the body of the oesophagus. Intraoesophageal pressure may be positive in relation to fundic pressure. The resting tone of the LOS may also be increased.

In contrast, in diffuse oesophageal spasm there is maintenance of some peristalsis, but an increase in the number of non-peristaltic, or simultaneous, contractions. Other irregularities frequently occur in the oesophageal body, e.g. high-amplitude contractions of prolonged duration, repetitive contractions, and spontaneous contractions. Abnormality may also occur in LOS function, e.g. incomplete relaxation or elevated sphincter pressure. Despite these various abnormalities and conflicting criteria for the diagnosis of diffuse oesophageal spasm, we concur with other investigators (Richter and Castell, 1984) that the term should be reserved for cases in which there is an increase in non-peristaltic contractions with preservation of some peristaltic function (Traube et al., 1983).

The introduction of the pneumohydraulic, low compliance infusion system for oesophageal manometry has been principally responsible for the discovery of patients with manometric tracings which differ from normal but which do not fit into the classic abnormalities of achalasia or of diffuse oesophageal spasm. Most of these patients have had normal peristaltic function with elevated contraction amplitude ('nutcracker' oesophagus) [Benjamin et al., 1979], but other disorders have also been described. Thus, newer, more inclusive classifications have been proposed for the motility disorders (Benjamin et al., 1983; Clouse and Staiano, 1983) and include patients with prolonged duration of contraction, but nonetheless do not independently classify the various permutations of abnormality in the oesophageal body and sphincter (Cohen, 1983).

Current nosology allows us to communicate about patients at the present level of knowledge although our understanding of the basic electrophysiology of the normal and abnormal oesophagus is limited. In this review a practical classification will be used (table I). Nevertheless, a word of caution is necessary: the presence of variation in investigators' measurements of peristalsis, in contractile amplitude and duration, and in sphincteric function suggests that the specific labelling of a patient's tracing as one abnormality or the other may require the demonstration of differences from normal subjects studied in the particular manometric laboratory.

Table I. Current practical classification of primary disorders of oesophageal motility

Achalasia
Diffuse oesophageal spasm
'Nutcracker' oesophagus (high-amplitude peristaltic contractions)
Contractions of prolonged duration
Isolated hypertensive lower oesophageal sphincter
Nonspecific disorders

3. Achalasia

3.1 Clinical Features and Diagnosis

Most patients with achalasia have dysphagia as their presenting symptom, although regurgitation, chest pain, weight loss or pneumonia may also be presenting complaints. Symptoms are often of insidious onset. Dysphagia results from the absence of peristalsis as well as from functional obstruction at the LOS because of failure of, or incomplete, relaxation of the LOS, which may or may not have elevated basal pressure.

The diagnostic approach to the patient should include roentgenographic examination, to exclude an anatomical basis for dysphagia, as well as a manometric study to clearly verify the presence of the motility disorder (Meshkinpour et al., 1982).

3.2 Management

The present therapeutic approaches to the patient with achalasia, other than reassurance, accommodation to softer diets, and elevation of the head of the bed, are all designed to decrease the level of LOS pressures without substantially changing oesophageal body function (table II). Although percentage LOS relaxation remains abnormal and unchanged, LOS pressure at the time of relaxation is less than that of pretreatment, thus causing less functional obstruction.

3.2.1 Pneumatic Dilatation

Various reports, as well-reviewed recently (Vantrappen and Hellemans, 1980; Vantrappen and Janssens, 1983), have described favourable results after pneumatic dilatation of the oesophagus. Results have generally been measured in terms of clinical response, although a recent report showed that a radionuclide-tagged sandwich could be used to document improved oesophageal emptying after treatment (Holloway et al., 1983).

Although most patients have been shown to have satisfactory results with single or, if necessary, repeated pneumatic dilatation, the technique varies between physicians, and the best technique still needs to be determined.

Some investigators have used a series of bags of increasing diameter which are used on successive dilatations until effective treatment was obtained (Vantrappen et al., 1971). The pneumatic dilator was insufflated to 200mm Hg for 1 minute and then to 300mm Hg for an additional minute. When clinical, manometric, and radiographic criteria indicated the need for further dilatation, a bag of larger diameter was used with the same pressure and time duration. The mean number of dilatations per patient was 3.2

Currently, most investigators use a single pneumatic bag of fixed diameter (e.g. Browne-McHardy dilator). Nevertheless, considerable variation exists in various aspects. There is a large range of pressures and durations of insufflation used (table III). Some investigators have advocated that identification of the site for placement of the dilator be done by fluoroscopy (Lishman and Dellipiani, 1982) or endoscopy (Fellows et al., 1983), while others have routinely used guide wires for ease in placement of the dilator (Fellows et al., 1983). Local pharyngeal anaesthesia and mild sedation are commonly used, but a recent report (Fellows et al., 1983) has advocated use of general anaesthesia with its advantages of prevention of pain and reduction of aspiration.

Table II. Treatment options for achalasia

Softer diet
Elevation of head of bed
Mercury-tipped bouginage
Pneumatic dilatation
Surgical or endoscopic myotomy
Pharmacological therapy

Table III. Variation of pressure and duration of insufflation in pneumatic dilatation of the oesophagus

References	Insufflation pressure (mm Hg)	Duration of insufflation
Fellows et al. (1983)	280-300	3 minutes
Lishman and Dellipiani (1982)	775	15 seconds; repeated once
Csendes et al. (1981)	620-775	3-5 seconds; repeated once
Okike et al. (1979)	150-200	Several seconds

It is our practice to premedicate fasting patients with 0.6mg atropine intramuscularly to reduce secretions. Intravenous administration of diazepam is reserved for anxious patients, but local pharyngeal anaesthesia is given to all. The dilator is passed without the use of guide wires or endoscopic intervention, unless the oesophagus is very dilated or 'sigmoid' (Holloway and McCallum, 1982). The position is confirmed fluoroscopically by the presence of a dumbbell shape of the sphincter straddling the dilator (fig. 2). Insufflation pressure ranges from 8 to 12 lb/sq. inch (about 400 to 600mm Hg), which is held for 45 to 60 seconds and usually repeated, depending on patient tolerance. Patients fast for 6 hours after the dilatation, and vital signs are monitored closely. Discharge from the hospital is usually possible on the following morning.

Oesophagograms are not routinely performed after dilatation but are performed if symptoms or

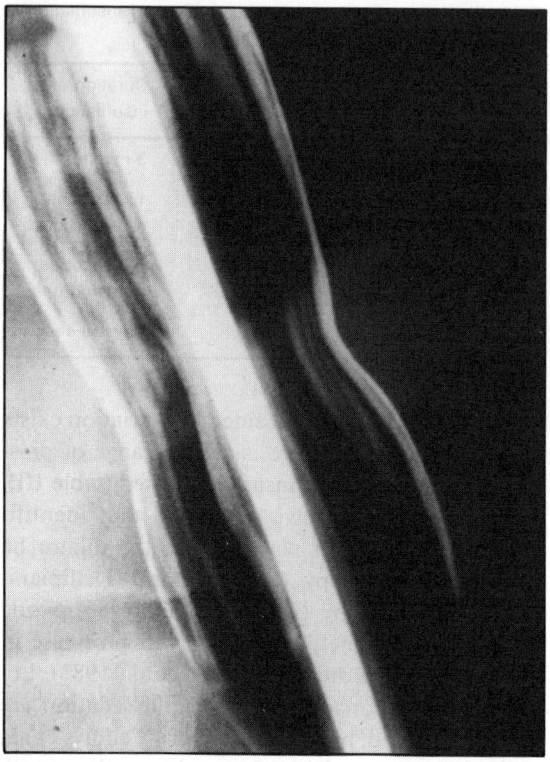

Fig. 2. Roentgenograph of a pneumatic bag dilator straddling the lower oesophageal sphincter. Note the typical dumbbell shape formed by the pressure of the sphincter against the dilated bag. This decreases with successful dilatation.

signs raise the suspicion of perforation. This complication ranges in frequency from 2 to 6% in various centres. If it occurs, we generally submit the patient to surgery, although some investigators have advocated a conservative approach (Vantrappen and Hellemans, 1980).

3.2.2 Surgical Myotomy

As with pneumatic dilatation, surgical myotomy has been shown in several series to be a successful method of treatment for achalasia. Variation in technique exists here as well.

Perhaps the largest reported series is that the Mayo Clinic (Okike et al., 1979), describing results of the Heller myotomy in 468 patients. 85% of the patients were considered to have excellent or good results after a mean follow-up of 6 years. In this series, repair of hiatal hernia was performed, but otherwise no antireflux procedure was performed prophylactically to prevent post-myotomy reflux oesophagitis.

More recently, some surgeons have argued for a formal antireflux procedure at the time of myotomy in order to reduce the likelihood of the long term complication of reflux oesophagitis (Vantrappen and Janssens, 1983). Black et al. (1976), for example, reported good to excellent relief of symptoms of dysphagia despite the paradoxical procedure which maintains sphincter tone, and found that reflux symptoms were seen less frequently in patients so treated compared with those not having an antireflux procedure. It seems that most surgeons perform some type of antireflux procedure along with the myotomy, but the actual type of operation varies from surgeon to surgeon.

A recent report (Hirashima et al., 1978) indicates a different approach: the myotomy is extended through the mucosa and the gap is covered with a gastric patch. This procedure is used in patients with advanced disease. The experience is primarily from Japan, and a wider experience would be required to judge relative efficacy compared to extramucosal myotomy.

3.2.3 Pneumatic Dilatation versus *Surgical Myotomy*

Although many series with pneumatic dilatation or surgical myotomy indicate favourable results, only a few papers have compared the two procedures with each other.

In the sole prospective study (Csendes et al., 1981) 18 patients were dilated pneumatically and 20 patients underwent surgical myotomy. Surgical treatment was accompanied by significantly better long term results compared with pneumatic dilatation. Nevertheless, the results of this study, using a dilatation procedure lasting only 3 to 5 seconds, cannot be extended to the more common method of dilating for a longer period (table III).

A retrospective study of the large number of patients seen at the Mayo Clinic (Okike et al., 1979) also indicated a greater success rate for myotomy than for dilatation. Here too, the dilatation was such that the pressure was sustained for several seconds only, and this could explain the poorer results with dilatation.

In a recent study from our institution indicating the use of the radionuclide oesophageal emptying test (Holloway et al., 1983), patients with achalasia successfully treated by myotomy or by dilatation had similar percentage reductions in retained isotope and similar subjective scores after treatment. This study was also retrospective and several of the surgical patients had previously undergone pneumatic dilatation. Nevertheless, our experience is such that sustained, long term relief was obtained by two-thirds of over 100 patients with achalasia treated by pneumatic dilatation. Therefore, our own preference is to begin treatment with pneumatic dilatation, thus avoiding the risks of general anaesthesia as well as prolonged hospitalisation. If poor results are obtained, one repeat dilatation may be performed, but a third dilatation does not seem to add much. Failures are referred for surgical treatment.

3.2.4 Non-Surgical Manipulative Therapy

Myotomy via the endoscope has recently been described in 17 patients with achalasia (Ortega et al., 1980). The electrical current used was chosen after experimentation in dogs, and the human data, using clinical and radiographic criteria, indicated satisfactory results. The follow-up was short (3 to 25 months) and the series of patients small; critical evaluation will need to await longer follow-up with a larger series of patients.

Repeated dilatation with mercury-filled bougies may also give relief of dysphagia. Selected patients, who are not candidates for either myotomy or pneumatic dilatation, may be appropriately treated in such a manner (Mandelstam et al., 1982).

3.2.5 Pharmacological Therapy

Successful therapy for achalasia depends on LOS pressure reduction; it does not generally affect function of the body of the oesophagus. It is thus not surprising that various agents which decrease LOS pressure have for years been studied for their effect in achalasia (Gelfond et al., 1982a). Hormones such as glucagon, secretin, and vasoactive intestinal peptide (VIP), which inhibit LOS pressure (Siegel et al., 1979), are not of practical value because of the necessity of parenteral administration. Nearly all drugs which have received wider interest belong to the following 4 groups: (a) nitrates; (b) anticholinergics; (c) adrenoceptor agonists; and (d) calcium antagonists. A few pertinent studies will be discussed.

Nitrates

In the largest and most recent study of nitrate treatment for achalasia, isosorbide dinitrate 5mg, given sublingually, significantly decreased LOS pressure and retention of an isotope-labelled meal in the oesophagus (Gelfond et al., 1982b). Although most patients had symptom relief, side effects limited the use of the drug, so that after an 8- to 14-month follow-up, only 5 of 15 patients continued with isosorbide dinitrate treatment.

Anticholinergic Agents

Studies with anticholinergic agents have presented either manometric or clinical data in achalasia patients (Gelfond et al., 1982a). These older reports gave no conclusive evidence for the clinical efficacy of anticholinergic agents and to our knowledge, no studies regarding this therapy have appeared in nearly a decade. Nevertheless, a role for nocturnal inhibition of oral secretions could be hypothesised.

Adrenoceptor Agonists

α-Adrenoceptor agonists cause LOS contraction, and β-adrenoceptor agonists, principally of the β_2 variety, cause LOS pressure reduction. In a recent dose-response study with carbuterol, a β_2-agonist, patients with achalasia had significant reductions in LOS pressure without substantial cardiovascular effects (DiMarino and Cohen, 1982). However, only manometric data were presented, and the clinical efficacy was not determined.

Calcium Antagonists

Currently, perhaps the most interest in pharmacological therapy of achalasia is in the use of the calcium antagonists. Sublingual nifedipine decreased LOS pressure in normal volunteers (Hongo et al., 1984a) and to a similar extent in a large series of patients with achalasia (Traube et al., 1984a). In a single-blind, placebo-controlled study of sublingual nifedipine 10 to 20mg before meals, the drug gave good results in a majority of the 20 patients studied (Bortolloti and Labo, 1981). On the other hand, another study showed that sublingual nifedipine 20mg did not alter the results of a radionuclide oesophageal emptying test (Gelfond et al., 1982b) and gave clinical results inferior to those obtained with nitrates. Side effects, however, were fewer with nifedipine. Experience with the other available calcium antagonists is more limited (Becker and Burakoff, 1983; Silverstein et al., 1982).

Currently, we give nifedipine 10 to 30mg sublingually taken 30 minutes before meals. Nifedipine is chosen because the capsule's liquid inner contents may be given sublingually, and the tablet form of the other currently available calcium antagonists does not allow for a sublingual approach. Oral administration of nifedipine may lead to delayed systemic absorption of the drug in patients with achalasia, who have delayed oesophageal emptying.

Clearly, various agents can decrease LOS pressure. The extent of reduction, however, may not be as great as that observed in more definitive therapy, unless higher doses are used, with the secondary problem of side effects. What is needed is an agent which has a relatively selective effect on oesophageal smooth muscle function with little or no effect on cardiovascular or other systems. Even so, the patient treated with medication must always be prepared to take the drug prior to scheduled or unscheduled meals. The considerations of limited efficacy data, of side effects, and of meal scheduling lead us to believe that more definitive therapy with pneumatic dilatation or myotomy should be considered first.

Drug therapy may be reserved for patients who are not considered candidates for other treatment or in patients who have failed or who refuse other therapy.

4. Diffuse Oesophageal Spasm

4.1 Clinical Features and Diagnosis

Most patients with diffuse oesophageal spasm complain of chest pain and/or dysphagia. Often patients will have been suspected as having coronary artery disease and are referred for further evaluation after appropriate cardiac studies.

The presence of dysphagia as a complaint requires roentgenographic and/or endoscopic examination to exclude an obstructive lesion. The roentgenographic finding of simultaneous contractions throughout the oesophagus is classic, but is neither sensitive nor specific for the disorder. The diagnosis should only be made by appropriate manometric examination, which, as discussed previously, should show an increase in non-peristaltic contractions of either normal or increased amplitude.

The cause(s) of diffuse oesophageal spasm remain for the most part unknown, although an association with gastro-oesophageal reflux has been known for a long time (Bennett and Hendrix, 1970). While the precise relationship between gastro-oesophageal reflux and dysmotility is unclear, the presence of diffuse oesophageal spasm should lead the clinician to consider the presence of reflux. If reflux is documented it should be vigorously treated; however, chest pain may persist after such therapy (Henderson, 1983).

4.2 Management

Perhaps of prime importance in the therapy of diffuse oesophageal spasm is the clinician's reassurance to the patient that the disease is a benign one (fig. 3). Patients will appreciate being convinced that their pain is not of cardiac origin and that their dysphagia is not of neoplastic origin. Nevertheless, some patients will need further therapy for relief of symptoms, and various measures are available.

4.2.1 Pharmacological Therapy

Over the last decade, nitrates have generated the most interest in the pharmacological therapy of

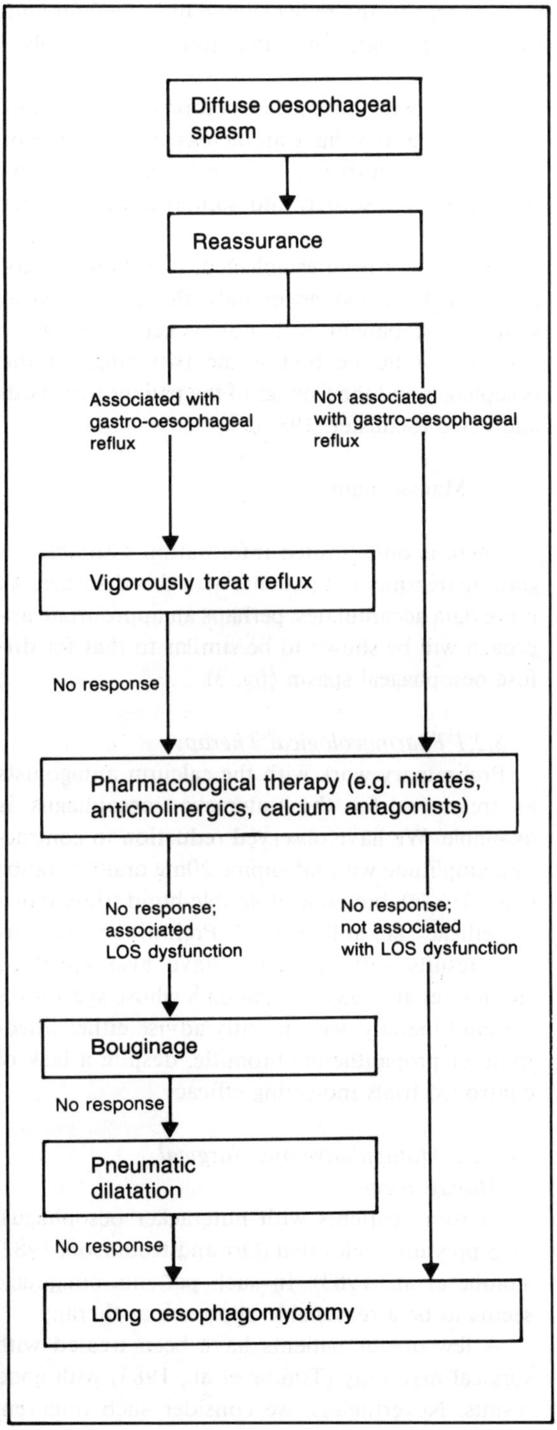

Fig. 3. Guide to therapy of diffuse oesophageal spasm.

diffuse oesophageal spasm. Sublingual glyceryl trinitrate (nitroglycerin) and long acting nitrates produced manometric and clinical improvement in those patients with diffuse oesophageal spasm not associated with gastro-oesophageal reflux (Swamy, 1977). The response was not uniformly good in patients with reflux-associated spasm; in such patients the prime treatment should be control of reflux, but nitrates may be used as adjunctive therapy.

Other pharmacological agents which have been used include anticholinergics and hydralazine (Mellow, 1982), although controlled trials are lacking.

In the last few years there has been intense interest in the use of calcium antagonists in the treatment of oesophageal motility disorders, including diffuse oesophageal spasm. Some reports of only small numbers of patients have shown a reduction in frequency of contractions (Weiser et al., 1978), reduction of amplitude of contractions (Blackwell et al., 1981; Weiser et al., 1978), or even a return of peristalsis (Nasrallah, 1982) after administration of nifedipine to patients with diffuse oesophageal spasm. Clinically, the patients had a reduction of frequency or severity of chest pain in some (Blackwell et al., 1981) but not other reports (Davies et al., 1982). In several patients nifedipine reportedly relieved acute episodes of pain although it had no prophylactic effect (Davies et al., 1982).

In the absence of definitive studies showing efficacy with the various pharmacological agents, our approach is conservative. Patients are advised to take glyceryl trinitrate 0.4mg sublingually or nifedipine 10 to 30mg sublingually (cracked capsule in mouth) at the onset of an attack. On occasion, for severe acute pain, atropine 0.6mg is given parenterally.

If pain occurs frequently, prophylaxis is attempted with long acting oral nitrates, nifedipine, or propantheline bromide singly or in combination (Hongo et al., 1984b).

4.2.2 Non-Surgical Manipulative Therapy

Only infrequently do we resort to manipulative, invasive therapy, and generally this is in patients who have either elevated LOS pressure or incomplete LOS relaxation in association with diffuse oesophageal spasm (DiMarino and Cohen, 1974). A large-diameter, mercury-filled bougie is passed at periodic intervals as necessary. Generally, relief of dysphagia, but not of chest pain, is the rule. In such patients, failure of bouginage should be followed by pneumatic dilatation of the oesophagus (Ebert et al., 1983).

4.2.3 Surgical Myotomy

Patients whose symptoms, particularly chest pain, are recalcitrant to the above measures are seen only infrequently in our experience but are referred for surgical myotomy. Variation exists in several aspects of surgical intervention: the proximal and distal extent of myotomy and whether an antireflux procedure should be included (Henderson, 1983). Extension of the myotomy to the sphincter is clearly indicated in the presence of LOS dysfunction; in its absence it is still performed by most surgeons. An antireflux procedure is included by most surgeons if the myotomy is extended to the sphincter.

5. 'Nutcracker' Oesophagus

5.1 Clinical Features

Over the past decade the 'nutcracker' oesophagus has been recognised as the most common motility disorder seen in patients referred for evaluation of non-cardiac chest pain (Benjamin et al., 1979; Brand et al., 1977; Herrington et al., 1983; Orr and Robinson, 1982; Traube et al., 1983). In the nutcracker oesophagus, contractions in the distal oesophagus are of increased amplitude, but normal peristaltic function is maintained. As with diffuse oesophageal spasm, patients may complain of chest pain or dysphagia.

The aetiology of this disorder remains unknown. However, an association with gastro-oesophageal reflux is suggested by an increased prevalence of positive Bernstein tests or other evidence of gastro-oesophageal reflux (Orr and Robinson, 1982; Traube et al., 1983). We believe this to be analogous to that of reflux-associated diffuse oesophageal spasm, and reflux should be looked for and treated in patients who have nutcracker oesophagus.

Patients with nutcracker oesophagus (and similar abnormalities) have an increased prevalence of psychiatric disturbance, primarily that of depression, anxiety disorder, and somatisation disorder (Clouse and Lustman, 1983). Although cause and effect have not been established, it certainly is appropriate to assess adequately the psychological state of the patient with nutcracker oesophagus. Therapy would be best if the twitchings of the oesophagus and the feelings of the patient were both addressed (Schuster, 1983).

5.2 Management

There is only limited information available regarding treatment of patients with this disorder. As more data accumulates, perhaps an appropriate approach will be shown to be similar to that for diffuse oesophageal spasm (fig. 3).

5.2.1 Pharmacological Therapy

Preliminary work with the calcium antagonists as treatment for the nutcracker oesophagus is available. We have observed reduction in contraction amplitude with nifedipine 20mg orally (Traube et al., 1984a), but clinical double-blind trials showing efficacy are still awaited. Preliminary, favourable results with diltiazem have also appeared (Richter et al., 1984). In patients whose symptoms demand therapy, we currently advise either nifedipine or propantheline bromide, despite a lack of controlled trials indicating efficacy.

5.2.2 Manipulative and Surgical Management

In some patients with nutcracker oesophagus, LOS pressure is elevated (Orr and Robinson, 1982; Traube et al., 1983). In such patients bouginage seems to be a reasonable approach at therapy.

A few of our patients have been treated with surgical myotomy (Traube et al., 1983) with good results. Nevertheless, we consider such intervention one of last resort.

6. Contractions of Prolonged Duration

Contractions in some patients with nutcracker oesophagus are of prolonged duration as well. In other patients, prolonged duration occurs in the absence of increased amplitude or other manometric abnormality (Herrington et al., 1984).

Various aspects of this disorder are similar to the nutcracker oesophagus. There is an overlap, since many patients with nutcracker oesophagus have contractions of prolonged duration. Both disorders are associated with chest pain and dysphagia. Elevated LOS pressure has been associated with both disorders (Herrington et al., 1984; Orr and Robinson, 1982; Traube et al., 1983). The psychiatric disturbances seen in patients with nutcracker oesophagus have also been seen in patients with contractions of prolonged duration (Clouse and Lustman, 1983).

In view of the present limited information regarding this disorder, our approach to therapy is similar to that of the nutcracker oesophagus.

7. Hypertensive Lower Oesophageal Sphincter

Most patients with elevated LOS pressure have other associated manometric abnormalities. Occasionally, however, patients with chest pain or dysphagia are seen in the motility laboratory to have an isolated abnormality of elevated LOS pressure. This disorder has recently been included in some manometric classifications (Benjamin et al., 1983; Herrington et al., 1983), although precise clinical description and the relationship of the disorder to symptoms are still awaited.

Since LOS pressure varies widely and may rise considerably from hour to hour even in normal subjects, we believe that the diagnosis should be made only if a thorough search excludes other causes for symptoms and a repeated manometric examination confirms the presence of an elevated LOS pressure. Under such circumstances, measures taken to decrease LOS pressure are indicated. Generally, pharmacological approaches, as previously discussed, or bouginage would be the treatments of choice, although on rare occasion we have resorted to pneumatic dilatation (Traube et al., 1984b).

8. Nonspecific Disorders

Other less well categorised disorders of the oesophageal body or LOS may be seen. Therapy must be individualised, since the lack of categorisation has hampered adequate description of the clinical presentations, manometric abnormalities, and appropriate approach to therapy.

Some of these abnormalities may be considered primary. Others may be related to diabetes mellitus, amyloidosis, intestinal pseudo-obstruction, Raynaud's phenomenon, scleroderma, and other connective tissue disorders, or the post-vagotomy state. In these latter conditions, however, it should be noted that motility disturbances are often incidental and not accompanied by symptoms. Clearly, such abnormalities will not require specific therapy.

9. Conclusions

Various oesophageal 'spastic' disturbances associated with chest pain and dysphagia should be considered by clinicians evaluating patients with such symptoms. Following confirmation of diagnosis, a rational approach, as reviewed herein, is available and may be taken in the management of such patients.

References

Becker, B.S. and Burakoff, R.: The effect of verapamil on the lower esophageal sphincter pressure in normal subjects and in achalasia. American Journal of Gastroenterology 78: 773-775 (1983).

Benjamin, S.B.; Gerhardt, D.C. and Castell, D.O.: High amplitude peristaltic esophageal contractions associated with chest pain and/or dysphagia. Gastroenterology 77: 478-483 (1979).

Benjamin, S.B.; Richter, J.E.; Cordova, C.M.; Knuff, T.E. and Castell, D.O.: Prospective manometric evaluation with pharmacologic provocation of patients with suspected esophageal motility dysfunction. Gastroenterology 84: 893-901 (1983).

Bennett, J.R. and Hendrix, T.R.: Diffuse esophageal spasm: A disorder with more than one cause. Gastroenterology 59: 273-279 (1970).

Black, J.; Vorbach, A.N. and Collis, J.L.: Results of Heller's operation for achalasia of the oesophagus. The importance of hia-

tal repair. British Journal of Surgery 63: 949-953 (1976).
Blackwell, J.N.; Holt, S. and Heading, R.C.: Effect of nifedipine on oesophageal motility and gastric emptying. Digestion 21: 50-56 (1981).
Bortolloti, M. and Labo, G.: Clinical and manometric effects of nifedipine in patients with esophageal achalasia. Gastroenterology 80: 39-44 (1981).
Brand, D.L.; Martin, D. and Pope, C.E. Esophageal manometrics in patients with angina-like chest pain. Digestive Diseases and Sciences 22: 300-304 (1977).
Clouse, R.E. and Lustman, P.J.: Psychiatric illness and contraction abnormalities of the esophagus. New England Journal of Medicine 309: 1337-1342 (1983).
Clouse, R.E. and Staiano, A.: Contraction abnormalities of the esophageal body in patients referred for manometry. Digestive Diseases and Sciences 28: 784-791 (1983).
Cohen, S.: Classification of the esophageal motility disorders. Gastroenterology 84: 1050-1051 (1983).
Cohen, S. and Green, F.: The mechanics of esophageal muscle contraction: Evidence of an inotropic effect of gastrin. Journal of Clinical Investigation 52: 2029-2040 (1973).
Csendes, A.; Velasco, N.; Braghetto, I. and Henriquez, A.: A prospective randomized study comparing forceful dilatation and esophagomyotomy in patients with achalasia of the esophagus. Gastroenterology 80: 789-795 (1981).
Davies, H.A.; Lewis, M.; Rhodes, J. and Henderson, A.: Nifedipine for relief of esophageal chest pain? (Letter.) New England Journal of Medicine 307: 1274 (1982).
deCarle, D.J.; Christensen, J.; Szabo, A.C.; Templemen, D.C. and McKinley, C.R.: Calcium dependence of neuromuscular events in esophageal smooth muscle of the opossum. American Journal of Physiology 232: E547-E552 (1977).
DiMarino, A.J. and Cohen, S.: Characteristics of lower eosphageal sphincter function in symptomatic diffuse esophageal spasm. Gastroenterology 66: 1-6 (1974).
DiMarino, A.J. and Cohen, S.: Effects of an oral beta$_2$-adrenergic agonist on lower esophageal sphincter pressure in normals and in patients with achalasia. Digestive Diseases and Sciences 27: 1063-1066 (1982).
Dodds, W.J.; Dents, J.; Hogan, W.J. and Arndorfer, R.C.: Effect of atropine on esophageal motor function in humans. American Journal of Physiology 240: G290-G294 (1981).
Ebert, E.C.; Ouyang, A.; Wright, S.H.; Cohen, S. and Lipshutz, W.H.: Pneumatic dilatation in patients with symptomatic diffuse esophageal spasm and lower esophageal sphincter dysfunction. Digestive Diseases and Sciences 28: 481-485 (1983).
Fellows, I.W.; Ogilvie, A.L. and Atkinson, M.: Pneumatic dilation in achalasia. Gut 24: 1020-1023 (1983).
Gelfond, M.; Rozen, and Gilat, T.: Is there a place for drug therapy in achalasia? P. in Weinbeck (Ed). Motility of the Digestive Tract, pp. 527-532 (Raven Press, New York 1982a).
Gelfond, M.; Rozen, P. and Gilat, T.: Isosorbide dinitrate and nifedipine treatment of achalasia: A clinical, manometric, and radionuclide evaluation. Gastroenterology 83: 963-969 (1982b).
Henderson, R.D.: Diffuse esophageal spasm. Surgical Clinics of North America 63: 951-962 (1983).
Herrington, J.P.; Burns, T.W. and Balart, L.A.: Chest pain, dysphagia, and high amplitude esophageal peristalsis: A clinical and manometric study. Southern Medical Journal 76: 599-602 (1983).
Herrington, J.P.; Burns, T.W. and Balart, L.A.: Chest pain and dysphagia in patients with prolonged peristaltic contractile duration of the esophagus. Digestive Diseases and Sciences 29: 134-140 (1984).
Hirashima, T.; Sato, H.; Hara, T.; Nakamura, H.; Kawamura, I. et al.: Results of esophagocardioplasty with gastric patch in the treatment of esophageal achalasia. Annals of Surgery 188: 38-42 (1978).
Holloway, R.H.; Krosin, G.; Lange, R.C.; Baue, A.E. and McCallum, R.W.: Radionuclide esophageal emptying of a solid meal to quantitate results of therapy in achalasia. Gastroenterology 84: 771-776 (1983).
Holloway, R.H. and McCallum, R.W.: Technique for pneumatic dilatation in achalasia complicated by 'sigmoid' esophagus. Journal of Clinical Gastroenterology 4: 123-125 (1982).
Hongo, M.; Traube, M.; McAllister, R.G. and McCallum, R.W.: Effects of nifedipine on esophageal motor function in humans: Correlation with plasma nifedipine concentration. Gastroenterology 86: 8-12 (1984a).
Hongo, M.; Traube, M. and McCallum, R.W.: Comparison of effects of nifedipine, propantheline bromide, and the combination on esophageal motor function in normal volunteers. Digestive Diseases and Sciences 29: 300-304 (1984b).
Liebermann-Meffert, D.; Allgower, M.; Schmid, P. and Blum, A.L.: Muscular equivalent of the lower esophageal sphincter. Gastroenterology 76: 31-38 (1979).
Lishman, A.L. and Dellipiani, A.W.: Management of achalasia of the cardia by forced pneumatic dilatation. Gut 23: 541-544 (1982).
Mandelstam, P.; Block, C.; Newell, L. and Dillon, M.: The role of bougienage in the management of achalasia – the need for reappraisal. Gastrointestinal Endoscopy 28: 169-172 (1982).
Mellow, M.D.: Effect of isosorbide and hydralazine in painful primary esophageal motility disorders. Gastroenterology 83: 364-370 (1982).
Meshkinpour, H.; Glick, M.E.; Sanchez, P. and Tarvin, J.: Esophageal manometry: A benefit and cost analysis. Digestive Diseases and Sciences 27: 772-775 (1982).
Nasrallah, S.M.: Nifedipine in the treatment of diffuse esophageal spasm. (Letter.) Lancet 2: 1285 (1982).
Okike, N.; Payne, W.S.; Neufeld, D.M.; Bernatz, P.E.; Pairolero, P.C. and Sanderson, D.R.: Esophagomyotomy versus forceful dilation for achalasia of the esophagus: Results in 899 patients. Annals of Thoracic Surgery 28: 119-125 (1979).
Orr, W.C. and Robinson, M.G.: Hypertensive peristalsis in the pathogenesis of chest pain: Further exploration of the 'nutcracker' esophagus. American Journal of Gastroenterology 77: 604-607 (1982).
Ortega, J.A.; Madureri, V. and Perez, L.: Endoscopic myotomy in the treatment of achalasia. Gastrointestinal Endoscopy 26: 8-10 (1980).
Richardson, B.J. and Welch, R.W.: Differential effect of atropine on rightward and leftward lower esophageal sphincter pressure. Gastroenterology 81: 85-89 (1981).
Richter, J.E. and Castell, D.O.: Diffuse esophageal spasm: A reappraisal. Annals of Internal Medicine 100: 242-245 (1984).
Richter, J.E.; Spurling, T.J.; Cordova, C.M. and Castell, D.O.: Effects of the oral calcium blocker, diltiazem, on esophageal contractions. Digestive Diseases and Sciences 29: 649-656 (1984).
Schuster, M.M.: Esophageal spasm and psychiatric disorder. New England Journal of Medicine 309: 1382-1383 (1983).
Siegel, S.R.; Brown, F.C.; Castell, D.O.; Johnson, L.F. and Said, S.I.: Effects of vasoactive intestinal peptide (VIP) on lower esophageal sphincter in awake baboons: Comparison with glucagon and secretin. Digestive Diseases and Sciences 24: 345-349 (1979).
Silverstein, B.D.; Kramer, C.M. and Pope, C.E.: Treatment of esophageal motor disorders with a calcium-blocker, diltiazem. (Abstract.) Gastroenterology 82: 1181 (1982).
Swamy, N.: Esophageal spasm. Clinical and manometric response to nitroglycerine and long acting nitrites. Gastroenterology 72: 23-27 (1977).
Traube, M.; Albibi, R. and McCallum, R.W.: High-amplitude peristaltic esophageal contractions associated with chest pain. J. American Med. Assoc. 250: 2655-2659 (1983).
Traube, M.; Hongo, M.; Huntoon, L. and McCallum, R.W.: Effects of nifedipine in achalasia and in patients with high-am-

plitude peristaltic esophageal contractions. Journal of the American Medical Association 252: 1733-1736 (1984a).
Traube, M.; Lagarde, S. and McCallum, R.W.: Isolated hypertensive lower esophageal sphincter: Treatment of a resistant case by pneumatic dilatation. Journal of Clinical Gastroenterology 6: 139-142 (1984b).
Vantrappen, G. and Hellemans, J.: Treatment of achalasia and related motor disorders. Gastroenterology 79: 144-154 (1980).
Vantrappen, G.; Hellemans, J.; Deloof, W.; Valembois, P. and Vandenbroucke, J.: Treatment of achalasia with pneumatic dilatations. Gut 12: 268-275 (1971).
Vantrappen, G. and Janssens, J.: To dilate or to operate? That is the question. Gut 24: 1013-1019 (1983).
Vantrappen, G.; Janssens, J.; Hellemans, J. and Coremans, G.: Achalasia, diffuse esophageal spasm, and related motility disorders. Gastroenterology 76: 450-457 (1979).
Weiser, H.F.; Lepsien, G.: Golenhofen, K. and Siewert, R.: Clinical and experimental studies on the effect of nifedipine on smooth muscle of the oesophagus and LES; in Duthie (Ed.) Gastrointestinal Motility in Health and Disease, pp. 565-572 (MTP Press, Lancaster 1978).

Address for correspondence and reprints: Associate Professor *Richard W. McCallum*, Gastroenterology Section, Yale University School of Medicine, 92 LMP, P.O. Box 3333, New Haven, CT 06510-8056 (USA).

Drugs 30: 78-84 (1985)
0012-6667/85/0700-0078/$03.50/0

Compliance and the Doctor-Patient Relationship

Connie L. Peck and *Neville J. King*
La Trobe University and Philip Institute, Bundoora

Non-compliance with medical regimens is one of the most important problems facing today's medical practitioner and a major obstacle to the provision of adequate medical care. A recent review by Sackett and Snow (1979) suggests that 20 to 30% of patients fail to follow short term medication regimens when the regimen is curative and 30 to 40% when the regimen is preventive. In long term regimens, non-compliance rates average around 50% and increase over time. Research on appointment-keeping shows that only 40 to 50% of patients keep appointments even for curative regimens. DiMatteo and DiNicola (1982) conclude that 'patient noncompliance thrives wherever and whenever medical recommendations are generated.'

The major consequences of non-compliance include poor patient health, renewed rounds of diagnostic testing, added discomfort for the patient, less preferred choice of treatment, increased cost to both the patient and the health care system, deterioration of the doctor-patient relationship, and inaccurate research results (DiMatteo and DiNicola, 1982).

Surprisingly, however, many medical practitioners remain unaware that their patients are not following their advice. Davis (1966) in a study of 131 junior and senior physicians found that only 11% of the doctors surveyed estimated accurate levels of compliance in their patients – most greatly overestimated compliance and 42% claimed that almost all of their patients were compliant. Moreover, practitioners were unable to recognise which patients were being non-compliant. Several more recent studies have reported similar findings (Caron and Roth, 1968; Moulding et al., 1970; Mushlin and Appel, 1977; Norell, 1981).

Why is it that physicians are so lacking in awareness of non-compliance? One reason appear to be that many do not ask their patients if they are following the regimen prescribed. A study by Inui et al. (1976) showed that compliance could be increased simply through physicians becoming aware of the magnitude of the problem. However, not only are many physicians unaware of the extent of the problem, but they are also unaware of the reasons for non-compliance. In the same survey by Davis, 61% of junior physicians and 67% of senior physicians stated that the patient's 'uncooperative personality' was the major cause of non-compliance. Social psychology research suggests that this tendency to 'blame' personality attributes is a well-known phenomenon when the observer does not have sufficient information. In contrast, compliance research has shown that it is not personality variables, but rather social, situational and environmental variables that are responsible for non-compliance. DiMatteo and DiNicola (1982) state that many factors have been shown to influence patient compliance, not the least of which is the health professional himself, and that the practitioner-patient relationship is the most important variable in the study of non-compliance.

Moreover, since issues related to the doctor-patient relationship are ones under the direct control of the practitioner, this area becomes the most accessible to change.

What, then, are some of the things which the practitioner can do to promote compliance in his or her patients?

1. Psychosocial Aspects

Davis (1982) has expressed the relationship between psychosocial problems and compliance:

> 'In the light of the complexity of this phenomenon known as illness, we are sometimes hard-pressed to define precisely what a patient is looking for when he or she seeks the help of a physician. ... Practitioner and patient are, however, quite often engaged in a *folie à deux.* The patient presents only the physical manifestations of the many stresses and conflicts he or she is experiencing, unaware of or hiding the emotional manifestations. The practitioner responds in kind to the medical issue from the framework he or she knows best. Yet the very crux of the matter may be overlooked, for in fact between 50 and 75% of patients who seek medical care have no positive physical findings – their problems are primarily psychosocial. Although these psychosocial issues are seldom addressed, patients are provided prescriptions for treatment. A large proportion of these recommendations (an average of 40%) are not followed.'

In other words, some patients do not receive what they need most from the medical practitioner (warmth and understanding) and do not want what they do receive (a prescription for medication).

2. Patient Participation in Treatment Planning

Including the patient as a full participant in decisions about and implementation of medical treatment will help to assure compliance. An authoritarian model where the doctor 'gives orders' and expects them to be carried out does not take into account the patient's difficulties in implementing these 'orders'. Moreover, when the practitioner's suggestions are given in this manner some patients may reject them, creating all the adverse consequences of non-compliance discussed above. Too often the professional expects the patient to accept his recommendations on his terms, while patients seek help on their own terms. Although it is true that the doctor may have more knowledge than the patient about the illness and the treatment being recommended, the patient has more knowledge about what the costs and benefits of a particular regimen are for him and about what obstacles he is likely to encounter in trying to follow such a programme, e.g. attitudinal, social, financial. Since each has knowledge necessary to the other, a 'mutual participation model' (Szasz and Hollender, 1956) or a 'contractual model' (Veatch, 1972) is more likely to benefit both the patient and doctor and lead to increased patient (and doctor) satisfaction and compliance.

In a study by Schulman (1979) in which hypertensive patients were assigned differing amounts of active orientation in their treatment, the group who were instructed to be most active showed better control of their blood pressure, adhered to treatment better, reported fewer side effects, were more likely to engage in health-enhancing behaviours, had an increased confidence in doctors and treatment, and believed that the benefits of treatment were greater than the costs.

3. Patients' Ideas of Illness and Treatment

Since patients quite often have their own beliefs about illness, severity, cause, prevention and treatment, and since it has been shown that these health beliefs can be related to compliance (Becker and Maiman, 1980), it is important for physicians to be aware of patient beliefs and the extent to which these are in agreement or disagreement with the physician's beliefs about the problem. Awareness of differences provides a starting point for negotiations which may result in the patient following through on recommendations rather than rejecting them because they are alien to his or her beliefs.

Kleinman et al. (1978) suggest that the following questions be asked:

1) What do you think has caused your problem?
2) Why do you think it started when it did?

3) What do you think your sickness does to you? How does it work?
4) How severe is your sickness? Will it have a short or long course?
5) What kind of treatment do you think you should receive?

4. Treatment Rationale

A large number of patients leave their doctor's office without an understanding of what to do to follow the treatment recommendations. Svarstad (1974, 1976) found that 50% of patients starting on a medication regimen could not identify how long they were supposed to take their medication, 17% did not know how often and 23% did not know the purpose of the medication. In a study by Waitzkin and Stoeckle (1972) where doctor-patient interviews were recorded, the practitioner was found to communicate information about the illness or treatment for an average of less than 1 minute out of an average 20-minute interview (i.e. less than 5% of the time). These same physicians, however, estimated that they spent 10 to 15 minutes on the topic (i.e. 50-75% of the time). In another study (Svarstad, 1976) in which consultations were recorded, doctors gave no verbal advice about how to use medication in 90% of drug-prescribing incidents and 60 of the 347 drugs prescribed were not even mentioned during the visit. This is particularly problematical when one considers the results of another study in which between 9 and 64% of patients who were asked to read labels on tablet bottles and describe how they would take the drugs made interpretive errors (Mazullo et al., 1974).

Written information has been found to be useful in increasing compliance in short term therapy (Linkewick et al., 1974; Sharpe and Mikeal, 1974). Specifying treatment recommendations in written form can provide the patient with information which he or she can study and absorb in the more relaxed atmosphere of the home environment. According to Morris and Halperin (1979), written instructions enhance the probability that important information will be attended to, understood, accepted and recalled. They suggest, however, that although it may be a necessary condition for compliance, it may not be a sufficient one.

When doctors do make diagnoses and treatment recommendations explicit, however, they do not always communicate in 'jargon-free' language which the patient can understand. DiMatteo and DiNicola (1982) provide the following example: 'You have essential hypertension. I'd like you to take hydrochlorothiazide bid to eliminate fluid retention. You should also reduce your sodium intake.' They suggest that patients are often afraid to ask what specific terms mean for fear that the doctor will think they are uneducated or unintelligent and thus do not question instructions even when they obviously do not understand. A number of studies have shown that many patients do not comprehend terms which doctors agreed were appropriate to use in consultations, such as 'respiratory', 'malignant', 'terminal' or 'tendon' (Samora et al., 1961; Segall and Roberts, 1980). Moreover, patients seldom ask questions or inform their doctors when they do not understand. Patients asked questions only 7% of the time in a study conducted by Stiles et al. (1979).

Also, some authors suggest that doctors may label patients who ask too many questions as 'bad patients' and ignore them, prematurely medicate them or be more likely to refer them to psychiatrists (Lorber, 1975; Taylor, 1979). In a study by Roter (1977) patients were trained by health educators to write down their questions and ask them during the consultation. These patients were subsequently more compliant and their medical interviews took less time per visit than those in the untrained group.

Furthermore, a patient is more likely to follow a treatment recommendation if he understands the rationale for the recommendation. Baekeland and Lundwall (1975) reviewed factors affecting why patients dropped out of treatment and found that many did so because they did not understand the rationale behind their treatment. Thus, if patients understand what the treatment is, how it is to be followed and why it has been suggested, they are more likely to adhere to it.

5. Relevance of Attitudes and Beliefs

In a mutual participation or contractual model, one of the issues which should be resolved is discrepancies which exist between the patient's and doctor's beliefs and attitudes about illness and treatment. Differences in social status, education, family background, willingness to engage in preventive health behaviours, future perspectives and knowledge of other patient problems are some of the factors which cause doctors and patients to feel differently about the importance of health, disease, prevention and treatment.

Since there is a reciprocal relationship between beliefs and behaviours, it is likely that the patient will behave in accordance with his or her belief system. Thus it may be necessary in some cases for the doctor to attempt to influence or change the patient's beliefs and attitudes. For example, provision of facts and statistics on the prevalence of lung cancer as a result of smoking and information on the course of lung cancer may influence the patient's beliefs about susceptibility and severity. Moreover, a realistic appraisal of the benefits of treatment *versus* the costs may also affect his or her attitude toward treatment (Becker and Maiman, 1980). Physicians who are liked by the patient, appear knowledgeable, inspire trust and confidence, are enthusiastic and expect positive results from their patients are more likely to succeed in influencing their patient's belief systems. (For a further discussion of strategies for changing beliefs, see DiMatteo and DiNicola, 1982.)

6. Treatment Recommendations

Research has repeatedly shown that the more different types of treatment or medication prescribed, the lower the compliance rate (Haynes et al., 1979). Although this has been found in all patients, the problem is particularly acute with older patients where memory problems may further complicate the picture. Thus, success will be maximised when treatment suggestions are kept simple.

7. Patient Commitment

Studies have shown that the effect of the patient's stated intention to comply can enhance compliance. Thus a simple verbal commitment, a written promise or a written contract, usually known as a 'contingency contract' in which the patient and doctor agree that the patient will be rewarded for compliance, can all be effective. (In a contingency contract, the patient can reward him- or herself or can be rewarded by a family member or the doctor.) A number of studies have shown that both simple contracts and contingency contracts are effective in maintaining compliance even in previously non-compliant patients (Haynes et al., 1979).

8. Support for the Patient

Another area which should be explored with the patient is the presence or absence of support from the patient's social environment (i.e. family and friends). If the patient is likely to be punished, scolded or ridiculed for following a particular regimen, he is unlikely to do so. On the other hand, if the family reminds, encourages and praises him for adhering to treatment, he is more likely to follow through. Attempting to predict which patients will have problems and trying to resolve these in advance can be important in the initiation and maintenance of compliance. Involvement of a family member in the treatment plan can be a useful idea. Various studies have found that family support can enhance behavioural compliance with treatment recommendations (Carpenter and Davis, 1976; McElveen, 1972; Oakes et al., 1970). Farquhar (1978) advocated using a contract which is co-signed by the patient and a supportive third person who promises to be a 'helper'.

9. Self-Monitoring

Ideally, self-monitoring involves a simple recording of information by the patient about his or her adherence to the treatment plan. Self-monitoring is most likely to be useful if it is worked out in conjunction with the patient and if its importance and rationale are well explained. Self-monitoring is in effect a diary of treatment behaviour which is noted every time treatment occurs.

Several studies have demonstrated that self-monitoring can increase compliance (Epstein and Masek, 1978; Gabriel et al., 1977). A good self-monitoring record can serve as a reminder to engage in the treatment behaviour and can provide a feeling of satisfaction when the patient records that he or she did indeed comply. Moreover, self-monitoring serves as a feedback loop to the doctor, who can use the self-monitoring schedule on subsequent visits to praise the patient for compliance and to work out together what the conditions are which cause the patient to fail to be compliant. For example, if a housewife doesn't take her medication as regularly on weekends when her husband and children are home, it may suggest that she has more difficulty remembering when she is very busy and could profit from the use of reminders. Alternatively, it could indicate that her family discourages her from taking her medication and may indicate that the doctor should involve the husband in the treatment programme. Through self-monitoring, both the patient and the doctor can explore what obstacles might be preventing compliance.

In the case of chronic diseases such as epilepsy or hypertension, doctors may assume after a period of successful self-monitoring that the patient is now compliant and that self-monitoring may, therefore, be dispensed with. However, since chronic diseases have been shown to be some of the most difficult to treat in terms of ensuring long term compliance, continual self-monitoring may be advisable. This will, however, mean that the doctor should attend to the patient's records at each visit in order to give the message to the patient that this is an important component of treatment.

10. The Forgetful Patient

Ley and Spelman (1965) have suggested that memory failure accounts for some patients' non-compliance. Several strategies have been found to be useful in aiding patients who are forgetful. Providing the patient with written instructions which can be referred to later has been shown to be effective, especially in short term regimens (Morris and Halperin, 1979). Tailoring, which refers to coordination of the patient's treatment with his daily schedule, has also been useful (Dunbar et al., 1979); scheduling an exercise programme for the same time period each day, such as when the patient first arrives home from work, is an example of tailoring. Reminders and cues are also helpful (Schmidt, 1979): examples include putting a reminder on the salt shaker that one is not to eat salt, or placing the tablet bottle next to one's toothbrush. Drug packaging has also been used successfully (Eshelman and Fitzloff, 1976; Linkewick et al., 1974). In a study by Azrin and Powell (1969) a tablet bottle with an auditory cue (a tone) which would not terminate until the tablet bottle was opened was more effective than a short reminder tone or no tone in getting patients to take their medication on schedule. Such a device is now available commercially in various parts of the world.

Even though many of these strategies are simple, patients often do not think of them spontaneously. A few minutes of discussion to work out a simple programme for cueing can be very effective with the patient who is non-compliant through forgetfulness.

11. Reward System

Anyone who has ever tried to keep up a diet, an exercise programme or remember to take drugs on schedule knows how arduous it can be. Since it is essential that benefits outweigh costs if patients are to comply on a regular basis, praise and rewards should be an important part of any programme aimed at promoting good compliance. Many doctors feel that good health should be reward enough and therefore fail to praise the patient or help him structure his own rewards. However, in matters of health the rewards may be long term ones which come later, whereas the aversion to the regimen may be short term. Abundant research in self-control suggests that short term consequences

Table I. Summary of strategies that may be used to enhance patient compliance

1. Be sensitive to the patient's psychosocial problems
2. Involve the patient as an active participant in planning his or her treatment
3. Ask the patient to explain his or her ideas about the illness, its cause and treatment
4. Communicate diagnosis and treatment recommendations in language the patient can understand
5. Attempt to resolve differences in beliefs and attitudes toward treatment
6. Keep treatment recommendations simple
7. Obtain a commitment from the patient that he or she will adhere to treatment
8. Enlist help from the patient's social environment, e.g. family and friends
9. Teach the patient how to self-monitor adherence to the treatment programme
10. Help the forgetful patient learn to use reminders
11. Reward compliant behaviour
12. Work with the patient to overcome obstacles to compliance

are more salient than long term ones. Thus even though good health may be a reward for the patient, it may not be strong enough by itself to overcome the objectionable short term consequences of complying with the treatment programme. It is therefore important that other rewards be built into the patient's programme to maximise success.

Self-reinforcement has been shown to be very powerful and it may be useful to recommend to patients that they reward themselves in a small way after each episode of compliance. Examples of small self-rewards include having a cup of coffee or a favourite item of food, listening to music, taking a break from work, taking a bath, going for a walk, or ringing a friend. Rewards need to be tailored to what the patient enjoys and are limited only by one's imagination. They work best when given immediately and it is often better to use a variety of rewards so that the patient doesn't become bored.

Praise is also an important reward for most people. Praise from the doctor for compliant behaviour can be very powerful. Of course, characteristics which make patients like their doctors (such as warmth, friendliness and sensitivity) enhance the importance of the doctor's praise.

12. Obstacles to Compliance

Scolding or punishing patients for non-compliant behaviour returns the doctor-patient relationship to an authoritarian parent-child interaction and detracts from the mutual participatory relationship which is ultimately more likely to be capable of solving the problems of non-compliance. A re-examination of the various obstacles to non-compliance, e.g. different patient and doctor agendas, differences in beliefs and attitudes, punishing consequences from the patient's social environment, the patient's inability to remember the treatment regimen, lack of sufficient rewards, and costs which outweigh benefits, can be carried out in a joint exercise. Good communication skills are necessary to probe and interpret the patient's responses, and trust is essential for patients to be truly forthcoming about their problems.

13. Conclusion

Research suggests that instead of looking for the source of non-compliance in the patient's uncooperative personality, we should turn to the doctor-patient relationship to be certain that the patient's needs are being met, that we are communicating productively with the patient, and that we are engaging in the necessary negotiation and programming to help the patient overcome the obstacles to compliance which are present in his or her environment. Attention to communication skills are at the heart of this process. DiMatteo and DiNicola (1982) state: 'Noncompliance is often a visible manifestation of dysfunctional communication between practitioner and patient.'

Enhancing patient compliance begins with the doctor's first contact with the patient – including how quickly the patient is seen after referral, how long the patient has to wait in the waiting room, and whether the doctor introduces himself – and continues throughout the doctor-patient relationship. While laying the foundation for compliance may take slightly more time in the first instance, more patients would get well and fewer would go treatment-shopping; ultimately this would leave the physician with more time, since patient demand would be less. Doctors would obtain more job satisfaction, more leisure time to respond to their own psychosocial needs, and 'burnout' would probably be reduced. Understanding how to minimise noncompliance should benefit the entire health care system.

References

Azrin, N.H. and Powell, J.: Behavioral engineering: The use of response priming to improve prescribed self-medication. Journal of Applied Behavioral Analysis 2: 39-42 (1969).

Baekeland, F. and Lunwall, L.: Dropping out of treatment: A critical review. Psychological Bulletin 82: 738-783 (1975).

Becker, M.H. and Maiman, L.H.: Strategies for enhancing patient compliance. Journal of Community Health 6: 113-135 (1980).

Caron, H.S. and Roth, H.P.: Patients' cooperation with a medical regimen. J. Americ. Med. Assoc. 203: 922-926 (1968).

Carpenter, J.O. and Davis, L.J.: Medical recommendation – followed or ignored? Factors influencing compliance in arthritis. Arch. Physic. Med. Rehab. 57: 241-246 (1976).

Davis, M.S.: Variations in patients' compliance with doctors' orders: Analysis of congruence between survey responses and results of empirical investigations. Journal of Medical Education 41: 1037-1048 (1966).

Davis, M.S.: Foreword; in DiMatteo and DiNicola (Eds) Achieving Patient Compliance (Pergamon Press, New York 1982).

DiMatteo, M.R. and DiNicola, D.D. (Eds): Achieving Patient Compliance (Pergamon Press, New York 1982).

Dunbar, J.M.; Marshall, G.D. and Hovell, M.F.: Behavioral strategies for improving compliance; in Haynes et al. (Eds) Compliance in Health Care (Johns Hopkins University Press, Baltimore 1979).

Epstein, L.H. and Masek, B.J.: Behavioral control of medicine compliance. J. Applied Behav. Analysis 11: 1-9 (1978).

Eshelman, F.N. and Fitzloff, J.: Effects of packaging on patient compliance with an antihypertensive medication. Current Therapeutic Research 20: 215-219 (1976).

Farquhar, J.W.: The American Way of Life Need Not Be Hazardous to Your Health (W.W. Norton, New York 1978).

Gabriel, M.; Gagnon, J.I. and Bryan, C.K.: Improving patient compliance through use of a daily drug reminder chart. American Journal of Public Health 67: 968-969 (1977).

Haynes, R.B.; Taylor, D.W. and Sackett, D.L. (Eds): Compliance in Health Care (Johns Hopkins University Press, Baltimore 1979).

Inui, J.F.; Yourtee, E.L. and Williamson, J.W.: Improved outcomes in hypertension after tutorials. Annals of Internal Medicine 84: 649-651 (1976).

Kleinman, A.; Eisenberg, L. and Good, B.: Culture, illness and care: Clinical lessons from anthropologic and cross-cultural research. Annals of Internal Medicine 88: 251-258 (1978).

Ley, P. and Spelman, M.S.: Communication in an outpatient setting. Brit. J. Soc. Clin. Psych. 4: 114-116 (1965).

Linkewick, J.A.; Catalano, R.B. and Flack, H.L.: The effect of packaging and instruction on outpatient compliance with medication regimens. Drug Intelligence and Clinical Pharmacy 8: 10-15 (1974).

Lorber, J.: Good patients and problem patients: Conformity and deviance in a general hospital. Journal of Health and Social Behavior 16: 213-225 (1975).

MacElveen, P.M.: Cooperative triad in hemodialysis care and patient outcomes. Com. Nurs. Res. 5: 135-147 (1972).

Mazullo, J.M.; Lasagna, L. and Griner, P.F.: Variations in interpretations of prescription instructions. Journal of the American Medical Association 227: 929-930 (1974).

Morris, L.A. and Halperin, J.A.: Effects of written drug information on patient knowledge and compliance. American Journal of Public Health 29: 47-52 (1979).

Moulding, T.S.; Onstad, G.D. and Barbaro, J.A.: Supervision of outpatient drug therapy with the medication monitor. Annals of Internal Medicine 73: 559-564 (1970).

Mushlin, A.I. and Appel, F.A.: Diagnosing patient noncompliance. Archives of Internal Medicine 137: 318-321 (1977).

Norell, S.E.: Accuracy of patient interviews and estimates by clinical staff in determining medication compliance. Social Science and Medicine 15: 57-61 (1981).

Oakes, T.B.; Ward, J.R.; Gary, R.M. et al.: Family expectations and arthritis patient compliance to a hand resting splint regimen. Journal of Chronic Disease 22: 757-764 (1970).

Roter, D.L.: Patient participation in the patient-provider interaction: The effect of patient question asking on the quality of interaction satisfaction and compliance. Health Education Monographs 5: 281-315 (1977).

Sackett, D.L. and Snow, J.C.: The magnitude and measurement of compliance; in Taylor and Sackett (Eds) Compliance in Health Care (Johns Hopkins University Press, Baltimore 1979).

Samora, J.; Saunders, L. and Larson, R.F.: Medical vocabulary knowledge among hospital patients. Journal of Health and Human Behavior 2: 83-89 (1961).

Schmidt, J.P.: A behavioral approach to patient compliance. Postgraduate Medicine 65: 39-42 (1979).

Schulman, B.A.: Active patient orientation and outcomes in hypertensive treatment: Applications of a socio-organizational perspective. Medical Care 17: 267-280 (1979).

Segall, A. and Roberts, L.W.: A comparative analysis of physician estimates of levels of medical knowledge among patients. Sociology of Health and Illness 2: 317-334 (1980).

Sharpe, T.J. and Mikeal, R.L.: Patient compliance with antibiotic regimens. Americ. J. Hosp. Pharmacy 31: 479-484 (1974).

Stiles, W.B.; Putnam, S.M.; Wolf, M.H. and James, S.A.: Verbal response mode profiles of patients and physicians in medical screening interviews. J. Med. Ed. 54: 81-89 (1979).

Svarstad, B.: The doctor-patient encounter: An observational study of communication and outcome. Doctoral Dissertation, University of Wisconsin (1974).

Svarstad, B.: Physician-patient communication and patient conformity with medical advice; in Mechanic (Ed.) The Growth of Bureaucratic Medicine (John Wiley and Sons, New York 1976).

Szasz, T.S. and Hollender, M.H.: A contribution to the philosophy of medicine. The basic models of the doctor-patient relationship. Archives of Internal Medicine 97: 585-592 (1956).

Taylor, S.E.: Hospital patient behavior: Reactance, helplessness or control? Journal of Social Issues 35: 156-184 (1979).

Veatch, R.: Models for ethical medicine in a revolutionary age. Hastings Center Report 2: 5 (1972).

Waitzkin, H. and Stoeckle, J.D.: The communication of information about illness. Clinical, sociological and methodological considerations. Advances in Psychosomatic Medicine 8: 180-215 (1972).

Address for correspondence and reprints: Dr *C.L. Peck*, Senior Lecturer, Department of Psychology, La Trobe University, Bundoora, Victoria 3083 (Australia).

Drugs 30: 85-126 (1985)
0012-6667/85/0008-0085/$21.00/0

Pirenzepine
A Review of its Pharmacodynamic and Pharmacokinetic Properties and Therapeutic Efficacy in Peptic Ulcer Disease and Other Allied Diseases

A.A. Carmine and *R.N. Brogden*

ADIS Drug Information Services, Auckland

Various sections of the manuscript reviewed by: ***H. Abrahamsson***, Division of Gastroenterology, Sahlgren's Hospital, Göteborg, Sweden, ***S. Bank***, Long Island Jewish-Hillside Medical Center, New Hyde Park, New York, USA; ***G. Bianchi Porro***, Gastrointestinal Unit, Ospedale L. Sacco, Milano, Italy; ***N. Birdsall***, National Institute for Medical Research, Mill Hill, London, England; ***G. Dobrilla***, Ospedale Generàle Regionale di Bolzano, Allgemeines Regional Krankenhaus Bezon, Italy; ***D.G. Colin-Jones,*** Queen Alexandra Hospital, Cosham, Portsmouth, England; ***B.H. Jaup***, Division of Gastroenterology, Sahlgrens Hospital Göteborg, Sweden; ***M.J.S. Langman***, Department of Therapeutics, University Hospital, Nottingham, England; ***J.J. Misiewicz***, Department of Gastroenterology and Nutrition, Central Middlesex Hospital, Acton Lane, London, England; ***D.W. Piper***, Royal North Shore Hospital, St Leonards, New South Wales, Australia; ***R. Stockbrügger***, Division of Gastroenterology, Sahlgren's Hospital, Göteborg, Sweden; ***E.C. Texter,*** Division of Gastroenterology, University of Arkansas for Medical Sciences, Little Rock, Arkansas, USA; ***J.G. Williams***, Royal Naval Hospital, Haslar, Gasport Hants, England; ***R.P. Walt,*** Department of Therapeutics, University Hospital, Nottingham, England.

Contents

Summary 86
1. Pharmacology 89
1.1 Muscarinic Receptor Selectivity 89
1.2 Anticholinergic Activity 90
1.2.1 Effect on Salivation 90
1.2.2 Effect on the Cardiovascular System 91
1.2.3 Effect on Ocular Function 91
1.2.4 Effect on the Central Nervous System 91
1.2.5 Effect on Urinary Function 92
1.2.6 Effect on Gastrointestinal Motility 92
1.3 Effect on Gastric Acid Secretion 92
1.3.1 Animal Studies 92
1.3.2 Human Studies 93
1.4 Prevention of Experimental Gastroduodenal Mucosal Damage 98
1.5 Effect on Serum Gastrin 99
1.6 Effect on Gastrointestinal Hormones 99
1.7 Effect on Pancreatic Secretion 99

1.8 Effect on Gastric Mucus Secretion 100
1.9 Effect on Pepsin Output 100
1.10 Effect on Endocrine Function 100
1.11 Effect on Lower Oesophageal Sphincter Pressure 101
1.12 Effect on Intragastric Bacteria and Nitrate 101
1.13 Toxicity Studies 101
2. Pharmacokinetic Studies 102
2.1 Absorption 102
2.2 Distribution 103
2.3 Elimination 103
2.3.1 Metabolism and Excretion 103
2.3.2 Half-Life 103
2.4 Plasma Concentration and Clinical Effects 103
2.5 Dialysability of Pirenzepine 104
3. Therapeutic Trials 104
3.1 Treatment of Duodenal Ulcer 104
3.1.1 Pirenzepine Compared with Placebo 106
3.1.2 Pirenzepine Compared with Cimetidine 106
3.1.3 Pirenzepine Compared with Other Therapy 109
3.2 Prevention of Duodenal Ulcer Recurrence 110
3.3 Treatment of Gastric Ulcer 111
3.3.1 Pirenzepine Compared with Placebo 111
3.3.2 Pirenzepine Compared with Other Therapy 112
3.4 Non-Ulcerous Dyspepsia 113
3.5 Zollinger-Ellison Syndrome 113
3.6 Treatment and Prevention of Other Conditions 114
4. Side Effects 115
4.1 Adverse Clinical Effects 115
4.2 Abnormal Laboratory Tests 117
5. Dosage and Administration 117
6. The Role of Pirenzepine in Peptic Ulcer Disease 118

Summary

Synopsis: *Pirenzepine*[1] *is a 'selective' antimuscarinic agent which, unlike classic anticholinergic agents, inhibits gastric acid secretion at lower doses than are required to affect gastrointestinal motility, salivary, central nervous system, cardiovascular, ocular and urinary functions. On a weight basis, pirenzepine has one-tenth to one-eighth the potency of atropine in inhibiting stimulated gastric acid secretion in humans. Extensive controlled trials utilising endoscopy in outpatients with duodenal ulcers indicate that patient response to pirenzepine is dose related. Doses of 100 to 150 mg/day are superior to placebo in promoting duodenal ulcer healing and in diminishing day and night pain and supplementary antacid consumption. At such doses, the efficacy of pirenzepine appears to be superior to that of gefarnate 300 mg/day and generally not significantly different from that of cimetidine 1 g/day in treating duodenal ulcers. A beneficial effect of pirenzepine in the prevention of duodenal ulcer recurrence was apparent in preliminary studies in small numbers of patients, but its efficacy in this regard needs further confirmation and the optimum dosage determined. Less extensive data on the treatment of benign gastric ulcers suggest that pirenzepine 100 to 150 mg/day is superior to placebo and gefarnate 300 mg/day and does not differ significantly from cimetidine 1 g/day in promoting gastric ulcer healing.*

1 'Gastrozepin', 'Gastrozepina', 'Gastropin', 'Bisvanil' (Boehringer Ingelheim); 'Gastrozepin' (Boots, Thomae); 'Leblon', 'Leblun' (De Angeli); 'Maghen' (Cristalfarma); 'Ulcosan' (Dompe).

Pirenzepine is well tolerated by most patients, with a low incidence of typical antimuscarinic effects on the gastrointestinal tract, genitourinary system or heart being reported in clinical studies. However, dry mouth and blurred vision are the more common side effects with clinically effective doses. Thus, pirenzepine appears to have relatively selective antimuscarinic activity, although controlled studies comparing pirenzepine and conventional antimuscarinics in patients with peptic ulcer disease have not been reported.

Pharmacodynamic Studies: Studies in animals have shown pirenzepine to be a competitive inhibitor of acetylcholine at muscarinic receptor sites, having one-hundredth to one-tenth the potency of atropine on a molar basis. Unlike classic anticholinergic agents, at low doses pirenzepine selectively blocks muscarinic receptors controlling gastric secretion, whereas higher doses are required to affect salivary, central nervous system, cardiovascular, ocular, urinary and gastrointestinal motility functions. In man, pirenzepine inhibits basal gastric acid secretion and that stimulated by pentagastrin, histamine and normal meals, having about one-tenth to one-eighth the potency of atropine (weight-for-weight) in healthy subjects and in patients with duodenal ulcer. In healthy subjects, single oral doses of pirenzepine 50 and 100mg reduced total acid output by 32% and 41%, respectively, whereas a 1-week regimen of 75 and 150mg daily reduced 24-hour acidity by 20% and 29%, respectively. In patients with duodenal ulcer, pirenzepine 25mg thrice daily administered orally reduced basal and pentagastrin-stimulated gastric acid output by 51% and 41%, respectively, over 4 weeks. Pirenzepine significantly decreased nocturnal acid output compared with placebo.

Pirenzepine at one-twentieth to one-tenth the dose (weight-for-weight) of cimetidine inhibited basal and pentagastrin-stimulated acid secretion to a similar or somewhat lesser degree, although pirenzepine appeared to have a longer duration of action. The addition of pirenzepine to cimetidine or ranitidine inhibits gastric secretion to a much greater degree than the individual drugs alone in healthy subjects, and in patients with duodenal ulcers or Zollinger-Ellison syndrome.

In healthy subjects and in patients with duodenal ulcer, usual doses of pirenzepine did not affect serum levels of gastrin, somatostatin, neurotensin, vasoactive intestinal peptide, secretin, gastric inhibitory polypeptide, trypsin, lipase, glucagon or insulin, or gastric mucus secretion, although enteroglucagon, pancreatic polypeptide, and basal motilin levels were significantly reduced. Parenteral doses reduced pepsin output and lower oesophageal sphincter pressure dose-dependently. Pirenzepine generally had no effect on the secretion of prolactin or of growth hormone.

Pharmacokinetics: After oral administration, peak plasma concentrations were achieved within 2 to 3 hours. Single oral doses of pirenzepine 25 and 50mg produced peak plasma concentrations of 24 to 32 μg/L and 51 to 62 μg/L, respectively. The reported bioavailability after single doses was between 20 and 30%, although this may decrease to 10 to 20% when pirenzepine is taken with food. No significant 'first-pass' hepatic metabolism occurred. The apparent volume of distribution of pirenzepine in the central compartment (14L) is equivalent to the extracellular water space. In healthy subjects, the cerebrospinal fluid concentration of pirenzepine was one-tenth that in plasma sampled at the same time. Pirenzepine was 12% protein bound. Very little pirenzepine is metabolised, and the small amount of the desmethyl metabolite formed is pharmacologically inactive. Over a period of 96 hours after oral administration, 10% of pirenzepine was excreted unchanged in the urine, and 90% in the faeces. Because of its hydrophilicity, no tubular reabsorption occurs. Total plasma clearance was about 15 L/h, renal clearance is equivalent to the glomerular filtration rate, and hepatic clearance is about 7.5 L/h. The mean elimination half-life of pirenzepine is 11 hours in healthy subjects. A plasma concentration of 70 to 165 μg/L was required for optimum inhibition of meal-stimulated gastric acid. However, since dosages needed to produce such plasma concentrations also cause anticholinergic side effects, lower dosage regimens are used in clinical practice.

Therapeutic Trials: Results from numerous double-blind, randomised, placebo-controlled studies in outpatients with endoscopically verified duodenal ulcers indicate that ulcer healing with pirenzepine is dose related. In general, pirenzepine 100 to 150 mg/day significantly improves healing rates compared with placebo, but smaller doses do not. Overall, duodenal ulcers usually healed in 32 to 57% of patients treated with placebo, in 45 to 75% of those taking less than 100 mg/day of pirenzepine and in 70 to 90% of patients taking pirenzepine 100 to 150 mg/day over a 4-week period. Day and night pain, and antacid consumption, were usually decreased in pirenzepine-treated patients compared with placebo controls.

Duodenal ulcer healing with pirenzepine 100 to 150 mg/day did not usually differ significantly from that achieved with cimetidine 1 g/day in numerous double- or single-blind outpatient studies, some of which were relatively large. However, in one double-blind study in 96 patients, ulcer healing following 6 weeks' treatment with cimetidine 1 g/day was superior to that with pirenzepine 100 mg/day. Most studies found that symptoms such as day and night pain, and antacid requirements, were reduced to a similar degree by the end of treatment with pirenzepine or cimetidine, although some results indicated that remission of symptoms occurred faster with cimetidine.

Duodenal ulcer healing with pirenzepine 100 or 125 mg/day was superior to that achieved with gefarnate 300 mg/day ($p < 0.01$) in 2 relatively large double-blind studies.

Small studies comparing long term prophylactic therapy with low doses of pirenzepine (30 to 50 mg/day) with placebo or cimetidine 400 mg/day have not consistently demonstrated any statistically significant differences in duodenal ulcer recurrence rates. The superiority of pirenzepine 100 mg/day over placebo in one double-blind 12-month study requires confirmation in well-designed studies, as the patient groups differed in age.

The efficacy of pirenzepine in treating benign gastric ulcers has been less extensively studied than that in duodenal ulcers. Pirenzepine 150 mg/day was superior to placebo in promoting ulcer healing and minimising ulcer symptoms in a small double-blind study. When compared with other drugs, ulcer healing with pirenzepine 100 to 150 mg/day did not differ significantly from that with cimetidine 1 g/day in a large non-blinded study. Similarly, pirenzepine 50 to 75mg daily was not significantly different from carbenoxolone 200 to 300mg daily in several small double-blind studies in outpatients. However, pirenzepine 75 to 150 mg/day was superior to gefarnate 300 mg/day in large double-blind studies in hospitalised patients and outpatients.

Controlled comparisons of pirenzepine and placebo or cimetidine have also been conducted in patients with non-ulcerous dyspepsia, duodenitis and/or gastritis. Pirenzepine 100 mg/day was superior to placebo in improving the endoscopic appearance of the gastric or duodenal mucosa and in providing relief from dyspepsia in patients with non-ulcerous dyspepsia.

The addition of pirenzepine to short or long term therapy with cimetidine or ranitidine in a few patients with Zollinger-Ellison syndrome has yielded some favourable results.

Side Effects: In short term controlled studies, pirenzepine was tolerated well by most patients and seldom discontinued (2%) because of adverse effects. Dry mouth (14%), blurred vision (2%), constipation (3%), diarrhoea (3%), headache (2%) and mental confusion (1.5%) were the most frequently reported side effects, upon questioning, following daily dosages of 100 to 150mg. The incidence of blurred vision appeared to be dose dependent (1% with 100 mg/day, 5.6% with 150 mg/day). The side effect profile of pirenzepine and cimetidine differed in that central nervous system, allergic and endocrine reactions occurred less frequently with pirenzepine, but dry mouth and blurred vision seemed to be less frequent with cimetidine.

Dosage: The usual adult dosage in the treatment of duodenal or benign gastric ulceration is 100mg daily in 2 divided doses at bedtime and in the morning before meals. Treatment should be continued until the ulcer has healed, or if endoscopic reassessment is not possible, for 4 to 8 weeks. Unlike classic anticholinergic drugs, pirenzepine is not contraindicated in glaucoma or prostatic hypertrophy.

1. Pharmacology

Pirenzepine (fig. 1) is a pyrido-benzodiazepine anticholinergic compound which is structurally similar to imipramine. It is largely devoid of central activity because of its poor penetration into the central nervous system. Unlike classic anticholinergic agents, pirenzepine appears to be selective in its binding to muscarinic receptors. As pirenzepine inhibits gastric secretion by blocking its high affinity to muscarinic receptors, it inhibits basal and stimulated gastric acid secretion at doses lower than are needed to affect cardiovascular, ocular, and urinary function, salivation and gastrointestinal motility.

1.1 Muscarinic Receptor Selectivity

Pirenzepine has been tested *in vitro* on broken cell preparations from peripheral tissues and regions of the brain and in intact isolated tissues in rats, guinea-pigs and rabbits. Pirenzepine receptor sites have been detected in competitive binding experiments employing the radioligands ^{3}H-N-methylscopolamine (Hammer, 1980), ^{3}H-quinuclidinylbenzilate and ^{3}H-propylbenzilylcholine (Hammer et al., 1980a), and directly using ^{3}H-pirenzepine as a marker ligand (Birdsall et al., unpublished data), although it has been suggested that differences in rat cerebral cortex binding of ^{3}H-pirenzepine and ^{3}H-quinuclidinylbenzilate may be partially accounted for by differences in receptor isomerisation (Luthin and Wolfe, 1984).

In both subcellular and intact tissue studies, radiolabelled pirenzepine manifested a 23- to 50-fold variation in its affinity for individual tissues (Brown et al., 1980; Hammer, 1978, 1982; Hammer et al., 1980a; Watson et al., 1983a,b), in contrast to atropine, propantheline and emepronium, which demonstrated only a 3- to 7-fold variation (Birdsall et al., 1980a,b; Burgen et al., 1974; Kloog et al, 1979; Nilvebrant and Sparf, 1982).

In *in vitro* binding studies with pirenzepine, it was possible to distinguish muscarinic receptor sites of high affinity ('A' or 'M_1' receptors) in the peripheral sympathetic ganglia, hippocampus, corpus striatum, and cerebral cortex from those of medium affinity ('B' receptors) in the salivary glands, medulla-pons, and lachrymal glands, and low affinity ('C' or 'M_2' receptors) in the heart, cerebellum, urinary bladder, and ileum smooth muscle (Giachetti et al., 1982; Hammer, 1980; Hammer et al., 1980a,b; Watson et al., 1983a,b). These 3 receptor sites have dissociation constants differing overall by a factor of 40 (Hammer et al., 1980a). Atropine can distinguish between muscarinic receptors in the cerebral cortex and myocardium but by only a relatively small factor ($\approx$4) [Birdsall et al., 1980b]. In contrast, affinity for muscarinic receptors varied by no more than 3-fold in studies involving radiolabelled N-methyl-hyoscine (scopolamine) [Hammer, 1980; Hammer et al., 1980a], and little or not at all with radiolabelled atropine (Beld et al., 1975; Nilvebrant and Sparf, 1982), ipratropium bromide (Beld et al., 1975), propantheline and emepronium (Nilvebrant and Sparf, 1982). In contrast to findings with pirenzepine, it was not possible to distinguish between the 3 muscarinic receptor subclasses with any the latter mentioned anticholinergic drugs. The atypical heterogeneity of pirenzepine's muscarinic receptor binding correlates well with its selective pharmacological activity in animal and human studies (see sections 1.2.1 to 1.2.6).

The exact location of the high affinity muscarinic receptors through which pirenzepine inhibits gastric secretion is unclear. Some investigators have reported that receptors in the central nervous system, the sympathetic ganglia, and the parietal cell itself are not responsible (Hammer, 1982; Rosenfeld, 1983). Hammer (1980, 1982) has suggested that it is most likely that the intramural plexus of

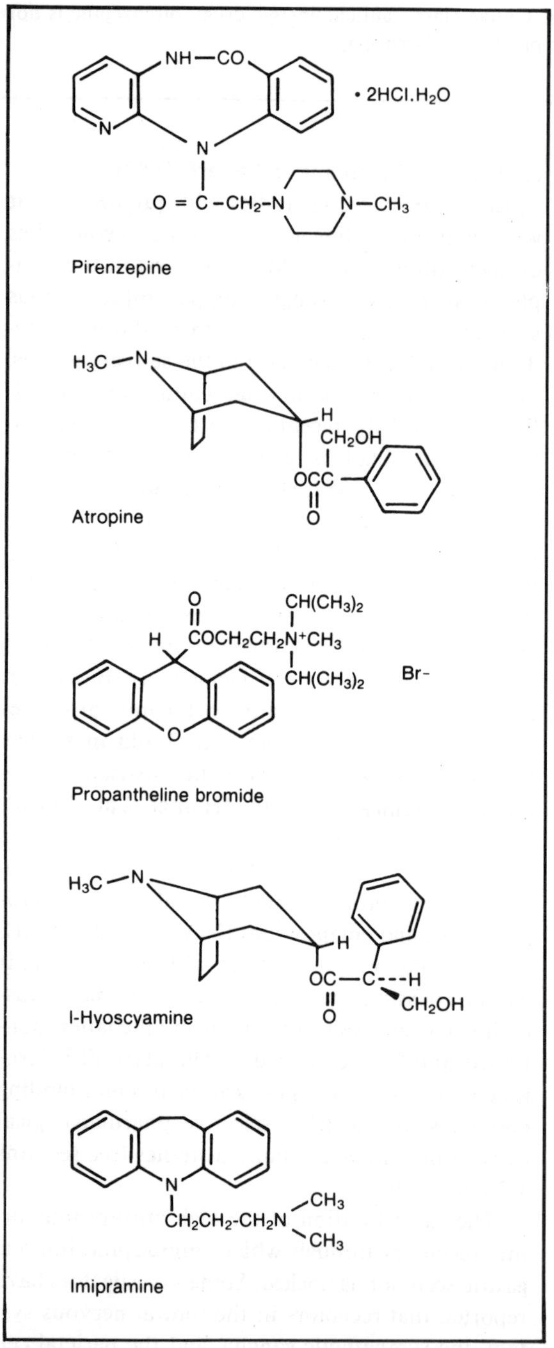

Fig. 1. Structural formulae for pirenzepine, the anticholinergic agents atropine sulphate, propantheline bromide and l-hyoscyamine, plus the structurally related tricyclic antidepressant imipramine.

the gastrointestinal tract, which is known to contain muscarinic synapses (Brown and Adams, 1980), could be selectively affected by pirenzepine.

Recent data, however, suggest that pirenzepine may influence gastrointestinal function through ganglia of the peripheral nervous system (Watson et al., 1984; Yamamura et al., 1984).

Pirenzepine does not appear to have muscarinic agonist or partial agonist activity (Hammer et al., 1980a), or histamine H_2-receptor blocking activity (Kuhn et al., 1977c; Parsons et al., 1978).

1.2 Anticholinergic Activity

Pirenzepine, like other antimuscarinic drugs, exhibits dose-related anticholinergic activity in animals and in man. However, at dosages which inhibit gastric acid secretion (section 1.3), pirenzepine has less effect than equipotent antisecretory doses of l-hyoscyamine on salivation, heart rate, ocular function, urinary bladder function, gastrointestinal motility and on the central nervous system (table I). The relatively lesser anticholinergic activity of pirenzepine is reflected in the low incidence of anticholinergic side effects in therapeutic trials (section 4.1).

1.2.1 Effect on Salivation

In patients with duodenal ulcers, a dose-related reduction in salivation occurred after therapeutic doses of pirenzepine administered intravenously, although it was less marked and shorter lasting (1 to 2 hours *vs* several hours) than that occurring after equipotent antisecretory doses of atropine (Konturek et al., 1980).

In a 4-day double-blind comparative trial in which salivary secretion was quantified in healthy subjects, oral pirenzepine 50mg twice daily was associated with a 26% reduction in maximum salivary capacity 2 hours after dosing (when peak plasma drug concentrations were present), and no significant reduction was noted at 4 hours (Jaup et al., 1980; Jaup and Dotevall, 1981). In contrast, l-hyoscyamine twice daily resulted in a reduction of maximum salivary capacity of 43% at 2 hours, and of 37% at 4 hours after administration. Inhibition of salivation was significantly greater and longer lasting with l-hyoscyamine ($p < 0.01$). In one study, however, pirenzepine 5 and 10mg intravenously inhibited bethanechol-stimulated gastric acid secretion and salivation to a similar extent (Dobrilla et al., 1983).

1.2.2 Effect on the Cardiovascular System

Single doses of pirenzepine 10 to 20mg intravenously have generally had no significant effect on heart rate (Bron and Infante, 1978; Brunner et al., 1978; Fritsch et al., 1980; Stenquist et al., 1982). However, in a few single-dose studies, a small transient decrease in heart rate (by 7 to 10 beats/min) was noted (Baldi et al., 1983a,b; Stacher et al., 1978a). It is unclear why this may occur, although these small decreases in heart rate are unlikely to be of clinical significance in most patients. However, after an intravenous dose of 40mg (twice that required for 50% inhibition of gastric acid secretion), pirenzepine produced a moderate rise in pulse rate and blood pressure. Nevertheless, these changes were less marked and of shorter duration than those occurring after atropine 1.5 and 3mg (Konturek et al., 1980). When administered orally, usual therapeutic doses of pirenzepine do not increase heart rate significantly (Fink and Irwin, 1980; Jaup et al., 1980), thus differing from propantheline (Hurwitz et al., 1977), methantheline (Hawkins et al., 1953), and atropine (Fritsch, 1978).

1.2.3 Effect on Ocular Function

In mice and rats (Heathcote and Parry, 1980; Parry and Heathcote, 1982), pupil diameter was affected by intravenous pirenzepine at 3 to 4 times the antisecretory dose, in contrast to the anticholinergics atropine, glycopyrronium, propantheline, poldine, benzhexol and isopropamide, which affected pupil size at doses similar to or lower than antisecretory doses. Similarly, in healthy subjects (Jaup and Dotevall, 1981; Jaup et al., 1980; Shimizu et al., 1980; Tauber, 1977) and in patients with duodenal ulcer (Chierichetti et al., 1979; Konturek et al., 1980), oral pirenzepine has demonstrated a low selectivity for the eye. Thus, in a 4-day comparative study, oral pirenzepine 50mg twice daily, like placebo, was associated with no ocular symptoms, whereas an equipotent antisecretory regimen of oral l-hyoscyamine 0.6mg twice daily produced blurred vision in 67% of subjects and increased pupil diameter by 13 to 25% (Jaup and Dotevall, 1981; Jaup et al., 1980). The near vision distance was not altered in the pirenzepine group, but that in l-hyoscyamine recipients increased 19 to 33% ($p < 0.05$) throughout each study day. However, pirenzepine 40mg administered intravenously produced blurred near vision in patients with duodenal ulcer, although visual effects were less marked and of shorter duration (1 to 2 hours *vs* several hours) than those of atropine 1.5 and 3mg (Konturek et al., 1980).

When taken at a low therapeutic dosage of 25mg thrice daily for 1 week, pirenzepine did not change intraocular pressure in subjects with open- or closed-angle glaucoma (Shimizu et al., 1980; Tauber, 1977), or induce abnormalities in the conjunctiva, cornea, iris or anterior chamber (Tauber, 1977).

1.2.4 Effect on the Central Nervous System

Despite the structural similarity of pirenzepine to tricyclic antidepressants (fig. 1), pirenzepine does not exhibit central effects, as its hydrophilic properties and low lipid solubility largely prevent penetration into the central nervous system. Thus, in animal studies, pirenzepine exerted no effect on central serotonergic synapses (Rogóz et al., 1981; Spánková et al., 1975), or against levodopa-induced hypermotility (Rogóz et al., 1981) and reserpine-induced hypotension (Kaehling et al., 1974). At dosages which inhibit gastric acid secretion, pirenzepine did not exhibit psychotropic activity in animals when administered parenterally (Eberlein et al., 1977; Hammer et al., 1977a,b; Kuhn et al., 1977b; Leitold et al., 1977) or intracerebrally (Eberlein et al., 1977; Leitold et al., 1977).

Similarly, in placebo-controlled trials in healthy subjects, single therapeutic doses of pirenzepine 25 to 150mg administered orally (Fink and Irwin, 1980; Itil, 1977), and 8mg administered intramuscularly (Kuhn et al., 1977a), were not associated with changes in the electroencephalogram (EEG) nor any significant changes in reaction time, visual motor coordination or critical flicker test threshold. However, pirenzepine 0.3 mg/kg administered intramuscularly reduced the power density in the faster α-range and increased the relative spectral density in the θ-range in a manner indistinguishable from that produced by atropine 1mg administered by the same route (Stacher et al., 1978b). As EEG effects from pirenzepine are unexpected (*vide supra*), Stacher et al. (1978b) have suggested that they may arise indirectly, via effects on peptidergic neurons and hormonal peptides.

In 10 duodenal ulcer patients, a therapeutic dosage of oral pirenzepine (25mg twice daily) was not associated with significant changes in anxiety, depression or appetite scores, compared with placebo (Kuhn and Honzak, 1980).

1.2.5 Effect on Urinary Function

In anaesthetised dogs, even at high doses intravenous pirenzepine had little effect on electrically stimulated urinary bladder contraction. On the other hand, intravenous atropine inhibited bladder contraction at a dosage much closer to that required to inhibit gastric acid secretion (Jennewein, 1978). In patients with prostatic hypertrophy, oral pirenzepine 37.5 to 75mg daily did not affect residual urine volume, bladder emptying, or tone of the bladder wall (Gleissner and Mielenz, 1977).

1.2.6 Effect on Gastrointestinal Motility

At usual therapeutic doses, oral pirenzepine did not slow the gastric emptying of a semisolid (Corinaldesi et al., 1982; Stacher et al., 1982) or a liquid meal in healthy subjects (Bianchi Porro et al., 1982c; Corinaldesi et al., 1982; Jaup and Dotevall, 1981; Mignon et al., 1982), thus differing from propantheline (Brömster et al., 1969; Hurwitz et al., 1977), 1-hyoscyamine (Brömster et al., 1969; Jaup and Dotevall, 1981), atropine and hyoscine butylbromide (Brömster et al., 1969). However, gastric emptying was slowed significantly ($p < 0.05$) more than placebo by an intramuscular dose (0.5 mg/kg) 2 to 3 times that required for an antisecretory effect but not by lower doses (Mignon et al., 1982).

Pirenzepine appears to influence colonic motility at lower doses than are required to decrease gastric emptying, neostigmine-stimulated sigmoid colonic motor activity being inhibited ($p < 0.05$) by pirenzepine 0.15 mg/kg intramuscularly. Pirenzepine 0.3 mg/kg intramuscularly, like atropine 1mg, reduced the amplitude of meal-induced colonic contractions by 21 to 25% (Stacher et al., 1978a). Pirenzepine 5mg intravenously reduced human sigmoid motility for 30 minutes when plasma drug concentrations were above 55 μg/L, while an equipotent antisecretory dose of atropine reduced motility for 90 minutes (Stockbrügger et al., 1984).

Interdigestive gastrointestinal motility was influenced by oral administration of pirenzepine 50mg daily, increasing the gastric component of the migrating motor complexes (MMCs). In contrast, atropine 1mg 4-hourly decreased the total number of MMCs but did not change the gastrointestinal/intestinal MMC ratio. Cimetidine 1000mg daily had no motility effects in the same 6 subjects (Lederer et al., 1982). In 10 healthy subjects, equipotent antisecretory regimens of pirenzepine 50mg and 1-hyoscyamine 0.6mg, each administered orally twice daily for 4 days, lowered mean basal oesophageal peristaltic amplitude, although the effect of 1-hyoscyamine was 3-fold greater (51% *vs* 15%; Jaup et al., 1982a,b). Primary oesophageal peristalsis induced by swallowing was significantly ($p < 0.05$) reduced by 1-hyoscyamine, but not pirenzepine. Gastrointestinal transit time was significantly decreased by pirenzepine 100mg given orally in 20 healthy subjects, while equipotent antisecretory doses of hyoscyamine increased transit time. Benzilonium bromide did not influence the transit time (Stockbrügger et al., 1984).

1.3 Effect on Gastric Acid Secretion

1.3.1 Animal Studies

The effectiveness of pirenzepine in inhibiting gastric acid secretion has been investigated *in vivo* in anaesthetised dogs (Daly et al., 1982) and rats (Del Soldata and Pagani, 1982; Pagani et al., 1984; Parry and Heathcote, 1982), dogs with a Heidenhain pouch (Bonfils et al., 1982; Del Tacca et al., 1982; Fujiwara et al., 1982; Jennewein, 1978; Matsuo and Seki, 1979), dogs, cats and rats with a gastric fistula (Del Tacca et al., 1982; Browning and Heathcote, 1983; Kitagawa et al., 1978, respectively), and *in vitro* in isolated mouse stomach (Müller-Lissner et al., 1982). In all studies, pirenzepine whether administered orally, subcutaneously, or intravenously, produced dose-related inhibition of gastric secretion stimulated by insulin, bombesin, tetragastrin, oxotremorine, pentagastrin, histamine, bethanechol, or a test meal.

Pirenzepine has about one-hundredth to one-tenth the potency of atropine on a molar basis (Heathcote and Parry, 1980, 1982; Müller-Lissner et al., 1982), and one-tenth to one-eighth the potency of atropine on a weight-for-weight basis (Engelhorn, 1982), depending on the experimental model, the secretory stimulant, and the route of administration. The secretory dose-response curves to carbachol (Parsons et al., 1978; Rosenfeld, 1983) and bethanechol (Szelenyi, 1982) were displaced to the right by pirenzepine and atropine without depressing the maximum response, indicating competitive inhibition. Carbachol inhibition of gastrin and somatostatin was likewise competitively inhibited by piperazine, suggesting it may affect gastric acid secretion via these effects on gastric hormone regulation (Sue et al., 1983). However, if pirenzepine's selectivity for gastric secretion is to be demonstrated it is necessary for functional autonomic ganglia to be involved in the stimulation of the gastric secretion (Browning and Henman, 1983). Intraduodenal pirenzepine was about one-third as potent as propantheline bromide on a weight-for-weight basis (when tested over 4 weeks) in inhibiting basal and pentagastrin- and histamine-stimulated gastric secretion in gastric fistula in rats, and in inhibiting the gastric secretion of pylorus-ligated rats (Okabe et al., 1982).

The inhibition of acid secretion through alteration of mucosal blood flow can be ruled out because the antisecretory effect of pirenzepine can also be demonstrated *in vitro* in the absence of any blood supply (Sachs et al., 1978).

1.3.2 Human Studies

The effect of pirenzepine on gastric acid secretion has been studied in healthy volunteers and in patients with a duodenal ulcer after either intravenous, intramuscular or oral administration. Its effect has been studied on basal secretion as well as secretion stimulated by pentagastrin, histamine, peptone, insulin, sham feeding, caffeine and normal meals. In several studies, pirenzepine has been compared with other anticholinergic agents, cimetidine, ranitidine, gefarnate, and proglumide in healthy subjects and in patients with duodenal ulcer. Pirenzepine is more potent in inhibiting neuronally stimulated gastric acid secretion than that stimulated by exogenous muscarinic agonists.

Non-Comparative Studies

In most studies with pirenzepine, the reduction in acid secretion appeared to be due to a decrease in the volume of secretion rather than acid concentration (Bertoglio et al., 1982; Fritsch, 1978; Konturek et al., 1980; Kuhn et al., 1977a; Scholten et al., 1982a), as is characteristic of an anticholinergic agent (Konturek et al., 1980), but in two studies, decreases in acid concentration approached those occurring in volume (Corinaldesi et al., 1980; Jaup et al., 1980).

In healthy subjects, intravenous pirenzepine produces a dose-related inhibition of gastric acid secretion stimulated by pentagastrin and insulin (Bianchi Porro et al., 1979). Similarly, single and multiple oral doses of pirenzepine produce a dose-related inhibition of basal acid secretion (Dammann et al., 1982; Etienne and Bron, 1982; Heller et al., 1978a,b; Jain et al., 1979; Stockbrügger et al., 1977, 1979, 1982a) and gastric acid secretion stimulated by histamine (Eugenides et al., 1982), pentagastrin (Galmiche et al., 1980; Heller et al., 1978a,b; Jain et al., 1979; Stockbrügger et al., 1979), insulin (Jain et al., 1979), and modified sham feeding (Stockbrügger et al., 1977, 1979, 1982). Pirenzepine markedly inhibits gastric acid secretion which is vagally induced (e.g. sham-feeding, insulin-induced hypoglycaemia, fundic distention, peptone, and electrical vagal stimulation), as would be expected for an anticholinergic drug, but causes a less marked inhibition of the effects of more direct stimuli such as histamine and pentagastrin and is

Table I. Comparison of the anticholinergic effects of 4 days' treatment with pirenzepine 50mg twice daily and l-hyoscyamine 0.6mg twice daily in 10 healthy subjects studied under double-blind conditions (after Jaup et al., 1982b)

Anticholinergic effect	l-Hyoscyamine	Pirenzepine
Gastric secretion	↓**	↓**
Salivary secretion	↓**	↓*-0
Gastric emptying	↓**	0
Oesophageal pressure	↓**	0
Ocular accommodation (nearpoint distance)	↑**	0
Pupil	↑*	0

Key: ↓ = decrease; ↑ = increase; * significant change, $p < 0.05$; ** significant change, $p < 0.01$; 0 = no change.

without significant effect on sham feeding-induced gastric acid secretion in vagotomised patients (Biancho Porro et al., 1983).

Following oral administration, peak antisecretory effects were generally noted at 2 hours, whereas the duration of action varied from 5 to 12 hours, depending on the dose given. In healthy subjects, pirenzepine 50 and 100mg given orally reduced total nocturnal acid output by 32% and 41%, respectively (Dammann et al., 1982). In a placebo-controlled trial (Etienne and Bron, 1982), 24-hour acidity was reduced by 20% and 29%, respectively ($p < 0.001$), after 1 week's therapy with pirenzepine 75 and 150mg daily administered orally, although pirenzepine 50mg twice daily had no significant effect on nocturnal secretory volume or acid output in another study (Mahachai et al., 1984a).

In patients with confirmed duodenal ulcer, pirenzepine administered intravenously or orally produced dose-related inhibition of basal acid secretion (Corinaldesi et al., 1980, 1981; D'Imperio et al., 1979; Einig, 1977; Jaup et al., 1978), and that stimulated by pentagastrin (D'Imperio et al., 1979; Einig, 1977; Jaup and Dotevall, 1978; Sarosiek et al., 1982; Wegmann et al., 1979), caffeine (Bixquert et al., 1982), L-amino acids (Bertoglio et al., 1982), betazole (Einig, 1977), and insulin (Jaup and Dotevall, 1978). Pirenzepine 50mg reduced nocturnal acid secretion to a significantly greater degree than placebo ($p < 0.01$; mean 21%) from 2 to 9 hours after administration (Corinaldesi et al., 1981). Acid secretion was still 44% below control 8 hours after administration. Basal and pentagastrin-stimulated gastric acid output was significantly lower than control (by 51% and 42%, respectively; ($p < 0.01$) after 4 weeks' treatment with 25mg thrice daily (Sternini et al., 1980).

In patients with gastric ulcers, oral pirenzepine significantly ($p < 0.02$ to 0.05) reduced basal acid secretion (Tatsuta et al., 1981) and that stimulated by meals (Tatsuta et al., 1981), pentagastrin (Wegmann et al., 1979) and histamine (Laureta et al., 1979). Thus, 1 hour after a single 50mg dose, basal gastric acid output fell by 71% and meal-stimulated output by 51% (Tatsuta et al., 1981). Pirenzepine 100mg daily had no cumulative or long term effect on the acid-secreting cells as evidenced by the lack of suppression of basal or histamine-stimulated acid secretion 12 hours after the last dose of a 4-week treatment period (Laureta et al., 1979).

Antisecretory doses of pirenzepine produced little or no elevation in gastric pH in healthy subjects (Bianchi Porro et al., 1979; Jain et al., 1979; Laureta et al., 1981; Lederer et al., 1982), or in patients with duodenal ulcers (Bertoglio et al., 1982; Bianchi Porro et al., 1979; Corinaldesi et al., 1981) or gastric ulcers (Laureta et al., 1979).

Comparisons with Anticholinergic Agents

In comparative studies in healthy subjects (Lederer et al., 1982) and in patients with duodenal ulcer (table I), pirenzepine has been demonstrated to have one-tenth to one-eighth the potency (on a weight-for-weight basis) of the tertiary anticholinergic atropine, and about one-tenth the potency of the quaternary agent benzilonium bromide. In healthy subjects, twice daily regimens of oral pirenzepine 50mg and l-hyoscyamine 0.6mg, administered for 4 days, inhibited basal acid output to a similar extent (a reduction of 54% *vs* 57%), but pirenzepine tended to be more effective in inhibiting pentagastrin-stimulated acid output (31% *vs* 22%) [Jaup et al., 1980]. 12-Hour basal antral pH remained greater

Table II. Relative activity of pirenzepine (P) and the anticholinergic agents methantheline bromide (MB), atropine (A), and benzilonium bromide (BB) in inhibiting gastric acid secretion in patients with duodenal ulcer

Reference	No. of patients	Secretory stimulant	Dose (route)	% Inhibition	
				stimulated secretion	basal secretion
Fritsch (1978)	. . .[a]	Pentagastrin 5 μg/kg	P 25mg MB 50mg (oral)	36 No change	38 . . .[a]
Fritsch et al. (1980)	17	Pentagastrin 0.15 μg/kg/h × 3h	P 0.24 mg/kg/h × 1h + 5mg A 0.03 mg/kg/h × 1h + 1mg (IV)	70 80	
	13	Electrical stimulation of vagus nerve	P 0.24 mg/kg/h × 1h + 5mg A 0.03 mg/kg/h x 1h + 1mg (IV)	≈ 45 ≈ 45	
Konturek et al. (1980)	12	Sham feeding	P 20mg 40mg A 1.5mg 3mg (IV)	46 75 62 90	
Stenquist et al. (1982)	6	Sham feeding	P 10mg BB 1mg (IV)	48 73	75 75

a Data not given.

than 4 for a shorter time with oral pirenzepine 25mg twice daily than with atropine 1mg, given 4-hourly (Lederer et al., 1982). In duodenal ulcer patients side effects were shorter after pirenzepine than after a dose of atropine causing similar antisecretory effects (Konturek et al., 1980)[table II].

Comparisons with Cimetidine

Most comparative trials with cimetidine have evaluated single intravenous doses of both drugs in healthy subjects (Bron and Infante, 1978; Brunner et al., 1978; Winter et al., 1978) and in patients with duodenal ulcer. Pirenzepine, when administered orally at a dose one-twentieth to one-eighth and intravenously at one-tenth the dose of cimetidine, generally inhibited basal and pentagastrin-stimulated acid secretion to a lesser extent than cimetidine (table III). However, in one study in healthy subjects, reduction of pentagastrin-stimulated acid secretion 7 hours after drug administration was greater with pirenzepine 20mg (52%) than with cimetidine 400mg (10%; Bron and Infante, 1978). In 22 duodenal ulcer patients, infusions of pirenzepine and cimetidine at a 1 : 10 dose ratio reduced the volume of secretion to a similar degree (67% and 74%, respectively), but pirenzepine had a much smaller inhibitory effect on gastric acid concentration (20% *vs* 95%, respectively) [Fritsch et al., 1980].

In critically or acutely ill patients in whom pre-

Table III. Relative activity of pirenzepine (P) and cimetidine (C) in inhibiting gastric acid secretion in patients with duodenal ulcer

Reference	No. of patients	Secretory stimulant	Dosage (route)	% Inhibition	
				stimulated secretion	basal secretion
Fritsch et al. (1980)	22	Pentagastrin 0.15 μg/kg/h × 3h	P 0.24 mg/kg/h × 1h + 5mg	70	
			C 2.4 mg/kg/h × 1h + 50mg (IV)	95	
	17	Electrical stimulation of vagus nerve	P 0.24 mg/kg/h × 1h + 5mg	≈ 45	
			C 2.4 mg/kg/h × 1h + 50mg	Variable[a]	
Giacosa et al. (1982)	60	Pentagastrin 6 μg/kg/h	P 100 mg/day × 4 weeks	11[b]	11[b]
			C 1000 mg/day × 4 weeks (oral)	33	37
Kamenisch (1978)	15	Pentagastrin[c]	P 50 mg/day × 4 weeks	29	31
			C 1000 mg/day × 4 weeks (oral)	. . .[d]	12[b]
Londong et al. (1980b)	5	Peptone 10% 250 to 300 ml/min	P 0.3 mg/kg	34	
			C 3 mg/kg	63	
			P + C (IV)	90	
Procacciante et al. (1984)	12	Pentagastrin 67 μg/kg/h	P 25mg	18,[e] 12[f]	44,[e] 36[f]
			P 50mg	35, 24	59, 20
			C 200mg	36, 31	85, 51
			C 400mg (oral)	59, 40	98, 57

a As the level of electrical vagal stimulation increased, the inhibitory effect of cimetidine decreased.
b Not significantly ($p > 0.05$) different from placebo.
c Dose not stated.
d A statistically insignificant increase actually was observed.
e Acid output.
f Volume.

vention of stress ulcer was sought, pirenzepine was less effective than cimetidine in maintaining a gastric pH above 4 (Dammann and Augustin, 1978; Höckerstedt et al., 1982). Where 24-hour acidity was measured, oral cimetidine 400mg 4 times daily reduced gastric pH by 28%, while pirenzepine 50mg twice daily resulted in no appreciable pH changes (Dammann and Augustin, 1978).

Several studies have noted that a combination of pirenzepine and cimetidine or ranitidine results in a markedly greater reduction in acid secretion than that with either agent used alone in healthy subjects (Lederer et al., 1982; Londong et al., 1979, 1980b), in critically ill patients (More et al., 1983) and in patients with duodenal ulcer (Londong et al., 1979, 1980b) or a history of duodenal ulceration (Deakin et al., 1984; Mahachai et al., 1984b) or Zollinger Ellison syndrome (Bonfils et al., 1979; Collen et al., 1982; Mignon et al., 1980). This potentiation of antisecretory effects, which is thought to be due to the simultaneous blockade of parietal cell histamine H_2-receptors by cimetidine and acetylcholine receptors by pirenzepine (Londong et al., 1980b), may be synergistic (Deakin et al., 1984), and has also been noted with other cimetidine/anticholinergic combinations (Feldman et al., 1977; Scholten et al., 1978; Venables et al., 1978). Thus, in 5 patients with Zollinger-Ellison syndrome, the addition of oral pirenzepine 75 to 125mg daily to a high dose regimen of cimetidine (1.8 to 7.2g daily) further reduced gastric acid secretion by 20 to 25% (Collen et al., 1982). The addition of therapeutic dosages of probanthine or isopropamide to cimetidine regimens resulted in similar potentiation of acid reduction in these patients but, unlike with pirenzepine, anticholinergic side effects necessitated discontinuation of therapy. Similarly, in small groups of patients with severe forms of Zollinger-Ellison syndrome, coadministration of high dose cimetidine with large dosages of pirenzepine administered intravenously (72mg daily; Mignon et al., 1980) or intramuscularly (1.5 mg/kg/day; Bonfils et al., 1979) over 4 to 14 days has resulted in significantly greater reductions in basal acid output and volume of secretion than administration of cimetidine alone.

Comparisons with Ranitidine

Pirenzepine 0.15 to 0.6 mg/kg/h administered by infusion inhibits pentagastrin-stimulated acid secretion to about one-half the degree of ranitidine 0.1 to 0.9 mg/kg/h given by the same route (Gabryelewicz et al., 1980; table IV). Pirenzepine 50 and 100mg orally administered for 4 weeks produced significantly ($p < 0.001$) less inhibition of stimulated gastric acid secretion than oral ranitidine 150 and 300mg (Giacosa et al., 1982). However, addition of pirenzepine to ranitidine regimens has markedly increased the percentage inhibition of pentagastrin- and peptone-stimulated gastric acid secretion, and the duration of antisecretory effects, both in healthy subjects (Londong et al., 1981, 1983) and patients with duodenal ulcer (Gabryelewicz et al., 1982; Scholten et al., 1982b).

Comparisons with Proglumide and Gefarnate

In 6 patients with 'various gastrointestinal complaints', pirenzepine 8mg was markedly more potent than the gastrin-receptor antagonist proglum-

Table IV. Relative activity of pirenzepine (P) and ranitidine (R) in inhibiting gastric acid secretion in patients with duodenal ulcer

Reference	No. of patients	Secretory stimulant	Dosage (route)	% Inhibition	
				stimulated secretion	basal secretion
Gabryelewicz et al. (1980)	20	Pentagastrin 2 μg/kg/h × 3h	P 0.15 mg/kg/h	35	
			0.3 mg/kg/h	44	
			0.6 mg/kg/h	57	
			R 0.1 mg/kg/h	69	
			0.3 mg/kg/h	93	
			0.9 mg/kg/h	98	
			(IV)		
Giacosa et al. (1982)	61	Pentagastrin 6 μg/kg/h	P 100 mg/day × 28 days	11[a]	11[a]
			R 300 mg/day × 28 days	46	65
			(oral)		
Scholten et al. (1982b)[b]	7	Peptone 200ml	P 50mg	29	
			R 150mg	78	
			P + R	88	
			(oral)		

a Not significantly ($p > 0.05$) different from placebo.
b Nocturnal acid secretion measured (6pm to 7am).

ide 400mg in reducing pentagastrin-stimulated acid output (47% *vs* 7%) and secretion volume (50% *vs* 12%) [Kuhn et al., 1977a]. In an 8-week comparative trial in 33 patients with duodenal ulcer, oral gefarnate 300mg daily produced no significant changes in basal acid output or volume of secretion, whereas pirenzepine 125mg daily reduced these measurements by 38% and 34%, respectively (Ishimori and Yamagata, 1982c). Reduction of basal acid output by pirenzepine in patients whose ulcers healed was double that which occurred in patients with unhealed ulcers (46% *vs* 23%).

1.4 Prevention of Experimental Gastroduodenal Mucosal Damage

In rats, pirenzepine administered orally, subcutaneously or intraduodenally produced dose-related inhibition of the formation of Shay ulcers and gastric ulcers induced by stress, histamine, aspirin, indomethacin, phenylbutazone, diclofenac, naproxen, and ibuprofen (Engelhorn, 1982; Engelhorn et al., 1980; Kitagawa et al., 1978; Meeroff, 1980; Okabe et al., 1978), and gastrointestinal haemorrhage associated with intracranial lesions (Tritthart, 1984). The potency of oral pirenzepine, relative to other orally administered antiulcer agents, varied with the type of experimental ulcer. Thus, in the prevention of gastric ulceration in rats induced by thermocoagulation plus cortisone, pirenzepine was similar in potency to propantheline (Inatomi et al., 1979), 8 times more potent than sucralfate against indomethacin-induced ulceration (Okabe et al., 1978), 2 to 3 times more active than carbenoxolone against gastric wall ulcers induced by chronic cauterisation and acetic acid (Leitold and Engelhorn, 1977), and equipotent with cimetidine in preventing stress-induced ulceration (Meeroff, 1980). In the prevention of experimentally induced duodenal ulceration in guinea-pigs, oral pirenzepine was less potent (7.7%) than atropine sulphate, but 7 times more effective than propantheline or metiamide against stress-induced lesions and similar to propantheline in inhibiting formation of ulcers induced by cysteamine (Leitold and Engelhorn, 1977).

A possible cytoprotective effect of pirenzepine has been demonstrated in rats (Bernardini et al., 1984; Guslandi and Del Soldato 1984; Konturek et al., 1982a; Rovati et al., 1982; Varin et al., 1984), but has not been clearly shown in healthy subjects (Konturek et al., 1982b; Stockbrügger et al., 1983b). Thus, at dosages less than those required to inhibit gastric acid secretion, oral pirenzepine significantly reduced the incidence of aspirin-, ethanol-, serotonin-, taurocholate- and hydrochloric acid-induced gastric ulcers and the size of erosions in rats by at least one-third, although atropine and prostaglandin E_2 were more effective in this regard (Rovati et al., 1982). Recent experiments suggest that the increase in gastric mucosal blood flow and mucosal volume, and the preservation of gastric prostaglandin synthesis associated with pirenzepine administration, contribute to the cytoprotective effect (Jeremy and Dandona, 1984; Kawamura et al., 1984). In man, pirenzepine 20mg daily in 4 divided doses administered orally had no effect on aspirin-induced gastric bleeding or deoxyribonucleic acid loss in 10 healthy subjects (Konturek et al., 1982b); but in another study, aspirin-induced inflammation, bleeding tendency and erosions of the duodenum were decreased by oral administration of pirenzepine 50mg twice daily (Stockbrügger et al., 1983b). These indices of aspirin-induced mucosal damage in the stomach were not influenced by pirenzepine. Prostaglandin E_2 0.5mg and a higher antisecretory dosage of pirenzepine (25mg), each given 4 times daily, reduced both measurements significantly ($p < 0.05$) [Konturek et al., 1982b]. As changes in the mucosal generation of prostaglandins were not observed with the higher dosage of pirenzepine, it was suggested that any protective effect was most likely due to the drug's antisecretory activity.

Single doses of pirenzepine 10 to 30mg administered intravenously increased the gastric transmural electric potential difference in a dose-related manner (Kleist et al., 1979, 1980), with similar elevations being noted after pirenzepine 10mg and hyoscine 40mg. In 58 healthy subjects, the dose ratio of pirenzepine to atropine required to induce a maximum increase in potential difference was

10 : 1 on a molar basis (Kleist et al., 1980).

1.5 Effect on Serum Gastrin

Atropine administration or vagotomy has been shown to result in increased serum gastrin levels. Pirenzepine seems to generally have a minimal effect on serum gastrin concentrations. Thus, no significant effect on serum gastrin in the basal state or after stimulation with peptone, pentagastrin, insulin, betazole or sham feeding was noted in healthy subjects following single oral doses of 25 to 100mg (Bianchi Porro et al., 1982c; Heller et al., 1978a,b) and intravenous doses of 10 to 20mg (Arnold et al., 1978; El-Sabbagh et al., 1980a; Höckerstedt et al., 1982; Londong et al., 1979, 1980a,b, 1981; Vantini et al., 1978), or in patients with duodenal ulcer treated with 20mg intravenously (Konturek et al., 1980, 1982c). However, single doses of pirenzepine 35 to 40mg administered intravenously inhibited basal gastrin secretion (Fritsch et al., 1982) and that stimulated by sham feeding in patients with duodenal ulcer (Konturek et al., 1980) and in healthy subjects (Mignon et al., 1982).

Basal gastrin levels increased in some studies (Giacosa et al., 1982; Maleev et al., 1982) but not in others (Fritsch et al., 1982; Kamenisch, 1978; Sternini et al., 1980) in which duodenal ulcer patients were given pirenzepine 25 to 125mg daily orally for 1 to 4 weeks. In a placebo-controlled trial in 120 patients with duodenal ulcer, pirenzepine 100mg daily administered orally for 4 weeks doubled basal gastrin levels, whereas cimetidine 1000mg daily, ranitidine 300mg daily, and placebo produced no significant changes (Giacosa et al., 1982). A reason for the greater gastrin response occurring after prolonged gastric acid inhibition by pirenzepine, but not histamine H_2-receptor antagonists, has not been explored.

In patients with gastric ulcers, a single oral dose of pirenzepine 50mg reduced basal gastrin levels by 52% and the meal-stimulated gastrin response by 67% (Tatsuta et al., 1981). As in patients with duodenal ulcer, basal and meal-stimulated gastrin values increased after 7 days' treatment with pirenzepine 25mg 4 times daily.

A high intravenous dose of pirenzepine 100mg had no effect on already increased serum gastrin levels in patients with pernicious anaemia (Brunner et al., 1977).

Long term treatment with pirenzepine in rats leads to a significant decrease in the number of parietal cells and gastrin cells in the stomach. In contrast, the somatostatin cell population is not affected (Lehy et al., 1978).

1.6 Effect on Gastrointestinal Hormones

Pirenzepine whether administered intravenously, intramuscularly or orally had no significant effect on the secretion of somatostatin, neurotensin, vasoactive intestinal polypeptide (El-Sabbagh et al., 1980a; Heller et al., 1978b), or secretin (Londong, 1980). However, 10mg administered intravenously reduced basal and postprandial levels of enteroglucagon ($p < 0.025$ to 0.05) and basal ($p < 0.05$), but not postprandial, motilin levels (El-Sabbagh et al., 1980a). Like intravenous atropine 1mg and oral cimetidine 400mg, intravenous pirenzepine 20mg did not alter basal levels of gastric inhibitory polypeptide or those stimulated by sham feeding (Arnold et al., 1978).

1.7 Effect on Pancreatic Secretion

In healthy subjects, single doses of pirenzepine 10 and 20mg intravenously (Arnold et al., 1978; El-Sabbagh et al., 1980a), 8mg intramuscularly (Heller et al., 1978b), or 50mg orally (Heller et al., 1978b) did not significantly affect basal or postprandial concentrations of serum insulin or glucagon. In patients with duodenal ulcer, intravenous administration of pirenzepine 20mg and atropine 1 to 1.5mg reduced basal secretion of pancreatic polypeptide and that stimulated by sham feeding (Konturek et al., 1980), reflecting their anticholinergic activity, whereas cimetidine 400mg given orally did not alter secretion of this hormone (Arnold et al., 1978; Konturek et al., 1980).

A single oral dose of pirenzepine 100mg had no effect on the output of trypsin and lipase in one study in 10 healthy subjects (Brunner et al., 1977), but in 10 patients with 'various abdominal disorders', pirenzepine 30mg intravenously decreased secretion of trypsin, lipase, amylase and chymotripsin by 19%, 26%, 44% and 24%, respectively, and increased bicarbonate secretion by 18% (Kuntzen and Kaess, 1978). In a comparative trial, pirenzepine 100mg orally and 20mg intravenously produced an increase in pancreatic bicarbonate secretion (7 and 67%, respectively) less than that with atropine 1mg intravenously (82%). Similarly, the decrease in pancreatic volume was less pronounced with pirenzepine than with atropine (Huchzermeyer, 1978).

1.8 Effect on Gastric Mucus Secretion

Intravenous administration of single doses of pirenzepine 0.15, 0.3 and 0.5 mg/kg/h decreased gastric mucus output by 27%, 33% and 42%, respectively, in 10 duodenal ulcer patients (Sarosiek et al., 1982). Pirenzepine 100mg daily given orally for 4 weeks (Guslandi, 1979) or 6 weeks (Guslandi et al., 1980) did not affect gastric mucin fractions in the gastric juice of patients with duodenal ulcer. In one 6-week comparative trial (Guslandi et al., 1980), the neutral glycoprotein to acid mucoprotein ratio of gastric mucin ('mucoprotective index') was unaltered by pirenzepine 100mg daily, but was reduced significantly ($p < 0.001$) by cimetidine 1000mg daily. Nevertheless, endoscopic ulcer healing rates were similar in this study. Pirenzepine did not alter the content of tyrosine or N-acetylneuraminic acid in gastric mucus in the treatment of duodenal ulcer patients (Molinari et al., 1980), nor did a single 50mg oral dose significantly affect gastric mucus viscosity or sialic acid content under basal conditions or pentagastrin stimulation (Stefenelli, 1978).

1.9 Effect on Pepsin Output

A dose-dependent decrease in pepsin output has been reported in healthy subjects (Cesnik, 1982; Sheers and Roberts, 1982) and in patients with duodenal ulcer (Cesnik, 1982; El-Sabbagh et al., 1980b; Gabryelewicz et al., 1980, 1982; Konturek et al., 1980) following single doses of pirenzepine administered intravenously. As with atropine (Konturek et al., 1980), cimetidine (Brogden et al., 1978) and ranitidine (Brogden et al., 1982), the fall in pepsin output was due mainly to a decrease in volume of gastric secretion rather than to a decrease in pepsin concentration (Konturek et al., 1980). Pirenzepine reduced basal and stimulated secretion of pepsin to a lesser degree than acid secretion when administered intravenously (El-Sabbagh et al., 1980b; Konturek et al., 1980) or orally (Stockbrügger et al., 1983a). As would be expected, vagally stimulated pepsin secretion was inhibited to a greater degree than that stimulated by exogenous agents.

Thus, in healthy subjects, insulin-induced pepsin secretion (a vagally mediated stimulus) was decreased more markedly by pirenzepine than by an equipotent antisecretory dose of ranitidine (49% *vs* 7%; Sheers and Roberts, 1982). However, pirenzepine had a weaker effect than ranitidine against pepsin secretion stimulated by histamine (34% *vs* 79%) and pentagastrin (24% *vs* 83%). In patients with duodenal ulcers or Zollinger-Ellison syndrome who had undergone proximal selective ragotomy, intravenous pirenzepine 40mg produced a more marked reduction in pepsin and pepsinogen output than cimetidine 400mg, although it was not ascertained whether this was statistically significant. In 'hypersecretory' duodenal ulcer patients, pirenzepine 0.15 mg/kg administered intravenously 1 hour after an infusion of ranitidine 0.05 mg/kg/h potentiated the maximum fall in pentagastrin-stimulated pepsin secretion from 63% to 84% (Gabryelewicz et al., 1982).

No data are available on the effects of orally administered pirenzepine on pepsin secretion.

1.10 Effect on Endocrine Function

As with atropine (Levenston and Cryer, 1980), single antisecretory doses in healthy subjects of pirenzepine administered intravenously (Londong et al., 1978, 1981), intramuscularly (Heller et al., 1978b) or orally (Heller et al., 1978b; Masala et al., 1982) generally had no effect on basal secretion of prolactin or that induced by thyrotropin-releasing hormone (Masala et al., 1982). Similarly, in comparative trials, pirenzepine and ranitidine, and their combination, did not alter prolactin secretion (Londong et al., 1981), whereas cimetidine increased it by more than 100% (Londong et al., 1980b). However, in one trial in which endocrine effects were evaluated according to sex, oral pirenzepine 75 and 100mg significantly ($p < 0.01$) reduced serum prolactin concentrations in females by 41 to 51% over the 3-hour period following administration (Masala et al., 1982). In contrast, no changes were noted in male subjects. The long term clinical significance of these differential findings is unclear.

Single doses of pirenzepine 50mg administered orally, and 8mg administered intramuscularly, had no effect on the secretion of growth hormone in 6 healthy subjects (Heller et al., 1978b).

1.11 Effect on Lower Oesophageal Sphincter Pressure

A dose-related decrease in mean lower oesophageal sphincter pressure generally occurred in healthy subjects and patients with dyspepsia following single doses of pirenzepine 10 to 16mg administered intravenously (Erckenbrecht et al., 1982; Pandolfo et al., 1981, 1982), and 0.2 to 0.5 mg/kg administered intramuscularly (Denis et al., 1982; Stacher et al., 1979). Mean lower oesophageal sphincter pressure decreased by 25 to 59%, the number of oesophageal contractions by 44 to 53%, peristaltic amplitude by 29 to 75%, and duration of oesophageal contractions by 8 to 23%. Maximal changes in these parameters occurred 2 to 10 minutes after intravenous injection (when peak plasma pirenzepine concentrations were much higher than that which would be achieved after usual oral doses; see section 2.1), and a return to normal values generally occurred within 50 to 90 minutes. The decrease in the amplitude of oesophageal peristalsis following pirenzepine 10mg intravenously was shorter, but slightly more marked (maximum 75 *vs* 66%) than that occurring after an equipotent antisecretory dose of atropine 0.5mg (Jaup et al., 1982a, 1983). In patients with duodenal ulcer who received pirenzepine by infusion at dosages which maintained plasma concentrations at or below 110 μg/L (Da Broi Gian et al., 1982; Dent et al., 1983), and in healthy subjects in whom serum plateau levels of 51 and 135 μg/L were achieved (Dent, 1984), there was no significant effect on any oesophageal measurement.

Pirenzepine 25 to 75mg daily administered orally had no effect on oesophageal function in healthy subjects (Abrahamsson et al., 1983; Blackwell et al., 1984; Castell et al., 1984; Denis and Galmiche, 1982; Jaup et al., 1983; Lederer et al., 1984), whereas higher doses (100 and 150mg daily) significantly reduced the supine oesophageal peristaltic pressure by 17 and 23% ($p < 0.05$), respectively, in one study (Abrahamsson et al., 1983), increased in two others (Malhotra et al., 1983; Texter et al., 1982, 1984) but had no effect in that of Denis and Galmiche (1982).

1.12 Effect on Intragastric Bacteria and Nitrate

Medium term (6 weeks) treatment of duodenal ulceration with cimetidine 1000mg daily causes intragastric bacterial overgrowth and nitrate formation (Stockbrügger et al., 1982b). Short term administration (4 days) of pirenzepine 100mg daily in healthy subjects did not alter intragastric bacterial counts or nitrate concentration of gastric fluid, whereas these variables were both influenced by benzilonium 70mg daily, which caused a greater inhibition of gastric acid secretion than did pirenzepine (Stockbrügger et al., 1984). The effect on bacterial count and nitrate formation of longer term administration of pirenzepine is not known.

1.13 Toxicity Studies

The histological characteristics of parietal cells were monitored over 4 weeks in 55 patients with duodenal ulcer who received oral pirenzepine 100mg daily or cimetidine 1g daily and attained similar healing rates with each drug (Zangger et al., 1982). Unlike cimetidine treatment, pirenzepine was associated with a moderate reduction in the number of fundic mucosal parietal cells, thickened lamina propria, sparse mitochondria, small or collapsed intracellular canaliculi, and fewer dense-cored vesicles in the oligoaxonal nerve fibre. These ultrastructural changes, which were reversible on stopping treatment, were thought to reflect antimuscarinic-induced depression of parietal cell function. At 6 months, no differences were noted in the structure of the fundic mucosa in patients who had been treated with pirenzepine or cimetidine. In another study (Oleksy et al., 1982) in patients with duodenal ulcer, a lower dosage of oral pirenzepine (50mg daily) for 4 weeks resulted in no significant changes in parietal cell number or morphology.

2. Pharmacokinetic Studies

The pharmacokinetics of single doses of pirenzepine have been studied after intravenous, intramuscular and oral administration in healthy subjects. Steady-state pharmacokinetics have been reported in healthy subjects receiving therapeutic doses of the drug. The pharmacokinetics of pirenzepine in ulcer patients have not been reported.

2.1 Absorption

Peak plasma concentrations of pirenzepine are usually attained 2 to 3 hours after oral administration (fig. 2) and increase linearly with dosage. Thus, in healthy subjects the mean peak plasma concentration was 12 μg/L after a 12.5mg dose (Ohashi et al., 1980) and 24 μg/L (Hammer et al., 1977a) to 32 μg/L (Ohashi et al., 1980) after a single 25mg dose. Mean peak plasma concentrations of 51 to 62 μg/L (Bozler and Hammer, 1980; Ohashi et al., 1980) and 210 μg/L (Ohashi et al., 1980) were attained after oral doses of 50 and 150mg, respectively. In all instances, the higher values were obtained in patients with a low bodyweight (54 to 61kg).

With multiple oral administration of 25 or 50mg 3 times daily for 4 days the plasma concentration increased for the first 3 days but remained constant thereafter (Ohashi et al., 1980). No accumulation of pirenzepine was observed after repeated administration in man (Ohashi et al., 1980) or in animals (Hammer et al., 1977b; Kobayashi et al., 1981).

The mean bioavailability of pirenzepine administered orally as tablets and aqueous solutions is 26% (range, 20 to 30%), as determined by comparing the area under the plasma concentration-time curve (AUC) after intravenous and oral administration (Hammer et al., 1977a). Absorption was said to fall to 10 to 20% when pirenzepine was taken with food, although no 'raw' data were given supporting this (Hammer and Koss, 1978).

After intramuscular injection, pirenzepine is rapidly and completely absorbed from the muscle. The plasma concentration reaches a peak of around

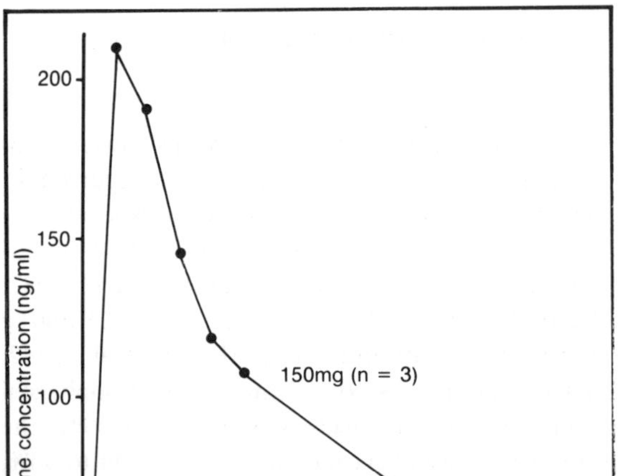

Fig. 2. Mean plasma concentrations of pirenzepine in healthy subjects given 12.5, 25, 50 and 150mg orally (after Ohashi et al., 1980).

90 μg/L 20 minutes after administration of 8mg. About 30 minutes after intramuscular injection the plasma concentration is similar to that attained at the same time after intravenous administration. Thereafter the plasma concentration declines at the same rate after both routes, but is about 20% higher after intramuscular administration (Hammer et al., 1977a).

2.2 Distribution

Audioradiographs in rats and baboons show that pirenzepine is very widely distributed in the body, being found in all internal organs and skeletal muscle, but not the brain (Hammer and Koss, 1979; Kobayashi et al., 1981). It does not readily pass across the placental barrier, no radioactivity having been noted in fetuses.

In healthy volunteers, the apparent volume of distribution of pirenzepine in the central compartment (14L) is equivalent to the extracellular water space, indicating that the drug rapidly equilibrates between the plasma water and extracellular fluids of the peripheral tissues (Hammer et al., 1977a). No information was given on the weights of the patients in this study.

Penetration into the central nervous system is limited (Hammer and Koss, 1979, 1980; Jaup and Blomstrand, 1980). Thus, in 5 volunteers given oral pirenzepine 50mg twice daily for 2 days, mean drug concentrations in serum and cerebrospinal fluid (CSF) were 45 and 4 μg/L, respectively, 2 hours after the last administration (Jaup and Blomstrand, 1980). The low CSF to serum ratio of 1 : 10 is to be expected because of the drug's poor lipid solubility and low plasma protein binding (*vide infra*).

Although no clinical data are available regarding the excretion of pirenzepine into human breast milk, milk to blood pirenzepine ratios in rats were approximately 1 : 10 after a single intravenous dose of 2 mg/kg (Kobayashi et al., 1981).

The extent of protein binding of pirenzepine in human plasma is about 12%, and the fraction bound is independent of plasma drug concentration (Hammer et al., 1977a).

2.3 Elimination

2.3.1 Metabolism and Excretion

Very little pirenzepine is metabolised, irrespective of the route of administration (Hammer et al., 1977a). Thus, within 24 hours after oral administration of radiolabelled pirenzepine 25mg, more than 85% of total radioactivity in the plasma is attributable to the original compound, while the inactive metabolite desmethylpirenzepine accounted for 4% (Hammer et al., 1977a).

Cumulative urinary excretion following administration of single oral doses of pirenzepine 12.5 to 150mg was 7 to 12% over a period of 96 hours (Ohashi et al., 1980). Similarly, Hammer et al. (1977a) reported 10% of a dose excreted unchanged in the urine by 96 hours after oral administration, with 90% being excreted in the faeces. Because of its hydrophilic properties, no tubular reabsorption occurs (Bozler and Hammer, 1980). After either intramuscular or intravenous administration of radiolabelled pirenzepine, 50% of a dose was excreted in the urine and 48% in the faeces over a period of 4 days (Hammer et al., 1977a).

Total plasma clearance (approximately 15 L/h) is low, and renal clearance corresponds with the glomerular filtration rate (Hammer et al., 1977a). Hepatic clearance, mostly biliary excretion, is about 7.5 L/h.

2.3.2 Half-Life

The mean elimination half-life of pirenzepine is 11 hours after single or repeated doses and is not influenced by the dose or route of administration (Bozler and Hammer, 1980; Hammer et al., 1977a; Ohashi et al., 1980).

2.4 Plasma Concentration and Clinical Effects

The relationship between plasma concentrations of pirenzepine and inhibition of gastric acid secretion has been studied in healthy subjects but not in patients with duodenal ulceration. Thus, Mignon et al. (1982) found that the pirenzepine plasma concentrations required for 50% (IC_{50}) and 80% inhibition (IC_{80}) of meal-stimulated gastric acid secretion were 200 and 300 μg/L, respectively. The IC_{50} value was said to be double that of ranitidine tested by these authors under identical conditions. However, as these concentrations have been associated with a bothersome level of dry mouth and blurred vision (Bozler and Hammer, 1980; Texter and Reilly, 1982), plasma pirenzepine concentrations of 70 to 165 μg/L have been suggested as producing optimal inhibition of gastric acid secretion with minimal anticholinergic side effects (Corinaldesi et al., 1982; Da Broi Gian et al., 1982; Huchzermeyer, 1978; Stockbrügger et al., 1977).

Jaup (1982) has predicted from receptor binding data that 70 to 85% of high affinity ('A') receptors for pirenzepine, but only 10% of lower affinity receptors (see section 1.1), will be blocked at a plasma concentration of 50 μg/L.

2.5 Dialysability of Pirenzepine

Pirenzepine is removed from the body by haemodialysis to a minor extent, the drug plasma concentration being decreased by 11 to 15% after a single dialysis session (Herrmann and Kuhlmann, 1978). The authors considered this decrease to be clinically insignificant. Pirenzepine plasma concentrations in 10 renal failure patients in this study remained 34 to 41% higher than drug concentrations in 10 normal control subjects (63 to 87 *vs* 37 to 57 μg/L), but they were not above the suggested therapeutic range (*vide infra*).

3. Therapeutic Trials

The efficacy of oral pirenzepine has been studied predominantly in the treatment and prevention of endoscopically verified duodenal ulcers, or in the treatment of benign gastric ulcers, in outpatients. Almost all such studies included a control group receiving placebo, cimetidine, ranitidine, gefarnate or carbenoxolone. Controlled studies have also been conducted in patients with non-ulcerous dyspepsia such as duodenitis and gastritis, and occasionally in patients with post-gastrectomy ulcers, or with gastric intolerance of non-steroidal anti-inflammatory drugs (NSAIDs). The prevention of gastrointestinal bleeding and stress ulcers has also been studied in a few specialised groups of patients at risk, and a small number of patients with Zollinger-Ellison syndrome have been treated with pirenzepine combined with cimetidine or ranitidine. The usual dosage in most conditions has been 100 mg/day given in 2 divided doses before meals, although dosages of between 50 and 150 mg/day given 2 to 4 times daily have also been studied.

3.1 Treatment of Duodenal Ulcer

Study design is particularly important in evaluating ulcer therapy because of the tendency for ulcer healing to occur spontaneously and to be affected by various patient, environmental and social factors. Placebo response is notably higher in the United States and Switzerland than in Europe in general (Baron, 1982; Wormsley, 1982), thus making it difficult to compare results obtained by investigators in different countries.

Most studies with pirenzepine in patients with duodenal ulcer have compared its efficacy with placebo or cimetidine, usually under double-blind or single-blind conditions over a 4-week period. These trials have been conducted mainly in Europe in outpatients who were advised to continue normal activity and diet, with moderate smoking, alcohol and coffee consumption. Only adequately reported studies in which duodenal ulcers were diagnosed and assessed by endoscopy have been reviewed. Ulcer healing was usually defined as complete re-epithelialisation of the lesion, or complete disappearance of the original ulcer crater with no new ulcers.

Some investigators attempted to check patient compliance, and nearly all reported comparability of treatment groups with regard to age, sex, history of ulcer disease, smoking and some aspects of the current episode such as symptom duration and severity prior to treatment. Comparability of groups within centres of multicentre trials was seldom established.

Supplementary consumption of antacids, if necessary for pain, was usually permitted and was quantified in most studies. While it is unlikely that

Table V. Therapeutic efficacy of pirenzepine (P) compared with that of placebo (pl) in patients with endoscopically verified duodenal ulcers

Reference	No. of patients	Dosage (mg/day)	Duration	Healing rate at completion of the study		Pain relief[a]		Antacids reduced
				pirenzepine	placebo	day	night	
Pirenzepine 50-75 mg/day								
Čerlek et al. (1981)	28	25 × 2	4 weeks	11/15 (73%)[b]	5/13 (39%)	P > pl		
Barbara et al. (1979a)	79	25 × 3 + 25 × 2	7 days + 21 days	23/44 (52%)	12/35 (34%)	P > pl	P > pl	P > pl
Gasbarrini et al. (1979)	21	25 × 3 + 25 × 2	10 days + 20 days	9/12 (75%)	4/9 (44%)	P > pl	P > pl	. . .[c]
Dobrilla et al. (1979)	26	25 × 3 + 25 × 2	7 days + 21 days	5/11 (45%)	8/15 (53%)	P = pl	P = pl	P > pl
Eichenberger et al. (1982)	43	75[d]	4 weeks[e]	11/22 (50%)	12/21 (57%)	P = pl	P = pl	P = pl
Pirenzepine 100-150 mg/day								
Barbara et al. (1979b)	92	100[f]	4 weeks	32/46 (70%)[g]	15/46 (32%)	P ⩾ pl	P = pl	P = pl
Do et al. (1982)	38	25 × 4	6 weeks	14/18 (78%)[h]	7/20 (35%)	P > pl	P > pl	P > pl
Gibinski et al. (1982)	121	50 x 2	4 weeks	45/58 (78%)	32/63 (51%)			
Hoffenberg (1983)	50	50 × 3 + 50 × 2	1 week + 3 weeks	12/25 (48%)	10/25 (40%)	P = pl		P = pl
Bianchi Porro et al. (1982a)	57	150[d]	4 weeks	21/29 (72%)[g]	10/28 (36%)	P > pl	P > pl	P > pl
D'Imperio et al. (1979)	20	50 × 3	4 weeks	9/10 (90%)	5/10 (50%)			
Laugier (1982)	100	50 × 3	4 weeks	31/50 (62%)	15/50 (30%)	P > pl		
Morelli et al. (1979)	29	50 × 3	6 weeks	11/14 (79%)[h]	2/15 (13%)	P > pl		P > pl
Pirenzepine 75 vs 150mg								
Osselladore et al. (1979)	45[i]	25 × 3 50 × 3	4 weeks	9/15 (60%) 13/15 (87%)[g]	6/15 (40%)	$P_{150} > P_{75} = pl$	$P_{150} < P_{75} < pl$	$P_{150} > P_{75} > pl$

a When differences in pain relief occurred they were usually after the first week.
b Statistically significant difference ($p < 0.05$), although report contained some deficiencies, e.g. pretrial group comparability not mentioned.
c Standardised antacid usage for all patients.
d Given in 4 doses with a double dose at bedtime (to preserve double-blind conditions with cimetidine – see table VII).
e Some patients were treated for 8 weeks.
f Given in 3 doses of 25, 25 and 50mg, respectively.
g Statistically significant difference ($p < 0.01$).
h Statistically significant difference ($p < 0.05$).
i Patients had severe duodenal ulcers.

the quantities of antacids consumed would have affected ulcer healing, they may well have influenced pain assessments, hence adding to the unreliability of this symptom as a criterion of efficacy of pirenzepine alone.

3.1.1 Pirenzepine Compared with Placebo

Results from numerous double-blind, randomised, placebo-controlled studies in outpatients with active endoscopically verified duodenal ulcers, indicate that ulcer healing with pirenzepine is dose related. In general, pirenzepine at dosages of 100 to 150 mg/day significantly improves healing rates but smaller doses do not (table V). The difference in healing rates according to dosage is well illustrated in a large multicentre trial in which patients received either the low or high dosage regimen for a period of 4 weeks. Ulcers were healed in 52% of patients treated with pirenzepine 50 to 75mg daily and in 70% of patients treated with 100 to 150mg daily. Placebo response did not vary (34% and 32%) between groups. Although Čerlek et al. (1981) found that significantly more ulcers were healed with pirenzepine 50 mg/day than with placebo (73% *vs* 39%), unfortunately it is not known whether the treatment groups were similar.

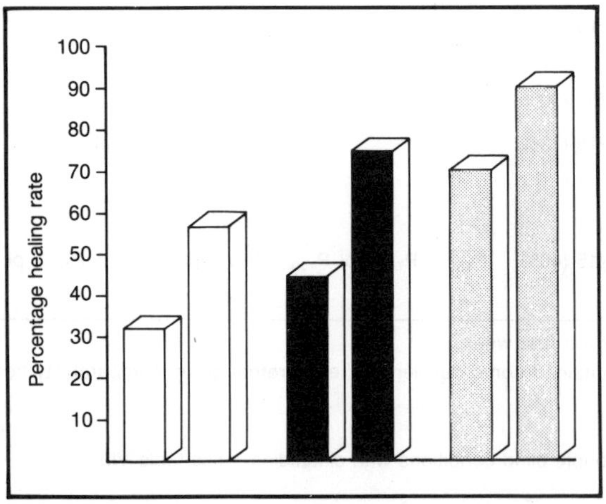

Fig. 3. Range of healing of duodenal ulcers in patients treated with placebo □ and with pirenzepine 50 to 75mg ■ or 100 to 150mg daily ▨ for a period of 4 weeks (for list of references see table V).

Overall, duodenal ulcers usually healed in 32 to 57% of patients taking placebo, in 45 to 75% of those treated with less than 100 mg/day of pirenzepine and in 70 to 90% of patients treated with pirenzepine 100 to 150 mg/day over a 4-week period (fig. 3). A similar conclusion regarding the dose-related efficacy of pirenzepine in the treatment of duodenal ulcer was reached by Texter and Reilly (1982) following statistical analysis of various published studies.

Interestingly, in most studies symptoms such as day and night pain persisted in fewer patients treated with pirenzepine than in those taking placebo (table V). Accordingly, antacid consumption was usually lower in patients treated with pirenzepine than in those receiving placebo.

Several studies comparing pirenzepine with cimetidine also included a placebo control group (Bianchi Porro et al., 1982a; Dobrilla et al., 1980; Eichenberger et al., 1982; Giacosa et al., 1982), but only those conducted under double-blind conditions have been included in table V.

3.1.2 Pirenzepine Compared with Cimetidine

Numerous studies, mostly in outpatients, have determined the relative efficacy and safety of pirenzepine 75 to 100 mg/day and cimetidine 1000 mg/day. Although most studies did not demonstrate a significant difference between healing rates, despite some studies being large enough to be expected to do so if small differences existed, in one double-blind study ulcer healing with cimetidine 1000 mg/day was superior to that with pirenzepine 100 mg/day (*vide infra*).

Important aspects of the design of the studies are summarised in table VI and only results from fully reported trials are discussed in this section of the review.

Owing to the difficulties in achieving and maintaining double-blind conditions for 2 tableted drugs given in different dosage schedules, many studies utilised a 'blind' endoscopist who was unaware of treatment received, thus providing single-blind conditions. Double-blind conditions were achieved in some studies by altering the dosage forms (to capsules) and schedules (to 4 times daily) [e.g.

Table VI. Summary of design of therapeutic trials comparing pirenzepine with cimetidine in patients with endoscopically verified duodenal ulcer

Reference	Double-blind	Single-blind[a]	No. of patients	Comparability of groups[b]	Definition of healing	Compliance checks
Ayoola (1983)		+	0[c]	+	+	+
Bianchi Porro et al. (1982a)	+		0[c]	±[d]	+	±[e]
Brunner (1982; 1984)		+	+	±[d]	0	0
Colley et al. (1982)	+		+	+	+	±[e]
Dobrilla et al. (1980)		+	0[c]	+	+	0
Eichenberger et al. (1982)	+		0[c]	±[d]	0	±[e]
Evreux et al. (1982)			0	±[d,f]	+	0
Fakunle et al. (1983)		+	0[c]	±	±	±[e]
Giorgi-Conciato et al. (1982)			+	±[d, f]	+	0
Guslandi et al. (1980)	+		0[c]	+	+	0
Henry et al. (1982)		+	0[c]	±[d]	–	0
Meunier et al. (1982)	+		0[c]	±[d]	0	+
Paoluzi et al. (1982)	+		+	±[d]	+	0

a Usually achieved by using an endoscopist unaware of treatment.
b Usually compared age, sex, history of ulcer disease, smoking and some aspects of current episode, e.g. duration and/or pretrial symptoms.
c Too few patients to detect any possible small differences between effective drugs.
d Comparability of groups within centres of multicentre trial not established.
e Compliance checked but results not reported.
f Significantly more patients randomly assigned to pirenzepine had a history of relapses (72% *vs* 66%).
Key: + = Adequate, specifically stated; ± = limited, incomplete; 0 = absent, not specifically mentioned, inadequate.

Bianchi Porro et al., 1982a; Eichenberger et al., 1982], but this could produce absorption characteristics *in vivo* which differ from those of the marketed dosage forms. For instance, Eichenberger et al. (1982) commented that serum concentrations of pirenzepine are lower when given in capsule rather than tablet form. As serum pirenzepine concentrations are also lower when the same daily dose is administered in 4 rather than 2 divided doses, the degree of suppression of acid secretion may be decreased during the 4-times-daily regimen.

Other difficulties in comparing these 2 drugs in a 'blind' study are that pirenzepine should be given prior to meals but cimetidine should be taken with meals and 'blindness' could be affected by the anticholinergic side effects of higher doses of pirenzepine. Although Brunner (1982) used the correct schedule, in most studies both drugs were prescribed either before or with meals (except for a bedtime dose).

Results from studies which compared pirenzepine 75 mg/day with cimetidine 1000 mg/day found that duodenal ulcers tended to heal more frequently with cimetidine than with pirenzepine, although statistically significant differences were not achieved, probably because of small patient groups (Dobrilla et al., 1980; Eichenberger et al., 1982).

Within each study, ulcer healing rates were usually similar following 4 or 6 weeks' treatment with pirenzepine 100 to 150 mg/day and cimetidine 1000

Table VII. Summary of studies comparing pirenzepine (P) with cimetidine (C) in patients with endoscopically verified duodenal ulcers

Reference	No. of patients	Dosage (mg/day)	Doses/ day	Healed at 4 weeks		Healed at 6 or 8 weeks		Pain relief		Antacid use
				P	C	P	C	day	night	
Ayoola (1983)	36	P 100 C 1000	2 4	13/17 (77%)	15/19 (80%)	14/17 (82%)[b]	17/19 (90%)[b]	P = C	P = C	. . .[c]
Bianchi Porro et al. (1982a)	57[a]	P 150 C 1000	4 4	21/29 (72%)	21/28 (75%)			P = C	P = C	P = C
Brunner (1982)	254	P 100 C 1000	2 4	81/126 (64%)	94/128 (73%)			P = C		
Colley et al. (1982)	121	P 100 C 1000	3 4			41/58 (71%)[d]	53/63 (84%)[d]	P = C[g]		
Dobrilla et al. (1980)	30	P 75 C 1000	3 4	5/13 (38%)	10/17 (59%)			P = C		P = C
Evreux et al. (1982)	71	P 150 C 1000	3 4	23/35 (71%)	21/36 (58%)				P > C[g]	. . .[c]
Eichenberger et al. (1982)	44[a]	P 75 C 1000	4 4	11/22 (50%)	16/22 (73%)	13/19 (68%)[b]	19/22 (86%)[b]	P = C	P = C	P = C
Fakunle et al. (1983)	30	P 100 C 1000	2 4			11/15 (73%)[d]	10/15 (67%)[d]			P = C
Giorgi-Conciato et al. (1982)	2905[e]	P 100-150[f] C 1000	3 4			742/1423 (52%)[d]	533/935 (57%)[d]	P = C[g]		P = C
Guslandi et al. (1980)	30	P 100 C 1000				9/15 (60%)[d]	8/15 (53%)[d]	P = C		
Henry et al. (1982)	47	P 100 C 1000	2 4	14/22 (64%)	17/25 (68%)	18/22 (82%)	22/25 (88%)	P = C	P = C	P ⩾ C
Meunier et al. (1982)	64	P 150 C 1200	3 4			25/33 (76%)	22/31 (71%)	P > C[g,i]		P > C
Paoluzi et al. (1982)	96	P 100 C 1000	3 4			15/46 (33%)[d]	28/50 (56%)[d]	P ⩽ C[h]		

a In addition, a placebo control group was also studied. See table V for results.
b Response after 8 weeks' treatment.
c Antacids not allowed.
d Response after 6 weeks' treatment.
e Total number of patients studied, but only 2358 were evaluated endoscopically.
f Most patients (82%) took 100 mg/day.
g Not specified as to whether day and/or night pain.
h See comments in section 3.1.2.
i Significantly different during weeks 5 and 6.

mg/day. Results between studies varied however, 52 to 73% of ulcers healing with pirenzepine and 53 to 84% healing with cimetidine (table VII). Paoluzi et al. (1982) demonstrated a significant difference in ulcer healing following 6 weeks' double-blind treatment with pirenzepine 100 mg/day or cimetidine 1000 mg/day. Complete anatomical healing (absence of lesions in the mucosa or wellepithelialised scars) occurred in 33% of 46 pirenzepine-treated patients and in 56% of 50 cimetidine-treated patients ($p < 0.05$), while incomplete healing (presence of residual linear, spotted or irregular erosions with disappearance of the typical ulcer crater) occurred in 35% and 34% of patients, respectively. Although the criteria for complete healing are strict, when disappeared of the ulcer crater with treatment is compared (i.e. complete plus incomplete healing rates), the difference between treatments is still statistically significant (67% *vs* 90%, $p < 0.025$). This study also found that the remission of unspecified symptoms was slower among pirenzepine-treated patients, although the clinical relevance of this observation is difficult to determine, as the comparability of treatment groups regarding initial symptoms was not reported. However, this and most other studies found that by the end of treatment, relief of pain and reduction in antacid consumption did not differ between treatment groups (table VII). Such reductions in antacid consumption were, however, significant only in the large multicentre study reported by Giorgi-Conciato et al. (1982).

Despite being a non-blinded study, results reported by Giorgi-Conciato et al. (1982) are included in table VII because of the very large number of patients (2905) studied. Following 6 weeks' treatment with pirenzepine 100mg (usually) to 150 mg/day or cimetidine 1000 mg/day, there were no clinically or statistically significant differences in endoscopically determined healing rates (52% *vs* 57%). In commenting on the relatively low response to treatment, the authors observed a marked geographical variation in healing rates, in that the number of patients with complete ulcer healing (in either group) was about 50% greater in northern Italy, compared with central and southern Italy.

Initial intravenous administration of pirenzepine 40 mg/day was compared with intravenous cimetidine 800 mg/day in a randomised non-blinded study in 28 hospitalised patients (Mittelstaedt et al., 1981). Following 5 days' intravenous therapy, patients were treated with oral pirenzepine 100 mg/day or cimetidine 1000 mg/day for 23 days. No significant differences in duodenal ulcer healing were detected after 14 or 28 days' treatment in this small study.

3.1.3 Pirenzepine Compared with Other Therapy

A few studies have compared pirenzepine with other drugs used in the treatment of duodenal ulcers, such as ranitidine – another H_2-receptor antagonist (Giacosa et al., 1982; Zangger et al., 1985) – gefarnate, a terpene compound (Ishimori and Yamagata, 1982b; Kohli et al., 1982) and propantheline bromide (Toussaint et al., 1982).

In a non-blinded, randomised study which compared pirenzepine 100 mg/day with ranitidine 300 mg/day and cimetidine 1 g/day, endoscopically verified ulcer healing was similar following 4 weeks' treatment with each drug (80%, 87%, 83% healed, respectively). Symptomatic relief at the end of treatment was also similar in each group of 30 patients, although symptoms (type not specified) resolved faster with ranitidine and cimetidine than with pirenzepine (3, 4, 13 days, respectively). Unfortunately pretrial comparability of treatment groups was not mentioned, neither was ulcer healing defined. Not unexpectedly, the efficacy of all 3 active drugs was significantly better than that with placebo (Giacosa et al., 1982). In another non-blind study in 102 outpatients with duodenal ulcer, endoscopic evidence of healing occurred in 75% (27 of 36) of patients treated with pirenzepine and in 88% (58 of 66) treated with ranitidine. Complete regeneration of the duodenal mucosa occurred more often with pirenzepine (48%) than with ranitidine (10%) [Zangger et al., 1985].

Two double-blind studies conducted in large groups of Japanese patients (130 to 230 per study) found endoscopically verified doudenal ulcer healing with pirenzepine 100 or 125 mg/day was superior to that achieved with gefarnate 300 mg/day after 4, 6 and 8 weeks of therapy. Following 8 weeks' treatment, ulcers healed in 83 to 84% of pirenzepine-treated patients compared with 54 to 67% of those receiving gefarnate ($p < 0.01$) [Ishimori and Yamagata, 1982b, Kohli et al., 1982].

No significant difference in healing rates in patients treated with either pirenzepine 150mg daily

Table VIII. Summary of studies of continuous maintenance treatment with pirenzepine in the prevention of duodenal ulcer recurrence (verified endoscopically)

Reference	Study design[a]	Duration (months)	No. of patients	Treatment[b] (mg/day)	Recurrence rate
Capria et al. (1983)	r	6	60	P 50 C 400	5/20 (25%)[c] 4/20 (20%)[c]
Cheli et al. (1982)	r	6	32	P 50 ...[d]	3/16 (19%) 10/16 (63%)
Cheli and Giacosa (1982)	r	12	47	P 50 R 150	9/23 (39%) 5/24 (21%)
Dal Monte et al. (1982[a])	db, r[e]	12	54	P 100 Placebo	15/26 (58%)[f] 27/28 (96%)
Eichenberger et al. (1982)	r	12	32	P 30 Placebo C 400	4/9 (44%) 8/12 (67%) 6/11 (55%)
Farini et al. (1983)	r	12	30	P 50 C 400	4/15 (27%) 5/15 (33%)
Ireland (1985)	db, r	6	89	P 50 C 400	9/43 (21%) 8/46 (17%)
Moshal et al. (1982)	db, r[g]	12	50	P 100 Placebo C 400	10/16 (62%) 14/17 (82%) 11/17 (65%)
Petrillo and Bianchi Porro (1980)	db, r	12	28	P 50 Placebo	7/15 (47%) 9/13 (69%)

a db = double-blind; r = randomised. Compliance rarely mentioned.
b P = pirenzepine; C = cimetidine.
c Recurrence rate includes patients with duodenal ulcer and/or erosive duodenitis.
d No treatment.
e Groups differed in age (see section 3.2).
f Significant difference ($p < 0.01$).
g Design deficiencies noted by authors: infrequent visits and too few patients.

or propantheline bromide 45mg daily was found by Toussaint et al. (1982). However, anticholinergic side effects occurred more frequently with propantheline.

3.2 Prevention of Duodenal Ulcer Recurrence

Double-blind or non-blinded comparative studies have been conducted with pirenzepine to determine ulcer recurrence rates during prophylactic administration of pirenzepine over 6- to 12-month periods following healing (table VIII).

Endoscopically verified recurrences of duodenal ulcers during low dose maintenance treatment with pirenzepine 30 to 50 mg/day (taken at night or twice daily) did not differ significantly from relapses in placebo-treated or untreated patients (Cheli et al., 1982; Eichenberger et al., 1982; Petrillo and Bianchi Porro, 1980). However, a trend toward a lower relapse rate with pirenzepine was apparent in these studies, and in one study in 47 patients the relapse rate with pirenzepine 50mg daily (39%) was not significantly different from that in patients treated with ranitidine 150mg daily (21%) [Cheli and Giacosa, 1982]. In addition, a significantly lower relapse rate occurred (25% *vs* 65%; $p < 0.01$) when pirenzepine 50mg at night was compared with antacids (liquid aluminium and magnesium compounds) taken when necessary, although the quantity of antacid consumed was not reported in this non-blinded study (Capria et al., 1983).

When a higher maintenance dose (100 mg/day) was used, one double-blind placebo-controlled study found significantly fewer ulcer recurrences with pirenzepine (58% *vs* 96%; Dal Monte et al., 1982a). However, treatment groups were not entirely comparable initially, in that patients randomly assigned to placebo were older than those given pirenzepine (44 *vs* 38 years; $p < 0.05$). However, this age-difference should not have been a confounding factor.

Recurrences rates following treatment with pirenzepine 30 to 100 mg/day or cimetidine 400mg at night did not differ significantly in several small studies (Capria et al., 1983; Eichenberger et al., 1982; Farini et al., 1983; Moshal et al., 1982; Visconti et al., 1983), or in a larger 6-month multicentre trial (Ireland et al., 1985).

In some studies the episode of duodenal ulceration prior to prophylactic therapy had been successfully treated with pirenzepine in all patients (Cheli et al., 1982; Petrillo and Bianchi Porro, 1980), while in other studies various drugs or placebo had been used (Dal Monte et al., 1982a; Eichenberger et al., 1982; Moshal et al., 1982; Visconti et al., 1983). Several authors attempted to correlate relapse rates with previous ulcer treatment (Dal Monte et al., 1982a; Eichenberger et al., 1982), but too few patients have been studied so far for conclusive results.

Additional studies have determined ulcer relapse rates using different treatment regimens from the above (Morelli et al., 1983, 1984; Vezzadini et al., 1982). In a brief preliminary report of a long term double-blind study in 81 patients, Morelli et al. (1983, 1984) indicated that intermittent treatment with pirenzepine 150 mg/day for two 6-week periods in spring and autumn significantly reduced ulcer relapse rates compared with placebo (10 of 21 pirenzepine patients relapsed within 20 months compared with 19 of 21 controls; $p < 0.01$).

In another double-blind study, 31 patients with duodenal ulceration were followed up 6 months after completing a 6-week course of pirenzepine 100 mg/day followed by 50 mg/day for the next 6 weeks, or cimetidine 1 g/day followed by 400 mg/day also given for 6-week periods. Recurrence rates did not differ significantly within 6 months of stopping either treatment (29% recurrence with pirenzepine *vs* 47% with cimetidine) [Vezzadini et al., 1982].

3.3 Treatment of Gastric Ulcer

The efficacy of pirenzepine in the treatment of benign gastric ulcers has been less extensively studied than has duodenal ulceration, and the results are less conclusive, probably because of the lesser role of acid hypersecretion in gastric compared with duodenal ulceration. Various dosages of pirenzepine, ranging from 50 to 150 mg/day, have been compared with placebo, cimetidine 1 g/day, carbenoxolone 200 to 300 mg/day and gefarnate 300 mg/day, usually in double-blind studies in outpatients.

3.3.1 Pirenzepine Compared with Placebo

Pirenzepine and placebo have been compared in outpatients and hospitalised patients with gastric ulcer (Gibiński et al., 1984; Schmid and Blaich, 1978). These studies employed a double-blind, randomised design, with gastric ulcer being verified and assessed endoscopically. Patients with malignant ulcers and those with previous gastric surgery or recent major surgery were usually not admitted to the studies, although in some studies exclusion criteria were not clearly defined.

A carefully conducted and well reported study by Morelli et al. (1979) in 20 outpatients found that gastric ulcer healing with pirenzepine 150 mg/day for 6 weeks was superior to that with placebo (90% *vs* 40%, $p < 0.05$). Pain relief was also significantly better in the pirenzepine group. Laureta and Lim (1981) also reported significantly better ulcer healing following 8 weeks' treatment with pirenzepine 150 mg/day than with placebo, despite pirenzepine-treated patients being older and hav-

Table IX. Summary of studies comparing pirenzepine (P) with cimetidine (Ci) or carbenoxolone (Ca) in outpatients with benign gastric ulcers

Reference	Study design[a]	No. of patients	Treatment (mg/day)	Doses/ day	Duration (weeks)	Healing rate		Pain relief		Antacids reduced
						pirenzepine	control	day	night	
Comparison with cimetidine (Ci)										
Giorgi-Conciato et al. (1982)	nb, r[b]	437	P 100-150 Ci 1000	3 4	6	135/269 (50%)	80/168 (48%)	P = Ci[c]		P = Ci
Comparisons with carbenoxolone (Ca)										
Barbara et al. (1979c)	db, r	21	P 75-50[d] Ca 300-200[d]	3-2 3-2	4	2/11 (18%)	4/10 (40%)	P = Ca	P = Ca	P = Ca
Gasbarrini et al. (1979)	db, r	21	P 75-50[d] Ca 300-200[d]	3-2 3-2	4	7/11 (64%)	7/10 (70%)	P = Ca	P = Ca	...[e]
Oselladore et al. (1979)	db, r	19	P 75 Ca 300	3 3	4	6/10 (60%)	6/9 (67%)	P = Ca	P ≥ Ca	P > Ca

a db = double-blind; nb = non-blinded; r = randomised.
b More patients assigned to pirenzepine had a history of relapses (52% *vs* 42%; $p < 0.05$).
c Not specified whether day or night pain.
d Dosage reduced after first 7 to 10 days' therapy.
e Standard amount of antacid prescribed.

ing a longer history of ulceration than those given placebo.

When a lower dose (50 mg/day) of pirenzepine was studied, ulcer healing was no better than with placebo, although in the report by Čerlek et al. (1981) on such a study, there was no mention of group comparability, healing criteria, or exclusion of malignant ulcers.

Two double-blind studies in hospitalised patients found that significantly more gastric ulcers were healed following 3 or 4 weeks' treatment with pirenzepine 50 or 100 mg/day than with placebo (Gibiński et al., 1982; Schmid and Blaich, 1978). However, since hospitalisation itself can result in healing of gastric ulcers, inpatients should ideally not be included in studies of ulcer healing.

3.3.2 Pirenzepine Compared with Other Therapy

The study design and results from adequately reported comparisons of pirenzepine and cimetidine or carbenoxolone in outpatients with benign gastric ulcers are summarised in table IX. Inclusion and exclusion criteria were similar to those employed in the placebo-controlled studies (see section 3.3.1). Patients were usually requested not to change their diet or normal activity, but to reduce smoking, plus coffee and alcohol consumption. Ulcer healing was normally defined as complete re-epithelialisation of the original ulcer crater without new ulcers or erosions being observed at endoscopy.

A few small studies (Gonvers et al., 1984; Knoblauch et al., 1984; Martínez Ruiz and Rodríguez, 1981; Mittelstaedt et al., 1981) and a large multicentre study (Giorgi-Conciato et al., 1982) have compared gastric ulcer healing in patients treated with pirenzepine or cimetidine. Ulcer healing following 6 weeks' treatment with pirenzepine 100 to 150 mg/day did not differ from that with cimetidine 1000 mg/day in the large non-blinded study reported by Giorgi-Conciato et al. (1982)

[table IX]. Pain and antacid consumption were significantly reduced during the study to a similar extent in both groups. Confirmation of these results in a well-designed study (currently in progress) is awaited. Smaller studies, some of which were available only in abstract form, likewise reported no significant difference in healing rates with pirenzepine 100 to 150mg daily or cimetidine 800mg daily.

Several small double-blind studies have been conducted in Italy comparing pirenzepine with carbenoxolone, a steroid-like compound which is a glycyrrhizinic acid derivative (table IX). In some studies the initial dose of each drug was reduced after the first 7 to 10 days, from 75 to 50 mg/day of pirenzepine or from 300 to 200 mg/day of carbenoxolone. No significant differences in ulcer healing were demonstrated, although the patient numbers involved were too small (table IX) to detect any except marked differences. Ulcer symptoms were usually reduced to a similar extent with both drugs, while in one study fewer supplementary antacid tablets were consumed by pirenzepine-treated patients at weeks 1, 2 and 3 (Oselladore et al., 1979).

Higher doses (100 to 150 mg/day) of pirenzepine are being compared with carbenoxolone, but results have not yet been fully reported (Barbara et al., 1979c; Bianchi Porro et al., 1982b).

Pirenzepine 75 to 150 mg/day was found to be superior to gefarnate 300 mg/day in 2 large double-blind studies conducted in Japan (Ishimori and Yamagata, 1982a; Miyoshi et al., 1980). Endoscopically confirmed gastric ulcer healing occurred in 71% and 51% ($p < 0.01$) of a total of 310 hospital inpatients and outpatients treated with pirenzepine 150 mg/day or gefarnate 300 mg/day, respectively, for 8 weeks. Significant differences in healing rates were evident both in inpatients (about two-thirds of the total) and in outpatients (Ishimori and Yamagata, 1982a).

3.4 Non-Ulcerous Dyspepsia

Controlled studies in patients with non-ulcerous dyspepsia, duodenitis, gastritis and gastroduodenitis have compared pirenzepine 50 to 150 mg/day with placebo or cimetidine 1 g/day (table X). Inclusion and exclusion criteria varied from study to study and could have influenced results. For instance, the use of antacids either as a standard dose (Gasbarrini et al., 1979), or as necessary (Giorgi-Conciato et al., 1982), could well affect the response rate assessed by symptomatic relief.

In a well-reported double-blind study (Dal Monte et al., 1982b), pirenzepine 100 mg/day was superior to placebo in eliminating symptoms (58% compared with 19%) and in improving the endoscopic appearance of the gastric or duodenal mucosa ($p < 0.001$) in 40 patients with non-ulcerous dyspepsia.

Interestingly, Fedeli et al. (1983) reported that neither pirenzepine nor cimetidine improved the histological appearance of the gastric mucosa despite endoscopic evidence of improvement. Studies to date comparing pirenzepine with cimetidine are limited by design deficiencies such as small patient groups or lack of blinding, and large variation in size of drug treatment groups (table X).

3.5 Zollinger-Ellison Syndrome

When Zollinger-Ellison syndrome is not adequately controlled medically with an H_2-histamine receptor antagonist alone, addition of an antimuscarinic agent to block another type of receptor involved in gastric acid secretion constitutes rational therapy. Hence, pirenzepine in combination with cimetidine or ranitidine has been used to treat a few patients with Zollinger-Ellison syndrome (Bonfils et al., 1979; Collen et al., 1982; Londong et al., 1982b; Mignon et al., 1980). Some cases had been unsatisfactorily treated with cimetidine alone (Mignon et al., 1980) or had experienced severe side effects with other anticholinergics (Collen et al., 1982).

Results from these preliminary studies indicate that symptoms were usually alleviated and/or gastric acid secretion further reduced (section 1.3.2) following short term parenteral administration of pirenzepine 72 mg/day and cimetidine 2.4 to 3.2 g/day to acute cases prior to total gastrectomy, and

Table X. Summary of studies comparing 4 weeks' treatment with pirenzepine (P), placebo (pl), cimetidine (C) or ranitidine (R) in patients with non-ulcerous dyspepsia

Reference	Condition	Study design[a]	No. of patients	Treatment (mg/day)	Endoscopic improvement	Clinical improvement		
						dyspepsia	day pain	night pain
Comparisons with placebo								
Dal Monte et al. (1982b)	Dyspepsia[b]	db, r	40	P 100 Placebo	P > pl	P > pl	P > pl	P = pl
Evreux and Jacquet (1984)	Oesophagitis	db, r	50	P 150 Placebo	P > pl	P > pl		
Hradsky and Wikander (1982)	Dyspepsia	db, r	48	P 50 Placebo	P > pl			
Gasbarrini et al. (1979)	Gastroduodenitis	db, r	55	P 75-50[c,d] Placebo[d]	P > pl	P > pl	P > pl	P > pl
Comparisons with cimetidine								
Fedeli et al. (1983)	Duodenitis	sb, r	35	P 100 C 1000	P = C	P = C		
	Gastritis - erosive or congestive	sb, r	23	P 100 C 1000	P = C	P ≥ C		
Giorgi-Conciato et al. (1982)	Duodenitis	nb	377[e]	P 100-150[f] C 1000[f]	P = C	P = C	P = C[g]	
	Gastritis	nb	426[e]	P 100-150[f] C 1000[f]	P = C	P = C	P = C[g]	
	Gastroduodenitis	nb	608[e]	P 100-150[f] C 1000[f]	P = C	P = C	P = C[g]	
Comparison with ranitidine								
Guslandi and Del Soldato (1984)	Erosive duodenitis	db, r	55	P 100 R 300	P > R	P = R	P = R	P = R

a db = double-blind; nb = non-blinded; r = randomised; sb = single-blind.
b Includes patients with 'chronic' (lasting for at least 3 months) epigastric pain temporally related to eating and relieved by food, milk or antacids and abnormal gastric or duodenal mucosa but no ulcerative or erosive lesions on endoscopy.
c Pirenzepine 75 mg/day for 10 days, followed by 50 mg/day for 20 days.
d All patients were also prescribed aluminium-magnesium hydroxide 400mg 4 times daily.
e Only about 20% of patients were treated with cimetidine.
f Supplementary antacid consumption was permitted (and measured).
g Not specified whether day or night pain.

following longer term (up to 6 months) oral administration of pirenzepine 75 to 125 mg/day plus cimetidine 1.8 to 7.2 g/day (Collen et al., 1982) or ranitidine 300 to 600 mg/day (Londong et al., 1982b). However, detailed data on more patients are required to clearly determine the efficacy and safety of such treatment.

3.6 Treatment and Prevention of Other Conditions

A few open and controlled studies have been conducted using pirenzepine to treat various other conditions such as postgastrectomy ulcers (Giorgi-Conciato et al., 1982), acute gastroduodenal haemorrhage (Fuentes del Toro et al., 1983; Höllerl, 1982; Höllerl et al., 1982) and gastric intolerance in patients receiving non-steroidal anti-inflammatory drugs (Adjan, 1979; Bach, 1980; Miehlke, 1980).

Use of pirenzepine in the prevention of recurrent bleeding from gastroduodenal lesions (Londong et al., 1982a) and the prevention of gastrointestinal bleeding and stress ulcers in polytraumatised or septic patients (Kelleher et al., 1984; Mattes et al., 1980; More et al., 1984; Tryba et al., 1983, 1984) or following severe head injuries or brain surgery (Klein and Deeg, 1982; Tritthart and Heppner, 1982), has also been reported recently. Tryba et al. (1983) conducted an analysis of risk factors for stress bleeding in 420 traumatised patients who received prophylactic treatment with cimetidine 800 or 1200mg daily intravenously, pirenzepine 30mg daily intravenously or oral antacids 2-hourly, alone or in different combinations. The incidence of bleeding, which correlated directly with the total risk score, was lower with combined therapy (cimetidine 1200mg plus pirenzepine and/or antacids) than with single-drug medication. In a later communication (Tryba et al., 1984) pirenzepine 50mg intravenously plus either cimetidine 2000mg intravenously or oral antacids 2-hourly appeared to be similarly effective in preventing stress ulcer bleeding. Combined treatment with pirenzepine 90mg daily intravenously and ranitidine 600mg daily by the same route was more effective than either drug alone at these dosages in preventing stress ulceration (More et al., 1984). While pirenzepine appeared to be beneficial in the treament or prevention of the above conditions, further data are required before conclusions can be drawn regarding the appropriateness of such therapy.

4. Side Effects

In short term controlled studies pirenzepine was tolerated well by most patients and seldom discontinued (2%) because of adverse effects. Dry mouth (14%), blurred vision (2%), constipation (3%), diarrhoea (3%), headache (2%) and mental confusion (1.5%) were the most frequently reported side effects. Hence, although pirenzepine was shown to have selective antimuscarinic effects in pharmacodynamic studies (see section 1.2), some antimuscarinic effects have occurred in patients treated with an effective dosage of 100 to 150 mg/day.

Most of the side effect data were obtained from a large multicentre post-marketing trial conducted in Italy (Giorgi-Conciato et al., 1982). Approximately 3300 patients with peptic ulcer or non-ulcerous diseases were treated with pirenzepine 100 to 150 mg/day for 4 to 6 weeks, during which time they were questioned with the aid of a checklist about specific effects. Thus, the incidence of side effects may be somewhat higher than in studies in which side effects were volunteered. The usual laboratory parameters were also monitored.

This non-blinded study included 1600 patients treated with cimetidine 1 g/day. Although differences in side effects were found between pirenzepine- and cimetidine-treated patients, the authors also reported that the incidences of cimetidine-related side effects elicited by direct questioning were higher than have been previously reported instudies where side effects were volunteered.

4.1 Adverse Clinical Effects

By far the most frequently reported side effect during treatment with pirenzepine 100 to 150 mg/day was dry mouth, which occurred in about 14% of patients. This was usually of mild (8%) to moderate (4%) severity, necessitating withdrawal of treatment in only 0.5% of patients. Although the overall incidence of this effect increased only slightly with increasing dose (table XI), the number of severe episodes doubled (1.1% *vs* 2.9%) and the effect occurred earlier with the higher dosage. Giorgi-Conciato et al. (1982) also reported that the incidence of dry mouth was higher in patients with reduced renal or hepatic function, as determined by blood urea nitrogen, creatinine and total bilirubin tests.

Blurred vision, another antimuscarinic effect of pirenzepine, was experienced by 1% of patients taking 100 mg/day and 5.6% of those on 150 mg/

Table XI. Percentage incidence of the most frequent adverse reactions with pirenzepine 100 mg/day (in 2881 patients) or 150 mg/day (in 448 patients) [after Giorgi-Conciato et al., 1982]

Adverse reaction	Incidence (%) with pirenzepine	
	100 mg/day	150 mg/day
Dry mouth	13.2	16.7
Blurred vision	1.1	5.6
Diarrhoea	3.4	3.8
Constipation	3.3	3.4
Headache	2.1	1.3
Mental confusion	1.6	0.5

day. Treatment was discontinued in 0.2 and 1.1% of the respective dosage groups (Giorgi-Conciato et al., 1982).

The clinical effect of pirenzepine on the gastrointestinal tract relative to its selective antimuscarinic action is unclear, as a similar proportion of patients reported constipation (3.3%) and diarrhoea (3.4%) upon questioning (Giorgi-Conciato et al., 1982). In this study, the authors observed a direct relationship between supplementary antacid intake and diarrhoea during the first week of treatment with pirenzepine 100 to 150 mg/day or cimetidine 1 g/day. However, Ishimori and Yamagata (1982a) reported a higher incidence of constipation (5.3%) than diarrhoea (1.3%) in 151 patients treated with pirenzepine 150 mg/day but no antacids. Only 0.5% of patients stopped treatment because of adverse gastrointestinal effects (Giorgi-Conciato et al., 1982).

Some central nervous system effects such as headache (1.9%) and mental confusion (1.5%) have been reported with pirenzepine, but rarely (0.4%) resulted in termination of treatment (Giorgi-Conciato et al., 1982).

Other infrequently reported adverse effects ($\leqslant$ 1%) include allergic skin reactions (Barbara et al., 1979b; Giorgi-Conciato et al., 1982), genitourinary effects (Barbara et al., 1979b; Giorgi-Conciato et al., 1982; Ishimori and Yamagata, 1982a), and appetite stimulation in both healthy subjects and patients (Einig, 1977; Schmid and Blaich, 1978).

Heart rate, blood pressure and bodyweight usually remained unchanged with low dosages of pirenzepine (< 100 mg/day) [Barbara et al., 1979a; Gasbarrini et al., 1979; Oselladore et al., 1979], and following higher dosages (Barbara et al., 1979b) in the few patients on whom this information was provided. However, in one double-blind study, tachycardia was reported (but no quantitative data provided) in 3 patients (12%) receiving pirenzepine and in 1 patient (4%) receiving placebo (Hoffenberg, 1983).

In general, increasing the dosage from 100 to 150 mg/day did not appear to increase the incidence of the most frequently reported side effects, other than blurred vision (table XI). Unfortunately, it is not possible to compare these results with those obtained from other, small studies using lower dosages and other methods of data collection. However, the incidence and type of side effects, except dry mouth, tended to be similar following either placebo or less than 100 mg/day of pirenzepine (Barbara et al., 1979a; Eichenberger et al., 1982; Gasbarrini et al., 1979).

When pirenzepine 100 to 150 mg/day and cimetidine 1 g/day were compared, the incidence of some side effects such as headache, dizziness, endocrine and allergic skin reactions was slightly but statistically significantly greater with cimetidine (fig. 4). The relative incidences of dry mouth and blurred vision were not reported in this study, although in another study (Brunner, 1982) both effects tended to occur more often with pirenzepine 100 mg/day, as would be expected. A preliminary report by Colley et al. (1982) indicated that adverse effects were more common with pirenzepine 100 mg/day than cimetidine 1 g/day ($p < 0.001$), but the nature of the side effects with these drugs was not specified.

Longer term studies (up to 12 months) with pirenzepine 50 to 100 mg/day in the prevention of duodenal ulcer recurrence in small groups of patients have not reported any clinically significant adverse effects (Capria et al., 1983; Cheli et al.,

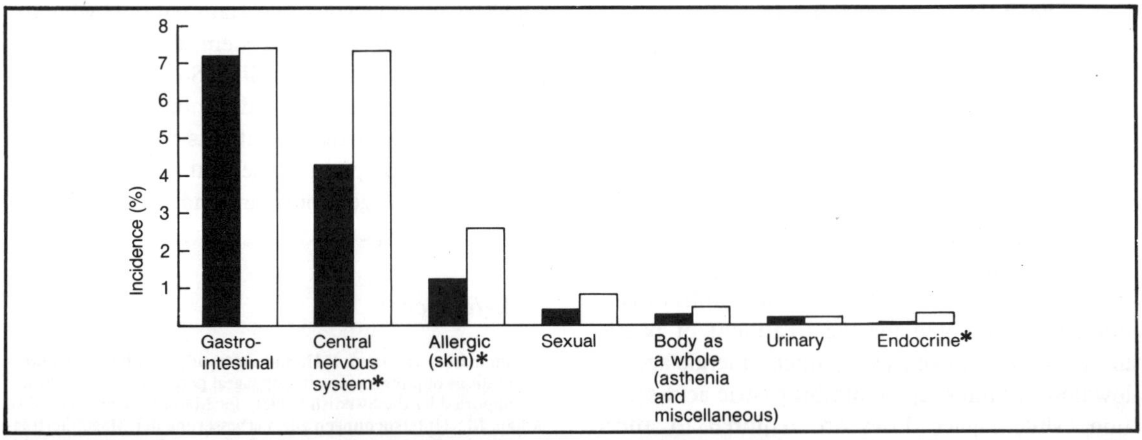

Fig. 4. Relative incidence of adverse effects (upon questioning) with pirenzepine (■) 100 to 150 mg/day in 3335 patients and cimetidine (□) 1 g/day in 1598 patients in a non-blinded study (data after Giorgi-Conciato et al., 1982). Also see section 4.1 regarding dry mouth and blurred vision.
* Significant difference between treatments ($p < 0.05$).

1982; Dal Monte et al., 1982a; Farini et al., 1983; Moshal et al., 1982; Petrillo and Bianchi Porro, 1980).

4.2 Abnormal Laboratory Tests

A detailed analysis of the usual laboratory parameters before and after short term treatment with pirenzepine 100 to 150 mg/day or cimetidine 1 g/day in a large number of patients showed only occasional deviations from the normal range in red and white blood cell counts, creatinine, blood urea nitrogen, total bilirubin and serum glutamic oxaloacetic or pyruvic transaminases [SGOT, SGPT (AST, ALT)]. 'Slight' increases occurred mainly in blood urea nitrogen (1.3 to 1.9% of patients) while more marked increases occurred in AST and/or ALT (0.1 to 0.5%) in both treatment groups.

Interestingly, red blood cell counts improved, together with ulcer healing or improvement, in 70% of patients who had very low pretreatment counts (< 3.5 million/μl) [Giorgi-Conciato et al., 1982]. Laboratory abnormalities were very rarely reported in individual studies which included such tests (e.g. Barbara et al., 1979a).

In duodenal ulcer patients, pirenzepine and atropine reduced potassium concentration in gastric juice by 40 to 45%, in contrast to cimetidine, which did not affect this measurement (Fritsch et al., 1980; Scholten et al., 1982a). Conventional anticholinergics, at dosages that suppress gastric acid secretion, also suppress electrolyte content of gastric juice (Piper and Steel, 1961). The clinical importance of this is doubtful, as serum potassium concentrations were not altered.

5. *Dosage and Administration*

The usual oral adult dosage of pirenzepine in the treatment of duodenal or benign gastric ulceration is 100mg daily in divided doses at bedtime and in the morning before meals. In more severe cases the total daily dose may be increased to 150mg in 2 divided doses. Treatment should be continued until ulcer healing occurs, or if endoscopic reassessment is not possible, then continued for 4 to 8 weeks.

The presence of malignant gastric neoplasm should be excluded before treating symptoms of gastric ulceration with pirenzepine.

Unlike previously available anticholinergic agents used in the treatment of peptic ulceration, pirenzepine is not contraindicated in glaucoma and prostatic hypertrophy.

6. The Role of Pirenzepine in Peptic Ulcer Disease

Anticholinergic agents have been accepted therapy for peptic ulcer disease for several decades, particularly before the development of histamine H_2-antagonists, although effective therapeutic dosing was often limited by secondary effects (Ivey, 1975; Littman and Pine, 1975; Londong, 1982). To date, pirenzepine is the first selective antimuscarinic agent promoted for the treatment of peptic ulcer disease. Unlike classic anticholinergic agents, low doses of pirenzepine inhibit gastric acid secretion, while higher doses are required to affect cardiovascular, ocular and urinary function, salivation and gastrointestinal motility. The efficacy of pirenzepine and the classic antimuscarinic propantheline bromide was comparable in peptic ulcer disease but pirenzepine had fewer anticholinergic side effects, thus confirming that pirenzepine is a relatively selective inhibitor of muscarinic receptors.

Numerous placebo-controlled trials, predominantly in outpatients with duodenal ulcers, have demonstrated that pirenzepine in daily doses of 100 to 150mg is effective in promoting healing of ulcers and in alleviating symptoms. Whether long term therapy will minimise ulcer recurrence has yet to be clearly demonstrated, but results from preliminary studies indicate that this is an area worthy of careful investigation. To date there are no studies of pirenzepine in patients with duodenal ulcer that did not heal during treatment with the H_2-receptor antagonists.

Pirenzepine is superior to gefarnate in the treatment of duodenal and benign gastric ulcers, and appears to be similar in efficacy to cimetidine in treating duodenal ulcers. Pirenzepine may be usefully combined with cimetidine or ranitidine, as this appears to potentiate the antisecretory effects of these latter drugs. Such combinations may also be of value in preventing stress-induced acute upper gastrointestinal bleeding and in the treatment of hypersecretory states.

As the side effect profile of pirenzepine differs somewhat from that of cimetidine, pirenzepine could be advantageous in certain patients who are prone to central nervous system, endocrine or allergic reactions with cimetidine. Some typical antimuscarinic side effects (e.g. dry mouth and blurred vision) have occurred in patients treated with effective doses of pirenzepine, but others (such as gastrointestinal, genitourinary and cardiac effects) were seldom reported.

References

Abrahamsson, H.; Jaup, B.H. and Dotevall, G.: Effects of different doses of pirenzepine on esophageal peristalsis in man. Study supported by the Swedish Society for Medical Sciences (1983).

Adjan, M.: Untersuchungen zur Verbesserung der Magenuerträglichkeit nichtsteroidaler Antiphlogistika. Therapiewoche 29: 5931-5932 (1979).

Arnold, R.; Ebert, L.; Koof, H. and Creutzfeldt, W.: Effect of atropine, pirenzepine and cimetidine on the secretion stimulated by sham-feeding of gastrin, pancreatic polypeptide and gastric inhibitory polypeptide. Paper presented at the First International Pirenzepine Symposium, Schwarzwald, Nov 10-11 (1978).

Ayoola, E.A.: Pirenzepine in duodenal ulcer: A double-blind controlled clinical trial in Nigerians. Current Therapeutic Research 33: 1029-1033 (1983).

Bach, G.L.: Beseitigung der unter Antiphlogistakatherapie auftretenden gastrointestinalen Nebenwirkungen durch Pirenzepin. Therapiewoche 30: 5960-5967 (1980).

Baldi, F.; Ferrarini, F.; Cassan, M.; Brunetti, G.; Borioni, D. and Miglioli, M.: Effect of pirenzepine on colonic motility in man. Current Therapeutic Research 33: 802-806 (1983a).

Baldi, F.; Ferrarini, F.; Cassan, M.; Brunetti, G.; Borioni, D. and Miglioli, M.: Pirenzepine inhibits prostigmine stimulated sigmoid motility in normal subjects (abstract). Gastroenterology 84 (Part 2): 1097 (1983b).

Barbara, L.; Belsasso, E.; Bianchi Porro, G.; Blasi, A.; Caenazzo, E. et al.: Pirenzepine in duodenal ulcer. A multicentre double-blind controlled clinical trial I. Scandinavian Journal of Gastroenterology 14 (Suppl. 57): 11-15 (1979a).

Barbara, L.; Belsasso, E.; Bianchi Porro, G.; Blasi, A.; Caenazzo, E. et al.: Pirenzepine in duodenal ulcer. A multicentre double-blind controlled clinical trial II. Scandinavian Journal of Gastroenterology 14 (Suppl. 57): 17-19 (1979b).

Barbara, L.; Belsasso, E.; Blasi, A.; Caenazzo, E.; Di Febo, G. et al.: Pirenzepine and carbenoxolone in gastric ulcer. Preliminary results of a multicentre double-blind controlled clinical trial. Scandinavian Journal of Gastroenterology 14 (Suppl. 57): 21-24 (1979c).

Baron, J.H.: Panel discussion. Scandinavian Journal of Gastroenterology 17 (Suppl. 80): 52 (1982).

Baumeister, M.: Comparative studies on the mutagenicity of pirenzepine with submammalian/bacterial and mammalian systems. Toxicology and Applied Pharmacology 54: 384-391 (1980).

Beld, A.J.; Van den Hoven, S.; Wouterse, A.C. and Zegers, M.A.P.: Are muscarinic receptors in the central and peripheral nervous system different? European Journal of Pharmacology 30: 360-363 (1975).

Bernardini, C.; Martinotti, E.; Del Tacca, M.; Soldani, G. and Bertelli, A.: Gastric cytoprotection by pirenzepine: Role of endogenous catecholamines. International Journal of Tissue Reactions 6 (2): 175 (1984).

Bertoglio, S.; Anfossi, A.; Arnulfo, G.; Valentini, P. and Berti Riboli, E.: Effect of pirenzepine on L-amino acids stimulated gastric acid secretion and serum gastrin levels in peptic ulcer disease in men. Scandinavian Journal of Gastroenterology 17 (Suppl. 72): 179-184 (1982).
Bianchi Porro, G.; Dal Monte, P.R.; Petrillo, M.; Giuliana Piccari, G.; D'Imperio, N. and Daniotti, S.: Pirenzepine *versus* cimetidine in duodenal ulcer. A double-blind, placebo-controlled, short-term clinical trial. Digestion 23: 110-115 (1982a).
Bianchi Porro, G.; Dobrilla, G.; Mazzacca, G.; De Pretis, G.; Sabbatini, F. and Prada, A.: Pirenzepine *vs* carbenoxolone for gastric ulcer. A double-blind trial. (Abstract no. 617.) Scandinavian Journal of Gastroenterology 17 (Suppl. 78): 155 (1982b).
Bianchi Porro, G.; Lazzaroni, M.; Mazzetti, A. and Daniotti, S.: Effects of pirenzepine, atropine and placebo on sham feeding-stimulated gastric secretion and serum gastrin in healthy volunteers and duodenal ulcer and vagotomised patients. Abstract of paper presented at the 2nd World Conference on Clinical Pharmacology and Therapeutics, July-August (1983).
Bianchi Porro, G.; Prada, A.; Parente, F.; Sangaletti, O. and Lazzaroni, M.: The effect of pirenzepine on meal-stimulated gastric acid secretion, gastrin release and gastric emptying. Scandinavian Journal of Gastroenterology 17 (Suppl. 72): 159-162 (1982c).
Bianchi Porro, G.; Prada, A.; Petrillo, M. and Grossi, M.: Inhibition of pentagastrin and insulin-stimulated gastric secretion by pirenzepine in healthy and duodenal ulcer subjects. Scandinavian Journal of Gastroenterology 14 (Suppl. 57): 63-67 (1979).
Birdsall, N.J.M.; Burgen, A.S.V.; Hammer, R.; Hulme, E.C. and Stockton, J.: Pirenzepine – A ligand with original binding properties to muscarinic receptors. Scandinavian Journal of Gastroenterology 15 (Suppl. 66): 1-4 (1980a).
Birdsall, N.J.M.; Hulme, E.C. and Burgen, A.: The character of the muscarinic receptors in different regions of the rat brain. Proceedings of the Royal Society of London 207: 1-12 (1980b).
Bixquert, M.; Rodrigo, J.M.; Crespo, M.; Garrigues, V.; Aparisi, L. et al.: Effect of pirenzepine on caffeine stimulated acid gastric secretion in patients with duodenal ulcer. (Abstract no. 452.) Scandinavian Journal of Gastroenterology 17 (Suppl. 78): 114 (1982).
Blackwell, J.N.; Dalton, C.B. and Castell, D.O.: Pirenzepine – a unique 'anticholinergic' on the esophagus. (Abstract.) Gastroenterology 86 (5) Part 2: 1029 (1984).
Bonfils, S.; Mignon, M. and Gratton, J.: Cimetidine treatment of acute and chronic Zollinger-Ellison syndrome. World Journal of Surgery 3: 597-604 (1979).
Bonfils, S.; Vatier, J.; De Mestier, P.; Accary, J.-P.; Kuan, T. and Bourgeois, M.: Pirenzepine inhibits meal-induced secretory and gastrin responses in dogs. Gastroenterologie Clinique et Biologique 6: 33-37 (1982).
Bozler, G. and Hammer, R.: An international pharmacokinetic study on pirenzepine following a single oral dose. Scandinavian Journal of Gastroenterology 15 (Suppl. 66): 27-33 (1980).
Brogden, R.N.; Carmine, A.A.; Heel, R.C.; Speight, T.M. and Avery, G.S.: Ranitidine: A review of its pharmacology and therapeutic use in peptic ulcer disease and other allied diseases. Drugs 24: 267-303 (1982).
Brogden, R.N.; Heel, R.C.; Speight, T.M. and Avery, G.S.: Cimetidine: A review of its pharmacological properties and therapeutic efficacy in peptic ulcer disease. Drugs 15: 93 (1978).
Brömster, D.; Carlberger, G.; Lundh, G.; Möller, J. and Rosén, A.: The effect of some oral anticholinergics on gastric emptying, pH and osmolarity in man. Scandinavian Journal of Gastroenterology 4: 185-192 (1969).
Bron, B. and Infante, F.: Pirenzepin: Ein wirksamer Hemmer der Magensekretion mit einer den Histamin-H_2-Rezeptorenblockern uberlegenen Wirkungsdauer. Paper presented at Forum de Recherche de Toulouse, Oct 13 (1978).
Brown, D.A. and Adams, P.R.: Muscarinic suppression of a novel voltage-sensitive K^+ current in a vertebrate neurone. Nature 283: 673-676 (1980).
Brown, D.A.; Forward, A. and March, S.: Antagonist discrimination between ganglionic and ileal muscarinic receptors. British Journal of Pharmacology 71: 362-364 (1980).
Browning, J.G. and Heathcote, B.U.: A comparison of pirenzepine and cimetidine inhibition of centrally-mediated gastric acid and pepsin secretion in the gastric-fistula cat. Archives Internationales de Pharmacodynamie et de Therapie 263: 288-296 (1983).
Browning, J.G. and Henman, F.D.: Peripheral ganglia – new ideas concerning possible sites of action for gastric antisecretory agents. Journal of Physiology 341: 68P (1983).
Brunner, H.: Pirenzepine and cimetidine in the treatment of peptic ulcer. Scandinavian Journal of Gastroenterology 17 (Suppl. 72): 207-209 (1982).
Brunner, H.; Dittrich, H.; Kratochvil, P.; Brandstätter, G.; Hentschel, E.; Schütze, K. et al.: Treatment of duodenal ulcer with pirenzepine and cimetidine. Gut 25: 206 (1984).
Brunner, H.; Veritá, M.; Polterauer, P. and Grabner, G.: Effect of pirenzepine, a new gastric acid-inhibiting agent on exocrine pancreatic secretion in man. Arzneimittel-Forschung 27: 684-687 (1977).
Brunner, H.; Winter, M. and Grabner, G.: Pattern of gastric acid secretion after intravenous injection of pirenzepine and cimetidine. Paper presented at the First International Pirenzepine Symposium, Schwarzwald, Nov 10-11 (1978).
Burgen, A.S.V.; Hiley, C.R. and Young, J.M.: The binding of (^{3}H)-propylbenzilycholine mustard by longitudinal muscle strips from guinea pig small intestine. British Journal of Pharmacology 50: 145-151 (1974).
Capria, A.; Bresci, G.; Polloni, A.; Rindi, G.; Geloni, M. and Del Tacca, M.: Pirenzepine in long term therapy for duodenal ulcer. International Journal of Clinical Pharmacology, Therapy and Toxicology 21: 422-424 (1983).
Castell, D.O.; Blackwell, J.N. and Dalton, C.B.: Pirenzepine: a unique 'antichinergic' on the esophagus. Paper presented at the International Gastroenterology Congress, Lisbon, Sep (1984).
Čerlek, S.; Papa, B.; Katičić, M.; Čolić-Curlje, V. and Mielenz, H.: Pirenzepine in gastric and duodenal ulcer: A double-blind trial. Journal of International Medical Research 9: 148-151 (1981).
Cesnik, H.: Pepsinogen in gastric juice, blood, and urine after proximal selective vagotomy, pirenzepine, and cimetidine. Paper presented at Conference on Pirenzepine, Stockholm, Jun 17 (1982).
Cheli, R. and Giacosa, A.: Prevention of duodenal ulcer relapses by means of long-term treatment with pirenzepine or ranitidine at low doses; in Dotevall (Ed.) Advances in Gastroenterology with the Selective Antimuscarinic Pirenzepine. Proceedings of the Stockholm Symposium, June 1982, pp. 246-250 (Excerpta Medica, Amsterdam 1982).
Cheli, R.; Giacosa, A. and Molinari, F.: Long term treatment of duodenal ulcer with pirenzepine. Scandinavian Journal of Gastroenterology 17 (Suppl. 72): 221-224 (1982).
Chierichetti, S.M.; Gaetani, M. and Petrin, G.: Pirenzepine in peptic ulcer. Introduction to clinical trials reports. Scandinavian Journal of Gastroenterology 14 (Suppl. 57): 7-10 (1979).
Collen, M.J.; Pandol, S.J.; Raufman, J.-P.; Allende, H.D.; Bissonnette, B.M. et al.: Beneficial effects of pirenzepine, a selective anticholinergic agent, in patients with Zollinger-Ellison syndrome. Gastroenterology 52 (par. 2): 1035 (1982).
Colley, S.; Howard, O.M.; Trotman, I.; Jarvis, L.; Chapman, R.; Jewell, C. et al.: A controlled trial of pirenzepine and cimetidine in the treatment of duodenal ulcer. (Abstract no. 398.) Scandinavian Journal of Gastroenterology 17 (Suppl. 78): 100 (1982).
Corinaldesi, R.; Galassi, A.; Giorgi-Conciato, M.; Hammer, R.;

Calamelli, R. and Barbara, L.: Effects of therapeutic doses of pirenzepine on the gastric emptying of a mixed meal: A double-blind crossover study; in Dotevall (Ed.) Advances in Gastroenterology with the Selective Antimuscarinic Compound Pirenzepine. Proceedings of the Stockholm Symposium, June 1982, pp. 58-63 (Excerpta Medica, Amsterdam 1982).

Corinaldesi, R.; Miglioli, M.; Daniotti, S.; Stanghellini, V.; Borghi, E. and Barbara, L.: Inhibition by pirenzepine of nocturnal acid secretion in duodenal ulcer patients. Abstract (no. 154) of paper presented at the 11th International Congress of Gastroenterology, Hamburg, Jun 8-13 (1980).

Corinaldesi, R.; Miglioli, M.; Danotti, S.; Stanghellini, V.; Borghi, E. and Barbara, L.: Inhibition by pirenzepine of nocturnal gastric acid secretion in duodenal ulcer patients. Scandinavian Journal of Gastroenterology 16: 929-931 (1981).

Da Broi Gian, L.; Sandro, A. and Sergio, D.: Effects of pirenzepine on lower esophageal sphincter (LES). (Abstract no. 520.) Scandinavian Journal of Gastroenterology 17 (Suppl. 78): 131 (1982).

Dal Monte, P.R.; Bianchi Porro, G.; Petrillo, M.; Giuliani-Piccari, G.; D'Imperio, N. and Daniotti, S.: Long term treatment of duodenal ulcer with pirenzepine. A double-blind, placebo-controlled trial. Scandinavian Journal of Gastroenterology 17 (Suppl. 72): 225-228 (1982a).

Dal Monte, P.R.; D'Imperio, N.; Accardo, P. and Daniotti, S.: Pirenzepine in non-ulcer dyspepsia. A double-blind, placebo controlled trial. Scandinavian Journal of Gastroenterology 17 (Suppl. 72): 247-250 (1982b).

Daly, M.J.; Humphray, J.M. and Stables, R.: Effects of H_2-receptor antagonists and anticholinoceptor drugs on gastric and salivary secretion induced by bethanechol in the anaesthetized dog. British Journal of Pharmacology 76: 361-365 (1982).

Dammann, H.-G. and Augustin, H.J.: The intragastric pH pattern in the 24-hour profile on oral and intravenous dosage of pirenzepine and cimetidine. Paper presented at the First International Pirenzepine Symposium, Schwarzwald, Nov 10-11 (1978).

Dammann, H.-G.; Simon, B; Müller, P. and Krüger, H.J.: Inhibition of nocturnal acid secretion by pirenzepine. Arzneimittel-Forschung 32: 309-310 (1982).

Deakin, M.; Ramage, J.K. and Williams, J.G.: Are pirenzepine and cimetidine additive or synergistic in combination? Abstract T25, Gut 25 (10): A1139 (1984).

Del Soldato, P. and Pagani, F.: Pharmacodynamic evaluation of selective antimuscarinic properties of pirenzepine in the rat. Pharmacological Research Communications 14: 279-288 (1982).

Del Tacca, M.; Soldani, G.; Polloni, A.; Bernardini, C. and Martinotti, E.: The effect of pirenzepine on gastric acid secretion and gastrin release induced by bombesin and meal in the dog. Scandinavian Journal of Gastroenterology 17 (Suppl. 72): 105-110 (1982).

Denis, P. and Galmiche, J.-P.: Effect of pirenzepine on human oesophageal motility. Scandinavian Journal of Gastroenterology 17 (Suppl. 78): 59 (1982).

Denis, P.; Galmiche, J.-P.; Gibon, J.-F.; Colin, R.; Pasquis, P. and Le Francois, R.: Effect of pirenzepine on human esophageal motility. Gastroenterologie Clinique et Biologique 6: 27-32 (1982).

Dent, J.: Muscarinic receptors and esophageal motor function. Trends in Pharmacological Sciences (Suppl. Jan 1984, p. 82).

Dent, J.; Bozler, G.; Heddle, R.; Barnes, B. and Lewis, I.: Evaluation of the selectivity of the antimuscarinic agent pirenzepine for inhibition of gastric secretion by comparison with atropine. (Abstract.) Gastroenterology 84 (Part 2): 1135 (1983).

D'Imperio, N.; Giuliani Piccari, G.; Lepore, A.M.; Sarti, F. and Dal Monte, P.R.: Pirenzepine in the treatment of duodenal ulcer. Scand. J. Gastroent. 14 (Suppl. 57): 41-44 (1979).

Do, D.; Martelli, S. and Daniotti, S.: Pirenzepine in duodenal ulcer A six week, double-blind study. Scandinavian Journal of Gastroenterology 17 (Suppl. 72): 211-214 (1982).

Dobrilla, G.; Filippini, M.; Valentini, M.; Bonoldi, M.C.; Felder, M.; Moroder, E. and Frizzera, S.: Pirenzepine in the treatment of active duodenal ulcer: Preliminary results. Acta Therapeutica 5: 359-364 (1979).

Dobrilla, G.; Felder, M.; Valentini, M. and Bonoldi, M.C.: Pirenzepine and cimetidine in the short-term treatment of duodenal ulcer: A drug *vs* placebo endoscopic controlled trial. Current Therapeutic Research 28: 371-376 (1980).

Dobrilla, G.; Lucchin, L.; Comberlato, M.; Coruzzi, G. and Bertaccini, G.: Pirenzepine and exocrine secretions: A selective agent for gastric glands? Hepato-gastroenterology 30: 246-248 (1983).

Eberlein, W.; Schmidt, G.; Reuter, A. and Kutter, E.: Anti-ulcer agent pirenzepine (L-S 519) – a tricyclic compound with particular physico-chemical properties. Arzneimittel-Forschung 27: 356 (1977).

Eichenberger, P.M.; Giger, M.; Mattle, W.; Pelloni, S.A.; Müller-Lissner, S.A. et al.: Treatment and relapse prophylaxis of duodenal ulcer with pirenzepine and cimetidine. Scandinavian Journal of Gastroenterology 17 (Suppl. 72): 197-206 (1982).

Einig, D.: A new secretion inhibitor: Results of a trial of efficacy and tolerance with Gastrozepin. Therapiewoche 27: 1630-1638 (1977).

El-Sabbagh, H.N.; Bloom, S.R.; Adrian, T.E.; Prinz, R.A.; Baron, J.H. and Welbourne, R.B.: The effect of pirenzepine on meal-stimulated gastrointestinal hormones. Scandinavian Journal of Gastroenterology 15 (Suppl. 66): 57-61 (1980a).

El-Sabbagh, H.N.; Prinz, R.A.; Welbourne, R.B. and Baron, J.H.: Influence of intravenous pirenzepine on gastric acid and pepsin in man. Scandinavian Journal of Gastroenterology 15 (Suppl. 66): 73-77 (1980b).

Engelhorn, R.: Evaluation of selectivity of two different antimuscarinic substances. Scandinavian Journal of Gastroenterology 17 (Suppl. 72): 49-57 (1982).

Engelhorn, R.; Hammer, R. and Koss, F.W.: On the pharmacology and therapeutic mechanism of pirenzepine. (Unpublished report, Feb 1, 1980).

Erckenbrecht, E.; Berges, W.; Sonnenberg, A.; Erckenbrecht, J. and Wienbeck, M.: The effect of pirenzepine on esophageal motility. Scandinavian Journal of Gastroenterology 17 (Suppl. 72): 185-190 (1982).

Etienne, A. and Bron, B.: The effect of pirenzepine on gastric pH. The interest of continuous recording to select the optimal therapeutical posology. Paper presented at Satellite Symposium: Advances in Gastroenterology with Selective Antimuscarinic Compounds, Stockholm, Jun 17 (1982).

Eugenides, N.; Stockbrügger, R.W.; Hobsley, M. and Cotton, P.B.: Effect of two doses of pirenzepine on histamine-stimulated gastric acid secretion in man. Scandinavian Journal of Gastroenterology 17 (Suppl. 72): 125-129 (1982).

Evreux, M.; Barthélémy, G.; Raillat, A. and Roberti, A.: Pirenzepine and cimetidine in the treatment of duodenal ulcer: A comparative controlled trial; in Dotevall (Ed.) Advances in Gastroenterology with the Selective Antimuscarinic Compound Pirenzepine. Proceedings of the Stockholm Symposium, June 1982, pp. 184-187 (Excerpta Medica, Amsterdam 1982).

Evreux, M. and Jacquet, N.: Pirenzepine in the treatment of oesophagitis. Paper presented at the International Gastroenterological Congress, Lisbon, Sept, 1984.

Fakunle, Y.M.; Malu, A.O. and Wali, S.S.: Clinical trial of pirenzepine (100mg daily) *versus* cimetidine (1gm daily) in duodenal ulcer healing in Nigerian patients. Current Therapeutic Research 34: 87-91 (1983).

Farini, R.; Vianello, F.; Di Mario, F.; Valentini, P.; Cannizzaro, R. et al: Pirenzepine and cimetidine in the long term treatment of duodenal ulcer. A controlled trial. Clinical Trials Journal 20: 71-76 (1983).

Fedeli, G.; Anti, M.; Rapaccini, G.L.; De Vitis, I.; Brighi, S.; Sabelli, C.; Caturelli, E. and Valentini, P.: Pirenzepine *versus* cimetidine in non ulcer-associated gastritis and duodenitis. Clinical Trials Journal 20: 104-114 (1983).

Feldman, M.; Richardson, C.T.; Peterson, W.L.; Walsh, J.H. and Fordtran, J.S.: Effect of low-dose propantheline on food-stimulated gastric acid secretion. New England Journal of Medicine 297: 1427-1430 (1977).

Fink, M. and Irwin, P.: EEG and behavioral effects of pirenzepine in normal volunteers. Scandinavian Journal of Gastroenterology 15 (Suppl. 66): 39-46 (1980).

Finkbeiner, A.E.; Bissada, N.K. and Welch, L.T.: Uropharmacology: Part VI. Parasympathetic depressants. Urology 10: 503-510 (1977).

Fritsch, W.-P.: Anticholinergic inhibition of secretion with atropine, methantheline bromide and pirenzepine. Paper presented at the First International Pirenzepine Symposium, Nov 10-11 (1978).

Fritsch, W.-P.; Schacht, U.; Scholten, Th.; Hengels, K.-J.; Müller, J. and Strasser, K.: Effects of cimetidine and pirenzepine on peroperative electrical vagal stimulation of gastric acid secretion. Scandinavian Journal of Gastroenterology 15 (Suppl. 66): 95-100 (1980).

Fritsch, W.-P.; Scholten, Th.; Müller, J.; Hengels, K.-J. and Hanrath, K.-D.: The effect of a 100mg pirenzepine-treatment on acid secretion and serum gastrin. Scandinavian Journal of Gastroenterology 17 (Suppl. 72): 173-178 (1982).

Fuentes del Toro, S.; Echeverria, J.; Argueta, V.L.; Salinas, J. and Díaz de León, M.: Analisis comparativo de pirenzepina (LS519) *vs* alcalinizacion gastrica sobre la erosion aguda de mucosa gastroduodenal, asociada a sepsis y trauma. Investigación Médica Internacional 10: 407 (1983).

Fujiwara, T.; Nakamura, M.; Matsumoto, H.; Okada, Y.; Shirakawa, T. et al.: Experimental studies of the specificity of pirenzepine in inhibition of gastric acid secretion. (Abstract no. 1091.) Scandinavian Journal of Gastroenterology 17 (Suppl. 78): 275 (1982).

Gabryelewicz, A.; Laszewicz, W. and Sarosiek, J.: The influence of various secretory inhibitors on peptic activity. Scandinavian Journal of Gastroenterology 15 (Suppl. 66): 79-85 (1980).

Gabryelewicz, A.; Sarosiek, J.; Laszewicz, W. and Piotrowski, J.: The effect of combined application of ranitidine/RN/ and pirenzepine/PZ/ on gastric mucus, hydrochloric acid and pepsin secretion stimulated with peptavlon/P/ in duodenal ulcer/DU/ patients. (Abstract no. 52.) Scandinavian Journal of Gastroenterology 17 (Suppl. 78): 13 (1982).

Galmiche, J.P.; Lerebours, E. and Colin, R.: The effect of pirenzepine on basal and pentagastrin stimulated gastric acid secretion in healthy man. Medecine et Chirurgie Digestives 9: 331-334 (1980).

Gasbarrini, G.; Giorgi-Conciato, M.; D'Anchino, M.; Di Tommaso, B.; Pesa, O. et al.: Pirenzepine in the treatment of benign gastroduodenal diseases. A double-blind controlled clinical trial. Scandinavian Journal of Gastroenterology 14 (Suppl. 57): 25-31 (1979).

Giachetti, A.; Giraldo, E.; Montagna, E. and Hammer, R.: Muscarinic receptor subtypes: M_1 and M_2. Paper presented at Satellite Symposium on Pirenzepine: Advances in Gastroenterology with Selective Antimuscarinic Compounds, Stockholm, Jun 17 (1982).

Giacosa, A.; Cheli, R.; Molinari, F. and Parodi, M.C.: Comparison between ranitidine, cimetidine, pirenzepine and placebo in the short term treatment of duodenal ulcer. Scandinavian Journal of Gastroenterology 17 (Suppl. 72): 215-219 (1982).

Gibiński, K.; Gabryelewicz, A.; Novak, A.; Hasik, J. and Marlicz, K.: Healing rate and rapidity of healing in pirenzepine-treated gastric and duodenal ulcers; in Dotevall (Ed.) Advances in Gastroenterology with the Selective Muscarinic Compound Pirenzepine. Proceedings of the Stockholm Symposium June, 1982, pp. 179-183 (Excerpta Medica, Amsterdam, 1982).

Giorgi-Conciato, M.; Daniotti, S.; Ferrari, P.A.; Gaetani, M.; Petrin, G. et al.: Efficacy and safety of pirenzepine in peptic ulcer and in non ulcerous gastroduodenal diseases. A multicentre controlled clinical trial. Scandinavian Journal of Gastroenterology 17 (Suppl. 81): 1-42 (1982).

Gleissner, O. and Mielenz, H.: Zur Frage der Beeinflussung des Entleerungs-mechanismus der Blase durch Gastrozepin. Therapiewoche 27: 1673-1675 (1977).

Gonvers, J.-J.; Realini, S.; Bretholz, A.; Arnold, J.; Voirol, M.; Capitaine, Y. et al.: Gastric ulcer: A double-blind comparison of 100mg pirenzepine *versus* 800mg cimetidine. Abstract of paper presented at the International Gastroenterology Congress, Lisbon, Sept. 1984.

Guslandi, M.: Pirenzepine and gastric mucus. Scandinavian Journal of Gastroenterology 14 (Suppl. 57): 57 (1979).

Guslandi, M. and Del Soldato, P.: Gastroduodenal erosions: An overview of clinical and pathogenetic problems and of some experiences with pirenzepine. Paper presented at the International Gastroenterology Congress, Lisbon, Sept. 1984.

Guslandi, M.; Testoni, P.A.; Fesce, E.; Ballarin, E. and Tittobello, A.: Behaviour of gastric mucin during pirenzepine treatment: A double-blind controlled study *versus* cimetidine. Current Therapeutic Research 27: 714-718 (1980).

Hammer, R.: Muscarinic-receptor binding studies with pirenzepine. Report presented at the First International Pirenzepine Symposium, Schwarzwald, Nov 10-11 (1978).

Hammer, R.: Muscarinic receptors in the stomach. Scandinavian Journal of Gastroenterology 15 (Suppl. 66): 5-11 (1980).

Hammer, R.: Subclasses of muscarinic receptors and pirenzepine: Further experimental evidence. Scandinavian Journal of Gastroenterology 17 (Suppl. 72): 59-67 (1982).

Hammer, R. and Koss, F.W.: Human and animal pharmacokinetics after oral and parenteral administration of pirenzepine. Paper presented at the First International Pirenzepine Symposium, Schwarzwald, Nov 10-11 (1978).

Hammer, R. and Koss, F.W.: The pharmacokinetic profile of pirenzepine. Scandinavian Journal of Gastroenterology 14 (Suppl. 57): 1-6 (1979).

Hammer, R. and Koss, F.W.: Zum Wirkungsmechanismus des Magensekretionshemmers Pirenzepin. Fortschritte der Therapie 98: 549-554 (1980).

Hammer, R.; Berrie, C.P.; Birdsall, N.J.M.; Burgen, A.S.V. and Hulme, E.C.: Pirenzepine distinguishes between different subclasses of muscarinic receptors. Nature 283: 90-92 (1980a).

Hammer, R.; Bozler, G.; Zimmer, A. and Koss, F.W.: Pharmacokinetics and metabolism of Gastrozepin in man. Therapiewoche 27: 1575-1593 (1977a).

Hammer, R.; Kaubisch, N.; Kopitar, Z.; Prox, A.; Zimmer, A. and Koss, F.W.: Pharmacokinetic and metabolic investigations with LS-519-Cl_2 (Pirenzepin) in rats, rabbits and dogs. Therapiewoche 27: 1567-1574 (1977b).

Hammer, R.; Mielenz, H. and Koss, F.W.: Pirenzepine, an original tricyclic agent with selective antimuscarinic properties; in Morck (Ed.) Offizinpharmazie, Band 2, pp. 50-54 (Thieme, Stuttgart 1980b).

Hawkins, G.K.; Margolin, S. and Thompson, J.J.: Gastric emptying time: Comparative studies with placebos, prantal and banthine. Gastroenterology 24: 193-199 (1953).

Heathcote, B.V. and Parry, M.: Pirenzepine selectively inhibits gastric acid secretion: A comparative pharmacological study between pirenzepine and seven other antiacetylcholine drugs. Scandinavian Journal of Gastroenterology 15 (Suppl. 66): 15-24 (1980).

Heathcote, B.V. and Parry, M.: A comparison of the effects of pirenzepine and atropine on gastric acid secretion, salivary secretion and pupil diameter in the rat. (Abstract no. 304.) Scandinavian Journal of Gastroenterology 17 (Suppl. 78): 77 (1982).

Heller, G.; Neubauer, M.; Althoff, P.; Karn, U. and Schoeffling,

K.: Pirenzepine: Investigations of its mode of action in man. Paper presented at the 6th World Congress of Gastroenterology, Madrid, Jun 5-9 (1978a).

Heller, G.; Neubauer, M.; Althoff, P.H. and Schoeffling, K.: The effect of pirenzepine on gastric secretion and release of gastrointestinal hormones. Paper presented at the First International Pirenzepine Symposium, Schwarzwald, Nov 10-11 (1978b).

Henn, R.M.; Isenberg, J.I.; Maxwell, V. and Sturdevant, R.A.L.: Inhibition of gastric acid secretion by cimetidine in patients with duodenal ulcer. New England Journal of Medicine 293: 371-375 (1975).

Henry, D.A.; Hawkey, C.; Somerville, K.; Burnham, W.R.; Bell, G.D. and Langman, M.J.S.: Pirenzepine and cimetidine in duodenal ulcer: a comparative study; in Dotevall (Ed.) Advances in Gastroenterology with the Selective Antimuscarinic Compound Pirenzepine. Proceedings of the Stockholm Symposium, June 1982 pp. 214-216 (Excerpta Medica, Amsterdam 1982).

Herrmann, M. and Kuhlmann, H.: Dialysability and serum concentration of pirenzepine. Paper presented at the First International Pirenzepine Symposium, Schwarzwald, Nov 10-11 (1978).

Höckerstedt, K.; Ahonen, J.; Kauste, A.; Kostamo, T. and Lalla, M.: Effect of cimetidine and pirenzepine on gastric acid output in critically ill patients. (Abstract no. 840.) Scandinavian Journal of Gastroenterology 17 (Suppl. 78): 211 (1982).

Hoffenberg, P.: Tratamiento de la ulcera duodenal con pirenzepina. Revista Medica de Chile 11: 419-423 (1983).

Höllerl, G.: Treatment of upper GI-bleeding with pirenzepine. (Abstract no. 845.) Scandinavian Journal of Gastroenterology 17 (Suppl. 78): 212 (1982).

Höllerl, G.; Stadler, H. and Tscheliessnigg, K.H.: Die Behandlung akut blutender gastroduodenaler Läsionen mit Pirenzepin. Medizinische Klinik 77: 367-370 (1982).

Hradsky, M. and Wikander, M.: Effect of pirenzepine in the treatment of non ulcer dyspepsia: a double-blind study; in Dotevall (Ed.) Advances in Gastroenterology with the Selective Antimuscarinic Compound Pirenzepine. Proceedings of the Stockholm Symposium, June 1982, pp. 170-172 (Excerpta Medica, 1982).

Huchzermeyer, H.: Excretory pancreatic function after oral administration of pirenzepine and atropine. Paper presented at the First International Pirenzepine Symposium, Schwarzwald, Nov 10-11 (1978).

Hurwitz, A; Robinson, R.G. and Herrin, W.F.: Prolongation of gastric emptying by oral propantheline. Clinical Pharmacology and Therapeutics 22: 206-210 (1977).

Inatomi, N.; Ishihara, Y. and Okabe, S.: Pirenzepine in the healing of experimental ulcers. Japanese Journal of Pharmacology 29: 486 (1979).

Ireland, A.; Gear, P.; Golding, P.L.; Jarvis, L.J.; Clark, R.J.; Williams, J.G.; Henry, D.A. et al.: Pirenzepine and cimetidine in the prevention of duodenal ulcer relapse: A multicentre trial (In press, 1985).

Ishimori, A. and Yamagata, S.: Therapeutic effect of pirenzepine dihydrochloride on gastric ulcer evaluated by a double-blind controlled clinical study. Arzneimittel-Forschung 32: 556-565 (1982a).

Ishimori, A. and Yamagata, S.: Double-blind controlled clinical study of pirenzepine in patients with duodenal ulcer. (Abstract no. 400.) Scandinavian Journal of Gastroenterology 17 (Suppl. 78): 101 (1982b).

Ishimori, A. and Yamagata, S.: Double-blind controlled clinical study of pirenzepine in gastric and duodenal ulcer; in Dotevall (Ed.) Advances in Gastroenterology with the Selective Antimuscarinic Compound Pirenzepine. Proceedings of the Stockholm Symposium June 1982 pp. 188-204 (Excerpta Medica, Amsterdam 1982c).

Itil, T.M.: EEG effects of single doses of pirenzepine, amitriptyline, cyproheptadine, and placebo in healthy volunteers (Preprint HZI-103, April 1977).

Ivey, K.J.: Anticholinergics: Do they work in peptic ulcer? Gastroenterology 68: 154-166 (1975).

Jain, A.K.; La Corte, W.; Haugue, D.; McMahon, F.G. and Ryan, J.R.: Gastric antisecretory activity of LS-519: A controlled study. (Abstract.) Clinical Pharmacology and Therapeutics 25: 231 (1979).

Jaup, B.H.: Results of clinical pharmacology of selective antimuscarinic compounds: Introduction and summary. Paper presented at Satellite Symposium on Pirenzepine: Advances in Gastroenterology with Selective Antimuscarinic Compounds, Stockholm, Jun 17 (1982).

Jaup, B.H.; Abrahamsson, H. and Dotevall, G.: Comparison of the effects of classical and selective antimuscarinic drugs on oesophageal motility. (Abstract no. 17.) Gut 24: A358 (1983).

Jaup, B.H.; Abrahamsson, H.; Virtanen, R. and Iisalo, E.: Effect of pirenzepine compared with atropine and L-hyoscyamine on esophageal peristaltic activity in humans. Scandinavian Journal of Gastroenterology 17: 233-239 (1982a).

Jaup, B.H. and Blomstrand, Ch.: Cerebro-spinal fluid concentrations of pirenzepine after therapeutic dosage. Scandinavian Journal of Gastroenterology 15 (Suppl. 66): 35-37 (1980).

Jaup, B.H.; Dotevall, G. and Stockbrügger, R.: The effect of pirenzepine on pentagastrin- and insulin-stimulated gastric secretion in patients with duodenal ulcer. Paper presented at the First International Pirenzepine Symposium, Schwarzwald, Nov 10-11 (1978).

Jaup, B.H. and Dotevall, G.: The effect of pirenzepine and L-hyoscyamine on gastric emptying and salivary secretion in healthy volunteers. Scandinavian Journal of Gastroenterology 16: 769-773 (1981).

Jaup, B.H.; Stockbrügger, R.W. and Dotevall, G.: Comparison between the effects of pirenzepine and L-hyoscyamine in man. Scandinavian Journal of Gastroenterology 17 (Suppl. 72): 119-122 (1982b).

Jaup, B.H.; Stockbrügger, R.W. and Dotevall, G.: Comparison of the action of pirenzepine and L-hyoscyamine on gastric acid secretion and other muscarinic effects. Scandinavian Journal of Gastroenterology 15 (Suppl. 66): 89-94 (1980).

Jennewein, H.M.: Pharmacological differences between pirenzepine and atropine. Paper presented at the First International Pirenzepine Symposium, Schwarzwald, Nov 10-11 (1978).

Jeremy, J.Y. and Dandona, P.: The effect of pirenzepine on *in vitro* prostaglandin synthesis by human and rat gastric tissue. Paper presented at the International Gastroenterology Congress, Lisbon, Sept. 1984.

Kaehling, J.H.; Ziegler, H. and Ballhause, H.: Central nervous system profile of pirenzepine. (Internal report of Boehringer Ingelheim, 1974).

Kamenisch, W.: Comparative investigation of the effect of cimetidine and pirenzepine on serum gastrin, gastric secretion and the healing of gastroduodenal ulcers. Paper presented at the First International Pirenzepine Symposium, Schwarzwald, Nov 10-11 (1978).

Kawamura, T.; Torii, A.; Nozawa, H.; Onizawa, N. and Kameda, H.: Comparison of effects on gastric mucosal blood flow and mucus between pirenzepine and other anti-ulcer agents. Paper presented at the International Gastroenterology Congress, Lisbon, Sept. (1984).

Kelleher, D.; O'Connor, M.; O'Driscoll, M.; Keeling, P.W.N. and Weir, D.G.: A controlled trial of pirenzepine in the prophylaxis of stress ulcer haemorrhage. Paper presented at the International Gastroenterology Congress, Lisbon, Sept. (1984).

Kitagawa, H.; Kurahashi, K.; Fujiwara, M. and Kohei, H.: Antiulcerogenic effect of a pyrido-benzodiazepine derivative (L-S 519) on experimental ulcers. Arzneimittel-Forschung 28: 2122-2127 (1978).

Klein, H.J. and Deeg, W.: Treatment of gastrointestinal haemorrhages following neurosurgical operations; in Dotevall (Ed.) Advances in Gastroenterology with the Selective Antimuscarinic compound Pirenzepine. Proceedings of the Stockholm Symposium June 1982 pp. 154-157 (Exerpta Medical Amsterdam 1982).

Kleist, D.; Staud, R.; Stopik, D. and Hampel, K.E.: The behaviour of the transmural gastric potential difference (PD) under pirenzepin, atropin and hyoscin-N-butylbromid. Extracta Gastroenterologica 9: 135-141 (1980).

Kleist, D.; Stopik, D.; Staud, R. and Hampel, K.E.: Measurement of the transmural gastric potential difference by endoscopy after intravenous administration of pirenzepin and glucagon. Aktuel Gastrologie 8: 603-612 (1979).

Kloog, Y.; Egozi, Y. and Sokolovsky, M.: Characterization of muscarinic acetylcholine receptors from mouse brain: Evidence for regional heterogenicity and isomerization. Molecular Pharmacology 15: 545-558 (1979).

Knoblauch, M.; Corrodi, P.; Fumagalli, I.; Funk, C.; Gassmann, R.; Schmid, E. and Gonvers, J.J.: Gastric ulcer: A double-blind comparison of 150mg pirenzepine *versus* 800mg cimetidine. Abstract of paper presented at the International Gastroenterology Congress, Lisbon, Sept. (1984).

Kobayashi, S.; Kyui, S.; Yoshida, T.; Nagakura, A.; Oiwa, Y.; Matsumura, R. and Kohei, H.: Absorption, distribution and excretion of ^{14}C-pirenzepine in rats. Arzneimittel-Forschung 31: 679-690 (1981).

Kohli, Y.; Takino, T. and Masuda, M.: Clinical evaluation of the use of pirenzepine dihydrochloride on duodenal ulcers. Double blind controlled clinical study in multiple institutes. Drugs under Experimental and Clinical Research 8: 103-114 (1982).

Konturek, S.J.; Brzozowski, T.; Radecki, T. and Piastucki, I.: Gastric cytoprotection by pirenzepine: Role of endogenous prostaglandins. Scandinavian Journal of Gastroenterology 17 (Suppl. 72): 255-259 (1982a).

Konturek, S.J.; Kwiecień, N.; Obtulowicz, W. and Oleksy, J.: Cytoprotective effects of pirenzepine. Paper presented at Satellite Symposium on Pirenzepine: Advances in Gastroenterology with Selective Antimuscarinic Compounds, Stockholm, Jun 17 (1982b).

Konturek, S.J.; Kwiecień, N.; Obtulowicz, W.; Swierczek, J.; Kopp, B. and Oliesky, J.: Paper presented at Satellite Symposium on Pirenzepine: Advances in Gastroenterology with Selective Antimuscarinic Compounds, Stockholm, Jun 17 (1982c).

Konturek, S.J.; Obtulowicz, W.; Kwiecień, N.; Dobrzańska, M.; Swierczek, J. et al.: Effects of pirenzepine and atropine on gastric secretory and plasma hormonal responses to sham-feeding in patients with duodenal ulcer. Scandinavian Journal of Gastroenterology 15 (Suppl. 66): 63-69 (1980).

Kuhn, E. and Honzak, R.: Psychometric studies of pirenzepine. Scandinavian Journal of Gastroenterology 15 (Suppl. 66): 47-53 (1980).

Kuhn, E.; Brodan, V.; Anděl, M. and Veselková, A.: Einige metabolische und physiologische Wirkungen von LS 519 im akuten Experiment. Therapiewoche 27: 1594-1606 (1977c).

Kuhn, E.; Honzák, R.; Hnídková, A.; Brodan, V. and Anděl, M.: Central effects of a single administration of LS 519. Therapiewoche 27: 1608-1619 (1977b).

Kuhn, E.; Skála, I.; Fučiková, E.; Šlygin, G.K. and Vasilevskaja, L.S.: The effect of Gastrozepin – A new preparation with antiulcerative activity on the gastric secretion of human beings and dogs. Therapiewoche 27: 1620-1629 (1977a).

Kuntzen, O. and Kaess, H.: Effect of intravenously injected pirenzepine on pancreatic exocrine function. Paper presented at the First International Pirenzepine Symposium, Schwarzwald, Nov 10-11 (1978).

Laugier, R.: Pirenzepine *versus* placebo in the treatment of duodenal ulcer; in Dotevall (Ed) Advances in Gastroenterology with the Selective Antimuscarinic Compound Pirenzepine. Proceedings of the Stockholm Symposium June 1982, pp. 177-178 (Excerpta Medica, Amsterdam 1982).

Laureta, H.C. and Lim, V.: Pirenzepine in the treatment of benign gastric ulcer. A double-blind short-term clinical trial. Philippine Journal of Internal Medicine 19: 102-108 (1981).

Laureta, H.C.; Sanchez, J.T.; Payot, C.D. and Ablan, D.N.: Determination of the optimum dose of parenteral Gastrozepin. Philippine Journal of Internal Medicine 19: 243-249 (1981).

Laureta, H.C.; Villamayor, C.B.; Calubiran, O.V. and Gonzales, R.B.: Evaluation of LS 519, a new tricyclic compound for benign gastric ulcer. 1. Its effects on basal gastric acid secretion and basal and maximum acid output in man. Philippine Journal of Internal Medicine 17: 145-154 (1979).

Lederer, P.C.; Thiemann, R.; Ellermann, A. and Radeck, J.: Differential effects of pirenzepine on esophageal interdigestive and sigmoid motility. (Abstract.) Gastroenterology 86 (5) part 2: 1156 (1984).

Lederer, P.C.; Thiemann, R.; Femppel, J.; Domschke, W. and Lux, G.: Influence of atropine, pirenzepine and cimetidine on nocturnal gastrointestinal motility and gastric acid secretion. Scandinavian Journal of Gastroenterology 17 (Suppl. 72): 131-136 (1982).

Lehy, T.; Lewin, M.J.M. and Bonfils, S.: Long term administration of pirenzepine to rats induces parietal and gastrin hypoplasia; in Blum and Hammer (Eds) Die Behandlung de Ulcus pepticum mit Pirenzepin pp. 35 (Karl Demeter - Verlag, Gräfelfins 1978).

Leitold, M. and Engelhorn, R.: Pharmacological investigations of the antiulcerative effect of 5,11-dihydro-11-[(4-methyl-piperazinyl) acetyl]-6H-pyrido [2,3-b] [1,4] benzodiazepin-6-one dihydrochloride (LS 519). Therapiewoche 27: 1532-1548 (1977).

Leitold, M.; Engelhorn, R.; Ballhause, H.; Kuhn, F.J. and Ziegler, H.: General pharmacodynamic properties of the secretion and ulcer inhibitor Gastrozepin: 3rd communication. Therapiewoche 27: 1551-1564 (1977).

Levenston, S.A. and Cryer, P.E.: Endogenous cholinergic modulation of growth hormone secretion in normal and acromegalic humans. Metabolism 29: 703-706 (1980).

Littman, A. and Pine, B.H.: Antacids and anticholinergic drugs. Annals of Internal Medicine 82: 544-551 (1975).

Londong, W.: Discussion after El-Sabbagh and Konturek. Scandinavian Journal of Gastroenterology 15 (Suppl. 66): 71 (1980).

Londong, W.: Anticholinergics for peptic ulcer – A Renaissance? Hepatogastroenterology 29: 40-46 (1982).

Londong, W.; Hasford, J.; Sander, R.; Sommerlatte, Th.; Uberla, K. et al.: Prophylaxis of recurrent bleeding from gastroduodenal lesions by combination of cimetidine and pirenzepine: A double-blind and multicentre trial. (Abstract no. 834.) Scandinavian Journal of Gastroenterology 17 (Suppl. 78): 210 (1982a).

Londong, W.; Londong, V.; Eberl, H.; Pöch, G.; Bozler, G. and Gugler, R.: Interaction of pirenzepine and ranitidine – Pharmacodynamic secretory studies in man. Gut 24: A974 (1983).

Londong, W.; Londong, V. and Pfeifer, K.J.: New approach of a differential treatment of patients with Zollinger-Ellison syndrome. (Abstract no. 1008.) Scandinavian Journal of Gastroenterology 17 (Suppl. 78): 254 (1982b).

Londong, W.; Londong, V.; Prechtl, R. and Eversmann, T.: Comparative investigations of the effects of pirenzepine and cimetidine on peptone-stimulated acid secretion and serum gastrin in man. Paper presented at the First International Pirenzepine Symposium, Schwarzwald, Nov 10-11 (1978).

Londong, W.; Londong, V.; Prechtl, R. and Schwanner, A.: Almost complete inhibition of gastric acid secretion by combined application of pirenzepine and cimetidine. Abstract of paper presented at the 13th Scandinavian Congress on Gastroenterology and 5th Scandinavian Meeting on Gastrointestinal Endoscopy, p. 83, Espoo, Finland, Aug 23-25 (1979).

Londong, W.; Londong, V.; Prechtl, R. and Schwanner, A.: Studies on effectiveness of cimetidine, pirenzepine and synthetic secretin on stimulated gastric acid secretion. Zeitschrift für Gastroenterologie 18: 306-313 (1980a).

Londong, W.; Londong, V.; Prechtl, R.; Weber, Th. and Von Werder, K.: Interactions of cimetidine and pirenzepine on peptone-stimulated gastric acid secretion in man. Scandinavian Journal of Gastroenterology (Suppl. 66): 103-112 (1980b).

Londong, W.; Londong, V.; Ruthe, C. and Weizert, P.: Complete inhibition of food-stimulated gastric acid secretion by combined application of pirenzepine and ranitidine. Gut 22: 542-548 (1981).

Luthin, G.R. and Wolfe, B.B.: [^{3}H] Pirenzepine and [^{3}H] quinuclidinyl benzilate binding to brain muscarinic cholinergic receptors. Molecular Pharmacology 26: 164 (1984).

Mahachai, V.; Jamali, F.; Reilly, P. and Thomson, A.B.R.: Pharmacokinetics and effect of pirenzepine on gastric acid secretion in duodenal ulcer disease. (Abstract.) Gastroenterology 86 (May part 2): 1171 (1984a).

Mahachai, V.; Jamali, F.; Reilly, P. and Thomson, A.B.R.: Pirenzepine potentiates inhibitory effects of cimetidine on gastric pH in duodenal ulcer disease. (Abstract 121.) Annales of Royal College of Physicians and Surgeons of Canada 17 (4): 314 (1984b).

Maleev, A.; Krastev, Z.; Deredjian, S.; Ivantchev, T.; Vradjaliev, J. et al.: Serum gastrin values before and after short term treatment of duodenal ulcer with cimetidine and pirenzepine. (Abstract no. 437.) Scandinavian Journal of Gastroenterology 17 (Suppl. 78): 110 (1982).

Malhotra, A.; Patel, G.K.; Texter, E.C.; Morrison, E.; Baskin, B. and Williams, A.D.: Pirenzepine, a muscarinic antagonist, increases lower esophageal sphincter pressure 2-3 fold for a prolonged period. Abstract. Gastroenterology 84 (5 part 2): 1238 (1983).

Martínez Ruiz, E. and Rodríguez, H.Z.: Valoracion clinica de la pirenzepina. Investigación Médica Internacional 8: 400-412 (1981).

Masala, A.; Alagna, S.; Devilla, L.; Rovasio, P.P.; Rassu, S. et al.: Muscarinic receptor blockade by pirenzepine: Effect on prolactin secretion in man. Journal of Endocrinological Investigation 5: 53-55 (1982).

Matsuo, Y. and Seki, A.: Actions of pirenzepine-dihydrochloride (LS-519 Cl) on gastric juice secretion, gastric motility and experimental gastric ulcer. Arzneimittel-Forschung 29: 1028-1035 (1979).

Mattes, P.; Peros, G.; Belohlavek, D.; Malfertheiner, P. and Herfarth, Ch.: Stressulkus-Prophylaxe mit Pirenzepin-eine kontrollierte Studie. Zeitschrift für Gastroenterologie 18: 325-327 (1980).

Meeroff, J.C.: Pirenzepine, meperidine, glucagon, secretin and cimetidine are equally effective in preventing experimental stress induced hemorrhagic gastritis. (Abstract.) Gastroenterology 78 (Part 2): 1220 (1980).

Meunier, P.; Martin, F.; Williams, C.N.; Poleski, M. and Reilly, P.A.: Double-blind comparison of pirenzepine and cimetidine in the short-term treatment of duodenal ulcer: an interim report; in Dotevall (Ed.) Advances in Gastroenterology with the Selective Antimuscarinic Compound Pirenzepine. Proceedings of the Stockholm Symposium, June 1982, pp. 232-237 (Excerpta Medica, Amsterdam 1982).

Miehlke, K.: Verbesserte Magenverträglichkeit nichtsteroidaler Antiphlogistika durch Pirenzepin (Gastrozepin®). Ergebnisse klinischer Doppelblind-Studien und experimenteller Versuche. Aktuelle Rheumatologie 5: 175-179 (1980).

Mignon, M.; Vallot, T.; Galmiche, J.P.; Dupas, J.L. and Bonfils, S.: Interest of a combined antisecretory treatment, cimetidine and pirenzepin, in the management of severe forms of Zollinger-Ellison Syndrome. Digestion 20: 56-61 (1980).

Mignon, M.; Vatier, J.; Bauer, P. and Bonfils, S.: Effect of pirenzepine on meal-stimulated acid secretion and gastrin release in normal man. Scandinavian Journal of Gastroenterology 17 (Suppl. 72): 145-151 (1982).

Mittelstaedt, A.; Zilly, A.; Verhoeven, A. and Mielenz, H.: Ergebnisse einer Kontrollierten Vergleichsstudie zwischen Cimetidin und Pirenzepin, Bei 60 Patienten mit Ulcera ventriculi oder duodeni. Fortschritte der Medizin 99: 1761-1768 (1981).

Miyoshi, A.; Ohe, K.; Inoue, M.; Takemoto, T.; Kawamura, S.; Kita, S. et al.: Effect of pirenzepine on gastric ulcer with randomized double-blind method. Japanese Archives of Internal Medicine 27: 33-48 (1980).

Molinari, F.; Caielli, E.; Bocchini, R.; Parodi, M.C.; Giacosa, A. and Cheli, R.: Total mucus secretion and NANA content in gastric juice of duodenal ulcer patients treated with pirenzepine. Abstract (no. 158) of a paper presented at the 11th International Congress of Gastroenterology, Hamburg, Jun 8-13 (1980).

More, D.G.; Raper, R.F.; Munro, I.; Watson, C.J.; Boutagy, J. and Shenfield, G.M.: Combination therapy with ranitidine and pirenzepine for stress ulcer prophylaxis in the critically ill. Abstract. Anaesthesia and Intensive Care 12: 85 (1984).

Morelli, A.; Narducci, F.; Pelli, M.A.; Farroni, F.; Daniotti, S. and Del Soldato, P.: Seasonal prophylactic treatment with pirenzepine to prevent duodenal ulcer recurrence. Correspondence. Lancet 2: 1157 (1984).

Morelli, A.; Pelli, A.; Narducci, F. and Spadacini, A.: Pirenzepine in the treatment of gastric ulcer. A double-blind short-term clinical trial. Scandinavian Journal of Gastroenterology 14 (Suppl. 57): 51-55 (1979).

Morelli, A.; Gaetani, M.; Pelli, M.A.; Narducci, F.; Daniotti, S. et al.: Prevention of duodenal ulcer relapse by seasonal treatment with pirenzepine. II. Results of a long-term follow-up in a double-blind trial. Gastroenterology 84: 1253 (1983).

Moshal, M.G.; Spitaels, J.-M.; Khan, F. and Manion, G.C.: Pirenzepine, cimetidine and placebo in the long-term treatment of duodenal ulceration. South African Medical Journal 62: 12-14 (1982).

Müller-Lissner, S.A.; Szelenyi, I.; Engler, H. and Blum, A.L.: Pirenzepine inhibits acid and pepsinogen secretion by the isolated perfused mouse stomach. Scandinavian Journal of Gastroenterology 17 (Suppl. 72): 101-103 (1982).

Nilvebrant, L. and Sparf, B.: Muscarinic receptor binding in the parotid gland. Different affinities of some anticholinergic drugs between the parotid gland and ileum. Scandinavian Journal of Gastroenterology 17 (Suppl. 72): 69-76 (1982).

Ohashi, I.; Otani, M. and Kohei, H.: The plasma level and urinary excretion of pirenzepine dihydrochloride (LS 519) in man. Japanese Journal of Clinical Pharmacology and Therapeutics 11: 153-159 (1980).

Ojewole, J.A.O.: Anticholinergic action of pirenzepine (Gastrozepin) on isolated gastrointestinal tract smooth muscles. Methods and Findings of Experimental and Clinical Pharmacology 5: 171-175 (1983).

Okabe, S.; Nosaka, A.; Matsumoto, M. and Kawahara, Y.: Effects of pirenzepine probanthine bromide or ulcerlmin on experimental peptic ulcers in rats. Pharmacometrics 15: 1235-1240 (1978).

Okabe, S.; Tabata, K. and Kawakami, M.: Effects of prolonged treatment of pirenzepine 2HCl on gastric secretion and plasma gastrin levels in rats. Arzneimittel-Forschung 32: 664-668 (1982).

Oleksy, J.; Taborska-Buczek, M.; Zyss, R. and Dabros, W.: The influence of pirenzepine on gastric mucosa morphometry and gastric secretion in duodenal ulcer patients and controls. (Abstract no. 462.) Scandinavian Journal of Gastroenterology 17 (Suppl. 78): 116 (1982).

Oselladore, D.; Chierichetti, S.M.; Norberto, L. and Vibelli, C.: Pirenzepine (LS 519) in severe duodenal ulcer and in gastric ulcer. A double-blind clinical trial. Scandinavian Journal of Gastroenterology 14 (Suppl. 59): 33-39 (1979).

Pagani, F.; Schiavone, A.; Monferini, E.; Hammer, R. and Giach-

etti, A.: Distinct muscarinic receptor subtypes (M_1 and M_2) controlling acid secretion in rodents. Trends in Pharmacological Sciences Suppl. January 1984, p.66.
Pandolfo, N.; Borgonovo, G.; Nebiacolombo, C. and Daniotti, S.: Effects of pirenzepine on esophageal peristalsis in humans. (Abstract no. 519.) Scandinavian Journal of Gastroenterology 17 (Suppl. 78): 130 (1982).
Pandolfo, N.; Borgonovo, G.; Torre, G.C.; Nebiacolombo, C. and Daniotti, S.: Response to pirenzepine to the human lower esophageal sphincter. Current Therapeutic Research 30: 38-43 (1981).
Paoluzi, P.; Ricotta, G.; Iafrancesco, G.; Zaccardelli, E.; Ripoli, F. and Carratu, R.: Pirenzepine and cimetidine in the treatment of duodenal ulcer: Results of a double-blind trial. Italian Journal of Gastroenterology 14: 225-227 (1982).
Parry, M. and Heathcote, B.V.: A comparison of the effects of pirenzepine and atropine on gastric acid secretion, salivary secretion and pupil diameter in the rat. Life Sciences 31: 1465-1471 (1982).
Parsons, E.; Bunce, T.; Blakemore, C. and Rasmussen, C.: Pharmacological studies on the gastric anti-secretory agent, pirenzepine. Paper presented at the First International Pirenzepine Symposium, Schwarzwald, Nov 10-11 (1978).
Petrillo, M. and Bianchi Porro, G.: Maintenance treatment of recurrent duodenal ulceration with pirenzepine. Hepato-Gastroenterology 27: 369-371 (1980).
Piper, D.W. and Steel, M.C.: The effect of anticholinergic drugs on the electrolyte content of gastric juice. Gut 2: 230-232 (1961).
Pounder, R.E.; Williams, J.G.; Milton-Thompson, G.J. and Misiewicz, J.J.: Effect of cimetidine on 24-hour intragastric acidity in normal subjects. Gut 17: 133-138 (1976).
Procacciante, F.; Citone, G.; Montesani, C. and Ribotta, G.: Antisecretory activity of pirenzepine *versus* cimetidine in man: a controlled study. Gut 25: 178 (1984).
Rogóz, Z.; Skuza, G. and Sowińska, H.: Central action of pirenzepine. Polish Journal of Pharmacology and Pharmacy 33: 615-626 (1981).
Rosenfeld, G.C.: Pirenzepine (LS 519): A weak inhibitor of acid secretion by isolated rat parietal cells. European Journal of Pharmacology 86: 99-101 (1983).
Rovati, V.; Foschi, D.; Ferrante, F.; Del Soldato, P.; Daniotti, S. and Varin, L.: Cytoprotection by PGE_2, atropine, pirenzepine and vagotomy in rats. Scandinavian Journal of Gastroenterology 17 (Suppl. 72): 261-264 (1982).
Sachs, G.; Kasbekar, D.K. and Berglindh, T.: The mechanism of action of pirenzepine on gastric secretion. Paper presented at the First International Pirenzepine Symposium, Schwarzwald, Nov 10-11 (1978).
Sarosiek, J.; Gabryelewicz, A. and Laszewicz, W.: A dose-related pirenzepine/PZ/inhibition of gastric mucus and hydrochloric acid secretion stimulated with peptavlon in duodenal ulcer/ DU/patients. (Abstract no. 454.) Scandinavian Journal of Gastroenterology 17 (Suppl. 78): 114 (1982).
Schmid, E. and Blaich, E.: Einfluss von Pirenzepin auf die Heilung des Magengeschwürs. Doppelblindstudie an stationär behandelten Patienten. Zeitschrift für Gastroenterologie 16: 778-780 (1978).
Scholten, T.; Fritsch, W.-P.; Müller, J.-E. and Hengels, K.-J.: The inhibition of vagal stimulated acid secretion by pirenzepine and cimetidine. Scandinavian Journal of Gastroenterology 17 (Suppl. 72): 169-171 (1982a).
Scholten, T.; Hengels, K.-J.; Fritsch, W.-P. and Hausamen, T.V.: Langzeitsuppression der H^+-Sekretion durch Kombination von Cimetidin mit Methanthelinbromide und Pirenzepin-Dihydrochlorid (Abstract No. 60); in Crentzfeldt and Classen (Eds) Ergebnisse der Gastroenterologie (Demeter, Gräfelfing 1978).
Scholten, T.; Schuchert, A.; Fritsch, W.-P.; Müller, J.-E. and Hengels, K.-J.: Inhibition of postprandial nocturnal gastric acid secretion by pirenzepine, ranitidine and combined therapy. (Abstract no. 51.) Scandinavian Journal of Gastroenterology 17 (Suppl. 78): 13 (1982b).
Sheers, R. and Roberts, N.B.: The effects of pirenzepine and ranitidine on pepsin secretion. Paper presented at Satellite Symposium on Pirenzepine: Advances in Gastroenterology with Selective Antimuscarinic Compounds, Stockholm, Jun 17 (1982).
Shimizu, N.; Shimizu, Y. and Kawabe, K.: Clinical trial of LS519 (pirenzepine dihydrochloride) in patients with glaucoma. Clinical Report 14: 1726-1732 (1980).
Spánková, H.; Kuhn, E.: Ryšánek, K. and König, J.: The effect of LS 519 CL_2 on the level and uptake of serotonin by thrombocytes. Activitas Nervosa Superior 17: 264-265 (1975).
Stacher, G.; Bauer, P.; Schmierer, G. and Steinringer, H.: The effect of intramuscular pirenzepine on esophageal contractile activity and lower esophageal sphincter pressure under fasting conditions and after a standard meal. A double-blind study. International Journal of Clinical Pharmacology and Biopharmacy 17: 442-448 (1979).
Stacher, G.; Havlik, E.; Bergmann, H.; Schmierer, G. and Winklehner, S.: Effects of oral pirenzepine on gastric emptying and antral motor activity in healthy man. Scandinavian Journal of Gastroenterology 17 (Suppl. 72): 153-158 (1982).
Stacher, G.; Steinringer, H.; Bauer, P.; Ehn, I. and Schmierer, G.: The effect of intramuscular pirenzepine, atropine and placebo on the meal-stimulated motility of the colon. A double-blind study. Paper presented at the First International Pirenzepine Symposium, Schwarzwald, Nov 10-11 (1978a).
Stacher, G.; Steinringer, H.; Bauer, P.; Schmierer, G. and Ehn, I.: Central nervous effects of intramuscularly administered pirenzepine. A double-blind study. Paper presented at the First International Pirenzepine Symposium, Schwarzwald, Nov 10-11 (1978b).
Stefenelli, N.: Viscosity of the gastric mucus on pirenzepine. Paper presented at the First International Pirenzepine Symposium, Schwarzwald, Nov 10-11 (1978).
Stenquist, B.; Haglund, U.; Lind, T. and Olbe, L.: The effect of different anticholinergics on the gastric acid response to sham feeding in man. Scandinavian Journal of Gastroenterology 17 (Suppl. 72): 165-167 (1982).
Sternini, C.; Ferri, G.L.; Bonora, G.; Salvi, M. and Vezzadini, P.: The effect of pirenzepine on gastric acid secretion and serum gastrin in duodenal ulcer patients. Abstract (no. 153) of paper presented at the 11th International Congress of Gastroenterology, Hamburg, Jun 8-13 (1980).
Stockbrügger, R.W.; Jaup, B.H.; Abrahamsson, H. and Dotevall, G.: Clinical pharmacology of muscarinic antagonists. Trends in Pharmacological Sciences (Suppl. Jan): 74 (1984a).
Stockbrügger, R.W.; Jaup, B.H. and Dotevall, G.: Pirenzepine – A new antisecretory drug. Scandinavian Journal of Gastroenterology 12 (Suppl. 45): 103 (1977).
Stockbrügger, R.W.; Jaup, B.H.; Lundqvist, G. and Dotevall, G.: Gastric acid and pepsin secretion, serum gastrin, and side effects after pirenzepine and benzilonium bromide. (Abstract.) Scandinavian Journal of Gastroenterology 18 (Suppl. 86): 83 (1983a).
Stockbrügger, R.W.; Jaup, B.H. and Dotevall, G.: The effect of different doses of pirenzepine on gastric secretion stimulated by modified sham feeding in man. Scandinavian Journal of Gastroenterology 17 (Suppl. 72): 111-117 (1982a).
Stockbrügger, R.; Jaup, B.; Hammer, R. and Dotevall, G.: Inhibition of gastric acid secretion by pirenzepine (LS 519) in man. Scandinavian Journal of Gastroenterology 14: 615-620 (1979).
Stockbrügger, R.W.; Kindblom, L.-G. and Dotevall, G.: Pirenzepine in the prevention of ASA-induced gastro-duodenal damage. (Abstract.) Scandinavian Journal of Gastroenterology 18 (Suppl. 86): 84 (1983b).
Stockbrügger, R.W.; Seeberg, S.; Hellner, L.; Jaup, B.H. and Dotevall, G.: Intragastric bacteria and nitrate after short-term

treatment with different doses of antimuscarinic drugs. Scandinavian Journal of Gastroenterology 19: 14 (1984b).

Sue, R.; Toomey, M.L.; Soll, A. and Yamada, T.: Pirenzepine sensitive muscarinic receptors regulate somatostatin and gastrin secretion from isolated perfused rat stomachs. (Abstract.) Gastroenterology 84 (5 part 2): 1326 (1983).

Szelenyi, I.: Does pirenzepine distinguish between 'subtypes' of muscarinic receptors? British Journal of Pharmacology 77: 567-569 (1982).

Tatsuta, M.; Itoh, T.; Okuda, S.; Tamura, H.; Baba, M. and Yamamura, H.: Inhibition of gastrin secretion by pirenzepine (LS 519) in treatment of gastric ulcer. Scandinavian Journal of Gastroenterology 16: 269-271 (1981).

Tauber, O.: Ocular effects of pirenzepine in glaucoma patients. Arzliche Praxis 29: 3918 (1977).

Texter, E.C.; Navab, F.; Boyd, C.M. and Rayford, P.L.: Differential effects of oral pirenzepine and atropine on oesophageal function and gut peptides. (Abstract.) Gastroenterology 86 (5) part 2: 1279 (1984).

Texter, E.C.; Patel, G.K.; Malhotra, A.; Morrison, E.; Rayford, P.L. and Boyd, C.M.: Comparison of the effect of oral atropine and pirenzepine on lower esophageal sphincter pressure, oesophageal emptying and gastroesophageal reflux: a preliminary report; in Dotevall (Ed.) Advances in Gastroenterology with the Selective Antimuscarinic Piperazine. Proceedings of the Stockholm Symposium, June 1982 pp. 50-57 (Excerpta Medica, Amsterdam 1982).

Texter Jr., E.C. and Reilly, P.A.: The efficacy and selectivity of pirenzepine: Review and commentary. Scandinavian Journal of Gastroenterology 17 (Suppl. 72): 237-246 (1982).

Toussaint, J.; Van der Veken, J. and Cremer, M.: A comparative double-blind trial of-pirenzepine and propantheline bromide in duodenal ulcer; in Dotevall (Ed.) Advances in Gastroenterology with the Selective Antimuscarinic Compound Pirenzepine. Proceedings of the Stockholm Symposium, June 1982, pp. 223-231 (Excerpta Medica, Amsterdam 1982).

Tritthart, H.: Gastrointestinal hemorrhage associated with intracranial lesions in rats: Effect of pirenzepine. Paper presented at the International Gastroenterology Congress, Lisbon, Sept. (1984).

Tritthart, H. and Heppner, F.: Pirenzepine as prophylaxis for gastrointestinal bleeding in neurosurgical patients. (Abstract no. 844.) Scandinavian Journal of Gastroenterology 17 (Suppl. 78): 212 (1982).

Tryba, M.; Huchzermeyer, H.; Török, M.; Zenz, M. and Pahlow, J.: Single-drug and combined medication with cimetidine, antacids and pirenzepine in the prophylaxis of acute upper gastrointestinal bleeding. Hepato-Gastroenterology 30: 154-157 (1983).

Tryba, M.; Levounou, F.; Grabhoefer, P.; Seifert, V. and Török, M.: Prophylaxe abuter Stressblutungen des oberen gastrointestinaltraktes mit pirenzepin and antazida. Anasthesie Intensivtherapie Notfallmedizin 19: 240 (1984).

Tsunenari, Y.; Kast, A.; Honma, M.; Fujii, M.; Nishikawa, J.; Shibata, T. and Yabe, T.: Toxicity studies with pirenzepine (LS 519 Cl_2) in rats and mice. Iyakuhin Kenkyu 11: 328-343 (1980).

Vantini, I.; Cavallini, G.; Ederle, A.; Piubello, W.; Benini, L.; Benini, P.; Di Giacomo, G. and Scuro, L.A.: Effect of pirenzepine on meal-stimulated serum gastrin in man. Italian Journal of Gastroenterology 10: 235-237 (1978).

Varin, L.; Del Soldato, P.; Foschi, D. and De Rosa, M.: Further evidences on gastric cytoprotection exerted by pirenzepine. Pharmacological Communications 16: 653 (1984).

Venables, C.W.; Stephen, J.G.; Blair, E.L.; Reed, J.D. and Saunders, J.D.: The effect of combined cimetidine and poldine in duodenal ulcer patients; in Wastell and Lance (Eds) Cimetidine – The Westminster Hospital Symposium, pp. 13-27 (Churchill Livingstone, Edinburgh 1978).

Vezzadini, P.; Sternini, C.; Bonora, G.; Botti, P.L.; Lugli, C. and Labò, G.: Relapse rates of duodenal ulcer after healing with pirenzepine or cimetidine: A double-blind study. (Abstract no. 399.) Scandinavian Journal of Gastroenterology 17 (Suppl. 78): 100 (1982).

Visconti, G.P.; Spotti, D.; Grasso, G.A.; Papetti, G. and Marini, U.: Long term trial of pirenzepine, cimetidine and placebo in the management of duodenal ulcer. Current Therapeutic Research 34: 853-856 (1983).

Watson, M.; Roeske, W.R.; Johnson, P.C. and Yamamura, H.I.: [3H] Pirenzepine identifies putative M_1 muscarinic receptors in human stellate ganglia. Brain Research 290: 179 (1984).

Watson, M.; Yamamura, H.I. and Roeske, W.R.: Direct evidence for M_1 and M_2 muscarinic receptor subtypes using ^3H pirenzepine. (Abstract no. 5012.) Federation Proceedings 42: 1147 (1983a).

Watson, M.; Yamamura, H.I.; Roeske, W.R.: A unique regulatory profile and regional distribution of [^3H] pirenzepine binding in the rat provide evidence for distinct M_1 and M_2 muscarinic receptor subtypes. Life Sciences 32: 3001-3011 (1983b).

Wegmann, R.; Bliem, J.; Löffelmann, K. and Lujf, A.: Experiences with pirenzepine in the therapy of peptic ulcers. Wiener Medizinische Wochenschrift 129: 513-516 (1979).

Wormsley, K.G.: Problems in the treatment of peptic ulcer. Scandinavian Journal of Gastroenterology 17 (Suppl. 80): 43-48 (1982).

Yamamura, H.I.; Watson, M.; Wamsley, J.K.; Johnson, P.C. and Roeske, W.R.: Light microscopic autoradiographic localization of [3H] pirenzepine and [3H](-) quinuclidinyl benzilate binding in human stellate ganglia. Life Sciences 35: 753 (1984).

Zangger, J.; Taufer, M.; Kratochvil, P.; Brandstätter, G. and Auböck, L.: Morphology in the duodenal ulcer scar after treatment with pirenzepine and cimetidine. Paper presented at Satellite Symposium on Pirenzepine: Advances in Gastroenterology with Selective Antimuscarinic Compounds, Stockholm, Jun 17 (1982).

Zangger, J.; Taufer, M.; Kratochvil, P. Brandstätter, G. and Auböck, L.: Pirenzepine versus ranitidine in duodenal ulcer treatment. Scar formation, relapse rate and behaviour of the parietal cell; in Bettarello (Ed.) Proceedings of Symposium on Pirenzepine: New Aspects in Research and Therapy, Lisbon, 18 Sept, 1984 (Excerpta Medica, Amsterdam 1985).

Authors' address: *Rex Brogden*, ADIS Drug Information Services, P.O. Box 34-030, Birkenhead, Auckland 10 (New Zealand).

Drugs 30: 127-144 (1985)
0012-6667/85/0008-0127/$09.00/0

Nabilone
A Preliminary Review of its Pharmacological Properties and Therapeutic Use

A. Ward and *B. Holmes*

ADIS Drug Information Services, Auckland

Various sections of the manuscript reviewed by: ***O.E. Akwari,*** Department of Surgery, Duke University Medical Center, Durham, North Carolina, USA; ***D.N. Bateman,*** Department of Pharmacological Sciences, University of Newcastle upon Tyne, Newcastle upon Tyne, England; ***H.L. Borison,*** Department of Pharmacology and Toxicology, Dartmouth Medical School, Hanover, New Hampshire, USA; ***J.R.B.J. Brouwers,*** General Hospital de Tjongerschans, Heerenveen, The Netherlands; ***L.A. Cone,*** Eisenhower Medical Center, Rancho Mirage, California, USA; ***L.E. Einhorn,*** Indiana University Department of Medicine, Indianapolis, Indiana, USA; ***D. Greene,*** Eisenhower Medical Center, Rancho Mirage, California, USA; ***P.R. Jackson,*** Department of Therapeutics, Hallamshire Hospital, Sheffield, England; ***R. Johansson,*** Department of Radiotherapy and Oncology, University of Kuopio, Kuopio, Finland; ***S.E. Jones,*** Cancer Center, University of Arizona, Tucson, Arizona, USA; ***J. Laszlo,*** Duke University Medical Center, Durham, North Carolina, USA; ***M. Levitt,*** Manitoba Cancer Treatment and Research Foundation, Winnipeg, Canada; ***J.-R. Malagelada,*** Gastroenterology Unit, Saint Mary's Hospital, Rochester, Minnesota, USA; ***E.E. Müller,*** Dipartimento di Farmacologia, Chemoterapia e Tossicologia Medica, Universita Degli Studi di Milano, Milan, Italy; ***G.L. Wampler,*** Division of Haematology and Oncology, Virginia Commonwealth University, Richmond, Virginia, USA.

Contents

Summary 128
1. Pharmacodynamic Studies 129
 1.1 Antiemetic Activity 129
 1.2 Cardiovascular Effects 130
 1.3 Respiratory Effects 131
 1.4 Behavioural Effects 131
  1.4.1 Animal Models 131
  1.4.2 Anxiety States in Man 132
 1.5 Opiate Activity and Abuse Potential 132
 1.6 Effects on Intraocular Pressure 133
 1.7 Development of Tolerance 133
 1.8 Toxicology Studies 134
2. Pharmacokinetic Studies 135
3. Therapeutic Trials 136
 3.1 Use as an Antiemetic During Cancer Chemotherapy 136
  3.1.1 Open Studies 136

3.1.2 Comparisons with Placebo 137
3.1.3 Comparisons with Prochlorperazine 138
3.1.4 Comparison with Chlorpromazine....... 140
3.1.5 Combination with Metoclopramide....... 140
4. Side Effects 140
5. Dosage and Administration 142
6. Place of Nabilone in Therapy 142

Summary

Synopsis: *Nabilone*[1] *is a new orally active cannabinoid for the treatment of severe gastrointestinal toxicity associated with cancer chemotherapy. The pharmacological profile of nabilone suggests that it acts primarily by preventing emesis controlled by the medulla oblongata, although its secondary mild anxiolytic activity may contribute to the overall efficacy. Nabilone 2mg twice daily starting 12 hours prior to, and continued for the duration of, chemotherapy produces significant reduction in the severity and duration of nausea and the frequency of vomiting in about 50 to 70% of patients with severe symptoms refractory to conventional therapy. Nabilone has proven to be more effective in controlling symptoms and preferred by more patients than prochlorperazine 10mg 2 to 4 times daily in a limited number of studies, despite a higher incidence of side effects. Comparative trials against other new antiemetic agents, such as high dose metoclopramide, and use of nabilone in combination with other antiemetics remain to be undertaken. The incidence of side effects is high with nabilone; drowsiness, dizziness and/or vertigo occur in 60 to 70% of patients, but rarely lead to drug withdrawal, although more troublesome effects, such as postural hypotension, ataxia, vision disturbance and toxic psychoses, may cause discontinuation of therapy. Thus, nabilone offers an effective alternative to the treatment options available in a difficult therapeutic area – those patients with severe gastrointestinal side effects from cancer chemotherapy who are refractory to conventional therapy.*

Pharmacodynamic Studies: The antiemetic activity of nabilone has been demonstrated in anaesthetised and unanaesthetised cats. Nabilone was more potent than prochlorperazine in preventing emesis due to intravenous cisplatin (cis-diamminedichloroplatinum), nitrosureas, mechlorethamine and other emetogenic agents. Less activity was seen against apomorphine-induced emesis and no activity was seen against intravenous nicotine-induced emesis, suggesting these effects of nabilone may occur at the level of the vomiting control mechanism in the medulla oblongata. Nabilone usually produces marked reduction in blood pressure in cats, rabbits and rats (but not in monkeys or dogs). However, there is some evidence that cardiovascular and behavioural effects are intimately linked, and that repeated administration is associated with tolerance to the cardiovascular effects of nabilone. Mild anxiolytic activity has been seen with 'lower' doses both in animal models and in man, and at high doses nabilone is associated with locomotor disturbance and sedation. Nabilone possesses little or no opiate-like activity, does not induce development of a withdrawal syndrome and *may* be associated with a lower incidence of euphoria than Δ^9-tetrahydrocannabinol, although evidence of abuse potential for nabilone has been demonstrated.

Pharmacokinetic Studies: Only very limited data are available on the disposition of nabilone in man. Oral doses are rapidly absorbed and the bioavailability is about 96%. Nabilone has an elimination half-life of about 2 hours and is extensively metabolised to a mixture of isomeric alcohols, with extended half-lives (up to 35 hours). Toxicity in dogs led to a withdrawal of nabilone from clinical trials until it was discovered that metabolism of the drug in dogs was different to that in man and other species.

1 'Cesamet' (Lilly).

Therapeutic Trials: Nabilone has been used as an oral antiemetic agent in the treatment of gastrointestinal toxicity in patients undergoing cancer chemotherapy. Significant reduction of the duration and severity of nausea and frequency of vomiting is usually seen after nabilone 2mg 2 or 3 times daily in about 50 to 70% of patients, many of whom have been refractory to conventional antiemetics. In a limited number of comparative studies, nabilone has produced significantly greater reduction of symptoms than prochlorperazine, and reduced the necessity for supplemental parenteral therapy. Despite a higher incidence of side effects, nabilone has also been preferred to prochlorperazine as treatment of choice in the majority of cases (40 to 75% *vs* 15 to 23%), although in 2 of 3 placebo-controlled studies less than 20% of patients elected to continue with nabilone therapy. Patients with more severe symptoms [induced by cisplatin, doxorubicin (adriamycin), cyclophosphamide] appear to respond equally well as those with less severe symptoms, and thus comprise the preferred treatment group for therapy with nabilone. Further therapeutic studies are needed with nabilone, particularly to clarify its efficacy compared with high dose metoclopramide and other antiemetic agents, and its use in combination with other antiemetic agents.

Side Effects: Nabilone is associated with a high incidence of mild or moderate side effects, the most common being drowsiness, dizziness and vertigo (60 to 70%), and dry mouth (29%). More severe effects such as postural hypotension, ataxia, visual disturbance and some toxic psychoses are occasionally seen, and may necessitate treatment withdrawal. Nabilone produces a higher incidence of side effects than prochlorperazine, but they may lessen in severity during continued therapy.

Dosage and Administration: The usual therapeutic dose of nabilone for use as an antiemetic agent in patients undergoing cancer chemotherapy is 2mg twice daily commencing 12 hours prior to, and continuing until one dose after, chemotherapy.

1. Pharmacodynamic Studies

Nabilone is a new synthetic cannabinoid derivative used as an antiemetic drug in the control of nausea and vomiting in patients undergoing cancer chemotherapy. Along with Δ^9-tetrahydrocannabinol, the active principal of marijuana, nabilone belongs to the chemical group known as dibenzo (b,d) pyrans. The presence of a ketone group at position 9 of the dibenzopyran nucleus and a dimethylheptyl side chain (fig. 1) are believed to be responsible for the differing pharmacological profiles of nabilone and Δ^9-tetrahydrocannabinol.

1.1 Antiemetic Activity

Using a technique of measuring thoracic pressure pulses (generated by the somatic muscles of ventilation) and the emetic end-point, the effects of nabilone, N-methyl-levonantradol and prochlorperazine on the latency, frequency and duration of emetic action of intravenous cisplatin were determined in unanaesthetised cats. Nabilone (25 to 100 μg/kg) and N-methyl-levonantradol (3 to 20 μg/kg) demonstrated dose-dependent antiemetic activity, affording complete protection at the highest doses, or increased latency to the first emetic episode and reduced the number of episodes at lower doses compared with control observations (table I). The effective doses in 50% of animals (ED_{50}) of these cannabinoids were 54 and 4.8 μg/kg, respectively, with prochlorperazine affording only minimal protection by comparison (McCarthy and Borison, 1981). In another study in anaesthetised cats where severity and repetition of vomiting were not assessed, intravenous nabilone 100 μg/kg abolished the vomiting associated with intravenous carmustine [1,3-bis-(2-chlorethyl)-1-nitrosurea] 10 to 20 mg/kg, and markedly reduced the vomiting associated with intravenous mustine (mechloretha-

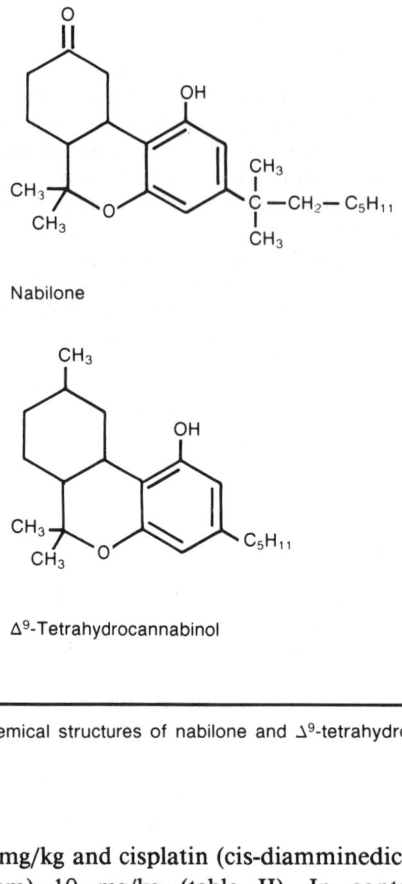

Fig. 1. Chemical structures of nabilone and Δ^9-tetrahydrocannabinol.

mine) 5 mg/kg and cisplatin (cis-diamminedichloroplatinum) 10 mg/kg (table II). In contrast, prochlorperazine 1 to 4 mg/kg afforded no protection against vomiting induced by mustine. Intravenous nabilone 25 to 200 μg/kg also resulted in a dose-related (but less potent) inhibition of emesis produced by intracerebroventricular apomorphine 0.25mg and intravenous deslanoside 0.12 to 0.16 mg/kg (ED_{50} 75 and 150 μg/kg, respectively), but showed no activity against intravenous bolus or infusion of nicotine (20 to 50 μg/kg and 50 to 100 μg/kg, respectively) [London et al., 1979].

Correlation of these results with studies in dogs which showed that prochlorperazine was highly effective in blocking apomorphine-induced emesis, whereas nabilone was ineffective (Stark, 1982a), suggests that the antiemetic action of nabilone occurs at a central nervous system (CNS) site which is not mediated primarily by a dopaminergic pathway, although some activity at the chemoreceptor trigger zone may occur. The emetic suppressant action of nabilone is possibly effected in the forebrain in association with its psychotropic influence to cause an inhibition of the vomiting control mechanism in the medulla oblongata through descending connections (London et al., 1979; Stark, 1982a).

1.2 Cardiovascular Effects

Intravenous nabilone, N-methyl-levonantradol and Δ^9-tetrahydrocannabinol consistently produced a rapid dose-related reduction in blood pressure and heart rate in anaesthetised healthy intact and vagotomised cats. In contrast to the respiratory effects of the drugs, cardiovascular effects were response limited (section 1.3) and did not progress ultimately to failure. There was no spontaneous reversal or indication of tachyphylaxis of either cardiovascular or respiratory effect upon repeated exposure to the drugs over a 6-hour period. The results indicate a direct decelerator action on the cardiac pacemaker and a central vagotonic action of these cannabinoids, and are in contrast to the tachycardia and slight hypertension which has been observed in unanaesthetised humans following exposure to other cannabinoids. These differences may be due to: species variation; state of anaes-

Table I. Effects of nabilone on the mean emesis latency period and number of emetic events in cats treated with cisplatin 7.5 mg/kg (after McCarthy and Borison, 1981)

Nabilone dose (μg/kg)	No. of cats vomiting	Mean time to first event (mins)	Mean no. of events
Control	7/7	71	3.7
25	2/2	123	2.0
50	4/6	140	1.5
100	0/6	NR	NR

NR = No result; complete protection from cisplatin-induced emesis.

Table II. Effect of pretreatment with intravenous nabilone (100 μg/kg) on the incidence of early vomiting induced by intravenous carmustine, mustine and cisplatin in cats (after London et al., 1979)

Drug	Dose (mg/kg)	Frequency of vomiting	
		control	nabilone-treated
Carmustine	10	5/13	0/10
	20	6/9	0/4
Mustine	5	5/5	2/8
Cisplatin	10	5/6	2/11

thesia; dose levels; and, importantly, to prior exposure to cannabis in man (Doherty et al., 1983). In another study, the cardiovascular effects of nabilone, canbisol, Δ^9-tetrahydrocannabinol and chlordiazepoxide were studied in unanaesthetised rabbits, dogs, rhesus monkeys and hypertensive rats. No consistent haemodynamic effects were seen with nabilone or the other cannabinoids; modest hypotensive activity was seen in rabbits and hypertensive rats, and variable effects in rhesus monkeys and dogs. The authors concluded that cardiovascular effects were linked closely to behavioural effects (Stark and Dews, 1980a).

The effects of nabilone on heart rate and standing and supine mean arterial blood pressures in healthy subjects and asthmatic patients did not differ significantly from placebo in one study (Gong et al., 1983) whilst in another, small but significant increases in pulse rates were seen in healthy subjects (Mendelson and Mello, 1984). Profound effects on standing blood pressure occurred initially in another study in healthy volunteers, however this effect became less marked upon repeated administration (Lemberger and Rowe, 1975; section 1.6).

1.3 Respiratory Effects

In experiments using isolated guinea-pig bronchus, neither nabilone (0.1 mmol/L) nor Δ^9-tetrahydrocannabinol (0.5 mmol/L) influenced the response to carbachol, histamine, potassium chloride, prostaglandin $F_{2\alpha}$ or caused relaxation in submaximally contracted tissues, or influenced the antigen-induced responses in tissues from ovalbumin-sensitised guinea-pigs. These compounds therefore did not display any direct action on respiratory smooth muscle or act by inhibiting mediator release. Thus, the bronchodilatory activity observed in man (see below) may be of indirect or central origin (Orzelek-O'Neil et al., 1980).

The outstanding respiratory depressant effect of nabilone (25 to 500 μg/kg), N-methyl-levonantradol and Δ^9-tetrahydrocannabinol in intact anaesthetised cats was an elevation of resting alveolar concentration of carbon dioxide (F_ACO_2) with little or no effect on the tidal volume (V_T). These effects were even more pronounced in vagotomised, anaesthetised cats.

The relative potency of N-methyl-levonantradol, nabilone, and Δ^9-tetrahydrocannabinol with regard to the elevation of F_ACO_2 was in the order of 100 : 10 : 1. Apneustic respiration was not observed, even in vagotomised cats. These results were consistent with depression of respiratory frequency, indicating a direct central depression of the respiratory rhythm centre in the lower medulla (Doherty et al., 1983).

In a comparative study, oral doses of nabilone 2mg, terbutaline 5mg and placebo were administered to 6 healthy volunteers and 6 stable asthmatics. There were no significant changes in respiratory rate, forced vital capacity or forced expiratory volume with any drug in healthy subjects, but terbutaline and, to a lesser extent, nabilone increased specific airways conductance to a greater degree than placebo. In asthmatic subjects only terbutaline produced significant increases in forced vital capacity, forced expiratory volume or specific airways conductance (through 1 to 6 hours). Nabilone produced small, but not significant, increases in indices of respiratory function (Gong et al., 1983).

1.4 Behavioural Effects

1.4.1 Animal Models

The anxiolytic activity of nabilone was first detected as a dose-related taming of hyper-reactivity seen in rats with mechanically destroyed medial and lateral areas of the septum (Stark and Henderson, 1966). In the muricidal rat assay, which is considered to be primarily a predictor of antidepressant and secondarily of anxiolytic activity, a dose-related decrease in muricidal activity was seen (Stark and Dews, 1980b).

In the mouse activity test, which measures exploratory behaviour (which may be a partially cognitive function), nabilone had the effect of lowering the typically high early activity (first 30 minutes), but raising the late activity, while the total activity remained relatively constant (Stark and Dews, 1980b). CNS stimulants typically increase counts at all time intervals, whereas depressants have the opposite effect.

A subjective evaluation of the behavioural effects of nabilone 25 to 100 μg/kg and N-methyl-levonantradol 3 to 20 μg/kg in cats showed some disturbance of posture and movement with both drugs at lower doses. However, at the higher doses N-methyl-levonantradol produced moderate ataxia and occasional startle responses whereas nabilone produced severe locomotor disturbance, ataxia and catalepsy. Prochlorperazine 4 mg/kg also produced marked behavioural changes and at this dose produced only minimal antiemetic effects (McCarthy and Borison, 1981). Behavioural effects seen in cats after nabilone 25 to 200 μg/kg were the same as seen in the previous study with, additionally, frank hypothermia in 1 animal at a dose of 500 μg/kg (London et al., 1979).

Handling-induced convulsions in mice have been reported to be both increased and decreased by cannabinoids. Convulsions were produced following intraperitoneal injection of nabilone 10 mg/kg and Δ^9-tetrahydrocannabinol 10 to 80 mg/kg (dose related) in one study. Maximal effects occurred 1 to 3 hours after dosing, and were abolished by diazepam 1.25 mg/kg. Convulsive responses were also reduced by phenobarbitone 48 mg/kg and ethanol 2 g/kg but not by phenytoin 20 mg/kg. Tolerance to the convulsant effects of Δ^9-tetrahydrocannabinol developed after a single dose, but pretreatment with cannabinol or cannabidiol had no effect on the response (Craigmill, 1979).

1.4.2 Anxiety States in Man

In 2 double-blind studies in anxious neurotic patients, nabilone 2 to 5 mg/day was found to be significantly more effective than placebo in reducing many of the anxiety ratings employed (Hamilton Anxiety Scale, Clinical Global Assessment Scale, SCL-56 scale) after 4 to 7 days of therapy. The most commonly reported side effects were dry mouth, dry eyes, drowsiness, dizziness and reduced blood pressure, including some cases of orthostatic hypotension (Fabre and McLendon, 1981; Fabre et al., 1978; Ilaria et al., 1981).

In contrast, when single oral doses of nabilone 1 to 5mg were administered to 8 anxious volunteers in a single-blind Latin square design study, only 2 subjects experienced significant antianxiety effects and these were only observed using the lower doses (1 to 2mg). Other patients experienced no significant alleviation of their subjective anxiety rating (Profile of Mood States), or significant effects on a continuous avoidance procedure of behavioural tasks, despite significant levels of sedation. High doses of nabilone (4 to 5mg) additionally produced orthostatic hypotension and mild increases in heart rate (Glass et al., 1980, 1981). These results are in agreement with those in a study in 36 volunteers who underwent 2 non-traumatic anxiety-producing procedures which avoided measuring effects on psychomotor or cognitive functions. Nabilone 2mg produced only mild (non-significant) antianxiety effects, whereas diazepam 5mg significantly alleviated anxiety (Nakano et al., 1978).

Subsequent antiemetic studies with nabilone in patients undergoing cancer chemotherapy revealed several cases of hallucinosis, at similar doses to those producing antianxiety effects. These findings along with the lack of data showing good antianxiety activity have led to withdrawal of the use of nabilone in alleviation of anxiety.

1.5 Opiate Activity and Abuse Potential

The 'chronic spinal' dog (spinal cord transection at T-10 under phenobarbitone anaesthesia followed by a 1-month recovery period) is a useful model in the study of opiate-like activity. Both morphine-dependent and non-dependent dogs have been used in studies with nabilone. In otherwise normal chronic spinal dogs, nabilone, nantradol, Δ^9-tetrahydrocannabinol and morphine all depressed the flexor reflex elicited by electrical stimuli (4.5 to 18psi), with the order of potency being nantradol (35) : Δ^9-tetrahydrocannabinol (5) : nabilone (1) : morphine (1). Nantradol, Δ^9-tetrahydrocannabinol and morphine also increased the latency of the skin twitch reflex, whereas nabilone did not. All cannabinoids produced a slightly increased startle response and mydriasis, in contrast to morphine which elicited miosis. Δ^9-Tetrahydrocannabinol was the only drug which did not reduce rectal temperature. Naltrexone failed to antagonise the effects of the cannabinoids on flexor reflex, skin twitch, miosis, rectal temperature and startle response, whereas all morphine-induced changes were reversed. In morphine-dependent chronic spinal dogs, cannabinoids showed partial suppression of signs of morphine withdrawal, but administration of naltrexone exaggerated the startle response. These results suggest that despite some similarities with the response to morphine, it is unlikely that the effects of nabilone and other cannabinoids are mediated via classic opiate receptors (Gilbert, 1981). In studies using rats, nabilone did not substitute for codeine or morphine and its activity was not antagonised by naloxone. The removal of nabilone after prolonged administration did not precipitate withdrawal symptoms (Stark, 1982a). However, in an antiemetic study in cats, naloxone reversed the blocking action of nabilone against apomorphine- and deslanoside-induced vomiting (McCarthy and Borison, 1977).

Δ^9-Tetrahydrocannabinol has been shown to have abuse potential of the cannabis type (of which it is the principal pharmacological constituent) producing euphoria or a 'high'. In 2 double-blind studies, healthy subjects who were experienced cannabis users received both nabilone and Δ^9-tetrahydrocannabinol to assess the abuse potential of the former drug. In one study intravenous and oral nabilone (0.25 and 2mg, respectively) produced lower degrees of 'high' (rating 2.5 and 2.3, respectively, according to the Cornell Medical Index rating) than did intravenous and oral Δ^9-tetrahydrocannabinol (2.2mg and 17.5mg doses produced ratings of > 4.5 and 3.3, respectively; Lemberger et al., 1982). However, in the other study using oral nabilone 2, 4 and 8mg and Δ^9-tetrahydrocannabinol 5, 10 and 20mg, both drugs produced similar, dose-related increases in symptoms such as euphoria, sedation and 'liking' the drug, with nabilone producing a high degree of dysphoria. It was estimated that nabilone was 7 times more potent than Δ^9-tetrahydrocannabinol (weight-for-weight) in producing these effects and consequently had abuse potential (Johnson et al., 1983).

1.6 Effects on Intraocular Pressure

Decreased intraocular pressure has been observed in man following smoking of marijuana (Hepler et al., 1972) and after oral and intravenous administration of Δ^9-tetrahydrocannabinol (Green et al., 1977). In a single-dose study, oral nabilone 0.5 to 2mg reduced the intraocular pressure by an average of 40% (from 32.5 to 19.5mm Hg) in 18 patients with open angle glaucoma or raised intraocular pressure. Peak effects were seen at 2 to 6 hours after a dose. In albino rabbits a 0.2% nabilone solution was topically applied to eyes and produced a 25% reduction in intraocular pressure at 30 to 150 minutes, although longer term studies indicated a tolerance to these effects after 6 days (Newell et al., 1979).

1.7 Development of Tolerance

Administration of nabilone in single oral doses of 1 to 5mg resulted in dose-related pharmacological effects in healthy volunteers in a single-blind study. While all doses induced relaxant and sedative effects, 1mg doses of nabilone did not produce euphoria, dry mouth, tachycardia or blood pressure changes. At 5mg doses nabilone produced marked postural (but not supine) hypotension, euphoria, dry mouth and increased heart rate (fig. 2). These effects were evident within 60 to 90 minutes and persisted for 8 to 12 hours. However, repeated

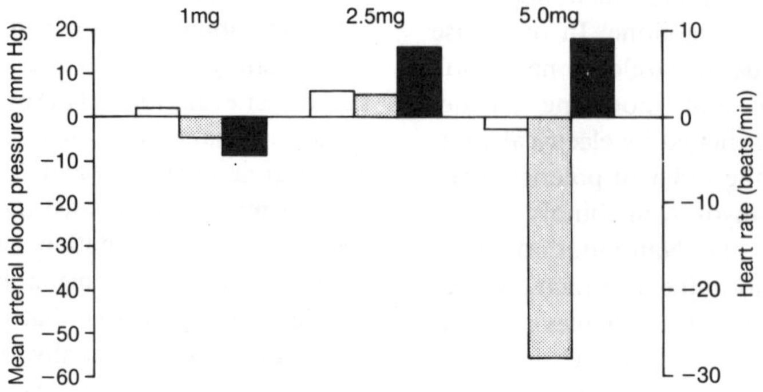

Fig. 2. Dose-response effect of nabilone on the change in mean supine (□) and upright (▨) arterial blood pressure and heart rate (■) compared with placebo in healthy volunteers (after Lemberger and Rowe, 1975).

administraton of nabilone 1 to 2mg twice daily resulted in adverse symptoms in the first 2 days which subsequently decreased until virtually absent at 6 and 7 days, without a concomitant reduction in the degree of relaxation.

Tolerance to these effects was confirmed when challenge with single doses of nabilone 5mg after this period resulted in a much reduced incidence of adverse effects compared with patients who had received placebo for 7 days (Lemberger and Rowe, 1975).

1.8 Toxicology Studies

Toxicological studies have been carried out in several species. Little or no acute toxicity occurred in the rat, mouse, dog or monkey, and long term studies of oral nabilone (90 days; no dose given) revealed no major untoward effects in dogs or rats. However, subsequent long term studies in dogs showed that seizures and deaths occurred as early as 56 days after nabilone 2 mg/kg/day and 5 months after nabilone 0.5 mg/kg/day. This observation prompted an immediate suspension of all studies with nabilone. In contrast, a subsequent 1-year pharmacokinetic and toxicological study in monkeys given oral nabilone 0.5 to 2 mg/kg/day revealed no deaths and considerably less toxicity than in dogs. The difference in toxicity observed between dogs and primates was found to be due to the species differences in the pharmacokinetic handling of nabilone. Dogs were observed to metabolise nabilone to an SSS-carbinol metabolite which they are unable to eliminate, leading to rising plasma concentrations. In monkeys and humans, the plasma concentrations of this metabolite are 25 to 30 times lower than in dogs (Archer et al., 1981).

In reproduction studies, nabilone (as the polyvinylpyrrolidine coprecipitate) was fed to rat and rabbit dams prior to mating and throughout gestation and lactation at doses of 1 to 12 mg/kg and 0.7 to 3.3 mg/kg, respectively. Fertility was unaffected but nabilone produced a dose-related decrease in live-born litter size in both species (19% and 31%, respectively, at the highest doses). No teratogenic effects were seen when given to rats from gestation day 6 to 15 and to rabbits at up to 3.3 mg/kg from gestation day 6 to 18. Doses of 25 mg/kg given to male rats had no significant effects on reproduction (Markham et al., 1979). When nabilone 12 mg/kg was administered from gestation day 14 through to postpartum day 20 in rats, live-born litter size and neonatal survival were reduced by 23% and 82%, respectively (Markham et al., 1979; Moss et al., 1979).

2. Pharmacokinetic Studies

Radiolabelled nabilone was readily absorbed from the gastrointestinal tract in man when administered orally as a coprecipitate with polyvinylpyrrolidine to healthy volunteers (fig. 3). Measurements of the area under the serum concentration time curve (AUC) values were 345 and 90 μg/L • hour after nabilone 2mg orally and nabilone 0.5mg intravenously. Thus, allowing for the differences in dose and assuming the kinetics were independent of dose and route of administration, the bioavailability of the oral dose was 95.8% (Rubin et al., 1977). Indeed, subsequent studies in 4 healthy adult volunteers did show the AUC to increase linearly over a dose range of 1 to 4mg, with a plasma clearance of 2.9 L/h, although large interindividual variation in the results was noted (Desante et al., 1983). After both oral and intravenous administration the absorbed drug disappeared rapidly, due to extensive tissue distribution and rapid metabolism, and the parent compound had a plasma elimination half-life of approximately 2 hours. However, total plasma radioactivity (due to circulating metabolites) persisted for a considerably longer period (half-lives of 20.6 and 35 hours after intravenous and oral doses) [fig. 3].

The major metabolites were found to be a mixture of isomeric alcohols (carbinols) produced by the reduction of the ketone group in the 9-position of nabilone. Nabilone and its isomeric carbinol metabolites were detected in plasma and faeces, but not in urine. The compounds discovered in the urine were not identified, but were highly polar and acidic with no evidence of glucuronide or sulphate conjugates being found. In addition a nabilone diol compound was detected in the faeces, the formation of which was attributed to a reduction of the 9-keto group plus oxidation at the penultimate carbon of the dimethylheptyl side chain by bacterial biotransformation in the gut. Most of the radioactivity from an oral or intravenous dose is eliminated in the faeces and urine (about 67% and 23% after 7 days, respectively). Bacterial degradation in the gut is suggested by the elimination of a small amount (< 1%) of radioactivity as respiratory $^{14}CO_2$ (Rubin et al., 1977). In *in vitro* studies 44% of over 350 bacterial isolates were capable

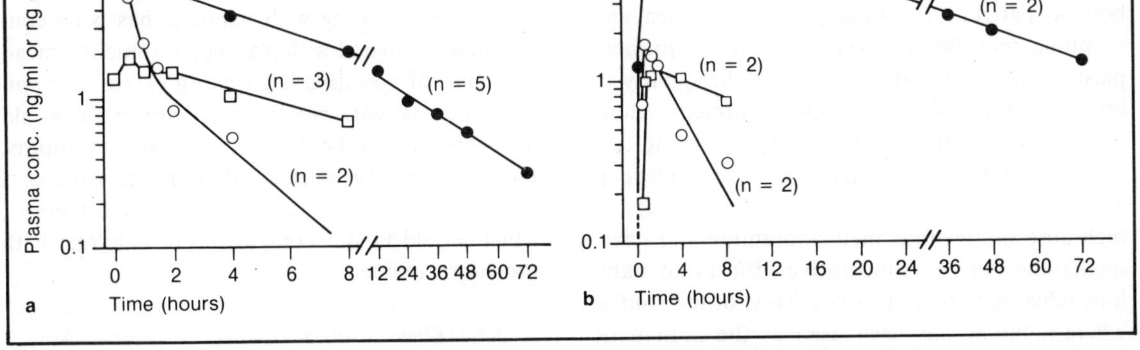

Fig. 3. Plasma concentrations of total radioactivity, nabilone, and the carbinol metabolite after intravenous (0.5mg or 12μCi) **[a]** or oral administration as a polyvinylpyrrolidine coprecipitate (2.0mg or 48μCi) **[b]** to healthy volunteers (after Rubin et al., 1977).

Table III. Overall data on the number of patients receiving different types of chemotherapeutic regimens and with different types of cancer treated in controlled studies using nabilone as the antiemetic agent

	Einhorn (1982)	Jones et al. (1982)	Wada et al. (1982)	Levitt (1982)	Cone et al. (1982)	Johansson et al. (1982)	Ahmedzai et al. (1983)	Steele et al. (1980)	Einhorn et al. (1981)
Chemotherapeutic regimen[a]									
Doxorubicin-based	28	25	39	0	...[c]	8	34	0	5
Cisplatin-based	28	14	43	23	...[c]	15	0	25	73
Other combinations	5	12	32	35[b]	...[c]	3	0	12	2
Cancer type									
Lung	...[c]	7	23	21	15	2	34	...[c]	0
Breast	...[c]	15	18	10	8	1	0	...[c]	0
Ovarian	...[c]	8	16	11	4	15	0	...[c]	0
Lymphoma	...[c]	12	12	0	2	2	0	...[c]	4
Other		12	45	16	21	6	0	...[c]	76[d]

a Cisplatin takes precedence over doxorubicin where both used in combination.
b Includes doxorubicin-based regimens.
c Not given.
d 70 patients with testicular cancer.

of modifying nabilone (Archer et al., 1979).

The extended pharmacological duration of action of nabilone despite its rapid and extensive metabolism suggests that its action, at least in part, may be attributed to one or more active metabolites.

3. *Therapeutic Trials*

3.1 Use as an Antiemetic During Cancer Chemotherapy

Gastrointestinal toxicity is frequently a limiting factor in the acceptability of cancer chemotherapy both to patients and to physicians. Nausea and vomiting may be so severe with some antineoplastic drugs as to adversely affect the quality of life and reduce compliance with treatment. Along with nabilone, other antiemetic agents being currently evaluated in these patients are prochlorperazine (with which nabilone has been compared) and high dose intravenous metoclopramide and dexamethasone (whose comparative efficacy to nabilone remains to be evaluated). Most of the studies where nabilone has been used as the antiemetic have been in patients being treated primarily with those agents causing the greatest degree of gastrointestinal toxicity, namely cisplatin and doxorubicin (adriamycin), and usually in patients where standard antiemetic therapy had failed to control vomiting and nausea (though which drugs had previously been used were not usually stated). The most commonly treated cancers have been located in the lung, breast, ovaries, and in one study, the testes (table III).

In assessing studies conducted with nabilone, there are a number of shortcomings of trial design which should be noted. The subjective use of 'good' relief has been used in many trials without standardisation. Indeed, in most studies although reduction of vomiting with nabilone has been considerable compared with placebo, in some the mean incidence of vomiting has been in excess of 7 episodes per patient, which many authorities would not consider to be 'good' relief of symptoms. Patients were also selected often on the basis of a poor response to standard phenothiazine therapy, which would favour comparison of nabilone with prochlorperazine.

3.1.1 Open Studies

In 2 non-blind, non-comparative studies, patients' received a variety of moderate to highly emetogenic drugs (including doxorubicin, cisplatin, streptozocin and mustine). 'Good' to complete relief of nausea and vomiting was seen in 33 of 52 patients following nabilone 1 to 2mg twice daily (Cone et al., 1982; 'good' relief being defined as at least 50% more effective than previous antiemetic therapy) and in 10 of 13 patients after nabilone 1 to 2mg 3 times daily (Herman et al., 1977; subjective rating scale in patients previously refractory to prochlorperazine and other conventional antiemetics). All 7 patients who received a daily dose of nabilone 2.5 mg/m^2 or more had 'good to complete' relief, whereas only 3 of 6 patients receiving nabilone 2.0 mg/m^2 or less had good or excellent clinical responses (Herman et al., 1977).

In another study of 20 patients undergoing treatment with various chemotherapeutic regimens, and who had experienced inadequate relief from nausea and vomiting after (low dose) prochlorperazine 4mg 4 times daily, nabilone 1 or 2mg twice daily produced 'good' or 'excellent' responses in 85% of patients (Niamatali et al., 1984).

3.1.2 Comparisons with Placebo

Four double-blind randomised crossover trials have compared nabilone 2mg twice daily with placebo according to a protocol designed by Stark (1982b). Each patient received 2 identical cycles of chemotherapy for the double-blind portions of the studies. The first dose of nabilone (or placebo) was given the evening prior to chemotherapy; the second doses were given 1 to 3 hours before chemotherapy, and all patients received at least 3 doses of nabilone.

Nabilone was clearly superior to placebo in all trials in terms of reducing the frequency of vomiting and severity of nausea, and in patient preference (table IV). The severity of the symptoms varied considerably between trials but did not seem to affect the efficacy of nabilone. Patients who vomited frequently, experienced proportionally as much relief compared with placebo [58% (Einhorn, 1982); 62% (Jones et al., 1982)] as those with less severe vomiting [60% (Levitt, 1982); 41% (Wada et al., 1982)], although whether relief in patients with over 5 episodes of vomiting can be considered

Table IV. Summary of clinical data from 4 double-blind crossover studies[a] comparing nabilone 2mg twice daily with placebo in patients undergoing cancer chemotherapy

Reference	No. of patients entered	No. of patients evaluated	Terminations due to adverse effects	Overall mean frequency of vomiting		Mean severity of nausea		Patient preference (%)			Mean change in S/D blood pressure (mm Hg)	Continued with open label nabilone
				nabilone	placebo	nabilone	placebo	nabilone	placebo	none		
Einhorn (1982)	61	50	6	9.65	22.9	1.48[b]	2.46[b]	90			−15/−9[c]	39
Jones et al. (1982)	54	24	11	7 .2	18.8	2.0	2.8	67	8	25		
Levitt (1982)	58	36	5	2.97	7.47	1.03	2.25	78	8	14	−16/−4[d]	11
Wada et al. (1982)	114	84	8	4.19	7.08[e]	1.22	1.96	70	22	8		22

a All study regimens according to the protocol of Stark (1982b).
b Day 1 only.
c Increase in blood pressure (6/5mm Hg) with placebo.
d No change in blood pressure with placebo.
e 5 patients excluded because of continuous vomiting.

'good' is debatable. Nabilone decreased the severity of nausea by 29 and 54% compared with placebo (table IV). Patients clearly preferred nabilone to placebo, with 64% of patients electing to continue with nabilone on an open-label basis in one study (Einhorn, 1982). However, in two of the other studies only 19% continued with nabilone therapy (Levitt, 1982; Wada et al., 1982). This observation did not appear to be linked to the termination rates due to adverse effects (10%, 9% and 7%, respectively) or mean change in blood pressure (table IV).

3.1.3 Comparisons with Prochlorperazine

An overall summary of the studies comparing the efficacy of nabilone with prochlorperazine in patients undergoing cancer chemotherapy is difficult because of the inconsistency of dosage regimens, patient populations and chemotherapy regimens. Having made that qualification it would appear that nabilone does have a greater effect than oral prochlorperazine in reducing nausea and vomiting associated with chemotherapy, and although the incidence of side effects is also higher, patients prefer nabilone therapy. However, in some cases, the doses of prochlorperazine used are now considered suboptimal.

In a double-blind comparative study in 37 patients receiving a variety of chemotherapeutic regimens, single oral doses of nabilone 2mg and prochlorperazine 10mg (slow release preparation) significantly reduced both the duration and severity of nausea and the duration and frequency of vomiting. Overall responses for nabilone were slightly better than those with prochlorperazine, but not significantly so. The duration of nausea after nabilone therapy decreased in accordance with the expected intensity of emetic stimulus [high dose cisplatin 120 mg/m^2 ± vindesine 3 mg/m^2 > low dose cisplatin 45-70 mg/m^2 ± vindesine 3 mg/m^2 or doxorubicin 45 mg/m^2 > mustine, streptozocin, actinomycin D and dacarbazine (DTIC)-based chemotherapy]. However, no such relationship was seen with either drug in relation to severity of nausea or duration or frequency of vomiting. It should be borne in mind when assessing the merit of this single-dose study that the prochlorperazine dose was suboptimal, some patients received sedatives or analgesics, and 13 of 16 patients guessed their therapy correctly from their side effect profiles, thus losing some of the 'blindness' of the study (Steele et al., 1980).

In two early double-blind crossover trials (reported in the same paper), 113 patients who had experienced severe nausea and vomiting during chemotherapy completed treatment with either (what is now considered to be high dose) oral nabilone 2mg, 3 or 4 times daily or oral prochlorperazine 10mg 3 or 4 times daily. 70 of these patients with testicular carcinoma received cisplatin daily for 5 days along with vinblastine and bleomycin, and received antiemetic therapy for 5.5 days. 12 patients with non-Hodgkin's lymphomas treated with cyclophosphamide, doxorubicin, vincristine and prednisone, and 11 patients with Hodgkin's lymphomas treated with nitrogen mustard, vincristine, procarbazine and prednisone, received antiemetic therapy for 1.5 days after each injection. 20 patients received other chemotherapeutic regimens including actinomycin D, dacarbazine, 5-fluorouracil, melphalan and nitrosurea compounds. 72% of patients had a partial response to nabilone and 8% experienced complete relief of symptoms, while prochlorperazine produced partial relief in only 36% of patients. There were significantly fewer and less severe episodes of vomiting with nabilone. 9 patients discontinued therapy due to side effects; 5 withdrew from nabilone (1 orthostatic hypotension and lethargy, 4 toxic psychoses); and 4 withdrew from prochlorperazine (severe somnolence, dry mouth, blurred vision). The predominant side effects were qualitatively similar with the 2 drugs, but occurred about twice as often with nabilone. Nearly all patients receiving nabilone experienced somnolence and dizziness and many had some degree of discoordination. In spite of these adverse effects 75% of patients chose to continue with nabilone therapy compared with only 15% preferring to continue with prochlorperazine (Herman et al., 1979). Subsequent reports of the same data also outline greater therapeutic efficacy (fig. 4) but also a higher incidence of decreased blood pressure and postural hypotension with nabilone than with prochlorperazine in these patients (Einhorn et al., 1981; Einhorn, 1982).

Nabilone 2mg twice daily was compared with oral prochlorperazine 10mg 3 times daily in a double-blind crossover study of 34 patients with small cell bronchial carcinoma. Most patients had not received previous chemotherapy but groups were otherwise poorly matched. All patients received chemotherapy which consisted of two 21-day cycles of cyclophosphamide 1 g/m^2, doxorubicin 40 mg/m^2 and etoposide 100 mg/m^2 on day 1, etoposide 100 mg/m^2 on days 2 and 3 vincristine 2mg with methotrexate 50 mg/m^2 on day 10 followed by folinic acid rescue. Antiemetic agents were administered for 3 days starting the day prior to cancer chemotherapy. 26 patients completed the study. Nabilone was shown to produce significant improvements in the subjective analysis of symptoms such as anorexia, nausea, retching and vomiting (fig. 5). The most severe symptoms were recorded on day 1 although the greatest number of episodes of symptoms occurred on day 2 in both nabilone- and prochlorperazine-treated patients. The mean number of vomiting episodes per patient during the 3 days of nabilone therapy (1.3, 2.0, 0) was significantly lower than with prochlorperazine (3.0, 2.6, 2.0). No patient required extra parenteral antiemetic therapy while receiving nabilone, whereas 4 of 30 patients receiving prochlorperazine required intravenous or intramuscular metoclopramide 10mg or chlorpromazine 50mg. 16 patients preferred nabilone therapy and 3 preferred prochlorperazine, however when adverse effects were taken into account 12 patients wished to continue with nabilone and 7 patients with prochlorperazine. Side effects were more prevalent with nabilone than with prochlorperazine (see section 4) with the most common effect of drowsiness occurring in 57% and 27%, and dizziness in 35% and 4%, respectively. There were no significant effects on blood pressure (Ahmedzai et al., 1983).

Twice-daily nabilone 2mg and oral prochlorperazine 10mg were administered in a double-blind crossover manner to 26 patients with various carcinomas undergoing chemotherapy with a number of agents (doxorubicin-based in 8; doxorubicin plus cisplatin-based in 14; other in 4). Antiemetic drugs were given for 4 consecutive doses (at least 3 doses to be evaluable). Efficacy was assessed in 18 patients, with nabilone being associated with a lesser severity of nausea (1.44 *vs* 2.06), significantly fewer episodes of vomiting (11.3 *vs* 23.7) or dry

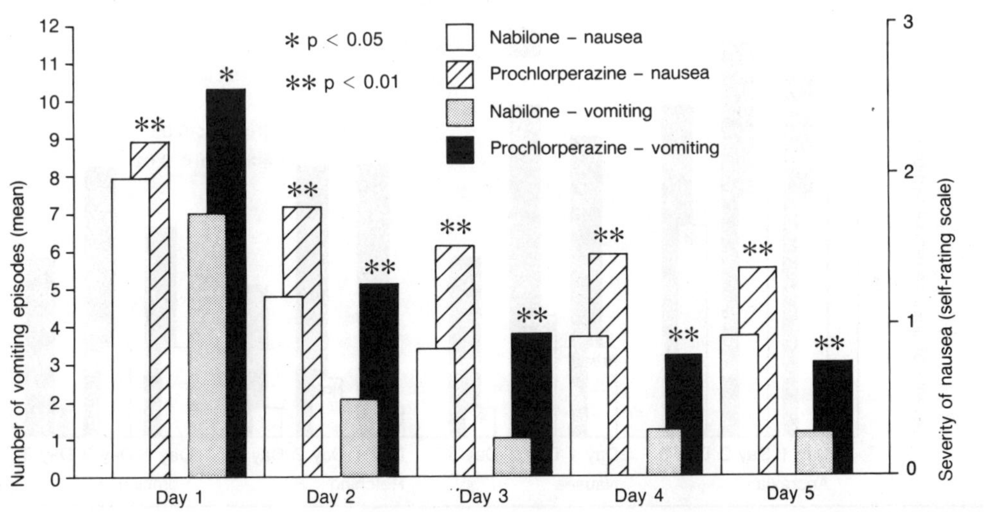

Fig. 4. Evaluation of effects of oral nabilone 2mg 4 times daily and oral prochlorperazine 10mg 3 times daily on the nausea and vomiting in 80 patients undergoing cancer chemotherapy (after Einhorn et al., 1981; Einhorn, 1982).

retching (7.1 *vs* 15.0), and greater patient preference (72% *vs* 17%) and overall therapeutic effect than prochlorperazine. However, patients experienced worse symptoms during their second crossover cycle of chemotherapy with both drugs. On the first and second cycles, the mean number of vomiting episodes during nabilone therapy was 6.7 and 14.2, and during prochlorperazine was 18.8 and 31.3, respectively. Side effects were observed in 54% of patients taking nabilone and in 39% receiving prochlorperazine (table V): severe postural hypotension occurred in 7 patients (causing withdrawal of nabilone treatment in 3 patients) and a further patient was withdrawn due to vertigo and headache. Decisions regarding patient preference were found to be based more on therapeutic efficacy than on side effects (Johansson et al., 1982).

3.1.4 Comparison with Chlorpromazine

In a randomised double-blind study in 20 patients with advanced gynaecological cancer who were receiving cisplatin-based chemotherapy, oral nabilone 3mg 3 times daily commencing the day prior to chemotherapy was compared with intramuscular chlorpromazine 12.5mg given 15 minutes before chemotherapy. There were no significant differences between treatments in reducing the frequency of vomiting (9.5 *vs* 11.4 episodes, respectively), however patients preferred nabilone therapy (10 *vs* 5) [George et al., 1983].

3.1.5 Combination with Metoclopramide

11 patients who received a 12-cycle cisplatin-based course of chemotherapy for a variety of malignancies also received antiemetic therapy consisting of a 'standard' metoclopramide dose (undefined) plus nabilone 1.5 to 3.0mg in divided doses. Six patients (58%) had fewer than 3 vomiting episodes and 9 patients (82%) had fewer than 5 vomiting episodes, compared with 46% and 27% of historical controls who received only 'standard' metoclopramide (Meyer et al., 1984).

4. Side Effects

Overall incidences of many of the reported side effects were difficult to quantitate due to the overlap in terminology used to describe them, and to widely differing methods of obtaining data. The most commonly reported side effects in studies with

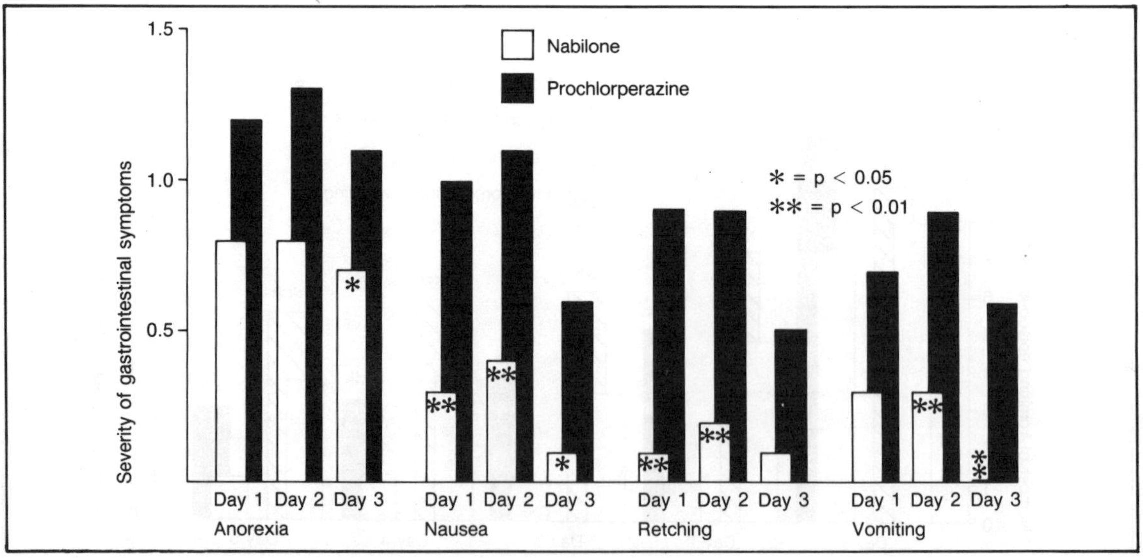

Fig. 5. Severity of gastrointestinal symptoms during cancer chemotherapy following 3-day antiemetic therapy with oral nabilone 2mg twice daily or oral prochlorperazine 10mg 3 times daily (n = 26) [after Ahmedzai et al., 1983].

Table V. Adverse experiences (%)[a] reported in crossover and open-label studies of over 20 patients during therapy with nabilone 2mg twice daily

Adverse experience	Ahmedzai et al. (1983)	Cone et al. (1982)	Einhorn (1982)	Johansson et al. (1982)	Jones et al. (1982)	Levitt (1982)	Wada et al. (1982)	Unpublished review
Number of patients evaluated	28	52	61	26	49	51	104	436
Drowsiness	57	40	89	4	51	61	34	65
Dizziness	53[b]	12		23[c]	65		49[b]	
Dysphoria	7	14	23				10	
Euphoria	14		18		6		25	7
Mood elevation	19[d]		7	8				27[d]
Decreased concentration			10			8		10
Disorientation	11					16	6	
Inebriated feeling	18					10		
Depersonalisation						35		6
Depression			7					10
Anxiety						8		
Vertigo			66[e]			67		65
Vision disturbance						10		9
Headache			34			10		9
Sleep disturbance			18		8	6		7
Dry mouth	11	6	62		31	24	28	29
Ataxia					8		9	13
Nausea			10		8	10		
Postural hypotension			8	42			5	5
Tachycardia	7							

a Only those side effects occurring in at least 4% of patients.
b Includes light-headedness.
c Include vertigo.
d Termed 'high'.
e Includes ataxia.

nabilone at usual therapeutic doses were drowsiness (4 to 89%), dizziness (12 to 65%) and dry mouth (6 to 62%) [table V]. In an unpublished review of cumulated data from 436 patients who had received nabilone during cancer chemotherapy (no dosage data), drowsiness (65%), vertigo (65%), dry mouth (29%) and 'high' (27%) were the most commonly seen adverse effects (data on file, Lilly). The incidence of side effects has been significantly higher with nabilone than prochlorperazine (occurring about twice as often) but there may be some similarities in type and severity of side effects (Ahmedzai et al., 1983; Herman et al., 1979; Johansson et al., 1982). Most side effects with nabilone are mild or moderate in severity and the severity of symptoms usually lessened progressively with continued treatment (Ahmedzai et al., 1983). However, they are occasionally severe enough to warrant early treatment termination.

In one study 10 of 18 patients receiving nabilone 2mg twice daily experienced significant psychotropic side effects, 5 of whom were withdrawn from treatment (Cornbleet et al., 1982). Exaggerated mood states were commonly reported, although the pattern of effects was not consistent, with euphoria and mood elevation occurring in some patients, whereas depression, toxic psychosis, depersonalisation and anxiety were reported in others (table V). In 2 studies, vertigo occurred in two-thirds of patients (Einhorn, 1982; Levitt, 1982) whereas this was not reported in other trials. Indeed, these studies also reported the highest overall side effect profiles, the only instances of headache, and along with Jones et al. (1982) the only sleep disturbances.

Postural hypotension is potentially one of the most troublesome adverse effects seen with nabilone, and has been observed in over 5% of patients on several occasions (Einhorn, 1982; Steele et al., 1980; Wada et al., 1982) and in one study was recorded in 42% (Johansson et al., 1982), although other studies have reported no blood pressure changes (Ahmedzai et al., 1983). Other side effects which have occasionally been reported include tachycardia (Ahmedzai et al., 1983), and more seriously, ataxia (Einhorn, 1982; Jones et al., 1982; Wada et al., 1982) and vision disturbance (Levitt, 1982).

Levels of β-human chorionic gonadotropin (an important 'marker' in the monitoring of treatment of testicular cancer) were unaffected by nabilone 2mg twice daily for 6 days in 6 patients with testicular teratoma who were also receiving combination chemotherapy with intravenous cisplatin, bleomycin and vinblastine (Hogan et al., 1983).

5. *Dosage and Administration*

Variations in the degree of therapeutic response and adverse effects necessitates the adjustment of nabilone dosage according to individual requirements. However, the currently recommended initial regimen is 2mg orally twice daily with the first dose being given 12 hours before the start of cancer chemotherapy. The duration of nabilone therapy depends on the chemotherapy regimen employed but usually continues for 1 dose after chemotherapy has been completed. Additional studies are required to better define optimal dosage recommendations for the various circumstances encountered in these patients.

6. *The Place of Nabilone in Therapy*

In moderate to severe nausea and vomiting associated with cancer chemotherapy, clinical trials with nabilone have clearly demonstrated its therapeutic efficacy in reducing nausea and vomiting, even in patients who were unresponsive to previous therapy with conventional agents such as phenothiazines, dopamine antagonists and antihistamines. Preliminary studies indicate that nabilone may be more effective than prochlorperazine, although the use of widely varying doses of both drugs makes interpretation of efficacy and toxicity difficult. Its efficacy and tolerability compared with that of other antiemetic therapies, such as high dose intravenous metoclopramide and dexamethasone, remains to be studied. Nabilone has not been studied in patients who have been treated with chemotherapeutic regimens associated with milder gastrointestinal effects where its high incidence of side effects probably makes it a less suitable alternative to conventional treatment. Initial studies showing some antianxiety activity were not pursued because of side effects, however this property may be advantageous in the anxious cancer chemotherapy patient. It is unlikely that nabilone will be used on a 'long term' basis, as the nature of cancer chemotherapy is itself intermittent. Therefore the possible abuse potential of nabilone is unlikely to be of clinical importance. Cautious use of nabilone should be advised in all patients upon first exposure, and special attention paid to the elderly and those with known cardiac disease.

Nabilone offers an effective alternative in the treatment of patients who experience either considerable nausea or frequent vomiting during cancer chemotherapy which is refractory to conventional therapy, provided the likelihood of side effects is outweighed by the expected therapeutic benefit in the individual patient.

References

Ahmedzai, S.; Carlyle, I.T. and Moran, F.: Anti-emetic efficacy and toxicity of nabilone, a synthetic cannabinoid, in lung cancer chemotherapy. British Journal of Cancer 48: 657-663 (1983).

Archer, R.A.; Fukuda, D.S.; Kossoy, A.D. and Abbott, B.J.: Microbiological transformations of nabilone, a synthetic cannabinoid. Applied and Environmental Microbiology 37: 965-971 (1979).

Archer, R.A.; Hanasono, G.K.; Lemburger, L. and Sullivan, H.R.: Update of nabilone research: The relationship of metabolism to toxicity in dogs; in Poster et al. (Eds) Treatment of Cancer Chemotherapy Induced Nausea and Vomiting, pp. 119-127 (Masson, New York 1981).

Cone, L.A.; Greene, D.S. and Helm, N.A.: Use of nabilone in the treatment of chemotherapy-induced vomiting in an outpatient setting. Cancer Treatment Reviews 9 (Suppl. B): 63-70 (1982).

Cornbleet, M.A.; Hamilton, D.A.; Christian, P. and Smyth, J.F.: Evaluation of nabilone as an anti-emetic. British Journal of Cancer 46: 492-493 (1982).

Craigmill, A.: Cannabinoids and handling-induced convulsions. Research Communications in Psychology, Psychiatry and Behaviour 4: 51-63 (1979).

Desante, K.; Wolen, K.; Bergstrom, R.; Hatcher, B.; Spradlin, C. and Lemberger, L.: Determination of the bioavailability and dose proportionality of nabilone using stable isotope technology. Proceedings of the 2nd World Conference on Clinical Pharmacology and Therapeutics, p. 48 (Washington, 1983).

Doherty, P.A.; McCarthy, L.E. and Borison, H.L.: Respiratory and cardiovascular depressant effects of nabilone, N-methyllevonantradol and Δ^9-tetrahydrocannabinol in anaesthetised cats. Journal of Pharmacology and Experimental Therapeutics 227: 508-516 (1983).

Einhorn, L.: Nabilone: An effective antiemetic agent in patients receiving cancer chemotherapy. Cancer Treatment Reviews 9 (Suppl. B): 55-61 (1982).

Einhorn, L.H.; Nagy, C.; Furnas, B. and Williams, S.D.: Nabilone: An effective anti-emetic in patients receiving cancer chemotherapy. Journal of Clinical Pharmacology 21: 64S-69S (1981).

Fabre, L.F. and McLendon, D.: The efficacy and safety of nabilone (a synthetic cannabinoid) in the treatment of anxiety. Journal of Clinical Pharmacology 21: 377S-382S (1981).

Fabre, L.F.; McLendon, D.M. and Stark, P.D.: Nabilone, and cannabinoid, in the treatment of anxiety: An open-label and double-blind study. Current Therapeutic Research 24: 161-169 (1978).

George, M.; Pejovic, M.H.; Thuaire, M.; Kramar, A. and Wolff, J.P.: Essai comparatif randomisé d'un nouvel anti-émétique: La nabilone, chez des maladies cancéreuses traitées par le cisplatinum. Biomedicine and Pharmacotherapy 37: 24-27 (1983).

Gilbert, P.E.: A comparison of THC, nantradol, nabilone and morphine in the chronic spinal dog. Journal of Clinical Pharmacology 21: 311S:319S (1981).

Glass, R.M.; Uhlenhuth, E.H.; Hartel, F.W.; Schuster, L.R. and Fischman, M.W.: A single dose study of nabilone, a synthetic cannabinoid. Psychopharmacology 71: 137-142 (1980).

Glass, R.M.; Uhlenhuth, E.H.; Hartel, F.W.; Shuster, C.R. and Fischman, M.W.: Single-dose study of nabilone in anxious volunteers. Journal of Clinical Pharmacology 21: 383-396 (1981).

Gong, H.; Tashkin, D.P. and Calvarese, B.: Comparison of bronchial effects of nabilone and terbutaline in healthy and asthmatic subjects. Journal of Clinical Pharmacology 23: 127-133 (1983).

Green, J.; Bigger, J.F.; Kim, K. et al.: Canabinoid action on the eye as mediated through the central nervous system and local adrenergic activity. Experimental Eye Research 24: 189-196 (1977).

Hepler, R.S.; Frank, I.M. and Ungerleider, J.T.: Pupillary constriction after maijuana smoking. American Journal of Ophthalmology 74: 1185-1190 (1972).

Herman, T.S.; Einhorn, L.H.; Jones, S.E.; Nagy, C.; Chester, A.B. et al.: Superiority of nabilone over prochlorperazine as an anti-emetic in patients receiving cancer chemotherapy. New England Journal of Medicine 300: 1295-1297 (1979).

Herman, T.S.; Jones, S.E.; Dean, J.; Leigh, S.; Dorr, R. et al.: Nabilone: A potent anti-emetic cannabinol with minimal euphoria. Biomedicine 27: 331-334 (1977).

Hogan, P.; Sharpe, M.; Smedley, H. and Sikora, K.: Cannabinoids and LCG levels in patients with testicular cancer. Lancet 2: 1144 (1983).

Ilaria, R.L.; Thornby, J.I. and Fann, W.E.: Nabilone, a cannabinol derivative, in the treatment of anxiety neurosis. Current Therapeutic Research 29: 943-949 (1981).

Johansson, R.; Kilkku, P. and Groenroos, M.: A double-blind, controlled study of nabilone *vs* prochlorperazine for refractory emesis induced by cancer chemotherapy. Cancer Treatment Research 9 (Suppl. B): 25-33 (1982).

Johnson, R.E.; Jasinski, D.R.; Boren, J.J. and Kocher, T.R.: Abuse potential of nabilone. Proceedings of the 2nd World Conference on Clinical Pharmacology and Therapeutics, p. 90 (Washington, DC, Jul-Aug 1983).

Jones, S.E.; Durant, J.R.; Greco, F.A. and Robertone, A.: A multi-institutional phase III study of nabilone *vs* chemotherapy-induced nausea and vomiting. Cancer Treatment Reviews 9 (Suppl. B): 45-48 (1982).

Lemberger, L. and Rowe, H.: Clinical pharmacology of nabilone, a cannabinol derivative. Clinical Pharmacology and Therapeutics 18: 720-726 (1975).

Lemberger, L.; Rubin, A.; Wolen, R.; DeSante, K.; Rowe, H. et al.: Pharmacokinetics, metabolism and drug-abuse potential of nabilone. Cancer Treatment Reviews 9 (Suppl. B): 17-23 (1982).

Levitt, M.: Nabilone *vs* placebo in the treatment of chemotherapy-induced nausea and vomiting in cancer patients. Cancer Treatment Reviews 9 (Suppl. B): 49-53 (1982).

London, S.W.; McCarthy, L.E. and Borison, H.L.: Suppression of cancer chemotherapy-induced vomiting in the cat by nabilone, a synthetic cannabinoid. Proceedings of the Society for Experimental Biology and Medicine 160: 437-440 (1979).

McCarthy, L.E. and Borison, H.L.: Antiemetic action of nabilone against apomorphine- and deslanoside-induced vomiting. Pharmacologist 19: 230 (1977).

McCarthy, L.E. and Borison, H.L.: Antiemetic activity of N-methyllevonantradol, and nabilone in cisplatin-treated cats. Journal of Clinical Pharmacology 21: 30S-37S (1981).

Markham, J.K.; Hanasono, G.K.; Adams, E.R. and Owen, N.V.: Reproduction studies on nabilone, a synthetic 9-ketocannabinoid. Toxicology and Applied Pharmacology 48: A119 (1979).

Mendelson, J.H. and Mello, N.K.: Reinforcing properties of oral Δ^9-tetrahydrocannabinol, smoked marijuana, and nabilone: Influence of previous marijuana use. Psychopharmacology 83: 351-356 (1984).

Meyer, B.R.; Reidenberg, M.M.; Drayer, D.E.; Pasmantier, M. and Lewin, M.: Initial trial of metoclopramide and nabilone combination anti-emetic therapy. Clinical Research 32: 688A (1984).

Moss, C.L.; Markham, J.K. and Hanasono, G.K.: Studies on the mechanism of neonatal toxicity in rats induced by nabilone, a synthetic 9-ketocannabinoid. Toxicology and Applied Pharmacology 48: A20 (1979).

Nakano, S.; Gillespie, H.K. and Hollister, L.E.: A model for evaluation of antianxiety drugs with the use of experimentally induced stress: Comparison of nabilone and diazepam. Clinical Pharmacology and Therapeutics 23: 54-62 (1978).

Newell, F.W.; Stark, P.; Jay, W.M. and Schanzlin, D.J.: Nabilone: A pressure-reducing synthetic benzopyran in open-angle glaucoma. Ophthalmology 86: 156-160 (1979).

Niamatali, C.; Fallon, S.D. and Egan, E.L.: Nabilone in the management of prochlorperazine resistant cancer chemotherapy induced emesis. Irish Medical Journal 77: 276-277 (1984).

Orzelek-O'Neil, R.M.; Goodman, F.R. and Forney, R.B.: The effects of Δ^9-tetrahydrocannabinol and nabilone on the isolated guinea pig bronchus. Toxicology and Applied Pharmacology 54: 493-500 (1980).

Rubin, A.; Lemberger, L.; Warrick, P.; Crabtree, R.E.; Sullivan, H. et al.: Physiologic disposition of nabilone, a cannabinol derivative, in man. Clin. Pharmacol. Therap. 22: 85-91 (1977).

Stark, P.: The pharmacologic profile of nabilone: A new anti-emetic agent. Cancer Treatment Reviews 9 (Suppl. B): 11-16 (1982a).

Stark, P.: Study design for the evaluation of the efficacy and safety of nabilone. Cancer Treatment Reviews 9 (Suppl. B): 35-37 (1982b).

Stark, P. and Dews, P.B.: Cannabinoids II. Cardiovascular Effects. Journal of Pharmacology and Experimental Therapeutics 214: 131-138 (1980a).

Stark, P. and Dews, P.B.: Cannabinoids I. Behavioural Effects. Journal of Pharmacology and Experimental Therapeutics 214: 124-130 (1980b).

Stark, P. and Henderson, J.K.: Increased reactivity in rats caused by septal lesions. International Journal of Neuropharmacology 5: 379-383 (1966).

Steele, N.; Gralla, R.J.; Braun, D.W. and Young, C.W.: Double-blind comparison of the anti-emetic effects of nabilone and prochlorperazine on chemotherapy-induced emesis. Cancer Treatment Reports 64: 219-224 (1980).

Wada, J.K.; Bogbon, D.L.; Gunnell, J.C.; Hum, G.J.; Gota, C.H. and Rieth, T.E.: Double-blind, randomized, crossover trial of nabilone *vs* placebo in cancer chemotherapy. Cancer Treatment Reviews 9 (Suppl. B): 39-44 (1982).

Authors' address: *Alan Ward,* ADIS Drug Information Services, P.O. Box 34-030, Birkenhead, Auckland 10 (New Zealand).

Drugs 30: 145-155 (1985)
0012-6667/85/0008-0145/$05.50/0

Drugs and Folate Metabolism

David G. Lambie and *Ralph H. Johnson*
Wellington Clinical School of Medicine, Wellington

Summary

Folates are a group of compounds which are required in the diet and are important in DNA, amino acids and possibly also amine metabolism. The biologically active folates are in the tetrahydro form. Tetrahydrofolates are produced from unreduced dietary folates by the enzyme dihydrofolate reductase. A number of drugs such as aminopterin, methotrexate (amethopterin), pyrimethamine, trimethoprim and triamterene act as folate antagonists and produce folate deficiency by inhibiting this enzyme. With other drugs which produce low serum and tissue concentrations of folate such as anticonvulsants, antituberculosis drugs, alcohol and oral contraceptives, the mechanism of this effect is uncertain. Possible mechanisms include reduced absorption, prevention of release of folate from tissue stores, altered plasma protein binding, or increased folate metabolism in the liver.

Treatment with folic acid antagonists such as methotrexate readily causes megaloblastic anaemia; this can be prevented by therapy with folinic acid (5-formyltetrahydrofolate). The role of other drugs in producing megaloblastic anaemia is less certain, e.g. it occurs in less than 0.75% of patients receiving anticonvulsants. The possible neurological and psychiatric effects of folate deficiency are also uncertain. However, in patients with folate deficiency who have neuropsychiatric symptoms, neuropathy or myelopathy, and normal vitamin B_{12} levels, it may be of value to try therapy with folic or folinic acid.

Folate deficiency is generally due to dietary factors or is seen physiologically during pregnancy. However, in recent years a number of drugs have been reported to cause folate deficiency. In some instances, e.g. the treatment of malignancy with methotrexate (amethopterin), the mechanism of folate deficiency is known to be inhibition of the enzyme dihydrofolate reductase. In other instances, e.g. with anticonvulsant drug administration, the mechanism is uncertain. In addition, there is controversy about the haematological and neuropsychiatric manifestations of drug-induced low folate concentrations. In this review, the possible mechanisms whereby this deficiency may occur are discussed and the clinical significance assessed.

1. Absorption and Metabolism of Folate

1.1 Absorption of Folate

Folic acid (pteroylglutamic acid) is the parent compound of a large group of naturally occurring structurally related compounds, called collectively 'folates'. Folate compounds are synthesised by higher plants as well as by micro-organisms and occur abundantly in yeasts, fresh green vegetables, as well as in liver. Dietary folates are absorbed mainly through the duodenum and jejunum; little is absorbed from the ileum, and none from the large bowel (Halsted, 1980; Hepner et al., 1968). Natural folates usually bear 1 to 6 or more additional glutamyl residues and these folate polyglutamates are deconjugated to monoglutamates by the enzyme folate conjugase which is present in saliva, succus entericus and in the small intestinal mucosa. The next step in metabolism is the reduction of the absorbed monoglutamates in the dihydrofolate form to the tetrahydrofolate derivative by the enzyme dihydrofolate reductase. Formylated and other non-methylated folates in the diet are converted, also in the intestinal cell, to the 5-methyl derivative (Perry and Chanarin, 1970). The 5-methyltetrahydrofolate passes via the portal circulation to the liver. Though dietary folates are well absorbed at low doses (50% with a dose of 200μg), at higher doses the proportion absorbed falls due to the rate-limiting transfer of compounds across the luminal cell surface membrane (Hepner et al., 1968).

1.2 Transport of Folate

Serum folate arises by displacement of endogenous folate from the liver by newly absorbed folate. About two-thirds of the 5-methyltetrahydrofolate in serum is loosely attached to proteins (L_2-macroglobulin, albumin or transferrin) [Markkanen et al., 1973b].

Folates enter bone marrow by an active uptake process into rapidly proliferating primitive red blood cells. Entry into the cerebrospinal fluid (CSF) from the blood involves a carrier-mediated transport process in the choroid plexus. The CSF folate level in man is about 3 times higher than the serum concentration (Wells and Casey, 1967) and is probably in the form of 5-methyltetrahydrofolate (Levitt et al., 1971). When folic acid is given orally, the serum folate concentration rises rapidly but CSF folate increases only slowly (Alperin and Haggard, 1970). Folate concentrations in the CSF may increase more rapidly with oral folate therapy if this is given in the form of folinic acid (5-formyltetrahydrofolate; 'Leucovorin') [Martinez Figueroa et al., 1980; Mattson et al., 1973].

1.3 Interconversion of Folates

The biologically active folates are the tetrahydro forms which are involved in the transfer of single carbon groups in amino acid metabolism and synthesis of purines and pyrimidines (for review see Blakley, 1969). The enzyme dihydrofolate reductase converts dihydrofolic acid and, much less effectively, folic acid to the tetrahydrofolate form. The attached carbon unit may be methyl ($-CH_3$), methylene ($-CH_2-$), formyl (–CHO) or formimino (–CH=NH) at the N_5 or N_{10} or $N_{5\text{-}10}$ positions of the folate molecule.

Various enzymes are present in mammalian tissues which are involved in interconversion of these groups. Folate antagonists such as methotrexate inhibit dihydrofolate reductase; however, there are no drugs in clinical use which are known to affect other steps in folate metabolism. 5-Methyltetrahydrofolate is the predominant tissue and serum form of folate. Folinic acid is one of the most chemically stable of the reduced folates and is used clinically to reverse the effects of certain antifolate drugs.

1.4 Metabolic Functions of Folate

1.4.1 Purine and Pyrimidine Synthesis

Folates are concerned in two stages in purine synthesis which involve insertion of carbon atoms in the purine ring. They are also involved in one reaction of pyrimidine synthesis, i.e. the methylation of deoxyuridylate monophosphate to thymidylate monophosphate. This latter reaction is rate-limiting for DNA synthesis in mammalian tissues. The enzyme system is coupled with dihydrofolate reductase and is sensitive to folate antagonists. The use of methotrexate in malignant conditions is based on its action in inhibiting DNA synthesis and hence cell division. Vitamin B_{12} is thought to be concerned in the provision of folate for formation of thymidylate monophosphate. The most likely explanation for its role is the 'methyl folate trap' (Scott and Weir, 1981).

1.4.2 Amino Acid Metabolism

The folate-dependent enzyme serine hydroxymethyltransferase catalyses the interconversion of serine and glycine. Its major role appears to be the production of glycine, which generates methyl groups which are used in the conversion of homocysteine to methionine. This latter reaction is also catalysed by a folate-dependent methyltransferase. One of the important uses for the methionine formed from homocysteine is its conversion to S-adenosyl-L-methionine (SAM), the primary methyl donor in mammalian metabolism. Vitamin B_{12} is required for methionine synthesis. In vitamin B_{12} deficiency, neuropathy may result from deficiency of S-adenosyl methionine required for methylation reactions in myelin synthesis (Hoffbrand, 1983; Scott and Weir, 1981). Folate therapy in patients with pernicious anaemia might lead to worsening of neurological symptoms by increasing cell division and thus incorporation of methionine into protein synthesis, so depriving methylation reactions of the limited amounts of methionine.

A folate-dependent enzyme is also involved in the histidine degradation pathway. Glutamate formiminotransferase acts to salvage formino groups for the 1-carbon pool by attaching these to tetrahydrofolate. A reduced supply of tetrahydrofolate in deficiency of folate or vitamin B_{12} results in a characteristic manifestation of these deficiencies – an increase in urinary excretion of N-formimino-L-glutamate (FIGLU), the other substrate of the reaction.

1.4.3 Amine Metabolism

Several methyl transferases are of importance in the metabolism of amines (Cantoni, 1975; Turner, 1977). For example, the biosynthesis of adrenaline (epinephrine) and inactivation of histamine involve N-methylation reactions, whereas the formation of melatonin and the inactivation of catecholamines involve O-methylation processes. Laduron (1972) proposed that 5-methyltetrahydrofolate may be the methyl donor for biogenic amines. However, Meller et al. (1975) reported that 5-methyltetrahydrofolate is not a direct methyl donor for biogenic amines and that S-adenosyl methionine functions as a methyl donor in the N-methylation of dopamine to adrenaline.

2. *Diagnosis of Folate Deficiency*

In a patient with megaloblastic anaemia and a serum vitamin B_{12} level which is normal, it is likely that folate deficiency is present. Folate deficiency may be confirmed by a therapeutic trial. In the non-anaemic patient, direct laboratory tests are necessary.

Measurement of serum folate is a reliable guide to the presence of folate deficiency. It is subnormal in all patients with folate deficiency and is normal or raised in vitamin B_{12}-deficient patients who are not also folate deficient. However, the serum folate concentration does not indicate the severity of folate deficiency since it may be equally low in grossly anaemic patients and in patients without anaemia.

A more reliable index of tissue depletion of folate is measurement of red cell folate. This is subnormal in patients with significant tissue depletion of folate, with or without megaloblastic anaemia, but is normal in patients with normoblastic haemopoiesis even if the serum folate is low (Hoffbrand et al., 1966). However, red cell folate may be low in about 60% of patients with megaloblastic anaemia due to vitamin B_{12} deficiency (Cooper and Lowenstein, 1964). Also, normal red cell folate concentrations may occur in patients with severe folate deficiency who have had a blood transfusion in the few weeks previously, since the folate in mature red cells is not released until the cells die. Most

Table I. Drugs causing folate deficiency

Drug mechanism	Therapeutic category
Inhibition of dihydrofolate reductase	
Methotrexate Aminopterin	Chemotherapeutic agents, immunosuppressives, antipsoriatics
Pryimethamine	Antimalarial
Trimethoprim	Antibacterial
Triamterene	Diuretic
Uncertain mechanism	
Phenytoin Phenobarbitone Primidone	Anticonvulsants
Ethinyloestradiol/ norethisterone acetate	Oral contraceptive
Cycloserine	Antituberculosis drug
Alcohol	

laboratories therefore carry out tests and report results of serum and red cell folate levels simultaneously.

3. Drugs Affecting Folate Metabolism (table I)

3.1 Folic Acid Antagonists

These are a group of compounds with a chemical structure similar to folic acid. Early studies revealed that a number of these drugs inhibit the growth of many bacteria. The most potent inhibitors are methotrexate, aminopterin and reduced derivatives of these compounds, and the 2,4-diaminopyrimidines (pyrimethamine). They usually act by inhibition of the enzyme dihydrofolate reductase, resulting in blockade of the production of tetrahydrofolate and its derivatives.

3.1.1 Aminopterin and Methotrexate

These drugs are used as folate antagonists in the treatment of leukaemias and related conditions and for the treatment of severe psoriasis (Weinstein, 1983). They inhibit dihydrofolate reductase by combining irreversibly with it. The megaloblastic change can be treated with folinic acid, which is already reduced and is thus beyond the step that is blocked.

3.1.2 Pyrimethamine

This drug also inhibits dihydrofolate reductase and has been shown to cause megaloblastic anaemia (Waxman and Herbert, 1969). It is widely employed as an antimalarial.

3.1.3 Trimethoprim

Trimethoprim, which was introduced as an antibacterial agent in combination with sulphonamides such as sulphamethoxazole, is also an inhibitor of dihydrofolate reductase. There have been reports of an association between trimethoprim use and megaloblastic anaemia (Chan et al., 1980) but Girdwood (1973) found that in a series of patients treated with the drug there was no evidence for the production of anaemia, and the serum and erythrocyte folate levels did not fall.

3.1.4 Sulphasalazine

Folate absorption from the intestine may be inhibited to a minor degree by sulphasalazine (salazosulfapyridine) [Halsted et al., 1981]. This may lead to megaloblastic anaemia when other factors, such as severe nutritional deficiency or coeliac disease, lead to folate deficiency (Longstreth and Green, 1983; Swinson et al., 1981).

3.2 Anticonvulsants

Investigations of megaloblastic anaemias not associated with low serum vitamin B_{12} showed that in some cases this was related to anticonvulsant therapy and that the effect was due to a secondary fall in serum folate (Druskin et al., 1962; Kohn et al., 1961). Subsequent studies of non-anaemic patients receiving anticonvulsants showed that low serum folate concentrations are present in a large percentage of the epileptic population, varying from 27 to 91% (Reynolds, 1973; Rose and Johnson, 1978). Subnormal serum folate concentrations are accompanied by a lowering of folate in red blood cells (Preece et al., 1971) and in the CSF (Reynolds et al., 1969; Wells and Casey, 1967). Low folate concentrations have been related to treatment with phenytoin, phenobarbitone or primidone, and Reynolds et al. (1966) found that the incidence rose with the number of drugs that the patient was receiving.

The proposed mechanisms for lowered serum folate in patients receiving anticonvulsants include an inhibition of the deconjugation of polyglutamates (Hoffbrand and Necheles, 1968). Although this has not been confirmed (Baugh and Krumdieck, 1969), there is evidence that phenytoin inhibits the absorption of the monoglutamate by the intestinal epithelium (Ariel et al., 1982; Gerson et al., 1972). Displacement of folate from serum proteins by anticonvulsants (Markkanen et al., 1973b) would lower serum folate concentrations but would probably not account for the reduction in red blood cell folate also observed.

Low serum folate may also be related to an effect of anticonvulsants on the drug-metabolising system in the liver (Chanarin, 1979; Labadarios et al., 1978; Maxwell et al., 1972). Folate is a cofactor for certain hydroxylations by hepatic microsomal enzymes and the reduction of serum folate in patients on long term anticonvulsant therapy may be the result of an increased metabolic requirement for folate. Studies in rats have shown that administration of phenobarbitone or phenytoin significantly increases the liver activities of glutamate formimino transferase and methylene tetrafolate dehydrogenase – enzymes involved in folate metabolism (Spray and Burns, 1972; Williams and Spray, 1976).

Other drugs which induce microsomal enzymes, such as phenothiazines or tricyclic antidepressants, may also reduce serum and tissue concentrations of folate. Patients in long term institutional care, who commonly have low dietary intake of folate, are likely to be at particular risk of folate deficiency when receiving anticonvulsants or other enzyme-inducing drugs (Labadarios et al., 1978).

3.3 Oral Contraceptives

The effects of oral contraceptives in causing lowered folate concentrations in serum and erythrocytes and an increased FIGLU excretion have been reported (Grace et al., 1982; Martinez and Roe, 1977; Shojania, 1982); other workers, however, have failed to confirm these observations (Spray, 1968; Stephens et al., 1972). Megaloblastic anaemia due to folate deficiency has been reported in a few women taking oral contraceptives (Necheles and Snyder, 1970; Paton, 1969; Streiff, 1970) but in some cases a contributing factor such as dietary deficiency or masked malabsorption was present.

It has been suggested that oral contraceptives may interfere with the absorption of pteroylpolyglutamates (Streiff, 1969), and Necheles and Snyder (1970) described lower rises in serum folate concentrations after treatment with polyglutamates in 2 women taking oral contraceptives than when therapy had been discontinued. Streiff and Greene (1970) suggested that oral contraceptives might cause malabsorption of dietary folate by inhibition of jejunal folate conjugase, but this was not confirmed by *in vitro* studies (Stephens et al., 1972). Shojania et al. (1975) found that oral contraceptive users have normal folate absorption but show increased serum clearance and urinary excretion of folates; they suggested that one possible mechanism for increased folate excretion would be a change in serum binding proteins for folate.

Low serum folate in oral contraceptive users may also be due to enzyme induction in the liver (Maxwell et al., 1972).

3.4 Antituberculosis Drugs

Low serum folate concentrations were found in 15 of 29 patients with tuberculosis who were being treated with isoniazid and cycloserine, but in only 2 of 55 patients receiving isoniazid alone (Klipstein et al., 1967). These results suggest that cycloserine can interfere with folate metabolism. The mechanism is unknown.

3.5 Alcohol

Megaloblastic anaemia is common in alcoholic patients. A study of patients with alcoholic cirrhosis (Lindenbaum and Lieber, 1969) showed that more than half had low liver and serum folate concentrations. It is likely that the cause of the deficiency is multiple. Poor intestinal absorption and liver storage of folate and inadequate dietary intake are likely to be important, but an acute effect of alcohol on folate metabolism may also play a role (Halsted, 1980; Wu et al., 1975). Alcohol has been shown to accelerate the appearance of folate deficiency in subjects with relatively normal folate stores by rapidly depressing the serum folate concentration (Eichner and Hillman, 1973; McGuffin et al., 1975). Short term exposure to alcohol has been suggested to block the release of 5-methyltetrahydrofolate from liver stores to bile for recirculation to tissues (Hillman and Steinberg, 1982; Lane et al., 1976), but there is a lack of evidence for this mechanism in primates; increased urinary and faecal losses may be of greater importance (Tamura and Halsted, 1983).

A role of folate in the ocular toxicity of methanol has been suggested. The toxic effects of methanol in primates may be related to formate accumulation. In monkeys, the severity of methanol toxicity and the accumulation of formate were found to be reduced by administration of folinic acid (Noker and Tephly, 1980).

4. Effects of Drug-Induced Folate Deficiency (table II)

4.1 Megaloblastic Anaemia

Treatment with folate antagonists such as aminopterin and methotrexate readily causes megaloblastic anaemia, but anaemia with other drugs associated with folate deficiency is relatively uncommon. Megaloblastic anaemia was first reported as a rare complication of anticonvulsant therapy by Mannheimer and colleagues in 1952. Since then there have been several reports which, as reviewed by Reynolds (1972), indicate that: (a) megaloblastic anaemia occurs in less than 0.75% of all patients receiving anticonvulsant drugs; (b) it is usually due to phenytoin, phenobarbitone or primidone, either alone or in combination; and (c) it is due to folate deficiency and always responds to treatment with folic acid.

4.2 Psychiatric Effects

Low serum folate concentrations have been reported in 10 to 50% of patients admitted to psychiatric hospitals (Shulman, 1979). It is not certain that this is evidence for folate deficiency as a cause of mental illness, as in most cases the deficiency appears to be the result of the illness – for dietary, drug or other reasons. However, insomnia, forgetfulness and irritability have been reported to be a result of folate deficiency (Herbert, 1962b; del Ser Quijano et al., 1983) as well as depression and schizoid psychosis (Botez et al., 1979a; Coppen and Abou-Saleh, 1982; Reynolds et al., 1966). Other reports link nutritional and drug-induced folate deficiency to mental deficiency (Anand, 1964; Hurdle and Picton-Williams, 1966; Strachan and Henderson, 1967; Trimble et al., 1980) and this may be responsive to folate therapy (Ahmed, 1972; Carney and Sheffield, 1970; Fehling et al., 1974). Also, mental retardation is a feature of some inborn errors of folate metabolism (Allen et al., 1983; Freeman et al., 1975; Tauro et al., 1976).

Table II. Clinical effects of folate deficiency

1. *Megaloblastic anaemia*
2. *Psychiatric*
Insomnia
Irritability
Forgetfulness
Depression
Schizoid psychosis
Mental deficiency
3. *Neurological*
Peripheral neuropathy
Myelopathy
Spinal cord syndromes
Restless legs
Decreased frequency of seizures?

Controlled trials of personality changes in patients with anticonvulsant-induced folate deficiency have, however, shown no clear relationship (Grant and Stores, 1970; Jensen and Olesen, 1970; Mattson et al., 1973). Studies in post-weanling rats showed an increase in learning performance with folate oversupplementation (Bachevalier and Botez, 1979). Dietary deficiency of folate resulted in impaired learning capacity, which was reversible by administration of folic acid (Bachevalier et al., 1981).

4.3 Neuropathy

Initial reports of neuropathies associated with folate deficiency included those of Arakawa et al. (1963), Hibbard and Smithels (1965), Strachan and Henderson (1967), Pincus et al. (1972), Fehling et al. (1974), Manzoor and Runcie (1976) and Su (1976), but there has been little study of the electrophysiological signs of polyneuropathy. A study of folic acid therapy associated with phenytoin use showed no effect on neuropathy as measured clinically or by nerve conduction measurements (Horwitz et al., 1968). However, a trial which we carried out of folinic acid therapy over a period of

1 month in patients receiving anticonvulsants showed significant reversal of abnormalities in motor and sensory nerve distal latencies (Martinez Figueroa et al., 1980). In a study of 28 patients receiving phenytoin, 6 patients who were found to have abnormalities of sensory nerve conduction had a significantly higher incidence of previous or current folate deficiency (Shorvon, 1979). Other workers have also found some evidence of improvement in nerve conduction velocities and sensory response after folate therapy in patients with folate deficiency and neuropathy associated with intestinal disease (Botez et al., 1978; Fehling et al., 1974).

Spinal cord syndromes, identical with those of subacute combined degeneration of the cord, have been described in patients with folate deficiency (Ahmed, 1972; Botez et al., 1976; Grant et al., 1965; Manzoor and Runcie, 1976; Pincus et al., 1972). It has been suggested that the pathological changes of the spinal cord are identical to those seen with posterolateral column degeneration seen with vitamin B_{12} deficiency (Robertson et al., 1971).

4.4 Folate Status and Seizure Control in Epilepsy

Many epileptic patients on phenytoin, phenobarbitone and primidone therapy have low serum and CSF folate concentrations. It has therefore been postulated that the anticonvulsant effect of these drugs may in some way be linked with the low folate concentrations. Administration of folate to epileptic patients increased the frequency of seizures as folate concentrations returned to normal (Dennis and Taylor, 1969; Lanzkowsky et al., 1969; Reynolds, 1967a; Wells, 1968). Neubauer (1970) in a further trial reported that administration of vitamin B_{12} and folate in such patients improved seizure control but seizures were more frequent when folate was given alone. However, these were uncontrolled observations, and controlled trials of folate administration in folate-deficient epileptics were unable to substantiate these findings (Gibberd et al., 1981; Grant and Stores, 1970; Jensen and Olesen, 1970; Mattson et al., 1973; Norris and Pratt, 1971; Ralston et al., 1970). It is possible that some of the reports of a worsening in seizure frequency may be accounted for by a lowering of the phenytoin serum concentrations when folate is given to these patients (Jensen and Olesen, 1970; Lambie, 1977; Mattson et al., 1973).

4.5 Neural Tube Defects

There is evidence of low blood folate concentrations in women who are pregnant with a child with a neural tube defect (Smithells et al., 1976), and a trial of folic acid therapy immediately before and during early pregnancy suggested that this could prevent neural tube defects (Laurence et al., 1981). Pregnant women receiving drugs which cause folate deficiency may be at particular risk of having a child with a neural tube defect. Aminopterin used to procure therapeutic abortions was reported to cause several cases of anencephaly (Thiersch, 1952).

5. *Metabolic Effects of Folate Deficiency*

5.1 Anticonvulsant Metabolism

Several workers (Baylis et al., 1971; Furlanut et al., 1978; Jensen and Olesen, 1970; Lambie, 1977; Mattson et al., 1973) have reported a fall in serum phenytoin concentrations in patients receiving folic acid therapy. Folate may be involved as a cofactor in drug hydroxylation and it is likely that the effect of folic acid treatment in reducing phenytoin concentrations is due to an increased metabolism of the drug. Kutt et al. (1966) demonstrated accelerated metabolism of phenytoin to *p*-hydroxyphenytoin in a patient with phenytoin intoxication. It is possible therefore that the low serum folate concentrations in patients on anticonvulsant therapy may slow metabolism of the drugs.

5.2 Amine Metabolism

5-Methyltetrahydrofolate may be involved in the synthesis of biogenic amines such as dopamine and serotonin (5-hydroxytryptamine), either as a direct methyl donor or in the synthesis of S-adenosyl methionine. This raises the possibility that the effect of anticonvulsants in reducing serum and tissue concentrations of folate may cause altered monoamine metabolism. There is evidence from animal studies that anticonvulsants may produce changes in monoamine metabolism (Bonnycastle et al., 1957; Botez et al., 1979b; Chase et al., 1969) and this may be related to their effects. Studies in man of homovanillic acid and 5-hydroxyindoleacetic acid (the metabolites of dopamine and serotonin, respectively) in CSF from folate-deficient patients have shown evidence of reduced concentrations in some studies (Garelis and Sourkes, 1973; Papeschi et al., 1972), but this has not been a universal finding (Chadwick et al., 1975; Lambie, 1977). It has been suggested that 5-hydroxyindoleacetic acid concentrations are low only in a subgroup of folate-deficient patients with neuropsychiatric symptoms which respond to folate therapy (Botez et al., 1982).

6. Clinical Implications

Drug-induced folate deficiency in some instances requires replacement therapy, as the patient may rapidly develop megaloblastic anaemia. Hence, with methotrexate therapy it is customary to treat the patients simultaneously with folinic acid. In women of child-bearing age who have low serum folate concentrations associated with anticonvulsant or other drug therapy, folate supplementation would appear to be a reasonable measure to prevent the development of congenital abnormalities (Hiilesmaa et al., 1983).

There are several reports of neurological disorders responsive to folic acid therapy (Botez et al., 1976; Manzoor and Runcie, 1976; Su, 1976). These include peripheral neuropathy (Botez et al., 1978; Grant et al., 1965), spinal cord syndromes (Anand, 1964; Hansen et al., 1964; Long et al., 1963), dementia (Strachan and Henderson, 1967), and neuropathic and myelopathic syndromes identical with those of subacute combined degeneration of the spinal cord (Manzoor and Runcie, 1976; Pincus et al., 1972), including the same pathological changes (Robertson et al., 1971). Folate deficiency seems to be responsible for these lesions as judged by such criteria as low serum folate and normal vitamin B_{12} concentrations and, in some patients, a gratifying response to treatment with folic acid. It seems reasonable therefore to suggest that serum folate estimations be obtained in patients with neuropsychiatric illness, myelopathy or neuropathy when the cause is not obvious. If vitamin B_{12} deficiency is excluded and the serum folate concentration is low, treatment with folic acid should be tried. Any benefit may be expected within a few weeks. In some instances of congenital folate deficiency (Su, 1976) and in patients with low folate concentrations secondary to treatment with drugs inhibiting dihydrofolate reductase, injections of folinic acid may be indicated rather than folic acid administration.

References

Ahmed, M.: Neurological disease and folate deficiency. British Medical Journal 1: 181 (1972).

Allen, R.J.; DiMauro, S.; Coulter, D.L.; Papadimitriou, A. and Rothenberg, S.P.: Kearns-Sayre syndrome with reduced plasma and cerebrospinal fluid folate. Annals of Neurology 13: 679-682 (1983).

Alperin, J.B. and Haggard, M.E.: Cerebrospinal fluid folate and the blood brain barrier. Clinical Research 18: 40 (1970).

Anand, M.P.: Iatrogenic megaloblastic anaemia with neurological complications. Scottish Medical Journal 9: 388-390 (1964).

Arakawa, T.; Ohara, K. and Kudo, Z.: Hyperfolic-acidemia with formiminoglutamic-aciduria following histidine loading. Suggested for a case of congenital deficiency in formiminotransferase. Tohoku Journal of Experimental Medicine 80: 370-382 (1963).

Ariel, M.; Eilam, Y.; Jablonska, M. and Grossowicz, N.: Effect of phenytoin on folic acid uptake in isolated intestinal epithelial cells. Journal of Pharmacology and Experimental Therapeutics 233: 224-226 (1982).

Bachevalier, J. and Botez, M.I.: Behavioral effects of folic acid deficiency and folate oversupplementation in postweanling rats; in Botez and Reynolds (Eds) Folic Acid in Neurology, Psychiatry, and Internal Medicine (Raven Press, New York 1979).

Bachevalier, J.; Botez, M.I. and Maag, V.: Learning deficits in folate-deficient rats reversible with folic acid or thiamine replacement therapy. Nutrition Reports International 23: 617-627 (1981).

Baugh, C.M. and Krumdieck, C.L.: Effects of phenytoin on folic-acid conjugases in man. Lancet 2: 519-521 (1969).

Baylis, E.M.; Crowley, J.M.; Preece, J.M.; Sylvester, P.E. and Marks, V.: Influence of folic acid on blood-phenytoin levels. Lancet 1: 62-64 (1971).

Blakley, R.L.: The Biochemistry of Folic Acid and Related Pteridines (North Holland Publishing Company, Amsterdam 1969).

Bonnycastle, D.D.; Giarman, N.J. and Paasonen, M.K.: Anticonvulsant compounds and 5-hydroxytryptamine in rat brain. British Journal of Pharmacology 12: 228-231 (1957).

Botez, M.I.; Botez, T.; Léveillé, J.; Bielmann, P. and Cadotte, M.: Neuropsychological correlates of folic acid deficiency: Facts and hypotheses; in Botez and Reynolds (Eds) Folic Acid in Neurology, Psychiatry, and Internal Medicine, pp. 435-461 (Raven Press, New York 1979a).

Botez, M.I.; Cadotte, M.; Beaulieu, R.; Pickette, L.P. and Pison, C.: Neurologic disorders responsive to folic acid therapy. Ca-

nadian Medical Association Journal 115: 217-223 (1976).
Botez, M.I.; Peyronnard, J.M.; Bachevalier, J. and Charron, L.: Polyneuropathy and folate deficiency. Archives of Neurology 35: 581-584 (1978).
Botez, M.I.; Young, S.N.; Bachevalier, J. and Gauthier, S.: Folate deficiency and decreased brain 5-hydroxytryptamine synthesis in man and rat. Nature 278: 182-183 (1979b).
Botez, M.I.; Young, S.N.; Bachevalier, J. and Gauthier, S.: Effect of folic acid and vitamin B_{12} deficiencies on 5-hydroxyindoleacetic acid in human cerebrospinal fluid. Annals of Neurology 12: 479-484 (1982).
Cantoni, G.L.: Biological methylation: Selected aspects. Annual Review of Biochemistry 44: 435-451 (1975).
Carney, M.W.P. and Sheffield, B.F.: Associations of subnormal serum folate and vitamin B_{12} values and effects of replacement therapy. Journal of Nervous and Mental Disease 150: 404-412 (1970).
Chadwick, D.; Jenner, P. and Reynolds, E.H.: Amines, anticonvulsants and epilepsy. Lancet 1: 473-476 (1975).
Chan, M.K.; Beale, D. and Moorhead, J.F.: Acute megaloblastosis due to cotrimoxazole. British Journal of Clinical Practice 34: 187-188 (1980).
Chanarin, I.: Effects of anticonvulsant drugs; in Botez and Reynolds (Eds) Folic Acid in Neurology, Psychiatry, and Internal Medicine, pp. 75-80 (Raven Press, New York 1979).
Chase, T.N.; Katz, R.I. and Kopin, I.J.: Effect of anticonvulsants on brain serotonin. Transactions of the American Neurological Association 94: 236-238 (1969).
Cooper, B.A. and Lowenstein, L.: Relative folate deficiency of erythrocytes in pernicious anaemia and its correction with cyanocobalamin. Blood 24: 502-521 (1964).
Coppen, A. and Abou-Saleh, M.T.: Plasma folate and affective morbidity during long-term lithium therapy. British Journal of Psychiatry 141: 87-89 (1982).
Corcino, J.; Waxman, S. and Herbert, V.: Mechanism of triamterene-induced megaloblastosis. Annals of Internal Medicine 73: 419-424 (1970).
Dennis, J. and Taylor, D.C.: Epilepsy and folate deficiency. British Medical Journal 4: 807-808 (1969).
Druskin, M.S.; Wallen, M.H. and Bonagura, L.: Anticonvulsant-associated megaloblastic anaemia. New England Journal of Medicine 267: 483-485 (1962).
Eichner, E.R. and Hillman, R.S.: Effect of alcohol on serum folate level. Journal of Clinical Investigation 52: 584-591 (1973).
FAO/WHO Expert Group: Requirements of ascorbic acid, vitamin D, vitamin B_{12} folate and iron. World Health Organization Technical Report (WHO, Geneva 1970).
Fehling, C.; Jägerstad, M.; Lindstrand, K. and Elmqvist, D.: Folate deficiency and neurological disease. Archives of Neurology 30: 263-265 (1974).
Freeman, J.M.; Finkelstein, J.D. and Mudd, S.H.: Folate-responsive homocystinuria 'schizophrenia'. A defect in methylation due to deficient 5,10-methylenetetrahydrofolate reductase activity. New England Journal of Medicine 292: 491-496 (1975).
Furlanut, M.; Benetello, P.; Avogaro, A. and Dainese, R.: Effects of folic acid on phenytoin kinetics in healthy subjects. Clinical Pharmacology and Therapeutics 24: 294-297 (1978).
Garelis, E. and Sourkes, T.L.: Factors affecting monoamine metabolite concentrations in the cerebrospinal fluid. Neurology 22: 1151-1159 (1973).
Gerson, C.D.; Hepner, G.W.; Brown, N.; Cohen, N.; Herbert, V. and Janowitz, H.D.: Inhibition by diphenylhydantoin of folic acid absorption in man. Gastroenterology 63: 246-251 (1972).
Gibberd, F.B.; Nicholls, A. and Wright, M.G.: The influence of folic acid on the frequency of epileptic attacks. European Journal of Clinical Pharmacology 19: 57-60 (1981).
Girdwood, R.H.: Trimethoprim/sulphamethoxazole: Long-term therapy and folate levels. Medical Journal of Australia (Special Supplement): 34-36 (June 1973).
Grace, E.; Emans, J. and Drum, D.E.: Hematologic abnormalities in adolescents who take oral contraceptive pills. Journal of Pediatrics 101: 771-774 (1982).
Grant, H.C.; Hoffbrand, A.V. and Wells, D.G.: Folate deficiency and neurological disease. Lancet 2: 763-767 (1965).
Grant, R.H.E. and Stores, O.P.R.: Folic acid in folate-deficient patients with epilepsy. British Medical Journal 4: 644-648 (1970).
Halsted, C.H.: Intestinal absorption and malabsorption of folates. Annual Review of Medicine 31: 79-87 (1980).
Halsted, C.H.; Gandhi, G. and Tamura, T.: Sulfasalazine inhibits the absorption of folates in ulcerative colitis. New England Journal of Medicine 305: 1513-1517 (1981).
Hansen, H.A.; Nordqvist, P. and Sourander, P.: Megaloblastic anemia and neurologic disturbances combined with folic acid deficiency: Observations on an epileptic patient treated with anticonvulsants. Acta Medica Scandinavica 176: 243-251 (1964).
Hepner, G.W.; Booth, C.C.; Cowan, J.; Hoffbrand, A.V. and Mollin, D.L.: Absorption of crystalline folic acid in man. Lancet 2: 302-306 (1968).
Herbert, V.: Minimal daily adult folate requirement. Archives of Internal Medicine 110: 649-652 (1962a).
Herbert, V.: Experimental nutritional folate deficiency in man. Transactions of the Association of American Physicians 125: 307-320 (1962b).
Hibbard, E.D. and Smithels, R.W.: Folic acid metabolism and human embryopathy. Lancet 1: 1254 (1965).
Hiilesmaa, V.K.; Teramo, K.; Granström, M.L. and Bardy, A.H.: Serum folate concentrations during pregnancy in women with epilepsy: Relation to antiepileptic drug concentrations, number of seizures, and fetal outcome. British Medical Journal 287: 577-579 (1983).
Hillman, R.S. and Steinberg, S.E.: The effects of alcohol on folate metabolism. Annual Review of Medicine 33: 345-354 (1982).
Hoffbrand, A.V.: Pernicious anaemia. Scottish Medical Journal 28: 218-227 (1983).
Hoffbrand, A.V. and Necheles, T.F.: Mechanism of folate deficiency in patients receiving phenytoin. Lancet 2: 528-530 (1968).
Hoffbrand, A.V.; Newcombe, B.F.A. and Mollin, D.L.: Method of assay of red cell folate activity and the value of the assay as a test for folate deficiency. Journal of Clinical Pathology 19: 17-28 (1966).
Horwitz, S.J.; Klipstein, F.A. and Lovelace, R.E.: Relation of abnormal folate metabolism to neuropathy developing during anticonvulsant drug therapy. Lancet 1: 563-565 (1968).
Hunter, R.; Barnes, J.; Curzon, G.; Kantamaneni, B.D. and Duncan, C.: Effect of folic acid by mouth on cerebrospinal fluid homovanillic acid and 5-hydroxyindoleacetic acid concentration. Journal of Neurology, Neurosurgery and Psychiatry 34: 571-575 (1971).
Hurdle, A.D.F. and Picton-Williams, T.C.: Folic acid deficiency in elderly patients admitted to hospital. British Medical Journal 2: 202-205 (1966).
Jensen, O.N. and Olesen, O.V.: Subnormal serum folate due to anticonvulsive therapy: A double-blind study of the effect of folic acid treatment in patients with drug-induced subnormal serum folates. Archives of Neurology 22: 181-182 (1970).
Klipstein, F.A.; Berlinger, F.G. and Reed, L.J.: Folate deficiency associated with drug therapy for tuberculosis. Blood 29: 697-712 (1967).
Kohn, J.; Mollin, D.L. and Rosenbach, L.M.: Conventional voltage electrophoresis for formiminoglutamic-acid determination in folic acid deficiency. Journal of Clinical Pathology 14: 345-350 (1961).
Kutt, H.; Winter, W. and McDowell, F.H.: Depression of parahydroxylation of diphenylhydantoin by antituberculosis therapy. Neurology 16: 594-602 (1966).
Labadarios, D.; Dickerson, J.W.T.; Parke, D.V.; Lucas, E.G. and Obuwa, G.H.: The effects of chronic drug administration on

hepatic enzyme induction and folate metabolism. British Journal of Clinical Pharmacology 5: 167-173 (1978).

Laduron, P.: N-methylation of dopamine to epinephrine in brain tissue using N-methyltetrahydrofolic acid as methyl donor. Nature (New Biology) 238: 212-213 (1972).

Lambie, D.G.: Anticonvulsant drugs: Their therapeutic and biochemical effects in epileptic patients (Ph.D Thesis, University of Glasgow, 1977).

Lane, F.; Goff, P.; McGuffin, R.; Eichner, E.R. and Hillman, R.S.: Folic acid metabolism in normal, folate deficient and alcoholic man. British Journal of Haematology 34: 489-500 (1976).

Lanzkowsky, P.; Erlandson, M.E. and Bezan, A.I.: Isolated defect of folic acid absorption associated with mental retardation and cerebral calcification. Blood 34: 452-456 (1969).

Laurence, K.M.; James, N.; Miller, M.H.; Tennant, G.B. and Campbell, H.: Double-blind randomised controlled trial of folate treatment before conception to prevent recurrence of neural-tube defects. British Medical Journal 282: 1509-1511 (1981).

Levitt, M.; Nixon, P.F.; Pincus, J.H. and Bertino, J.R.: Transport characteristics of folates in cerebrospinal fluid; A study utilizing doubly labeled 5-methyltetrahydrofolate and 5-formyltetrahydrofolate. Journal of Clinical Investigation 50: 1301-1308 (1971).

Lindenbaum, J. and Lieber, C.S.: Hematologic effects of alcohol in man in the absence of nutritional deficiency. New England Journal of Medicine 281: 333-338 (1969).

Long, M.T.; Childress, R.H. and Bond, W.H.: Megaloblastic anemia associated with the use of anticonvulsant drugs: Report of a case and review of the literature. Neurology 13: 697-702 (1963).

Longstreth, G.F. and Green, R.: Folate status in patients receiving maintenance doses of sulfasalazine. Archives of Internal Medicine 143: 902-904 (1983).

McGuffin, R.; Goff, P. and Hillman, R.S.: The effect of diet and alcohol on the development of folate deficiency in the rat. Journal of Haematology 31: 185-192 (1975).

Mannheimer, E.; Pakesch, F.; Reimer, E.E. and Vetter, H.: Die hematologischen komplikationen der epilepsiebehandlung mit Hydantoinkorpem. Medizinische Klinik 47: 1397 (1952).

Manzoor, M. and Runcie, J.: Folate-responsive neuropathy: Report of 10 cases. British Medical Journal 1: 1176-1178 (1976).

Markkanen, T.; Himanen, P.; Pajula, R.L. and Molnar, G.: Binding of folic acid to serum proteins: II. The effect of diphenylhydantoin and of various diseases. Acta Haematologica 50: 284-292 (1973a).

Markkanen, T.; Pajula, R.L.; Himanen, P. and Virtanen, S.: Serum folate activity (*L. casei*) in Sephadex gel chromatography. Journal of Clinical Pathology 26: 486-493 (1973b).

Martinez, O. and Roe, D.A.: Effect of oral contraceptives on blood folate levels in pregnancy. American Journal of Obstetrics and Gynecology 128: 255-261 (1977).

Martinez Figueroa, A.; Johnson, R.H.; Lambie, D.G. and Shakir, R.A.: The role of folate deficiency in the development of peripheral neuropathy caused by anticonvulsants. Journal of the Neurological Sciences 48: 315-323 (1980).

Mattson, R.H.; Gallagher, B.B.; Reynolds, E.H. and Glass, D.: Folate therapy in epilepsy. Archives of Neurology 29: 78-81 (1973).

Maxwell, J.D.; Hunter, J.; Steward, D.A.; Ardeman, S. and Williams, R.: Folate deficiency after anticonvulsant drugs: An effect of hepatic enzyme induction? British Medical Journal 1: 297-299 (1972).

Meller, E.; Rosengarten, H.; Friedhoff, A.J.; Stebbins, R.D. and Silber, R.: 5-Methyltetrahydrofolic acid is not a methyl donor for biogenic amines: Enzymatic formation of formaldehyde. Science 187: 171-173 (1975).

Moir, A.T.B.; Halliday, J. and Williams, I.R.: Lack of effect of folic-acid administration on cerebral metabolism. Lancet 2: 798-800 (1971).

Necheles, T.F. and Snyder, L.M.: Malabsorption of folate polyglutamates associated with oral contraceptive therapy. New England Journal of Medicine 282: 858-859 (1970).

Neubauer, C.: Mental deterioration in epilepsy due to folate deficiency. British Medical Journal 2: 759-761 (1970).

Noker, P.E. and Tephly, T.R.: The role of folates in methanol toxicity. Advances in Experimental Medicine and Biology 132: 305-315 (1980).

Norris, J.W. and Pratt, R.F.: A controlled study of folic acid in epilepsy. Neurology 21: 659-664 (1971).

Papeschi, R.; Molina-Negro, P.; Sourkes, T.L. and Erba, G.: The concentration of homovanillic and 5-hydroxyindoleacetic acids in ventricular and lumbar CSF: Studies in patients with extrapyramidal disorders, epilepsy, and other diseases. Neurology 22: 1151-1159 (1972).

Paton, A.: Oral contraceptives and folate deficiency. Lancet 1: 418 (1969).

Perry, J. and Chanarin, I.: Intestinal absorption of reduced folate compounds in man. British Journal of Haematology 18: 329-339 (1970).

Pincus, J.; Reynolds, E.H. and Glaser, G.H.: Subacute combined system degeneration with folate deficiency. Journal of the American Medical Association 221: 496-497 (1972).

Preece, J.; Reynolds, E.H. and Johnson, A.L.: Relation of serum to red cell folate concentrations in drug-treated epileptic patients. Epilepsia 12: 335-350 (1971).

Ralston, A.J.; Snaith, R.P. and Hinley, R.P.: Effects of folic acid on fit-frequency and behaviour in epileptics on anticonvulsants. Lancet 1: 867-868 (1970).

Reynolds, E.H.: Effects of folic acid on the mental state and fit-frequency of drug-treated epileptic patients. Lancet 1: 1086-1088 (1967a).

Reynolds, E.H.: Schizophrenia-like psychoses of epilepsy and disturbances of folate and vitamin B_{12} metabolism induced by anticonvulsant drugs. British Journal of Psychiatry 113: 911-919 (1967b).

Reynolds, E.H. Diphenylhydantoin: Hematologic aspects of toxicity; in Woodbury et al. (Eds) Antiepileptic Drugs, pp. 247-262 (Raven Press, New York 1972).

Reynolds, E.H.: Anticonvulsants, folic acid, and epilepsy. Lancet 1: 1376-1378 (1973).

Reynolds, E.H.; Chadwick, D.; Jenner, P. and Chanarin, I.: Folate and monoamine metabolism in epilepsy. Journal of the Neurological Sciences 26: 605-615 (1975).

Reynolds, E.H.; Chanarin, I.; Milner, G. and Mathews, D.M.: Anticonvulsant therapy, folic acid and vitamin B_{12} metabolism and mental symptoms. Epilepsia 7: 261-270 (1966).

Reynolds, E.H.; Preece, J. and Chanarin, I.: Folic acid and anticonvulsants. Lancet 1: 1264-1265 (1969).

Robertson, D.M.; Dinsdale, H.B. and Campbell, R.J.: Subacute combined degeneration of the spinal cord – no association with vitamin B_{12} deficiency. Archives of Neurology 24: 203-209 (1971).

Rose, M. and Johnson, I.: Reinterpretation of the haematological effects of anticonvulsant treatment. Lancet 1: 1349-1350 (1978).

Scott, J.M. and Weir, D.G.: The methyl folate trap. Lancet 2: 337-340 (1981).

del Ser Quijano, T.; Pareja, F.B.; Muñoz-Garcia, D. and Sánchez, A.P.: Psychological disturbances and folic acid in chronic epileptic outpatients. Epilepsia 24: 588-596 (1983).

Shojania, A.M.: Oral contraceptives: Effects on folate and vitamin B_{12} metabolism. Canadian Medical Association Journal 126: 244-247 (1982).

Shojania, A.M.; Hornady, G. and Barnes, P.H.: Oral contraceptives and serum-folate level. Lancet 1: 1376-1377 (1968).

Shojania, A.M.; Hornady, G.J. and Barnes, P.H.: The effect of oral contraceptives on folate metabolism. American Journal of Obstetrics and Gynecology 111: 782-791 (1971).

Shojania, A.M.; Hornady, G.J. and Scaletta, D.: The effect of oral

contraceptives on folate metabolism. III. Plasma clearance and urinary folate excretion. Journal of Laboratory and Clinical Medicine 85: 185-190 (1975).
Shorvon, S.D.: Anticonvulsant therapy and peripheral neuropathy: in Botez and Reynolds (Eds) Folic Acid in Neurology, Psychiatry, and Internal Medicine, pp. 335-347 (Raven Press, New York 1979).
Shulman, E.R.: An overview of folic acid deficiency and psychiatric illness: in Botez and Reynolds (Eds) Folic Acid in Neurology, Psychiatry, and Internal Medicine, pp. 433-474 (Raven Press, New York 1979).
Smithels, R.W.: Sheppard, S. and Schorah, C.J.: Nutritional deficiencies and neural tube defects. Archives of Disease in Childhood 51: 944-950 (1976).
Spray, G.H.: Oral contraceptives and serum-folate levels. Lancet 2: 110-111 (1968).
Spray, G.H. and Burns, D.G.: Folate deficiency and anticonvulsant drugs. British Medical Journal 2: 167 (1972).
Stephens, M.E.M.; Craft, I.; Peters, T.J. and Hoffbrand, A.V.: Oral contraceptives and folate metabolism. Clinical Science 42: 405-414 (1972).
Strachan, R.W. and Henderson, J.G.: Dementia and folate deficiency. Quarterly Journal of Medicine 36: 189-204 (1967).
Streiff, R.R.: Malabsorption of polyglutamic acid secondary to oral contraceptives. Clinical Research 17: 345 (1969).
Streiff, R.R.: Folate deficiency and oral contraceptives. Journal of the American Medical Association 214: 105-108 (1970).
Streiff, R.R. and Greene, B.: Drug inhibition of folate conjugase. Clinical Research 18: 418 (1970).
Su, P.C.: Congenital folate deficiency. New England Journal of Medicine 294: 1128 (1976).
Swinson, C.M.: Perry, J.; Lumb, M. and Levi, A.J.: Role of sulphasalazine in the aetiology of folate deficiency in ulcerative colitis. Gut 22: 456-461 (1981).
Tamura, T. and Halsted, C.H.: Folate turnover in chronically alcoholic monkeys. Journal of Laboratory and Clinical Medicine 101: 623-628 (1983).
Tauro, G.P.; Danks, D.M.; Rowe, P.B.; Van der Weyden, M.B.; Schwart, M.A.; Collins, V.L. and Neal, B.W.: Dihydrofolate reductase deficiency causing megaloblastic anemia in two families. New England Journal of Medicine 294: 466-470 (1976).
Thiersch, J.B.: Therapeutic abortions with a folic antagonist, 4-aminopteroylglutamic acid (4-amino PGA) administered by the oral route. American Journal of Obstetrics and Gynecology 63: 1298-1304 (1952).
Trimble, M.R.; Corbett, J.A. and Donaldson, D.: Folic acid and mental symptoms in children with epilepsy. Journal of Neurology, Neurosurgery and Psychiatry 43: 1030-1034 (1980).
Turner, A.J.: The roles of folate and pteridine derivatives in neurotransmitter metabolism. Biochemical Pharmacology 26: 1009-1014 (1977).
Waxman, S. and Herbert, V.: Mechanism of pyrimethamine-induced megaloblastosis in human bone marrow. New England Journal of Medicine 280: 1316 (1969).
Weinstein, G.D.: Commentary: Three decades of folic acid antagonists in dermatology. Archives of Dermatology 119: 525-527 (1983).
Wells, D.G.: Folic acid and neuropathy in epilepsy. Lancet 1: 146 (1968).
Wells, D.G. and Casey, H.J.: *Lactobacillus casei* CSF folate activity. British Medical Journal 3: 834-836 (1967).
Williams, D.L. and Spray, G.H.: The effect of some anticonvulsant drugs on depletion of folate in rats on a vitamin B_{12} deficient diet. British Journal of Haematology 33: 273-278 (1976).
Wu, A.; Chanarin, I.; Slavin, G. and Levi, A.J.: Folate deficiency in the alcoholic – its relationship to clinical and haematological abnormalities, liver disease and folate stores. British Journal of Haematology 29: 469-478 (1975).

Address for correspondence and reprints: Prof. *R.H. Johnson*, Wellington Clinical School of Medicine, Wellington Hospital, Wellington 2 (New Zealand).

Drugs 30: 156-173 (1985)
0012-6667/85/0008-0156/$09.00/0

Paget's Disease of Bone
An Update on Management

D.J. Hosking

Department of Medicine, University Hospital, Nottingham

Summary

The essential requirement for effective treatment of Paget's disease of bone is that the characteristic abnormality of bone remodelling is predictably corrected without the occurrence of significant side effects. Although the ideal agent is not currently available, appropriate use of the calcitonins or diphosphonates goes a long way to achieving this goal. Calcitonin (50 to 100 MRC units subcutaneously daily or 3 times weekly) will generally reduce bone turnover by approximately 50% within 6 months. However, very active disease will not be controlled and bone turnover will generally increase once treatment is withdrawn. Calcitonin is without significant side effects, although some patients will develop antibody-mediated resistance to the exogenous calcitonin species. An advantage of calcitonin is that there is radiographic evidence of a return to normal bone remodelling during treatment.

Although a number of diphosphonates (now more correctly termed bisphosphonates) are available for experimental use, only the first generation compound, disodium etidronate (EHDP) is commercially available. It too will reduce bone turnover by about 50% within 6 months when given in a dose of 5 mg/kg daily. Unlike calcitonin, it results in a more sustained control of bone turnover while having the additional advantage that it can be given by mouth. Although larger doses are more effective in controlling very active disease, there is a real risk of causing defective bone mineralisation which may result in the development of atraumatic long bone fractures or diffuse bone pains. Combinations of calcitonin and disodium etidronate in conventional dosage seem to result in an additive suppressant effect on bone turnover and may be indicated for more active disease. Advances in treatment are progressing rapidly and it seems likely that in the next few years the introduction of new agents for the control of Paget's disease will more nearly approach the ideal goal of treatment.

Paget's disease (osteitis deformans) is characterised by an increase in the rate of bone turnover coupled with qualitative changes in the remodelling process. This leads to characteristic clinical symptoms and structural abnormalities. The ideal treatment should effect a permanent cure of the primary cellular abnormality without the risk of significant side effects. Although such an ideal agent is not generally available, advances in the last decade make it likely that this goal could soon be realised. In the meantime, it is important to make the best use of current preparations. In essence, this means a choice between the calcitonins and diphosphonates used either alone or in combination. In this review the use of these agents, and their clinical effectiveness, are assessed against the background of the basic pathological changes in bone turnover.

Table I. Indications for treatment of Paget's disease

Surgical	
	Complete fracture (internal fixation, external splinting)
	Relief of neurological compression syndromes
	Correction of deformity
	Associated degenerative joint disease
Medical	
Common	
	Control of bone pain
	Immobilisation hypercalciuria or hypercalcaemia
	Neurological compression symptoms
Doubtful	
	High output cardiac failure
	Improvement of deafness
	Reduction in bone blood flow before surgery
Unproven	
	Rapid osteolysis in weight-bearing bones
	Prevention of deformity in relatively young patients
	Prevention of long bone fractures or malignant change

1. Prevalence and Pathophysiology of Paget's Disease

Although early descriptins of single cases were given by Saucerotte (1801), Rullier (1812), Wilks (1869) and Czerney (1973), the most complete account of osteitis deformans was given by Sir James Paget on 14th November 1876 to the Medical and Chirurgical Society of London. It is a relatively common condition in the United Kingdom, Europe, Australasia and the United States, although it is rare in Scandinavia, Switzerland, Africa and the Middle East (Barry, 1969).

The disease begins by an acceleration of bone resorption as a consequence of a primary abnormality of osteoclasts. Since resorption and formation are linked, this results in secondary changes in remodelling with the development of woven bone, marrow fibrosis and increased vascularity (Singer et al., 1978). A unique feature of the osteoclasts of Paget's disease (and one not seen in other bone cell lines nor in osteoclasts from other high turnover bone diseases) is that they contain inclusion bodies within the nucleus or cytoplasm (Rebel et al., 1976). These bear a morphological resemblance to the nucleocapsids of a paramyxovirus. However, although it is possible that Paget's disease may be due to a slow virus infection, this is as yet unproven and remains an area of intense study.

As a consequence of the progressive loss of the normal skeletal architecture the bones become painful, deformed and liable to fracture. This in turn accelerates degenerative changes in adjacent joints and may also lead to neurological compression symptoms. However, Paget's disease is rarely associated with significant mortality and only about 5% of affected individuals have symptoms directly attributable to the condition (Collins, 1976). Thus, treatment involves an element of selection; the main indications for treatment are listed in table I in an approximately descending order of responsiveness and clinical priority.

2. General Principles of Treatment

Bone pain is one of the commonest symptoms of Paget's disease and in the early stages it is often intermittent, perhaps only occurring after exercise or at night. Initial treatment should be with simple analgesics or non-steroidal anti-inflammatory drugs, irrespective of the level of bone turnover. If pain is not controlled and bone turnover is increased then specific treatment with the calcitonins or diphosphonates is appropriate.

Indications for surgical treatment include fixation of fractures, correction of deformity or relief of symptoms due to secondary osteoarthritis or compression of nervous tissue. This aspect of management has recently been reviewed (Stevens, 1981) and will not be considered further.

3. Drugs Used to Control Abnormal Bone Turnover

Fluoride (Riggs and Jowsey, 1972), glucagon (Condon, 1971) and mithramycin (Ryan, 1977) have all been used to reduce bone turnover in Paget's disease but only the calcitonins and diphosphonates have found an established place in treatment. Before considering the effects of these latter two compounds in Paget's disease, their structure and effects on bone will be briefly reviewed.

3.1 Calcitonin

Calcitonin is a 32 amino acid peptide hormone secreted by the parafollicular cells of the thyroid (Foster et al., 1964). Secretion may also occur in extrathyroidal sites, notably the pituitary (Deftos et al., 1978), lung and thymus, but the presence of immunoreactive material in a variety of other tissues probably represents receptor-bound hormone originating from the main site of secretion (Silva et al., 1981).

3.1.1 Structure-Activity Relationships

Calcitonin has now been isolated from a large number of species and synthetic preparations of the human, porcine, salmon and eel hormone have been produced for therapeutic purposes. A common feature of all the calcitonins is the 32 amino acid sequence with a ring closure between 2 cystine residues at positions 1 and 7 (fig. 1). Although 7 of the first 9 residues are common to all species, there is considerable variability in the composition of the rest of the molecule. However, there is no simple relationship between the amino acid sequence of the different calcitonins and their potency (Guttman, 1981). Thus, although human and rat calcitonin only differ with respect to 2 amino acids, they have very different potencies (table II). In contrast, human and porcine calcitonin (which have similar biological effects) differ with respect to 18 residues. It may be that the overall shape and size of the molecule is more important for activity

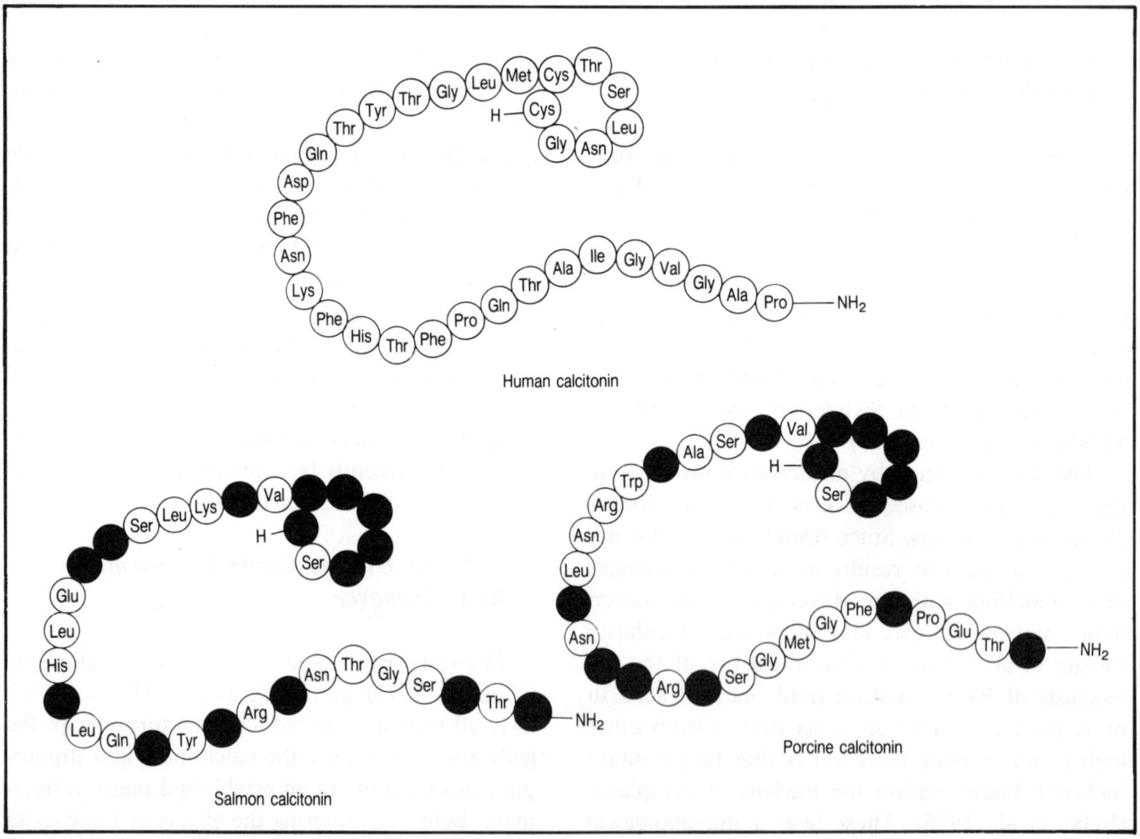

Fig. 1. Amino acid sequence of human calcitonin. Common residues in salmon and porcine calcitonin are shown as solid circles (after Guttman, 1981).

Table II. Relative potencies of different calcitonin species (after Guttman, 1981)

Species	Hypocalcaemic activity (MRC units/mg)
Salmon, Chicken	4000-6000
Eel	2000-4000
Rat	400
Beef, Sheep, Pig, Man	100-200

than the presence of isolated residues or sequences. For example, salmon calcitonin is more hydrophilic than the less active calcitonins and the greater preponderance of leucine residues in the mid-portion of the molecule may enhance α helix formation. Both of these properties could increase receptor binding, and *in vitro* studies using renal and skeletal membranes (Marx et al., 1972) have confirmed that this is at least partly true for salmon calcitonin. However, the duration of action of calcitonin may be determined more by its rate of renal inactivation rather than its receptor affinity (Newsome et al., 1973).

3.1.2 Effects on Bone

Calcitonin reduces the efflux of calcium out of bone (Grubb et al., 1977), but the cell type which is primarily responsible for this effect is still uncertain. Although the use of calcitonin in the treatment of Paget's disease depends on its inhibitory effect on osteoclastic bone resorption (Friedman and Raisz, 1965), it has not yet been established that it modulates physiological bone remodelling in man (Talmage et al., 1983). Osteoclasts have receptors for calcitonin (Warshawsky et al., 1980) and respond to the hormone by increasing cyclic AMP production (Holtrop et al., 1974). Within minutes of an injection osteoclasts show a decrease in the area of their ruffled border in contact with bone (Holtrop et al., 1974), while cells incubated on glass, which show pseudopodial motility under these circumstances, become inactive (Chambers and Magnus, 1982). Unfortunately, this inhibitory effect of calcitonin on osteoclasts is not sustained (Wener et al., 1972). This may be due either to down-regulation of calcitonin receptors (Tashjian et al., 1978) or to the emergence of a new population of resistant cells. Such a mechanism may underly the transient effect of calcitonin when used in the treatment of osteolytic bone diseases such as hyperparathyroidism or the hypercalcaemia of malignancy, and the failure to restore normal bone turnover in many patients with Paget's disease (De Rose et al., 1974).

An alternative view suggests that the main target cell for the action of calcitonin is the lining cell-osteocyte complex on the surface of bone (Grubb et al., 1977; Talmage et al., 1981). This seems to be supported by morphological studies showing contraction of lining cells and their underlying osteocytes within minutes of calcitonin injection (Matthews et al., 1972), as does the appearance of electron-dense material in the bone extracellular fluid surrounding the osteocytes. These changes may be relevant to a proposed physiological role of calcitonin during feeding (Cooper et al., 1981). It is suggested in this model that the inhibition of calcium mobilisation from bone by calcitonin offsets the rise in extracellular fluid calcium produced by intestinal absorption. This in turn limits the suppression of parathyroid hormone (PTH) which would otherwise have occurred and preserves its stimulatory effect on renal tubular calcium reabsorption, thereby ensuring that the absorbed calcium is retained within the body rather than being lost by renal excretion

At a cellular level, it is suggested that calcitonin enhances mitochondrial calcium uptake thereby lowering cytosolic calcium and its efflux from the cell (Borle, 1973). Phosphate, which increases the capacity of the mitochondria to accumulate calcium, would enhance this effect. However, calcitonin is known to increase total cell calcium (Harell et al., 1973) and this implies that the inhibition of calcium efflux from the cell is transiently greater than any inhibition of calcium influx. Thus, the overall consequence of these cellular events could be a reduction in transcellular calcium transport and an inhibition of calcium mobilisation from bone.

3.2 Diphosphonates (Bisphosphonates)

3.2.1 Structure-Activity Relationships and Pharmacokinetic Properties

It has been recognised for some time that pyrophosphate may play an important biological role in protecting the soft tissues from calcification, as well as regulating the deposition and dissolution of bone mineral (Fleisch et al., 1966). Unfortunately, it is not possible to utilise these properties therapeutically to modify bone remodelling because pyrophosphate is rapidly hydrolysed after administration. The diphosphonates (more properly termed bisphosphonates) which are characterised by a P-C-P bond (fig. 2) are resistant to hydrolysis but share many of the properties of pyrophosphate, including its high affinity for apatite.

Diphosphonates are not found in nature; since there are no enzymes which cleave the P-C-P bond they tend to be absorbed, stored, and excreted unchanged. Pharmacokinetic studies have been limited by the lack of sensitive quantitative assays for these compounds in biological tissues and most of the available data relates to disodium etidronate (disodium ethane-1-hydroxy-1,1-diphosphonate; EHDP). Intestinal absorption is poor (about 1 to 10%) and is reduced by food and antacids (Recker and Saville, 1973). Diphosphonates disappear rapidly from plasma. About half the absorbed dose is deposited in bone and the remainder is excreted in the urine; only very small amounts can be recovered from the soft tissues (Michael et al., 1972). Thus, the plasma half-life is very short, perhaps of the order of minutes, but the half-life within the skeleton is prolonged and depends on the rate of remodelling.

3.2.2 Effects on Bone

The selectivity of the diphosphonates' effect on bone reflects their pattern of clearance. Absorption to amorphous calcium phosphate at sites of active mineralisation inhibits this process directly, while deposition in fully mineralised bone only inhibits resorption when this bone is subsequently mobilised.

The main reason for the interest in the diphosphonates in the treatment of Paget's disease is their ability to inhibit bone resorption. The mechanism by which this is brought about is uncertain. Since there is no correlation between their *in vitro* and *in vivo* activity this might suggest that factors other

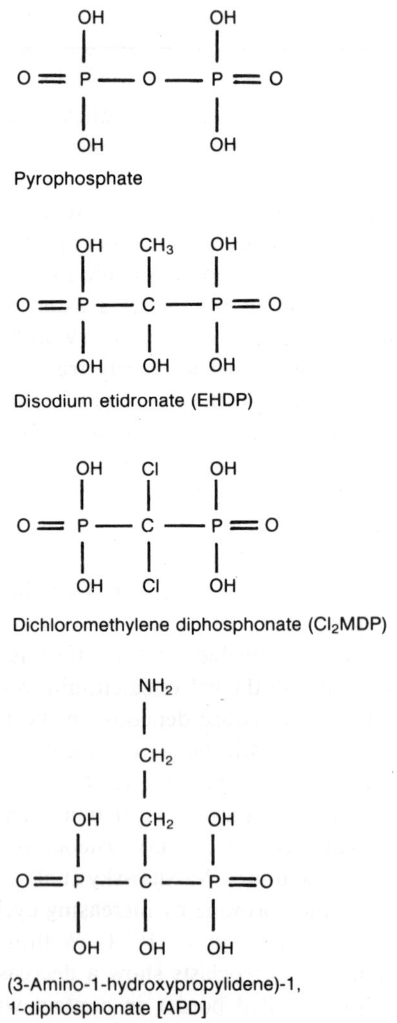

Fig. 2. Structure of pyrophosphate and the diphosphonates in clinical use.

than physicochemical binding to hydroxyapatite are important. Diphosphonates seemed to be able to enter mammalian cells (Fast et al., 1978) and may be accumulated within specific cellular compartments. Cells with phagocytic properties take up these compounds with special avidity, particularly if they are bound to apatite crystals (Chambers, 1980). This perhaps explains why osteoclasts are the target cells for these compounds and why they may show morphological changes after *in vitro* and *in vivo* diphosphonate exposure (Schenk et al., 1973). An indirect piece of evidence supporting a cellular action of the diphosphonates is the observed increase in renal tubular phosphate reabsorption seen with disodium etidronate (Walton et al., 1975), although this is not a feature of Cl_2MDP (dichloromethylene diphosphonate) or APD ([3-amino-1-hydroxypropylidene]-1, 1-diphosphonate) [Frijlink et al., 1979].

Although a variety of cellular changes have been described which might form the basis of diphosphonate action, there is no effect which is common to all the compounds tested (Fleisch et al., 1983). Thus, glycolysis and lactate production, which may be involved in mineral dissolution, are inhibited by disodium etidronate and Cl_2MDP but not by APD. Similar variability in effect is seen with respect to prostaglandin production, although the inhibition of lysozomal enzyme activity seems to be a more general phenomenon. Although confusing in a conceptual sense, the differences in the mechanisms which may underly diphosphonate action provide the possibility of selecting agents which control specific remodelling functions.

Inhibition of Bone Mineralisation

The inhibition of bone mineralisation by the diphosphonates is unwanted but it is surprising that there is not a close correlation between *in vitro* and *in vivo* effects (Treschel et al., 1977). For example, Cl_2-MDP and APD are very potent inhibitors of crystalisation, yet they do not seem to produce a mineralisation defect *in vivo* (Reitsma et al., 1980; Schenk et al., 1973). This is of practical importance because what is needed is a compound with as large a margin as possible between the dose inhibiting resorption and that impairing mineralisation. It is unfortunate, therefore, that there is a degree of overlap between these wanted and unwanted effects with disodium etidronate, the only commercially available preparation. Disodium etidronate also produces a number of other effects on the calcium homeostatic system. For example, high-dose (20 mg/kg/day) disodium etidronate therapy producing a mineralisation defect is associated with a fall in calcium absorption (Gasser et al., 1972) and 1,25-dihydroxycholecalciferol production (Hill et al., 1973). Conversely, doses which preferentially reduce resorption and induce a positive calcium balance are associated with an increase in circulating 1,25-dihydroxycholecalciferol. It seems likely that these changes are indirect and reflect adaptation to changes in calcium requirement, a view which is supported by *in vitro* studies of renal cell 1α-hydroxylase activity which did not show a direct diphosphonate effect (Treschel et al., 1979).

4. *Clinical Efficacy of the Calcitonins and Diphosphonates in Paget's Disease*

The response to these agents will be considered under 3 headings: relief of symptoms, control of bone turnover, and correction of abnormal skeletal architecture.

4.1 Relief of Symptoms

Comparison of the clinical effectiveness of the calcitonins and diphosphonates is hindered by the fact that pain, which is the usual indication for treatment, is so difficult to evaluate objectively. Although other symptoms such as neurological entrapment, immobilisation, hypercalciuria or high-output cardiac failure are more susceptible to quantitation and critical assessment, they are relatively uncommon. Moreover, since skull and long bone disease respond better to treatment than hip or back pain (Evans, 1977; Khairi et al., 1977; Plehwe et al., 1977) the number of patients experiencing clinical improvement within a particular study is critically dependent on the pattern of skeletal involvement.

4.1.1 Calcitonins

There has been only 1 double-blind study of the effects of calcitonin (Bouvet, 1977) but it showed that 50% of those treated with salmon calcitonin experienced symptomatic improvement compared with only 15% given placebo.

Relief of Pain

Given the complexity of the pathogenesis of pain and the uncontrolled nature of the remaining studies, it is not surprising that the clinical response is reported to vary from 30 to 100% (Burkhardt et al., 1977; De Rose et al., 1974; Grunstein et al., 1981; Hamilton, 1974; Kanis et al., 1974; Martin et al., 1977; Plehwe et al., 1977; Singer et al., 1977; Sturtridge et al., 1977). Symptomatic improvement generally begins within 4 to 6 weeks of starting treatment, although in some patients this may occur earlier. Since bone blood flow may begin to decrease within a week of starting calcitonin (Wooton et al., 1978), some of the early pain relief could be due to a reduction in intramedullary pressure.

In the studies cited above, the dose of calcitonin (porcine or salmon hormone) varied from 150 to 1400 MRC units/week, but the optimum dose probably lies in the region of 50 to 100 MRC units (0.5mg in the case of human calcitonin) per injection given on 3 to 7 days per week. It has been suggested that divided doses are more effective than a single injection (Chapuy et al., 1980) but the individual responses are so variable that this is difficult to confirm. The use of 100 MRC units porcine or salmon calcitonin thrice weekly is particularly convenient because it combines an adequate, and generally well tolerated, dose with the minimum number of injections.

Relationship Between Clinical Response and Reduction of Bone Turnover

There is no clear relationship between the clinical responses and the reduction in bone turnover. This is particularly obvious when treatment is stopped, at which time alkaline phosphatase and hydroxyproline invariably return to pretreatment levels within 6 months (Hosking, 1981a; Kanis et al., 1974; Martin et al, 1977), even though at least 50% of the patients stay in clinical remission for at least a year (Avramides et al., 1976; Evans, 1977; Martin et al., 1977). This may be a consequence of the normal bone remodelling which occurred during treatment (Meunier, 1975; Rasmussen and Bordier, 1974).

Reduction of Neurological Symptoms

Neurological symptoms due to distortion or compression of nervous tissue reflect the predisposition of Paget's disease for the axial skeleton (Friedman et al., 1971). Deafness is particularly common but evaluating the effect of calcitonin is difficult because the rate of progression of hearing loss is slow, and since most of these patients are elderly they may be deaf for other reasons. Although there have been some reports of improvement in hearing loss after calcitonin (Moffatt et al., 1974; Shai et al., 1971), these were small studies and a beneficial response has not been found by others (Grimaldi et al., 1975; Menzies et al., 1975). In the absence of major symptoms such as pain there seems little evidence that calcitonin should be given for deafness alone.

Chronic neurological compression symptoms involving the cranial nerves or spinal cord may respond well to calcitonin (Chen et al., 1979; De Rose et al., 1974; Melick et al., 1976; Shai et al., 1971), although myelographic evidence of improvement is variable (De Rose et al., 1974; Melick et al., 1976). In some cases the improvement in neurological symptoms was so rapid that it was suggested that calcitonin acts by reducing vertebral bone blood flow, thereby increasing the blood supply to the spinal cord (Herzberg and Bayliss 1980).

Improvement of Mechanical Properties of Bone

Calcitonin has been advocated for use prior to elective orthopaedic surgery in order to improve the mechanical properties of bone (Dove, 1980), and to avoid the problems of operative bleeding (Bowie and Kanis, 1977; Stevens, 1981) and immobilisation of hypercalcaemia (Nagant de Deuxchaisnes and Krane, 1964). However, there is no evidence that calcitonin improves the mechanical properties of bone in the short term, but bone blood flow may be significantly reduced within a week or so (Wooton et al., 1978) and there is some evidence that a short period of preoperative treatment is of benefit (Meyers and Singer, 1978). Since hypercalcaemia and hypercalciuria are uncommon and respond rapidly to calcitonin (Woodhouse, 1972) it seems best to treat this problem if it arises, particularly since calcitonin does not impair fracture healing (Evans and Slee, 1977) and therefore is not contraindicated in the postoperative phase.

Improvement of High-Output Cardiac Failure

Extensive skeletal involvement is usually accompanied by an increase in bone blood flow, a high cardiac output (Woodhouse et al., 1975), and may be complicated by heart failure. Although this usually responds to conventional diuretic therapy, resistant cases occasionally occur and may benefit from treatment with calcitonin (De Rose et al., 1974; Shai et al., 1971).

Avoidance of Adverse Effects

Side effects (Grunstein et al., 1981) which include nausea (37%), flushing (17%), urinary frequency (10%) and diarrhoea (4%) are generally mild and tend to improve with time. They are rarely severe enough to warrant withdrawal of treatment; rare occurrences include urticaria (De Rose et al., 1974), a pruritic rash (Plehwe et al., 1977) and tetany (Zeigler et al., 1977). The common side effects are dose-dependent and are more marked after intramuscular injections which produce higher peak concentrations than the subcutaneous route. The inconvenience that they produce can be minimised by giving the injection subcutaneously immediately before bed combined, if necessary, with 25 to 50mg of promethazine or 10mg of metoclopramide orally. Most patients, even those who are elderly, can usually be taught to give their own injections. If side effects are troublesome it may help to switch to a different calcitonin species (Grunstein et al., 1981).

4.1.2 Disodium Etidronate

The clinical effects of disodium etidronate are well supported by double-blind controlled studies (Canfield et al., 1977; Khairi et al., 1974). Clinical benefit can be expected in 60% of those treated with 5 to 20 mg/kg/day, compared with 34% given placebo or 2.5 mg/kg/day. Maximum improvement is achieved within 6 months and there seems no advantage to more prolonged treatment. Clinical benefit persists for some time after the withdrawal of etidronate and up to 50% of patients may remain in remission for up to 2 years (Johnston et al., 1980; Khairi et al., 1974). But the length of remission does not seem to correlate with the dose or duration of treatment (Finerman et al., 1976).

Relationship of Dosage to Occurrence of Treatment Complications

Although early studies suggested that 20 mg/kg/day produced better responses than 5 mg/kg/day (Altman et al., 1973; Khairi et al., 1974) this has not been confirmed in other studies (Khairi et al., 1977). Moreover, 20% of those given doses of 10 to 20 mg/kg/day felt less well after 6 months of treatment because of the development of new symptoms (Canfield et al., 1977; Stein et al., 1977). These usually took the form of severe incapacitating pain, often, but not exclusively, at sites of Pagetic involvement. The pains were diffuse and showed a predilection for the lower limbs so that physical activity was limited (Canfield et al., 1977; Fromm et al., 1975; Khairi et al., 1977). This 'bone pain syndrome' usually developed after 6 months' treatment with doses of 10 to 20 mg/kg/day but occasionally appeared earlier and at lower doses, perhaps reflecting variations in drug absorption (Recker et al., 1973). Bone radiographs showed no specific changes but when iliac crest bone biopsies were performed there was evidence of defective mineralisation (Fromm et al., 1975; Khairi et al., 1977). The risk of developing this complication does not seem to relate to the initial disease activity but symptoms generally improve within 3 months of stopping treatment, although the mineralisation defect may take longer to recover (Canfield et al., 1977; Khairi et al., 1977).

The accumulation of unmineralised bone is associated with delay in fracture healing, although both processes recover when the drug is withdrawn

(Khairi et al., 1977). A minor manifestation of this may be the appearance of callus at the site of unsuspected fractures when treatment is stopped. A more serious problem of high, but not low, dose therapy (Johnston et al., 1980) is the development of long bone fractures. These may occur in the absence of trauma at the site of fissure fractures (Canfield et al., 1977; Finerman et al., 1976; Kantrowitz et al., 1975). Both fractures and the bone pain syndrome seriously restrict the use of high-dose disodium etidronate, although it has been suggested that short courses of cyclical therapy may be of value in maintaining existing remissions (Siris et al., 1980).

Reduction of Neurological Symptoms

There has been less experience with the diphosphonates than with calcitonin in the management of neurological entrapment syndromes but preliminary reports are encouraging (Douglas et al., 1981). Benefit was found in 8 of the 10 patients treated with disodium etidronate or Cl_2MDP for spinal cord dysfunction. Improvement in symptoms was surprisingly rapid, developing within days in 1 patient, but becoming clinically obvious in the remainder within 3 weeks. Several of these patients had relapsed following an earlier surgical decompression but, as with calcitonin, myelographic evidence of improvement could not be demonstrated in most patients.

4.1.3 Combination Therapy

Combinations of calcitonin and disodium etidronate usually need to be given for 1 to 2 months before there is appreciable evidence of a clinical response (Bijvoet et al., 1978; Hosking et al., 1976). However, prolonged treatment for periods of up to 2 to 3 years has been given which seems capable of maintaining both a clinical and biochemical remission without the development of defective mineralisation or the bone pain syndrome. Unfortunately, these studies and those using the newer diphosphonates APD (Frijlink et al., 1979) and Cl_2MDP (Douglas et al., 1980; Meunier et al., 1979) suffer from a lack of appropriate controls. This makes it difficult to assess whether the clinical responses which are achieved differ in any significant respect from those obtained with calcitonin or disodium etidronate alone.

4.2 Control of Bone Turnover

4.2.1 Calcitonins

Changes in serum alkaline phosphatase and urinary hydroxyproline levels remain the cornerstone of objective assessments of the response to treatment. Calcitonin generally reduces bone turnover by about 50% and there appears to be no important qualitative or quantitative difference between porcine, salmon and human calcitonins in this respect (table III). However, at any given level of bone turnover there is considerable individual variation in response (Hosking, 1981a). This makes it difficult to define the minimum dose of calcitonin needed to produce a maximum reduction in disease activity. Very small doses of salmon calcitonin (e.g. 50 MRC units weekly) are clearly insufficient (Avramides et al., 1975) and the optimum dose seems to lie in the region of 50 to 100 MRC units thrice weekly (De Rose et al., 1974; Martin, 1979; Woodhouse, et al., 1977). Double this dose of porcine calcitonin is probably required for a maximum effect (De Rose et al., 1974). Comparable figures for human calcitonin are difficult to assess because of a recent improvement in purity of the current preparation, but 0.5mg thrice weekly seems as effective as larger doses (table III).

Patterns of Response

Several patterns of response are seen during calcitonin therapy (fig. 3). Although some patients remain unaffected (primary non-response) this is rare (De Rose et al., 1974; Evans, 1977; Hamilton, 1974), and most patients experience a 40 to 50% fall in alkaline phosphatase and hydroxyproline levels which is invariably achieved within 6 months, further reductions thereafter being unusual (De Rose et al., 1974; Evans, 1977; Kanis et al., 1974; Martin et al., 1977). However, as soon as calcitonin is withdrawn bone turnover increases rapidly and the extent to which this occurs is independent of the dose given, the duration of treat-

Table III. Biochemical response to calcitonins

Reference	No. of patients	Dose (MRC units/week)[a]	Duration of treatment (months)	Initial values		Response (% pretreatment)	
				AP (× ULN)	HYPRO (μmol/day)	AP	HYPRO
Porcine calcitonin							
Dube et al. (1972)	5	280-420	12-24			80	
De Rose et al. (1974)	21	1400	6-14	4.6	1080	41	67
Kanis et al. (1975)	12	1120	0-6	4.1	520	67	64
Nagant de Deuxchaisnes et al. (1977)	5	160-2240	3-10	18.6		55	
Plehwe et al. (1977)	24	320-2240	1-40	21.5		65	
Martin et al. (1977)	38	560	3-42	16.6	1015	64	60
Salmon calcitonin							
Haddad et al. (1972)	15	234-6120	3-7.5			49	
Goldfield et al. (1972)	3	350	3-4	3.7	1294	50	19
De Rose et al. (1974)	28	150-700	4-27	8.2	2355	52	48
Hamilton (1974)	16	175-3500	3-20	2.9	406	54	62
Kanis et al. (1974)	15	204-450	1-9	5.8		67	
Avramides et al. (1975)	9	50	10-16	4.5	1295	72	82
Nagant de Deuxchaisnes et al.	2	150-350	4	12.2		60	
(1977)	8	175-700	3	4.9		60	
Hadjipavlou et al. (1977)	13	700	3-36				30
Woodhouse et al. (1977)	28	200-700	9-42	6	1250	50	57
Sturtridge et al. (1977)	12	300	7-12	7.8	1764	52	36
Williams et al. (1978)	31	300	6	4.9	801	57	71
Hosking et al. (1981)							
Human calcitonin							
Woodhouse et al. (1971)	5	7.0[a]	4-12	2.5	655	40	33
Singer et al. (1977)	7	1.75-3.0	2-30			50	50
Evans et al. (1977)	33	7.0	12			60	62
Nagant de Deuxchaisnes et al. (1977)	2	7.0	4	12.2		29	
Haymovits et al. (1977)	6	3.5-7.0	3	12.6	294[b]	63	55
Burckhardt et al. (1977)	13	2.5-3.5	5-20	3.1	97[b]	67	57
Ziegler et al. (1977)	17	7.0	6			50	50
Epstein et al. (1977)	12	3.5-7.0	6	4.4	1682	69	54
Murphy et al. (1980)	6	3.5	6	5.9	199[b]	45	41

a Human calcitonin dose in mg/wk.
b mg/g creatinine.
Abbreviations: AP = mean alkaline phosphatase [expressed as a multiple of upper limit of normal (ULN) range]; HYPRO = hydroxyproline.

ment or the degree of suppression achieved (Avramides et al., 1976; Evans et al., 1980; Hosking, 1981a; Kanis et al., 1975). Thus, at a cellular level there is probably no fundamental difference between those who achieve normal bone turnover and those with more active disease in whom residual activity persists (plateau response); in neither case is the underlying process controlled.

The plateau response is not due to insufficient dosage (De Rose et al., 1974; Haddad and Caldwell, 1972; Singer et al., 1972) or to the secondary hyperparathyroidism engendered by the hypocalcaemic effect of calcitonin (Burkhardt et al., 1973; De Rose et al., 1974; Sturtridge et al., 1977). It seems to be a fundamental property of the cellular action of calcitonin which is probably reflected *in vitro* by the phenomenon of 'escape' (Wener et al., 1972), whereby the suppressive effect of calcitonin on osteoclastic resorption diminishes with time. However, it is clear that osteoclasts are not entirely unresponsive during the plateau phenomenon because histological and radiological studies show that bone remodelling continues to be regulated (Meunier, 1975; Nagant de Deuxchaisnes et al., 1977) and this is underlined by the increase in turnover once treatment is withdrawn. Although down-regulation of calcitonin receptors undoubtedly occurs during treatment, a significant number remain to elicit an almost maximal response (Tashjian et al., 1978). The cellular basis for the plateau phenomenon thus remains an enigma.

Development of Resistance

Antibodies develop in 30 to 60% of patients treated with porcine or salmon calcitonin because of the structural differences which exist between these peptides and human calcitonin (De Rose et al., 1974; Haddad and Caldwell, 1972; Hosking, 1981b; Singer et al., 1972, 1980; Sturtridge et al., 1977). Although the development of antibodies does not correlate with the dose of calcitonin used, their concentration tends to rise with time (Hosking, 1981b; Woodhouse et al., 1977). Since clinical resistance (fig. 3) is largely a phenomenon of high antibody titres, generally above 1 : 1500 (Singer et al., 1980), it is more of a problem of prolonged treatment and this may account for the wide variation (5 to 40%) in its reported prevalence (De Rose et al., 1974; Haddad and Caldwell 1972; Singer et al., 1980). The diagnosis of resistance should be based on the presence of high antibody titres and the demonstration that control of bone turnover can be re-established by changing to a calcitonin species to which antibodies are absent (Haddad and Caldwell, 1972; Singer et al., 1972, 1980). It is now recognised that the rat bioassay system and acute hypocalcaemic responses to calcitonin in man (Hosking, 1981b; Martin, 1979; Singer et al., 1972, 1980) may be misleading and have probably contributed to an overestimate of the prevalence of resistance in the past.

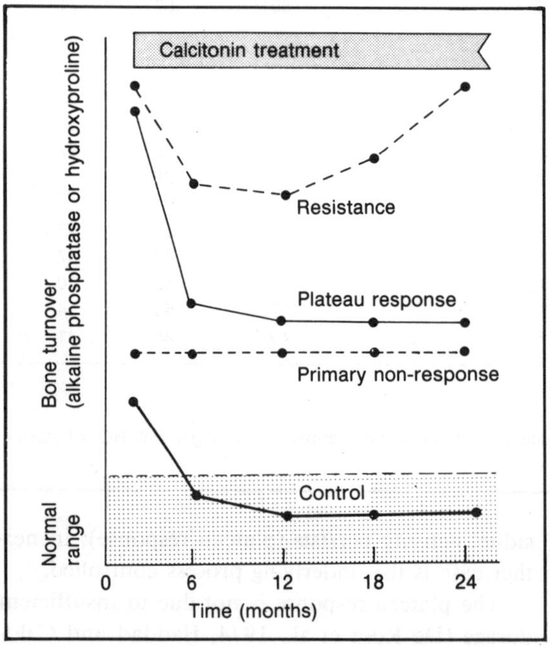

Fig. 3. Patterns of biochemical response to calcitonin in Paget's disease.

4.2.2 Disodium Etidronate

As with calcitonin, there is considerable variation in the reduction of bone turnover which can be achieved with disodium etidronate (table IV). This may reflect variations both in the susceptibility of bone cells and in drug absorption. As discussed above, effective doses lie in the region of 5 to 20 mg/kg bodyweight per day. The larger doses produce the greatest reduction in bone turnover in the shortest period (Khairi et al., 1977) but are also accompanied by the greatest risk of important side effects. If assessments are made after 3 to 6 months' treatment, by which time the response is usually at a maximum, there seems to be little difference between the 5 and 20 mg/kg doses in terms of control of bone turnover (Altman et al., 1973; Canfield et al., 1977; DeVries and Bijvoet, 1974; Finerman et al., 1976).

Table IV. Biochemical response to disodium etidronate (EHDP)

Reference	No. of patients	EHDP dose (mg/kg/day)	Duration of treatment (months)	Initial values		Response (% pretreatment)	
				AP (× ULN)	HYPRO (μmol/day)	AP	HYPRO
Russell et al. (1974)	7	5	6	3.3	565	77	66
Khairi et al. (1974)	8	5	6	3.3	650	41	49
Canfield et al. (1977)	5	5	6	6.6	1461	44	43
DeVries et al. (1974)	6	7.5	6	6.1	1070	45	40
Russel et al. (1974)	10	10	6	9.6	1717	35	23
Khairi et al. (1974)	11	10	6	4.5	725	65	51
Canfield et al. (1977)	14	10	6	7.0	1800	62	34
DeVries et al. (1974)	7	15	3	5.9	1039	67	53
Guncaga et al. (1974)	3	20	3	5.5	1558	68	40
Meunier et al. (1975)	7	20	3	4.8	163[a]	35	41
Reiner et al. (1975)	8	20	3	4.3	1293	54	17
Fromm et al. (1975)	37	20	5			63	47
Russell et al. (1974)	15	20	6	4.4	995	60	42
Khairi et al. (1974)	8	20	6	5.4	1050	21	14
Guncaga et al. (1974)	5	20	6-8	5.0	1446	39	25
Meunier et al. (1975)	4	20	6	5.6	170[a]	52	23
Jung et al. (1976)	8	20	6	5.4	2117	26	17
Finerman et al. (1976)	17	20	6			33	24
Canfield et al. (1977)	44	20	6	6.3	890	30	16
Stein et al. (1977)	13	20	6			21	16

a μg/g creatinine.

Abbreviations: AP = mean alkaline phosphatase [expressed as a multiple of upper limit of normal (ULN) range]; HYPRO = hydroxyproline.

Patterns of Response

Treatment with disodium etidronate produces an immediate reduction in hydroxyproline which is subsequently followed by a decline in alkaline phosphatase (Altman et al., 1973; Canfield et al., 1977; DeVries and Bijvoet, 1974; Guncaga et al., 1974). This may represent a temporary uncoupling of bone resorption and formation and may account for the transiently positive calcium balance found at this time (DeVries and Bijvoet, 1974; Guncaga et al., 1974). At the point of maximum response the reduction in hydroxyproline usually exceeds that of alkaline phosphatase (table IV) and distorts the usual correlation between these two variables, which is a feature of the untreated disease (Franck et al., 1974; Siris et al., 1980). Reactivation of abnormal bone turnover once disodium etidronate is withdrawn is slower than that seen after the discontinuation of calcitonin. The rate of relapse is largely a function of the dose of disodium etidronate rather than its duration (Khairi et al., 1977), although the level of pretreatment bone turnover is also an important factor. Thus, moderately active disease is usually easy to control and stays in prolonged remission once treatment is withdrawn, while very active disease is less easy to control and relapses more rapidly (Finerman et al., 1976; Siris et al., 1980; Stein et al., 1977). A feature of post-treatment relapse is that the suppression of hydroxyproline generally outlasts that of alkaline phosphatase (DeVries and Bijvoet, 1974; Khairi et al., 1977; Meunier, 1975), again emphasising the dominance of the effect of disodium etidronate on the osteoclast. Because of the variables involved it is difficult to quantify the rate of relapse with any precision but bone turnover can be expected to increase by at least 20% within the first 6 months off treatment. However, many patients will remain in clinical remission, and despite the increase in bone turnover, a sustained reduction at 50 to 60% below pretreatment levels is often achieved (Altman et al., 1973; Finerman et al., 1976; Khairi et al., 1977; Stein et al., 1977).

An important observation is that should retreatment become necessary, subsequent responses are just as good as those achieved with the first course (Finerman et al., 1976; Johnston et al., 1980; Siris et al., 1980; Stein et al., 1977). Repeated cycles of treatment may thus permit sustained control, particularly in those with mild to moderate disease (Siris et al., 1980, 1981).

4.2.3 Combination Therapy

The use of disodium etidronate and calcitonin in combination results in a synchronised decrease in hydroxyproline and alkaline phosphatase (Bijvoet et al., 1978; Hosking et al., 1976) which contrasts with the delayed suppression of alkaline phosphatase seen with disodium etidronate alone (Canfield et al., 1977) and the delayed effect of calcitonin on hydroxyproline (Hosking, 1981a). With combined treatment, bone turnover declines in a roughly exponential fashion with a half-time of approximately 6 weeks. Using 7.5 mg/kg of disodium etidronate in combination with various doses of human and salmon calcitonin (all of which were in the optimal dose range) normal bone turnover was achieved in 83% of the patients, many of whom had very active disease (Bijvoet et al., 1978). The time taken to achieve control was proportional to the initial activity but despite prolonged treatment, for up to 2 years in some cases, there was no evidence of defective mineralisation.

The variability of the response to treatment makes it difficult to assess from a relatively small number of patients whether combined treatment has real advantages. Although there is probably little difference between comparable doses of disodium etidronate alone and in combination on bone resorption (hydroxyproline), there is enhanced suppression of bone formation (alkaline phosphatase). Combined treatment is clearly superior to the effect of calcitonin alone, particularly with respect to the reduction in hydroxyproline. Although many patients treated with the disodium etidronate/calcitonin combination stay in a prolonged remission once treatment is withdrawn, a strict comparison with either agent alone must include matching for variables such as dose and initial disease activity which affect the propensity of bone turnover to increase. At present, there is insufficient published material to make such a comparison. However, the observation that 72% of those treated with the combination still had normal bone turnover 6 months after stopping treatment is encouraging, particularly since some were still in remission 2 years later (Bijvoet et al., 1978).

4.2.4 The Newer Diphosphonates

Two of the newer diphosphonates, APD and Cl_2MDP have been used in Paget's disease but unfortunately neither agent is currently commercially available. Both are potent inhibitors of bone turnover which is reduced by about 80%, many patients achieving normal or near normal values within the first 6 months of treatment (Douglas et al., 1980; Frijlink et al.; 1979; Meunier et al., 1979). Moreover, normal bone turnover seems to persist when treatment is stopped. The great advantage of these compounds is that they do not appear to inhibit skeletal mineralisation, although APD may cause a transient fever in the first few days of treatment in about half the patients.

APD also causes a transient lymphopenia, particularly of those cells bearing receptors for the Fc fragment of IgM, and it has been suggested that it acts on the mononuclear phagocyte system (Bijvoet et al., 1980).

4.3 Effects on Skeletal Architecture

The effects of treatment on skeletal architecture can be assessed radiographically and histologically, while the relationship between bone formation and resorption can be measured by balance techniques or radioisotope kinetic analysis.

4.3.1 Radiographic Assessment

Calcitonin

Skeletal radiography is the only technique which provides information about structural changes at a macroscopic level and is probably the most relevant parameter when considering the impact of treatment on mechanical complications of the disease. Spontaneous improvement in the radiographic appearances does not occur (Woodhouse et al., 1972) but the beneficial effects of treatment are slow to develop and meticulous radiographic technique is essential if films taken at different times are to be compared (Doyle et al., 1974; Nagant de Deuxchaisnes et al., 1977). It is much easier to assess improvement in lytic rather than sclerotic lesions and several studies have shown that calcitonin has a beneficial effect in this respect (Doyle et al., 1974; Murphy et al., 1980; Nagant de Deuxchaisnes et al., 1977; Woodhouse et al., 1977). The progression of the resorption front in long bones may be arrested or even reversed, although comparable changes in the skull (osteoporosis circumscripta) are more resistant to improvement (Woodhouse et al., 1977). Intracortical or other lytic areas may become consolidated and there may be a general trend towards a more normal architectural appearance. Although changes have been reported after as little as 2 to 4 months' calcitonin treatment (Nagant de Deuxchaisnes et al., 1977), the usual pattern in response is towards a slower evolution of improvement over 8 to 12 months (Doyle et al., 1974; Murphy et al., 1980). An interesting observation, and one of considerable theoretical importance, is that radiographic remodelling continues during the plateau phase when biochemical indices of bone turnover are static (Nagant de Deuxchaisnes et al., 1977; Woodhouse et al., 1972), indicating a persisting hormonal influence on bone cells.

Disodium Etidronate

There is much less information about the radiographic changes produced by disodium etidronate except with respect to major complications such as fractures (Canfield et al., 1977; Finerman et al., 1976; Khairi et al., 1977; Stein et al., 1977). However, trabecular reconstruction and consolidation of lytic lesions does not seem to occur and there may even be evidence of deterioration (Canfield et al., 1977; Finerman et al., 1976; Nagant de Deuxchaisnes et al., 1979). The addition of calcitonin appears to protect the bone to some extent from these adverse effects but the radiographic changes are not as good as those seen with calcitonin alone (Nagant de Deuxchaisnes et al., 1979). Furthermore, when combined treatment is stopped, the adverse effects associated with the disodium etidronate alone may appear for the first time, presumably because disodium etidronate remains absorbed on the bone surface and is only slowly removed.

4.3.2 Histological Assessment

Assessment of the changes produced by calcitonin and disodium etidronate at a cellular level must be tempered by an awareness of the patchy nature of the skeletal involvement in Paget's disease. This is accentuated by limitation of biopsy sites to the iliac crest where it has been shown that disease activity can vary considerably between adjacent areas (Martin et al., 1977; Rasmussen and Bordier, 1974). Thus it may sometimes be difficult to distinguish changes produced by treatment from those due to this regional variation.

Calcitonin reduces osteoclast size and numbers and the extent of active resorption surfaces (Haymovits et al., 1977; Rasmussen and Bordier, 1974; Singer et al., 1977). There may also be a reduction in the number of osteoclast nuclei, although this has not been a universal finding (Meunier, 1975; Rebel et al., 1977; Woodhouse et al., 1971). Osteoclastic activity is suppressed in the involved areas but does not disappear entirely, and together with control of abnormal bone formation may result in replacement of woven bone by lamellar bone (Meunier, 1975; Woodhouse et al., 1971).

Disodium etidronate is capable of producing a much more profound inhibition of bone turnover than that seen with calcitonin. The effect is dose dependent but with the 20 mg/kg/day dose the calcification rate is reduced to subnormal levels

(Johnston et al., 1980). The accumulation of osteoid which develops in the first 3 months of treatment (Reiner et al., 1975) does not seem to be a progressive phenomenon. It may reflect an immediate inhibition of mineralisation and a less rapid inhibition of matrix production by osteoblasts (Talmage and Anderson, 1974) but the bone which is formed under these circumstances is lamellar in type. The dose at which defective mineralisation becomes a problem seems variable and is probably due to vagaries in drug absorption. However, there seems to be general agreement that this is not a common problem with 5 mg/kg/day doses (although the cellular suppressant effects are not as impressive as those seen at the larger doses).

The addition of calcitonin seems to protect against the defective mineralisation seen with disodium etidronate alone, and both osteoclastic and osteoblastic activity returns to normal or near normal levels (Bijvoet et al., 1978; Hosking et al., 1976). However, abnormal osteoclastic activity may persist in some patients whose biochemical indices of turnover have returned to normal, and this may be a factor predisposing towards later relapse.

4.3.3 Other Assessment Techniques

Changes in calcium balance and 47-calcium kinetic studies reflect temporal imbalances between the suppression of osteoclastic resorption and osteoblastic formation together with the effects of remineralisation of the excess osteoid (which is a feature of the high bone turnover of untreated Paget's disease). Both calcitonin and disodium etidronate alone, and in combination, produce a positive calcium balance but this is only transient and most patients will have returned to an equilibrium state by 6 months (Avramides et al., 1974; Bijvoet et al., 1978; DeVries et al., 1974; Guncaga et al., 1974; Woodhouse et al., 1971). The extent of this calcium retention is much more marked with the newer diphosphonates such as APD where there is a significant uncoupling of resorption and formation (Frijlink et al., 1979).

Calcium kinetic studies (Bijvoet et al., 1978; Guncaga et al., 1974; Hosking et al., 1981) support these observations by showing a greater reduction in mobilisation than accretion in the early stage of treatment. However, kinetic measurements, unlike other indices of turnover may not return to normal because the exchangeable pool is increased by the presence of woven bone which is only slowly remodelled to the less exchangeable lamellar type. Kinetic studies are of interest because they illustrate the basic processes underlying the disordered bone turnover of Paget's disease, although they contribute little to routine management.

5. Conclusions

Although current treatment for Paget's disease is not perfect, many of the pathological processes which contribute to the varied symptomatology of this condition can be controlled by an appropriate choice of treatment. Advances in this field have been considerable over the last few years and new therapeutic agents may soon become generally available. The hope is that they will not only control abnormal bone turnover but also promote skeletal reconstruction so that the long term mechanical complications of Paget's disease can be avoided.

References

Altman, P.D.; Johnson, C.C.; Khairi, M.R.A.; Wellman, H.N.; Serafini, A.N. and Sankey, R.R.: Influence of disodium etidronate on clinical and laboratory manifestations of Pagets disease of bone (osteitis deformans). New England Journal of Medicine 289: 1379-1384 (1973).

Avramides, A.; Baker, R.K. and Wallach, S.: Metabolic effects of synthetic salmon calcitonin in Pagets disease of bone. Metabolism 23: 1037-1046 (1974).

Avramides, A.; Flores, A.; De Rose, J. and Wallach, S.: Treatment of Pagets disease of bone with once a week injections of salmon calcitonin. British Medical Journal 3: 632 (1975).

Avramides, A.; Flores, A.; De Rose, J. and Wallach, S.: Pagets disease of bone: Observations after cessation of long term synthetic salmon calcitonin treatment. Journal of Clinical Endocrinology and Metabolism 42: 459-463 (1976).

Barry, H.C.: Paget's Disease of Bone (Livingstone, Edinburgh 1969).

Bijvoet, O.L.M.; Frijlink, W.B.; Jie, K.; van der Linden, H.; Meijer, C.J.L.M. et al.: APD in Paget's disease of bone: Role of the mononuclear phagocyte system? Arthritis and Rheumatism 23: 1193-1204 (1980).

Bijvoet, O.L.M.; Hosking, D.J.; Frijlink, W.B.; TeVelde, J. and Vellenga, C.J.L.R.: Treatment of Paget's disease with combined calcitonin and diphosphonate (EHDP). Metabolic Bone Disease and Related Research 1: 251-261 (1978).

Borle, A.B.: Calcium metabolism at the cellular level. Federation Proceedings. 32: 1944-1950 (1973).

Bouvet, J.P.: Traitement de la maladie de Paget par la thyrocalcitonine de saumon. Etude coöperative en double insu. Nouvelle Presse Médicale 6: 1447-1450 (1977).
Bowie, H.C. and Kanis, J.A.: Calcitonin in the assessment and preparation of patients with Paget's disease for surgery; in Kanis (Ed.) Bone Disease and Calcitonin, pp. 61-69 (Armour Pharmaceutical, Eastbourne 1977).
Burckhardt, P.; Ducommun, J. and Hessler, C.: Treatment of Paget's disease with human calcitonin; in MacIntyre (Ed.) Human Calcitonin and Paget's disease, pp. 155-166 (Hans Huber, Berne 1977).
Burckhardt, P.M.; Singer, F.R. and Potts Jr, J.T.: Parathyroid function in patients with Paget's disease treated with salmon calcitonin. Clinical Endocrinology 2: 15-22 (1973).
Canfield, R.; Rosner, W.; Skinner, J.; McWhorter, J.; Resnick, L. et al.: Diphosphonate therapy of Paget's disease of bone. Journal of Clinical Endocrinology and Metabolism 44: 96-106 (1977).
Chambers, T.J.: The cellular basis of bone resorption. Clinical Orthopaedics and Related Research 151: 283-293 (1980).
Chambers, T.J. and Magnus, C.J.: Calcitonin alters behaviour of isolated osteoclasts. Journal of Pathology 136: 27-39 (1982).
Chapuy, M.C.; Meunier, P.J. and Alexandre, C.: Comparison of the acute effects of human and salmon calcitonin in Pagetic patients in relation with plasma calcitonin levels. Metabolic Bone Disease and Related Research 2: 93-98 (1980).
Chen, J.R.; Rhee, R.S.C.; Wallach, S.; Avramides, A. and Flores, A.: Neurologic disturbances in Paget's disease of bone. Responses to calcitonin. Neurology 29: 448-457 (1979).
Collins, D.H.: Pagets disease of bone incidence and subclinical forms. Lancet 2: 51-57 (1976).
Condon, J.R.: Glucagon in the treatment of Paget's disease of bone. British Medical Journal 4: 719-721 (1971).
Cooper, C.W.; Peng, T.-C.; Toverud, S.U.; Vander-Wiel, C.J. and Talmage, R.V.: Calcitonin and feeding; in Cohn et al. (Eds) Hormonal Control of Calcium Metabolism, Internal Congress Series 511, pp. 271-280 (Excerpta Medica, Amsterdam 1981).
Deftos, L.J.; Burton, D.; Catherwood, B.D.; Bone, H.G.; Parthemore, J.G. et al.: Demonstration by immunoperoxidase histochemistry of calcitonin in the anterior lobe of the rat pituitary. Journal of Clinical Endocrinology and Metabolism 47: 457-460 (1978).
De Rose, J.; Singer, F.R.; Avramides, A.; Flores, A.; Dziadiw, R. et al.: Response of Paget's disease to porcine and salmon calcitonins. American Journal of Medicine 56: 858-866 (1974).
DeVries, H.R. and Bijvoet, O.L.M.: Results of prolonged treatment of Paget's disease of bone with disodium ethane-1-hydroxy-1,1-diphosphonate (EHDP). Netherlands Journal of Medicine 17: 281-297 (1974).
Douglas, D.L.; Duckworth, T.; Kanis, J.A.; Preston, D.; Beard, D.J. et al.: Biochemical and clinical responses to dichloromethylene diphosphonate (Cl_2MDP) in Paget's disease of bone. Arthritis and Rheumatism 23: 1185-1192 (1980).
Douglas, D.L.; Kanis, J.A.; Duckworth, T.; Beard, D.J.; Paterson, A.D. and Russell, R.G.G.: Paget's disease. Improvement of spinal cord dysfunction with diphosphonates and calcitonin. Metabolic Bone Disease and Related Research 3: 327-335 (1981).
Dove, J.: Complete fractures of the femur in Paget's disease of bone. Journal of Bone and Joint Surgery 62B: 12-17 (1980).
Doyle, F.R.; Pennock, J.; Greenberg, P.B.; Joplin, G.F. and MacIntyre, I.: Radiological evidence of a dose related response to longterm treatment of Paget's disease with human calcitonin. British Journal of Radiology 47: 1-8 (1974).
Dube, W.J.; Goldsmith, R.S.; Arnaud, S.B. and Arnaud, C.D.: Hyperparathyroidism secondary to long-term therapy of Paget's disease of bone with calcitonin; in Talmage and Munson (Eds) Calcium, Parathyroid hormone and the Calcitonins, pp. 113-115 (Excerpta Medica, Amsterdam 1972).
Epstein, S. and Owen, G.: Paget's disease of bone (osteitis deformans) treated with human synthetic calcitonin. South African Medical Journal 51: 133-137 (1977).
Evans, G.A. and Slee, G.A.: Calcitonin for multiple fractures in Paget's disease. British Medical Journal 1: 357 (1977).
Evans, I.M.A.: Human calcitonin in the treatment of Paget's disease; long term trial; in MacIntyre (Ed.) Human Calcitonin and Paget's Disease, pp. 111-123 (Hans Huber, Berne 1977).
Evans, I.M.A.; Banks, L.; Doyle, F.H.; Joplin, G.F.; Pennock, J. et al.: Paget's disease of bone – the effect of stopping long term human calcitonin and recommendations for future treatment. Metabolic Bone Disease and Related Research 2: 87-92 (1980).
Fast, D.K.; Felix, R.; Dowse, C.; Neuman, W.F. and Fleisch, H.: The effects of diphosphonates on the growth and glycolysis of connective-tissue cells in culture. Biochem. J. 172: 97 (1978).
Finerman, G.A.M.; Gonick, H.C.; Smith, R.K. and Mayfield, J.M.: Diphosphonate treatment of Paget's disease. Journal of Clinical Orthopaedics and Related Research 120: 115-124 (1976).
Fleisch, H.: Bisphosphonates; mechanisms of action and clinical applications; in Peck (Ed.) Bone and Mineral Research Annual 1, pp. 319-357 (Excerpta Medica, Amsterdam 1983).
Fleisch, H.; Russell, R.G.G. and Straumann, T.: Effect of pryophosphate on hydroxyapatite and its implications in calcium homeostasis. Nature 212: 901-903 (1966).
Foster, G.V.; MacIntyre, I. and Pearse, A.G.E.: Calcitonin production and the mitochondrion rich cells of the dog thyroid. Nature 203: 1029-1030 (1964).
Franck, W.A.; Bress, N.M.; Singer, F.R. and Krane, S.M.: Rheumatic manifestations of Paget's disease of bone. American Journal of Medicine 56: 592-603 (1974).
Friedman, J. and Raisz, L.G.: Thyrocalcitonin, inhibitor of bone resorption in tissue culture. Science 150: 1465-1467 (1965).
Friedman, P.; Sklaver, N. and Klawans, H.L.: Neurological manifestations of Paget's diseases of the skull. Disease of the Nervous System 32: 809-817 (1971).
Frijlink, W.B.; Bijvoet, O.L.M.; TeVelde, J. and Heynen, G.: Treatment of Paget's disease with (3-amino-1-hydroxypropylidene)-1,1-biphosphonate (APD). Lancet 1: 799-803 (1979).
Fromm, G.; Schajowicz, E. and Mautalen, C.A.: Disodium ethane-1-hydroxy-1,1-diphosphonate (EHDP) in Paget's disease. Lancet 2: 666 (1975).
Gasser, A.B.; Morgan, D.B.; Fleisch, H.A. and Richell, L.J.: The influence of two diphosphonates on calcium metabolism in the rat. Clinical Science 43: 31-45 (1972).
Goldfield, E.B.; Braiker, B.M.; Prendergast, J.J. and Kolb, F.O.: Synthetic salmon calcitonin: Treatment of Paget's disease and osteoporosis imperfects. Journal of the American Medical Association 221: 1127-1129 (1972).
Grimaldi, P.M.G.B.; Mohamedally, S.M. and Woodhouse, N.J.Y.: Deafness in Paget's disease: Effect of salmon calcitonin. British Medical Journal 2: 726-727 (1975).
Grubb, S.A.; Markham, T.C. and Talmage, R.V.: Effect of calcitonin infusion on plasma concentrations of recently administered radiocalcium. Calcified Tissue Research 24: 201-208 (1977).
Grunstein, H.; Clifton-Bligh, O. and Posen, S.: Pagets disease of bone; experiences with 100 patients treated with salmon calcitonin. Medical Journal of Australia 2: 278-280 (1981).
Guncaga, L.; Lauffenburger, T.; Lentner, C.; Dambacher, M.A. and Haas, H.G.: Diphosphonate treatment of Paget's disease of bone. Hormone and Metabolic Research 6: 62-69 (1974).
Guttman, S.: Chemistry and structure – activity relationship of natural and synthetic calcitonins; in Pecile (Ed.) Calcitonin 1980: Chemistry, Physiology, Pharmacology and Clinical Aspects pp. 11-24 (Excerpta Medica, Amsterdam 1981).
Haddad, J.G. and Caldwell, J.G.: Calcitonin resistance: Clinical and immunologic studies in subjects with Paget's disease of bone treated with porcine and salmon calcitonin. Journal of Clinical Investigation 51: 3133-3141 (1972).

Hadjipavlou, A.G.; Tsoukas, G.M.; Siller, T.N.; Danias, S. and Greenwood F.: Combination drug therapy in treatment of Paget's disease of bone. Journal of Bone and Joint Surgery 59A: 1045-1051 (1977).

Hamdy, R.C.: Paget's Disease of Bone, pp. 1-3 (Praeger Scientific, New York (1981)

Hamilton, C.R.: Effect of synthetic salmon calcitonin in patients with Paget's disease of bone. American Journal of Medicine 56: 315-322 (1974).

Harell, A.; Binderman, I. and Rodan, G.A.: The effect of calcium concentration on calcium uptake by bone cells treated with thyrocalcitonin (TCT) hormone. Endocrinology 92: 550-555 (1973).

Haymovitis, A.; Zluizek, V.; Ling, A.S.C.; Hobitz, J. and Fotino, M.: Studies on short term therapy with human calcitonin and ultrastructural, immunological and genetic observations on the aetiology of Paget's disease; in MacIntyre (Ed.) Human Calcitonin and Paget's Disease, pp. 138-154 (H. Huber, Bern 1977).

Herzberg, L. and Bayliss, E.: Spinal cord syndrome due to non-compressive Pagets disease of bone: A spinal artery steal phenomenon reversible with calcitonin. Lancet 2: 13-15 (1980).

Hill, L.F.; Lumb, G.A.; Mawer, E.B. and Stanbury, S.W.: Indirect inhibition of the biosynthesis of 1,25-dihydroxycholecalciferol in rats treated with a diphosphonate. Clinical Science 44: 335-347 (1973).

Holtrop, M.E.; Raisz, L.G. and Simmons, H.A.: The effects of parathyroid hormone, colchicine and calcitonin on the ultrastructure and activity of osteoclasts in organ culture. Journal of Cell Biology 60: 346-355 (1974).

Hosking, D.J.: Calcitonin and diphosphonate in the treatment of Paget's disease of bone. Metabolic Bone Disease and Related Research 3: 317-326 (1981a).

Hosking, D.J.: Clinical significance of calcitonin antibodies; in Pecile (Ed.) Calcitonin 1980, pp. 365-377 (Excerpta Medica, Amsterdam 1981b).

Hosking, D.J.; Bijvoet, O.L.M.; Van Aken, J. and Will, E.J.: Paget's bone disease treated with diphosphonate and calcitonin. Lancet 1: 615-617 (1976).

Hosking, D.J.; Vennart, W. and Huddlestone, L.B.: Bone turnover in Paget's disease. Biochemical and kinetic measurements during salmon calcitonin therapy. Calcified Tissue International 31: 471-476 (1981).

Johnston, C.C.; Khairi, M.R.A. and Meunier, P.J.: Use of etidronate (EHDP) in Paget's disease of bone. Arthritis and Rheumatism 23: 1172-1176 (1980).

Jung, A.; Merillod, B.; Schenk, R.; Courvoisier, B.; Burckhardt, P.; Epiney, J. and Fleisch, H.: Traitement de 10 cas symptomatiques de maladie de Paget par l'etidronte (EHDP). Schweiz. Med. Woch. 106: 1667-1673 (1976).

Kanis, J.A.; Fitzpatrick, K. and Strong, J.A.: Treatment of Paget's disease with porcine calcitonin. Clinical and metabolic responses.. British Medical Journal 44: 399-413 (1975).

Kanis, J.A.; Horn, D.B.; Scott, R.D.M. and Strong J.A.: Treatment of Paget's disease of bone with synthetic salmon calcitonin. British Medical Journal 3: 727-731 (1974).

Kantrowitz, F.G.; Byrne, M.H.; Schiller, A.L. and Krane, S.M.: Clinical and biochemical effects of diphosphonates in Paget's disease of bone. Arthritis and Rheumatism 18: 407 (1975).

Khairi, M.R.A.; Altman, R.D.; DeRosa, G.P.; Zimmerman, J. et al.: Sodium etidronate in the treatment of Paget's disease of bone. A study of long term results. Annals of Internal Medicine 87: 656-663 (1977).

Khairi, M.R.A.; Johnston, C.C.; Altman, R.D.; Wellman, H.N.; Serafani, A.N. and Sankey, R.R.: Treatment of Paget's disease of bone (osteitis deformans). Results of one year study with sodium etidronate. Journal of the American Medical Association 230: 562-567 (1974)

Martin, T.J.: Treatment of Paget's disease with calcitonins. Australian and New Zealand Journal of Medicine 9: 36-43 (1979).

Martin, T.J.; Jerums, G.; Melick, R.A.; Xipell, J.M. and Arnott, R.: Clinical, biochemical and histological observations on the effect of porcine calcitonin in Pagets disease of bone. Australian and New Zealand Journal of Medicine 7: 36-43 (1977).

Marx, S.J.; Woodward, C.J. and Aurbach, G.D.: Calcitonin receptors of kidney and bone. Science 178: 999-1000 (1972).

Mathews, J.L.; Martin, J.H.; Collins, E.J.; Kennedy, J.W. and Powell, E.L.: Immediate changes in the ultrastructure of bone cells following thyrocalcitonin administration; in Talmage and Munson (Eds.) Calcium, Parathyroid Hormone and the Calcitonins. International Congress Series 243, pp. 375-382 (Excerpta Medica, Amsterdam 1972).

Melick, R.A.; Ebeling, P. and Hjorth, R.J.: Improvement in paraplegia and vertebral Paget's disease treated with calcitonin. British Medical Journal 1: 626-628 (1976).

Menzies, M.A.: Greengerg, P.B. and Joplin, G.F.: Otological studies in patients with deafness due to Paget's disease before and after treatment with synthetic human calcitonin. Acta Otolaryngologica 79: 378-383 (1975).

Meunier, P.: Paget's disease of bone. Quantitative histology, histopathogenesis and therapeutic prospects. Lyon Médical 233: 839-853 (1975).

Meunier, P.; Chapuy, M.C.; Alexandre, C.; Bressot, C.; Edouard, C. et al.: Effects of disodium dichloromethylene diphosphonate on Paget's disease of bone. Lancet 2: 489-492 (1979).

Meunier, P.; Chapuy, M.C.; Courpron, P.; Vignon, E.; Edouard, C. and Bernard, J.: Effects cliniques, biologiques et histologiques de l'ethane-1-hydroxy 1, 1 diphosphonate (EHDP) dans la maladie de Paget. Revue du Rheumatisme 42: 699-705 (1975).

Meyers, M.H. and Singer, F.R.: Osteotomy for tibia vara in Paget's disease under cover of calcitonin. Journal of Bone and Joint Surgery 60A: 810-814 (1978).

Michael, W.R.; King, W.R. and Wakim, J.M.: Metabolism of disodium ethane-1-hydroxy-1, 1-diphosphonate (disodium etidronate) in the rat, rabbit, dog and monkey. Toxicology and Applied Pharmacology 21: 503-515 (1972).

Moffatt, W.H.; Morrow, J.D. and Simpson, N.: Effect of calcitonin therapy in deafness associated with Paget's disease of bone. British Medical Journal 4: 203 (1974).

Murphy, W.A.; Whyte, M.P. and Haddad, J.G.: Paget's bone disease: Radiologic documentation of healing with human calcitonin therapy. Radiology 136: 1-4 (1980).

Nagant de Deuxchaisnes, C. and Krane, S.M.: Paget's disease of bone. Clinical and metabolic observations. Medicine (Baltimore) 43: 233-266 (1964).

Nagant de Deuxchaisnes, C.; Rombouts-Lindermans, C.; Huaux, J.P.; Malgham, J. and Maldague, B.: Roentgenologic evaluation of the efficacy of calcitonin in Paget's disease of bone; in MacIntyre and Szelke (Eds) Molecular Endocrinology, pp. 213-233 (Elsevier/North Holland Biomedical Press, Amsterdam 1977).

Nagant de Deuxchaisnes, C.; Rombouts-Lindemans, C.; Huaux, J.P.; Devogelaer, J.P.; Malgham, J. and Maldague, B.: Roentgenologic evaluation of the action of the diphosphonate EHDP and of combined therapy (EHDP and calcitonin) in Pagets disease of bone; in MacIntyre and Szelke (Eds) Molecular Endocrinology, pp. 405-433 (Elsevier/North Holland Biomedical Press, Amsterdam 1979).

Newsome, F.E.; O'Dor, R.K.; Parkes, C.O. and Copp, D.H.: A study of stability of calcitonin biological activity. Endocrinology 92: 1102-1106 (1973).

Plehwe, W.E.; Hudson, J.; Clifton-Bligh, P. and Posen, S.: Porcine calcitonin in the treatment of Paget's disease of bone. Medical Journal of Australia 1: 577-581 (1977).

Rasmussen, H. and Bordier, P.: Primary disorders of bone cell function; in The Physiological and Cellular Basis of Metabolic Bone Disease, pp. 292-303 (Williams and Wilkins, Baltimore 1974).

Rebel, A.; Basle, M.; Minard, M.F. and Malakani, K.: Actions de la calcitonine sur les osteoclasts de la maladie de Paget au cours d'un traitement de longue durée. Pathologie Biologie 25: 611-616 (1977).

Rebel, A.; Malkani, K.; Basle, M. and Bregeon, C.: Osteoclast ultrastructure in Paget's disease. Calcified Tissue Research 20: 187-199 (1976).

Recker, R.R. and Saville, P.D.: Intestinal absorption of disodium ethane-1-hydroxy-1, 1-diphosphonate (disodium etidronate) using a deconvolution technique. Toxicology and Applied Pharmacology 24: 580-589 (1973).

Reiner, M. Jung, A.; Seiler, A.; Schenk, R. and Fleisch, H.: Le traitement de la maladie de Paget par les diphosphonates. Schweiz. Med. Woch. 105: 1701-1703 (1975).

Reitsma, P.H.; Bijvoet, O.L.M.; Verlinden-Ooms, H. and Van der Wee-Pals, L.J.A.: Kinetic studies of bone and mineral metabolism during treatment with (3-amino-1-hydroxypropylidene)-1,1-bisphosphonate (ADP) in rats. Calcified Tissue International 32: 145-147 1980).

Riggs, L. and Jowsey, J.: Treatment of Paget's disease with fluoride. Seminars in Drug Treatment 2: 65-75 (1972).

Russell, R.G.G.; Smith, R.; Preston, C.; Walton, R.J. and Woods, C.G.: Diphosphonates in Paget's disease. Lancet 1: 894-898 (1974).

Ryan, W.G.: Treatment of Paget's disease of bone with mithramycin. Clinical Orthopaedics and Related Research 127: 106-110 (1977).

Schenk, R.; Merz, W.A.; Muhlbauer, R.; Russel, R.G.G. and Fleisch, H.: Effect of ethane-1-hydroxy-1,1-diphosphonate (EHDP) and dichloromethylene diphosphonate (Cl_2MDP) on the calcification and resorption of cartilage and bone in the tibial epiphysis and metaphysis of rats. Calcified Tissue Research 11: 196-214 (1973).

Shai, F.; Baker, R.K. and Wallach, S.: The clinical and metabolic effects of porcine calcitonin on Pagets disease of bone. Journal of Clinical Investigation 50: 1927-1940 (1971).

Silva, O.L. and Becker, K.L.: Immunoreactive calcitonin in extrathyroidial tissues; in Pecile (Ed.) Calcitonin 1980. Chemistry, Physiology, Pharmacology and Clinical Aspects, pp. 144-153 (Excerpta Medica, Amsterdam 1981).

Singer, F.R.; Aldred, J.P.; Neer, R.M.; Krane, S.M.; Potts Jr, J.T. and Bloch, K.J.: An evaluation of antibodies and clinical resistance to salmon calcitonin. Journal of Clinical Investigation 51: 2331-2338 (1972).

Singer, F.R.; Fredericks, R.S. and Minkin, C.: Salmon calcitonin therapy for Paget's disease of bone. The problem of acquired clinical resistance. Arthritis and Rhematism 23: 1148-1154 (1980).

Singer, F.R.; Rude, R.K. and Mills, B.G.: Studies of the treatment and aetiology of Paget's disease of bone; in MacIntyre, (Ed.) Human Calcitonin and Paget's Disease, pp. 93-110 (H. Huber, Bern 1977).

Singer F.R.; Rude, R.K. and Mills, B.G.: Paget's disease of bone; in Avioli and Krane (Eds) Metabolic Bone Disease, pp. 489-575 (Academic Press, New York 1978).

Siris, E.S.; Canfield, R.E.; Jacobs, T.P. and Baquiran, D.C.: Long term therapy of Paget's disease of bone with EHDP. Arthritis and Rheumatism 23: 1177-1184 (1980).

Siris, E.S.; Canfield, R.E.; Jacobs, T.P.; Stoddart, K.E. and Spector, P.J.: Clinical and biochemical effects of EHDP in Paget's disease of bone: Patterns of response to initial treatment and to long term therapy. Metabolic Bone Disease and Related Research 3: 301-308 (1981).

Stein, I.; Shapiro, B.; Ostrum, B. and Beller, M.: Evaluation of sodium etidronate in the treatment of Paget's disease of bone. Clinical Orthopaedics and Related Research 122: 347-358 (1977).

Stevens, J.: Orthopaedic aspects of Paget's disease. Metabolic Bone Disease and Related Research 3: 271-278 (1981).

Sturtridge, W.C.; Harrison, J.E. and Wilson, D.R.: Long term treatment of Paget's disease of bone with salmon calcitonin. Canadian Medical Association Journal 117: 1031-1034 (1977).

Talmage, R.V. and Anderson, J.J.B.: Parathyroid hormone effects in rats treated with diphosphonates. Science 183: 661-663 (1974).

Talmage, R.V.; Cooper, C.W. and Toverud, S.U.: The physiological significance of calcitonin; in Peck (Ed.) Bone and Mineral Research Annual 1, pp. 74-143 (Excerpta Medica, Amsterdam 1983).

Talmage, R.V.; Hirsch, P.F. and Van der Weil, C.J.: Calcitonin, feeding and calcium conservation; in Pecile (Ed.) Calcitonin 1980. Chemistry, Physiology, Pharmacology and Clinical Aspects, pp. 96-109 (Excerpta Medica, Amsterdam 1981).

Tashjian, A.H.; Wright, D.R.; Ivey, J.L. and Pont, B.: Calcitonin binding sites in bone: Relationships to biological response and escape. Recent Progress in Hormone Research 34: 285-334 (1978).

Treschsel, U.; Bonjour, J.-P. and Fleisch, H.: Regulation of the metabolism of 25-hydroxyvitamin D_3 in primary cultures of chick kidney cells. Journal of Clinical Investigation 64: 206-217 (1979).

Treschsel, U.; Schenk, R.; Bonjour, J.-P.; Russell, R.G.G. and Fleisch, H.: Relation between bone mineralization, Ca absorption, and plasma Ca in phosphonate-treated rats, American Journal of Physiology 232: E298-E305 (1977).

Walton, R.J.; Russel, R.G.G. and Smith, R.: Changes in the renal and extrarenal handling of phosphate induced by disodium etidronate (EHDP) in man. Clinical Science and Molecular Medicine 49: 45-56 (1975).

Warshawsky, H.; Goltzman, D.; Rouleau, M.F. and Bergeron, J.J.M.; Direct *in-vivo* demonstration by radioautography of specific binding sites for calcitonin in skeletal and renal tissues of the rat. Journal of Cell Biology 85: 682-694 (1980).

Wener, J.A.; Gorton, S.J. and Raisz, L.G.: Escape from inhibition of resorption in cultures of foetal bone treated with calcitonin and parathyroid hormone. Endocrinology 90: 752-759 (1972).

Williams, C.P.; Meachim, G. and Taylor, W.H.: Effect of calcitonin treatment on osteoclast counts in Pagets disease of bone. Journal of Clinical Pathology 31: 1212-1217 (1978).

Woodhouse, N.J.Y.: Paget's disease of bone. Journal of Clinical Endocrinology and Metabolism 1: 125-141 (1972).

Woodhouse, N.J.Y.; Bordier, P.; Fisher, M.; Joplin, G.F.; Reiner, M. et al.: Human calcitonin in the treatment of Paget's disease. Lancet 1: 1139-1143 (1971).

Woodhouse, N.J.Y.; Crosbie, W.A. and Mohamedally, S.M.: Cardiac output in Paget's disease: Response to long term salmon calcitonin therapy. British Medical Journal 4: 686 (1975).

Woodhouse, N.J.Y.; Joplin, G.F.; MacIntyre, I. and Doyle, F.H.: Radiological regression in Paget's disease treated by human calcitonin. Lancet 2: 992-994 (1972).

Woodhouse, N.J.Y.; Mohamedally, S.M.; Saed-Nejad, L.F. and Martin, T.J.: Development and significance of antibodies to salmon calcitonin in patients with Paget's disease on long term treatment. British Medical Journal 2: 927-929 (1977).

Wooton, R.; Reeve, J.; Spellacy, E. and Tellez-Yudilevich, M.: Skeletal blood flow in Paget's disease of bone and its response to calcitonin therapy. Clinical Science and Molecular Medicine 54: 69-74 (1978).

Zeigler, R.; Holz, G.; Rave, F.; Minne, H. and Delling, G.: Therapeutics studies with human calcitonin; in MacIntyre (Ed.) Human Calcitonin and Paget's Disease, pp. 167-173 (H. Huber, Bern 1977).

Address for correspondence and reprints: Dr *D.J. Hosking*, Department of Medicine, University Hospital, Queen's Medical Centre, Nottingham NG7 2UH (England).

General Information

Publication data: Two volumes of *Drugs* are published annually. Each volume comprises six 96-page issues. The annual subscription price is US$320.00/Sw.F.750/Aust$390.00 including postage. *Drugs* is published by ADIS Press Limited, P.O. Box 34-030, Birkenhead, Auckland 10, New Zealand.

Editorial matter is prepared by our own professionally qualified editorial staff and by honorary specialist consultants from all fields of medicine. While great care has been taken in compiling and checking the information contained in *Drugs*, the publisher cannot accept responsibility or be in any way liable for errors or omissions. The inclusion or exclusion of any product does not mean that the publisher advocates or rejects its use either generally or in any particular field or fields.

Drug nomenclature: Approved names of the British Pharmacopoeia Commission are used throughout the text. When the Commission has not adopted a name for the drug under discussion, the United States Adopted Name (USAN – United States Pharmacopeial Convention Inc.) or the International Non-Proprietary Name (INN – WHO) is used. When available, all three names are given at the head of the 'Drug Evaluations' and 'Review Articles' sections, and elsewhere in the text as appropriate. Other synonyms (e.g. research code names of new drugs) are also given.

Manuscripts: Information on the preparation of manuscripts will be provided to authors.

Drugs 30: 175-181 (1985)
0012-6667/85/0009-0175/$03.50/0

Pharmacokinetic Properties of the Newer Cephalosporins
A Valid Basis for Drug Selection?

James T. Noble and *Michael Barza*

Section of Infectious Diseases, Boston University School of Medicine, Carney Hospital, Boston; and Tufts University School of Medicine, New England Medical Center Hospitals, Boston

The past few years have seen a plethora of new β-lactam antibiotics. The most striking example is that of the 'third generation' cephalosporins, a group which includes cefotaxime, ceftizoxime, latamoxef (moxalactam), cefoperazone, ceftazidime and ceftriaxone [see reviews by Brogden et al., 1981; Carmine et al., 1983a,b; Richards and Brogden, 1985; Richards and Heel, 1985; Richards et al., 1985]. The availability of these agents has confronted physicians with difficult choices. Ideally, the decision to use one of these drugs in preference to another should be based on the results of randomised, comparative studies. Such studies are lacking, and decisions must therefore be made by inference from other data.

1. Criteria for Selection of an Individual Agent

One basis for selection is the antibacterial spectrum. By and large, all of these drugs are highly active against the Enterobacteriaciae, although cefoperazone is weaker in this regard. Most have only modest activity against *Pseudomonas aeruginosa*, although cefoperazone shows moderate activity and ceftazidime excellent activity against this organism. Only latamoxef shows marked activity against *Bacteroides fragilis*. The new cephalosporins are generally less active than older agents against Gram-positive cocci. Of course individual isolates, particularly of Gram-negative bacilli, may show great variations in susceptibility from one drug to another.

The physician's choice of a third generation cephalosporin may also be influenced by concern about adverse effects. Latamoxef and, to a lesser extent, cefoperazone may cause prolongations in the prothrombin time (Andrassy et al., 1982) and a disulfiram-like intolerance reaction with alcohol (Neu and Prince, 1980). Latamoxef in high doses may also impair platelet aggregation (Weitekamp and Aber, 1983), whereas cefoperazone has a tendency to cause diarrhoea.

A third basis for choosing among third generation cephalosporins relates to their pharmacokinetic properties. Although the third generation drugs have a number of features in common, including poor oral absorption, longer serum half-lives and better penetration of the inflamed meninges than older cephalosporins, they also exhibit marked diversity, particularly in serum half-life and route(s) of elimination. These may have important consequences in terms of cost, ease of administration, and usefulness in particular situations.

Table I. Summary of important pharmacokinetic properties of the third generation cephalosporins

Drug	Protein binding (%)	Metabolism	Serum half-life (h)	Primary route of excretion	Dose altered in renal failure	CSF levels[a] (% peak serum)	References
Cefotaxime	30-50	Yes	1.0-1.2	Renal (GFR + TS)	Yes	5-15	1, 2
Ceftizoxime	30	No	1.3-2.1	Renal (GFR + TS)	Yes	0-10	2, 3
Latamoxef	43-52	No	2.0-2.5	Renal (?TS, GFR)	Yes	5-15	2, 4
Cefoperazone	90	No	1.9	Biliary (25% renal)	No	3	5, 6, 7
Ceftazidime	17	No	1.8	Renal (GFR)	Yes	5-25	6, 8, 9, 10
Ceftriaxone	83-96	No	6.0-8.0	Renal (60%) Biliary (40%)	No	3-6	10, 11, 12

a In patients with meningitis.

Abbreviations: TS = tubular secretion; GFR = glomerular filtration.

Key to references: 1 LeFrock et al. (1982); 2 Neu (1982); 3 Neu (1984); 4 Fitzpatrick and Staniford (1982); 5 Bundtzen et al. (1980); 6 Coombs (1982); 7 Funk and Strasbaugh (1982); 8 Gower and Hobbs (1981); 9 Kemmerich et al. (1983); 10 Norrby (1984); 11 Demos (1982); 12 Patel and Kaplan (1984).

2. Possible Clinical Relevance of Pharmacokinetic Differences

It is far easier to identify pharmacokinetic differences among these drugs than it is to evaluate the clinical importance of these differences. Nevertheless, given the similar structures and modes of action of the agents, it seems justifiable to draw some comparisons. We will focus on 4 clinically relevant points. The first is the serum half-life (table I): this may be of importance in determining the dosing interval. As a rough approximation, it seems reasonable to suggest that doses (commonly 2g) be given at intervals of 4 times the serum half-life for serious infections and 6 times the serum half-life for mild to moderate infections. For a peak serum concentration of 100 mg/L, subsequent concentrations would be 6.25 and 1.6 mg/L after 4 and 6 half-lives, respectively. Clearly, a variety of other factors could be weighed in the choice of a dosing interval, including the degree of susceptibility of the infecting organism, the extent of serum protein binding of the antibiotic, the duration of the post-antibiotic effect, and the toxicity of the drug. Nevertheless, one has to start somewhere. The schedule suggested above has the merit that it applies a single standard to all of the members of a closely related group of drugs and results in recommendations which are in the usual range for these agents.

The second point that we will consider is penetration of the cerebrospinal fluid (CSF) in meningitis (table I). Although other factors are important, CSF penetration appears to be inversely related to serum protein binding of drugs in this group (Barza and Butler, 1980).

The third point relates to biliary concentration of the antibiotic (table II). A high concentration of an antibiotic in the bile is desirable up to a point, in that it may facilitate therapy of biliary tract infection. Extensive biliary secretion may also eliminate the need for dosage modification in renal failure. Very high bile levels, however, may predispose to diarrhoea and to marked alterations in the intestinal flora. Although it is not proven that changes in the normal faecal flora have adverse effects in humans, animals in which the intestinal flora are suppressed show a tendency to become colonised with exogenous micro-organisms (Hentges, 1983). Furthermore, although controversial, it has been proposed that inhibition of the normal faecal flora leads to a decrease in synthesis of vitamin K precursors, leading to the hypoprothrombinaemia seen in patients treated with drugs such as latamoxef and cefoperazone (Conly et al., 1984).

The fourth point to be considered is the ease of dosage adjustments of the various drugs in the presence of renal insufficiency. As mentioned above, the greater the degree of biliary excretion, the less the adjustment required as renal function decreases.

3. *Implications of Pharmacokinetic Properties for Clinical Use*

3.1 Cefotaxime

Cefotaxime has the shortest serum half-life of the new cephalosporins - about 1 hour (table I). The short half-life may be due in part to the fact that the drug is actively secreted by the renal tubule; however, ceftizoxime (which has a longer serum half-life) is also actively secreted. The main reason for the short half-life of cefotaxime is that, uniquely among the third generation cephalosporins, it is metabolised by the liver to a less active compound. About 50 to 60% of an administered dose appears in the urine unchanged and 15 to 20% as desacetylcefotaxime, the principal metabolite (LeFrock et al., 1982). The situation is complicated by the fact that the metabolite, although less active than cefotaxime, has moderate antimicrobial activity and actually shows synergy with the parent compound against some isolates (Jones et al., 1982). Furthermore, the metabolite has a longer serum half-life (about 1.6 hours) than cefotaxime itself (Neu, 1982). Because of these factors, it has been argued that cefotaxime can be administered on an 8- or 12-hourly basis (Chin and Neu, 1984). However, we are not aware of studies in seriously ill patients to validate this concept. On the basis of clinical trials and the apparent half-life of 1.0 to 1.2 hours as measured by bioassay, we would suggest that the dose of 2g be given every 4 to 6 hours to adults with serious infections, and every 6 to 8 hours to those with moderate infections.

Cefotaxime penetrates body tissues and fluids readily, as would be expected from its low degree of serum protein binding (about 30 to 50%). Levels in the CSF in meningitis are about 10% of peak serum concentrations (table I), and are adequate for the treatment of meningitis. Biliary concentrations of 34 to 82 mg/L have been reported during therapy (LeFrock et al., 1982). However, faecal lev-

Table II. Biliary concentrations, effects on faecal flora and propensity to cause hypoprothrombinaemia of the third generation cephalosporins

Drug	Biliary concentrations (mg/L)	Effect on faecal flora		Hypoprothrombinaemia	References
		aerobes	anaerobes		
Cefotaxime	34-82	++	0	No	Guggenbicher and Kofler (1984); LeFrock et al. (1982)
Ceftizoxime	11-70	++	0	No	Cunha et al. (1982); Lode et al. (1981)
Latamoxef	38-65	+++	+++	Yes	Malmborg et al. (1983); Shimada and Ueda (1982)
Cefoperazone	400-6000	++++	++++	Yes	Alestig et al. (1983); Greenfield et al. (1983)
Ceftazidime	5-45	+++	0	No	Kemmerich et al. (1983); Ruf (1982)
Ceftriaxone	25-4366	++++	+++	No	Bodey et al. (1983); Owens et al. (1982)

els are low and there is no significant effect on the intestinal flora (Guggenbicher and Kofler, 1984). Hypoprothrombinaemia has not been described with this agent.

Cefotaxime does not accumulate in renal failure; however, the half-life of the desacetyl metabolite is prolonged (Neu, 1982). This likely accounts for the widely discrepant results of cefotaxime serum concentrations measured by bioassay in patients with renal failure. The manufacturer recommends that the dosage be halved when creatinine clearance falls below 20 ml/min. Thus, dosage adjustments in renal failure should be relatively simple to calculate. Liver dysfunction does not seem to alter the elimination of cefotaxime, but more data are needed to be certain. The serum half-life of cefotaxime has been reported to be doubled in patients with ascites (Moreau et al., 1980).

3.2 Ceftizoxime

This agent is identical to cefotaxime except that it lacks the side chain at the 3 position which is metabolised in cefotaxime. Thus, the serum half-life of ceftizoxime is about 1.9 hours (range 1.3 to 2.1 hours) [Neu, 1984], which is longer than that of cefotaxime, but similar to that of cefoperazone, latamoxef and ceftazidime. 80% of a dose is recovered unchanged in the urine (Neu, 1984). Based on the serum half-life and on clinical studies, ceftizoxime should be given in a dosage of 2g every 6 to 8 hours for serious infections and every 8 to 12 hours for moderate infections in adults with intact renal function.

Ceftizoxime penetrates the meninges readily to produce CSF concentrations slightly lower than those of cefotaxime (Ruf, 1982). Biliary levels of up to 70 mg/L have been reported (Cunha et al., 1982), which are well above the minimum inhibitory concentrations for most biliary pathogens. There are minimal effects on the faecal flora (Lode et al., 1981), and hypoprothrombinaemia has not been reported.

Ceftizoxime is eliminated mainly by renal glomerular filtration, but there is probably some degree of tubular secretion insofar as the serum half-life is prolonged by concomitant administration of probenecid (Neu, 1982). The manufacturer recommends that the drug be administered 12-hourly in patients with a creatinine clearance of 5 to 50 ml/min and once daily in patients with a creatinine clearance of less than 5 ml/min. Ceftizoxime is removed by haemodialysis (Shah et al., 1982) and a 1 to 2g dose should be given after dialysis. Dosage modification does not appear to be necessary in patients with hepatic dysfunction.

3.3 Latamoxef

The serum half-life of latamoxef (moxalactam; lamoxactam) is 2.0 to 2.5 hours (table I), in the typical range for this class of compound. The drug is not metabolised, and 70 to 90% of a dose is excreted unchanged in the urine (Parsons et al., 1981). Based on the serum half-life and *in vitro* activity of the drug, latamoxef should be given in a dose of 2g every 8 hours to adults with serious infections and every 12 hours to patients with moderate infections. Clinical data support the former dosing interval, but more data are needed to substantiate the latter.

Consistent with its relatively low degree of serum protein binding (table I), latamoxef penetrates the CSF in meningitis as readily as cefotaxime. However, latamoxef is not as active as cefotaxime against Gram-positive cocci (Fitzpatrick and Staniford, 1982) and should not be used for therapy of meningitis caused by these organisms.

Significant amounts of latamoxef are found in the bile (Shimada and Ueda, 1982), presumably accounting for the marked alteration of the faecal flora found with this drug (Malmborg et al., 1983). Although diarrhoea is infrequent with latamoxef, hypoprothrombinaemia is a well-recognised side effect. The mechanism of this adverse reaction is controversial. Some evidence supports the hypothesis that the drug inhibits the synthesis of vitamin K precursors by intestinal bacteria in patients who are already nutritionally deficient (Bang et al., 1981; Conly et al., 1984). Other data point to a warfarin-like effect of the methyltetrazolethiol side chain (MTT), which is also found in cefamandole and cefoperazone. MTT inhibits carboxylation of pre-prothrombin (Lipsky, 1984), resulting in decreased prothrombin activity. MTT may also inhibit the epoxide reductase enzyme which is needed to recycle vitamin K. The manufacturer recommends that all patients treated with latamoxef be given 10mg of vitamin K weekly to prevent hypoprothrombinaemia.

Latamoxef is eliminated in the urine chiefly by glomerular filtration and the half-life is markedly prolonged in renal insufficiency (LeRoy et al., 1981). The following dosage adjustments have been recommended: for a creatinine clearance of 25 to 50 ml/min, one-half the usual dose; for a creatinine clearance of 2 to 25 ml/min, one-quarter the usual dose; and in anuria, 2 to 3g as a loading dose, then 1g daily as a maintenance dose, and 2 to 3g following each haemodialysis.

3.4 Cefoperazone

Cefoperazone has a serum half-life of 1.9 hours, which is similar to that of latamoxef, leading to similar dosing recommendations. However, in the case of cefoperazone, abundant clinical data are available to support its efficacy on a 12-hourly dosing schedule for moderate infections (Swarz et al., 1982). In our opinion, the drug should be given every 8 hours for more serious infections.

Several features distinguish cefoperazone from the other drugs discussed so far. It is highly bound to serum proteins (greater than 90%), which contributes to its low CSF penetration (Funk and Strasbaugh, 1982). Thus, it is not recommended for the treatment of meningitis. More importantly, three-quarters of a single dose is excreted unchanged in bile. Bile concentrations as high as 6000 mg/L have been reported (Greenfield et al., 1983) and appreciable amounts have been found despite complete biliary obstruction, which is not the case with other cephalosporins (Bundtzen et al., 1980). However, a consequence of the enormous biliary excretion is that the normal faecal flora is virtually eliminated in patients given cefoperazone intravenously (Alestig et al., 1983). Diarrhoea is a frequent problem with this drug but, surprisingly, colonisation and superinfection have not been a problem to date. Hypoprothrombinaemia has been described less frequently than with latamoxef but, presumably on the same basis, the manufacturer recommends monitoring of the prothrombin time in patients who are at particular risk of vitamin K deficiency, and administration of vitamin K in cases of prolongation.

3.5 Ceftazidime

The serum half-life of ceftazidime is 1.8 hours, leading to a suggested dosing interval of 6 to 8 hours for serious infections and 8 to 12 hours for moderate infections. Over 80% of a dose has been recovered in the urine and no metabolites have been identified (Luthy et al., 1981).

Ceftazidime is negligibly protein bound (table I). Penetration into the CSF is excellent where levels of up to 25% of serum concentrations can be achieved (Norrby, 1984), making this a promising agent for therapy of many types of meningitis. However, clinical studies will be needed to confirm the efficacy of this agent in meningitis. Biliary excretion in animals is minimal; however, concentrations in bile of up to 45 mg/L have been measured in man (Saito, 1983), presumably accounting for the reported reduction in the aerobic faecal flora (Kemmerich et al., 1983). Hypoprothrombinaemia has not been described with this drug.

It has been proposed that the dose of ceftazidime be halved for patients with a creatinine clearance of less than 30 ml/min, with further reductions at very low levels of renal function (Gower and Hobbs, 1981).

3.6 Ceftriaxone

Ceftriaxone has a half-life of 6 to 8 hours (Patel and Kaplan, 1984), longer than that of any other cephalosporin antibiotic. Renal elimination is relatively inefficient because the drug is not actively secreted and its high degree of serum protein binding (> 90%; Neu, 1982) sharply limits the amount that can be filtered by the glomerulus. Biliary excretion, although it eventually disposes of about

40% of a dose, must be relatively slow or the drug would have a half-life similar to that of cefoperazone. Ceftriaxone is not metabolised.

Based on the long serum half-life and accumulating clinical data, a dosage interval of 24 hours can be recommended for most infections. This schedule lends itself to outpatient therapy and is a uniquely attractive feature of ceftriaxone.

As with cefoperazone, extensive protein binding limits access to the CSF, and the penetration of ceftriaxone is only 3 to 6% of peak serum concentrations (Demos, 1982). However, unlike cefoperazone, the minimum inhibitory concentrations of ceftriaxone for *Streptococcus pneumoniae, Neisseria meningitidis,* and *Haemophilus influenzae* are so low that successful therapy of meningitis caused by these organisms is possible. The same is probably true of meningitis caused by susceptible Gram-negative bacilli, but clinical data are needed to prove this. Meningitis caused by the 3 major meningeal pathogens has been successfully treated on a once daily treatment schedule in a small scale study (Martin and Guggi, 1984) and further work is in progress. For less susceptible organisms, twice daily therapy may be more appropriate.

Biliary concentrations can exceed 4000 mg/L (Owens et al., 1982), and profound changes in the faecal flora, similar to those seen with cefoperazone, have been noted (Bodey et al., 1983). Diarrhoea has been reported in 3 to 6% of recipients (Moskovitz, 1984) but hypoprothrombinaemia has not been attributed to this agent.

Because of its dual mechanism of excretion, dosage modification is not necessary with ceftriaxone except in patients with severe hepatic *and* renal failure. In this situation, serum concentrations of the drug should be monitored.

4. Conclusions

The third generation cephalosporins exhibit a number of pharmacokinetic advantages over earlier agents. These include a longer serum half-life, better CSF penetration and, in some cases, prodigious biliary excretion. Pharmacokinetic differences provide rational reasons for certain preferences among these drugs. The unique half-life of ceftriaxone is convenient when parenteral treatment is necessary for outpatients, and may afford cost savings for inpatients as well. The extensive biliary excretion of cefoperazone may be useful in patients with infection of an obstructed biliary tract. Whether the very high biliary concentrations produced by cefoperazone and ceftriaxone are of benefit in treating infections of the patent biliary tract remains to be shown; in such cases most of the cephalosporins exhibit effective biliary concentrations. However, the administration of cefoperazone or ceftriaxone has a disconcerting effect on the faecal flora, although this usually results in no more than diarrhoea.

The other pharmacokinetic differences among the third generation cephalosporins are more subtle. Cefotaxime should probably be given at shorter intervals than the other drugs because of its shorter serum half-life. Cefoperazone is not recommended for the treatment of meningitis. Physicians who are inexperienced in adjusting the dosage of drugs in patients with renal failure will find cefoperazone or ceftriaxone easier to use than the other agents in this class.

References

Alestig, K.; Carlberg, H.; Nord, C.E. and Trollfors, B.: Effect of cefoperazone on fecal flora. Journal of Antimicrobial Chemotherapy 12: 163-167 (1983).

Andrassy, K.; Koderisch, J. and Ritz, E.: Influence of cefotaxime, cefoperazone, and lamoxactam on hemostasis; in Proceedings of the 22nd ICAAC, Abstract 523 (American Society for Microbiology, Washington, DC 1982).

Bang, N.U.; Tessler, S.S.; Heidenreich, R.O.; Marks, C.A. and Mattler, L.E.: Effects of moxalactam on blood coagulation and platelet function. Reviews of Infectious Diseases 4 (Suppl.): S546-S554 (1981).

Barza, M. and Butler, E.: The penetration of penicillins and cephalosporins into selected sites of clinical interest; in Weinstein and Fields (Eds) Seminars in Infectious Diseases, Vol. III, pp. 193-224 (Thieme-Stratton, New York 1980).

Bodey, G.P.; Fainstein, V.; Garcia, I.; Rosenbaum, B. and Wong, Y.: Effect of broad-spectrum cephalosporins on the microbial flora of recipients. Journal of Infectious Diseases 148: 892-897 (1983).

Brogden, R.N.; Carmine, A.; Heel, R.C.; Morley, P.A.; Speight, T.M. and Avery, G.S.: Cefoperazone: A review of its *in vitro* antimicrobial activity, pharmacological properties and therapeutic efficacy. Drugs 22: 423-460 (1981).

Bundtzen, R.; Craig, W.; Toothaker, R. et al.: Cefoperazone: Single-dose pharmacokinetics; in Proceedings of the 20th ICAAC, Abstract 112 (American Society for Microbiology, Washington, DC 1980).

Carmine, A.A.; Brogden, R.N.; Heel, R.C.; Speight, T.M. and Avery, G.S.: Cefotaxime. A review of its activity, pharmacological properties and therapeutic use. Drugs 25: 223-289 (1983a).
Carmine, A.A.; Brogden, R.N.; Heel, R.C.; Romankiewicz, J.A.; Speight, T.M. and Avery, G.S.: Moxalactam (latamoxef): A review of its antibacterial activity, pharmacokinetic properties and therapeutic use. Drugs 26: 279-333 (1983b).
Chin, N. and Neu, H.C.: Cefotaxime and desacetylcefotaxime: An example of advantageous antimicrobial metabolism. Diagnostic Microbiology and Infectious Diseases 2: 215-225 (1984).
Conly, J.M.; Ramotar, K.; Chubb, H.; Bow, E.J. and Louie, T.J.: Hypoprothrombinemia in febrile, neutropenic patients with cancer: Association with antimicrobial suppression of intestinal microflora. J. Infect. Dis. 150: 202-212 (1984).
Coombs, J.D.: Metabolism and pharmacokinetics of new cephalosporin agents; in Neu (Ed.) New Beta Lactam Antibiotics: A Review from Chemistry to Clinical Efficacy of the New Cephalosporins, pp. 177-214 (College of Physicians of Philadelphia, Philadelphia 1982).
Cunha, B.; Ristuccia, A. and Jonas, M.: Tissue penetration characteristics of ceftizoxime and cefazolin in human bile and gallbladder wall. Journal of Antimicrobial Chemotherapy 10 (Suppl. C): 117-120 (1982).
Demos, P.: Clinical aspects of ceftriaxone; in Neu (Ed.) New Beta Lactam Antibiotics: A Review from Chemistry to Clinical Efficacy of the New Cephalosporins, pp. 263-274 (College of Physicians of Philadelphia, Philadelphia 1982).
Fitzpatrick, B.J. and Staniford, H.C.: A comparative evaluation of moxalactam. Pharmacotherapy 2: 197-212 (1982).
Funk, E.A. and Strasbaugh, L.J.: Antimicrobial activity, pharmacokinetics, adverse reactions, and therapeutic indications of cefoperazone. Pharmacotherapy 2: 188-189 (1982).
Gower, P.E. and Hobbs, P.M.: The kinetics of ceftazidime in renal impairment; in Program and Abstracts of the 12th ICC, Florence, Italy (1981).
Greenfield, R.A.; Gerber, A.U. and Craig, W.A.: Pharmacokinetics of cefoperazone in patients with normal and impaired renal function. Reviews of Infectious Diseases 5 (Suppl.): S127-S136 (1983).
Guggenbicher, J.P. and Kofler, J.: Influence of third-generation cephalosporins on aerobic intestinal flora. Journal of Antimicrobial Chemotherapy 14 (Suppl. B): 67-70 (1984).
Hentges, D.J.: Role of the intestinal microflora in host defense against infection; in Hentges (Ed.) Human Intestinal Microflora in Health and Disease, pp. 311-331 (Academic Press, New York 1983).
Jones, R.N.; Barry, A.L. and Thornsberry, C.: Antimicrobial activity of desacetylcefotaxime alone and in combination with cefotaxime: Evidence of synergy. Reviews of Infectious Diseases 4 (Suppl.): S366-S373 (1982).
Kemmerich, B.; Warns, H.; Lode, H.; Borner, K.; Koeppe, P. and Knothe, H.: Multiple-dose pharmacokinetics of ceftazidime and its influence on fecal flora. Antimicrobial Agents and Chemotherapy 24: 333-338 (1983).
LeFrock, J.L.; Prince, R.A. and Leff, R.D.: Mechanism of action, antimicrobial activity, pharmacology, adverse effects, and clinical efficacy of cefotaxime. Pharmacotherapy 2: 177 (1982).
LeRoy, A.; Humbert, G. and Filastre, J.P.: Pharmacokinetics of moxalactam in subjects with normal and impaired renal function. Antimicrob. Agents Chemoth. 19: 965-971 (1981).
Lipsky, J.J.: Mechanisms of the inhibition of the gamma-carboxylation of glutamic acid by N-methylthiotetrazole containing antibiotics. Proceedings of the National Academy of Sciences 81: 2893-2987 (1984).
Lode, H.; Warns, H.; Kemmerich, B.; Knothe, H. and Koeppe, P.: Ceftizoxime: Multiple-dose pharmacokinetics and their effect on fecal flora; in Proceedings of the 21st ICAAC, Abstract 37 (American Society for Microbiology, Washington, DC 1981).
Luthy, R.; Blaser, J.; Bonetti, A.; Simmon, H.; Wise, R. and Sigenthaler, W.: Comparative multiple-dose pharmacokinetics of cefotaxime, moxalactam, and ceftazidime. Antimicrobial Agents and Chemotherapy 21: 567-575 (1981).
Malmborg, A.S.; Kager, L. and Nord, C.E.: Effect of moxalactam on bowel flora in patients undergoing colorectal surgery; in Proceedings of the 23rd ICAAC, Abstract 127 (American Society for Microbiology, Washington, DC 1983).
Martin, E. and Guggi, T.: Single daily dose short course treatment of pediatric meningitis with ceftriaxone; in Proceedings of the 24th ICAAC (American Society for Microbiology, Washington, DC 1984).
Moreau, L.; Durand, H. and Biclet, P.: Cefotaxime concentrations in ascites. J. Antimicrob. Chemoth. 6 (Suppl. A): 121-122 (1980).
Moskovitz, B.L.: Clinical adverse effects during ceftriaxone therapy, American J. Med. 77 (Suppl. 4C): 84-88 (1984).
Neu, H.C.: The new beta-lactamase stable cephalosporins. Annals of Internal Medicine 97: 408-419 (1982).
Neu, H.C.: Ceftizoxime: A beta-lactamase-stable, broad-spectrum cephalosporin. Pharmacotherapy 4: 51 (1984).
Neu, H.C. and Prince, A.S.: Interactions between moxalactam and alcohol. Lancet 1: 1422 (1980).
Norrby, S.R.: The place of cephalosporins in the treatment of bacterial meningitis in adults; in Moellering and Neu (Eds) Advances in Cephalosporin Therapy: Beyond the Third Generation (Health Projects International, Phoenix 1984).
Owens, N.J.; Nightingale, C.H.; Quintiliani, R. and Hickingbotham, J.M.: Ceftriaxone penetration pharmacokinetics in serum, bile, and gallbladder wall; in Proceedings of the 22nd ICAAC (American Society for Microbiology, Washington, DC 1982).
Parsons, J.; Romano, J. and Levison, M.: Pharmacology of a new 1-oxa-beta-lactam in normal volunteers. Antimicrobial Agents and Chemotherapy 19: 302-305 (1981).
Patel, I. and Kaplan, S.: Pharmacokinetic profile of ceftriaxone in man. American J. Med. 77 (Suppl. 4C): 17-25 (1984).
Richards, D.M. and Brogden, R.N.: Ceftazidime: A Review of its antibacterial activity, pharmacokinetic properties and therapeutic use. Drugs 29: 105-161 (1985).
Richards, D.M. and Heel, R.C.: Ceftizoxime. A review of its antibacterial activity, pharmacokinetic properties and therapeutic use. Drugs 29: 281-329 (1985).
Richards, D.M.; Heel, R.C.; Brogden, R.N.; Speight, T.M. and Avery, G.S.: Ceftriaxone. A review of its antibacterial activity, pharmacological properties and therapeutic use. Drugs 27: 469-527 (1984).
Ruf, B.: Penetration of ceftizoxime (FK 749) into the cerebrospinal fluid. Infection 10: 76-80 (1982).
Saito, A.: Studies on absorption, distribution, metabolism, and excretion of ceftazidime in Japan. Journal of Antimicrobial Chemotherapy 12 (Suppl. A): 255-262 (1983).
Shah, P.M.; Knobloch, M. and Haag, R.: Pharmacokinetics of ceftizoxime in patients undergoing hemodialysis. Methods in Experimental and Clinical Pharmacology 4: 185-188 (1982).
Shimada, J. and Ueda, Y.: Moxalactam: Absorption, excretion, distribution, and metabolism. Reviews of Infectious Diseases 4 (Suppl.): S569-S580 (1982).
Swarz, H.; Fay, D.; Siemans, A.J. and Fishman, S.K.: The clinical aspects of cefoperazone; in Neu (Ed.) New Beta Lactam Antibiotics: A Review from Chemistry to Clinical Efficacy of the New Cephalosporins, pp. 243-262 (College of Physicians of Philadelphia, Philadelphia 1982).
Weitekamp, M.R. and Aber, R.C.: Prolonged bleeding times and bleeding diathesis associated with moxalactam administration. Journal of the American Medical Association 249: 69-71 (1983).

Address for correspondence and reprints: Dr *Michael Barza*, Tufts University School of Medicine, New England Medical Center Hospitals, 171 Harrison Avenue, Boston, MA 02111 (USA).

Drugs 30: 182-274 (1985)
0012-6667/85/0009-0182/$46.50/0

Nifedipine
A Review of Its Pharmacodynamic and Pharmacokinetic Properties, and Therapeutic Efficacy, in Ischaemic Heart Disease, Hypertension and Related Cardiovascular Disorders

E.M. Sorkin, S.P. Clissold and *R.N. Brogden*

ADIS Drug Information Services, Auckland

Various sections of the manuscript reviewed by: ***U. Elkayam,*** Department of Medicine, University of Southern California, Los Angeles, California, USA; ***H. Emanuelsson,*** Department of Medicine I, University of Göteborg, Göteborg, Sweden; ***K. Fox,*** National Heart Hospital, London, England; ***W.H. Frishman,*** Hospital of the Albert Einstein College of Medicine, Bronx, New York, USA; ***M.D. Guazzi,*** Cattedra di Cardiologia, Università Degli Studi de Milano, Milan, Italy; ***J.R. Hampton,*** University Hospital, Queen's Medical Centre, Nottingham, England; ***C.H. Kleinbloesem,*** Sylvius Laboratories, Leiden, The Netherlands; ***O. Lederballe Pedersen,*** Department of Internal Medicine I, Aarhus Amtssygehus, Aarhus, Denmark; ***P. Lichtlen,*** Medizinische Hochschule Hannover, Department of Cardiology and Cardiovascular Surgery, Hannover, Federal Republic of Germany; ***R.G. McAllister,*** Veterans Administration Medical Center Research Service, Lexington, Kentucky, USA; ***P.W. Serruys,*** Erasmus Universiteit Rotterdam, Rotterdam, The Netherlands; ***A.L. Soward,*** Erasmus Universiteit Rotterdam, Rotterdam, The Netherlands.

Contents

Summary 184
1. Pharmacodynamic Properties 188
  1.1 Electrophysiological Effects of Calcium Antagonists 188
    1.1.1 Electrophysiological Effects of Nifedipine 189
  1.2 Haemodynamic Effects 190
    1.2.1 Effect on Blood Pressure 191
    1.2.2 Effect on Heart Rate 193
    1.2.3 Effect on Cardiac Haemodynamics 193
    1.2.4 Haemodynamic Effects of Nifedipine Compared with, and in Combination with, Other Cardiovascular Drugs 197
    1.2.5 Effect on Exercise Tolerance in Patients with Angina Pectoris 199
  1.3 Effect on Coronary Circulation and Myocardial Oxygen Consumption 201
  1.4 Cardioprotective Effect 202
  1.5 Effect on Peripheral Vascular Circulation 203
  1.6 Effect on Non-Vascular Smooth Muscle 205
    1.6.1 Gastrointestinal Tract 205
    1.6.2 Urinary and Uterine Smooth Muscle 205
  1.7 Effect on Platelets 206
  1.8 Effect on Blood Glucose Concentrations and Insulin Release 207

1.9 Renal Effects 208
1.9.1 Effect on Renal Blood Flow, Renovascular Resistance and Glomerular Filtration Rate 208
1.9.2 Effect on Plasma Renin Activity, Angiotensin and Aldosterone 208
1.9.3 Other Renal Effects 209
1.10 Other Effects 210
1.10.1 Effects on Hepatic Blood Flow 210
1.10.2 Effects on the Sympathetic Nervous System 210
1.10.3 Effects on Histamine Release and Airway Conductance 210
1.11 Mechanism of Action 211
2. Pharmacokinetic Properties 214
2.1 Absorption 215
2.2 Distribution 218
2.3 Metabolism 219
2.3.1 Half-Life 219
2.3.2 Elimination 220
2.4 Effect of Disease on Pharmacokinetics 220
2.5 Relationship of Plasma Concentration and Clinical Effects 220
3. Therapeutic Use in Ischaemic Heart Disease 221
3.1 Use in Stable Angina 222
3.1.1 Placebo-Controlled Trials 222
3.1.2 Comparisons with β-Blockers, and Their Use in Combination 223
3.1.3 Comparative Efficacy of Calcium Antagonists 226
3.1.4 Medium to Long Term Trials 227
3.2 Use in Variant (Prinzmetal's) Angina 227
3.2.1 Open Studies 228
3.2.2 Comparisons with Placebo 228
3.2.3 Comparisons with Isosorbide Dinitrate 229
3.2.4 Comparative Efficacy of Calcium Antagonists 229
3.2.5 Long Term Trials 230
3.3 Use in Unstable Angina 231
3.3.1 Open Studies 232
3.3.2 Controlled Trials 232
3.4 Use in Acute Myocardial Infarction 234
3.4.1 Prevention or Attenuation of Myocardial Infarction 234
3.4.2 Post-Myocardial Infarction 234
3.5 Use in Coronary Artery Bypass Surgery 235
4. Therapeutic Use in Systemic Hypertension 235
4.1 Acute Studies 236
4.1.1 Comparative Trials 236
4.1.2 Hypertensive Crisis 237
4.1.3 Hypertension Associated with Pregnancy 238
4.1.4 Hypertension During Coronary Artery Bypass Surgery 239
4.1.5 Hypertension After Surgery 239
4.1.6 Hypertension in Renal Patients 239
4.2 Medium to Long Term Studies 240
4.2.1 Comparisons with Other Antihypertensive Drugs 240
4.2.2 Nifedipine in Combination with Other Antihypertensive Drugs 241
4.2.3 Long Term Trials 244
5. Other Therapeutic Uses 245
5.1 Congestive Heart Failure 245
5.2 Hypertrophic Cardiomyopathy 246
5.3 Pulmonary Hypertension 247
5.4 Raynaud's Phenomenon 248
5.4.1 Controlled Comparisons with Placebo 248

5.4.2 Other Studies 250
6. Side Effects 250
7. Dosage and Administration 253
8. Drug Interactions 254
9. Place of Nifedipine in Therapy 255

Summary

Synopsis: *Nifedipine*[1] *is an antagonist of calcium influx through the slow channel of the cell membrane and has been shown to be an effective and relatively well-tolerated treatment for stable, variant and unstable angina, mild to severe hypertension and Raynaud's phenomenon. Although its exact mechanism of action in these various diseases has not been precisely described, the potent coronary and peripheral arterial dilator properties of nifedipine, with concomitant improvements in oxygen supply/demand and reductions in systemic vascular resistance, are of major importance.*

Clinical trials support the view that nifedipine can be considered a first-line choice in all grades of angina, especially when coronary vasospasm is the underlying cause or when hypertension and/or congestive heart failure are added complications. Nifedipine also appears to be particularly useful in clinical situations when a rapid lowering of elevated blood pressure is needed, and there is growing evidence that it is an effective and safe choice for the longer term management of patients with mild to moderate hypertension. However, the majority of data have been from medium term studies, and confirmation of its long term usefulness in well-designed trials is still required. Additionally, nifedipine has convincingly been shown to be a useful adjunct for controlling blood pressure in patients refractory to conventional treatment with β-blockers, diuretics and various vasodilators. Nifedipine reduces the number, duration and severity of vasospastic attacks in more than 60% of patients with Raynaud's phenomenon of varying aetiology, and in individual cases it apparently facilitates the healing of digital ulcers.

Side effects appear to be dose related and occur in approximately 20% of patients. These effects, most of which are manifestations of the drug's potent vasodilating activity, include headache, flushing and dizziness.

Thus, nifedipine is a worthwhile alternative to other drugs available for the treatment of the various forms of angina, acute episodes of hypertension, mild to severe hypertension (alone or in combination) and Raynaud's phenomenon. While further well-designed clinical trials are needed to clarify its relative place in the long term management of mild to moderate hypertension, it is clear that nifedipine is now a well established agent in cardiovascular therapeutics.

Pharmacodynamic Properties: Nifedipine inhibits the slow inward current of calcium in normal cardiac tissues, its major effects being on the sinoatrial and atrioventricular nodes. In contrast to diltiazem or verapamil, nifedipine *in vivo* either has no effect on, or enhances, sinus or paced atrioventricular nodal conduction. Nifedipine also reduces atrioventricular nodal functional and effective refractory periods and atrioventricular nodal Wenckebach cycle lengths, and may be preferable to diltiazem or verapamil in patients with symptomatic ischaemic heart disease and depressed atrioventricular nodal function.

Sublingual or oral administration of nifedipine may lower mean arterial blood pressure at rest and after exercise by 20% or more. The onset of this reduction after both oral and sublingual administration occurs within 30 minutes and may last up to 5 hours. Intravenous nifedipine 1 to 4mg has produced significant decreases in blood pressure of up to 34% in patients with various cardiac disorders, with greater reductions in blood pressure seen in patients with hypertension than in normotensive individuals.

The effect of nifedipine on heart rate depends on its rate of input into the body. Oral capsule administration has not been associated with significant increases in heart rate,

1 'Adalat', 'Adalat Retard' (Bayer); 'Procardia' (Pfizer).

while sublingual, intravenous and intracoronary administration increase heart rate by up to 28%.

The reduction in systemic vascular resistance produced by sublingual nifedipine causes significant increases in cardiac output and decreases in left ventricular filling pressure due to afterload reduction, especially in patients with impaired left ventricular function. Intravenous nifedipine may produce decreases in left ventricular end-diastolic pressure and increases in cardiac index; however, intracoronary nifedipine may increase left ventricular end-diastolic pressure while decreasing systolic blood pressure. Thus, in contrast to intracoronary administration, the direct negative inotropic effect of intravenous nifedipine is overridden by reflex increases in heart rate and contractility that result from lowered blood pressure. In addition, both pulmonary vascular resistance and mean pulmonary arterial pressures decrease after nifedipine administration. Concomitant increases in cardiac index that are associated with these pulmonary effects further indicate that nifedipine has a selective effect on arterial resistance vessels.

By virtue of its strong arterial dilating ability, in patients with angina pectoris nifedipine produces favourable haemodynamic effects such as decreases in systemic vascular resistance and left ventricular afterload, and also decreases in systolic, diastolic and mean arterial pressure while maintaining cardiac inotropy and chronotropy in patients with left ventricular dysfunction. In such patients nifedipine is comparable to diltiazem, verapamil, β-blockers or nitrates in improving clinical status and reducing electrocardiographic signs of myocardial ischaemia on exercise or atrial pacing.

Greater reductions in blood pressure are achieved with the combination of nifedipine and β-blockers than result from either drug used separately in volunteers and patients with angina pectoris and hypertension. Reflex increases in heart rate and acute increases in plasma renin activity produced by nifedipine are blocked by β-blockade, and increases in total peripheral resistance produced by β-blockers are decreased by nifedipine.

Although hydralazine may be more suitable than nifedipine in patients with severe congestive heart failure when left ventricular afterload reduction is required, nifedipine produces more pulmonary vasodilatation than hydralazine and has a more balanced overall vasodilating effect. The combinations of nifedipine and captopril, and nifedipine and digoxin or dobutamine, produce greater decreases in blood pressure and increases in cardiac index, respectively, than when these drugs are used alone. Nifedipine may also produce comparable improvements in cardiac performance as nitrates in patients with heart failure secondary to acute myocardial infarction, and in combination with nitrates may produce greater decreases in systemic vascular resistance and increases in cardiac index than sole nitrate therapy. Nitroprusside may be preferable to nifedipine in the single-dose treatment of severe congestive heart failure because it produces less reduction in blood pressure and greater increases in cardiac index.

The administration of nifedipine to patients with coronary artery disease results in an increase in coronary blood flow, especially to myocardial tissue served by stenotic coronary arteries, with little change in myocardial oxygen consumption. Nifedipine may protect the myocardium during subsequent reperfusion after cardiac surgery, and may also limit the extent of ischaemic injury after myocardial infarction, although further studies in humans are needed to define the exact degree of benefit that may be obtained in such patients.

Other pharmacodynamic effects of nifedipine include increased peripheral blood flow and decreased peripheral vascular resistance (especially in hypertensive subjects), inhibition of platelet aggregation, decreased lower oesophageal sphincter pressure and inhibition of peristalsis. In short term studies a reduction in glucose tolerance has been reported, but no such effects occurred in longer studies.

Nifedipine produces little effect on renal blood flow but its effect on renovascular resistance and glomerular filtration rate has been varied. Angiotensin II and acute plasma renin activity concentrations increase after nifedipine administration, possibly due to increases in sympathetic discharge induced by the drug; however, plasma aldosterone concentrations do not appear to be affected. Varying increases in hepatic blood flow have been reported with nifedipine use, possibly due to arterial vasodilatation produced by the drug.

Pharmacokinetic Properties: Close to 100% of a single oral dose of nifedipine is absorbed, although only about 45 to 68% of the drug reaches the systemic circulation. Considerable variations in peak plasma nifedipine concentrations after oral and sublingual administration, and the time required to reach these peaks, have been measured, presumably due to interindividual differences in the rate of drug absorption and/or variability in the extent of first-pass hepatic extraction and metabolism.

The steady-state volume of distribution of nifedipine in man after oral and intravenous administration is 1.32 and 0.62 to 1.12 L/kg, respectively. Nifedipine protein binding to albumin is concentration dependent and has ranged from 92 to 98%. Nifedipine undergoes almost complete (95%) hepatic oxidation to 3 pharmacologically inactive metabolites which are excreted in the urine.

The elimination half-life of nifedipine is apparently dependent upon the dosage form in which it is administered, with half-lives of 6 to 11 hours, 2 to 3.4 hours and 1.3 to 1.8 hours measured after oral tablet, oral capsule and intravenous administration, respectively. The total systemic and intrinsic clearances of nifedipine from plasma have ranged from 27 to 66 L/h and 33 to 37 L/h, respectively. Renal impairment does not significantly alter nifedipine pharmacokinetics.

Despite the difficulties involved in establishing a direct relationship between nifedipine plasma concentrations and clinical effects, some studies have shown plasma nifedipine concentrations to correlate significantly with changes in blood pressure, heart rate and lower oesophageal sphincter pressure. In addition, improved exercise tolerance and decreases in the frequency and occurrence of ischaemic attacks in patients with angina pectoris have also been shown to be directly related to nifedipine plasma concentrations.

Therapeutic Trials: Nifedipine has been shown to be effective in stable exercise-induced angina as assessed by decreases in anginal frequency and glyceryl trinitrate (nitroglycerin) consumption, and improvements in objective parameters such as work performance and time to onset of ST segment changes during exercise. Comparative trials in patients with stable angina have generally been of short duration in small numbers of patients and have failed to identify any consistent differences in efficacy between nifedipine and alternative first-line drugs such as β-blockers or other calcium antagonists. In those studies where nifedipine and a β-blocker were used together, the combination produced more favourable results without any significant deterioration of left ventricular function.

Approximately 80% of patients with variant (Prinzmetal's) angina had a greater than 50% reduction in angina frequency (almost half gained complete remission from anginal attacks) when treated with nifedipine. Similar response rates were reported during short and long term (up to 6 years) trials, although some authors cited the need for additional antianginal drugs such as nitrates and β-blockers to help control symptoms. Comparative studies in patients with variant angina have not identified any consistent advantages or disadvantages for nifedipine over other drugs used, such as isosorbide dinitrate, diltiazem or verapamil.

Open trials in patients with unstable angina refractory to conventional therapy have shown that addition of nifedipine to their treatment regimen produced a favourable response in 47 to 89% of those treated. In comparative studies in patients with unstable angina, nifedipine was significantly superior to placebo and of equivalent efficacy as propranolol – alone, or combined with isosorbide dinitrate. Combination of nifedipine with propranolol in patients who did not benefit from monotherapy greatly increased the rate of successful responses. In terms of mortality, incidence of infarction, infarct size or extent of myocardial necrosis, nifedipine did not offer any advantages over placebo when administered to patients threatened by an acute myocardial infarction. In contrast, nifedipine was extremely useful for reducing or eliminating recurring episodes of ischaemic pain immediately after myocardial infarction.

A number of case studies have demonstrated the efficacy of sublingual or intracoronary nifedipine, alone or in combination with glyceryl trinitrate for preventing coronary artery spasm during coronary artery bypass surgery.

Nifedipine, administered by various routes, has been shown to be a relatively safe and effective drug for rapidly lowering elevated blood pressure in a number of clinical settings such as during or after surgery, in haemodialysis patients, and in hypertensive crises. In a comparative single-dose trial, nifedipine produced a faster reduction of blood pressure than prazosin in patients with uncontrolled hypertension. Prazosin, on the other hand, lowered blood pressure by a greater amount 2 to 3 hours after administration, although this was associated with a high incidence of postural hypotension.

In numerous therapeutic trials in patients with mild to severe hypertension, the antihypertensive efficacy of nifedipine has been maintained for periods of up to 3 or 4 years. Comparative medium term studies in patients with mild to moderate hypertension have shown nifedipine to be of equivalent efficacy as traditional first-line agents such as β-blockers and diuretics. Nifedipine has also been found to be an extremely useful adjunct for controlling blood pressure in patients refractory to conventional 2- or 3-drug regimens. Recently, a sustained release formulation of nifedipine, allowing twice daily administration, has been introduced to improve compliance. Therapeutic trials to date demonstrate that this preparation maintains 24-hour control of blood pressure at least as well as the conventional capsule formulation of nifedipine.

Nifedipine has been used in patients with Raynaud's phenomenon of varying aetiology and has produced subjective improvement in the number, duration and severity of vasospastic attacks in more than 60% of patients. In some individuals nifedipine apparently facilitated the healing of cutaneous ulceration and relieved the frequency and severity of migraine associated with Raynaud's phenomenon. Clinical evaluation of nifedipine in other therapeutic areas such as congestive heart failure, pulmonary hypertension and hypertrophic cardiomyopathy have been of a preliminary nature. Firm conclusions regarding its relative efficacy awaits further research, although some encouraging individual results have been reported.

Side Effects: Side effects from nifedipine are dose related and occur in approximately 20% of patients. The most common side effects occur secondary to the vasodilating properties of nifedipine and include headache (7%), flushing (5 to 7%) and dizziness (3 to 12%). The character, severity and incidence of side effects with nifedipine use is no greater during long term (> 6 months) treatment with the drug than during shorter courses of therapy. These side effects may be mitigated by reducing the nifedipine dose or by combining the drug with a β-blocker. This combination of nifedipine and β-blockers has not been found to place patients at greater risk than sole nifedipine therapy and thus may be advantageous in the treatment of angina pectoris or hypertension in patients with compromised cardiovascular function. Discontinuance of the drug due to side effects has been necessary in 2 to 6% of patients, while the occurrence of a true 'withdrawal syndrome' has not been noted.

Drug Interactions: Most studies suggest that nifedipine has no effect on plasma digoxin concentrations, although some studies have reported increased concentrations and clinical effects of digoxin. Nifedipine does not alter the pharmacokinetics of metoprolol, atenolol, nadolol or propranolol, but a few case reports have described severe hypotension or cardiac failure associated with nifedipine/β-blocker use in high risk patients with severe angina pectoris, triple-vessel disease, impaired left ventricular function and a prior history of myocardial infarction.

Dosage and Administration: For the clinical management of patients with angina pectoris, hypertension or Raynaud's phenomenon, nifedipine dosage should be individualised. The current recommendation is for a starting dosage of one 10mg capsule 3 times daily, during or after meals, and this can be carefully titrated up to 20mg 3 times daily in patients with hypertension or Raynaud's phenomenon and up to 90 to 120 mg/day (in divided doses) in patients with angina. If an immediate effect is required the capsules should be bitten open and the liquid contents allowed to remain in the mouth for faster sublingual absorption. A sustained release tablet formulation of nifedipine is now available for the treatment of hypertension, the recommended dosage of which is 20mg twice daily, after food, increased if necessary to 40mg twice daily. Recently, injectable (intravenous injection or infusion) preparations of nifedipine have been introduced for treating coronary vasospasm and/or acute hypertensive episodes. An intracoronary formulation is also available for treating coronary vasospasm that occurs during diagnostic or therapeutic interventions. It is imperative that these products are protected from light.

Nifedipine, a dihydropyridine derivative (fig. 1), is one of a group of compounds thought to act by blocking the transmembrane inward movement of calcium. Nifedipine and these other compounds, often referred to as calcium antagonists, have been used frequently as tools for the elucidation of calcium-dependent regulatory mechanisms. More importantly though, these compounds have in themselves been found to possess many important therapeutic properties useful in the management of certain cardiovascular and related disorders in man. This review will concentrate solely on the effects of nifedipine in man and its application in the treatment of angina, hypertension and related cardiovascular disorders.

1. Pharmacodynamic Properties

1.1 Electrophysiological Effects of Calcium Antagonists

The electrophysiological basis of action of calcium blockers has been extensively reviewed (Ant-

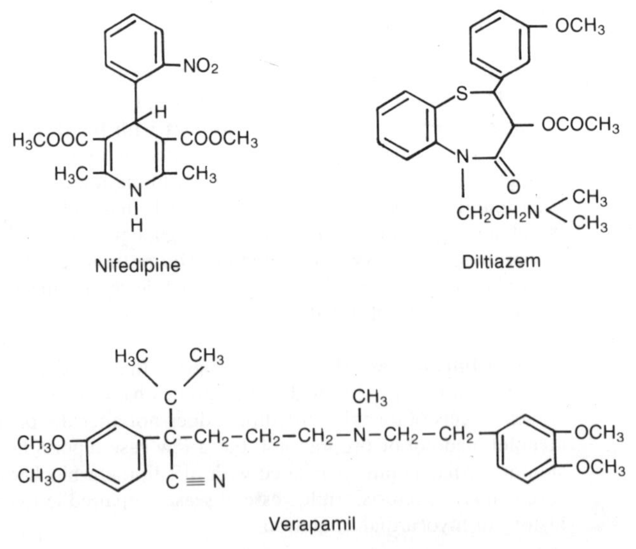

Fig. 1. Chemical structures of nifedipine (a dihydropyridine derivative), diltiazem (a benzothiazepine derivative) and verapamil (a papaverine derivative).

Table I. Clinical electrophysiological properties of some calcium antagonists (adapted from Singh et al., 1983)

	Nifedipine	Diltiazem	Verapamil
R-R interval	↓	↑↓	↑↓
QRS	0	0	0
P-R	0	↑	↑
A-H	0	↑	↑
H-V	0	0	0
Atrial ERP	0	0	0
AV node ERP	↑↓	↑	↑↑
AV node FRP	↑↓	↑	↑↑
Ventricular ERP	0	0	0
His-Purkinje ERP	0	0	0
Bypass tract ERP	0	?	↑↓
SNRT	0	0[a]	0[a]
Ventricular automaticity	0	0	0

a Prolonged in sick sinus syndrome.
Key and abbreviations: 0 = no effect; ↓ = decrease; ↑ = increase; ↑↓ = variable effect; ERP = effective refractory period; FRP = functional refractory period; SNRT = sinus node recovery time.

man et al., 1980b; Mitchell et al., 1982; Singh et al., 1982, 1983, 1984). Briefly, normal cardiac tissues may be separated into 2 groups (slow and fast channel tissues) based upon their action potential characteristics (Mitchell et al., 1982; Singh et al., 1982, 1983, 1984) [fig. 2]. In the slow channel dependent tissues, which include the sinoatrial and atrioventricular nodes, the major cationic species traversing the cell membrane is calcium. Thus, the effects of slow channel blocking agents such as the calcium blockers are most evident in these tissues (Singh et al., 1982, 1983, 1984; Wit and Cranefield, 1974; Zipes and Fischer, 1974). Although these slow channel blockers may have an effect in diseased fast channel tissues which are dependent upon the slow channel for remaining function (Mitchell et al., 1982), few or no changes are expected in the electrophysiological characteristics of normal fast channel tissues in man (Furlanello et al., 1980; Kawai et al., 1981; Mitchell et al., 1982).

A summary of the clinical electrophysiological properties of nifedipine and other frequently used calcium channel blocking agents is presented in table I.

1.1.1 Electrophysiological Effects of Nifedipine

Sinus nodal function may be assessed by measurement of spontaneous heart rate, maximal corrected sinus nodal recovery time following overdrive suppression by atrial pacing, and sinoatrial conduction time (which indicates the conduction characteristics of perinodal tissues). Although nifedipine may induce a statistically significant increase in heart rate (section 1.2.2; table II), it does not produce clinically significant changes in either the maximal corrected sinus nodal recovery time or sinoatrial conduction time in patients with normal sinus function (Franchi and Padeletti, 1981; Furlanello et al., 1980; Kawai et al., 1981; Padeletti et al., 1979; Vey et al., 1984). However, in patients with sinus node disease, nifedipine may have a variable and unpredictable effect on the maximal corrected sinus nodal recovery time (Furlanello et al., 1980).

Atrioventricular function is assessed electrophysiologically by measurement of atrioventricular conduction time and refractoriness characteristics. Atrioventricular conduction times are measured by the AH and VA intervals during anterograde and retrograde conduction, respectively. Refractoriness of the AV node is estimated by the effective and functional refractory periods and the shortest cycle length (Wenckebach cycle length) conducted with Wenckebach periodicity during atrial pacing (Mitchell et al., 1982). In contrast to diltiazem and verapamil, nifedipine either has no effect on or enhances sinus or paced AV nodal conduction (Furlanello et al., 1980; Kawai et al., 1981; Krikler and Rowland, 1980; Mitchell et al., 1982; Padeletti et al., 1979; Rowland et al., 1979) [fig. 3]. The lack of a direct suppressant effect on AV nodal conduction may occur because of the low doses of nifedipine used (one-tenth that of diltiazem or verapamil) and reflex increases in sympathetic tone as a result of a fall in blood pressure (Kawai et al., 1981). In fact, increases in sympathetic tone have

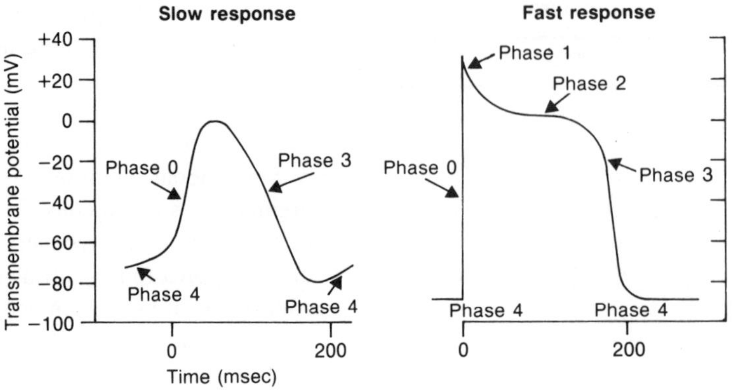

Predominant ion movement during phase 0	*Calcium*	*Sodium*
Where found	Sinoatrial and atrioventricular nodes, mitral and tricuspid valves and coronary sinus	Atria, ventricles, His-Purkinje fibres
Conduction velocity	0.01 to 0.1 msec	0.5 to 5 msec
Activation and inactivation kinetics	Sluggish	Fast
Activation potential	−40 to −50mV	−60 to −70mV
Selective blocking agents	Manganese, cobalt and calcium channel blocking agents	Tetrodotoxin and local anaesthetics

Fig. 2. Characteristics of fast and slow response action potentials in cardiac muscle (after Sobel, 1981).

been confirmed by the measurement of increased plasma noradrenaline (norepinephrine) concentrations after nifedipine administration (section 1.10.2). As compared to diltiazem and verapamil, nifedipine may also have no effect on or may reduce AV nodal functional and effective refractory periods and AV nodal Wenckebach cycle lengths (Bexton et al., 1983; Furlanello et al., 1980; Kawai et al., 1981; Padeletti et al., 1979). Thus, in patients with depressed AV nodal function, nifedipine may be preferable to diltiazem or verapamil in the treatment of symptomatic ischaemic heart disease.

As expected, nifedipine does not cause measurable changes in conduction or refractoriness of normal fast channel tissues (i.e. high right atrial to low septal right atrial conduction times or His-Purkinje conduction times) either in spontaneous sinus rhythm or in constant rate atrial paced rhythm (Franchi and Padeletti, 1981; Furlanello et al., 1980; Kawai et al., 1981; Padeletti et al., 1979; Rowland et al., 1979; Singh et al., 1984; Vey et al., 1984). Nifedipine has also had no effect on the QRS duration or on the QT_c interval of the 12-lead electrocardiogram (Furlanello et al., 1980; Singh et al., 1984); it may, however, significantly reduce ST segment depression in the process of lessening the occurrence of ischaemia in myocardial tissue after physical exercise (Brügmann et al., 1983; Cassera et al., 1976; Majid and De Jong, 1982; sections 1.2.5 and 3.1.1).

1.2 Haemodynamic Effects

The haemodynamic effects of nifedipine have been investigated utilising invasive techniques with Swan-Ganz catheters to allow continuous monitoring of right atrial and pulmonary artery pressures. Cardiac output has been determined by thermodilution method, and arterial and venous pressures by direct and indirect techniques. Results obtained from these procedures have then been used to derive indices of myocardial function, including stroke work, cardiac index and pulmonary vascular resistance. Clinical and acute haemodynamic evaluations have been done both in cardiac patients with varying disorders and in normal volunteers. Acute haemodynamic effects after sublingual administration are summarised in table III.

1.2.1 Effect on Blood Pressure

As can be seen from table III, nifedipine may lower mean arterial blood pressure at rest and after exercise by up to 20% or more. Significant reductions ($p < 0.001$) in blood pressure occur within 30 minutes after administration of both the oral and sublingual dosage forms (Bonaduce et al., 1983), and may last up to 5 hours (Banzet et al., 1983). Intravenous nifedipine 1 to 4mg produces significant decreases in blood pressure of up to 34% in patients with hypertension, coronary artery disease or hypertrophic obstructive cardiomyopathy (Murphy et al., 1982; Pfeiffer et al., 1983; Pfisterer and Burkart, 1982; Schanzenbächer et al., 1982). Although Kurnik et al. (1984) showed that decreases in mean arterial pressure were greater in patients with impaired left ventricular function than

Table II. Effects of short term administration of nifedipine on the sinus and atrioventricular (AV) nodes and fast channel tissues (after Mitchell et al., 1982)

References	No. of patients	Diagnosis	Dose (mg) [route]	Time[a] (min)	ΔCSRT	AH int		AV FRP/ AV ERP	AV WCL	Sinus HRA-LSRA/ Sinus HV int	A-FRP/ A-ERP
						sinus	paced				
Bexton et al. (1983)	5	Denerv	? IV	5		−6.6		±/±	±		
Franchi and Padeletti (1981)	36	Misc	20 SL	NG	±	±		±/±		±/±	±/±
Furlanello et al. (1980)	20	Misc	20 SL	15-30	±	±		Short/ short	Short	NG/±	±/±
Kawai et al. (1981)	8	Misc	1 IV	NG	−25	−4		−13/ −17	−7	NG/±	
Padeletti et al. (1979)	10	Misc	20 SL	20	±	±	±	±/±		±/±	+11/±
Rowland et al. (1979)	11	EHD	7.5 μg/kg IV	5		±				NG/±	
Vey et al. (1984)	32	Misc	20 SL	15	±	±				NG/±	

a Interval between drug administration and electrophysiological reassessment.

Abbreviations: ΔCSRT = percentage change in maximal corrected sinus nodal recovery time; AH int = percentage change in AH conduction time determined in spontaneous sinus rhythm (sinus) and in constant rate atrial paced rhythm (paced); AV FRP = percentage change in AV nodal function refractory period; AV ERP = percentage change in AV nodal effective refractory period; AV WCL = percentage change in AV nodal Wenckebach cycle length; HRA-LSRA = high right atrial to low septal right atrial conduction time (intra-atrial conduction time); HV int = His-Purkinje conduction time; A-FRP = right atrial functional refractory period; A-ERP = right atrial effective refractory period; Denerv = cardiac transplant recipients; Misc = patients from several diagnostic categories; EHD = electrical heart disease; IV = intravenous; SL = sublingual; Short = refractory period shortening; NG = not given.

All values reported are in percentages and are reported as statistically significant changes from control values; ± = no change and refers to no statistically significant change from control values.

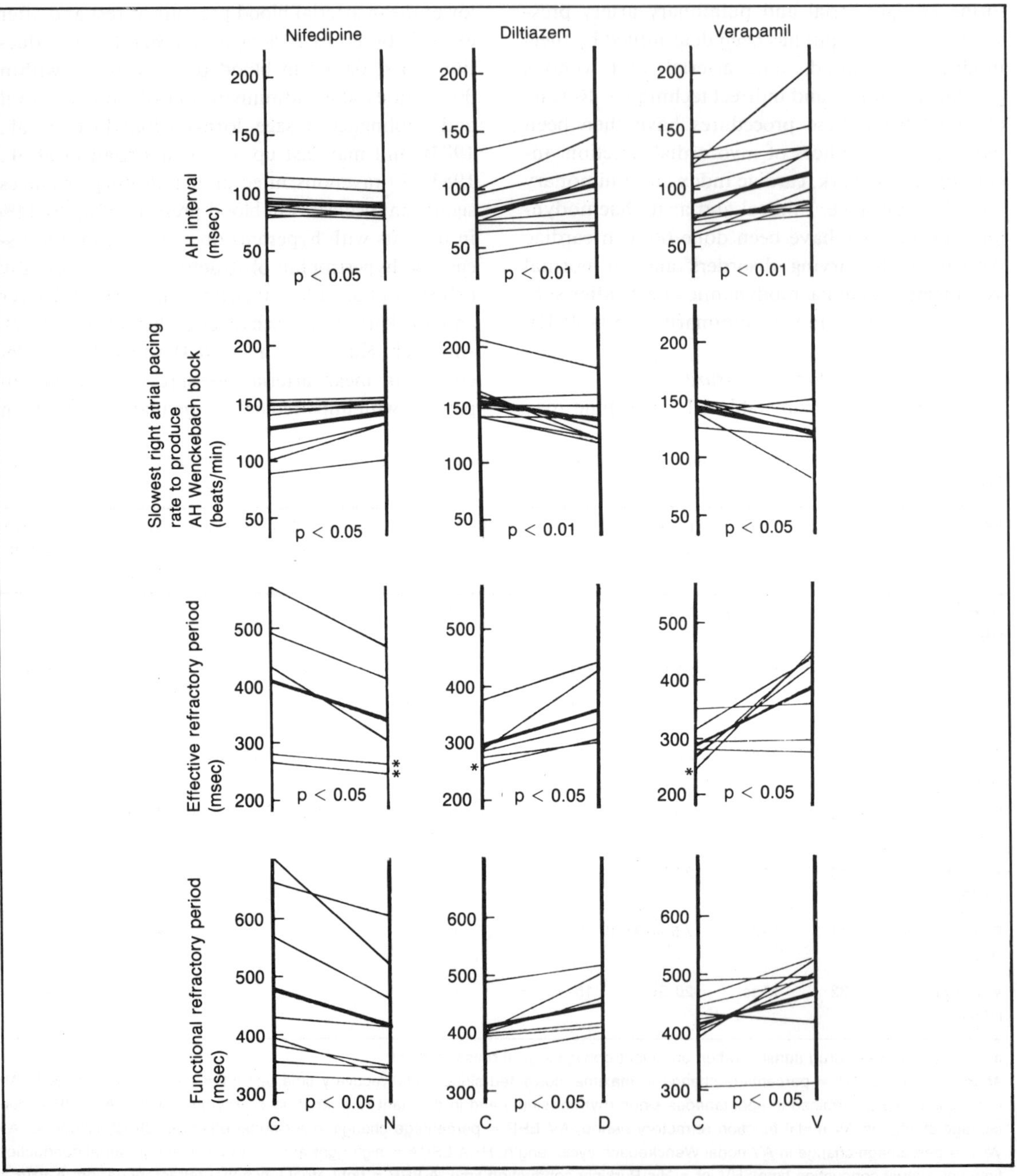

Fig. 3. Effects of intravenous nifedipine 1mg (n = 8), diltiazem 10 to 20mg (n = 10) and verapamil 10mg (n = 13) on AH intervals, Wenckebach periodicity, and the effective and functional refractory periods of the AV node in patients with atrial septal defects or arrhythmias (pre-excitation syndrome, paroxysmal supraventricular tachycardia or accelerated idioventricular rhythm). Thick lines denote mean values; C = control; * = cases in which failure of atrial capture by extrastimulus preceded; therefore, atrial value is lower than that shown in the figure [from Kawai et al. (1981), with permission from the American Heart Association Inc.].

in those with normal function, this has not always been shown to be the case (Ludbrook et al., 1982; Nelson et al., 1984b). However, nifedipine does produce a greater reduction in blood pressure in patients with hypertension compared with normotensive individuals (Corea et al., 1979a; Emanuelsson et al., 1984a; Kiowski et al., 1983; MacGregor et al., 1982, 1983; Magometschnigg, 1983); in 29 normotensive subjects and 33 patients with essential hypertension, oral nifedipine 5mg lowered mean blood pressure by 4.7 and 10.4%, respectively ($p < 0.01$ between the 2 groups of subjects) [MacGregor et al., 1983].

1.2.2 Effect on Heart Rate

Kleinbloesem et al. (1984c) showed that the rate of input of nifedipine is an important determinant of its effects. Nifedipine, given by slow osmotic rectal infusion at a zero-order rate (1.3 mg/h for 24 hours) in 6 healthy subjects, lowered blood pressure but did not alter heart rate. Since the increase in heart rate after vasodilation is mediated by baroreflex (Lederballe Pedersen and Mikkelsen, 1978), these findings imply that this reflex can be avoided by slow rates of drug input. Thus, it may be possible to dissociate the effects of nifedipine on blood pressure and heart rate by administering the drug so it is absorbed at a relatively low rate (Kleinbloesem et al., 1984c), which may include giving the drug with food (Hirasawa et al., 1985; section 2.1).

The acute administration of sublingual nifedipine has been shown to increase heart rate in cardiac patients and normal volunteers (table III). The increases in heart rate have ranged between statistically non-significant changes and increases of up to 28% over control values, and have been shown to be due to a baroreceptor-mediated increase in β-adrenergic tone secondary to systemic vasodilatation (Lederballe Pedersen and Mikkelsen, 1978). In contrast to the significant increases in heart rate produced by nifedipine in subjects at rest and during mild and moderate exercise, changes in heart rate during maximal exercise or atrial pacing are less marked (Andersen and Vik-Mo, 1984; Magorien et al., 1983) [table III]. This may possibly be due to the fact that complete sympathetic stimulation may already occur during peak exercise or atrial pacing before the nifedipine is administered (Andersen and Vik-Mo, 1984).

Interestingly, there have been no significant increases in heart rate following acute or long term (up to 12 months) oral administration of nifedipine capsules (Bellocci et al., 1982; Corea et al., 1981a; Ekelund et al., 1982; Elkayam et al., 1983, 1984a,b,c; Littler et al., 1983; Lund-Johansen and Omvik, 1983; Olivari et al., 1984; Saadjian et al., 1984), whereas oral administration of nifedipine tablets in doses of 20 to 60mg in hypertensive individuals has been associated with increases in heart rate of between 29 and 38% (Banzet et al., 1983).

The intravenous and intracoronary administration of nifedipine has been associated with significant increases in heart rate of 5 to 15 minutes duration in healthy subjects and in cardiac patients both at rest and during exercise (Amende et al., 1983; Kaltenbach et al., 1979; Kleinbloesem et al., 1984a; Murphy et al., 1982; Pfisterer and Burkart, 1982; Schanzenbächer et al., 1982; Schulz et al., 1978; Serruys et al., 1981b).

1.2.3 Effect on Cardiac Haemodynamics

Sublingual nifedipine may elicit significant increases in cardiac output and decreases in left ventricular filling pressure as a result of the reductions in systemic vascular resistance it may produce (Kurnik et al., 1984) [table III]. These increases in cardiac output and reductions in systemic vascular resistance are due to direct arteriolar vasodilatation and therefore to reductions in impedance to left ventricular ejection (Andersen and Vik-Mo, 1984; Cantelli et al., 1983; Klugman et al., 1980; Matsumoto et al., 1980). Relatively greater increases in cardiac output measured in subjects at rest compared with after exercise or atrial pacing are due to the significant increases in heart rate produced after nifedipine administration under rest conditions; however, significant reductions in arterial pressure maintain the rate-pressure product equal to or below those of the pretreatment levels (Fioretti et al., 1983; Hanrath et al., 1982; Kelly et al., 1982; section 1.2.2). Decreases in left ventric-

Table III. Summary of some single-dose haemodynamic studies of sublingually administered nifedipine in volunteers and patients with cardiovascular disease

References	Patient population [no. of subjects]	Dose (mg)	Patient status	Statistically significant percentage changes from baseline															
				MAP	MBP	SBP	DBP	HR	CI	SVI	SVR	PVR	RAP	MPAP	LVFP (PCWP)	LVEDP	LVEF	LVESV	LVEDV
Cantelli et al. (1981)	HF (AMI) [13]	10	Rest		−9	−12	±	±	+15	+17	−25	±	±	−13	−21				
Cantelli et al. (1983)	CHF [12]	10	Rest		−10	−9	−11	±	+30	+28	−36	±	±	±	−18				
Emanuelsson and Holmberg (1983)	AP [14]	10	Rest		−6	−13	±	+9	+14	+8	−18	−18		±					
Fioretti et al. (1983)	AIS [14]	20	Rest					+12	+16		−29					−50			
			Atrial pacing[a]					±	±		±					−64			
			Atrial pacing[b]					±	±		−19					−44			
Hanrath et al. (1982)	LVD (CAD) [14]	30	Rest	−10				+7	+24	+15	−26	−22		±					
			Exercise	−7				±	+20	+16	−22	−25		−15					
Kelly et al. (1982)	AP [15]	20	Rest	−18				+15	+33	+13	−35						+8	±	±
			Exercise	−21				+10	+7	±	−32						+10	−11	−26
Klugmann et al. (1980)	CHF [11]	20	Rest	−21					+47	+45	−44	±	−22	−26	−34	−37	+58	−23	−7
Ludbrook et al. (1982)	IHD [19]	20	Rest[c]	−10		−13	−17		+16	±	−33	−40				±	+14		
			Rest[d]	−12		−11	−13		±	±	−14	±				±	+9		
			Rest[e]	±		±	−19		+25	±	−41	±				−18	+34		
Matsumoto et al. (1980)	CHF [8]	20	Rest		−10	−11	−17	+10	+16	±	−21	±		±	±				
Naeije et al. (1982)	Volunteers [8]	20	Rest[f]	−7				+28	+24		−27	±	±	±	±				
			Rest[g]	±				+17	+15		−14	+56	±	+21	±				
Nelson et al. (1984a)	AP [9]	20	Rest[h]	−6				+14											
			Exercise[h]	−9				+7											
			Rest[i]	−10				±											
			Exercise[i]	−7				−2											

Olivari et al. (1984)	PPH [7]	20	Rest	≈−14			±	+31		−38	−35	±	≈−12	±	
Paulus et al. (1983)	NHC [10]	10	Rest	±			+5			−31		±			−18
Polese et al. (1979)	HCD [7]	10	Rest		−20	−22	±	+34		−39	−23			−36	
	PCD [7]	10	Rest		±	−16	±	+39		−39	−40			−33	
	RHDAS [5]	10	Rest		±	±	+11	+37		−34	−47			−35	
	RHDMR [5]	10	Rest		−19	−22	±	+29		−34	−34			−26	
Schartl et al. (1985)	CAD [10]	20	Rest	−17			+10	+12	±				±		±
			Exercise	−8			±	+9	±				−18		−19

a 92 beats/min.
b 114 beats/min.
c All patients in study.
d Patients with LVEDP ⩽ 20mm Hg and/or end-diastolic volume ⩽ 90 ml/m^2.
e Patients with LVEDP > 20mm Hg and/or end-diastolic volume > 90 ml/m^2.
f Normoxic conditions.
g Acute inspiratory hypoxic conditions.
h Patients with LVEDV < 20mm Hg.
i Patients with LVEDV > 20mm Hg.

Abbreviations: MAP = mean arterial pressure; MBP = mean blood pressure; SBP = systolic blood pressure; DBP = diastolic blood pressure; HR = heart rate; CI = cardiac index; SVI = stroke volume index; SVR = systemic vascular resistance; PVR = pulmonary vascular resistance; RAP = right atrial pressure; MPAP = mean pulmonary artery pressure; LVFP (PCWP) = left ventricular filling pressure (pulmonary capillary wedge pressure); LVEDP = left ventricular end-diastolic pressure; LVEF = left ventricular ejection fraction; LVESV = left ventricular end-systolic volume; LVEDV = left ventricular end-diastolic volume; HF = heart failure; AMI = acute myocardial infarction; CHF = congestive heart failure; AP = angina pectoris; AIS = aortic insufficiency; LVD = left ventricular dysfunction; CAD = coronary artery disease; IHD = ischaemic heart disease; PPH = primary pulmonary hypertension; NHC = nonobstructive hypertrophic cardiomyopathy; HCD = hypertensive cardiac disease; PCD = primary cardiac disease (not defined); RHDAS = rheumatic heart disease (aortic insufficiency); RHDMR = rheumatic heart disease (mitral regurgitation); ± = no statistically significant changes from control values.

ular filling pressure may be related to an improvement in ventricular emptying due to afterload reduction (Andersen and Vik-Mo, 1984; Klein et al., 1984).

Intravenous administration of nifedipine produces significant decreases and increases of left ventricular end-diastolic pressure and cardiac index, respectively (Amende et al., 1983; Kaltenbach et al., 1979; Pfisterer and Burkart, 1982; Pfisterer et al., 1983; Schanzenbächer et al., 1982; Serruys et al., 1981b). However, intracoronary administration of nifedipine 0.1mg has a profound depressant effect on global and regional left ventricular function in patients with coronary artery disease, as left ventricular end-diastolic pressure increases while systolic pressure decreases. Thus, Serruys et al. (1981b) suggested that the direct negative inotropic effect of intravenous nifedipine is overridden by reflex increases in heart rate and contractility that result from lowered blood pressure.

Reductions in pulmonary vascular resistance associated with increases in the cardiac index further suggest a selective effect of nifedipine on arterial resistance vessels (Bonaduce et al., 1983). Afterload reduction has also been demonstrated by the consistent lowering of left ventricular end-systolic and diastolic volumes (Fioretti et al., 1983; Kelly et al., 1982; Klugmann et al., 1980).

The magnitude of the decreases in systemic vascular resistance due to nifedipine administration has been inversely correlated with initial values, indicating that basal vascular tone is very important in modulating the response to arterial vasodilatation (Fioretti et al., 1983; Klugmann et al., 1980). Greater decreases in systemic vascular resistance have also been observed in patients with abnormal left ventricular function than in those with normal left ventricular function (Kurnik et al., 1984; Ludbrook et al., 1982).

Nifedipine also reduces left and right ventricular end-diastolic pressures in patients with impaired left ventricular function (Bellocci et al., 1981; Klugmann et al., 1980; Kurnik et al., 1984; Losardo et al., 1982; Majid and De Jong, 1982; Polese et al., 1979; Taggart and Zelis, 1982) but does not alter the filling pressures of those with normal left ventricular function (Kurnik et al., 1984; Ludbrook et al., 1982; Majid and De Jong, 1982; Matsumoto et al., 1980; Naeije et al., 1982). Nifedipine may also effect a striking improvement in the left ventricular ejection fraction and ejection rate both in subjects with normal or with impaired left ventricular function (Kelly et al., 1982; Klugmann et al., 1980; Ludbrook et al., 1982; Weiss et al., 1984). Likewise, cardiac output has increased significantly in patients with impaired left ventricular function but it unchanged in those with normal left ventricular function (Debaisieux et al., 1980; Kurnik et al., 1984; Ludbrook et al., 1982). Thus, the reduction of left ventricular preload by nifedipine is not due to venous pooling but rather to improved left ventricular systolic function in response to afterload reduction, especially in patients with impaired left ventricular function (Kurnik et al., 1984).

Ren et al. (1985) determined the effects of posture on the haemodynamic responses to nifedipine (10mg orally) in 10 patients with congestive heart failure. Compared with values obtained when the patients were in the supine position, nifedipine demonstrated greater afterload-reducing properties when measured in patients in the upright position, as manifested by the additional augmentation of cardiac output and stroke volume index, with a further reduction in systemic vascular resistance.

Pulmonary vascular resistance and mean pulmonary arterial pressures decrease after nifedipine administration, with pulmonary arterial pressures being significantly more affected during exercise than in the resting state and in those patients whose initial pressures are elevated (Hanrath et al., 1982; Kennedy et al., 1984; Magometschnigg, 1983) [table III]. In hypoxaemic patients with pulmonary hypertension secondary to aggravated chronic obstructive pulmonary disease, in stable patients with chronic obstructive pulmonary disease during rest and exercise, and in patients with cor pulmonale from cystic fibrosis, nifedipine has dilated pulmonary vessels (Kennedy et al., 1984; Michael et al., 1984; Simonneau et al., 1981). However, in normal volunteers nifedipine has been unable to abolish hypoxic pulmonary vasoconstriction (Naeije et al., 1982), and Simonneau et al. (1981)

have suggested that nifedipine may not dilate pulmonary vessels when their initial tone is low.

Nifedipine has had no adverse haemodynamic effects in patients with angina pectoris given the drug both at rest and during exercise. A 20mg sublingual dose given to 18 patients with stable angina pectoris significantly decreased systemic vascular resistance, systolic and diastolic blood pressure and mean arterial pressures at rest and exercise without further impairing the cardiac pumping activity in angina patients with severe left ventricular dysfunction (Nelson et al., 1984b). Furthermore, the strong arterial dilating ability of nifedipine has increased cardiac performance in patients with congestive heart failure by reducing the left ventricular afterload while maintaining adequate preload (Elkayam et al., 1984a; Kurnik et al., 1984; Klugmann et al., 1980; Matsumoto et al., 1980).

1.2.4 Haemodynamic Effects of Nifedipine Compared with, and in Combination with, Other Cardiovascular Drugs

Other Calcium Antagonists

The haemodynamic effects of nifedipine have been evaluated in comparison, and in combination, with many cardiovascular drugs. In a comparative study to evaluate the haemodynamic effects of single doses of nifedipine, diltiazem and verapamil in patients with recent myocardial infarctions (fig. 4), the 3 calcium blockers differed in their effects on heart rate and cardiac index. Nifedipine, compared with baseline, significantly increased these parameters while both diltiazem and verapamil either decreased or had no effect on them (Théroux et al., 1980). In further comparisons, Silke et al. (1984) and Chaitman et al. (1984) also found that nifedipine caused an increase in heart rate of 12 to 16% ($p < 0.01$) while verapamil had no statistically significant effect and diltiazem decreased heart rate by 7% ($p < 0.05$). All 3 drugs significantly decreased blood pressure to a similar degree, although the more rapid reduction after nifedipine administration resulted in the reflex increase in heart rate. Similar results were reported by Lehmann and Hochrein (1985). The increase in cardiac output after nifedipine, and the absence of any increase in resting left ventricular stroke volume (as with verapamil) [Lehmann and Hochrein, 1985; Silke et al., 1984] indicates that nifedipine may therefore be valuable in patients with angina pectoris who have a low cardiac output.

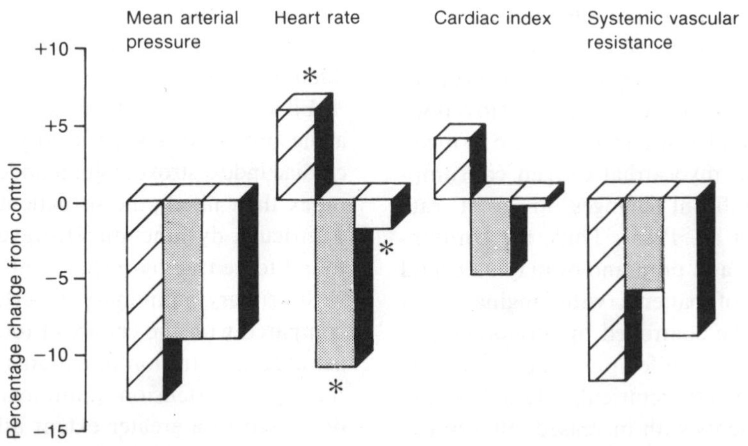

Fig. 4. Comparative haemodynamic effects of single doses of orally administered nifedipine 20mg (▨; n = 12), diltiazem 120mg (▩; n = 12) and verapamil 160mg (□; n = 10) in patients with recent myocardial infarctions. Significantly different from values of the other 2 drugs: * $p < 0.01$ (after Théroux et al., 1980).

β-Blockers

The haemodynamic effects of combined nifedipine and β-adrenoceptor blockade have also been examined in several studies. The additive effects on blood pressure of the combination in volunteers and in patients with angina pectoris and hypertension have resulted in greater blood pressure reductions than those achieved with either drug used separately (Bassan et al., 1982; Ekelund et al., 1982; Esper et al., 1980; Koch, 1980; Landmark et al., 1983; Pfisterer et al., 1982). Esper et al. (1980) found that in volunteers, nifedipine 20mg sublingually, acebutolol 200mg orally and the combination of the two decreased systolic and diastolic arterial pressures by a mean value of 7, 14 and 22% and 8, 14 and 18%, respectively. Reflex increases in heart rate and in plasma renin produced by nifedipine are blocked by the β-adrenoceptor blockers; conversely, increases in total peripheral resistance produced by β-blockade are decreased by nifedipine (Bassan et al., 1982; Choong et al., 1983; Corea et al., 1980; Findlay et al., 1983; Koch, 1980; Landmark et al., 1983; Nelson et al., 1984a; Pfisterer et al., 1982).

In 12 patients with angiographically documented coronary artery disease, intravenous nifedipine 1mg was administered 10 minutes after intravenous propranolol 0.1 mg/kg was given. Compared to results obtained from propranolol alone, the addition of nifedipine produced a transient increase in coronary blood flow and a reduction in coronary vascular resistance and the coronary arteriovenous oxygen difference, and a sustained decrease in mean aortic pressure and myocardial oxygen consumption without significant changes in heart rate (Schanzenbächer et al., 1985). Thus, the combination of nifedipine and propranolol may be useful in the treatment of patients with angina when symptoms cannot be controlled by monotherapy.

The combination of nifedipine and β-blockers may also improve left ventricular function and compliance in patients with increased left ventricular end-diastolic pressures. The combination does not significantly depress left ventricular function (Findlay et al., 1983) and may further decrease left ventricular peak systolic pressures (Landmark et al., 1983). It thus appears that left ventricular haemodynamics are distinctly improved when nifedipine is added to β-blockade, both in patients with normal left ventricular function and in patients with high left ventricular filling pressures (Findlay et al., 1983; Koch, 1980; Landmark et al., 1983; Pfisterer et al., 1982; Rowland et al., 1983; Winniford et al., 1982b) – the negative effects of acute β-blockade on cardiac index, resting ejection fraction and total peripheral resistance are balanced by the vasodilatory actions of nifedipine.

Hydralazine

Nifedipine and hydralazine have produced similar effects on pulmonary artery wedge pressure and right atrial pressure (Elkayam et al., 1984b; Fisher et al., 1984; Olson et al., 1984; Rich et al., 1983). However, nifedipine worsened the haemodynamic status in 4 of 15 patients with congestive heart failure in whom systemic vascular resistance was reduced by less than 25%, whereas hydralazine had no such adverse effects while decreasing systemic vascular resistance by at least 25% in all patients (Elkayam et al., 1984b). This suggests that nifedipine may have clinically important negative inotropic effects in congestive heart failure that are only partially offset by its strong arteriolar dilatory effect. Therefore, hydralazine may be more suitable than nifedipine in patients with severe congestive heart failure when left ventricular afterload reduction is required.

Elkayam et al. (1984b) also found that hydralazine produced a significantly ($p < 0.05$) higher cardiac index, stroke volume index and stroke work index than nifedipine in patients with severe left ventricular dysfunction. However, the reverse was found to be true by Fisher et al. (1984) in patients with primary pulmonary hypertension. Moreover, compared with the changes produced after hydralazine administration in patients with primary pulmonary hypertension, pulmonary artery pressures decreased to a greater extent after nifedipine and the pulmonary artery diastolic to mean pulmonary artery wedge pressure gradient also tended to decrease after nifedipine, suggesting more pulmonary vasodilation from nifedipine (Fisher et al., 1984).

Furthermore, the ratio of pulmonary to systemic vascular resistances was unchanged after nifedipine but increased after hydralazine, indicating a more balanced vasodilatory effect of nifedipine (Fisher et al., 1984; Rich et al., 1983).

Other Drugs

The combination of digoxin or dobutamine with nifedipine has produced greater increases in cardiac index than with either drug alone; however, while left ventricular filling pressures decreased to a greater extent with the combination of nifedipine and digoxin, no further decrease in left ventricular filling pressure was seen when nifedipine was combined with dobutamine both in patients with congestive heart failure and heart failure following myocardial infarction (Bellocci et al., 1984; Cantelli et al., 1983).

In 9 patients with essential hypertension, administration of captopril 25mg orally 3 times daily, nifedipine 10mg orally 3 times daily, or the combination of the 2 drugs for 7 days showed that the combination decreased blood pressure to a greater extent than either drug alone ($p < 0.005$). Heart rate increased after administration of nifedipine, but when nifedipine was combined with captopril no increase in heart rate was observed (Stornello et al., 1983).

Nifedipine has been shown to produce comparable improvements in cardiac performance as nitrates in patients with heart failure secondary to acute myocardial infarction. In an acute study in 13 patients, nifedipine 10mg sublingually was compared with 5mg sublingual isosorbide dinitrate. Isosorbide dinitrate was more effective than nifedipine in decreasing left ventricular filling pressures, right atrial pressures ($p < 0.01$ each) and mean pulmonary arterial pressures ($p < 0.005$), but nifedipine was more effective in increasing cardiac index ($p < 0.02$) and decreasing systemic vascular resistance ($p < 0.01$) [Cantelli et al., 1981]. Similarly, the addition of nifedipine 10mg orally to glyceryl trinitrate (nitroglycerin) ointment (20mg, or 4cm) in 10 patients with acute myocardial infarction significantly decreased systemic vascular resistance (25%; $p < 0.001$) and increased cardiac index (13%; $p < 0.01$) compared with values resulting from glyceryl trinitrate treatment alone (Mori et al., 1982).

Compared with nitroprusside in doses matched to decrease systemic vascular resistance by 27 to 28%, nifedipine produced a significantly greater ($p < 0.05$) hypotensive effect, but lesser beneficial effects on right and left ventricular filling pressures, cardiac output and left ventricular function (Elkayam et al., 1984c). The smaller decreases in blood pressure (8 *vs* 17%) and greater increases in cardiac index (40 *vs* 18%) after nitroprusside suggests that for the acute treatment of severe congestive heart failure, nifedipine may be less satisfactory than nitroprusside (Elkayam et al., 1984c).

1.2.5 Effect on Exercise Tolerance in Patients with Angina Pectoris

In virtually all single-dose or short term studies involving patients with angina pectoris, oral or sublingual administration of nifedipine in doses of 5 to 40mg has significantly increased exercise tolerance and total workload capacity by up to 30 to 88% and up to 112%, respectively (Ardissino et al., 1983; Coronelli et al., 1983; Faris et al., 1980; Gibelli et al., 1983; Grandjean and Valenti, 1978; Romano et al., 1981; Van der Wall et al., 1983; Vuori et al., 1977). Onset of increased exercise tolerance occurred within 1 hour of nifedipine administration and lasted for up to 6 hours (Ardissino et al., 1983).

Nifedipine may also abolish or significantly delay the onset of anginal pain at pacing rates or exercise levels previously associated with angina (Cherchi et al., 1975; Choong et al., 1984; Corbalan et al., 1981; Emanuelsson and Holmberg, 1983; Romano et al., 1981), and may significantly reduce ST segment depression and the time required to reach this depression after both pacing-induced tachycardia and exercise (Ardissino et al., 1983; Brügmann et al., 1982; Cherchi et al., 1975; Choong et al., 1984; Corbalan et al., 1981; Lorell et al., 1981; Romano et al., 1981; Schreiner et al., 1983; Van der Wall et al., 1983). The effects of nifedipine on ST segment depression appear to be dose related, with statistically insignificant reductions seen 5 hours after 10 and 20mg oral doses, but significant ($p < 0.005$) reductions of 20% still present 5 hours after 30mg doses (Brügmann et al., 1982). Intravenous and intracoronary nifedipine, at doses of 1.0mg and 0.1mg, respectively, have significantly reduced ST segment depression at rest and after exercise in patients with angina pectoris (Kaltenbach et al., 1979; Schreiner et al., 1983; Schulz et al., 1978, 1981). The duration of the anti-ischaemic effects after intravenous administration was up to 60 minutes (Kaltenbach et al., 1979).

Interestingly, Schulz et al. (1985) have reported that the antianginal effect of nifedipine is influenced by underlying coronary pathomorphological characteristics. In 36 patients with chronic stable angina pectoris or with stable and vasospastic components of angina pectoris, oral nifedipine 20mg was given. Exercise testing 60 minutes after the nifedipine administration revealed that mean ischaemic ST segment depression was reduced 21% ($p < 0.05$) in the patients with single stenotic coronary arteries, but was not significantly altered in the patients with occluded coronary arteries that had collateralised to varying degrees. The occurrence of angina pectoris paralleled these changes in ST segment depression. Thus, it was suggested that nifedipine may not be effective in providing relief of myocardial ischaemia if occluded but collateralised coronary arteries are present.

Comparisons, and Combinations, with Other Antianginal Drugs

In patients with angina pectoris, nifedipine has been shown to be comparable to verapamil, diltiazem, β-blockers and nitrates in the ability to increase exercise tolerance and reduce electrocardiographic signs of ischaemia due to atrial pacing or exercise (Bassan et al., 1983; Daly et al., 1982; DePonti et al., 1981; Hopf et al., 1983; Pinto et al., 1981; Rizzon et al., 1983; Silke et al., 1984; Tolins et al., 1984; Vuori et al., 1977). Significant increases in exercise time by at least 50% are observed within the first hour after administration of nifedipine, verapamil or isosorbide dinitrate, and persist for up to 6 to 8 hours (Bassan et al., 1983). In patients receiving long term treatment with β-blocking drugs or isosorbide dinitrate, the addition of nifedipine has further significantly prolonged the pacing time to angina, increased the working capacity and reduced the magnitude of ST segment depression (Bassan et al., 1983; Choong et al., 1983; Daly et al., 1982; DePonti et al., 1981; Findlay et al., 1984; Hopf et al., 1983; Pinto et al., 1981; Rizzon et al., 1983; Tolins et al., 1984). However, in 9 of 16 patients with stable angina pectoris, exercise tolerance was reduced by the 3-drug combination of oral nifedipine 20mg, isosorbide dinitrate 20mg and propranolol (≥ 160mg daily), compared with the 2-drug combination of nifedipine and propranolol (Tolins et al., 1984). Thus, although in an individual patient the combination of nifedipine, β-blocker and isosorbide dinitrate may not offer optimal therapy, it appears that the combinations of nifedipine and β-blocker, and nifedipine and isosorbide dinitrate, may provide significant improvements in exercise tolerance and significant reductions in electrocardiographic signs of ischaemia.

In a double-blind, randomised, placebo-controlled study, Chaitman et al. (1984) compared the effects of single doses of sublingual nifedipine 20mg, oral diltiazem 120mg, oral propranolol 80mg and sublingual glyceryl trinitrate 0.6mg on exercise tolerance in 15 patients with stable angina pectoris. Maximal increases in exercise tolerance were most marked at 3 hours after drug administration for nifedipine, diltiazem and propranolol, but were also significant at 1 hour for nifedipine and at 8 hours for diltiazem. Mean exercise time was increased 14% by nifedipine, 31% by diltiazem and 30% by propranolol (all $p < 0.05$). The onset of ST segment depression ≥ 0.1mV was delayed by 189, 203, 120 and 79 seconds (all $p < 0.05$) by nifedipine, diltiazem, propranolol and glyceryl trinitrate, respectively.

Thus, nifedipine may improve exercise performance to an extent comparable to that of other calcium-blocking drugs, nitrates and β-blockers. Additionally, in cases where the use of β-adrenoceptor blocking drugs is contraindicated, the combination of nifedipine and nitrates may provide a valuable therapeutic alternative.

Table IV. Summary of some studies of the effect of nifedipine (N) on coronary circulation and myocardial oxygen consumption (MVO_2) in patients with coronary artery disease

References	No. of patients	Dose (mg) [route]	Patient status	MBF	CVR	$\Delta A\text{-}VO_2$	RPP	MVO_2
Amende et al. (1983)	8	0.1 [IC]	Resting	+31				
Emanuelsson and Holmberg (1983)	14	10 [SL]	Resting	±	−18.8	−15.5		±
			Atrial pacing	±	−18.6	−10.1		±
Engel and Lichtlen (1981)	10	20 [SL]	Resting	+18.4			−21.8	
			Atrial pacing	±				
Gunther et al. (1981)	10	10 [SL]	Resting	±	±	±		±
			Cold pressor test	+27	−10	±		±
Kramer et al. (1984)	11	20 [PO]	Rest	±	−25	−17	±	±
			Subanginal pacing[a]	±	−21	−13	−13	±
			Anginal pacing	±	±	−6	−9	−10
Malacoff et al. (1981)	11	10 [PO]	Cold pressor test	+13.5			±	
Malacoff et al. (1982)	18	10 or 20 [SL]	Resting	+17.4	−14.5		±	
Schanzenbächer et al. (1983)	10	1 [IV]	Resting	+41.9	−43.8		±	±
		0.1 [IC]	Resting	+67.8	−41.3			−19.6
Serruys et al. (1983a)	10	0.15 [IC]	Resting	+50.5	−42.6	−50.4		−27.6
Simonsen and Nitter-Hauge (1978)	8	10 [SL]	Resting	+16	−18	±		±
			Atrial pacing	±	±	±		±
Stone et al. (1983a)	12	20 [SL]	Resting	±	±	−11.6		±
			Atrial pacing	±	±	−9		±

a Supraventricular pacing at a rate 50% higher than resting heart rate.

Abbreviations: MBF = myocardial blood flow; CVR = coronary vascular resistance; Δ A-VO_2 = arterial-coronary sinus oxygen difference; RPP = rate-pressure product; IC = intracoronary; SL = sublingual; PO = oral; IV = intravenous. All values reported are in percentages and are reported as statistically significant changes from pre-N values; ± = no statistically significant changes from pre-N values.

1.3 Effect on Coronary Circulation and Myocardial Oxygen Consumption

Intravenous and intracoronary administration of nifedipine may increase coronary sinus oxygen saturation and coronary artery diameter in normal and post-stenotic segments (Kober et al., 1979; Schulz et al., 1981, 1983; Serruys et al., 1980). The dilation of large epicardial coronary arteries after intracoronary nifedipine is prolonged and suggests that nifedipine predominantly results in a sustained relaxation of the epicardial conductance vessels, while intramural arterioles are only transiently dilated (Schanzenbächer et al., 1983; Schulz et al., 1981).

Many studies have shown that administration of nifedipine to patients with coronary artery disease results in increases in coronary blood flow (table IV). The greatest increases appear to occur following intracoronary administration, followed by intravenous, sublingual and oral administration, in that order. Using thermodilution or xenon-washout techniques, nifedipine has increased coronary flow to myocardial tissue served both by normal and stenotic coronaries (Engel and Lichtlen, 1981; Lichtlen et al., 1979a,b; Serruys et al., 1983a). Relative to baseline, percentage increases in coronary flow to myocardial tissue served by stenotic coronaries were greater than those in tissues served by normal coronaries. As these increases occurred both under conditions of rest and continuous atrial pacing, a more uniform distribution of perfusion throughout the heart at higher levels of activity was observed (Engel and Lichtlen, 1981; Lichtlen et al., 1979a,b; Serruys et al., 1983a). In fact, improvements in myocardial perfusion have occurred after nifedipine administration: exercise-induced perfusion defects as detected by thallium-201 perfusion scintigraphy have been significantly reduced after nifedipine administration (Lichtlen et al., 1979a,b; Zacca et al., 1982).

The improvement in coronary blood flow after nifedipine administration in patients with coronary artery disease is due to a dilation of coronary resistance vessels and is often associated with decreases in coronary vascular resistance (table IV). Decreases in coronary vascular resistance in patients with coronary artery disease of up to 44, 43 and 18% have resulted from intravenous, intracoronary and sublingual nifedipine administration, respectively (Emanuelsson and Holmberg, 1983; Gunther et al., 1981; Malacoff et al., 1981, 1982; Serruys et al., 1983a; Simonsen and Nitter-Hauge, 1978). However, nifedipine decreased coronary blood flow and increased coronary vascular resistance in patients with *normal* coronary arteries, leading Malacoff et al. (1982) to suggest that the beneficial effect of nifedipine on coronary blood flow in patients with coronary artery disease may be related to a decrease in resting coronary vascular tone.

Nifedipine has had little effect on coronary sinus flow or myocardial oxygen consumption either at rest, during rapid atrial pacing or during cold pressor tests; however, a decrease in myocardial oxygen extraction indicated coronary vasodilatation (Amende et al., 1980; De Ponti et al., 1979; Moskowitz et al., 1979; Mueller and Chahine, 1981; Stone et al., 1980a; Zacca et al., 1982) [table IV]. Since the protective effects of nifedipine under these conditions have been unaccompanied by significant changes in myocardial oxygen consumption in most cases, nifedipine thus appears to exert selective vasodilation on the coronary vasculature (Gunther et al., 1981; Simonsen and Nitter-Hauge, 1978).

Decreases in myocardial oxygen consumption have, however, been seen after the intracoronary injection of nifedipine 0.1mg (Schanzenbächer et al., 1983; Serruys et al., 1983a). These decreases may result from a direct negative inotropic effect of nifedipine, since it has been shown that the intracoronary injection of nifedipine 0.1mg does not induce systemic haemodynamic changes (Kaltenbach et al., 1979).

Thus, the overall effects of nifedipine are consistent with a mild coronary vasodilatory action, reduced coronary arteriolar resistance and increased myocardial blood flow, usually without a significant reduction in myocardial oxygen consumption (Hugenholtz et al., 1981) [table IV].

Nifedipine also reverses vasoconstriction induced by ergonovine (Gunther et al., 1981; Tiefenbrunn et al., 1981). This and the ability of nifedipine to attenuate the coronary haemodynamic alterations induced by other provocative measures such as the cold pressor test may provide a rational basis for the use of nifedipine in vasospastic ischaemic myocardial syndromes (Singh and Phil, 1982).

1.4 Cardioprotective Effect

Myocardial ischaemia and subsequent reperfusion may lead to an accumulation of excess cytosolic calcium and result in inhibition of adenosine triphosphate (ATP) production by the mitochondria. In turn, this depression of ATP synthesis can eventually affect the sodium and calcium pumps and ultimately cause additional calcium accumulation in the cytoplasm and mitochondria, thus further decreasing the ATP-generating capacity of the mitochondria (Frey et al., 1980; Shen and Jennings, 1972). Increased intracellular calcium appears to be partly responsible for ischaemic myocardial cell death (Katz and Reuter, 1979), with the net result of this process being an irreversible loss of mechanical and electrical activity within the cells of the ischaemic myocardium. Inhibition of the inward transport of calcium by means of calcium antagonism may therefore prevent mitochondrial calcium overload and consequently preserve the structure and function of myocardial cells while protecting against the deleterious effects of hypoxia and ischaemia (Braunwald, 1982; Fleckenstein et al., 1983; Henry, 1980; Nayler, 1980, 1983; Nayler and Grinwald, 1981; Nayler et al., 1980; Stone et al., 1980b; Winniford et al., 1982c).

There have been few studies investigating the cardioprotective effect of nifedipine in man. However, nifedipine may protect the myocardium during reperfusion after cardiac surgery in humans. During postischaemic reperfusion, nifedipine (0.2 to 0.9mg, given by the intracoronary route by direct injection or as part of a cardioplegic solution) decreased lactic acid accumulation and prevented both the entry of calcium and significant decreases in ATP or creatine phosphate concentrations in myocardial tissue (Elert, 1983; Serruys et al., 1983b).

The total incidence of acute low cardiac output death in cardiac surgery patients treated with cardioplegic solution has ranged between 4 and 10% in patients treated by nifedipine and between 11 and 18% in those not so treated. Postoperative evidence of left ventricular injury in these same groups as assessed by ^{99}technetium pyrophosphate scans has ranged from 0 to 20% and 15 to 29%, respectively (Clark and Magovern, 1983; Clark et al., 1981, 1983, 1985a). Nifedipine-treated patients also had significantly ($p < 0.05$) greater postoperative cardiac and stroke work indices than the untreated group (Clark and Magovern, 1983; Clark et al., 1981, 1983). However, the total benefit or lack thereof of continuation of nifedipine in the postoperative phase is unknown (Clark et al., 1985b).

Although many animal studies have shown that nifedipine augments collateral flow into the ischaemic myocardium after coronary occlusion and decreases infarct size while preserving ventricular function (Clark et al., 1979; Hattori et al., 1980; Henry, 1979a; Maroko, 1980; Millard et al., 1982; Nayler and Grinwald, 1981; Perez et al., 1979; Schmier et al., 1976; Selwyn et al., 1979), there are conflicting data regarding the effect of nifedipine in limiting the extent of ischaemic injury after acute myocardial infarction in humans. In 32 such patients, with and without congestive heart failure, nifedipine 10mg sublingually given later than 48 hours after the onset of symptoms reduced ST segment elevations by an average of 66%. In the subgroup of patients with congestive heart failure ($n = 10$), ST segment elevations were decreased by 90% (Hayashi et al., 1984). However, Sirnes et al. (1984) and the Norwegian Nifedipine Group found that early (less than 12 hours after suspected myocardial infarction) and continued nifedipine treatment had no influence on the infarct size (assessed by myocardial band isoenzyme levels) in 227 patients with suspected myocardial infarctions.

It is likely that other mechanisms may contribute to the cardioprotective effect of nifedipine. Other possible mechanisms may include inhibition of calcium-dependent platelet aggregation and release reactions *in vitro* and *ex vivo* (section 1.7), the effect of nifedipine on coronary haemodynamics and myocardial oxygen supply (section 1.3), and the ability of nifedipine to retard and/or prevent the onset of arrhythmias associated with ischaemia (Parratt and Coker, 1983).

1.5 Effect on Peripheral Vascular Circulation

Although it is thought that nifedipine increases the distensibility of peripheral veins in muscle and skin (Linhart, 1981), significant venous pooling in the periphery does not occur (Lederballe Pedersen and Mikkelsen, 1978; Mostbeck et al., 1976; Robinson et al., 1980). In healthy volunteers or patients with hypertension or cardiac disease, nifedipine has been shown to increase blood flow and decrease vascular resistance in peripheral vascular areas (table V). Sublingual or oral administration of nifedipine 10 to 20mg in man has resulted in increases in forearm blood flow and decreases in

Table V. Results of some single-dose studies reporting the maximal effects of nifedipine (N) on peripheral vascular circulation as determined by venous occlusion plethysmography or ^{133}xenon clearance

References	No. of pts (diagnosis)	N dose (mg) [route]	Results		
			FBF	FVR	BF
Forearm blood flow and vascular resistance					
Ferguson and Dorsey (1985)	14 (vol)	20 [SL] or 30 [PO]	+46*	±	
Kurnik et al. (1984)	21 (cp)	20 SL	+25.8***	−31.4***	
Lederballe Pedersen et al. (1980b)	11 (vol)	10 or 20 [SL]		−17.2[a]	
Lederballe Pedersen and Mikkelsen (1978)	17 (hyp)	10 or 20 [SL]	+20*	−35***	
McLeay et al. (1983)	9 (hyp)	10 [PO][b]	+19*	−30**	
Robinson et al. (1980)	5 (vol) 6 (vol)	10 [SL] 0.4-6.4 μg/min [IA]	+75* +220[a]		
Cerebral circulation					
Angelino et al. (1975)[c]	20 (5 vol + 15 cp)	1 [IV]			±
Lydtin et al. (1975a)	7 (vol)	15 μg/kg [IV]			±
Skin blood flow					
Mostbeck et al. (1975b)	15 (vol)	20 [SL]			+87***
Lower limb flow					
Lydtin et al. (1975a)	5 (vol)	15 μg/kg [IV]			+150[a]
Lydtin et al. (1975b)	5 (vol)	20 [SL]			+100[a]
Mostbeck et al. (1975b)	15 (vol) 15 (vol)	20 [SL] 20 [SL]			+67* +111***

a Level of significance not reported.
b N given thrice daily for 4 months.
c Heart-to-brain mean circulating time assessed.
d Blood flow to feet.

Abbreviations: FBF = forearm blood flow; FVR = forearm vascular resistance; BF = blood flow to area being studied; hyp = patients with essential hypertension; vol = healthy volunteers; cp = cardiac patients; SL = sublingual; PO = oral; IA = intra-arterial infusion; IV = intravenous injection. All values reported are in percentages and are reported as statistically significant changes from baseline parameters; ± = no significant change from baseline values; * = $p < 0.05$; ** = $p < 0.01$; *** = $p < 0.005$.

forearm vascular resistance of 19 to 75% and 17 to 35%, respectively (Kurnik et al., 1984; Lederballe Pedersen et al., 1980a; Lederballe Pedersen and Mikkelsen, 1978; McLeay et al., 1983; Robinson et al., 1980). The vasodilating effect of nifedipine has tended to be stronger in hypertensive than in normotensive individuals (Lederballe Pedersen et al., 1980b). While both cerebral and fingertip blood flow have been shown to increase marginally though non-significantly, fingertip vascular resistance has decreased significantly ($p < 0.05$) [Angelino et al., 1975; Creager et al., 1984; Lydtin et al., 1975a]. However, it has been shown that *in vivo*, nifedipine does exert a preferential action on cerebral vessels, vasodilating large arteries and arterioles (Payen et al., 1984). This action appears to be more powerful if the vessels are already vasoconstricted.

Blood flow to the skin and lower limbs has been shown to increase by 67 to 111% after sublingual administration of nifedipine 20mg, and 150% after intravenous injection of 15 μg/kg (Lydtin et al., 1975a, 1975b; Mostbeck et al., 1975b), while the oral administration of 0.2 mg/kg to 8 patients with congestive heart failure produced increases in limb blood flow of 15% (Leier et al., 1984). However, in patients with peripheral arterial insufficiency, neither blood flow nor local peripheral resistance in the calf and forefoot was shown to change significantly after the administration of sublingual nifedipine 10mg (Lorentsen and Landmark, 1983).

In isolated human mesenteric arteries and veins, nifedipine has been shown to produce a concentration-dependent and long-lasting relaxation of noradrenaline (norepinephrine)-induced contractions (Mikkelsen et al., 1979). In addition, *in vitro* nifedipine has been shown to be ineffective in reversing constrictions in forearm resistance vessels induced by noradrenaline but effective in reversing constrictions induced by potassium (Robinson et al., 1980).

1.6 Effect on Non-Vascular Smooth Muscle

1.6.1 Gastrointestinal Tract

The role of extracellular and intracellular calcium in smooth muscle contraction has recently been reviewed (Forman, 1984). *In vitro* studies have shown that both acetylcholine-induced and electrically induced contractions of human colonic muscle are comparably, but only partially, antagonised by nifedipine, prompting Zar and Gooptu (1983) to suggest that nifedipine acts directly on the smooth muscle. Antman et al. (1980b) postulated that the inhibitory effect of nifedipine on transmembrane calcium flux, which is responsible for electromechanical coupling in smooth muscle, determines the spasmolytic effect of nifedipine on the oesophagus.

The effect of nifedipine in decreasing lower oesophageal sphincter pressure may be due to blockage of the calcium transmembrane influx, which determines the lower oesophageal sphincter tone (Fox and Daniel, 1978). In healthy volunteers and patients with achalasia, diffuse oesophageal spasm and 'nutcracker oesophagus', nifedipine significantly decreases lower oesophageal sphincter pressures (by 18 to 56%) as well as the amplitude (5 to 59%) and duration (16 to 33%) of peristaltic spasms (Blackwell et al., 1981; Bortolotti and Labò, 1981; Danielides et al., 1984; Gelfond et al., 1982; Hongo et al., 1984a,b; Nasrallah et al., 1985; Richter et al., 1984; Traube et al., 1984). In patients with diffuse oesophageal spasm, the amplitude and frequency of non-peristaltic contractions were also significantly reduced ($p < 0.05$) by 39 and 59%, respectively (Blackwell et al., 1979). Blackwell et al. (1981) have suggested that the reduction in lower oesophageal sphincter pressure in patients with spasms may be proportionately smaller than in normal subjects, but this has yet to be substantiated. Hongo et al. (1984a) noted that the effect of nifedipine on sphincter pressure required a lower dose and was more marked than that on contraction amplitude.

1.6.2 Urinary and Uterine Smooth Muscle

Nifedipine has been shown to inhibit both spontaneous and drug-induced ($PGF_{2\alpha}$ oxytocin, vasopressin and potassium) contractile activity in isolated human pregnant myometrium at midterm, term and in the immediate postpartum period, and uterine activity in menstruating, pregnant, postpartum and dysmenorrhagic females (Andersson and Ulmsten, 1978; Andersson et al., 1979; Forman et al., 1979, 1982a,b; Maigaard et al., 1983; Sandahl et al., 1979; Ulmsten et al., 1978, 1980).

Nifedipine has also been shown to inhibit the contractile responses to potassium and barium chloride in the isolated human bladder and ureter, but not to have any effect on bladder or urethral tone *in vivo* (Forman et al., 1978). However, nifedipine reduced the frequency and amplitude of uninhibited detrusor contractions in women with urge incontinence, and also increased bladder capacity (Rud et al., 1979).

1.7 Effect on Platelets

Platelets are involved in the genesis and expression of coronary heart disease in several ways. Firstly, platelets release specific mitogenic proteins that may induce the smooth muscle cell intimal hyperplasia that is commonly seen in arteriosclerosis (Burns and Frishman, 1983). Secondly, transient or permanent coronary occlusion with subsequent myocardial ischaemia or infarction may result from platelet tendencies to adhere and aggregate (Haerem, 1974). And thirdly, platelets produce vasoactive amines and prostaglandin endoperoxides, such as serotonin and thromboxane A_2, during aggregation that can stimulate coronary vasospasm and result in ischaemia (Ellis et al., 1976; Lewy et al., 1980).

Calcium in turn is essential for many platelet functions. Baumgartner (1979) showed that removal of calcium ions by high concentrations of sodium citrate or ethylenediaminetetraacetic acid (EDTA) reduced platelet membrane adhesion by 80% and inhibited platelet spreading and release. Each step in the normal physiological function of platelets is dependent on either extracellular calcium (aggregation), or calcium mobilisation from intracellular storage sites (shape change, thromboxane synthesis and granule release) [Burns and Frishman, 1983; Han and Ardlie, 1974; Holmsen and Day, 1971]. Therefore, if nifedipine inhibits the transport of calcium across the platelet membrane, it may influence platelet reactivity.

Adenosine diphosphate (ADP)-induced primary platelet aggregation has been shown to be inhibited both *in vitro* and *in vivo* by nifedipine (Dale et al., 1983; Han et al., 1983; Hiroki et al., 1982; Johnsson, 1981; Kiyomoto et al., 1983; Latta et al., 1983; Ono and Kimura, 1981; Takahara et al., 1985). Dale et al. (1983) found that after nifedipine administration mean maximal rates of *in vivo* primary platelet aggregation were reduced by 26, 23 and 20% when initiated by ADP in concentrations of 0.7, 1.7 and 3.5 μmol/L, respectively (fig. 5). However, Johnsson (1981) found that, *in vitro*, nifedipine concentrations of 8 to 16 mg/L inhibited ADP-induced primary aggregation, while concentrations *in vivo* as low as 1.5 mg/L were enough to inhibit this aggregation.

In vitro, nifedipine concentrations of less than 4 mg/L had no effect on either adrenaline- or arachidonic acid-induced platelet aggregation; however, concentrations greater than 8 mg/L produced inhibition (Johnsson, 1981). Other investigators have also found nifedipine to inhibit platelet aggregation induced by adrenaline (Addonizio et al., 1980; Latta et al., 1983; Ono and Kimura, 1981; Takahara et al., 1985), arachidonic acid (Davì et al., 1982; Han et al., 1983; Latta et al., 1983) and thrombin (Davì et al., 1982) in a concentration-dependent manner.

Collagen-induced secondary platelet aggregation is also inhibited by nifedipine (Ono and Kimura, 1981; Takahara et al., 1985). Dale et al. (1983) found that a single 20mg oral dose of nifedipine given to 20 patients with coronary heart disease reduced collagen-induced aggregation by 23% (fig. 5), while Johnsson (1981) found that *in vitro* and *in vivo* nifedipine concentrations of 8 to 16 and 1.5 mg/L, respectively, were capable of inhibiting this aggregation.

Although neither platelet count nor adhesiveness were significantly affected by nifedipine *in vivo*, bleeding time was shown to increase by 12%, or 36 seconds, by Dale et al. (1983) [fig. 5]. This effect on bleeding time, however, was not observed by Burns and Frishman (1983).

The effect of nifedipine in reducing platelet aggregation implies that nifedipine inhibits the transport of calcium across the platelet cell membrane, as aggregation is dependent on extracellular calcium but adhesion is not (Holmsen and Day, 1971). However, in contrast to the effect of aspirin on platelets (Mielke, 1981), the inhibitory effect of nifedipine on platelet aggregation is reversible and thus dependent on nifedipine concentrations in the plasma (Johnsson, 1981). Furthermore, the discovery that nifedipine inhibits *in vivo* thromboxane synthesis induced by thrombin, but not by arachidonic acid, implies that nifedipine does not affect platelet cyclo-oxygenase but rather exerts its action by interfering with arachidonic acid release from platelet membrane phospholipids (Davì et al., 1982).

Nifedipine has also been found to potentiate the inhibitory actions of propranolol on platelets (Han et al., 1983). It is possible that this synergistic effect may contribute to the therapeutic efficacy of this combination in stable angina (section 3.1.2) [Ekelund and Orö, 1979; Itoh et al., 1975; Kenmure and Scruton, 1976].

The inhibitory effect of nifedipine on platelet function may therefore serve to potentiate the effect of the drug on the clinical manifestations of coronary heart disease by preventing platelet clumping, thromboxane release and therefore thromboxane-induced coronary artery spasm.

1.8 Effect on Blood Glucose Concentrations and Insulin Release

Animal studies have shown that nifedipine inhibits calcium net uptake and glucose-induced insulin release in pancreatic islets without affecting glucose oxidation and calcium efflux (Malaisse and Boschero, 1977; Malaisse and Sener, 1981). These findings are compatible with the idea that nifedipine inhibits calcium entry into the pancreatic B cells (Malaisse and Boschero, 1977; Malaisse and Sener, 1981).

Several investigators (Bhatnager et al., 1984; Charles et al., 1981; Ferlito et al., 1981; Giugliano et al., 1980; Petralito et al., 1979; Sando et al., 1983) have reported that the short term (less than 1 month) effects of nifedipine on carbohydrate metabolism and insulin secretion in subjects with or without cardiovascular disease and normal or decreased glucose tolerance have shown it to be potentially diabetogenic. While insulin concentrations have seemed to demonstrate a tendency to decrease after nifedipine administration, associated with delays in the response and resynthesis of insulin (Charles et al., 1981; Ferlito et al., 1981), glucose-induced glucagon suppression also appears to be inhibited (Ferlito et al., 1981).

Nifedipine may also decrease glucose tolerance

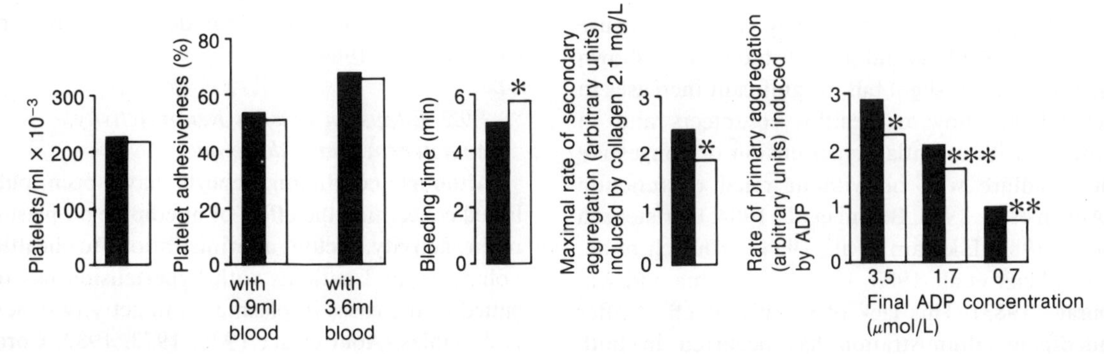

Fig. 5. Platelet counts, adhesiveness, maximal rate of primary and secondary platelet aggregation induced with ADP and collagen, and bleeding time in 20 patients with coronary heart disease before (■) and 1 hour after (□) a single oral dose of nifedipine 20mg. Significantly different from pre-nifedipine values: * $p \leq 0.02$; ** $p < 0.01$; *** $p < 0.002$ (after Dale et al., 1983).

by increasing the release of catecholamines secondary to vasodilation-induced activation of the sympathetic nervous system (Ebner et al., 1983; Greenwood, 1982; Koch, 1977). It is also possible that the changes in circulating insulin concentrations observed after nifedipine treatment may be the consequence of regional changes in splanchnic blood flow and distribution (Giugliano et al., 1980).

In contrast, many other single-dose, short term and long term (i.e. greater than 1 month) studies using nifedipine in standard recommended doses have shown it to have no significant effect on glucose tolerance in healthy volunteers and in those with impaired glucose tolerance or diabetes (Abadie and Passa, 1984; Andersen et al., 1982; Bonetti et al., 1979; Brauman et al., 1984; Dean and Kendall, 1983; Deedwania et al., 1984; Delahaye et al., 1979; Donnelly and Harrower, 1980; Ebner, 1977; Greenwood, 1982; Hausmann, 1983; Joffe et al., 1983; Kanatsuna et al., 1985; Lacchè et al., 1981; Murphy et al., 1983b; Nicita-Mauro et al., 1980; Raffestin et al., 1984; Ravens, 1981; Ueda et al., 1978; Vessby et al., 1983). Thus, it is probably more accurate to conclude that nifedipine has no true diabetogenic potential.

1.9 Renal Effects

1.9.1 Effect on Renal Blood Flow, Renovascular Resistance and Glomerular Filtration Rate

Nifedipine has been shown to rarely cause marked renal effects and several studies have shown that it produces slight but insignificant increases in renal blood flow in healthy volunteers and in patients with essential hypertension or congestive heart failure with or without renal dysfunction (Austin et al., 1983; Bellini et al., 1984; Christensen et al., 1982; Elkayam et al., 1984d; Klütsch et al., 1972; Leier et al., 1983, 1984; Yokoyama and Kaburagi, 1983). This lack of significant effect after nifedipine administration has occurred in both healthy subjects and hypertensive patients on regular and on sodium-restricted diets (Bellini et al., 1984).

Since several studies seem to indicate that renal blood flow is virtually unchanged in hypertensives and normotensives after nifedipine administration, decreases in blood pressure in hypertensives are associated with significant reductions in renal vascular resistance. This is in contrast to the effect on renal vascular resistance seen in normotensives and can be explained by an exaggerated effect of nifedipine on the vascular smooth muscle of hypertensives (Ishii et al., 1980; Lederballe Pedersen et al., 1978; Yokoyama and Kaburagi, 1983). Renal vascular resistance is also reduced in patients with congestive heart failure given nifedipine (Leier et al., 1983).

There are conflicting data regarding the effect of nifedipine on glomerular filtration rate. Glomerular filtration rate in healthy volunteers and in those with heart failure has been shown to be little affected by nifedipine administration (Austin et al., 1983; Bellini et al., 1984; Elkayam et al., 1984d; Yokoyama and Kaburagi, 1983). However, in patients with uncomplicated severe hypertension treated for 5 weeks with nifedipine alone or in combination with methyldopa, or in patients with essential hypertension and in patients with glomerulonephritis and hypertension, nifedipine has increased glomerular filtration rate by 11, 46, and 12.5%, respectively (Guazzi et al., 1980; Yokoyama and Kaburagi, 1983). In contrast, in another study in hypertensive patients both on regular and low sodium diets, glomerular filtration rate was significantly ($p < 0.01$ and $p < 0.001$, respectively) reduced after an oral 10mg dose of nifedipine (Bellini et al., 1984).

1.9.2 Effects on Plasma Renin Activity, Angiotensin and Aldosterone

Although conflicting reports have been published concerning the effect of nifedipine on plasma renin activity, acute administration to healthy volunteers and patients with hypertension has resulted in increases in plasma renin activity in several studies (Aoki et al., 1976, 1978, 1982; Corea et al., 1979, 1980; Ekelund et al., 1982; Hiramatsu et al., 1982; Kiowski et al., 1983; Lederballe Pedersen et al., 1979; Leonetti et al., 1982; Resnick et al., 1982; Streifler et al., 1983). The increases in plasma renin activity appear to be directly related to sodium intake and basal plasma renin activity and inversely related to the age of the patient (Bellini et al., 1984; Hiramatsu et al., 1982; Lederballe Pedersen et al., 1979). Administration of β-blocking drugs such as metoprolol has been shown to reverse increases in plasma renin activity induced by nifedipine alone (Corea et al., 1980; Ekelund et al., 1982).

It is thought that increases in plasma renin activity due to nifedipine may be partly related to increases in sympathetic discharge (Bellini et al., 1984). However, no correlation was found between the haemodynamic and neurohumoral changes produced by nifedipine in 15 patients with congestive heart failure, where increased plasma renin concentrations after nifedipine administration did not correlate with increases in sympathetic discharge (Elkayam et al., 1985). Consistent with this, long term administration of nifedipine for 3 to 6 weeks did not produce uniform changes in renin activity, with both increases and decreases having been reported (Corea et al., 1980; Kiowski et al., 1983; Lederballe Pedersen et al., 1979). Thibonnier et al. (1980) were unable to demonstrate an alteration of plasma renin activity after short term nifedipine administration, while Olivari et al. (1979) also reported no changes in plasma renin activity after 3 weeks of drug administration.

This discrepancy in the effect of nifedipine on plasma renin activity during acute and long term treatment may be explained by a diminishing sympathetic tone after repeated administration of the drug (Lederballe Pedersen et al., 1979). Since the reductions in blood pressure due to nifedipine are of the same magnitude during both acute and chronic treatment, blood pressure variations are thus not responsible for the varying plasma renin activity results. This concept is supported by the fact that β-adrenoceptor blockade abolishes the rise in plasma renin activity after acute nifedipine administration (Corea et al., 1980).

Increases in plasma renin activity reported with the use of nifedipine have not been paralleled by changes in plasma aldosterone concentrations (Bellini et al., 1984; Hiramatsu et al., 1982; Lederballe Pedersen et al., 1979; Millar and Reid, 1983; Resnick et al., 1982; Streifler et al., 1983). While aldosterone concentrations have not been significantly affected by nifedipine administration, angiotensin II concentrations have been shown to increase, particularly in younger normotensive or hypertensive individuals (Hiramatsu et al., 1982). Therefore, similar to the relationship of nifedipine-induced increases in plasma renin activity, increases in angiotensin II concentrations appear to be directly related to basal angiotensin II concentrations and inversely related to age (Hiramatsu et al., 1982).

The failure of aldosterone concentrations to increase after nifedipine administration, despite increasing concentrations of angiotensin II, is an unexpected finding. However, since calcium is required for aldosterone secretion from the adrenal cortex (Fakunding et al., 1979), a possible explanation to account for this finding is that the effect of angiotensin II on aldosterone secretion is inhibited by nifedipine through its calcium antagonising action (Hiramatsu et al., 1982; Millar and Reid, 1983).

1.9.3 Other Renal Effects

Diuretic and natriuretic effects after the acute administration of nifedipine in healthy volunteers and patients with hypertension have been reported by several investigators (Christensen et al., 1982; Ene et al., 1984, 1985; Klütsch et al., 1972; Leonetti et al., 1982; Valdés et al., 1982, 1983; Yokoyama and Kaburagi, 1983). The changes in urinary volume and renal sodium excretion have been of greater magnitude in patients with essential hypertension than in those with glomerulonephritis with hypertension or in healthy volunteers (Yokoyama and Kaburagi, 1983).

Increases in the urinary excretion of potassium of 35 and 17%, respectively, have been reported in patients with essential hypertension and glomerulonephritis with hypertension given nifedipine (Yokoyama and Kaburagi, 1983).

Nifedipine also produced significant ($p \leq 0.01$) uricosuria in patients with moderate hypertension treated with β-blockers (Christensen et al., 1982).

The uricosuric effect appears to be directly related to the basal level of renal vascular resistance – the larger the nifedipine-induced fall in renal vascular resistance, the larger the increase in urate excretion (Christensen et al., 1982).

1.10 Other Effects

1.10.1 Effects on Hepatic Blood Flow

Although animal studies seem to indicate that nifedipine decreases hepatic blood flow as its blood concentration increases (Hamann et al., 1984), nifedipine seems to increase hepatic blood flow in humans, though the extent remains unresolved. In the study by Mostbeck et al. (1975a), 15 healthy volunteers were given sublingual nifedipine 20mg. Liver blood flow was assessed by the disappearance rate of intravenously injected colloidal ^{198}Au. It was found that while the average liver blood flow increased, the change was not statistically significant. However, Feely (1984) showed that nifedipine 10mg sublingually significantly ($p < 0.05$) increased apparent liver blood flow estimated by the indocyanine green method in 6 healthy volunteers. There was also a positive correlation between the decrease in arterial blood pressure and the percentage increases in liver blood flow. The author suggested that the increase in liver blood flow was due to arterial vasodilatation produced by nifedipine (Feely, 1984). Additionally, in patients with congestive heart failure, oral nifedipine increased hepatic blood flow and decreased hepatic vascular resistance by 9 to 11% and 19%, respectively (Leier et al., 1983, 1984).

1.10.2 Effects on the Sympathetic Nervous System

In vivo studies performed in rats and dogs have shown that nifedipine is devoid of β-adrenergic stimulant properties but interferes with the excitation of vascular α_2- but not α_1-adrenoceptors (Kroneberg, 1975b; Lappe et al., 1984; Saeed et al., 1983; Timmermans et al., 1983a,b,c; Van Meel et al., 1981, 1983a,b; van Zwieten et al., 1983). However, in a study utilising 6 healthy volunteers to determine whether nifedipine administration produced α-adrenoceptor antagonism in man, Murphy et al. (1984) reported that the pressor response to selective α_1- and α_2-agonists (methoxamine and α-methylnoradrenaline, respectively), and to angiotensin II were similar. Therefore, nifedipine is not thought to possess selective α-adrenoceptor antagonist activity in man.

Nifedipine has been shown to increase the concentration of plasma catecholamines after both short and long term administration (Corea et al., 1979b, 1981a, 1984; Kleinbloesem et al., 1984a; Lederballe Pedersen et al., 1979; Leonetti et al., 1982; Murphy et al., 1982; Olivari et al., 1984; Saris et al., 1984; Stein et al., 1984), with acute responses thought to occur as a result of a baroreceptor-mediated reflex increase in sympathetic activity (Corea et al., 1979b; Lederballe Pedersen et al., 1979; Leonetti et al., 1982). However, long term therapy (3 to 6 weeks) has resulted in smaller increases or significant decreases in plasma noradrenaline concentrations (Corea et al., 1979b, 1984; Lederballe Pedersen et al., 1979), possibly reflecting either diminished reflex sympathetic activity because of a resetting of the baroreceptors or an inhibitory effect of nifedipine on prejunctional noradrenaline release (Kiowski et al., 1983; Lederballe Pedersen et al., 1979).

Since the haemodynamic changes (section 1.2) produced by nifedipine occur in spite of increased plasma catecholamine concentrations, it may be inferred that they are not associated with a reduction of sympathetic activity (Emanuelsson et al., 1984b).

1.10.3 Effects on Histamine Release and Airway Conductance

The role of calcium in airway functions has been recently reviewed (Russi and Ahmed, 1984). Thus, contraction of bronchial smooth muscle and release of chemical mediators such as histamine and slow-reacting substance of anaphylaxis (SRS-A) result from the influx of calcium ions across cell membranes from the extracellular to the intracellular compartment of the mast cells and basophils (Foreman et al., 1977; Kirkpatrick, 1975; Middleton, 1980). *In vitro*, nifedipine has been shown to inhibit anaphylaxis in airway smooth muscles (Weiss and Markowicz, 1981) and also to prevent release of platelet-activating factor and SRS-A from human neutrophils (Cerrina et al., 1981b). Consequently, Bedard and Busse (1983, 1984), Jensen et al. (1983) and Norn et al. (1983) showed that basophil histamine release was inhibited by nifedipine both *in vivo* and *in vitro*. Drazen et al. (1983) performed *in vitro* studies on histamine-induced contractions of human trachealis muscle and found that nifedipine caused an approximate 10-fold increase in the histamine concentration required to produce 40% of the maximal constriction, while others showed that nifedipine provided a significant protective effect against histamine-induced bronchoconstriction in both normal and asthmatic patients (Malik et al., 1982; Williams et al., 1981). However, nifedipine has not consistently improved histamine reactivity in asthmatic patients (Patel and Al-Shamma, 1982).

Although nifedipine has been shown to inhibit airway smooth muscle constriction induced by cholinergic agents both *in vitro* and *in vivo* in man (Baronti et al., 1984; Gonzales et al., 1983; Henderson et al., 1983; Horio et al., 1984; Kneussl et al., 1983; Malik et al., 1982), nifedipine has not demonstrated bronchodilator effects of its own in most studies (Barnes et al., 1981; Cerrina et al., 1981a; Corris et al., 1983; Fanta et al., 1982; Gonzales et al., 1983; Henderson et al., 1983; Patel, 1981c; Svedmyr et al., 1984; Williams et al., 1981). These findings, however, were not supported by Patakas et al. (1983), who demonstrated a bronchodilator effect of nifedipine in the large airways only in patients with chronic asthma. Similarly, Ikeda et al. (1985) reported that nifedipine dilated the bronchial and tracheal smooth muscle in healthy volunteers and in patients with chronic obstructive lung disease. Nevertheless, nifedipine may prolong the bronchodilator action of salbutamol in patients with asthma (Lever et al., 1984).

Contradictory findings have also been reported regarding the effect of nifedipine on antigen-induced bronchoconstriction in asthmatic patients. Henderson et al. (1983) and Koppermann and Kaukel (1984) reported that nifedipine significantly reduced antigen-induced bronchoconstriction, while So et al. (1982) found that nifedipine failed to protect against allergen-induced asthma. Interestingly, in healthy volunteers, nifedipine and diltiazem were shown to inhibit ethanol-induced bronchoconstriction, while verapamil and flunarizine had no effect (Lombardi et al., 1985). Nifedipine has also been shown to exert a protective effect in exercise-induced asthma (Barnes et al., 1981; Cerrina et al., 1981a; Crimi et al., 1984; Koppermann and Kaukel, 1984; Patel, 1981b). However, controversy still exists as to whether nifedipine exerts its effects on bronchial muscle contractility rather than by stabilising mast cells (Barnes et al., 1981; Henderson et al., 1983; Kneussl et al., 1983; Patel, 1981a,b; Patel and Al-Shamma, 1982).

Nair et al. (1984) studied the effect of nifedipine 20mg sublingually on forced vital capacity, forced expiratory volume in 1 second (FEV_1) and forced expiratory flow at 25 to 75% of total volume in 60 subjects, including normal individuals and those with asthma, chronic obstructive pulmonary disease and angina. After 2 weeks of treatment, not only was there no adverse effect on the pulmonary function, but FEV_1 was significantly ($p < 0.05$) improved after nifedipine.

The salutary effects of nifedipine on ventilatory function in cardiac patients with concomitant chronic airway obstruction may thus be of significance in patients intolerant of β-blocking agents (Gonzales et al., 1983; Löfdahl et al., 1984; Lombardi et al., 1985; Jaiprakash et al., 1980; Patakas et al., 1983; Williams et al., 1981).

1.11 Mechanism of Action

Although the precise mechanism of action of nifedipine and other calcium channel blocking agents used in the treatment of angina pectoris, hypertension and other cardiovascular disorders is still unclear (Flaim et al., 1982), all calcium antagonists share the common mechanism of action of competitively blocking the cell membrane slow channels, resulting in a decreased influx of calcium into the cell during the active state (Fleckenstein et al., 1972).

Much has been written on the cellular and subcellular mechanism of action of calcium antagonists (Andersson and Högestätt, 1984; Antman et al., 1980b; Braunwald, 1982; Flaim et al., 1982; Fleckenstein, 1977; Fleckenstein et al., 1972; Henry, 1979b; Katz et al., 1984; Mannhold, 1984; Rahwan, 1983; Silver et al., 1984; Stone et al., 1980b). Thus, the concentration of myoplasmic calcium may be increased 3 ways: the slow inward current of calcium, the sodium-calcium exchange across the sarcolemma, and calcium release from the sarcoplasmic reticulum. The proteins actin and myosin slide across each other in an adenosine triphosphate-dependent mechanism that is inhibited by the regulatory proteins tropomyosin and troponin in myocardial cells, and calmodulin in smooth muscle cells. Increases in intracellular calcium in myocardial cells and smooth muscle cells permit the binding of calcium to troponin and calmodulin, respectively. In myocardial cells this results in an inhibition of the effect of troponin, which allows muscular contraction to occur. In smooth muscle cells, the calcium-calmodulin complex activates myosin kinase which phosphorylates the light chain of myosin and therefore allows myosin to interact with actin, thereby leading to contraction. The inhibition of calcium influx by nifedipine results in electromechanical decoupling, which effects an inhibition of contraction and permits relaxation of the cardiac or smooth muscle fibres. Therefore, calcium inhibition leads to negative inotropy of heart muscle and vasodilatation of the blood vessels (fig. 6).

In the treatment of angina pectoris, the efficacy of nifedipine is probably dependent upon its general abilities to increase myocardial oxygen supply and decrease myocardial oxygen demand (Théroux et al., 1983). Indeed, nifedipine may increase oxygen supply to the myocardium by relieving and preventing coronary artery spasm, decreasing coronary artery tone, decreasing coronary vascular resistance and causing a redistribution of regional blood flow to ischaemic areas (sections 1.3, 1.4 and table IV), which are all dependent, at least in part, on relaxation of coronary artery smooth muscle.

Factors which may cause a decrease in myocardial oxygen demand include vasodilatation, reduced blood pressure and afterload, a slowing of the heart rate and negative inotropy (Théroux et al., 1983). Although in humans nifedipine has neither a negative inotropic effect nor decreases the heart rate (sections 1.2.2 and 1.2.3), myocardial oxygen consumption, as measured by the rate-pressure product, is not significantly changed (section 1.3). This is due to the high degree of systemic vasodilatation that occurs after nifedipine administration which is manifested as decreases in mean arterial pressure and systemic vascular resistance (sections 1.2.1 and 1.2.3; fig. 6). Reduction of left ventricular afterload due to systemic vasodilatation usually reduces myocardial oxygen consumption providing blood pressure does not decrease to a level at which coronary perfusion is impaired (Scheidt, 1982).

Other possible modes of action of nifedipine in improving symptoms of ischaemic heart disease may include improved filterability and increased deformability of red blood cells (Cristal et al., 1982; Waller et al., 1984a) and the prevention of platelet clumping, thromboxane release and thromboxane-induced coronary artery spasm (section 1.7).

Inhibition of *in vivo* platelet activation has also been postulated as the mechanism of action of nifedipine in effecting subjective clinical improvement in patients with Raynaud's phenomenon (Malamet et al., 1985).

Inasmuch as it has been suggested that elevated intracellular free calcium concentration is an important factor for the maintenance of elevated blood pressure (Erne et al., 1984), it is not surprising that nifedipine has been used successfully in the treatment of hypertension (section 4). Thus, a direct relationship between decreases in intracellular free calcium concentrations and blood pressure has been observed after the administration of nifedipine in hypertensive patients (Erne et al., 1984). However, it is the decrease in peripheral arterial vascular tone and subsequent decrease in systemic vascular resistance due to inhibition of intracellular calcium influx that is directly responsible for the decrease in blood pressure seen after nifedipine administration (sections 1.2.1 and 1.2.3). The decrease in

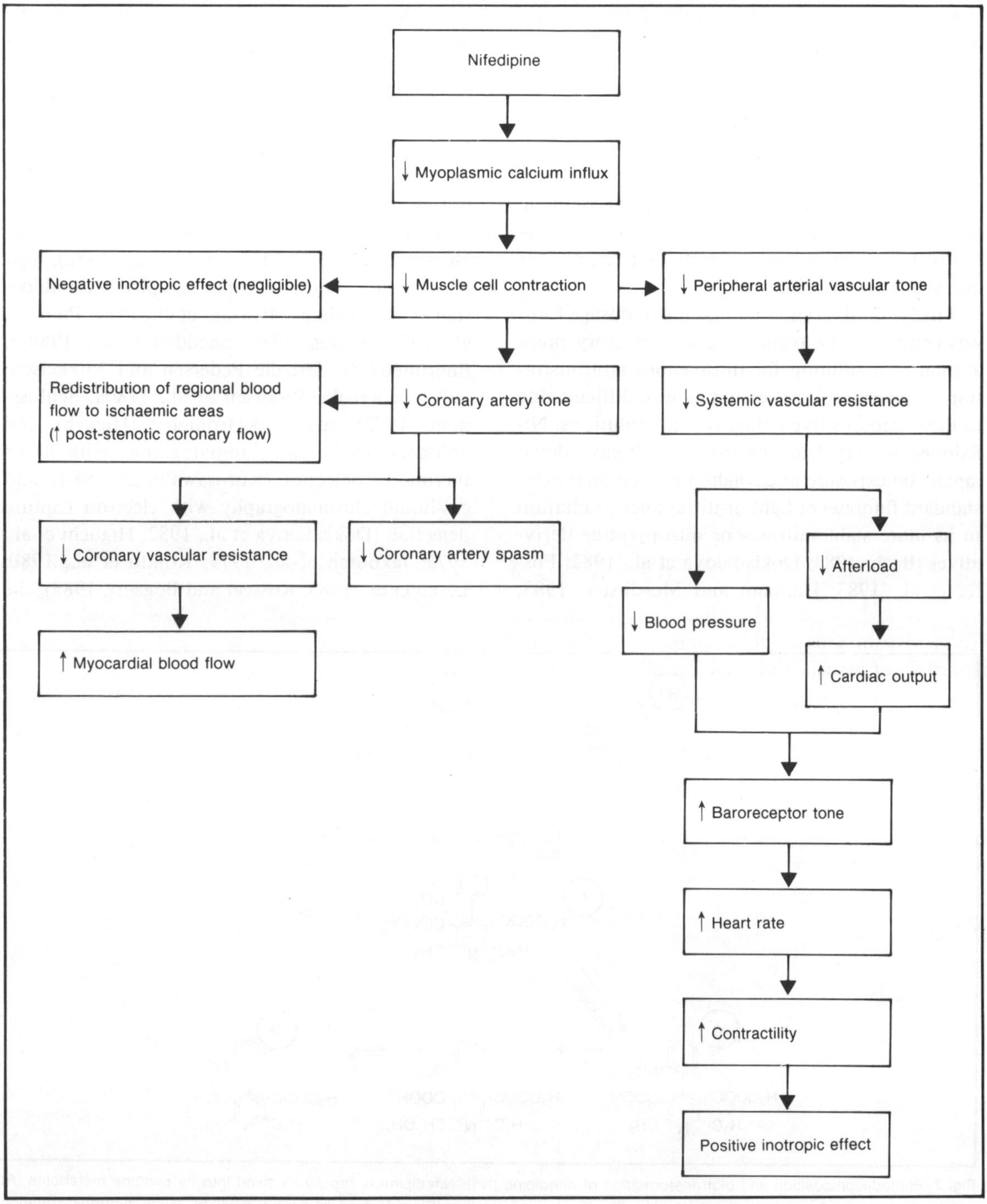

Fig. 6. Effect of nifedipine on the myocardium and the coronary and peripheral arterial systems; ↑ = increase; ↓ = decrease (after Lichtlen et al., 1984).

blood pressure produced by nifedipine is independent of adrenergic- or angiotensin-mediated systems (Murphy et al., 1984; section 1.10.2).

2. Pharmacokinetic Properties

Few well designed studies have been performed that adequately describe the pharmacokinetic properties of nifedipine. The paucity of information detailing the kinetic aspects of nifedipine is due primarily to 2 factors.

Firstly, until recently no parenteral dosage form was commercially available, and laboratory preparation of a solution for intravenous administration in pharmacokinetic studies was difficult due to the photosensitive nature of such solutions. Nifedipine is very light-sensitive and breaks down rapidly on exposure to daylight, tungsten-bulb light, standard fluorescent light or ultraviolet irradiation to its more stable nitroso- or nitropyridine derivatives (Bach, 1983; Dokladalova et al., 1982; Foster et al., 1983; Hamann and McAllister, 1983; Kleinbloesem et al., 1984b) [fig. 7]. Nifedipine is, however, stable when 'gold' fluorescent light is used (Hamann and McAllister, 1983).

Secondly, there have been problems in developing a sufficiently sensitive and specific method for the analysis of nifedipine plasma concentrations after therapeutic doses. Although the concentration of nifedipine in body fluids has been determined by radioisotope (Duhm et al., 1972; Horster et al., 1972; Medenwald et al., 1972), high performance liquid chromatography (Kleinbloesem et al., 1984a,b; Miyazaki et al., 1984; Pietta et al., 1981; Santos, 1980; Snedden et al., 1984a), fluorimetry (Lederballe Pedersen and Mikkelsen, 1978; Lederballe Pedersen et al., 1980a; Schlossman, 1972), mass spectrometry (Higuchi and Shiobara, 1978), gas chromatography with flame thermionic detection (Kurosawa et al., 1984), and gas-liquid chromatography with electron capture detection (Dokladalova et al., 1982; Higuchi et al., 1975; Jakobsen et al., 1979; Kondo et al., 1980; Lesko et al., 1983; Rosseel and Bogaert, 1983), the

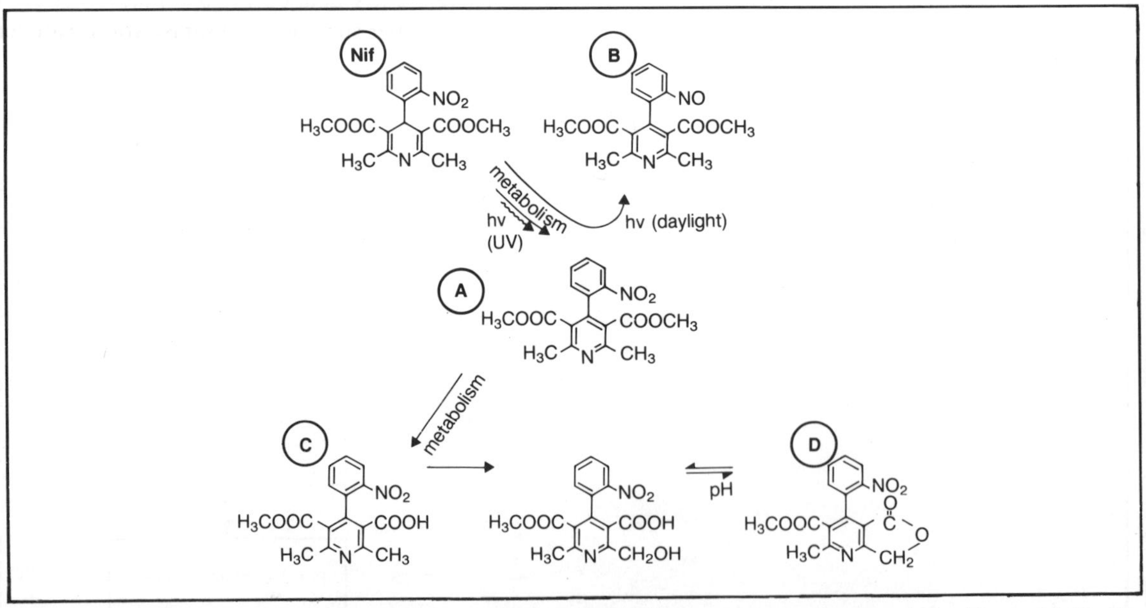

Fig. 7. Photodecomposition and biotransformation of nifedipine (Nif). Nifedipine is rapidly oxidised into its pyridine metabolite (A), which may also be formed in ultraviolet light. The 2-nitrosoderivative (B) is formed in normal daylight. Upon biotransformation, hydrolysis to an hydroxy carboxylic acid (C) and further oxidation to a methoxy carboxylic acid (D) derivative occurs (after Kleinbloesem et al., 1984b).

various discrepancies reported for nifedipine pharmacokinetic parameters may originate in part from the inefficiency of some of these assay techniques in distinguishing parent drug from its inactive metabolites and photodegradation products. Metabolites of nifedipine have been measured by thin layer and gas-liquid chromatography and ion-pair high performance liquid chromatography (Kleinbloesem et al., 1984b; Raemsch and Sommer, 1983).

Published pharmacokinetic studies of nifedipine to date have included normal volunteers, patients with hypertension and angina pectoris, and patients with chronic renal failure or on dialysis. Although most studies have been single-dose in nature and have investigated the kinetics of nifedipine from oral capsules and tablets, sublingual capsules and after intravenous and rectal administration (Aoki et al., 1982; Banzet et al., 1983; Bogaert et al., 1984; Foster et al., 1983; Kleinbloesem et al., 1984a,b,c; Nakashima et al., 1984; Ochs et al., 1984; Raemsch and Sommer, 1983; Spital and Scandling, 1983; Taburet et al., 1983), nifedipine kinetics have also been studied after repeated oral dosing (Raemsch and Sommer, 1983).

2.1 Absorption

Although nifedipine is absorbed over the whole length of the gastrointestinal tract, close to 100% of an oral dose is absorbed largely in the small intestine (Raemsch and Sommer, 1983; unpublished data on file, Bayer AG). However, there has been considerable variation among subjects in the manner and extent to which nifedipine is absorbed (table VI). The differences in measured plasma concentrations among subjects may be attributed to the rate of drug absorption and/or variability in the extent of first-pass hepatic extraction and metabolism (Foster et al., 1983; Jakobsen et al., 1979; Kleinbloesem et al., 1984a; McAllister, 1982; Nakashima et al., 1984; Snedden et al., 1984a, b; Stern et al., 1984). The specificity of the particular assay used in the studies may also contribute to the wide discrepancy in plasma concentrations obtained (see above).

Nifedipine plasma concentrations have been studied after oral administration in tablets and capsules, sublingual administration in capsules, and intravenous administration (fig. 8). Oral capsules produce peak plasma concentrations in 0.5 to 2.2 hours and are 45 to 68% bioavailable (Foster et al., 1983; Kleinbloesem et al., 1984a; Nakashima et al., 1984; Raemsch and Sommer, 1983). While some investigators have indicated that nifedipine is up to 90% absorbed after a single oral dose (Horster, 1975; Kleinbloesem et al., 1984a; McAllister, 1982), it has been theorised that substantial first-pass metabolism is responsible for the lower bioavailability of the drug (Kleinbloesem et al., 1984a; McAllister, 1982). However, no significant changes in absorption rate or saturation of presystemic metabolism occurred at doses between 5 and 20mg in fasted volunteers (Raemsch and Sommer, 1983). Additionally, the area under the plasma concentration-time curve (AUC) for nifedipine capsules increased proportionally to the dose administered, and its kinetics were linear in the 20 to 60mg dose range (Banzet et al., 1983; Raemsch and Sommer, 1983; Taburet et al., 1983).

There are few data on the pharmacokinetics of nifedipine after sublingual administration. Horster (1975) noted that only 10 minutes after administration of radiolabelled nifedipine to hospitalised patients, radioactivity was measured in the plasma. Peak plasma concentrations have occurred between 30 and 120 minutes after sublingual administration (Jakobsen et al., 1979; Raemsch and Sommer, 1983; Snedden et al., 1984a).

The rate of absorption from both oral and sublingual capsules varies widely among individuals. Several investigators have described 'fast' and 'slow' absorbers of nifedipine depending on the time required to reach maximum plasma concentrations, which has ranged from 30 minutes to 1 hour in the 'fast' group and from 2 to 4 hours in the 'slow' group (Foster et al., 1983; Jakobsen et al., 1979; Nakashima et al., 1984; Snedden et al., 1984b). Similarly, Kleinbloesem et al. (1984d) identified 'rapid metabolisers' as the principal phenotype describing the polymorphism that exists regarding the disposition kinetics of nifedipine, with AUCs < 500 $\mu g/L \cdot h$ and higher urinary excretions (25 to 70%)

Table VI. Summary of some pharmacokinetic values reported for nifedipine (healthy volunteers in all studies, except essential hypertension in the study by Banzet et al., 1983)

References	No. of subjects	Study design	Dose (mg)	C_{max} (μg/L)	T_{max} (h)	Vd (L/kg)	CL (L/h)	$t_{1/2}$ (h)	AUC (μg/L · h)	F	Assay method
Oral administration (tablet)											
Banzet et al. (1983)	8	r, db, co, sd	20	62.6	1.63		33.2	10.8	537		GLC-ED
			40	109.3	2.13		33.7	10.2	1170		
			60	170.1	1.75		34.8	9.7	1682		
Kleinbloesem et al. (1984a)	6	r, co, sd	20	25.9	4.2			11.1		0.52	HPLC
Ochs et al. (1984)	10	r, sd, db, co	40	44.6	2.7			5.9			GLC-ED
Oral administration (capsule)											
Foster et al. (1983)	12	r, co, sd	10	73.5[a]	0.57[a]	1.32[b]	36.9[b]	3.4	125	0.45[c]	GLC-ED
Kleinbloesem et al. (1984a)	6	r, co, sd	20	117	1.4			2		0.56	HPLC
Nakashima et al. (1984)	8	sd	10	100.6	2.17				704		GLC-ED
Raemsch and Sommer (1983)	5	sd, co	5							0.61	GLC-ED
			10							0.61	
			20							0.68	
	10	sd, co	10	153	0.5						GLC-ED
Sublingual administration (capsule)											
Raemsch and Sommer (1983)	10	sd, co	10	97.5	1.0						GLC-ED
Intravenous administration											
Foster et al. (1983)	12	r, co, sd	1	26	0.08	1.12[a]	46.7[a]	1.8[a]	26.4[a]		GLC-ED
Hamann and McAllister (1983)	12	sd	1	≈18.9			43.4[d]	1.8			GLC-ED
Kleinbloesem et al. (1984a)	6	r, co, sd	1			0.8	27	1.7			HPLC

Kleinbloesem et al. (1984b)	5	sd	4.5		0.78	33	1.76		HPLC
Raemsch and Sommer (1983)	7	sd	1	≈41	0.62	31.5[e]	1.26	36.04	GLC-ED
Rectal administration (infusion)									
Kleinbloesem et al. (1984c)	6	r, co	1.5 mg/h × 24h	21[f]		66	2		HPLC

a Results from 9 subjects.
b Results from 11 subjects.
c Results from 8 subjects.
d 10.3 ml/min/kg extrapolated to 70kg individuals.
e 7.5 ml/min/kg extrapolated to 70kg individuals.
f Mean steady-state concentration.

Abbreviations: C_{max} = maximum plasma concentration; T_{max} = time to reach maximum plasma concentration; Vd = volume of distribution; CL = clearance; $t_{1/2}$ = elimination half-life; AUC = area under the plasma concentration/time curve; F = mean systemic bioavailability; r = random; db = double-blind; co = crossover; sd = single dose; GLC-ED = gas-liquid chromatography with electron capture; HPLC = high performance liquid chromatography.

of the hydroxy carboxylic derivative (see section 2.3). Nakashima et al. (1984) have suggested that in 'fast' and 'slow' absorbers nifedipine is absorbed in the stomach and small intestine, respectively. Additionally, it has been reported that biting and swallowing the nifedipine *capsule* will achieve higher plasma concentrations more rapidly than standard oral or sublingual administration (Love et al., 1985).

Study of the pharmacokinetics of a single dose level of nifedipine capsules (10mg thrice daily) for 7 days has shown that, at this dose level, there is no cumulative effect or other changes in its pharmacokinetic behaviour (Raemsch and Sommer, 1983). Definitive studies of longer term nifedipine dosing and the linearity of its kinetics at other dose levels have yet to be done.

The absorption of nifedipine from oral tablets is delayed (t_{max} 1.6 to 4.2 hours) compared with that from capsules (t_{max} 0.5 to 2.17 hours), but the bioavailability of 52% (Kleinbloesem et al., 1984a) is similar to that for the capsule form. The plasma concentration-time curve produced after administration of nifedipine tablets is much flatter and longer than that after ingestion of capsules, with peak plasma concentrations being lower and half-life longer after tablet administration (table VI; fig. 8; section 2.3.1). The absorption of drug is slower than its elimination when nifedipine is given in tablet form. 24 to 32 hours after tablet administration, nifedipine may still be in the process of being absorbed, which may occur due to its precipitation in the intestinal mucosa (Kleinbloesem et al., 1984a; Raemsch and Sommer, 1983). Coingestion of food delays the peak serum concentration and may decrease or have no effect on the AUC of orally administered nifedipine tablets (Hirasawa et al., 1985; Ochs et al., 1984; Reitberg et al., 1985). Smoking has also been reported to lower nifedipine blood concentrations, though these decreases were not significant (Deanfield et al., 1984).

Studies of nifedipine kinetics after intravenous administration have revealed that a 1mg dose produces a maximum plasma concentration of 19 to 41 μg/L (Foster et al., 1983; Hamann and Mc-

Allister, 1983; Kleinbloesem et al., 1984a; Raemsch and Sommer, 1983). Foster et al. (1983) reported peak plasma concentrations after intravenous administration occurring 5 minutes after the end of the infusion; they postulated that this might have been due to a 'mixing time' phenomenon, which may have resulted from the inherent vasodilating actions of nifedipine causing venous pooling.

Rapid and complete absorption has also been reported following rectal infusions and rectal administration of suppositories containing nifedipine 10mg (Kleinbloesem et al., 1984c; Raemsch and Sommer, 1983).

2.2 Distribution

When administered to rats in doses of 0.03 to 3 mg/kg intravenously or orally, distribution patterns of nifedipine did not vary significantly between the intravenous and oral treatments after 1 hour. While liver, serum, kidneys and lungs contained higher concentrations of nifedipine, lower concentrations were found in the brain, skeletal muscle and testes (Duhm et al., 1972). In the blood of rats, nifedipine activity was mainly found in the serum, with concentrations 3 to 5 times higher than those in the erythrocytes (Duhm et al., 1972).

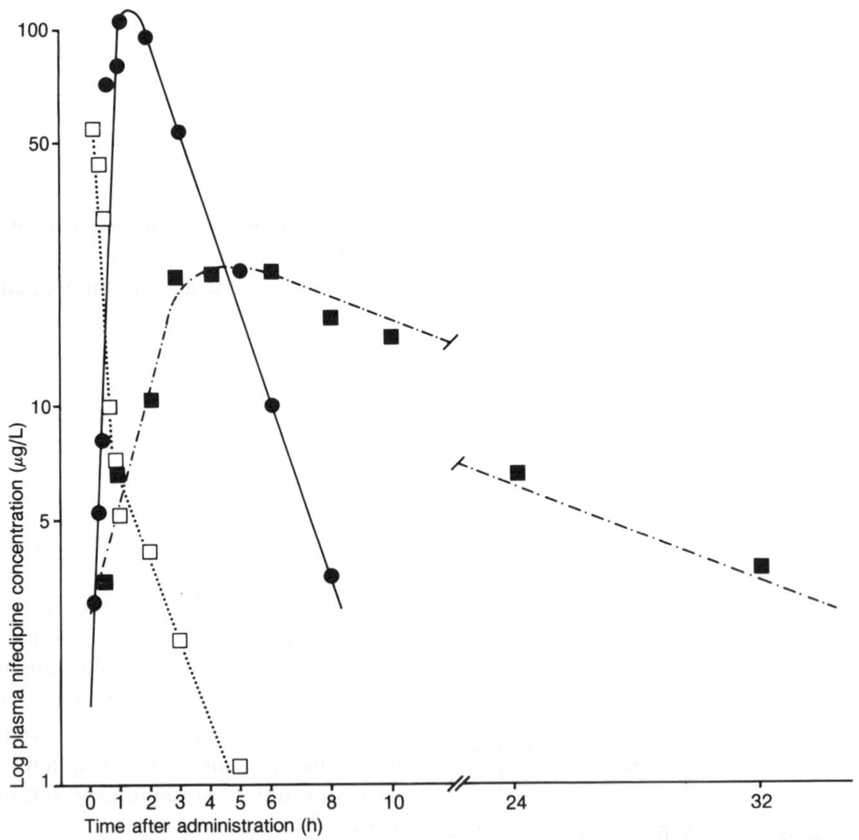

Fig. 8. Log plasma concentrations of nifedipine in a fasted healthy volunteer after oral administration of 20mg in capsules [2 × 10mg (●)], a 20mg tablet (■), and after intravenous administration of nifedipine 0.015 mg/kg bodyweight (□) [after Kleinbloesem et al., 1984a].

Rapid average distribution phase half-lives of 0.09 and 0.17 hours have been seen after the intravenous administration of nifedipine 1 and 4.5mg respectively, in human volunteers (Kleinbloesem et al., 1984a,b).

The steady-state volume of distribution of nifedipine in man after oral administration has been investigated in only 1 study and was found to be 1.32 L/kg (Foster et al., 1983). Estimations of the volume of distribution at steady-state after intravenous administration of nifedipine have ranged from 0.62 to 1.12 L/kg (Foster et al., 1983; Kleinbloesem et al., 1984a,b; Raemsch and Sommer, 1983). In the study by Kleinbloesem et al. (1984a), the steady-state volume of distribution was noted to be 0.8 L/kg, whereas the volume of the central or plasma compartment was only 0.25 L/kg. Since nifedipine is very highly bound to plasma proteins to the extent of 92 to 98% (Rosenkranz et al., 1974; Schlossman et al., 1975), this would appear to indicate that nifedipine undergoes extensive tissue distribution in man.

In man, nifedipine protein binding to albumin has been found to be dependent on the drug concentration. Schlossman et al. (1975) found that nifedipine protein binding in human serum increased from 92% to 98% as the total nifedipine concentration decreased from 20 to 0.2 mg/L.

The extensive binding of nifedipine to albumin is thought to contribute to the long duration of action of the drug (Schlossman et al., 1975). However, the main metabolite of nifedipine (section 2.3) is bound to a lesser extent than the parent compound, 54% being bound to human serum proteins (Rosenkrantz et al., 1974; Schlossman et al., 1975).

2.3 Metabolism

Animal studies have shown that nifedipine metabolism appears to involve hepatic enzyme systems other than the cytochrome P-450 monooxygenase (s), as phenobarbitone (phenobarbital) and SKF-525A neither induced nor inhibited nifedipine metabolism, respectively, in rats (Hamann et al., 1985).

Radiolabelled nifedipine has been found to undergo hepatic oxidation to 3 pharmacologically inactive metabolites which are excreted in the urine (Kroneberg and Krebs, 1980) [fig. 7]. Two of these metabolites, an hydroxy carboxylic acid derivative and a methoxy carboxylic acid derivative, contain 95% of the total detectable urinary radioactivity. Thus, this amount of nifedipine undergoes biotransformation; only traces of unchanged parent drug are excreted in the urine (Kondo et al., 1980; Kroneberg, 1975a; Raemsch and Sommer, 1983). In most cases, after a single dose of nifedipine more of the hydroxy than methoxy cardboxylic acid derivative is present in the plasma (Raemsch and Sommer, 1983). However, Waller et al. (1984b) found that the nitropyridine analogue of nifedipine, which is also formed from nifedipine by a photochemical reaction under ultraviolet light, shows a marked presence in the plasma after nifedipine is given orally, but is present only in trace amounts after intravenous administration in humans. Peak plasma concentrations and AUCs in the same study suggested that this nitropyridine analogue was a major first-pass metabolite of nifedipine.

Following enteric absorption of nifedipine, some drug (30 to 40%, if 100% absorption is assumed) is eliminated metabolically during the first pass through the liver and does not enter the systemic circulation (Raemsch and Sommer, 1983).

2.3.1 Half-Life

Although the elimination half-life of nifedipine is apparently dependent upon the dosage form in which it is administered (table VI), the prolonged half-life after oral tablets are administered may reflect more the absorption half-life than the elimination half-life of the drug (Taburet et al., 1983).

The elimination half-life of nifedipine after administration of oral tablets has been found to vary between 6 and 11 hours, which is about 2 to 3 times longer than previously reported after the administration of oral capsules (Banzet et al., 1983; Foster et al., 1983; Horster et al., 1972; Kleinbloesem et al., 1984a; Ochs et al., 1984; Taburet et al., 1983).

Elimination half-lives after intravenous administration and rectal infusions range from 1.3 to 2 hours, and are shorter than those reported after oral capsules (Foster et al., 1983; Hamann and McAllister, 1983; Kleinbloesem et al., 1984a,b,c; Raemsch and Sommer, 1983).

2.3.2 Elimination

After enteral and intravenous administration of radioactively labelled nifedipine, 70 to 80% of activity (in the form of highly water-soluble metabolites) is eliminated in the urine and 90% of this amount is eliminated after 24 hours (Horster et al., 1975; Raemsch and Sommer, 1983). The remainder is excreted in the faeces also in metabolised form (Raemsch and Sommer, 1983). Unchanged nifedipine is excreted in the urine in trace amounts approximating 0.1% of the total dose (Kondo et al., 1980; Kleinbloesem et al., 1984a).

The total systemic clearance (intravenous) of nifedipine from plasma ranges from 27 to about 66 L/h, while its intrinsic clearance (oral) ranges from 33 to 37 L/h (table VI). Kleinbloesem et al. (1984a,b) found the clearance of nifedipine after oral and intravenous administration in volunteers to be 27 to 33 L/h and suggested that the rate of nifedipine elimination depended on drug metabolising enzyme activity as well as on hepatic blood flow.

2.4 Effect of Disease on Pharmacokinetics

Nifedipine plasma concentrations in patients with severe renal dysfunction have been found to be slightly greater than those measured in normal subjects (Bogaert et al., 1984). However, this difference was not found to be significant, as AUCs 0 to 9 hours after oral administration of a single nifedipine 10mg capsule were 133 and 107 mg/kg • h in the renal patients and normal volunteers, respectively (Bogaert et al., 1984).

Pharmacokinetics of nifedipine were not significantly affected by either haemodialysis or continuous ambulatory peritoneal dialysis (Bogaert et al., 1984; Singlas et al., 1984; Spital and Scandling, 1983). The lack of a significant effect of dialysis on the plasma concentration-time curve of nifedipine is thought to be due in part to the high protein binding and high lipophilicity of the drug (section 2.2) [Bogaert et al., 1984].

As less than 2% of nifedipine is removed by peritoneal dialysis, no dosage modifications are necessary in patients undergoing this type of procedure (Singlas et al., 1984; Spital and Scandling, 1983).

2.5 Relationship of Plasma Concentration and Clinical Effects

It has been difficult to ascertain whether there is a relationship between nifedipine plasma concentrations and pharmacodynamic effects. Problems in making this sort of correlation with nifedipine have resulted from: a lack of hysteresis analyses and individual correlations; failure to investigate non-linear correlations; varying intervals between blood samplings and haemodynamic measurements; differing assay specificities and sensitivities (section 2); differences in administration methods, preparations and duration of treatment; and differing individual sensitivities to the drug. Although therapeutic serum concentrations of nifedipine are not known, several studies have intimated that plasma nifedipine concentrations may correlate significantly with changes in blood pressure, heart rate and other haemodynamic parameters known to be influenced by nifedipine (Aoki et al., 1982; Banzet et al., 1983; Gutierrez et al., 1984; Hirasawa et al., 1985; Kleinbloesem et al., 1984a; Taburet et al., 1983; Traube et al., 1985) [fig. 9]. Decreases in lower oesophageal sphincter pressure and in amplitude of contractions have also correlated well with plasma nifedipine concentrations (Hongo et al., 1984a). Kleinbloesem et al. (1984a) found that a minimal effective plasma nifedipine concentration of about 15 μg/L was required to produce the increases in heart rate and decreases of blood pressure seen with the drug. However, a relationship between nifedipine plasma concentrations and clinical effects has not been supported in other investigations (Lederballe Pedersen et al., 1979, 1980a; Reves et al., 1983).

The effect of nifedipine in improving exercise tolerance and decreasing the frequency and occurrence of ischaemic attacks in patients with angina pectoris has been shown to be related to plasma drug concentrations (Chaitman et al., 1984; Stern et al., 1984); 3 hours after administration of sublingual nifedipine 20mg to 15 patients with chronic stable angina pectoris, an increase in exercise time of more than 2 minutes was observed in all of the 7 patients with plasma nifedipine concentrations greater than 90 μg/L (Chaitman et al., 1984). In addition, side effects due to nifedipine may also be related to high peak plasma concentrations of the drug (Zylber-Katz et al., 1984a).

It has been suggested that since individual sensitivities to nifedipine clinical effects may vary markedly, routine plasma concentration measurements would not be advantageous; in these situations, involving either hypertensive patients or those with angina pectoris, it would therefore be necessary to titrate the nifedipine dose to the desired clinical effect (Pasanisi and Reid, 1983; Reves et al., 1983; Stern et al., 1984).

3. Therapeutic Use in Ischaemic Heart Disease

Ischaemic heart disease encompasses a wide spectrum of disorders which range in severity from mild forms of classic exercise-induced angina pectoris, variant angina and mixed angina, to serious unstable angina which may be prodromal to myocardial infarction. At present the indications are that the majority of ischaemic episodes result from

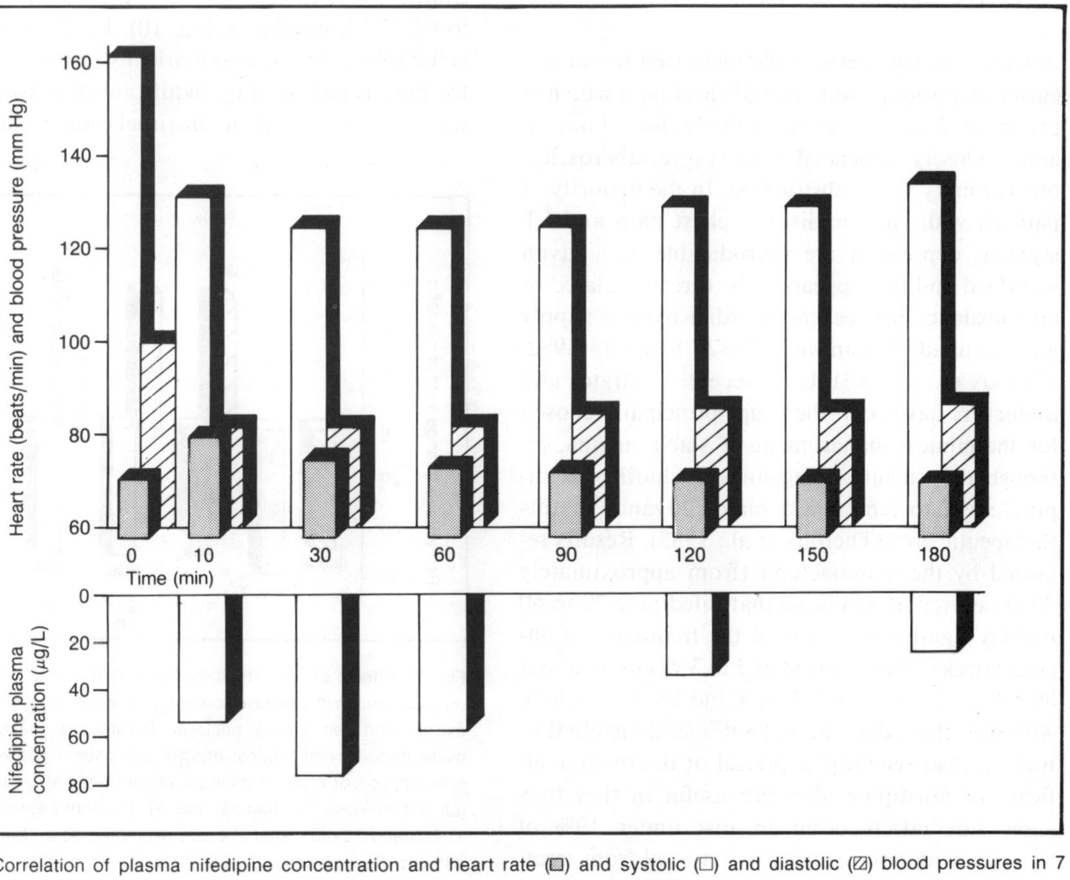

Fig. 9. Correlation of plasma nifedipine concentration and heart rate (▩) and systolic (□) and diastolic (▨) blood pressures in 7 patients with essential hypertension given nifedipine 5mg orally (after Aoki et al., 1982).

an imbalance between myocardial oxygen supply and demand. This imbalance can be directly related either to some degree of coronary artery atherosclerosis, which is characteristically insidious in onset and diffuse (but not necessarily uniformly spread), and/or to an alteration in coronary artery tone, which most seriously results in arterial spasm. Nifedipine has been used to treat patients suffering from all different forms of ischaemic heart disease, including those pre- and postinfarction, and in most instances (stable angina, variant angina, mixed angina and unstable angina) with a large degree of success. However, its efficacy compared with that of other drugs widely used to treat these diseases is not well-documented and needs to be clarified.

3.1 Use in Stable Angina

Classic stable angina is characterised by the occurrence of sudden retrosternal chest pain which is precipitated by exercise of relatively short duration and is closely associated with severe atherosclerotic coronary artery obstruction. In the majority of patients with chronic disease, chest pain and ST segment depression are reproducible at a given workload and this appears to be directly related to an imbalance between myocardial oxygen supply and demand (Braunwald, 1982; Scheidt, 1982; Théroux et al., 1983). Until recently, nitrates and β-blockers have been the drugs principally chosen for the clinical management of stable angina, although the calcium antagonists, including nifedipine, seem to represent a major advance in this therapeutic area (Théroux et al., 1983). Results reported by the manufacturer (from approximately 7000 case reports) indicate that nifedipine 30 to 60 mg/day significantly reduced the frequency of anginal attacks, after a period of 2 to 3 weeks, in about 80% of patients treated (Ebner and Donath, 1980). Although these data are not sufficiently explicit to make a clear scientific appraisal of the relative efficacy of nifedipine, they are useful in that they show side effects occur in just under 19% of patients, with 6% requiring withdrawal from treatment. Other trials with nifedipine have included controlled comparisons with placebo, β-blockers or alternative calcium antagonists, and they usually assessed efficacy by evaluating frequency of anginal attacks and glyceryl trinitrate consumption. In addition, some studies also measured objective parameters such as exercise duration, work performance and changes in ST segment depression in the electrocardiogram.

3.1.1 Placebo-Controlled Trials

In recent double-blind placebo-controlled studies nifedipine 30 to 60 mg/day for periods of up to 6 weeks was found to be significantly more effective than placebo in the management of stable angina (Mueller and Chahine, 1981; Sherman and Liang, 1983; Van der Wall, 1983). The incidence of anginal attacks and the consumption of glyceryl trinitrate tablets were reduced by approximately 50 to 60% with nifedipine (fig. 10). Furthermore, exercise tolerance was also markedly improved by nifedipine as indicated by significant increases in the time to onset of angina, maximal exercise duration

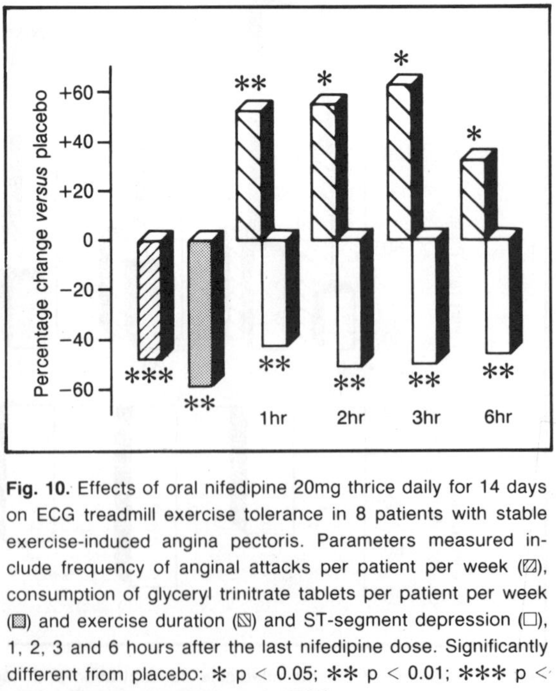

Fig. 10. Effects of oral nifedipine 20mg thrice daily for 14 days on ECG treadmill exercise tolerance in 8 patients with stable exercise-induced angina pectoris. Parameters measured include frequency of anginal attacks per patient per week (▨), consumption of glyceryl trinitrate tablets per patient per week (▩) and exercise duration (▧) and ST-segment depression (□), 1, 2, 3 and 6 hours after the last nifedipine dose. Significantly different from placebo: * $p < 0.05$; ** $p < 0.01$; *** $p < 0.001$ (after Van der Wall et al., 1983).

Table VII. Exercise performance and haemodynamic values during symptom-limited treadmill exercise following 6 weeks' treatment with nifedipine 30 to 60 mg/day or placebo in a double-blind crossover study in 23 patients with chronic stable angina (after Sherman and Liang, 1983)

Parameter	Placebo	Nifedipine
At the onset of angina		
Time to onset (sec)[a]	274	319*
Work performance (met)[a]	17.5	22.3*
ST segment depression (mV)[a]	0.11	0.09
Heart rate (beats/min)[b]	122	123
Blood pressure (mm Hg)[b]	159/87	154*/82*
RPP (mm Hg • beats/min × 10 ^{3})[b]	19.5	18.8
At maximal exercise		
Maximum duration of exercise (sec)[a]	440	490*
Work performance (met)[a]	38.2	45.3*
ST segment depression (mV)[a]	0.18	0.14*
Heart rate (beats/min)[b]	133	133
Blood pressure (mm Hg)	167/88	157*/80*
RPP (mm Hg • beats/min × 10 ^{3})[b]	22.4	20.9

a Results from 23 patients who entered the study.
b 17 patients whose exercise response was associated with typical anginal pain during both legs of the crossover.
Abbreviations: met = the energy expenditure at rest, equivalent to approximately 3.5ml of oxygen/kg bodyweight/min; RPP = rate pressure product (systolic BP × heart rate); * = significantly different from placebo, $p < 0.05$.

and work performance, at both the onset of angina and at maximal exercise (table VII). Sherman and Liang (1983) found that both systolic and diastolic blood pressures were significantly reduced at the onset of angina and at maximum exercise, whereas the rate-pressure product (indicative of myocardial oxygen consumption) was not. However, rate-pressure product was significantly lower in the nifedipine group compared with the placebo group during submaximal exercise. Myocardial ischaemia as reflected by ST segment depression at peak exercise was significantly reduced by nifedipine and there was a diminution in the magnitude of ST segment depression at specific levels of rate-pressure product during moderate to maximal exertion. These data suggest that in patients with chronic stable angina the vasodilator properties of nifedipine reduce afterload while heart rate remains relatively unchanged, and that the drug confers clinical benefits on such patients by decreasing myocardial oxygen demand. Additional evidence indicates that nifedipine may augment myocardial oxygen supply by direct coronary vasodilation, although this appears to be of lesser importance (Braunwald, 1982; Scheidt, 1982).

In the studies of Mueller and Chahine (1981) and Sherman and Liang (1983) the dose of nifedipine was titrated to obtain an optimal response and this seems to be of critical importance, since it has been shown that the therapeutic response to a range of doses of nifedipine (10 to 40mg 3 times daily) varies from patient to patient (Deanfield et al., 1983b; Fox et al., 1982). Fox et al. (1982) also investigated the effects of smoking on the response to nifedipine 60 mg/day in 10 patients with stable exercise-induced angina. ST segment depression was significantly reduced when patients on placebo stopped smoking, and an even greater reduction was noted when the nifedipine group stopped. Smoking increased resting and exercise heart rate in both groups and it was also associated with lower blood concentrations of nifedipine. In a comparative study it has been shown that smoking adversely affected the heart and interfered with the efficacy of antianginal drugs such as atenolol, propranolol and nifedipine (Deanfield et al., 1984). However, the efficacy of nifedipine was most influenced, with patients taking this calcium antagonist gaining the greatest benefit after they stopped smoking.

Nifedipine 10mg 3 times daily for 2 weeks has also been compared with placebo in patients with stable angina and coexisting chronic airways obstruction. Nifedipine was effective in controlling angina in 17 of 19 patients without adversely affecting respiratory function (Jaiprakash et al., 1980).

3.1.2 Comparisons with β-Blockers, and Their Use in Combination

Both nifedipine and β-blockers improve the relationship between myocardial oxygen demand and supply in patients with angina, but the mechanisms by which they achieve their effects are different. β-Blockers decrease left ventricular demands by reducing heart rate and myocardial contractility, particularly during exercise, while nifedipine as a potent vasodilator (see sections 1.2.3, 1.2.4) reduces systemic vascular resistance, including coronary vascular resistance (Geddes, 1983; Leon et al., 1985; Nelson et al., 1984a). Therapeutic studies with these 2 classes of drug have been designed to compare their relative efficacy and also to evaluate their use in combination, in patients with stable angina. Because they have different mechanisms of action it was hoped that when used together additional benefit would be gained, either in terms of increased efficacy or in a reduction of adverse effects, or both.

In practice, clinical trials performed to date have generally been inconclusive when comparing the relative efficacy of nifedipine with that of various β-blockers (table VIII). The reasons for this relate mainly to poor trial design. Thus, the studies summarised in table VIII have usually included too few patients and have been too short to fully compare drugs which are obviously of similar efficacy. Additionally, most trials did not titrate dosage to optimum levels for each patient, which has been shown to be of critical importance for achieving a beneficial response with nifedipine (see section 3.1.1). The overall trend has been for the β-blockers to be more effective than nifedipine, and if this is found to be true in better designed clinical trials, then in those patients with mild to moderate disease who require single-drug therapy it may be better to initiate treatment with a β-blocker and retain nifedipine for those patients who cannot tolerate or do not respond to β-blockade.

Studies in which nifedipine was used in combination with a β-blocker have demonstrated that the combination produced greater therapeutic benefit, as assessed by a decrease in the number of anginal attacks and glyceryl trinitrate consumption, than either drug used alone (table VIII). There have been fears that combining these 2 classes of drug (both having negative inotropic properties) may lead to profound haemodynamic depression which would be of major concern in patients with impaired left ventricular function. However, in the 3-week study of Findlay and Dargie (1983), combination of nifedipine with atenolol did not depress left ventricular function in patients with stable angina. Similarly, a combination of sublingual nifedipine 20mg and intravenous metoprolol 10mg, in a single-dose study in patients with chronic stable angina and depressed left ventricular function, was found to be haemodynamically more advantageous than either drug used alone, both at rest and during exercise (Nelson et al., 1984a). These results are obviously encouraging, but they are not sufficient on their own to establish the safety of combined long term treatment with nifedipine and a β-blocker in patients with stable angina and impaired left ventricular function. Further studies are essential to clarify the effects of these drugs when used in combination in such patients.

Apart from the above comparative trials a number of research groups have evaluated the clinical effects of adding nifedipine to the dosage regimen of patients treated with β-blockers (Braun et al., 1985; Ekelund and Orö, 1976; Fox et al., 1980; Jenkins and Nagle, 1982; Tirlapur and Mir, 1984; Tweddel et al., 1981; Young and Macdonald, 1982). All these studies arrived at a similar conclusion, that treatment with the combination is more beneficial than treatment with a β-blocker or a calcium antagonist alone. Interestingly, in 1 study using maximal propranolol doses the improvement with the combination was even more pronounced when propranolol dosage was halved, which may reflect the myocardial depressant effect of β-blockade in these patients with coronary heart disease, some of whom had poor left ventricular function. However, in contrast with the above findings, Katz et al. (1982) did not observe any significant improvement in exercise tolerance, anginal frequency or glyceryl trinitrate usage when nifedipine 60 mg/day was added to the dosage regimen of 10 patients receiving maximum doses of nitrates and propranolol in a 10-week placebo-controlled double-blind trial. Whether increased doses of nifedipine would have proved more beneficial was not evaluated.

The efficacy and tolerability of nifedipine 10mg 3 times daily was also evaluated in approximately 300 patients with stable angina who were poorly

Table VIII. Some recent studies comparing the therapeutic efficacy of nifedipine (N) with that of various β-blockers in patients with stable angina

References	No. of patients[a] (N group)	Study design	Dosage	Duration (weeks)	Parameters measured	Overall efficacy and comments
Bailey (1982)	13	db, co pc	N 10mg tid Prop 40mg tid	6 6	Anginal frequency, GTN usage, BP, HR	General practice study N ≡ Prop
Cocco et al. (1979)	40 (21)	r, sb, pc, pg	N 20 to 30 mg/day Pind 20 to 30 mg/day	6.4 6.4	Anginal frequency, GTN usage, exercise tolerance, ambulatory ECG monitoring	Antianginal activity N ≡ Pind but N ⩾ Pind in reducing asymptomatic myocardial ischaemia
Dargie et al. (1981)	16	r, db, co, pc	N 10 to 20mg tid Prop 80 to 160 tid N + Prop in combination at low and high dosages	2 2 2	Anginal frequency, GTN usage, precordial exercise ST segment mapping, ambulatory ECG monitoring, BP, HR	N + Prop > Prop ⩾ N, with the high dose combination of N + Prop (60 + 480) mg/day always producing the greatest improvement
De Buitleir et al. (1984)[b]	6	r, co	N 20mg tid At 100mg om Prop 160mg bid N + At combined N + Prop combined	2 2 2 2 2	Precordial exercise ST segment mapping, anginal frequency, duration of angina	N + Prop ⩾ N + At and this seemed to be related to higher plasma concentrations of Prop when administered in combination with N. However, none of the differences was statistically significant
Findlay and Dargie (1983)	14	r, db, pc, co	N 20mg tid At 100mg N + At combined	3 3 3	Anginal frequency, GTN usage, left ventricular ejection fraction (LVEF)	Antianginal efficacy N + At ⩾ AT ⩾ N and the combination did not depress LVEF at rest and significantly improved the response to exercise
Kenmure and Scruton (1979)	21	db, pc, co	N 10mg tid Prop 80mg tid N + Prop (10 + 40)mg tid	2 2 2	Anginal frequency, GTN usage, BP, HR	N + Prop ⩾ Prop ⩾ N
Keyriläinen et al. (1984)[b]	51	M, r, db, co	N 10mg tid Met 100mg bid N + Met combined	3 3 3	Anginal frequency, GTN usage, patient and physician subjective rating scores	Antianginal efficacy Met ⩾ N + Met > N. Subjective rating N + Met ⩾ Met > N and these results were in accordance with exercise results performed during study

a Number of patients who completed the study.
b Presented as an abstract with few details.
Abbreviations: Prop = propranolol; Pind = pindolol; At = Atenolol; Met = metoprolol; GTN = glyceryl trinitrate; db = double-blind; sb = single-blind; r = randomised; pc = placebo-controlled; pg = parallel groups; co = crossover; M = multicentre; tid = 3 times daily; bid = twice daily; om = in the morning; od = daily; BP = blood pressure; HR = heart rate; N ≡ Prop = the 2 drugs produced equivalent changes; N ⩾ signifies a trend in favour of N; N > indicates that N produced a significantly better response.

controlled by various β-blockers, including propranolol, atenolol and metoprolol, in a general practice setting (Young and Macdonald, 1982). Analysis of 234 patient cards at the completion of the 12-week trial indicated that the mean frequency of anginal attacks was decreased by 39% and the average consumption of nitrates by 46%. The antianginal efficacy of the combination increased progressively throughout the study and it was equally effective whether the patients had suffered a previous myocardial infarction or had elevated blood pressure. Indeed, in a subgroup of 36 patients with hypertension (blood pressure > 160/95mm Hg) the combination significantly lowered systolic blood pressure by 9.4% and diastolic pressure by 11.9%, which indicates that nifedipine may be particularly beneficial in patients in whom stable angina and hypertension coexist (Young and Macdonald, 1982).

Tirlapur and Mir (1984) noted that both isosorbide dinitrate and nifedipine (10 to 20mg 3 times daily) tended to reverse the reduction in forced expiratory volume in 1 second produced by nadolol alone and at low doses the combinations provided additional antianginal efficacy. The larger dose of isosorbide produced a further significant reduction in glyceryl trinitrate consumption and anginal frequency whereas nifedipine 20mg 3 times daily did not. The authors suggest that a combination of nifedipine and a long acting β-blocker (which increased arterial oxygen saturation and decreased summed ST segment depression) is preferable to combined administration of long acting nitrate and long acting β-blocker (which decreased arterial oxygen saturation and increased summed ST segment depression), especially in those patients with poor respiratory function or who have evidence of myocardial dysfunction. Another trial comparing nifedipine and isosorbide dinitrate, both given in combination with a β-blocker (propranolol), observed nifedipine to be significantly more effective in reducing anginal attacks and increasing exercise time, and it was better tolerated (Morse, 1983).

Thus, in the majority of patients with stable angina it would seem that a combination of nifedipine with a β-blocker can be used to gain additional benefit, even if left ventricular function is impaired. Nevertheless, care should be exercised when treating this latter group of patients, since the combination is not without risk and there have been isolated reports of hypotension and heart failure after the addition of nifedipine to patients being treated with a β-blocker (see section 8) [Anastassiades, 1980; Opie and White, 1980].

3.1.3 Comparative Efficacy of Calcium Antagonists

Clinical trials published to date comparing the efficacy of various calcium antagonists in patients with stable exercise-induced angina have failed to establish a consistent clinical advantage for any particular member of this group of drugs.

Johnston et al. (1985) recently evaluated the clinical efficacy of combining nifedipine (60 mg/day), diltiazem (240 mg/day) and verapamil (360 mg/day) to treatment with propranolol (160 mg/day) with or without isosorbide dinitrate in 21 patients with stable angina. The trial was a well-designed 4-weekly crossover study which found the 3 combinations to be equally effective, and they were all significantly superior to propranolol alone. Because of a lower incidence of adverse effects the authors suggest that the combination of diltiazem plus propranolol may be the first choice, although the combination with nifedipine did produce a greater reduction of ST segment depression and also had a lesser effect on P-R interval. At the end of the trial 7 patients requested the combination with diltiazem, 5 the combination with nifedipine and 2 the combination with verapamil. When administered alone, diltiazem 60mg 3 times daily was superior to nifedipine 10mg 3 times daily in improving work performance and reducing ST segment depression at submaximal effort in 20 patients with stable angina (Schurtz et al., 1983). Bala Subramanian et al. (1982) compared nifedipine 20mg 3 times daily with verapamil 120mg 3 times daily and recorded significant advantages with verapamil in increasing exercise tolerance, decreasing ST segment changes and increasing the time to onset of ST segment depression. Using the same dosages, Winniford et al. (1985) found that verapamil was more beneficial than nifedipine when added to the treatment of 16 patients with severe stable angina not adequately controlled by propranolol (180 to 360 mg/day). However, verapamil plus propranolol occasionally caused symptomatic bradycardia and this combination should be administered with caution. In contrast, Dawson et al. (1981) used the same fixed dosages of nifedipine and verapamil and found no difference in efficacy between them. A notable finding in the above studies was that nifedipine tended to produce a greater incidence of adverse effects, particularly those associated with vasodilatation.

As emphasised in section 3.1.1, to obtain optimal benefit with nifedipine the dosage should be carefully titrated to each individual patient's needs. In view of the fixed dosages of nifedipine, verapamil and diltiazem used in the above studies, a true reflection of the relative efficacy of these 3 calcium antagonists in the clinical situation may not have been presented. Additionally, the trials included too few patients (16 to 30) and were too short (1 to 4 weeks) to fully compare drugs which are obviously of similar efficacy. Firm conclusions with respect to the comparative value of the various calcium antagonists still await more definitive data from well-designed clinical trials in larger patient groups.

3.1.4 Medium to Long Term Trials

Only a few reports regarding the long term efficacy of nifedipine in patients with stable angina have been published and these have generally involved small groups of patients. Thus, in a 6-month open trial in 12 patients with exercise-induced angina, nifedipine produced a good or very good response in 8 patients, no improvement in 3 patients and a deterioration of the underlying disease in 1 patient, as assessed by the frequency of anginal attacks, need for glyceryl trinitrate, and exercise tolerance (Castilho et al., 1976). Similar results were reported in the 6-month open trial of Alvarado and Pineros (1976) which included 22 patients with stable angina who were treated with nifedipine 20 to 30 mg/day. A recent report of the long term use of nifedipine (titrated to response) in 27 patients with stable angina and inoperable coronary artery disease has been published (Rubenfire et al., 1984). The patients were refractory to nitrates and β-blockers and had angiographic evidence of diffuse disease and/or severe left ventricular dysfunction without a discrete aneurism. 19 patients (73%) responded to nifedipine therapy (angina attacks or glyceryl trinitrate usage reduced > 50%) and 7 (27%) did not, during a mean follow-up of 25 (range 1 to 43) months. Cumulative survival for the group after 3 years was 44%, with no difference between responders and non-responders; the authors conclude that in this type of patient nifedipine may provide symptomatic relief, but it does not seem to have a significant effect on cardiac morbidity and mortality.

3.2 Use in Variant (Prinzmetal's) Angina

Variant (Prinzmetal's) angina is a clinical syndrome characterised by episodes of spontaneous and unprovoked ischaemic cardiac pain at rest (usually at night or early morning) associated with ST segment elevation and relieved by sublingual glyceryl trinitrate (Ginsburg et al., 1982; Prinzmetal et al., 1959; Schroeder, 1982). Although the precise mechanisms are unknown, there is substantial evidence that coronary artery spasm (a transient narrowing of an epicardial coronary artery of sufficient severity to induce ischaemia) plays a major pathophysiological role in the ischaemia of variant angina (Braunwald, 1982; Théroux et al., 1983). Coronary anatomy, as assessed by coronary arteriography, has presented a wide spectrum of arterial obstruction, from normal to moderately severe occlusive atherosclerotic disease (Schroeder, 1982). Evaluation of patients with variant angina is made difficult by the variable course of the disease, by the wide range of clinical severity among patients, and because many attacks are asymptomatic (Théroux et al., 1983; Waters et al., 1981a). Provocative testing with ergonovine maleate has been used in a number of trials to assess objectively the clinical status of patients with variant angina, and to evaluate the efficacy of various drugs for treating the disease (Miller et al., 1983; Waters et al., 1981a; Winniford et al., 1983). However, Winniford et al. (1983) found this test to be inaccurate in predicting disease activity (see section 3.2.4) and others do not recommend routine ergonovine testing because serious complications, or even death, can result (Waters et al., 1981a).

3.2.1 Open Studies

The clinical efficacy of nifedipine for the treatment of variant angina has been extensively documented (see 1st, 2nd, 3rd, 4th and 5th International Adalat® Symposia, 1975 to 1983). Retrospective analysis of record cards from 439 patients with variant angina treated with nifedipine 10 to 160 mg/day for periods up to 6 years indicated that an overall 'success rate' of 87% was achieved (Ebner and Donath, 1980). Additionally, in a multicentre trial nifedipine 40 to 160 mg/day was added to the treatment regimen of 127 patients with severe recurrent angina at rest (with electrocardiographic and angiographic evidence of coronary artery spasm), in the majority of whom conventional antianginal therapy had failed (Antman et al., 1980a). 63% of the patients gained complete control of anginal attacks, and in 87% the frequency of angina was reduced by at least 50%, during a mean follow-up period of 9 (range 0.1 to 45) months (fig. 11). As an extension of this trial 389 patients with documented variant angina, 292 patients with 'mixed' angina (evidence of both classic exertional angina and coronary vasospasm), and 35 patients with classic exertional angina (all refractory to conventional therapy) were treated with nifedipine 10 to 200 mg/day, in addition to their usual drugs, for a mean period of 6.5 months (Stone et al., 1983b). Complete remission of anginal attacks or a reduction in anginal frequency of more than 50% was noted more often in patients with variant (42% and 83%, respectively) or 'mixed' (20% and 76%, respectively) angina than in those with stable angina (3% and 51%, respectively). These results indicate that nifedipine can be expected to produce a beneficial response in most patients with a vasospastic component to their angina. However, in the study of Stone et al. (1983b) a paradoxical exacerbation of anginal symptoms occurred in 13 to 29% of patients (most frequently in those with no evidence of vasospasm), so care is warranted when adding nifedipine to the dosage regimen of patients receiving maximally tolerated doses of conventional therapy.

3.2.2 Comparisons with Placebo

There have been few well-designed studies comparing nifedipine with placebo in patients with variant angina. This probably reflects the serious nature of the underlying disease and the potentially hazardous consequences of not actively treating such patients, since myocardial infarction and severe arrhythmias can be a complication during the active phase of the disease (Kimura et al., 1977; Maseri et al., 1978). In an appropriately designed multicentre trial, Schick et al. (1982) evaluated 38 patients with well-documented coronary artery spasm who responded to open label treatment with nifedipine. Following a 2-week single-blind phase in which nifedipine was maintained at prestudy levels, each patient was randomly allocated to continue with nifedipine (n = 19) or to receive placebo (n = 19) for a maximum of 4 weeks under double-

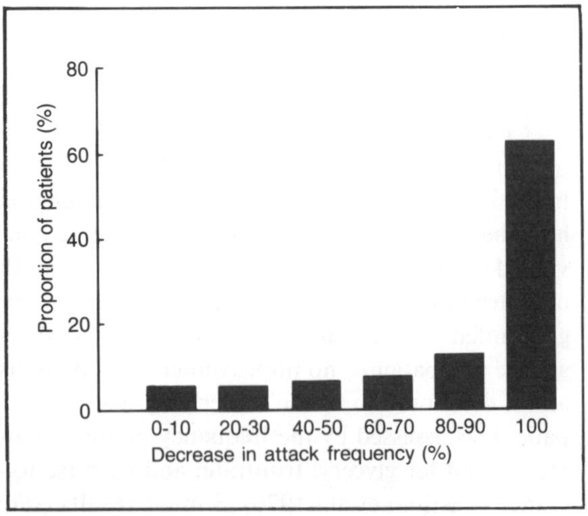

Fig. 11. Distribution of the decrease in anginal attack frequency in 127 patients with variant angina treated with nifedipine 40 to 160 (mean 64) mg/day for a mean of 9 months. Decrease in attack frequency was estimated from pretreatment level to that during the last week of treatment with nifedipine (adapted from Antman et al., 1980a).

blind conditions. During the double-blind phase an increase in median anginal frequency and glyceryl trinitrate usage occurred only in those patients on placebo, and 7/19 (37%) prematurely withdrew from the study because of an exacerbation of disease severity; only 1 patient in the nifedipine group experienced an increase in anginal frequency. Overall the treatment was considered effective in 16 patients (84%) receiving nifedipine but in only 3 patients (16%) taking placebo. This controlled trial confirms the short term efficacy of nifedipine in the treatment of coronary vasospasm and verifies previous open-label clinical experience with the drug.

3.2.3 Comparisons with Isosorbide Dinitrate

Long acting nitrates have traditionally been recognised as the most effective prophylactic treatment for patients with coronary artery spasm/variant angina, especially as β-blockade and coronary artery bypass surgery have proved to be unsatisfactory (Antman et al., 1980a; Schroeder, 1982; Schroeder et al., 1980). Controlled clinical trials comparing nifedipine with long acting nitrates in patients with variant angina have been limited, and those published have included too few patients (10 to 25) to be able to detect small differences in efficacy which may exist between the 2 drugs.

Nifedipine has been compared with isosorbide dinitrate, both drugs titrated up to a maximum of 30mg 4 times daily, in 2 double-blind crossover trials of 5 weeks duration (Ginsburg et al., 1982; Hill and Conti, 1983). In the study of Ginsberg et al. (1982) 11 patients completed the study and the results generally favoured nifedipine in terms of subjective improvements such as reduction of anginal frequency and glyceryl trinitrate consumption. With respect to patient preference, 64% preferred nifedipine while only 27% preferred isosorbide dinitrate. The authors concluded that nifedipine was more effective and produced fewer side effects than isosorbide dinitrate. Using similar parameters, Hill and Conti (1983) found no significant differences in efficacy between nifedipine and isosorbide dinitrate in 21 patients with variant angina. Both drugs produced a greater than 50% reduction of anginal frequency in approximately 70% of patients. Importantly, many patients responded differently to the 2 drugs so that when one was ineffective the other frequently induced a favourable response. Unfortunately, no patient characteristic was identified which could predict a likely positive outcome. In both of the above studies a small proportion of patients did not respond to nifedipine (13 to 17%) or to isosorbide dinitrate (24 to 27%). From the above results it is not possible to make a categorical statement regarding the relative efficacy of nifedipine and isosorbide dinitrate in patients with variant angina. However, it would seem reasonable to conclude that nifedipine is at least as effective as isosorbide dinitrate in the short term management of the disease.

3.2.4 Comparative Efficacy of Calcium Antagonists

Comparative evaluations between various calcium antagonists have mainly been reports of clinical experience rather than controlled therapeutic trials. Nifedipine, diltiazem and verapamil have been the calcium antagonists most frequently investigated in patients with variant angina, and studies to date have failed to identify any consistent trend in favour of any one of these drugs. The 3 drugs produce different responses in a large proportion of patients, so if one fails to be effective it would seem reasonable to try another, or a combination of 2 calcium antagonists, in an attempt to control angina symptoms.

There have been a number of surveys from various cardiology clinics in Japan reporting their experience with calcium-blocking drugs in patients with variant angina (Kimura and Kishida, 1981; Kishida and Kimura, 1980; Kishida et al., 1982). In the largest of these, Kimura and Kishida (1981) reported the combined data of 286 patients treated in 11 centres with nifedipine (mean dose 39mg, n = 149), diltiazem (mean dose 160mg, n = 87), verapamil (mean dose 228mg, n = 15) or other drugs including propranolol and anticoagulants. Over a mean treatment period of 24.8 (range 3 to 129) days, efficacy (complete elimination of angina after 2 days or a reduction of angina frequency to

< 50% of the baseline value) rates of 94.0, 90.8 and 85.7% were achieved by nifedipine, diltiazem and verapamil, respectively. The calcium antagonists were significantly more effective than other drugs used such as β-blockers and anticoagulants. In another uncontrolled trial of 1 year duration using the same 3 calcium antagonists, a 'good response' (> 50% decrease in angina attacks without a coronary event) was achieved in 29 of the 45 patients including: 11/16 on nifedipine (mean dose 68 mg/day), 9/13 on diltiazem (mean dose 240 mg/day) and 9/16 on verapamil (mean dose 419 mg/day) [Pepine et al., 1983]. Additional antianginal drugs were required in 20 (44%) of these patients and 17 (38%) patients experienced side effects (6 taking nifedipine, none of diltiazem, and 11 on verapamil). 16 patients did not respond to treatment with a calcium blocker; 3 died, 5 had a myocardial infarction and 8 required hospitalisation for other reasons. Even though treatment with calcium antagonists afforded excellent initial protection in the majority of patients with angina at rest, and this was sustained during the first year of therapy, morbid events still occurred – particularly in those patients with coronary artery disease.

As part of a clinical study, Waters et al. (1981b) evaluated the initial (3-day) response to treatment with nifedipine (80 mg/day), diltiazem (360 mg/day) and verapamil (480 mg/day) in 27 patients with variant angina, and correlated it to longer term efficacy. Provocative testing with ergonovine maleate was used to assess the initial response and all 3 drugs partially or totally blocked the provoked anginal episodes in most patients. However, in 12 of 27 patients the 3 calcium antagonists produced dissimilar effects and nifedipine and diltiazem were the preferred choice in 5 patients each, while verapamil was the preferred choice in the remaining two. Each patient was treated during follow-up with the drug that gave the best initial result and after a mean period of 7 (range 1 to 15) months, 14 of 15 (93%) patients receiving a drug that completely blocked the ergonovine response remained angina free. This compared with only 4 of 12 (33%) patients administered a drug which only (at best) partially blocked the ergonovine response. The findings of this study did not demonstrate a significant superiority for any one of the calcium antagonists.

Winniford et al. (1982a) compared verapamil (mean dose 450 mg/day) with placebo over a period of 9 months in 27 patients with variant angina and the first 23 patients to complete this phase went on to receive 2 months' treatment with nifedipine (mean dose 71 mg/day). The 2 calcium antagonists were found to be of similar efficacy and both were significantly superior to placebo in reducing the frequency of angina, glyceryl trinitrate consumption and ST segment deviation. In a subset of 10 patients with relatively normal left ventricular function neither nifedipine nor verapamil had an adverse influence on left ventricular volume or ejection fraction. As part of a separate report, efficacy was evaluated by ergonovine provocation and it was shown that this test did not accurately predict disease activity, since some patients had negative results at times of marked clinical and electrocardiographic activity while other patients had positive results at a time of little or no activity (Winniford et al., 1983). The authors concluded that subjective assessment of anginal frequency and ambulatory electrocardiographic monitoring were preferable to ergonovine provocation for accurately evaluating variant angina activity. Recently, the same group noted that combinations of verapamil or nifedipine with isosorbide dinitrate were significantly more effective than isosorbide dinitrate alone in reducing anginal frequency and ischaemic ECG changes in 9 patients with variant angina. Nifedipine (71 mg/day) and verapamil (453 mg/day) were equally effective when used in combination with isosorbide dinitrate (117 mg/day) [Winniford et al., 1984].

3.2.5 Long Term Trials

Various centres have reported long term (up to 6 years) clinical experience using nifedipine to treat patients with variant angina (Bertrand et al., 1981; Besse et al., 1980; Delahaye et al., 1980; Hill et al., 1983; Waters et al., 1983). Beneficial response rates ranged between 50 and 90% depending upon the criteria used to define a positive response. For example, Besse et al. (1980) reported the complete disappearance of anginal attacks in 56% of patients, whereas in the study of Hill et al. (1983) there was a greater than 50% decrease in the frequency of angina in 86% of patients. In this latter study additional antianginal drugs such as nitrates and β-blockers were frequently needed to control symptoms. Waters et al. (1983) followed 169 patients with variant angina who were treated with various antianginal drugs for a mean period of 15.3 (range 1 to 68) months. 14 (8%) of the patients died and 22 (13%) had myocardial infarction, with the majority of these adverse events occurring within the first 3 months. The strongest predictors of survival and survival without a myocardial infarction were absence of coronary artery disease, disease activity *per se,* and left ventricular function. The choice of drug did not influence the survival rate but it did affect the incidence of survival without a myocardial infarction. Thus, 87% of patients treated with nifedipine (n = 38), diltiazem (n = 32), or verapamil (n = 17) survived without a myocardial infarction after 1 year while the rate for patients treated with perhexiline maleate or nitrates was only 61% ($p < 0.008$). As expected, those patients with multivessel disease had the worst prognosis, and their survival was not affected by any treatment.

3.3 Use in Unstable Angina

Unstable angina (also termed coronary insufficiency, preinfarction angina or intermediate angina) is a clinical syndrome which is usually diagnosed when episodes of angina increase in either frequency, severity or duration, and such patients frequently report decreased responsiveness to antianginal medications or a need to use them more often (for recent reviews see Helfant, 1982; Schroeder, 1982; Théroux et al., 1983). The increased symptomatic manifestations of myocardial ischaemia, with pain occurring at rest (day or night), are often associated with reversible electrocardiographic changes in the ST segment and/or T wave. Although the vast majority of ischaemic episodes abate (with no enzyme abnormalities and the electrocardiogram returning to baseline), this is not always the case, and the disease can exacerbate and an acute myocardial infarction develop. Because unstable angina occurs across the wide spectrum of coronary artery disease, the patients by definition must represent a heterogeneous population. This has probably hindered attempts to define the exact pathophysiological mechanisms underlying this form of myocardial ischaemia, and has also contributed to the poor long term prognosis for such patients. There seems to be a growing appreciation that coronary vasospasm may play an important role in the onset of ischaemic attacks, and the interplay of this with other factors such as the severity of coronary artery thrombosis and severe obstruction, and changes in coronary artery tone, needs to be clarified – not only to develop a more rational means for treating patients with unstable angina but also to help elucidate the cause of the changing anginal threshold (Blaustein et al., 1983; Muller et al., 1984b; Schroeder, 1982).

Patients with unstable angina generally represent a high risk group and the usual treatment involves hospitalisation, bed rest and therapeutic intervention to help stabilise the disease. Normally the patients are sedated and nitrate therapy initiated (intravenous, oral or topical depending upon the severity of the angina). The use of β-blockers under these circumstances is more questionable and has not been the subject of rigorous scientific appraisal; however, most centres have maintained their usage because of past clinical experience (Helfant, 1982; Hugenholtz et al., 1981; Schroeder, 1982; Théroux et al., 1983). It is against this background that clinical trials with nifedipine have to be performed, and evaluation of the efficacy of the calcium antagonist is made all the more difficult by the unpredictable course of the disease and the heterogeneous nature of the patient groups studied. The increasing awareness of the importance of coronary vasospasm in the pathophysiology of certain patients with unstable angina suggests that the calcium antagonists may make a major contribution to their treatment. Most trials so far have been in patients refractory to conventional therapy and have evaluated the efficacy of nifedipine under open or controlled conditions as a second- or third-line choice to nitrates and β-blockers.

Table IX. Summary of open trials evaluating the efficacy of nifedipine (Nif) as a second- or third-line choice for the acute management of patients with unstable angina refractory to conventional treatment with β-blockers (β-B) and/or nitrates (N)

References	No. of patients	Previous therapy	No. of patients responding after addition of Nif (%)
Blaustein et al. (1983)	47	β-B + N	22 (47)
Hagemeijer et al. (1982)	35 47	β-B β-B + N	31 (89) 39 (83)
Moses et al. (1981)	19	β-B + N	14 (74)
Serruys et al. (1981a)	52	β-B + N	42 (81)

3.3.1 Open Studies

As can be seen in table IX, 47 to 89% of patients with unstable angina refractory to conventional therapy may be expected to respond successfully when nifedipine 30 to 240 mg/day is added to their treatment regimen during short term hospitalisation. The various studies used different criteria for defining a positive response but they generally required abolition of the symptoms of angina at rest following addition of the calcium antagonist. Because only small numbers of patients were included in these trials it is not possible to make absolute statements about the relative efficacy of nifedipine in the various subgroups treated. There is evidence that nifedipine may be more effective in those patients with less advanced coronary artery obstruction (Hagemeijer and van Mechelen, 1983; Hugenholtz et al., 1981; Serruys et al., 1981a), although Moses et al. (1981) could find no significant differences between responders and non-responders with respect to the clinical or angiographic characteristics of the underlying disease in the small number of patients included in their study.

In the largest of these trials nifedipine 10mg 6 times daily was found to produce short term stabilisation of unstable angina in greater than 80% of patients, although with longer term follow-up 7% of the group developed a myocardial infarction and 19% required coronary artery bypass surgery. After 2 years, nifedipine titrated to between 30 and 80 mg/day maintained excellent long term benefit in 49 patients (60%) [Hagemeijer et al., 1982]. Similar response rates were reported by Moses et al. (1981) in 19 patients with severe rest angina and obstructive coronary artery disease. However, less impressive long term efficacy was noted by Blaustein et al. (1983), with only 22 of 47 patients (47%) with unstable angina gaining a favourable response which allowed discharge from hospital or full in-hospital activity. Eight of these 22 patients developed a cardiac event (recurrent unstable angina, myocardial infarction, or death) within the first 4 months; 13 patients were discharged from hospital and during a follow-up period of 8 to 26 months only 1 had a cardiac event. The authors concluded that an initial favourable response with nifedipine did not improve long term prognosis, but it did control symptoms to a sufficient degree that coronary bypass surgery could be performed less urgently. Boden et al. (1983) recently reported results from 10 of their patients with unstable angina in whom nifedipine 60 to 120 mg/day produced a paradoxical increase in myocardial ischaemia when administered in combination with nitrates, alone or together with a β-blocker. All 10 patients developed a hypotensive response to combination treatment which may have provoked ischaemia by decreasing coronary perfusion. It was concluded that nifedipine should be added with caution to the treatment regimen of patients prone to hypotension.

3.3.2 Controlled Trials

Nifedipine has been compared with propranolol (Moll et al., 1984), 'conventional' therapy (Muller et al., 1984b) and with placebo (as an addition to conventional treatment) [Gerstenblith et al., 1982] in controlled randomised trials in patients with unstable angina.

Gerstenblith et al. (1982) compared the efficacy of nifedipine (n = 68) with that of placebo (n = 70) when either drug was added to the 'conventional' treatment regimen of patients with unstable angina. The addition of placebo was a failure (defined as bypass surgery, myocardial infarction or sudden death) in 61% of patients, while nifedipine failed in 44% of patients ($p = 0.003$). Active treatment was most successful in those patients with ST segment elevation during anginal attacks, with only 36% of such patients failing to respond to nifedipine compared with 67% of the placebo group. This may not be unexpected considering the impressive response rates reported for nifedipine in patients with coronary vasospasm/variant angina, who frequently exhibit ST segment elevation (see section 3.2). ST segment elevation is, however, much less frequently observed in patients with unstable angina admitted to coronary care units (Feldman et al., 1982).

Two separate reports of the above clinical trial first presented by Gerstenblith et al. (1982) have also been published. In the first of these, involving 104 patients who had undergone cardiac catheterisation, nifedipine was of greatest value in patients with the most advanced disease, as indicated by the severity of coronary artery disease (Brinker et al., 1983). Recently, 81 patients from the original double-blind trial entered a second study in which nifedipine and placebo were withdrawn, either 1 to 14 hours prior to coronary bypass surgery ($n = 39$) or following 2 years of continued treatment ($n = 42$) [Gottlieb et al., 1984]. In the surgical patients the incidence of perioperative myocardial infarction or other overt haemodynamic changes during the withdrawal phase did not differ between the nifedipine group and the placebo group. Similarly, in the 34 patients in whom the disease had stabilised during long term treatment with placebo or nifedipine (in addition to nitrates and propranolol) there was no significant difference during withdrawal. However, 8 patients continued having attacks of resting angina prior to entering this trial and in 5 (4 on nifedipine and 1 on placebo) there was a marked deterioration of their angina during the discontinuation phase. These preliminary results suggest that for the majority of patients with unstable angina who are to undergo bypass surgery or whose condition has stabilised on drug therapy, few acute adverse effects accompany nifedipine withdrawal. Such conclusions must be considered in light of the short duration of follow-up (a mean of 66 hours continual ECG monitoring) and apply only to patients who have been maintained on long acting nitrates and propranolol in addition to nifedipine, and not to those patients who may be controlled by nifedipine alone. Furthermore, it would appear unwise to withdraw nifedipine in those patients still experiencing episodes of angina at rest, since this group do seem to be at risk and should continue to be treated with a calcium antagonist.

In another short term (14-day) double-blind trial, nifedipine was compared with conventional treatment with propranolol and isosorbide dinitrate in 126 patients with unstable angina (Muller et al., 1984b). Appropriate treatment regimens were obtained by dose titration: 34 patients could not tolerate propranolol, and in these, nifedipine was compared with isosorbide dinitrate alone. Overall there was no significant difference in anginal symptoms between those patients treated with nifedipine and those receiving conventional anti-anginal drugs. Of 27 patients who were refractory to initial conventional ($n = 13$) or nifedipine ($n = 14$) treatment, 5 in each group became pain free when the treatments were combined. 67 patients received propranolol prior to randomisation, and addition of nifedipine was more effective in this subgroup than was an increase in conventional therapy ($p = 0.026$). In the subgroup who had not received previous propranolol ($n = 59$), conventional therapy produced a more rapid relief from pain than nifedipine ($p < 0.001$). Overall the results support the use of nifedipine alone in the initial medical management of unstable angina and they also confirm the added benefit of combining nifedipine and propranolol when monotherapy is not effective.

In a recent prospective randomised trial in 40 patients with unstable angina, nifedipine 80 to 120mg and propranolol 160 to 240mg were found to be equally effective in controlling episodes of angina (Moll et al., 1984). Both drugs stabilised the underlying unstable disease in 45% of patients, and in those who did not improve, a combination of nifedipine and propranolol increased the response rate to approximately 90%.

3.4 Use in Acute Myocardial Infarction

Before, during and after acute myocardial infarction one of the major aims of treatment must be to limit the spread of myocardial necrosis which can adversely affect short and long term prognosis. Thus, nifedipine has been used both prophylactically, in an attempt to attenuate threatened infarction, and therapeutically, to limit the extent of myocardial necrosis or to stabilise those patients with recurrent ischaemic pain immediately after infarction.

3.4.1 Prevention or Attenuation of Myocardial Infarction

In a well-designed clinical trial Muller et al. (1984a) compared nifedipine 20mg every 4 hours (10mg 4-hourly if side effects occurred) with placebo in patients with threatened myocardial infarction (n = 105) and in patients who had experienced an acute myocardial infarction (n = 66). Treatment was initiated a mean of 4.6 hours after the onset of chest pain and efficacy was evaluated in terms of mortality, incidence of infarction, infarct size, and extent of myocardial necrosis. The results indicated that nifedipine did not reduce the likelihood of a threatened myocardial infarction progressing into an acute event and neither did it limit infarct size in those who eventually had an acute myocardial infarction. At 6 months there was no significant difference between the placebo and nifedipine groups with regard to mortality. Contrasting with these results, during the first 2 weeks more patients treated with nifedipine died (n = 7) than did patients treated with placebo (n = 0; p = 0.018). When account was taken of the greater proportion of patients aged over 60 years in the nifedipine group (47% *vs* 38%) the significance of the mortality difference was reduced from p = 0.018 to p = 0.030. The authors were extremely surprised by the lack of deaths in the placebo group within 2 weeks of infarction and suggest this complicates interpretation of the data presented. The overall conclusion from the trial is that, under circumstances when treatment cannot be initiated earlier than about 5 hours, there seems to be little advantage in the routine use of nifedipine in patients with suspected myocardial infarction. Whether earlier intervention with nifedipine will be beneficial, as has been speculated for various β-blockers, needs to be evaluated.

3.4.2 Post-Myocardial Infarction

Immediately following an acute myocardial infarction a small group of patients may continue to experience episodes of ischaemic pain or develop persistent hypertension which may lead to an extension of existing areas of myocardial necrosis; a limited number of studies have assessed the efficacy of nifedipine in a small number of patients in this clinical setting.

Stone and Muller (1982) reported their experience in 11 patients with recurrent ischaemic pain a mean of 9.2 days after infarction. Episodes of ischaemia at rest stopped in 10 of the 11 patients treated with nifedipine (40 to 120 mg/day), although 2 of these continued to have attacks with minimal exertion. These 3 'failures' subsequently all underwent coronary artery bypass surgery. The 8 responders to nifedipine were clinically managed for a mean of 5.4 (range 1 to 12) months and remained pain-free on a combination of nifedipine, β-blockers and/or nitrates. The authors concluded that if this initial experience with nifedipine is confirmed in controlled trials, then it may eliminate the need for bypass surgery in some patients, and in others it may provide a period of clinical stability prior to operating.

Similar results were reported by Wertheimer et al. (1982) when nifedipine 30 to 120 mg/day was used to treat 18 patients with recurrent chest pain after myocardial infarction. Complete abolition of rest pain was achieved in 14 patients, 2 had a partial reduction in anginal episodes, and 2 did not respond. Of these latter 4 patients, 3 died within 1 month and 1 underwent successful bypass surgery, while of the 14 responders 6 remained pain free after a mean follow-up of 13 months, 3 stopped nifedipine after 2 to 4 months and remained pain free, 2 elected to undergo surgery, 2 died and 1 patient was lost to follow-up.

Hypertension after myocardial infarction is a complication which can adversely affect prognosis by placing at risk additional areas of the myocardium. In a short term haemodynamic study in 22 patients with hypertension complicating myocardial infarction, it was found that nifedipine 20mg sublingually and labetalol 1 mg/kg intravenously equally lowered mean blood pressure by about 18mm Hg. Only nifedipine reduced systemic vascular resistance ($p < 0.01$) and because of its acute haemodynamic effects the authors suggest it may be a suitable choice in those patients with low heart rate and low cardiac output (Taylor et al., 1983).

3.5 Use in Coronary Artery Bypass Surgery

It is thought that coronary artery spasm may play an important role in the sudden perioperative haemodynamic collapse associated with coronary artery bypass surgery (Kopf et al., 1982). Intravenous glyceryl trinitrate has usually been the treatment of choice under these circumstances although there is mounting evidence that nifedipine may be a useful alternative and/or addition.

Cohen et al. (1983) found nifedipine 30mg administered via a nasogastric tube to be beneficial when used adjunctively with intravenous glyceryl trinitrate in preventing further recurrences of coronary artery spasm in a patient with triple-vessel coronary artery disease undergoing coronary artery bypass surgery. Other case reports have shown that sublingual nifedipine 10 to 30mg quickly relieved coronary artery spasm which occurred during bypass surgery and was refractory to glyceryl trinitrate (Kopf et al., 1982; Lewis et al., 1982). In addition, it has been reported that injection of nifedipine 0.1 to 0.2mg directly into the affected coronary vessel quickly reversed electrocardiographic changes which were suggestive of coronary artery spasm in 2 patients undergoing coronary artery bypass surgery.

This latter finding is in agreement with the data of Bertrand et al. (1981) who showed that intracoronary administration of nifedipine 0.2mg suppressed spasm in 9 of 12 patients during coronary arteriography.

4. Therapeutic Use in Systemic Hypertension

Single-dose studies indicate that the antihypertensive effects of nifedipine are primarily mediated through peripheral arteriolar dilatation with an accompanying increase in sympathetic tone which results in parallel increases in heart rate (depending on the formulation administered), indices of left ventricular contractility, cardiac output and stroke work index (see sections 1.2.1 and 1.2.3). With longer term administration the increase in sympathetic tone seems to diminish as assessed by a reduction of the heart rate response and lower circulating noradrenaline concentrations (Lederballe Pedersen et al., 1979).

Until fairly recently, interest in the use of calcium antagonists in the various forms and grades of systemic hypertension has been limited, and reviews of the use of nifedipine in this therapeutic area have usually reached a general conclusion that it is likely to be a useful addition to the large number of antihypertensive drugs currently available, but that further clinical trials are needed to clearly define its overall position (Braunwald, 1982; Bühler et al., 1983; Frishman and Charlap, 1984; Frishman et al., 1984; Robinson, 1983; Schwartz et al., 1984b; Toggart and Zelis, 1982). Furthermore, there has been a trend away from the view that nifedipine is not indicated for the treatment of mild hypertension (Guazzi et al., 1983), and clinical data are accumulating rapidly supporting the view that nifedipine may be useful in all grades of hypertension.

In the treatment of acute episodes of severe hypertension, and particularly in hypertensive crisis, the efficacy and safety of nifedipine has been consistently reported. The advantages of a drug that can be administered orally or sublingually and still produce significant reductions of blood pressure within 5 to 10 minutes are obvious. Even though there have been few comparisons with existing first-line drugs, most authors consider nifedipine to be one of the drugs of choice in an emergency room setting. In combination with other antihypertensive drugs such as β-blockers, methyldopa and diuretics, nifedipine has been found to be a useful third-line agent in patients with refractory severe hypertension. Probably the greatest conflict surrounds the suitability of using nifedipine alone for the long term management of mild, moderate or severe hypertension. However, there have been a large number of comparative clinical studies published recently which indicate that nifedipine effectively lowers blood pressure in such patients, at least in short to medium term studies, and the optimism of most authors would seem justified. Nevertheless, further long term evaluation is necessary to clearly establish its efficacy and safety when used alone.

The difficulty in fully defining the role of nifedipine in the management of the various forms of systemic hypertension stems not only from the relatively recent evaluation of calcium antagonists in this clinical area, but also from the use of different formulations of the drug which clearly have different onsets and durations of action. Single-dose studies with the sustained release formulation have shown it to have a potent, dose-dependent, antihypertensive action which lasts longer than that of the conventional capsule preparation (Corvol et al., 1983). It remains to be seen however, whether this preparation (which offers the advantage of twice daily administration) will become the formulation of choice for the long term management of hypertensive patients.

4.1 Acute Studies

In single-dose studies in patients with mild to severe hypertension, nifedipine 10 to 20mg (orally or sublingually) has been shown to be a safe and effective drug for the rapid reduction of elevated blood pressure (Aoki et al., 1978; Beer et al., 1981; Guazzi et al., 1977; Haft et al., 1983; Huysmans et al., 1983b; Ito et al., 1984; Lederballe Pedersen and Mikkelsen, 1978; Yoshimura et al., 1983). The results from these studies and from trials in patients requiring emergency reduction of high blood pressure (see section 4.1.2) indicate that maximal hypotensive activity is generally achieved 20 to 45 minutes after sublingual administration and 30 to 60 minutes after oral administration. Blood pressure usually returned to pretreatment values between 4 and 8 hours later. Interestingly, the degree of reduction of blood pressure appears to be directly related to the pretreatment level, after both single and multidose (for 8 weeks) administration (Yoshimura et al., 1983). Nifedipine did not produce a precipitous fall in blood pressure, and postural hypotension was rarely encountered. Pulse rate was usually increased in parallel with the blood pressure response but tachycardia was never reported to be a clinical problem. These results suggest nifedipine may be useful for the acute lowering of severely elevated blood pressure, and many trials have investigated its efficacy in this setting.

4.1.1 Comparative Trials

There have been few comparative trials in patients with moderate to severe hypertension in whom a prompt reduction of blood pressure is required due to an acute rise in pressure resulting from the uncontrolled nature of the underlying disease.

Compared with placebo, sublingual nifedipine 10 to 20mg rapidly and significantly ($p < 0.001$) lowered blood pressure in 42 of 43 patients with moderate to severe hypertension (Beer et al., 1981). Nifedipine 10mg orally compared with prazosin 2mg orally for the acute management of 26 patients (2 groups of 13) with uncontrolled hypertension produced a more rapid and smoother reduction of blood pressure over the 3-hour observation period (Yagil et al., 1983b). Prazosin, on the other hand, lowered blood pressure by a significantly greater amount between 2 and 3 hours but this was associated with postural hypotension in 9 of the 13 patients. Overall, the rapid onset and smoother effect of nifedipine (still producing a sustained reduction of blood pressure) together with the absence of postural hypotension, appears to offer important advantages over prazosin. Despite different mechanisms of action, both slow release nifedipine 40mg 12-hourly and atenolol 100mg once

Table X. Results of some recent studies evaluating the clinical effectiveness of single doses of nifedipine for the acute management of hypertensive emergency

References	No. of patients	Nifedipine dose (mg) and route	Blood pressure (mm Hg)		Time to onset (min)	Time to maximal effect (min)
			pretreatment	post-treatment		
Bertel et al. (1983)	25	10 or 20 PO	221/126	152/89	10	30-40
Conen et al. (1982)	18	20 PO	220/122	150/86	5	20-30
De Los Reyes et al. (1982)	7	10 PO or SL	216/144	129/82	< 15 SL 20-40 PO	nd
Dilmen et al. (1983)	21[a]	0.25 to 0.5 mg/kg SL	181/136	132/98	nd	30
Erbel et al. (1983)	30	20 SL	235/123	170/91	5	20
Groth et al. (1984)	24[b]	10 SL	219/122	172/100	15	90
Haft and Litterer (1984)	43 20	10 SL 20 SL[c]	205/128 212/128	159/89 165/94	< 10 < 10	40 66[d]
Huysmans et al. (1983a)	10	10 or 20 SL	211/134	172/107	10	30
Lacché and Basaglia (1983)	40	20 SL	232/122	168/87	5	30-45
Magometschnigg and Pichler (1981)	7	20 PO	257/157	176/98	10	60
Takekoshi et al. (1981)	3 4 4	5 or 10 PO 3 to 10 SL 5 to 20 EN	241/120 235/128 210/123	155/85 173/101 150/81	nd nd nd	30-60 5-15 30

a Children aged from 8 to 16 years (mean 11.3 years).
b 18 patients with severe asymptomatic hypertension and 6 hypertensive emergencies.
c The second nifedipine dose was administered 20 minutes after the first dose if the response was inadequate.
d i.e. 46 minutes after the second dose.
Abbreviations: PO = oral; SL = sublingual; EN = enema; nd = no details.

daily were effective in 20 Black patients with uncomplicated malignant hypertension (grade 3 or 4 retinopathy and diastolic blood pressure > 120mm Hg). Blood pressure decreased more slowly after atenolol, although the maximum reductions (67/41mm Hg 5 hours after nifedipine and 64/40mm Hg 16 hours after atenolol) were comparable (Isles et al., 1984).

4.1.2 Hypertensive Crisis

Nifedipine 10 to 20mg has been administered by various routes for the rapid reduction of very high blood pressure during hypertensive emergency (table X). Generally, the severity of baseline blood pressure was suitably confirmed over a short period and patients had typical clinical manifestations of the disease, such as hypertensive encephalopathy, intracranial bleeding, unstable angina, acute myocardial infarction, congestive heart failure, severe headache, visual loss, fundal haemorrhage, disturbance of consciousness, or convulsions. Blood pressures were maximally reduced by 39-87/8-62mm Hg. Most authors concluded that nifedipine was a safe and effective drug for treating hypertensive crises and also suggested it is a reasonable first-line choice in this setting. Particular advantages include its rapid effect (significant reductions of blood pressure occurred within 5 to 10 minutes of sublingual administration), its ability to lower blood pressure without inducing hypercorrection, even in patients who had taken various other antihypertensive drugs (Haft et al., 1983; Haft and Litterer, 1984), and the absence of severe side effects. Additionally, several studies in small numbers of patients in hypertensive crisis with associated acute left ventricular failure have demonstrated that sublingual nifedipine 10mg significantly reduced systemic and pulmonary arterial pressures and relieved pulmonary oedema (Bartorelli et al., 1978; Guazzi et al., 1977; Polese et al., 1979). In 3 patients with disturbances of consciousness, nifedipine 10mg administered nasogastrically also caused a rapid reduction of blood pressure (Kuwajima et al., 1978). In each study the acute lowering of blood pressure was associated with a concomitant marked improvement of adverse symptoms. Heart rate was generally slightly increased, although in some studies nifedipine has been reported to reduce heart rate (Erbel et al., 1983; Lacché and Basaglia, 1983).

Nifedipine has also been used for the management of hypertensive emergency in 21 children of mean age 11.3 (range 8 to 16) years (Dilmen et al., 1983). The disease was of variable underlying aetiology although in most cases it was related to some form of renal damage. Sublingual nifedipine 0.25 to 0.5 mg/kg produced a maximal antihypertensive effect after 30 minutes and blood pressure was still significantly ($p < 0.001$) reduced 6 hours after administration. Mean heart rate increased from 108 to 117 beats/min after 30 minutes. Hypotension was not recorded, and facial flushing was observed in only 4 of the children. The data from these studies all seem to emphasise the usefulness of nifedipine in the treatment of acute hypertensive crisis. However, its efficacy relative to alternative first-line drugs such as diazoxide, hydralazine and sodium nitroprusside has not been documented to date.

4.1.3 Hypertension Associated with Pregnancy

Severe hypertension during pregnancy represents a major risk to both the mother and fetus. The drugs most commonly used for the rapid reduction of blood pressure during the gestational period have been parenterally administered diazoxide and hydralazine (Redman, 1980). These 2 drugs have the disadvantage of having to be administered by injection and of producing a high incidence of side effects, which has led to the evaluation of alternative drugs, including nifedipine, in this setting (Walters and Redman, 1984).

In a heterogeneous group of 21 women in an obstetrics department, nifedipine 5 or 10mg orally was used to treat 26 episodes of acute severe hypertension during pregnancy or puerperium. Within 20 minutes blood pressure was significantly reduced by an average of 26/20mm Hg and in those women already taking antihypertensive medications (including methyldopa, β-blockers, or vasodilators) nifedipine did not induce an exaggerated hypotensive effect. Mean pulse rate was only slightly raised after nifedipine in those patients already receiving other antihypertensive drugs, and only 1 patient had a pulse rate > 120 beats/min. The most common side effects were headache and facial flushing. Importantly, no adverse fetal effects were detected. The subsequent course of the pregnancy in these patients treated antenatally was considered consistent with the expectations for a group of women with complicated pregnancies. A preliminary study in 7 women with severe pre-eclampsia unresponsive to atenolol found that addition of nifedipine to their treatment regimen significantly reduced blood pressure ($p < 0.02$) from 175/99mm Hg after 32.6 weeks' gestation to a final reading before delivery of 141/81mm Hg (Rubin et al., 1984). Although laboratory indices of the pre-eclamptic process were not improved by nifedipine, fetal growth continued till birth and all babies were alive up to 1 year of age.

These preliminary results suggest nifedipine may have a place in the management of pregnancy-associated severe hypertension, but further controlled comparisons in larger numbers of women are needed to clarify its overall position.

4.1.4 Hypertension During Coronary Artery Bypass Surgery

Arterial hypertension is encountered in more than one-third of patients undergoing coronary artery bypass surgery (Hess et al., 1984). The intraoperative episodes of hypertension frequently occur after sternotomy and during manipulation of the aortic root, and increase the risk of myocardial ischaemia. In this context, intravenous nifedipine was compared with intravenous nitroprusside for controlling hypertensive episodes in 20 patients undergoing surgery (Hess et al., 1984). If, when moving the sternum or manipulating the aorta, mean arterial pressure increased to 110mm Hg, then 1 of the 2 drugs was infused into a central venous line. The mean dosage of nitroprusside for control of blood pressure was 0.75 (range 0.25 to 1.5) μg/kg/min, while nifedipine was started at a mean dose of 3.4 (range 1.8 to 5.3) μg/kg/min and maintained at a dosage of 1.7 (range 1.3 to 2.3) μg/kg/min. At these dosages both drugs reduced mean arterial pressure to baseline values within about 3 minutes. To achieve a comparable decrease of blood pressure nifedipine produced a more pronounced vasodilation, increased cardiac performance, and slightly (but significantly) increased heart rate. In contrast, nitroprusside did not affect cardiac performance but significantly decreased pulmonary artery, and right and left ventricular filling pressures. These data suggest that nifedipine primarily acts on the arteriolar vessels and does not significantly affect venous tone.

Another trial evaluated the relative efficacy of nifedipine (loading dose 5 μg/kg followed by an infusion of 0.7 μg/kg), verapamil (loading dose 70 μg/kg followed by an infusion of 10 μg/kg), glyceryl trinitrate (infused at 0.7 μg/kg), no additional vasodilator therapy, in 4 groups of 20 patients undergoing coronary artery bypass surgery. The results indicated that nifedipine was a suitable alternative to glyceryl trinitrate for controlling blood pressure during bypass surgery but the authors suggested verapamil should not be recommended because of its negative inotropic activity (Bovill et al., 1984).

4.1.5 Hypertension After Surgery

Following intranasal, sublingual or nasogastric administration of a single 10mg dose of nifedipine to 29 patients with postsurgical hypertension it was found to be a safe and effective drug for the acute lowering of raised blood pressure resulting from surgery (Sodeyama et al., 1983). The time to onset of action was most rapid in the intranasal group (2.1 min) followed by the sublingual group (5.2 min), and was slowest in the group administered the drug nasogastrically (12 min). Other parameters were not significantly different between the 3 groups; blood pressure fell by 26/23%, the effect lasted for 3 to 5 hours, and heart rate was not significantly increased. In 10 patients who underwent haemodynamic testing the reduction in mean arterial pressure (110 to 81mm Hg) was associated with marked decreases in systemic and pulmonary vascular resistances and increases in cardiac index and systemic oxygen transport.

4.1.6 Hypertension in Renal Patients

Hypertension is a considerable risk factor in patients with chronic renal failure and the acute antihypertensive efficacy of nifedipine has occasionally been investigated in this group of patients, particularly those requiring haemodialysis for survival (Eliahou et al., 1982; Garcia López et al., 1984 Kubo et al., 1983; Kusano et al., 1982, 1984). In these single-dose studies nifedipine 10 to 20mg administered orally or sublingually rapidly reduced blood pressure, and maximal decreases were generally noted within 30 to 60 minutes. Antihypertensive activity usually lasted about 3 hours, and in the study of Eliahou et al. (1982) the effects noted in renal patients were similar to those obtained in patients with essential hypertension. Thus, the decrease in blood pressure produced by nifedipine was positively correlated with pretreatment blood pressure in both groups of patients. Garcia López et al.

(1984) treated 3 patients with chronic renal failure (requiring peritoneal dialysis) with nifedipine 10 to 20mg for severe hypertensive crisis. Mean blood pressure dropped from 256/176mm Hg to 156/105mm Hg and nifedipine was extremely effective in all 3 patients. In a small group of patients (n = 9) nifedipine 10mg orally rapidly reduced elevated blood pressure during or following haemodialysis. Its antihypertensive efficacy was greatest in those patients with low cardiac preload which suggests that it may be most useful after dialysis when excess body fluid has been removed (Kubo et al., 1983).

4.2 Medium to Long Term Studies

In addition to its antihypertensive effects following acute administration (section 4.1), oral nifedipine 30 to 100 mg/day has been shown to maintain efficacy in medium term studies (up to 4 weeks) in patients with mild to moderate essential hypertension (Lederballe Pedersen and Mikkelsen, 1978; Masotti et al., 1984; Olivari et al., 1979) and in patients with renal failure (Ambroso et al., 1985; Eliahou et al., 1982; Kusano et al., 1984). As with single-dose administration, the antihypertensive response to continued treatment with nifedipine seems to be positively correlated with the pretreatment severity of hypertension and is also inversely correlated with plasma renin activity (Erne et al., 1983). Preliminary evidence indicates that nifedipine may be particularly beneficial in patients with lower plasma renin activity such as older subjects (for recent reviews see Bühler et al., 1983; Massie et al., 1984; Müller et al., 1984). These effects are similar to those produced by thiazide diuretics and unlike those produced by β-blockers and could, in the future, form the basis for a more rational pathophysiologically oriented method of treating patients with hypertension.

As emphasised earlier, it was only recently that extensive evaluation of the antihypertensive efficacy of nifedipine was initiated and the majority of studies to date fall into 2 main areas: studies comparing nifedipine alone with standard drugs in patients with mild to moderate hypertension, and studies comparing nifedipine plus other antihypertensive drugs with other drug combinations in more severe disease (particularly refractory hypertension). Nifedipine is available for the treatment of hypertension as a conventional capsule and as a sustained release tablet that was introduced in an attempt to improve compliance and decrease the frequency of side effects.

Therapeutic trials using a sustained release tablet formulation of nifedipine have generally shown that twice daily administration (40 to 120 mg/day) provides 24-hour control of blood pressure (Bonaduce et al., 1985; Grampa and Frazetti, 1984; Hornung et al., 1983; Sassano et al., 1983) which is at least as effective as that produced by a conventional capsule preparation (Bayley et al., 1982). Significantly lower blood pressures were observed throughout the day and also during isometric and dynamic exercise testing (Bonaduce et al., 1985; Hornung et al., 1983).

Contrasting with these findings, during a 20-week trial in 20 patients with essential hypertension, even though sustained release nifedipine 20 to 60mg twice daily significantly reduced blood pressure in all patients, 10 of them were withdrawn before completion of the study; 2 did not achieve a target blood pressure of 160/95mm Hg, 7 developed intolerable side effects and 1 patient had a cerebral infarct (Brennan et al., 1983). The authors conclude that the sustained release nifedipine preparation will have a limited role as monotherapy for essential hypertension. However, in comparative (section 4.2.1) and long term (section 4.2.3) trials the sustained release tablet formulation was as efficacious as drugs currently considered first-line choices for the treatment of hypertension, and its antihypertensive properties were maintained for up to 2 years.

4.2.1 Comparisons with Other Antihypertensive Drugs

The majority of comparative trials have been in patients with mild to moderate hypertension (World Health Organization class I to III) and the results of some of the more recent studies are presented in table XI. The trials have been of sufficient duration to evaluate the short to medium term efficacy of nifedipine and have usually been appropriately designed to reduce variation and bias. However, too few patients have generally been included to identify small differences, if they exist, between nifedipine and other active treatments such as other calcium antagonists, β-blockers and diuretics.

Another disadvantage in a large number of trials published to date has been the failure to titrate dosage to that optimal for individual patients. Despite such design problems, the large number of trials performed indicate that nifedipine is an effective antihypertensive drug in patients with mild to moderate hypertension and suggest that it may be a suitable alternative to β-blockers or diuretics as a first-line choice for the management of these patients. Obviously, well-designed long term comparative studies are required to clearly define its overall position amongst the large number of drugs currently available for the treatment of mild to moderate hypertension.

Guazzi et al. (1984a) compared nifedipine 10mg 6 hourly with captopril 25mg 6-hourly for treating 14 patients with severe essential hypertension (diastolic blood pressure > 120mm Hg). Both drugs rapidly reduced blood pressure (< 1 hour) but the magnitude and duration of the antihypertensive effect were greater following nifedipine. Additionally, the 2 drugs were also used together and in this short term trial (7 days) the combination proved to be more effective than either drug used alone. Similar results have recently been reported by MacGregor et al. (1985) in 15 patients with moderate essential hypertension treated with nifedipine and captopril, both separately and in combination.

Other studies have shown that nifedipine produced a greater diminution of elevated blood pressure than prazosin in patients with mild to moderate hypertension (Corea et al., 1981b), and was of similar antihypertensive efficacy as dihydroergotoxine mesylate in elderly patients (> 60 years) [Bellani et al., 1983]. However, in these elderly patients nifedipine more frequently caused side effects.

4.2.2 Nifedipine in Combination with Other Antihypertensive Drugs

Nifedipine is a potent vasodilator that has been successfully combined with various other drugs for the management of hypertension, particularly when the disease has proved to be refractory to conventional drugs such as β-blockers, diuretics, and vasodilators (for recent reviews see Schwartz et al., 1984b; Spivack et al., 1983; Toggart and Zelis, 1982). Since it reduces blood pressure by vasodilation, with an associated reflex stimulation of the sympathetic nervous system which usually results in an increased pulse rate, it is not surprising that nifedipine has been combined with various drugs such as methyldopa (Guazzi et al., 1980), captopril (Guazzi et al., 1984a), clonidine (Imai et al., 1980), mefruside (Lejeune et al., 1984), and various β-blockers (Aoki et al., 1981, 1982; Husted et al., 1982; Imai et al., 1980; Lederballe Pedersen et al., 1980a; Lejeune et al., 1985; Opie et al., 1982a,b; Yagil et al., 1983a), which may help attenuate this effect. Combination treatments including nifedipine have generally been safe and effective, although isolated drug interactions have been documented (see section 8).

Nifedipine (10mg 4 times daily) combined with methyldopa (250mg 4 times daily) in 23 patients with uncomplicated severe hypertension (diastolic blood pressure > 120mm Hg) lowered blood pressure by a greater amount than either drug used alone (Guazzi et al., 1980). The authors recently reported that 17 of these patients have been followed regularly for 3 years and the combination still lowered blood pressure as effectively as it did in the short term trial. Beneficial effects included improvement in fundi (13 cases), reduction in heart size (15 cases) and disappearance of ECG signs of left ventricular strain (15 cases) [Guazzi et al., 1983].

In combination with β-blockers such as propranolol, atenolol, acebutolol, pindolol or timolol, nifedipine has been shown to produce sustained reductions of blood pressure in patients with hypertension (usually severe), but if peripheral oedema was a problem then inclusion of a thiazide diuretic seemed to be of some benefit (Aoki et al., 1981,

Table XI. Some recent clinical trials comparing nifedipine (N) with alternative antihypertensive medications in patients with hypertension

References	No. of patients[a] (nifedipine grp)	Severity of disease	Study design	Duration of treatment (weeks)	Dosage	Reduction of blood pressure (%)[b]			Responders to treatment (%)[c]	Overall efficacy[d]
						supine	sitting	standing		
Comparisons with verapamil (V) and diltiazem (D)										
Erne et al. (1983)	91 (48)	Mild to moderate essential hypertension	o, pg	≈12	N 20 to 40mg SR bid V 240 to 720mg SR/day		16/19 11/14		85 60	N ⩾ V
Gould et al. (1983)	25 (9)	Essential hypertension DBP > 95mm Hg	o, pg	⩾6	N 20 to 60mg bid V 120 to 160mg tid	19/19 18/22		21/16 21/22		N ≡ V
Klein et al. (1983)	47 (24)	Mild to moderate essential hypertension	r, db, pg, pcri	8 8	N 30 to 60 mg/day D 180 to 270 mg/day		11/13 12/13		80[e] 80[e]	N ≡ D
Midtbø et al. (1982)	26	Mild to moderate essential hypertension	r, db, co	6 6	N 20mg SR bid V 80mg tid		11/13[f] 14/19[f]		54 81	N < V
Muiesan et al. (1982)	40 (12)	Mild to moderate essential hypertension	o, pg	8 16 8	N 10mg tid V 80mg tid V 160mg tid	11/12 13/10 25/20		9/14 11/11 25/20		N 10mg ≡ V 80mg
Schulte et al. (1984)	34 (nd)	Mild to moderate essential hypertension	r, db, pg, pcri	8 8	N 40 to 60mg SR/day D 180 to 270mg SR/day	12/16 11/13				N ≡ D
Comparisons with the β-adrenergic blocking drugs; acebutolol (A), metoprolol (M) and pindolol (P)										
De Divitiis et al. (1984)	15	Moderate hypertension DBP ⩾ 110mm Hg	r, db, co, pcri	4 4 4	N 10mg tid A 200mg tid N + A combined	11/12[g] 16/13[g] 24/22[g]		15/11[g] 16/12[g] 23/22[g]	27 33 60	N ≡ A N < N + A > A
Eggertsen and Hansson (1982)	22 (nd)	Essential hypertension	r, db, pg, pcri	12 12	N 10mg tid M 100mg bid	6/9 13/14				N ⩽ M
Tsukiyama et al. (1984)	25 (12)	Essential hypertension	o, pg	6 6	N 10 to 30mg bid P 5 to 10mg bid		14/14 9/10		50[e] 23[e]	N ⩾ P

Comparisons with mefruside (Mef) and bendrofluazide (bendroflumethiazide, B)								
Douglas-Jones and Mitchell (1984)	20	Mild to moderate hypertension	r, db, co, pcri, pcwo	8	N 20mg SR bid	13/13	13/9	N ≡ Mef
				8	Mef 25 mg/day	12/12	14/10	
Rosenthal (1983)	30 (10)	Mild to moderate essential hypertension	r, db, pg, pcri	4	N 20mg bid	13/18	13/18	N ≡ Mef
				4	Mef 25mg bid	12/16	12/15	≡ N + Mef
				4	N + Mef combined	13/16	14/18	
Hallin et al. (1983)	30 (nd)	Mild to moderate hypertension	r, db, pg, pcri	24	N 20mg bid	10/10	7/5	N ≡ B
				24	B 2.5mg bid	9/10	8/10	N < N + B
				24	N + B combined	14/12	11/11	> B

a Number of patients who completed the trial.
b Reduction in systolic/diastolic blood pressure at the end of each treatment, as compared with pretreatment values.
c Diastolic blood pressure ≤ 95mm Hg.
d In terms of antihypertensive efficacy.
e Blood pressure for responders not stated.
f Mean of supine, sitting and standing blood pressures.
g Approximate values extrapolated from a graphical presentation.
Abbreviations: r = randomised; db = double-blind; o = open; pg = parallel groups; co = crossover; pcri = placebo-controlled run-in; pcwo = placebo-controlled washout; nd = no details; N ≡ = equivalent to nifedipine; N > = nifedipine produced superior response; N ≥ = a trend in favour of nifedipine; bid = twice daily; tid = 3 times daily; SR = sustained release preparation; ≈ = approximately.

1982; Franz and Wiewel, 1984; Husted et al., 1982; Imai et al., 1980; Yagil et al., 1983a). Lejeune et al. (1985) recently demonstrated that a fixed combination of nifedipine 10mg plus acebutolol 100mg was as effective and safe as nifedipine 20mg monotherapy (both regimens administered once or twice daily) in 116 patients with essential hypertension. Antihypertensive effects were maintained over a 24-hour period and after physical exercise. In some trials that included patients with angina and associated hypertension the combination of nifedipine with a β-blocker gave improved blood pressure control but did not induce consistent significant improvement of anginal symptoms compared with β-blockade alone (Opie et al., 1982a,b).

Refractory Hypertension

Nifedipine has also been used in a number of studies as a third- or fourth-line choice for reducing blood pressure which is still considered high (diastolic blood pressure usually > 95 to 105mm Hg), despite intensive treatment with various other antihypertensive drugs (table XII). The results from all these trials, which have been up to a year in duration, indicate that nifedipine is a useful adjunct for the control of blood pressure refractory to conventional treatment.

A retrospective survey of 122 patients with resistant hypertension treated with nifedipine and an equivalent group of 102 patients treated with hydralazine (for up to 2 years) demonstrated that nifedipine 40 mg/day was of comparable antihypertensive efficacy and produced a similar side effect profile as hydralazine 86 mg/day (Murphy et al., 1984). Furthermore, in an 8-week multicentre study of 179 patients with severe hypertension (diastolic blood pressure ≥ 105mm Hg despite 2 drug therapy) there is evidence that nifedipine (30 to 80 mg/day) was a more effective third-line choice than hydralazine (75 to 200 mg/day), as assessed by antihypertensive efficacy and subjective improvement (Ueda and Murakami, 1983). In a small group of patients with refractory hypertension associated with congestive heart failure, addition of nifedipine to their treatment resulted in a marked re-

Table XII. Summary of some recent clinical trials using nifedipine (N) in combination with other antihypertensive drugs in patients with refractory hypertension

References	No. of patients[a]	Previous therapy[b]	Drug combination under evaluation	Nifedipine dosage (mg/day)	Duration of treatment	Supine blood pressure (mm Hg)		Responders to treatment[c] (%)
						pre-nifedipine	post-nifedipine	
Arguedas and Fuchs (1984)	5	S, D, V	B, D, N	30-90	15-90 days	DBP > 105	≤ 160/95	100
Bayley et al. (1982)	42	B or M, D	N added[d]	20-60	ND	165/106	141/97	
Brennan and Blake (1982)	21	B, D, and 1 other drug[e]	B, D, N	30-100	Up to 6 months	176/107[f]	143/88	86
Bursztyn et al. (1984)	19[g]	B, D, V	B, D, N	40-80 SR	Up to 6 months	195/114[h]	144/82[h]	100
Dean and Kendall (1983)	20	B, D, V	B, D, N	30-90	At least 1 year	173/104	148/93	85
Evans et al. (1984)	10	B, D, V, or C	V stopped; N started	20-100	3-8 weeks	194/111	145/85	80
Given et al. (1985)	8[i]	Various B, D, V	Various + N	40-120	Mean 16 weeks	222/116	143/77	75
Mimran and Ribstein (1985)	12	Ca or E, D	N added[d]	40-80 SR	Mean 2.6 months	172/111	133/85	
Murphy et al. (1983a)	15	B, D	B, D, N	30 60 90	2 weeks 2 weeks 2 weeks	155/97	144/91 142/88 132/81	93
Sloan and Beevers (1983)	10	B, D	B, D, N	30-40	Mean 5.7 months	180/108[j]	142/93[j]	60
	10	B, D, V	B, D, V, N	30-40	Mean 3.7 months	214/118[j]	177/102[j]	60

a Number entering the study.
b Which did not adequately control BP.
c In terms of adequate control of BP and who did not have to withdraw from the study because of adverse reactions.
d Nifedipine added to previous therapy.
e 15 patients were taking B and D while 6 patients failed to respond even with the addition of a third drug.
f Position for measuring BP not stated.
g 15 with uncontrolled BP and 4 with intolerable side effects.
h Approximate values derived from a bar graph.
i Patients with congestive heart failure and refractory hypertension.
j BP measured in the seated position.

Abbreviations: S = sympathetic blocking drug; D = diuretic; V = vasodilator; B = β-blocker; M = methyldopa; C = clonidine; Ca = captopril, E = enalapril, DBP = diastolic blood pressure; ND = no details; SR = sustained release.

duction of blood pressure in 6 of the 8 patients and the signs and symptoms of heart failure were greatly improved (Given et al., 1985).

4.2.3 Long Term Trials

Although only a limited number of patients have been evaluated during long term treatment (for about 12 months or more) with nifedipine, all the trials confirm that the antihypertensive properties of the calcium antagonist are maintained (Ambroso et al., 1985; Dean and Kendall, 1983; Englert, 1984; Guazzi et al., 1983; Landmark, 1985;

Maeda et al., 1982; Robinson, 1983; Ueda et al., 1984). In the majority of cases it has been used for multiple drug management of moderate to severe hypertension. Some of the authors report that nifedipine has been used for periods in excess of 3 to 4 years and that the initial blood pressure-lowering response was continued (Guazzi et al., 1983; Maeda et al., 1982; Robinson, 1983). In the study of Guazzi et al. (1983) brief interruptions in nifedipine therapy at 2, 8 and 24 months invariably caused blood pressure to rise, which suggests tolerance to the antihypertensive activity of nifedipine is not a problem. Side effects usually occurred during the initial phase of treatment and subsided with longer term use. However, ankle oedema is reported to be a common problem with nifedipine usage, occurring in as many as 20% of treated patients (Guazzi et al., 1983).

Sustained release nifedipine administered for 2 years to a small group of patients with mild to moderate hypertension significantly reduced mean blood pressure from a baseline value of 195/103mm Hg to 165/86mm Hg, 165/82mm Hg, and 157/81mm Hg after 4, 12 and 24 months of therapy, respectively (Englert, 1984). Landmark (1985) reported similar reductions of blood pressure in 16 men with mild to moderate essential hypertension given sustained release nifedipine 20mg twice daily for 48 weeks.

5. Other Therapeutic Uses

Apart from the abundance of data derived from treating patients with ischaemic heart disease and/or hypertension, there are also some data available, albeit very limited, resulting from clinical experience with nifedipine in patients with other diseases such as congestive heart failure, hypertrophic cardiomyopathy, pulmonary hypertension and Raynaud's phenomenon. In none of these areas is it possible to make categorical statements regarding the relative efficacy of nifedipine. However, in those diseases where previous therapeutic intervention has been particularly disappointing (pulmonary hypertension, Raynaud's phenomenon), nifedipine has produced sustained benefit in a small number of patients treated. Although these improvements do not seem overly impressive they are at least as useful as those produced by other drugs currently available, and nifedipine would seem worth a trial in patients with these disorders, especially if other treatments have failed. Obviously, further well-designed studies are essential to evaluate the efficacy of nifedipine in these therapeutic areas and to identify those patients likely to respond to the calcium antagonist.

5.1 Congestive Heart Failure

Congestive heart failure is a clinical syndrome with many underlying causes all of which result in the heart failing to maintain an adequate output, the major consequences of which are diminished blood flow to the tissues and congestion in the pulmonary and/or systemic circulation. As discussed in section 1.2, nifedipine has negative inotropic properties and there is real concern that a reduction in contractility may precipitate further decompensation in an already failing ventricle (for recent reviews see Charlap and Frishman, 1984; Colucci et al., 1985). However, in the limited number of trials published to date this has not been a serious problem since the potent vasodilatory properties of the calcium antagonist seem to have offset its negative inotropic effects, thus resulting in an increase in cardiac output (Packer, 1983; Toggart and Zelis, 1982).

Apart from the acute haemodynamic studies discussed in section 1.2 there have been few published clinical trials with nifedipine in patients with congestive heart failure. Those that have been reported involved small numbers of patients treated for short periods (Bellocci et al., 1982; Camerini et al., 1983; Corea et al., 1983, 1984; Guazzi et al., 1984). Thus, Camerini et al. (1983) compared nifedipine 80 mg/day with placebo in 8 patients with congestive cardiomyopathy and chronic heart failure who had previously responded during acute haemodynamic testing with the calcium antagonist. The study was designed as a randomised double-blind crossover trial with exercise tests performed at the end of each 3-week period. Six patients considered placebo to be more effective than nifedipine and the authors reported that active treatment did not seem to increase exercise tolerance or symptomatic improvement during long term administration. In contrast, in an open trial Moriyama et al. (1983) found nifedipine 10mg 3 times daily to be particularly beneficial during long term (1 month) treatment of patients with severe refractory heart failure associated with myocardial disease.

Corea et al. (1983) compared nifedipine 10mg 3 times daily with captopril 75mg 3 times daily in a randomised 2-week crossover trial in 12 patients with severe chronic congestive heart failure refractory to conventional therapy. Both drugs produced a similar decrease in peripheral vascular resistance associated with a marked increase in cardiac output. However, stroke index and ejection fraction were significantly higher ($p < 0.01$) on captopril. The different haemodynamic and humoral responses produced by the 2 drugs led the authors to conclude that, while nifedipine may be preferable for obtaining a very rapid haemodynamic improvement, captopril may prove to be the more beneficial during long term treatment because an increase in cardiac output is achieved at a lower heart rate and lower plasma noradrenaline concentration.

Recently, Guazzi et al. (1984b) compared the medium term (1 month) efficacy of nifedipine 20mg 4 times daily with that of verapamil 160mg 3 times daily in 29 patients with grade II to IV [New York Heart Association (NYHA)] hypertensive heart disease. Nifedipine persistently reduced systemic vascular resistance, mean arterial pressure, mean pulmonary wedge pressure and left ventricular diastolic diameter, and improved cardiac index and circumferential fibre shortening velocity. Mean NYHA classification decreased from 3.67 to 2.00 and all the patients had relief from dyspnoea and a reduction of heart size. Although verapamil reduced systemic vascular resistance and mean arterial pressure it did not have a significant effect on pulmonary wedge pressure, left ventricular diastolic diameter or fibre shortening velocity and it did not improve the clinical symptoms of the disease. These results indicate that nifedipine is significantly superior to verapamil in the failing enlarged hypertensive heart and further investigations are warranted to clearly define its place in therapy in patients with heart failure.

5.2 Hypertrophic Cardiomyopathy

Hypertrophic cardiomyopathy is a familial disease of low prevalence and low mortality (2 to 3% per year), and is characterised by cellular hypertrophy in the intraventricular septum, left ventricular free wall or right ventricle, either separately or combined (for recent reviews see Lorrell, 1985; Toggart and Zelis, 1982). As noted by these authors, haemodynamic studies have shown a wide spectrum of disease activity from large intraventricular pressure gradients, associated with outflow obstruction, to isolated angiographic disturbances without pressure gradients. Traditionally, medical treatment has consisted of β-blockers (to reduce heart rate and contractility and to prolong ventricular filling time) or surgical resection of hypertrophied myocardial tissue. Neither of these modes of therapy has been entirely successful; the mortality rate from surgery appears to be quite high (8 to 10%) and β-blockers, although reducing the symptomatology of the disease, have not made any major impact on the progress of cardiomyopathy or on the incidence of sudden death.

Clinical trials with nifedipine in hypertrophic cardiomyopathy have been extremely limited in terms of the small numbers of patients studied over short periods. A number of case reports have shown that nifedipine can have both beneficial (Katzenburg et al., 1982; Lee et al., 1983; Serfas et al., 1983) and deleterious (Katzenburg et al., 1982) effects in patients with hypertrophic cardiomyopathy. Two case reports have demonstrated that nifedipine 0.6 mg/kg/day (increased gradually to 0.9 mg/kg/day) produced immediate and sustained (up to 6 months) symptomatic improvement in neonates with hypertrophic cardiomyopathy (Dickinson et al., 1985). Although only limited objective evidence was available, the observed improvements in these infants (aged 3 weeks and 1 year) was encouraging, and nifedipine warrants further evaluation in this condition which normally has a poor prognosis. Acute haemodynamic evaluation of 6 patients with obstructive disease showed that nifedipine 3mg administered intravenously not only decreased outflow obstruction in 3 patients with intraventricular pressure gradients but also increased mean cardiac index (from 3.0 to 3.8 L/min/m^2) and mean oxygen saturation in the coronary sinus (from 29 to 54%) [Schanzenbächer et al., 1982].

In a randomised double-blind crossover comparison between nifedipine (mean dose 41 mg/day) and placebo in 11 patients with non-obstructive hypertrophic cardiomyopathy, long term treatment (4 weeks) with the calcium antagonist improved the functional status of 7 patients, produced no change in 2 and caused left ventricular failure in the remaining 2 (Ruddy et al., 1982). The final 2 patients could be identified by a previous history of biventricular failure and a lower peak ejection fraction after nifedipine. The improvement noted in 64% of the group is encouraging but was associated with a high incidence of side effects, which may limit the usefulness of nifedipine in this clinical setting.

A preliminary report of the long term (up to 30 months) therapeutic effects of β-blockers and calcium antagonists in 16 patients with hypertrophic cardiomyopathy did not reach any clearcut conclusions (Koide et al., 1981). At some stage during the study 11 patients were treated with a β-blocker, 13 with nifedipine and 4 with verapamil. Eight of the 16 patients were symptomatic at the start of the trial and there was an improvement in 50% of those receiving a β-blocker and in 33% receiving a calcium antagonist. However, those patients administered nifedipine or verapamil developed improved control of angina.

Recently, Strauer et al. (1984) demonstrated that long term treatment (mean 3.9 months) with large doses of nifedipine (mean 120 mg/day) improved left ventricular function and reduced established ventricular wall hypertrophy in small numbers of patients with hypertrophic non-obstructive cardiomyopathy and hypertensive heart disease.

5.3 Pulmonary Hypertension

Primary idiopathic pulmonary hypertension is a rare disease of unknown aetiology characterised by extreme increases in pulmonary artery pressure and pulmonary vascular resistance which can progress to right ventricular failure and ultimately death (Camerini et al., 1980; Rubin et al., 1983). Pulmonary hypertension can also occur as a secondary event, particularly in chronic obstructive pulmonary diseases such as cor pulmonale and hypoxia-induced pulmonary vasospasm (Kennedy et al., 1985; Toggart and Zelis, 1982). The finding of pulmonary arteriolar medial hypertrophy and muscular hyperplasia, suggestive of some degree of vasoconstriction, has been the premise for initiating treatment with various potent vasodilators – apparently with limited success (Rubin et al., 1983). Much of the early data relating to the use of nifedipine in patients with pulmonary hypertension comes from single-dose studies (El Allaf et al., 1982; Fisher et al., 1982) or case reports (Camerini et al., 1980; De Feyter et al., 1983; Lunde and Rasmussen, 1984; Ocken et al., 1983; Saito et al., 1983). Individual case reports in patients with mild to severe grades of the disease have recorded sustained periods (3 months to 2 years) of haemodynamic improvement (reduced pulmonary artery pressure and pulmonary vascular resistance) using dosages of 30 to 120 mg/day. It has been suggested that acute haemodynamic response is a useful indicator for identifying those patients likely to respond to long term treatment (Rozkovec et al., 1982). Apart from the above encouraging case reports, other clinicians have employed nifedipine with fatal consequences (Dalal et al., 1981; Farber et al., 1983) and these serve to highlight the difficulties encountered in treating patients with pulmonary hypertension.

Published studies in groups of patients with pulmonary hypertension have also been extremely limited in terms of the actual numbers included and the duration of treatment. Thus, in the trials of Fisher et al. (1983), McKenzie et al. (1983) and McLeod et al. (1981), a total of 34 patients with pulmonary hypertension (18 primary, 16 secondary) underwent acute haemodynamic evaluation with nifedipine, but only 10 (7 primary, 3 secondary) showed sustained symptomatic or haemodynamic benefit. Fisher et al. (1983) noted that the 4 responders in their study all had Raynaud's phenomenon, and they suggested that this may be a specific indicator for those patients with pulmonary vasospasm. In the most comprehensively reported trial to date, Rubin et al. (1983) evaluated the single-dose and long term effects of nifedipine in 9 patients with primary pulmonary hypertension. Single-dose sublingual nifedipine 10 to 20mg increased cardiac output (from 3.6 to 5.3 L/min) and reduced pulmonary vascular resistance (from 1605 to 1025 dyne • sec • cm^{-5}) but did not significantly reduce pulmonary arterial pressure. During long term treatment (4 to 14 months) with nifedipine 40 to 120 mg/day, haemodynamic improvement was maintained in 5 of the 6 patients.

Many of the authors who have studied patients with pulmonary hypertension, a disease with a poor prognosis, suggest that nifedipine should be considered as a potentially useful drug for the initial treatment of this condition. These conclusions must be tempered in light of the fatalities that have occurred and the minority of patients who have gained long term benefit. Preliminary acute haemodynamic evaluation of the effects of nifedipine in individual patients would seem to be obligatory if long term treatment is to be considered. Furthermore, careful monitoring and re-evaluation of patients is desirable to limit the incidence of morbid events and to check that the improved haemodynamic response is maintained.

5.4 Raynaud's Phenomenon

Raynaud's phenomenon is a peripheral vascular disorder characterised by intermittent attacks of vasospasm in the digital arteries which are frequently precipitated by exposure to cold or emotional stress. The vasospastic attacks usually result in blanching or cyanosis of the digits which is associated with numbness, tingling or burning and may last for minutes to hours. Raynaud's phenomenon is often idiopathic (Raynaud's disease) or can be secondary to various other conditions, particularly connective tissue disorders such as systemic sclerosis and systemic lupus erythematosus (Kahan et al., 1983c). In patients with long-standing disease, painful areas of ulceration or even gangrene may appear on the tips of the digits, although these occur less frequently in patients with idiopathic Raynaud's syndrome. Therapy of secondary forms of the disease depend on the recognition of the underlying disturbance but, as noted recently, treatment of primary and secondary peripheral vasospastic disease has generally been disappointing (Sarkozi et al., 1984b; Winston et al., 1983).

Since there appears to be no proven reliable technique for evaluating the severity of the symptoms associated with Raynaud's phenomenon, subjective assessment of changes in the frequency and severity of attacks, as recorded on patient symptom diary cards, has been the most extensively used method. Where objective methods of measurement have been used (usually digital blood pressure, blood flow or temperature response to cold provocation) they have generally failed to correlate with reported subjective improvement (Bravard and Moore, 1983; Douglas Smith and McKendry, 1982; Ettinger et al., 1984; Rodeheffer et al., 1983; Sarkozi et al., 1984a), although some studies in small numbers of patients have noted marked improvement in objective parameters (Kahan et al., 1983c; Myers et al., 1984; Nilsson et al., 1984; White et al., 1984).

5.4.1 Controlled Comparisons with Placebo

Because of the heterogeneous nature of most patient groups, the major influence of variables such as environmental temperature and emotional stress, and the lack of well defined objective criteria for assessment, clinical trials in patients with Raynaud's phenomenon are fraught with problems and are difficult to analyse. To minimise the influence of many of these factors the majority of clinical trials with nifedipine have been randomised double-blind crossover comparisons with placebo. The effects of environmental temperature are more problematical, since other factors (such as how often patients go out into the cold and for how long) are

Table XIII. Summary of some randomised double-blind clinical trials in which nifedipine (N) was compared with placebo (P) in patients with Raynaud's phenomenon (RP) of varying aetiology

References	No. of patients[a] (study design)	Patient diagnosis	Nifedipine dosage	Duration of treatment[b] (weeks)	Parameters measured	Overall efficacy and comments
Bravard and Moore (1983)	5 (co)	Systemic sclerosis	10mg tid	3	Patient preference, no. of attacks, cold provocation test	N ≡ P; 3 patients preferred N while the other 2 found no difference
Douglas Smith and McKendry (1982)	17 (co)	Moderate to severe RP of varying aetiology	10 mg qid	2	Diary card for no. and severity of attacks, skin temperature recovery to cold provocation	N > P with respect to subjective assessment but there was no difference in skin temperature recovery times
Ettinger et al. (1984)	19 (co)	RP of varying aetiology	20mg tid	2	Diary card for no. and severity of attacks, digital BP	N ≥ P regarding subjective improvement
Hawkins et al. (1984)	57 (co)	RP of varying aetiology	10mg qid	6	No. and severity of attacks, and effects on cellular function	N > P and seemed more effective in patients with depressed cellular function
Kahan et al. (1983c)	16 (co)	RP of varying aetiology	20mg	Single-dose	Cold provocation test	N > P effective protection in 14/16 patients
	30 (co)	RP of varying aetiology	20mg tid	1	No. of attacks	N > P and seemed to be more effective in patients with idiopathic disease
Myers et al. (1984)	6 (co)	RP[c]	10mg tid	3	Digital artery blood flw before and after cold provocation tests	N > P in 5/6 patients
Rodeheffer et al. (1983)	15 (co)	RP of varying aetiology	10-20mg tid	2	Diary card for vasospastic attacks, digital BP	N > P with respect to subjective improvement, particularly in patients with idiopathic disease
Sarkozi et al. (1984a)	39 (pg)	Idiopathic RP	10-20mg tid	10	Diary card for no. of attacks, photoplethysmography	N > P with respect to subjective improvement during the first 5 weeks of treatment
Sauza et al. (1984)	18 (pg)	RP of varying aetiology	30-60 mg/day	10	Diary card for no. and severity of attacks	N > P regarding reduction in the no. of attacks for the duration of the trial
Winston et al. (1983)	8 (co)	RP of varying aetiology	10-20mg qid	At least 3	No. and severity of vasospastic attacks	N > P regarding reduction in the no. of attacks and 4/5 had digital ulcer healing

a Number of patients who completed the trial.
b Duration of treatment of each phase if a crossover study.
c No further information regarding the patients admitted.
Abbreviations: co = crossover; pg = parallel groups; tid = 3 times daily; qid = 4 times daily; ≡ = equivalent to; N > = significant difference in favour of N; N ≥ = trend in favour of N; BP = blood pressure.

further variables that can influence the results obtained.

Taking into account any limitations imposed by the above, and also the less than satisfactory improvements achieved with various other treatments (see Douglas Smith and McKendry, 1982), the results from clinical trials with nifedipine in patients with Raynaud's phenomenon published to date (table XIII) must make it a rational first-line choice, especially if other therapies have failed. In these trials, nifedipine 30 to 80 mg/day usually produced a marked subjective improvement (reduced number, duration and severity of attacks of vasospasm) in 60 to 100% of patients for periods up to 10 weeks. There is some evidence that those patients with idiopathic disease have a better response to nifedipine than do patients with an underlying systemic disease (Kahan et al., 1983c; Lindsey et al., 1985; Rodeheffer et al., 1983). Indeed, Lindsey et al. (1985) reported no significant subjective improvement during treatment with nifedipine 20mg 3 times daily in 18 patients with Raynaud's phenomenon secondary to systemic sclerosis. Furthermore, nifedipine decreased peripheral blood flow and increased peripheral vascular resistance and these changes are potentially deleterious if they were to be sustained. A recent trial conducted by Hawkins et al. (1984) in 57 patients with severe Raynaud's phenomenon found that subjective improvement was significantly greater with nifedipine than with placebo ($p < 0.001$). However, the response to nifedipine was variable with the most benefit being experienced by a subgroup of 21 patients (number of vasospastic attacks fell by more than 70%) in whom nifedipine caused the greatest suppression of cellular function (as estimated by lymphocyte proliferation and neutrophil function).

5.4.2 Other Studies

In addition to the placebo-controlled trials described in section 5.4.1, nifedipine has been evaluated in various other trials in patients with Raynaud's phenomenon. Nilsson et al. (1984) found nifedipine to be a useful agent for reducing cold-induced digital vasospasm, and the degree of reduction was dose dependent (20mg 3 times daily for 2 weeks producing a significantly greater increase in digital blood pressure than 10mg 3 times daily). Other workers have reported that nifedipine may be useful in healing cutaneous ulceration in patients with progressive systemic sclerosis and severe Raynaud's phenomenon, although only small numbers of patients have been treated to date (Jaffe, 1982; Kahan et al., 1983a; Woo et al., 1984). Similarly, there is preliminary evidence that nifedipine is effective in reducing the frequency and severity of migraine when associated with Raynaud's phenomenon (Kahan et al., 1983b).

The results of a long term (average of 3 months) open trial with nifedipine 10mg 3 times daily were similarly positive to those of a controlled short term study with nifedipine 20mg 3 times daily in the same 30 patients with Raynaud's phenomenon, although 7 patients discontinued treatment because of side effects (Kahan et al., 1983c). The authors recently reported that many of the patients have since been treated with nifedipine (30 to 80 mg/day) for greater than 2 years with good therapeutic results (Kahan et al., 1984a). Sarkozi et al. (1984b) also noted that nifedipine can be efficacious with long term use (28 months) in a case report of a patient with rheumatoid arthritis with severe Raynaud's phenomenon associated with mixed connective tissue disease. In this patient, nifedipine reduced the incidence of vasospastic episodes and apparently facilitated healing of digital ulceration.

In a prospective double-blind crossover trial in 15 patients with Raynaud's phenomenon, each patient was treated with nifedipine 20mg 3 times daily for 1 week, prazosin 1mg 3 times daily for 1 week and placebo for 2 weeks in randomised order (Kahan et al., 1984b). Nifedipine produced the greatest protection against Raynaud's phenomenon by significantly reducing the number and severity of vasospastic attacks.

6. Side Effects

Analysis of composite studies of nifedipine usage worldwide has shown an overall incidence of side effects of about 20% (Lewis, 1983). These side ef-

Table XIV. Incidence (%) of the most common categories of adverse experiences in patients receiving nifedipine (after Ebner and Donath, 1980 and Terry, 1982) [CHF = congestive heart failure]

Adverse experience	Ebner and Donath (1980) [n = 4863]	Terry (1982)			
		total population [n = 3081]	CHF as concomitant diagnosis [n = 233]	concomitant β-blocker therapy [n = 1431]	long term therapy (≥ 6 months) [n = 795]
Headache	7.2	7.1	8.2	6.8	7.2
Facial flush, burning, heat sensitivity, numbness, reddening, tingling	5.3	7.4	5.2	5.7	9.4
Dizziness, giddiness, light-headedness	3.1	12.1	15.5	10.6	16.5
Gastrointestinal symptoms (nausea, vomiting, heartburn, dyspepsia)	5.2	7.5	8.2	8.0	9.3
Oedema, swelling, fluid retention	0.6	7.7	10.3	8.2	11.6

fects, which are generally extensions of the vasodilating effects of nifedipine, can be alleviated by either decreasing the nifedipine dose or by combining the drug with a β-blocker. Although most studies investigating the side effects of nifedipine have utilised oral or sublingual dosage forms, intravenous and intracoronary preparations have also been given. Side effects from nifedipine increase with increasing dosage (Covinsky and Hamburger, 1983); thus, the slower release of nifedipine from oral tablet formulations may minimise those side effects which are related to higher plasma concentrations (section 2.5).

An analysis of overall nifedipine side effects was presented by Ebner and Donath (1980) based on 4863 patients (table XIV). It was shown that side effects usually occurred within the first 14 days of treatment, with the vasodilating effects being dose related. Similarly, Terry (1982) tabulated side effect data from over 3000 patients and further divided them into 3 subsets. It can be seen from the table that the most frequent side effects from nifedipine use are headache (7.1-7.2%), flushing (5.3-7.4%), dizziness (3.1-12.1%), gastrointestinal symptoms (5.2-7.5%) and fluid retention and oedema (0.6-7.7%), particularly in the lower leg.

Terry (1982) also evaluated side effects related to cardiovascular function (table XV). Although the side effects of congestive heart failure or pulmonary oedema, preinfarction angina and myocardial infarction occurred slightly more frequently in the patients with a pretreatment diagnosis of congestive heart failure, the occurrence of congestive heart failure due to concomitant nifedipine and β-blockade was no higher than that of the total study population. Thus, the concomitant administration of nifedipine and β-blockers would appear to place the patient at no greater risk than nifedipine therapy alone. The incidence of hypotension appears to be dose related, occurring in 2.2 and 5% of patients receiving less than 60mg or greater than 120mg of nifedipine per day, respectively. In those patients on concurrent β-blockers, 2.3% of patients on nifedipine 60mg or less and 4.5% of those receiving nifedipine 120mg or more daily experienced hypotension.

Stone et al. (1983b) reviewed 716 cases of patients with refractory angina pectoris and noted that 100 (14%) of them experienced an increase in angina frequency during treatment with nifedipine. However, an exacerbation of anginal symptoms was more common in patients with classic exertional

Table XV. Incidence of cardiovascular side effects due to nifedipine [after Terry (1982) with permission]

Side effect	All patients[a] (n = 3081)	CHF as concomitant diagnosis[a] (n = 233)	Concomitant β-blocker therapy[a] (n = 1431)	Long term therapy[a] (≥ 6 months) (n = 795)
Hypotension	3.4	3.9	4.0	5.5
Preinfarction angina or MI	3.2	7.3	3.3	1.3
CHF or pulmonary oedema	1.3	5.2	1.3	0.9
Angina	1.2	0.9	1.3	1.5
TIA or CVA	0.3	0.4	0.2	0.4
Conduction disturbances	0.2	0	0.1	0.1
Syncope	0.2	0	0.07	0.4
Atrial arrhythmias	0.1	0	0.2	0.3
Ventricular tachycardia or arrest	0.1	0	0.1	0
Other ventricular arrhythmias	0.2	0	0.1	0.5

a Entries are patient incidences (percentage of patients demonstrating an adverse experience in the category at some time during treatment with nifedipine), as judged by the investigator.
Abbreviations: MI = myocardial infarction; CHF = congestive heart failure; TIA = transient ischaemic attack; CVA = cerebrovascular accident.

angina (29% of 35 patients) than in patients with either mixed angina (13% of 292 patients) or in patients with Prinzmetal's angina (14% of 389 patients). Paradoxical worsening of cardiac ischaemia due to nifedipine administration has also been described in several case reports of high risk patients (Abinader and Shahar, 1983; Boden et al., 1985; Jariwalla and Anderson, 1978; Itoh et al., 1975; Keidar et al., 1979; Manga and Vythilingum, 1984; Mysliwiec et al., 1983; Robson and Vishwanath, 1982; Rodger and Stewart, 1978; Schanzenbächer et al., 1984; Sia et al., 1985; Yokoyama et al., 1982), where the manifestations included chest pain accompanied by tachycardia with and without electrocardiographic changes. In addition, electrocardiographic changes without accompanying cardiac pain have been reported (Yagil et al., 1982). Similarly, the abrupt cessation of nifedipine in patients with stable, unstable or vasospastic angina has also precipitated coronary artery spasm or electrocardiographic changes with associated chest pain (Engelman et al., 1984; Kay et al., 1982; Lette et al., 1984; Strickland et al., 1982), but the occurrence of a true 'withdrawal syndrome' has been rejected by many authors (Bühler, 1983; Deanfield et al., 1983a; Guazzi et al., 1980; Nehring and Camm, 1983).

During the course of long term (≥ 6 months) treatment with nifedipine, the character, severity and incidence of specific side effects is similar to those experienced during shorter courses of therapy (Terry, 1982) [tables XIV and XV].

Other potentially serious side effects – the relationship to nifedipine of which has not always been clearly established – have been reported in a very few patients including the effect of nifedipine on glucose metabolism (section 1.8), its interactions with other drugs (section 8), allergic hepatitis and abnormal liver function tests (Abramson and Littlejohn, 1985; Davidson, 1980; Rotmensch et al.,

1980), rash (Ginsburg et al., 1982; Grunwald, 1982; Scoble et al., 1984), muscle cramps (Keidar et al., 1982; Macdonald, 1982), immune complex glomerulonephritis or nephrotic syndrome (Hall-Craggs et al., 1984; Scoble et al., 1984), acute reversible deteriorations in renal function in patients with chronic renal insufficiency (Diamond et al., 1984), acute psychosis (Ahmad, 1984a), increased asthmatic symptoms after cessation of therapy in patients with chronic obstructive lung disease (Eliraz et al., 1984; section 1.10.3) and cerebral and retinal ischaemia (Nobile-Orazio and Sterzi, 1981; Pitlik et al., 1983). Gum alterations (gingival hyperplasia) may occur in extremely rare cases during long term treatment; these regress completely after the treatment has stopped (Lederman et al., 1984; Ramon et al., 1984; Van der Wall et al., 1984).

The reported frequency with which side effects, most commonly those related to vasodilatation (dizziness, flushing and headache), require discontinuation of nifedipine has been reported to be 2 to 6% (Ebner and Donath, 1980; Gerstenblith et al., 1982; Pfisterer et al., 1982; Terry, 1982).

7. Dosage and Administration

For the prophylactic management of the various forms of angina and for the treatment of hypertension, the recommended starting dosage of nifedipine capsules is 10mg 3 times daily during or after meals. Dosage should then be carefully titrated to produce an optimal response; a 5mg capsule is available for this purpose. Typically, the usual optimal dosage is between 30 and 90 mg/day but, where required, this may be gradually increased to six 20mg capsules per day. An interval of at least 2 hours should be allowed between each individual dose of 20mg.

For the treatment of Raynaud's phenomenon the recommended starting dosage is 10mg 3 times daily with subsequent titration, according to response, to a maximum of 20mg 3 times daily.

A sustained release tablet formulation of nifedipine is now available for the treatment of hypertension, the recommended dosage of which is 20mg twice daily after food, increased if necessary to 40mg twice daily.

If for some reason an immediate effect is desired in patients with angina or hypertension, a capsule can be bitten open and the contents allowed to remain in the mouth, thus permitting sublingual absorption. This has been particularly useful in patients requiring rapid reduction of severe hypertension.

Recently, intravenous preparations (injection and infusion) of nifedipine have been made available for treating coronary vasospasm and/or acute episodes of hypertension. For the intravenous injection of nifedipine 1 mg/10ml, the recommended dosage is 0.5 to 1.0 mg/patient (0.007 to 0.015 mg/kg bodyweight) administered slowly (over about 3 min) at a constant rate – a total dose of 9 × 0.02 mg/kg bodyweight in 7 hours should not be exceeded. For the intravenous infusion of nifedipine 5 mg/50ml, the usual dosage is 5mg over 4 to 8 hours with a maximum of 15 to 30 mg/24 hours. This regimen may be repeated for up to 3 days but this total daily dosage should not be exceeded.

An intracoronary injection of nifedipine 0.2 mg/2ml is also available. This is used for treating coronary vasospasm that occurs during diagnostic or therapeutic interventions, e.g. percutaneous transluminal coronary angioplasty or recanalisation, and coronary artery bypass grafting. The usual dose is 0.1 to 0.2 mg/patient administered slowly (over 1.5 to 2 min) at a constant rate. Total dosage should not exceed 6 × 0.2 mg/patient over a 3-hour period. All 3 injectable preparations must be protected from light.

Nifedipine may be used in combination with β-blockers and other antihypertensive drugs, although the possibility of additive effects should be borne in mind. A small percentage of patients have reported an increase in ischaemic pain within 30 minutes of introducing nifedipine; in these patients the drug should be discontinued. Nifedipine should be used with caution in dialysis patients with malignant hypertension and irreversible kidney failure with hypovolaemia, and in patients with poor cardiac reserve. Nifedipine must not be used during pregnancy.

8. Drug Interactions

Conflicting reports have been published concerning the effect of nifedipine on the steady-state plasma concentrations and elimination of digoxin. In an acute trial nifedipine has been reported to elevate the plasma concentrations and to decrease the renal clearance of digoxin in healthy subjects by 45 and 30%, respectively, but the reduction in renal clearance was not of sufficient magnitude to explain the observed increases in plasma digoxin concentrations (Belz et al., 1980, 1983). Since the increases in plasma digoxin concentration were associated with increased glycoside effects, it was suggested that all patients receiving this drug combination should have their digoxin dose reduced by 40 to 50%, their plasma digoxin concentrations checked, and be monitored for signs and symptoms of digitalis toxicity (Auricchio, 1983; Belz et al., 1983).

Conversely, several single- and multiple-dose studies in cardiac patients and in healthy volunteers have indicated no significant pharmacokinetic interaction between nifedipine and digoxin or digitoxin (Garty et al., 1984; Hansen et al., 1984; Kuhlmann, 1985; Kuhlmann and Marcin, 1983; Kuhlmann et al., 1983, 1984; Pedersen et al., 1982; Schwartz and Migliore, 1984; Schwartz et al., 1984a; Zylber-Katz et al., 1984b). In fact, Perez-Olea and Quevedo (1984), using animal models, showed that pretreatment with nifedipine inhibited arrhythmias due to digitalis toxicity. Accordingly, it has also been suggested that neither digoxin dosage modifications nor more frequent than normal monitoring of plasma digoxin concentration monitoring are necessary in patients receiving both nifedipine and digoxin (Pedersen et al., 1982; Schwartz et al., 1984a; Schwartz and Migliore, 1984). Finally, although Hansen et al. (1984) found that nifedipine attenuates digoxin-induced inotropism, it is obvious that further research on the effect of nifedipine on digoxin pharmacokinetics and clinical effects is required.

Numerous studies indicate that the combination of nifedipine and β-blockers is safe (section 6) and may produce favourable clinical responses in patients with angina pectoris and hypertension (sections 3.1.2 and 4.2.2). Although no significant pharmacokinetic interactions between nifedipine and metoprolol, atenolol, nadolol and propranolol have been reported (Gangji et al., 1984; Kendall et al., 1984; Wilkins et al., 1985), several reports have appeared which describe severe hypotension or cardiac failure associated with the combined use of nifedipine and β-blockers (Anastassiades, 1980, 1982; Opie and White, 1980; Robson and Vishwanath, 1982; Staffurth and Emery, 1981). Each of these cases, with the exception of the one described by Opie and White (1980), involved high risk patients with severe angina pectoris, triple-vessel disease, impaired left ventricular function and a prior history of myocardial infarction. All had been on β-blockade for years, but because of a worsening of their angina, had nifedipine added to their drug regimens. Within 5 to 21 days they all developed dyspnoea, hypotension and heart failure. Ebner et al. (1983) have suggested that a possible explanation for these symptoms may involve pronounced decreases in blood pressure without corresponding increases in heart rate due to concomitant β-blockade, while Kleinbloesem et al. (1985) have concluded that the pharmacodynamic interaction between nifedipine and propranolol can most likely be explained by transient decreases in apparent liver blood flow when the 2 drugs are given together. A report of acute hypotensive episodes after the concomitant administration of nifedipine and prazosin has also been published (Jee and Opie, 1983).

Case reports of decreased plasma quinidine and increased plasma phenytoin and theophylline concentrations due to nifedipine administration have been reported (Ahmad, 1984b; Farringer et al., 1984; Green et al., 1983; Parrillo and Venditto, 1984). Nifedipine has also been reported to have a potentiating effect on terbutaline- and salbutamol-induced bronchodilatation in asthmatics (Lever et al., 1984; Löfdahl et al., 1984; Svedmyr et al., 1984).

While both ranitidine and cimetidine have been shown to significantly increase the bioavailability of nifedipine, cimetidine has additionally been shown to increase the hypotensive effect of nifedipine in healthy volunteers (Kirch et al., 1983, 1984,

1985). However, neither drug has been found to significantly affect the antianginal or other pharmacodynamic effects of nifedipine (Dylewicz et al., 1984; Kirch et al., 1983, 1984, 1985).

9. Place of Nifedipine in Therapy

Calcium ion flux from the extracellular space through the slow channel of the cell membrane plays an important role in several fundamental physiological processes in myocardial and vascular smooth muscle cells. Nifedipine blocks this influx of calcium into the cell which confers on it potent coronary and peripheral arteriodilator properties that are useful in various clinical areas. Most early experience was gained in patients with ischaemic heart disease in whom – along with β-blockers, nitrates and other calcium antagonists – it now represents one of the drugs of choice. Clinical trials to date support the view that nifedipine should be considered a first-line choice in patients with a predominant vasospastic component to their angina, i.e. variant or unstable disease, and in those patients whose angina is complicated by hypertension or congestive heart failure. There is also increasing evidence that nifedipine, used alone, may be a useful alternative in the clinical management of stable exertional angina. However, further well-designed comparative trials are necessary to fully define its position in relation to other available drugs such as β-blockers and nitrates, which are currently the most frequently used drugs in this clinical setting. In those studies where nifedipine and a β-blocker have been used together, the combination always produced more favourable results than monotherapy, without any significant deterioration of left ventricular function. However, if these drugs are to be used in combination in patients with impaired left ventricular function, care should be exercised, since there have been isolated reports of excessive negative inotropic or hypotensive effects.

Apart from being used in ischaemic heart disease, nifedipine has been used successfully in patients with various grades of hypertension. Many authors report that for those situations requiring acute reduction of blood pressure, sublingual nifedipine is possibly the drug of choice because of its convenient route of administration, and its rapid lowering of elevated blood pressure without overcorrection or excessive adverse effects. Nifedipine has also been shown to be an extremely useful adjunct for controlling blood pressure in patients refractory to conventional treatment regimens with combinations of β-blockers, diuretics, and various vasodilators. Greater conflict surrounds the suitability of nifedipine, used alone, in the long term management of patients with mild to moderate hypertension. Results from short to medium term comparative trials suggest that it may be considered an effective and reasonably safe alternative to β-blockers and diuretics, but confirmation in well-designed long term trials is still needed. To assist with compliance (a common problem in patients with mild to moderate hypertension), a sustained release formulation of nifedipine, allowing twice daily administration, has been marketed, and this preparation appears to maintain 24-hour control of blood pressure as well as the conventional capsule formulation of nifedipine.

Recently, nifedipine has been used in the management of Raynaud's phenomenon and produced subjective improvement in the number, duration and severity of vasospastic attacks in more than 60% of patients treated. Additionally, it was found to be useful in helping to heal cutaneous ulceration that occurred in some patients. In a preliminary trial, nifedipine more effectively reduced the symptoms of Raynaud's phenomenon than did prazosin and it would seem to be a rational first-line choice in this clinical setting, where drug intervention usually produces unsatisfactory improvements.

Clinical trials in other therapeutic areas such as congestive heart failure, hypertrophic cardiomyopathy and pulmonary hypertension have often been encouraging but are limited in terms of the total numbers of patients studied, and more information is needed to clarify any role nifedipine may have in treating such patients. The particularly beneficial effects of nifedipine in a few patients with pulmonary hypertension has led some authors to suggest that the calcium antagonist is well worth a trial in this group of patients, not only because of the marked long term improvement it can sometimes generate but also because of the poor results achieved with conventional treatment.

Thus, nifedipine has shown itself to be a useful addition to the drugs available to the clinician for the management of angina and/or hypertension. It may also be of particular benefit in patients with Raynaud's phenomenon and preliminary data suggest it may have a role in treating pulmonary hypertension, especially if some predictor for identifying those likely to respond can be found.

References

1st International Nifedipine (Adalat®) Symposium: New Therapy of Ischemic Heart Disease, Hashimoto et al. (Eds). Proceedings of the Symposium held in Tokyo, November 24-25, 1973 (University of Tokyo Press 1975).

2nd International Adalat® Symposium: New Therapy of Ischemic Heart Disease, Lochner et al. (Eds). Proceedings of the Symposium held in Amsterdam, October 4-5, 1974 (Springer, Berlin-Heidelberg-New York 1975).

3rd International Adalat® Symposium: New Therapy of Ischemic Heart Disease, Jatene and Lichtlen (Eds). Proceedings of the Symposium held in Rio de Janeiro, October 10-11, 1975 (Excerpta Medica, Amsterdam-Oxford 1976).

4th International Adalat® Symposium: New Therapy of Ischemic Heart Disease, Puech and Krebs (Eds). Proceedings of the Symposium held in Paris, October 19-20, 1979 (Excerpta Medica, Amsterdam-Oxford-Princeton 1980).

5th International Adalat® Symposium: New Therapy of Ischemic Heart Disease and Hypertension, Kaltenbach and Neufeld (Eds). Proceedings of the Symposium held in Berlin, May 12th-14th, 1982 (Excerpta Medica, Amsterdam-Oxford-Princeton 1983).

Abadie, E. and Passa, P.: Diabetogenic effects of nifedipine. British Medical Journal 289: 438 (1984).

Abinader, E. and Shahar, J.: Production of paradoxical chest pains by nifedipine. Irish Medical Journal 76: 180-181 (1983).

Abramson, M. and Littlejohn, G.O.: Hepatic reactions to nifedipine. Medical Journal of Australia 142: 47-48 (1985).

Addonizio, V.P.; Fisher, C.A. and Edmunds Jr, L.H.: Effects of verapamil and nifedipine on platelet activation. Circulation 62 (Suppl. III): III-326 (1980).

Ahmad, S.: Nifedipine-induced acute psychosis. Journal of the American Geriatrics Society 32: 408 (1984a).

Ahmad, S.: Nifedipine-phenytoin interaction. Journal of the American College of Cardiology 3: 1582 (1984b).

Alvarado, E. and Pineros, J.: The efficacy of Adalat in angina pectoris patients. Results of a 6-month trial; 3rd International Adalat Symposium, pp. 261-267 (1976).

Ambroso, G.C.; Como, G.; Scalamogna, A.; Citterio, A.; Casati, S. and Ponticelli, C.: Treatment of arterial hypertension with nifedipine in patients with chronic renal insufficiency. Clinical Nephrology 23: 41-45 (1985).

Amende, I.; Simon, R.; Hood Jr, W.P.; Hetzer, R. and Lichtlen, P.R.: Intracoronary nifedipine in human beings: magnitude and time course of changes in left ventricular contraction/relaxation and coronary sinus blood flow. Journal of the American College of Cardiology 2: 1141-1145 (1983).

Amende, I.; Simon, R. and Lichtlen, P.R.: Early effects of nifedipine on left ventricular diastolic function in man. (Abstract.) Circulation 62 (Suppl. III): III-259 (1980).

Anastassiades, C.J.: Nifedipine and beta-blocker drugs. British Medical Journal 281: 1251-1252 (1980).

Anastassiades, C.: Nifedipine and beta-blockade as a cause of cardiac failure. British Medical Journal 284: 506 (1982).

Andersen, K. and Vik-Mo, H.: Increased left ventricular emptying at maximal exercise after reduction in afterload. Circulation 69: 492-496 (1984).

Andersen, L.; Kolendorf, K. and Thorsteinsson, B.: Nifedipine does not decrease insulin secretion. Acta Endocrinologica 100 (Suppl. 247): 7 (1982).

Andersson, K.-E. and Högestätt, E.D.: On the mechanism of action of calcium antagonists. Acta Medica Scandinavica (Suppl. 681): 11-24 (1984).

Andersson, K.-E.; Ingemarsson, I.; Ulmsten, U. and Wingerup, L.: Inhibition of prostaglandin-induced uterine activity by nifedipine. British Journal of Obstetrics and Gynaecology 86: 175-179 (1979).

Andersson, K.- E. and Ulmsten, U.: Effects of nifedipine on myometrial activity and lower abdominal pain in women with primary dysmenorrhoea. British Journal of Obstetrics and Gynaecology 85: 142-148 (1978).

Angelino, P.F.; Tortore, P. and Algrananti, R.: Hemodynamic studies on the new coronary therapeutic drug nifedipine (BAY a 1040); 2nd International Adalat Symposium, pp. 128-139 (1975).

Antman, E.; Muller, J.; Goldberg, S.; MacAlpin, R.; Rubenfire, M. et al.: Nifedipine therapy for coronary-artery spasm. Experience in 127 patients. New England Journal of Medicine 302: 1269-1273 (1980a).

Antman, E.M.; Stone, P.H.; Muller, J.E. and Braunwald, E.: Calcium channel blocking agents in the treatment of cardiovascular disorders. Part I: Basic and clinical electrophysiologic effects. Annals of Internal Medicine 93: 875-885 (1980b).

Aoki, K.; Sato, K.; Kawaguchi, Y. and Yamamoto, M.: Acute and long-term hypotensive effects and plasma concentrations of nifedipine in patients with essential hypertension. European Journal of Clinical Pharmacology 23: 197-201 (1982).

Aoki, K.; Kondo, S.; Mochizuki, A.; Yoshida, T.; Kato, S. et al.: Antihypertensive effects of cardiovascular Ca^{2+}-antagonist in hypertension patients in the absence and presence of beta-adrenergic-blockade. American Heart Journal 96: 218-226 (1978).

Aoki, K.; Kondo, S.; Sato, K.; Kato, K.; Kawaguchi, Y. et al.: Hypotensive action of nifedipine (Ca^{2+}-antagonist) and propranolol in acute trials and its long-term therapy of hypertensive coronary heart disease patients. Japanese Heart Journal 22: 575-584 (1981).

Aoki, K.; Yoshida, T.; Kato, S.; Tazume, K.; Soto, I. et al.: Hypotensive action and increased plasma renin activity by calcium antagonist (nifedipine) in hypertensive patients. Japanese Heart Journal 17: 479-484 (1976).

Ardissino, D.; DeServi, S.; Salerno, J.A.; Specchia, G.; Previtali, M. et al.: Efficacy, duration and mechanism of action of nifedipine in stable exercise-induced angina pectoris. European Heart Journal 4: 873-881 (1983).

Arguedas, C. and Fuchs, J.R.: Nifedipine for refractory hypertension. Cardiovascular Reviews and Reports 5: 395 (1984).

Auricchio, R.J.: Digoxin interactions with calcium channel blockers. Drug Interactions Newsletter 3: 45-48 (1983).

Austin, M.B.; Robson, R.A. and Bailey, R.R.: Effect of nifedipine on renal function of normal subjects and hypertensive patients with renal functional impairment. New Zealand Medical Journal 96: 829-831 (1983).

Bach, P.R.: Determination of nifedipine in serum or plasma by reversed-phase liquid chromatography. Clinical Chemistry 29: 1344-1348 (1983).

Bailey, J.S.: The prophylaxis of angina pectoris in general practice. A placebo-controlled comparison of nifedipine and propranolol. Practitioner 226: 343-345 (1982).

Bala Subramanian, V.; Bowles, M.J.; Khurmi, N.S.; Davies, A.B.

and Raftery, E.B.: Randomized double-blind comparison of verapamil and nifedipine in chronic stable angina. American Journal of Cardiology 50: 696-707 (1982).

Banzet, O.; Colin, J.N.; Thibonnier, M.; Singlas, E.; Alexandre, J.M. and Corvol, P.: Acute antihypertensive effect and pharmacokinetics of a tablet preparation of nifedipine. European Journal of Clinical Pharmacology 24: 145-150 (1983).

Barnes, P.J.; Wilson, N.M. and Brown, M.J.: A calcium antagonist, nifedipine, modifies exercise-induced asthma. Thorax 36: 726-730 (1981).

Baronti, A.; Grieco, A.; Lelli, M.; Vibelli, C. and Virgili, G.: Reduction of airway hyperresponsiveness in allergic asthmatic and rhinitic patients by acute nifedipine. Current Therapeutic Research 35: 247-252 (1984).

Bartorelli, C.; Magrini, F.; Moruzzi, P.; Olivari, M.T.; Polese, A. et al.: Haemodynamic effects of a calcium antagonistic agent (nifedipine) in hypertension: Therapeutic implications. Clinical Science and Molecular Medicine 55: 291S-292S (1978).

Bassan, M.; Weiler-Ravell, D. and Shalev, O.: The additive antianginal action of oral nifedipine in patients receiving propranolol. Magnitude and duration of effect. Circulation 66: 710-716 (1982).

Bassan, M.M.; Weiler-Ravell, D. and Shalev, O.: Comparison of the antianginal effectiveness of nifedipine, verapamil, and isosorbide dinitrate in patients receiving propranolol: A double-blind study. Circulation 68: 568-575 (1983).

Baumgartner, H.R.: Effects of acetylsalicylic acid, sulfinpyrazone, and dipyridamole on platelet adhesion and aggregation in flowing native and anticoagulated blood. Haemostasis 8: 340-352 (1979).

Bayley, S.; Dobbs, R.J. and Robinson, B.F.: Nifedipine in the treatment of hypertension: Report of a double-blind controlled trial. British Journal of Clinical Pharmacology 14: 509-512 (1982).

Bedard, R.M. and Busse, W.W.: Nifedipine inhibition of human basophil histamine release. American Review of Respiratory Disease 127 (Suppl. 2): 70 (1983).

Bedard, R.M. and Busse, W.W.: Inhibition of basophil histamine release by the calcium channel antagonist nifedipine in asthma. American Review of Respiratory Disease 129 (Suppl. 2): A9 (1984).

Beer, N.; Gallegos, I.; Cohen, A.; Klein, N.; Sonnenblick, E. and Frishman, W.: Efficacy of sublingual nifedipine in the acute treatment of systemic hypertension. Chest 79: 571-574 (1981).

Bellani, M.; Meregalli, M.; Guffanti, E.; Bartucci, F.; Fiorella, G. et al.: Treatment of hypertension in the elderly: A controlled clinical trial of dihydroergotoxine mesilate in comparison with nifedipine. Current Therapeutic Research 34: 1014-1022 (1983).

Bellini, G.; Battilana, G.; Puppis, E.; Rigoni, A.; Cosenzi, A. et al.: Renal response to acute nifedipine administration in normotensive and hypertensive patients during normal and low sodium intake. Current Therapeutic Research 35: 974-981 (1984).

Bellocci, F.; Ansalone, G.; Santarelli, P.; Frustaci, A.; Scabbia, E. and Montenero, A.: Hemodynamic effects of dobutamine in patients with congestive heart failure receiving nifedipine. (Abstract.) European Heart Journal 5 (Suppl. 1): 35 (1984).

Bellocci, F.; Ansalone, G.; Santarelli, P.; Loperfido, F.; Scabbia, E. et al.: Oral nifedipine in the long-term management of severe chronic heart failure. Journal of Cardiovascular Pharmacology 4: 847-855 (1982).

Bellocci, F.; Ansalone, G.; Scabbia, E.; Affinito, V.; Santarelli, P. et al.: Sustained beneficial effect of nifedipine in chronic refractory heart failure. (Abstract.) American Journal of Cardiology 47: 407 (1981).

Belz, G.G.; Doering, W.; Munkes, R.; Aust, P.E. and Belz, G.: Effects of various calcium antagonists on blood level and renal clearance of digoxin. Circulation 64: 24 (1980).

Belz, G.G.; Doering, W.; Munkes, R. and Matthews, J.: Interaction between digoxin and calcium antagonists and antiarrhythmic drugs. Clinical Pharmacology and Therapeutics 33: 410-417 (1983).

Bertel, O.; Conen, D.; Radü, E.W.; Müller, J.; Lang, C. and Dubach, U.C.: Nifedipine in hypertensive emergencies. British Medical Journal 286: 19-21 (1983).

Bertrand, M.E.; Lablanche, J.M. and Tilmant, P.Y.: Treatment of Prinzmetal's variant angina. Role of medical treatment with nifedipine and surgical coronary revascularization combined with plexectomy. American Journal of Cardiology 47: 174-178 (1981).

Besse, P.; Casassus, J.; Page, A.; Colle, J.P. and Vallot, F.: Nifedipine in the treatment of Prinzmetal's variant of angina pectoris. 4th International Adalat Symposium, pp. 110-125 (1980).

Bexton, R.S.; Nathan, A.W.; Hellestrand, K.J.; Cory-Pearce, R.; Spurrell, R.A.J. et al.: The direct electrophysiological effects of nifedipine and verapamil. (Abstract.) Circulation 68 (Suppl. III): 275 (1983).

Bhatnagar, S.K.; Amin, M.M.A. and Al-Yusuf, A.R.: Diabetogenic effects of nifedipine. British Medical Journal 289: 19 (1984).

Blackwell, J.N.; Holt, S. and Heading, R.C.: Effect of nifedipine on oesophageal motility. Gut 20: A919 (1979).

Blackwell, J.N.; Holt, S. and Heading, R.C.: Effect of nifedipine on oesophageal motility and gastric emptying. Digestion 21: 50-56 (1981).

Blaustein, A.S.; Heller, G.V. and Kolman, B.S.: Adjunctive nifedipine therapy in high-risk, medically refractory, unstable angina pectoris. American Journal of Cardiology 52: 950-954 (1983).

Boden, W.E.; Korr, K.S. and Bough, E.W.: Nifedipine-induced hypotension may provoke myocardial ischaemia in unstable angina. (Abstract.) Circulation 68 (Suppl. II): III-367 (1983).

Boden, W.E.; Korr, K.S. and Bough, E.W.: Nifedipine-induced hypotension and myocardial ischemia in refractory angina pectoris. Journal of the American Medical Association 253: 1131-1135 (1985).

Bogaert, M.G.; Rosseel, M.T.; Joos, R. and Boelaert, J.: Plasma concentrations of nifedipine in patients with renal failure. Arzneimittel-Forschung 34: 307-308 (1984).

Bonaduce, D.; Canonico, V.; Mazza, F.; Nicolino, A.; Ferrara, N. et al.: Evaluation of the efficacy of slow-release nifedipine in systemic hypertension by ambulatory, intraarterial blood pressure monitoring. Journal of Cardiovascular Pharmacology 7: 145-151 (1985).

Bonaduce, D.; Ferrara, N.; Petretta, M.; Romano, E.; Postiglione, M. et al.: Hemodynamic study of nifedipine administration in hypertensive patients. American Heart Journal 105: 865-867 (1983).

Bonetti, A.; Del Prato, C.; Orlandini, G. and Zuliani, U.: Influenza della somministrazione acuta di un calcio-antagonista (nifedipina) sul metabolismo glico-lipidico. Giornale di Arteriosclerosia 4: 287-289 (1979).

Bortolotti, M. and Labò, G.: Clinical and manometric effects of nifedipine in patients with esophageal achlasia. Gastroenterology 80: 39-44 (1981).

Bovill, J.G.; Wezel, H.V.; Schuller, J. and Hoeneveld, M.: Comparison of nitroglycerine, verapamil and nifedipine in coronary artery surgery. Brit. J. Anaesth. 56: 804P (1984).

Brauman, A.; Golik, A.; Gilboa, Y. and Hertzianu, I.: Effect of nifedipine on metabolism of glucose and secretion of insulin in diabetic patients. Diabetologia 27: 260A (1984).

Braun, S.; Terdiman, R.; Berenfield, D. and Laniado, S.: Clinical and hemodynamic effects of combined propranolol and nifedipine therapy versus propranolol alone in patients with angina pectoris. American Heart Journal 3: 478-485 (1985).

Braunwald, E.: Mechanism of action of calcium-channel-blocking agents. New England Journal of Medicine 307: 1618-1627 (1982).

Bravard, P. and Moore, N.: Nifedipine for Raynaud's phenomenon. Lancet 1: 130-131 (1983).
Brennan, F.N. and Blake, S.: The use of nifedipine as a third-step agent in the treatment of refractory hypertension. Irish Medical Journal 75: 29-30 (1982).
Brennan, F.; Flanagan, M.; Blake, S. and Cannon, P.: Nifedipine in the treatment of hypertension. European Journal of Clinical Pharmacology 25: 713-715 (1983).
Brinker, J.A.; Ouyang, P.; Mellits, E.D. and Gerstenblith, G.: Influence of fixed disease on the response to nifedipine in patients with unstable angina. (Abstract.) Clinical Research 31: 170A (1983).
Brügmann, U.; Blasini, R. and Rudolph W.: Antiischämische Wirkung von Nifedipin in Retard-Form. Ergebnisse einer doppelblind, randomisiert, cross-over durchgeführten, placebokontrollierten Akustudie. Herz 8: 206-210 (1983).
Brügmann, U.; Dirschinger, J.; Blasini, R. and Rudolph, W.: Antiischämische Wirksamkeit unterschiedlicher Nifedipin-Dosen. Herz 7: 235-242 (1982).
Bühler, F.: Kalzium-Antagonisten: Kennt man ein Absetz-Syndrom? Münchener Medizinische Wochenschrift 125: 13 (1983).
Bühler, F.R.; Hulthén, U.L.; Kiowski, W. and Bolli, P.: β-Blockers and calcium antagonists: Cornerstones of antihypertensive therapy in the 1980s. Drugs 25 (Suppl. 2): 50-57 (1983).
Burns, E.R. and Frishman, W.H.: The anti-platelet effects of calcium channel blockers add to their anti-anginal properties. International Journal of Cardiology 4: 372-379 (1983).
Bursztyn, M.; Grossman, E. and Rosenthal, T.: Long acting nifedipine in the treatment of severe hypertension. European Journal of Clinical Pharmacology 27: 13-17 (1984).
Camerini, F.; Alberti, E.; Benussi, B.; Fioretti, P.; Klugmann, S. and Salvi, A.: Nifedipine as an afterload reducing agent; 5th International Adalat Symposium, pp. 64-80 (1983).
Camerini, F.; Alberti, E.; Klugmann, S. and Salvi, A.: Primary pulmonary hypertension: Effects of nifedipine. British Heart Journal 44: 352-356 (1980).
Cantelli, I.; Pavesi, P.C.; Naccarella, F. and Bracchetti, D.: Comparison of acute haemodynamic effects of nifedipine and isosorbide dinitrate in patients with heart failure following acute myocardial infarction. International Journal of Cardiology 1: 151-163 (1981).
Cantelli, I.; Pavesi, P.C.; Parchi, C.; Naccarella, F. and Bracchetti, D.: Acute hemodynamic effects of combined therapy with digoxin and nifedipine in patients with chronic heart failure. American Heart Journal 106: 308-315 (1983).
Cassera, J.C.; Menna, J.; Traina, M. and Ferreirós, E.: The effect of a single dose of Adalat during exercise in patients with coronary heart disease; 3rd International Adalat Symposium, pp. 123-127 (1976).
Castilho, F.; Goncalves, D.A. and Balbi, J.D.S.: Long-term treatment with a new coronary pharmacotherapeutic agent of ischaemic manifestations in chronic coronary insufficiency induced by exercise; 3rd International Adalat Symposium, pp. 247-254 (1976).
Cerrina, J.; Denjean, A.; Alexandre, G.; Lockhart, A. and Duroux, P.: Inhibition of exercise-induced asthma by a calcium antagonist, nifedipine. American Review of Respiratory Disease 123: 156-160 (1981a).
Cerrina, J.; Jouvin, E.; Duroux, P. and Beneveniste, J.: Inhibition of the release of platelet-activating factor and slow reactive substance from human neutrophils by the calcium antagonist nifedipine. American Review of Respiratory Disease 123 (Suppl. 4): 44 (1981b).
Chaitman, B.R.; Wagniart, P.; Pasternac, A.; Brevers, G.; Scholl, J.-M. et al.: Improved exercise tolerance after propranolol, diltiazem or nifedipine in angina pectoris: Comparison at 1, 3 and 8 hours and correlation with plasma drug concentration. American Journal of Cardiology 53: 1-9 (1984).
Charlap, S. and Frishman, W.H.: Nifedipine in heart failure. International Journal of Cardiology 6: 665-671 (1984).
Charles, S.; Ketelslegers, J.-M.; Buysschaert, M. and Lambert, A.E.: Hyperglycaemic effect of nifedipine. British Medical Journal 283: 19-20 (1981).
Cherchi, A.; Fonzo, R. and Bina, M.: Influence of nifedipine on the effort tolerance test in angina patients; 1st International Nifedipine 'Adalat' Symposium, pp. 85-96 (1975).
Choong, C.Y.P.; Roubin, G.S.; Harris, P.J.; Shen, W.F. and Kelly, D.T.: Effects of vasodilatation by nifedipine on the peripheral distribution of cardiac output during exercise and oxygen utilisation by working muscles. (Abstract.) Australian and New Zealand Journal of Medicine 14 (Suppl. 2): 557 (1984).
Choong, C.Y.P.; Roubin, G.S.; Tokuyasu, Y.; Shen, W.F.; Bautovich, G.J. et al.: Acute effects of nifedipine and combination with metoprolol on exercise capacity, haemodynamics and left ventricular function in patients with exertional angina. (Abstract.) Australian and New Zealand Journal of Medicine 13: 417 (1983).
Christensen, C.K.; Lederballe Pedersen, O. and Mikkelsen, E.: Renal effects of acute calcium blockade with nifedipine in hypertensive patients receiving beta-adrenoceptor-blocking drugs. Clinical Pharmacology and Therapeutics 32: 572-576 (1982).
Clark, R.E.; Christlieb, I.Y.; Ferguson, T.B.; Weldon, C.S.; Marburger, J.P. et al.: The first American clinical trial of nifedipine in cardioplegia. A report of the first 12 month experience. Journal of Thoracic and Cardiovascular Surgery 82: 848-859 (1981).
Clark, R.E.; Christlieb, I.Y.; Henry, P.D.; Fischer, A.E.; Nora, J.D. et al.: Nifedipine: A myocardial protective agent. American Journal of Cardiology 44: 825-831 (1979).
Clark, R.E.; Christlieb, I.Y. and Magovern, G.J.: Use of nifedipine during cardiac surgery for improved myocardial protection. American Journal of Medicine 78 (Suppl. 2B): 6-8 (1985a).
Clark, R.E.; Christlieb, I.Y.; Vanderwonde, J.C. and Henry, P.D.: Use of nifedipine to decrease ischemic-reperfusion injury in the surgical setting. American Journal of Cardiology 55: 125B-138B (1985b).
Clark, R.E. and Magovern, G.J.: Nifedipine cardioplegia experience: results of a 2-year cooperative clinical study. European Heart Journal 4 (Suppl. C): 89-90 (1983).
Clark, R.E.; Magovern, G.J.; Christlieb, I.Y. and Boe, S.: Nifedipine cardioplegia experience: Results of a 3-year cooperative clinical study. Annals of Thoracic Surgery 36: 654-663 (1983).
Cocco, G.; Strozzi, C.; Chu, D.; Amrein, R. and Castagroli, E.: Therapeutic effects of pindolol and nifedipine in patients with stable angina pectoris and asymptomatic resting ischemia. European Journal of Cardiology 10: 59-69 (1979).
Cohen, D.J.; Foley, R.W. and Ryan, J.M.: Intraoperative coronary artery spasm successfully treated with nitroglycerin and nifedipine. Annals of Thoracic Surgery 36: 97-100 (1983).
Colucci, W.S.; Fifer, M.A.; Lorell, B.H. and Wynne, J.: Calcium channel blockers in congestive heartfailure: Theoretic considerations and clinical experience. American Journal of Medicine 78 (Suppl. 2B): 9-17 (1985).
Conen, D.; Bertel, O. and Dubach, U.C.: An oral calcium antagonist for treatment of hypertensive emergencies. Journal of Cardiovascular Pharmacology 4 (Suppl. 3): 378-382 (1982).
Corbalan, R.; Gonzalez, R.; Chamorro, G.; Muñoz, M.; Rodriguez, J.A. and Casanegra, P.: Effect of a calcium inhibitor, nifedipine, on exercise tolerance in patients with angina pectoris. A double-blind study. Chest 79: 302-305 (1981).
Corea, L.; Alunni, G.; Bentivoglio, M.; Boschetti, E.; Cosmi, F. et al.: Acute and long-term effects of nifedipine on plasma renin activity and plasma catecholamines in controls and hypertensive patients before and after metoprolol. Acta Therapeutica 6: 177-187 (1980).
Corea, L.; Bentivoglio, M.; Cosmi, F. and Alunni, G.: Catecholamines plasma levels and haemodynamic changes induced by

nifedipine in chronic severe heart failure. Current Therapeutic Research 30: 698-707 (1981a).
Corea, L.; Bentivoglio, M.; Cosmi, F.; Alunni, G. and Carnovali, M.: Nifedipine versus prazosin in essential hypertension: A double-blind study. Current Therapeutic Research 30: 708-717 (1981b).
Corea, L.; Bentivoglio, M. and Verdecchia, P.: Captopril compared with nifedipine in the treatment of heart failure: A randomized study. Drugs Under Experimental and Clinical Research IX: 901-910 (1983).
Corea, L.; Bentivoglio, M. and Verdecchia, P.: Nifedipine in heart failure. Current Therapeutic Research 36: 951-958 (1984).
Corea, L.; Miele, N.; Bentivoglio, M.; Boschetti, E.; Agabiti-Rosei, E. and Muiesan, G.: Acute and chronic effects of nifedipine on plasma renin activity and plasma adrenaline and noradrenaline in controls and hypertensive patients. Clinical Science 57: 115S-117S (1979b).
Coronelli, M.; Zuzolo, V.; Tonti, M.; Carosi, M. and Teggia, L.: Antianginal activity of nifedipine in 5mg capsules for acute administration. Current Therapeutic Research 33: 639-645 (1983).
Corris, P.A.; Nariman, S. and Gibson, G.J.: Nifedipine in the prevention of asthma induced by exercise and histamine. American Review of Respiratory Disease 128: 991-992 (1983).
Corvol, P.; Marre, M.; Banzet, O.; Colin, J.N.; Thibonnier, M. et al.: Acute antihypertensive effects and pharmacokinetic parameters of a new galenic form of nifedipine; in 5th International Adalat Symposium, pp. 158-163 (1983).
Covinsky, J.O. and Hamburger, S.C.; Slow channel blockers. Southern Medical Journal 76: 55-64 (1983).
Creager, M.A.; Pariser, K.M.; Winston, E.M.; Rasmussen, H.M.; Miller, K.B. and Coffman, J.D.: Nifedipine-induced vasodilation in patients with Raynaud's phenomenon. American Heart Journal 108: 370-373 (1984).
Crimi, N.; Palermo, F.; Sorace, R.; Gibellino, F. and Mistretta, A.: Effect of a calcium antagonist, nifedipine, in exercise-induced asthma. Respiration 45: 262-264 (1984).
Cristal, N.; Slonim, A. and Shainkin-Kestenbaum, R.: Improved red cell filterability by nifedipine in coronary patients – therapeutic implications. (Abstract.) Asian Pacific Adalat Symposium, p. 11 (Tokyo, 23-24 October 1982).
Dalal, J.J.; Griffiths, B.E. and Henderson, A.H.: Primary pulmonary hypertension: Effects of nifedipine. British Heart Journal 46: 230-231 (1981).
Dale, J.; Landmark, K.H. and Myhre, E.: The effects of nifedipine, a calcium antagonist, on platelet function. American Heart Journal 105: 103-105 (1983).
Daly, K.; Bergman, G.; Rothman, M.; Atkinson, L.; Jackson, G. and Jewitt, D.E.: Beneficial effect of adding nifedipine to beta-adrenergic blocking therapy in angina pectoris. European Heart Journal 3: 42-46 (1982).
Danielides, I.C.; Basioukas, P. and Pouggouras, P.: Effects of nifedipine on primary esophageal motility disorders. (Abstract.) Gastroenterology 86: 1056 (1984).
Dargie, H.J.; Lynch, P.G.; Krikler, D.M.; Harris, L. and Krikler, S.: Nifedipine and propranolol: A beneficial drug interaction. American Journal of Medicine 71: 676-682 (1981).
Davi, G.; Novo, S.; Fiore, M.; Foderà, A.; Mattina, A. et al.: Effects by nifedipine on thromboxane synthesis *in vitro* and *in vivo*. Thrombosis Research 28: 837-842 (1982).
Davidson, A.R.: Lymphocyte sensitisation in nifedipine-induced hepatitis. British Medical Journal 281: 1354 (1980).
Dawson, J.R.; Whitaker, N.H.G. and Sutton, G.C.: Calcium antagonist drugs in chronic stable angina. Comparison of verapamil and nifedipine. British Heart Journal 46: 508-512 (1981).
Dean, S. and Kendall, M.J.: Nifedipine in the treatment of difficult hypertensives. European Journal of Clinical Pharmacology 24: 1-5 (1983).
Deanfield, J.E.; Selwyn, A.P.; Chierchia, S.; Maseri, A.; Ribeiro, P. and Krikler, S.: Myocardial ischaemia during daily life in patients with stable angina: Its relation to symptoms and heart rate changes. Lancet 1: 753-758 (1983a).
Deanfield, J.; Wright, C. and Fox, K.: Treatment of angina pectoris with nifedipine: Importance of dose titration. British Medical Journal 286: 1467-1470 (1983b).
Deanfield, J.; Wright, C.; Krikler, S.; Ribeiro, P. and Fox, K.: Cigarette smoking and the treatment of angina with propranolol, atenolol, and nifedipine. New England Journal of Medicine 310: 941-954 (1984).
Debaisieux, J.-C.; Theroux, P.; Waters, D.D. and Mizgala, H.F.: Hemodynamic effects of a single oral dose of nifedipine following acute myocardial infarction. Chest 78: 574-579 (1980).
De Buitleir, M.; Rowland, E. and Krikler, D.M.: Combination of nifedipine with atenolol or propranolol in chronic stable angina. (Abstract No. 546.) European Heart Journal 5 (Suppl. 1): 128 (1984).
De Divitiis, O.; Petitto, M.; Di Somma, S.; Fazio, S.; Galderisi, M. et al.: Acebutolol and nifedipine in the treatment of arterial hypertension: Efficacy and acceptability. Arzneimittel-Forschung 34: 710-715 (1984).
Deedwania, P.; Shah, J.; Robison, C.; Watson, P. and Hurks, C.: Effects of nifedipine on glucose tolerance and insulin release in man. Clinical Research 32: 46A (1984).
De Feyter, P.J.; Kerkkamp, J.J. and de Jong, J.P.: Sustained beneficial effect of nifedipine in primary pulmonary hypertension. American Heart Journal 105: 333-334 (1983).
Delahaye, J.P.; Touboul, P.; Gaspard, P.; Delaye, J. and Cassagnes, J.: Le traitement de l'angine de poitrine de prinzmetal par la nifedipine. Lyon Médical 241: 769-775 (1979).
Delahaye, J.P.; Touboul, P.; Cassagnes, J.; Gaspard, P. and Milon, H.: The long-term treatment of Prinzmetal's angina with nifedipine; 4th International Adalat Symposium, pp. 87-94 (1980).
De Los Reyes, M.P.; De Los Reyes, X.P.; Passalacqua, A.S.W.: Tratamiento de la encefalopatia hipertensiva aguda con nifedipina en 7 pacientes. Revista Medica de Chile 110: 1204-1206 (1982).
De Ponti, C.; De Biase, A.M.; Pirelli, S.; Cataldo, G.; Salvadé, P. et al.: Effects of nifedipine, acebutolol, and their association on exercise tolerance in patients with effort angina. Cardiology 68 (Suppl. 2): 195-199 (1981).
De Ponti, C.; Mauri, F.; Ciliberto, G.R. and Carù, B.: Comparative effects of nifedipine, verapamil, isosorbide dinitrate and propranolol on exercise-induced angina pectoris. European Journal of Cardiology 10: 47-58 (1979).
Diamond, J.R.; Cheung, J.Y. and Fang, L.S.T.: Nifedipine-induced renal dysfunction. Alterations in renal hemodynamics. American Journal of Medicine 77: 905-909 (1984).
Dickinson, D.F.; Wilson, N. and Curry, P.: Use of nifedipine in hypertrophic cardiomyopathy in infants. A report of two cases. International Journal of Cardiology 7: 159-160 (1985).
Dilmen, U.; Cağlar, M.K.; Senses, D.A. and Kinik, E.: Nifedipine in hypertensive emergencies of children. American Journal of Diseases of Children 137: 1162-1165 (1983).
Dokladalova, J.; Tykal, J.A.; Coco, S.J.; Durkee, P.E.; Quercia, G.T. and Korst, J.J.: Occurrence and measurement of nifedipine and its nitropyridine derivative in human blood plasma. Journal of Chromatography 231: 451-458 (1982).
Donnelly, T. and Harrower, A.B.D.: Effect of nifedipine on glucose tolerance and insulin secretion in diabetic and non-diabetic patients. Curr. Med. Res. Op. 6: 690-693 (1980).
Douglas-Jones, A.P. and Mitchell, A.D.: Comparison of nifedipine (retard formulation) and mefruside in the treatment of mild to moderate hypertension – a prospective randomized double-blind crossover study in general practice. Postgraduate Medical Journal 60: 529-532 (1984).
Douglas Smith, C. and McKendry, R.J.R.: Controlled trial of nifedipine in the treatment of Raynaud's phenomenon. Lancet II: 1299-1301 (1982).

Drazen, J.M.; Fanta, C.H. and Lacouture, P.G.: Effect of nifedipine on constriction of human tracheal strips *in vitro*. British Journal of Pharmacology 78: 687-691 (1983).

Duhm, B.; Maul, W.; Medenwald, H.; Patzschke, K. and Wegner, L.A.: Tierexperimentalle Untersuchungen zur Pharmakokinetik und Biotransformation von radioaktive markiertem 4-(2'nitrophenyl)-2, 6-dimethyl-l, 4-dihydropyridin-3, 5-dicarbonsäuredimethyl ester. Arzneimittel-Forschung 22: 42-52 (1972).

Dylewicz, P.; Kirch, W.; Benesch, L. and Ohnhaus, E.E.: Influence of cimetidine on exercise capacity of nifedipine treated patients. (Abstract No. 933P). UPHAR 9th International Congress of Pharmacology, London (1984).

Ebner, F.: Wirkung und Verträglichkeit von Adalat bei Kombinationen mit verschiedenen Medikamenten. Münchener Medizinishe Wochenschrift 119 (Suppl. 1): 69-76 (1977).

Ebner, F. and Donath, M.: Mode of action and efficacy of nifedipine; 4th International Adalat Symposium, pp. 25-37 (1980).

Ebner, F.; Leisten, L.; Lejeune, P.; Donath, M. and Rämsch, K.D.: Administration of nifedipine to patients treated with digitalisglycosides, anti-diabetic agents and beta-blockers; 5th International Adalat Symposium, pp. 328-338 (1983).

Eggertsen, R. and Hansson, L.: Effects of treatment with nifedipine and metoprolol in essential hypertension. European Journal of Clinical Pharmacology 21: 389-390 (1982).

Ekelund, L.-G.; Ekelund, C. and Rössner, S.: Antihypertensive effects at rest and during exercise of a calcium blocker, nifedipine, alone and in combination with metoprolol. Acta Medica Scandinavica 212: 71-75 (1982).

Ekelund, L.-G. and Orö, L.: Antianginal efficiency of nifedipine with and without a beta-blocker, studied with exercise test. A double-randomized subacute study. Clinical Cardiology 2: 203-211 (1979).

Ekelund, L.-G. and Orö, L.: Antianginal efficiency of Adalat with and without a beta-blocker. A subacute study with exercise tests; 3rd International Adalat Symposium, pp. 218-225 (1976).

El Allaf, D.; Garzaniti, N.; Cremers, S.; D'Orio, V.; Marcelle, R. and Carlier, J.: Nifedipine in secondary pulmonary hypertension. (Abstract No. 193.) Circulation 66: II-49 (1982).

Elert, O.: Myocardial protection with nifedipine in open heart surgery: 5th International Adalat Symposium, pp. 100-106 (1983).

Eliahou, H.E.; Iaina, A.; Schneider, R.; Cohen, D.; Goldfarb, D. and Gross, M.: Treatment of hypertension in dialysis and essential hypertension patients with nifedipine. Clinical and Experimental Dialysis and Apheresis 6: 299-236 (1982).

Eliraz, A.; Wishnitzer, R. and Fink, A.: Exacerbation of asthmatic symptoms after cessation of nifedipine therapy. Annals of Allergy 52: 125-127 (1984).

Elkayam, U.; Roth, A.; Hsueh, W.; Weber, L.; Freidenberger, L. and Rahimtoola, S.H.: Neurohumoral changes following arterial dilation with hydralazine and nifedipine in heart failure. (Abstract.) Clinical Research 33: 88A (1985).

Elkayam, U.; Weber, L.; Campese, V.M.; Massry, S.G. and Rahimtoola, S.H.: Renal hemodynamic effects of vasodilation with nifedipine and hydralazine in patients with heart failure. Journal of the American College of Cardiology 4: 1261-1267 (1984d).

Elkayam, U.; Weber, L.; McKay, C.R. and Rahimtoola, S.: Variable, unpredictable, and deleterious hemodynamic response to oral nifedipine in severe chronic heart failure: An experience in 32 patients. (Abstract.) Journal of the American College of Cardiology 3: 478 (1984a).

Elkayam, U.; Weber, L.; McKay, C.R. and Rahimtoola, S.H.: Differences in hemodynamic response to vasodilation due to calcium channel antagonism with nifedipine and direct-acting agonism with hydralazine in chronic refractory congestive heart failure. American Journal of Cardiology 54: 126-131 (1984b).

Elkayam, U.; Weber, L.; Torkan, B.; Berman, D. and Rahimtoola, S.H.: Acute hemodynamic effect of oral nifedipine in severe chronic congestive heart failure. American Journal of Cardiology 52: 1041-1045 (1983).

Elkayam, U.; Weber, L.; Torkan, B.; McKay, C.R. and Rahimtoola, S.H.: Comparison of hemodynamic responses to nifedipine and nitroprusside in severe chronic congestive heart failure. American Journal of Cardiology 53: 1321-1325 (1984c).

Ellis, E.F.; Oelz, O.; Robert, I.J.; Payne, N.A.; Sweetman, B.J. et al.: Coronary arterial smooth muscle contraction by a substance released from platelets: Evidence that is thromboxane A_2. Science 193: 1135-1137 (1976).

Emanuelsson, H.; Herlitz, J.; Hjalmarson, Å.; Holmberg, S.; Waagstein, F. et al.: Hemodynamic and clinical findings after combined therapy with metoprolol and nifedipine in acute myocardial infarction. Clinical Cardiology 7: 425-432 (1984a).

Emanuelsson, H.; Hjalmarson, Å.; Holmberg, S.; Waagstein, F. and Waldenström, A.: Effects of nifedipine on arterial concentration and myocardial extraction of catecholamines during pacing-induced angina pectoris. Journal of Cardiovascular Pharmacology 6: 224-232 (1984b).

Emanuelsson, H. and Holmberg, S.: Mechanisms of angina relief after nifedipine: A hemodynamic and myocardial metabolic study. Circulation 68: 124-130 (1983).

Ene, M.D.; Williamson, P.J.; Roberts, C.J.C. and Waddell, G.: Natriuretic effects of nifedipine and nitrendipine. British Journal of Clinical Pharmacology 17: 193P (1984).

Ene, M.D.; Williamson, P.J.; Roberts, C.J.C. and Waddell, G.: The natriuresis following oral administration of the calcium antagonists – nifedipine and nitrendipine. British Journal of Clinical Pharmacology 19: 423-427 (1985).

Engel, H.-J. and Lichtlen, P.R.: Beneficial enhancement of coronary blood flow by nifedipine. Comparison with nitroglycerin and beta blocking agents. American Journal of Medicine 71: 658-666 (1981).

Engelman, R.M.; Hadji-Rousou, I.; Breyer, R.H.; Whittredge, P.; Harbison, W. and Chircop, R.V.: Rebound vasospasm after coronary revascularization in association with calcium antagonist withdrawal. Annals of Thoracic Surgery 37: 469-472 (1984).

Englert, R.: Verlaufsbeobachtungen über 2 Jahre bei Hypertoniepatienten mit Adalat-retard. Wiener Medizinische Wochenschrift 134 (Suppl. 82): 7-8 (1984).

Erbel, R.; Brand, G.; Meyer, J. and Effert, S.: Emergency treatment of hypertensive crisis with sublingual nifedipine. Postgraduate Medical Journal 59 (Suppl. 3): 134-136 (1983).

Erne, P.; Bolli, P.; Bertel, O.; Hulthen, U.L.; Kiowski, W. et al.: Factors influencing the hypotensive effects of calcium antagonists. Hypertension 5 (Suppl. II): 97-102 (1983).

Erne, P.; Kiowski, W.; Bolli, P.; Bürgisser, E. and Bühler, F.R.: Reduction of elevated intracellular free calcium concentration in platelets and blood pressure in essential hypertension by chronic treatment with calcium antagonists. (Abstract.) Journal of Hypertension 2: 102-103 (1984).

Esper, R.J.; Caprarella, M.; Marcos, R.M. and Lythgoe, M.: Echophonocardiographic assessment of the effect of the vasodilator nifedipine and the β-blocking agent acebutolol, separately and simultaneously, on the heart; 4th International Adalat Symposium, pp. 154-175 (1980).

Ettinger, W.H.; Wise, R.A.; Schaffhauser, D. and Wigley, F.M.: Controlled double-blind trial of dazoxiben and nifedipine in the treatment of Raynaud's phenomenon. American Journal of Medicine 77: 451-456 (1984).

Evans, M.G.; Olanoff, L.S.; Hurwitz, G.; Cowart, T.D. and Conradi, E.C.: Use of nifedipine as an adjunct to current antihypertensive therapy. Archives of Internal Medicine 144: 985-987 (1984).

Fanta, C.H.; Venugopalan, C.S.; Lacouture, P.G. and Drazen, J.M.: Inhibition of bronchoconstriction in the guinea pig by a calcium channel blocker, nifedipine. American Review of Respiratory Disease 125: 61-66 (1982).

Fakunding, J.L.; Chow, R. and Catt, K.J.: The role of calcium in the stimulation of aldosterone production by adrenocorticotropin, angiotensin II, and potassium in isolated glomerulosa cells. Endocrinology 105: 327-333 (1979).

Farber, H.W.; Karlinsky, J.B. and Faling, L.J.: Fatal outcome following nifedipine for pulmonary hypertension. Chest 83: 708-709 (1983).

Faris, J.V.; Childress, R.H. and Watanabe, A.M.: Effect of nifedipine on exercise tolerance in coronary artery disease. (Abstract.) American Journal of Cardiology 45: 439 (1980).

Farringer, J.A.; Green, J.A.; O'Rourke, R.A.; Linn, W.A. and Clementi, W.A.: Nifedipine-induced alterations in serum quinidine concentrations. American Heart Journal 108: 1570-1572 (1984).

Feely, J.: Nifedipine increases and glyceryl trinitrate decreases apparent liver blood flow in normal subjects. British Journal of Clinical Pharmacology 17: 83-85 (1984).

Feldman, R.L.; Pepine, C.J. and Conti, C.R.: Nifedipine in unstable angina. (Correspondence.) New England Journal of Medicine 307: 627 (1982).

Ferguson, D.W. and Dorsey, J.K.: Effects of nifedipine on baroreflex modulation of vascular resistance in man. American Heart Journal 109: 55-62 (1985).

Ferlito, S.; Fichera, C.; Carrá, G.; Puleo, F.; Calafato, M. and Volpicelli, D.: Effect of nifedipine on blood sugar, insulin and glucagon levels after an oral glucose load. Panminerva Medica 23: 75-80 (1981).

Findlay, I.N. and Dargie, H.J.: The effects of nifedipine, atenolol and that combination on left ventricular function. Postgraduate Medical Journal 59 (Suppl. 2): 70-73 (1983).

Findlay, I.N.; Dargie, H.J.; Ford, M. and Elliott, A.T.: Left ventricular ejection fraction, blood pressure and heart rate response during treatment of angina pectoris with nifedipine and atenolol. (Abstract.) II World Conference on Clinical Pharmacology and Therapeutics, p. 20 (Washington, D.C., 31 July-5 August 1983).

Findlay, I.N.; Gillen, G.; Elliott, A.T. and Dargie, H.J.: The treatment of angina pectoris with calcium channel and beta blockers, efficacy and effect on cardiac function. (Abstract.) Journal of the American College of Cardiology 3: 482 (1984).

Fioretti, P.; Benussi, B.; Klugmann, S. and Camerini, F.: Acute hemodynamic effects of nifedipine at rest and during stress in severe aortic incompetence. European Heart Journal 4: 110-116 (1983).

Fisher, J.; Borer, J.S.; Moses, J.W.; Goldberg, H.L.; Niarchos, A. et al.: Pulmonary hypertension: Comparative effects of nifedipine versus hydralazine. (Abstract No. 194.) Circulation 66: II-49 (1982).

Fisher, J.F.; Borer, J.S.; Moses, J.W.; Goldberg, H.L.; Niarchos, A.P.; et al.: Hemodynamic effects of nifedipine *versus* hydralazine in primary pulmonary hypertension. American Journal of Cardiology 54: 646-650 (1984).

Fisher, J.; Mack, R.; Borer, J.S.; Pickering, T.; Niarchos, A. et al.: Nifedipine in pulmonary hypertension: Importance of Raynaud's phenomenon. Clinical Research 31: 696A (1983).

Flaim, S.F.; Irwin, J.M.; Ratz, P.H. and Swigart, S.C.: Differential effects of calcium channel blocking agents on oxygen consumption rate in vascular smooth muscle. American Journal of Cardiology 49: 511-518 (1982).

Fleckenstein, A.: Specific pharmacology of calcium in myocardium, cardiac pacemakers, and vascular smooth muscle. Annual Review of Pharmacology and Toxicology 17: 149-166 (1977).

Fleckenstein, A.; Frey, M. and Fleckenstein-Grün, G.: Consequences of uncontrolled calcium entry and its prevention with calcium antagonists. European Heart Journal 4 (Suppl. H): 43-50 (1983).

Fleckenstein, A.; Tritthart, H.; Döring, H.J. and Byon, K.Y.: BAY a 1040-ein hochaktiver Ca^{++}-antagonistischer Inhibitor der elektro-mechanischen Koppelungsprozesse im Warmblütermyokard. Arzneimittel-Forschung 22: 22-23 (1972).

Foreman, J.C.; Hallett, M.B. and Mongar, J.L.: The relationship between histamine secretion and $^{45}Ca^{++}$ uptake by mast cells. Journal of Physiology 271: 193-214 (1977).

Forman, A.: Calcium entry blockade as a therapeutic principle in the female urogenital tract. Acta Obstetrica et Gynecologica Scandinavica (Suppl. 121): 5-26 (1984).

Forman, A.; Andersson, K.-E.; Henriksson, L.; Rud, T. and Ulmsten, U.: Effects of nifedipine on the smooth muscle of the human urinary tract *in vitro* and *in vivo*. Acta Pharmacologica et Toxicologica 43: 111-118 (1978).

Forman, A.; Andersson, K.-E.; Persson, C.G.A. and Ulmsten, U.: Relaxant effects of nifedipine on isolated, human myometrium. Acta Pharmacologica et Toxicologica 45: 81-86 (1979).

Forman, A.; Gandrup, P.; Andersson, K.-E. and Ulmsten, U.: Effects of nifedipine on spontaneous and methylergometrine-induced activity post partum. American Journal of Obstetrics and Gynecology 144: 442-448 (1982a).

Forman, A.; Gandrup, P.; Andersson, K.-E. and Ulmsten, U.: Effects of nifedipine on oxytocin- and prostaglandin $F_{2\alpha}$-induced activity in the postpartum uterus. American Journal of Obstetrics and Gynecology 144: 665-670 (1982b).

Foster, T.S.; Hamann, S.R.; Richards, V.R.; Bryant, P.J.; Graves, D.A. and McAllister Jr, R.G.: Nifedipine kinetics and bioavailability after single intravenous and oral doses in normal subjects. Journal of Clinical Pharmacology 23: 161-170 (1983).

Fox, J.E. and Daniel, E.E.: The role of Ca^{++} in the genesis of lower esophageal sphincter (LES) tone and contraction. (Abstract.) Gastroenterology 74: 1082 (1978).

Fox, K.M.; Deanfield, J.; Selwyn, A.; Krikler, S. and Wright, C.: Treatment of chronic stable angina pectoris with nifedipine; 5th International Adalat Symposium, pp. 197-208 (1982).

Fox, K.; Jonathan, A. and Selwyn, A.P.: Combined high-dosage administration of nifedipine and propranolol in patients with angina pectoris; 4th International Adalat Symposium, pp. 147-153 (1980).

Franchi, F. and Padeletti, L.: Evaluation of the clinical electrophysiological effects of antianginal drugs without specific antiarrhythmic properties. Methods and Findings in Experimental and Clinical Pharmacology 3: 17-27 (1981).

Franz, I.-W. and Wiewel, D.: Antihypertensive effects on blood pressure at rest and during exercise of calcium antagonists, β-receptor blockers, and their combination in hypertensive patients. Journal of Cardiovascular Pharmacology 6: S1037-S1042 (1984).

Frey, M.; Keidel, J. and Fleckenstein, A.: Verhütung experimenteller Gefässverkalkungen (Mönckebergs Typ der Arteriosklerose) durch Calcium-Antagonisten bei Ratten; in Fleckenstein, A. and Roskamm, H. (Eds) Calcium-Antagonismus, pp. 258-285 (Springer, Berlin 1980).

Frishman, W.H. and Charlap, S.: Nifedipine in the treatment of systemic hypertension. Archives of Internal Medicine 144: 2335-2336 (1984).

Frishman, W.H.; Weinberg, P.; Peled, H.B.; Kimmel, B.; Charlap, S. and Beer, N.: Calcium entry blockers for the treatment of severe hypertension and hypertensive crisis. American Journal of Medicine 77: 35-45 (1984).

Furlanello, F.; Disertori, M.; Vergara, G. and Del Favero, A.: Study on the electrophysiological effects of nifedipine in man; 4th International Adalat Symposium, pp. 227-235 (1980).

Gangji, D.; Juvent, M.; Niset, G.; Wathieu, M.; Degreve, M. et al.: Study of the influence of nifedipine on the pharmacokinetics and pharmacodynamics of propranolol, metoprolol and atenolol. British Journal of Clinical Pharmacology 17: 29S-35S (1984).

Garcia López, E.; Treviño, A.; Avilés, C.; Vásquez, B. and Garcia, A.: Nifedipine in severe hypertensive crisis in chronic renal failure patients treated with peritoneal dialysis. Dialysis and

Transplantation 13: 700-704 (1984).
Garty, M.; Shamir, E. and Rosenfeld, J.B.: Nifedipine-digoxin noninteraction. (Abstract No. H11.) International Symposium on Calcium Entry Blockers and Tissue Protection, Rome 15-16 March, 1984, p. 124 (1984).
Geddes, J.S.: Calcium antagonists and beta blockade – a useful combination. Postgraduate Medical Journal 59 (Suppl. 2): 62-69 (1983).
Gelfond, M.; Rozen, P. and Gilat, T.: Isosorbide dinitrate and nifedipine treatment of achalasia: A clinical, manometric and radionuclide evaluation. Gastroenterology 83: 963-969 (1982).
Gerstenblith, G.; Ouyang, P.; Achuff, S.C.; Bulkley, B.H.; Becker, L.C. et al.: Nifedipine in unstable angina. A double-blind, randomized trial. New England Journal of Medicine 306: 885-889 (1982).
Gibelli, G.; Carnovali, M.; Orvieni, C.; Colombo, G. and De Vita, C.: Effect and duration of action of nifedipine 20mg tablets: Double-blind ergometric evaluation *versus* placebo. Current Therapeutic Research 33: 295-304 (1983).
Ginsburg, R.; Lamb, I.H.; Schroeder, J.S.; Hu, M. and Harrison, D.C.: Randomized double-blind comparison of nifedipine and isosorbide dinitrate therapy in variant angina pectoris due to coronary artery spasm. American Heart Journal 103: 44-48 (1982).
Giugliano, D.; Torella, R.; Cacciapuoti, F.; Gentile, S.; Verza, M. and Varricchio, M.: Impairment of insulin secretion in man by nifedipine. European Journal of Clinical Pharmacology 18: 395-398 (1980).
Given, B.D.; Lee, T.H.; Stone, P.H. and Dzau, V.J.: Nifedipine in severely hypertensive patients with congestive heart failure and preserved ventricular systolic function. Archives of Internal Medicine 145: 281-285 (1985).
Gonzales, J.M.; Morice, R.C.; Bloom, K.; Akers, S.; Raizner, A.E. and Stevens, P.M.: Inhibition of airway reactivity by nifedipine in patients with coronary artery disease. American Review of Respiratory Disease 127: 155-157 (1983).
Gottlieb, S.O.; Ouyang, P.; Achuff, S.C.; Baughman, K.L.; Traill, T.A. and Mellits, E.D.: Acute nifedipine withdrawal: Consequences of preoperative and late cessation of therapy in patients with prior unstable angina. Journal of the American College of Cardiology 4: 382-388 (1984).
Gould, B.A.; Hornung, R.S.; Mann, S.; Subramanian, V.B. and Raftery, E.B.: Nifedipine or verapamil as sole treatment of hypertension. An intraarterial study. Hypertension 5 (Suppl. II): 91-96 (1983).
Grampa, A. and Franzetti, I.: Evaluation of a delayed-action Ca^{++}-antagonist in the medium-term treatment of hypertension. Gazzetta Medica Italiana Archivio Per Le Scienze Mediche 143: 189-198 (1984).
Grandjean, T. and Valenti, P.: Effects of nifedipine on effort tolerance and left ventricular function during exercise in patients suffering from severe angina pectoris; in Lichtlen et al. (Eds) International Adalat Panel Discussion. New Experimental and Clinical Results, pp. 118-126 (Excerpta Medica, Amsterdam 1978).
Green, J.A.; Clementi, W.A.; Porter, C. and Stigelman, W.: Nifedipine-quinidine interaction. Clinical Pharmacy 2: 461-465 (1983).
Greenwood, R.H.: Hyperglycaemic effect of nifedipine. British Medical Journal 284: 50 (1982).
Groth, H.; Förster, E.-C.; Neyses, L.; Sigenthaler, W. and Vetter, W.: Nifedipine in hypertensive emergencies and severe hypertension. Journal of Hypertension 2: 106 (1984).
Grunwald, Z.: Painful edema, erythematous rash, and burning sensation due to nifedipine. Drug Intelligence and Clinical Pharmacy 16: 492 (1982).
Guazzi, M.D.; Cesare, N.D.; Galli, C.; Salvioni, A.; Tramontana, C. et al.: Calcium-channel blockade with nifedipine and angiotensin converting-enzyme inhibition with captopril in the therapy of patients with severe primary hypertension. Circulation 70: 279-284 (1984a).
Guazzi, M.D.; Cipolla, C.; Bella, P.D.; Fabbiocchi, F.; Montorsi, P. and Sganzerla, P.: Disparate unloading efficacy of the calcium channel blockers, verapamil and nifedipine, on the foiling hypertensive left ventricle. American Heart Journal 108: 116-123 (1984b).
Guazzi, M.D.; Fiorentini, C.; Olivari, M.T.; Bartorelli, A.; Necchi, G. and Polese, A.: Short and long-term efficacy of a calcium-antagonistic agent (nifedipine) combined with methyldopa in the treatment of severe hypertension. Circulation 61: 913-919 (1980).
Guazzi, M.; Olivari, M.T.; Polese, A.; Fiorentini, C.; Magrini, F. and Moruzzi, P.: Nifedipine, a new antihypertensive with rapid action. Clin. Pharmacol. Therap. 22: 528-532 (1977).
Guazzi, M.D.; Polese, A.; Fiorentini, C.; Bartorelli, A. and Moruzzi, P.: Treatment of hypertension with calcium antagonists: Review. Hypertension 5 (Suppl. II): 85-90 (1983).
Gunther, S.; Green, L.; Muller, J.E.; Mudge Jr, G.H. and Grossman, W.: Prevention by nifedipine of abnormal coronary vasoconstriction in patients with coronary artery disease. Circulation 63: 849-855 (1981).
Gutierrez, L.M.; Lesko, L.J.; Whipps, R.; Carliner, N. and Fisher, M.: Pharmacokinetics and pharmacodynamics of nifedipine after chronic administration. Clinical Pharmacology and Therapeutics 35: 245 (1984).
Haerem, J.W.: Mural platelet microthrombi and major acute lesions of main epicardial arteries in sudden coronary death. Atherosclerosis 19: 529-541 (1974).
Haft, J.I. and Litterer, W.E.: Chewing nifedipine to rapidly treat hypertension. Archives of Internal Medicine 144: 2357-2359 (1984).
Haft, J.I.; Litterer, W.E.; Perez, L.; Zawislak, W. and Burachinsky, A.: Chewing nifedipine in the acute treatment of hypertension. Clinical Research 31: 190A (1983).
Hagemeijer, F. and van Mechelen, R.: Effectiveness of nifedipine in unstable angina persisting despite conventional medical therapy: 5th International Adalat Symposium, pp. 255-265 (1983).
Hagemeijer, F.; van Mechelen, R. and Santoso, T.: Benefits from adding nifedipine to the treatment of unstable angina when beta-blockade and isosorbide dinitrate have proved inadequate. Herz 7: 126-131 (1982).
Hall-Craggs, M.; Light, P.D. and Peters, R.W.: Development of immune complex nephritis during treatment with the calcium channel-blocking agent nifedipine. Human Pathology 15: 691-694 (1984).
Hallin, L.; Andren, L. and Hansson, L.: Controlled trial of nifedipine and bendroflumethiazide in hypertension. Journal of Cardiovascular Pharmacology 5: 1083-1085 (1983).
Hamann, S.R.; Blouin, R.A.; Chang, S.L.; Kaltenborn, K.E.; Tan, T.G. and McAllister Jr, R.G.: Effects of hemodynamic changes on the elimination kinetics of verapamil and nifedipine. Journal of Pharmacology and Experimental Therapeutics 231: 301-305 (1984).
Hamann, S.R. and McAllister Jr, R.G.: Measurement of nifedipine in plasma by gas-liquid chromatography and electron-capture detection. Clinical Chemistry 29: 158-160 (1983).
Hamann, S.R.; Tan, T.G.; Kaltenborn, K.E.; Brouwer, K.L.R.; Blouin, R.A. et al.: Effects of phenobarbital and SKF-525A on *in vitro* hepatic metabolism of verapamil and nifedipine. Pharmacology 30: 121-128 (1985).
Han, P. and Ardlie, N.G.: The influence of pH, temperature and environmental pH and platelet function for *in vitro* studies in plasma. British Journal of Haematology 26: 373-389 (1974).
Han, P.; Boatwright, C. and Ardlie, N.G.: Effect of the calcium-entry blocking agent nifedipine on activation of human platelets and comparison with verapamil. Thrombosis and Haemostasis 50: 513-517 (1983).

Hanrath, P.; Kremer, P. and Bleifeld, W.: Influence of nifedipine on left ventricular dysfunction at rest and during exercise. European Heart Journal 3: 325-330 (1982).
Hansen, P.B.; Buch, J.; Rasmussen, O.Ø.; Waldorff, S. and Steiness, E.: Influence of atenolol and nifedipine on digoxin-induced inotropism in humans. British Journal of Clinical Pharmacology 18: 817-822 (1984).
Hattori, S.; Weintraub, W.W.; Agarwai, J.B.; Bodenheimer, M.M.; Banka, V.S. and Helfant, R.H.: The effects of nifedipine on ischemic myocardium: preservation of contraction during partial coronary occlusion. (Abstract.) American Journal of Cardiology 45: 485 (1980).
Hausmann, L.: Verhalten des Kohlenhydratstoffwechsels unter einer 16 wöchigen Therapie mit Nifedipin. Erfahrungen mit Adalat in Klinik und Praxis, Munich 23 October, 1982, pp. 37-42 (Fachbuch-Verlagsgesellschaft, Erlangen 1983).
Hawkins, S.; Forskitt, S.; Hall, N.D.; Maslen, C.; Maddison, P.J. et al.: Clinical and laboratory effects of nifedipine in the treatment of Raynaud's phenomenon. Annals of the Rheumatic Diseases 43: 110-111 (1984).
Hayashi, H.; Takumi, K.; Ishikawa, T.; Yabe, S.; Ohsugi, S. et al.: Limitation of myocardial ischemic injury by nifedipine in patients with acute myocardial infarction evaluated by body surface mapping. (Abstract.) European Heart Journal 5 (Suppl. 1): 221 (1984).
Helfant, R.H.: In patient treatment of unstable angina: Clinical perspective and sequential management. American Heart Journal 104: 697-701 (1982).
Henderson, A.F.; Heaton, R.W.; Dunlop, L.S. and Costello, J.F.: Effects of nifedipine on antigen-induced bronchoconstriction. American Review of Respiratory Disease 127: 549-553 (1983).
Henry, P.D.: Protection of ischemic myocardium by treatment with nifedipine; in Winbury, M.M. and Abiko, Y. (Eds) Ischemic Myocardium and Antianginal Drugs, pp. 129-142 (Raven Press, New York 1979a).
Henry, P.D.: Calcium antagonists: Mechanisms of action with special reference to nifedipine; in Kharasch, N. (Ed.) Trace Metals in Health and Disease, pp. 227-233 (Raven Press, New York 1979b).
Henry, P.D.: Comparative pharmacology of calcium antagonists: Nifedipine, verapamil, and diltiazem. American Journal of Cardiology 46: 1047-1058 (1980).
Hess, W.; Schulte-Sasse, U. and Tarnow, J.: Nifedipine versus nitroprusside for controlling hypertensive episodes during coronary artery bypass surgery. European Heart Journal 5: 140-145 (1984).
Higuchi, S.; Sasaki, H. and Sado, T.: Determination of a new cerebral vasodilator 2,6-dimethyl-4-(3-nitrophenyl)-1,4-dihydropyridine-3, 5-dicarboxylic acid 3-2-(N-benzyl-N-methylamino)-ethyl ester 5-methyl ester hydrochloride (YC-93) in plasma by election capture gas chromatography. Journal of Chromatography 110: 301-307 (1975).
Higuchi, S. and Shiobara, Y.: Quantitative determination of nifedipine in human plasma by selected ion monitoring. Biomedical Mass Spectrometry 5: 220-223 (1978).
Hill, J.A. and Conti, C.R.: Coronary spasm: Uses of nifedipine and isosorbide dinitrate. Primary Cardiology 9: 104-113 (1983).
Hill, J.A.; Feldman, R.L.; Conti, R.; Hill, C.K. and Pepine, C.J.: Long-term responses to nifedipine in patients with coronary spasm who have an initial favourable response. American Journal of Cardiology 52: 26-29 (1983).
Hiramatsu, K.; Yamagishi, F.; Kubota, T. and Yamada, T.: Acute effects of the calcium antagonist, nifedipine, on blood pressure, pulse rate, and the renin-angiotensin-aldosterone system in patients with essential hypertension. American Heart Journal 104: 1346-1350 (1982).
Hirasawa, K.; Shen, W.F.; Kelly, D.T.; Roubin, G.; Tateda, K. and Shibata, J.: Effect of food ingestion on nifedipine absorption and haemodynamic response. European Journal of Clinical Pharmacology 28: 105-107 (1985).
Hiroki, T.; Inoue, T.; Yoshida, T. and Arakawa, K.: Effect of the calcium antagonistic agent nifedipine on platelet aggregation response to exercise in patients with angina pectoris. Arzneimittel-Forschung 32: 1571-1574 (1982).
Holmsen, H. and Day, J.: Biochemistry and physiology of blood platelets. Annals of Clinical and Laboratory Science 1: 38-44 (1971).
Hongo, M.; Traube, M.; McAllister Jr, R.G. and McCallum, R.W.: Effects of nifedipine on esophageal motor function in humans: Correlation with plasma nifedipine concentration. Gastroenterology 86: 8-12 (1984a).
Hongo, M.; Traube, M. and McCallum, R.W.: Comparison of effects of nifedipine, propantheline bromide, and the combination on esophageal motor function in normal volunteers. Digestive Diseases and Sciences 29: 300-304 (1984b).
Hopf, R.; Pietruska, M.; Dowinsky, S. and Kaltenbach, M.: Combined administration of various doses of nifedipine and isosorbide dinitrate in patients with angina pectoris: 5th International Adalat Symposium, pp. 209-217 (1983).
Horio, S.; Kohrogi, H.; Ando, M.; Sugimoto, M. and Araki, S.: Preventive and reverse effects of nifedipine on human bronchoconstriction 'in vitro'. Archives Internationales de Pharmacodynamie et de Thérapie 267: 80-90 (1984).
Hornung, R.S.; Gould, B.A.; Jones, R.I.; Sonecha, T. and Raftery, E.B.: Nifedipine tablets for hypertension: A study using continuous ambulatory intra-arterial recording. Postgraduate Medical Journal 59 (Suppl. 2): 95-97 (1983).
Horster, F.A.: Pharmacokinetics of nifedipine-^{14}C in man; 2nd International Adalat Symposium, pp. 124-127 (1975).
Horster, F.A.; Duhm, B.; Maul, W.; Medenwald, H.; Patschke, K. and Wegner, L.A.: Klinische Untersuchungen zur Pharmakokinetik von radioaktif markierten 4-(2-Nitrophenyl)-2, 6-dimethyl-1, 4-dihydropyridin-3, 5-dicarbonsaure-dimethyl-ester. Arzneimittel-Forschung 22: 330-334 (1972).
Hugenholtz, P.G.; Michels, H.R.; Serruys, P.W. and Brower, R.W.: Nifedipine in the treatment of unstable angina, coronary spasm and myocardial ischemia. American Journal of Cardiology 47: 163-173 (1981).
Husted, S.E.; Nielsen, H.K.; Christensen, C.K. and Lederballe Pedersen, O.: Long-term therapy of arterial hypertension with nifedipine given alone or in combination with a beta-adrenoceptor blocking agent. European Journal of Clinical Pharmacology 22: 101-103 (1982).
Huysmans, F. Th.M.; Sluiter, H.E.; Thien, Th.A. and Koene, R.A.P.: Acute treatment of hypertensive crisis with nifedipine. British Journal of Clinical Pharmacology 16: 725-727 (1983a).
Huysmans, F. Th.M.; Thien, Th.A.; Sluiter, H.E. and Koene, R.A.P.: Acute treatment of hypertension with nifedipine. Netherlands Journal of Medicine 26: 256-261 (1983b).
Ikeda, H.; Takahashi, K.; Sasaki, H.; Ito, E. and Yasui, S.: Acute effects of nifedipine on patients with chronic obstructive lung disease. Arzneimittel-Forschung 35: 518-521 (1985).
Imai, Y.; Abe, K.; Otsuka, Y.; Irokawa, N.; Yasujima, M. et al.: Management of severe hypertension with nifedipine in combination with cloridine or propranolol. Arzneimittel-Forschung 30: 674-678 (1980).
Ishii, H.; Itoh, K. and Nose, T.: Different antihypertensive effects of nifedipine in conscious experimental hypertensive and normotensive rats. European Journal of Pharmacology 64: 21-29 (1980).
Isles, C.G.; Johnston, A.O.C. and Milne, F.J.: Slow release nifedipine and atenolol as initial therapy in Blacks with malignant hypertension. Journal of Hypertension 2: 559 (1984).
Ito, H.; Arakawa, M.; Shibasaki, T. and Hirakawa, S.: Acute antihypertensive effect of nifedipine by sublingual route in cases with clinically severe systolic hypertension. Arzneimittel-Forschung 34: 630-636 (1984).
Itoh, Y.; Tawara, I. and Itoh, T.: Clinical experience with nifed-

ipine; 1st International Nifedipine 'Adalat' Symposium, pp. 251-259 (1975).

Jaffe, I.A.: Nifedipine in digital ulceration in scleroderma. Arthritis and Rheumatism 25: 1267-1269 (1982).

Jaiprakash, S.S.; Chatterjee, S.S.; Sahay, J.N. and MacDonald, G.: Efficacy of nifedipine in the treatment of angina pectoris and chronic airways obstruction. Postgraduate Medical Journal 56: 624-628 (1980).

Jakobsen, P.; Lederballe Pedersen, O. and Mikkelsen, E.: Gas chromatographic determination of nifedipine and one of its metabolites using electron capture detection. Journal of Chromatography 162: 81-87 (1979).

Jariwalla, A.G. and Anderson, E.G.: Production of ischaemic cardiac pain by nifedipine. British Medical Journal 1: 1181-1182 (1978).

Jee, L.D. and Opie, L.H.: Acute hypotensive response to nifedipine added to prazosin in treatment of hypertension. British Medical Journal 287: 1514 (1983).

Jenkins, R.M. and Nagle, R.E.: The symptomatic and objective effects of nifedipine in combination with beta-blocker therapy in severe angina pectoris. Postgraduate Medical Journal 58: 697-700 (1982).

Jensen, C.; Skov, P.S. and Norn, S.: Inhibitory effect of calcium antagonists on histamine release from human leukocytes. *In vivo* and *in vitro* experiments. Allergy 38: 233-237 (1983).

Joffe, B.I.; Lamprey, J.M.; Shires, R.; Baker, S.; Viljoen, M. and Seftel, H.C.: Lack of hormonal effects of a single dose of nifedipine in healthy young men. Journal of Cardiovascular Pharmacology 5: 700-702 (1983).

Johnsson, H.: Effects by nifedipine (Adalat®) on platelet function *in vitro* and *in vivo*. Thrombosis Research 21: 523-528 (1981).

Johnston, D.L.; Lesoway, R.; Humen, D.P. and Kostuk, W.J.: Clinical and hemodynamic evaluation of propranolol in combination with verapamil, nifedipine and diltiazem in exertional angina pectoris: A placebo-controlled, double-blind, randomized, crossover study. American Journal of Cardiology 55: 680-687 (1985).

Kahan, A.; Amor, B. and Menkes, C.J.: Nifedipine treatment for Raynaud's phenomenon. Arthritis and Rheumatism 27: 959 (1984a).

Kahan, A.; Amor, B.; Menkes, C.J. and Weber, S.: Nifedipine in digital ulceration in scleroderma. Arthritis and Rheumatism 26: 809 (1983a).

Kahan, A.; Foult, J.; Weber, S.; Amor, B.; Menkes, C.J. and Degeorges, M.: Nifedipine and alpha-adrenergic blockade in Raynaud's phenomenon. (Abstract No. 599.) European Heart Journal 5 (Suppl. I): 139 (1984b).

Kahan, A.; Weber, S.; Amor, B.; Guerin, F. and Degeorges, M.: Nifedipine in the treatment of migraine in patients with Raynaud's phenomenon. New England Journal of Medicine 308: 1102-1103 (1983b).

Kahan, A.; Weber, S.; Amor, B.; Menkes, C.J.; Saporta, L.; et al.: Calcium entry blocking agents in digital vasospasm (Raynaud's phenomenon). European Heart Journal 4 (Suppl. C): 123-129 (1983c).

Kaltenbach, M.; Schulz, W. and Kober, G.: Effects of nifedipine after intravenous and intracoronary administration. American Journal of Cardiology 44: 832-838 (1979).

Kanatsuna, T.; Nakano, K.; Mori, H.; Kano, Y.; Nishioka, H.; et al.: Effects of nifedipine on insulin secretion and glucose metabolism in rats and in hypertensive type 2 (non-insulin dependent) diabetics. Arzneimittel-Forschung 35: 514-517 (1985).

Katz, A.M.; Hager, W.D.; Messineo, F.C. and Pappano, A.J.: Cellular actions and pharmacology of the calcium channel blocking drugs. American Journal of Medicine 77: 2-10 (1984).

Katz, A.M. and Reuter, H.: Cellular calcium and cardiac cell deth. American Journal of Cardiology 44: 188-190 (1979).

Katz, R.I.; Weintraub, W.S.; Bodenheimer, M.M.; Agarwal, J.B.; Banka, V.S. and Helfant, R.H.: Failure of low dose nifedipine to improve exercise tolerance in stable angina. (Abstract.) American Journal of Cardiology 49: 895 (1982).

Katzenberg, C.; Morrison, D.A. and Goldman, S.: Nifedipine in hypertrophic cardiomyopathy. Clinical Research 30: 13A (1982).

Kawai, C.; Konishi, T.; Matsuyama, E. and Okazaki, H.: Comparative effects of three calcium antagonists, diltiazem, verapamil, and nifedipine, on the sinoatrial and atrioventricular nodes: Experimental and clinical studies. Circulation 63: 1035-1042 (1981).

Kay, R.; Blake, J. and Rubin, D.: Possible coronary spasm rebound to abrupt nifedipine withdrawal. (Correspondence.) American Heart Journal 103: 308 (1982).

Keidar, S.; Binenboim, C. and Palant, A.: Muscle cramps during treatment with nifedipine. British Medical Journal 285: 1241-1242 (1982).

Keidar, S.; Marmor, A.; Grenadier, E. and Palant, A.: Nifedipine and Prinzmetal's angina. Circulation 59: 195 (1979).

Kelly, D.T.; Choong, C.Y.P.; Roubin, G.S.; Shen, W.F.; Bautovich, G.J.; et al.: Effects of nifedipine on exercise haemodynamics and left ventricular function in patients with exertional angina pectoris. (Abstract.) Abstracts of the Asian Pacific Adalat Symposium: 14 (Tokyo, 23-24 October 1982).

Kendall, M.J.; Jack, D.B.; Laugher, S.J.; Lobo, J. and Smith, S.R.: Lack of a pharmacokinetic interaction between nifedipine and the β-adrenoceptor blockers metoprolol and atenolol. British Journal of Clinical Pharmacology 18: 331-335 (1984).

Kennedy, T.P.; Michael, J.R.; Huang, C.-K.; Kallman, C.H.; Zahka, K.; et al.: Nifedipine inhibits hypoxic pulmonary vasoconstriction during rest and exercise in patients with chronic obstructive pulmonary disease. A controlled double-blind study. American Review of Respiratory Disease 129: 544-551 (1984).

Kennedy, T.P.; Michael, J.R. and Summer, W.: Calcium channel blockers in hypoxic pulmonary hypertension. American Journal of Medicine 78 (Suppl. 2B): 18-26 (1985).

Kenmure, A.C.F. and Scruton, J.H.: A double-blind controlled trial of the antianginal efficacy of nifedipine compared with propranolol; 3rd International Adalat Symposium, pp. 268-271 (1976).

Kenmure, A.C.F. and Scruton, J.H.: A double-blind controlled trial of the antianginal efficacy of nifedipine compared with propranolol. British Journal of Clinical Practice 33: 49-51 (1979).

Keyriläinen, O.; Bae, E.; Rytkönen, U.; Mathiesen, M.S. and Wendelin, H.: Metoprolol, nifedipine and the combination in effort angina pectoris. I Clinical effects. (Abstract No. 1464.) European Heart Journal 5 (Suppl. 1): 293 (1984).

Kimura, E.; Tanaka, K.; Mizuno, K.; Honda, Y. and Hashimoto, H.: Suppression of repeatedly occurring ventricular fibrillation with nifedipine in variant form of angina pectoris. Japanese Heart Journal 18: 736-742 (1977).

Kimura, E. and Kishida, H.: Treatment of variant angina with drugs: A survey of 11 cardiology institutes in Japan. Circulation 63: 844-848 (1981).

Kiowski, W.; Bertel, O.; Erne, P.; Bolli, P.; Hulthén, L.; et al.: Hemodynamic and reflex responses to acute and chronic antihypertensive therapy with the calcium entry blocker nifedipine. Hypertension 5 (Suppl. I): 70-74 (1983).

Kirch, W.; Janisch, H.D.; Heidemann, H.; Rämsch, K. and Ohnhaus, E.E.: Einfluss von Cimetidin und Ranitidin auf pharmakokinetik und antihypertensiven Effekt von Nifedipin. Deutsche Medizinische Wochenschrift 108: 1757-1761 (1983).

Kirch, W.; Hoensch, H.; Ohnhaus, E.E. and Janisch, H.D.: Ranitidin-Nifedipin Interaktion. Deutsche Medizinische Wochenschrift 109: 1223 (1984).

Kirch, W.; Ohnhaus, E.E.; Hoensch, H. and Janisch, H.D.: Ranitidine increases bioavailability of nifedipine. (Abstract.) Clinical Pharmacology and Therapeutics 37: 204 (1985).

Kirkpatrick, C.T.: Excitation and contraction in bovine tracheal smooth muscle. Journal of Physiology 244: 263-281 (1975).

Kishida, H. and Kimura, E.: The medical treatment of variant angina; 4th International Adalat Symposium, pp. 95-102 (1980).
Kishida, H.; Otsu, F.; Kusama, Y.; Takayama, M.; Hayakawa, H. and Kimura, E.: Effects of calcium antagonists, especially nifedipine, on variant angina, resting angina, and unstable angina. Japanese Heart Journal 23: 871-881 (1982).
Kiyomoto, A.; Sasaki, Y.; Odawara, A. and Morita, T.: Inhibition of platelet aggregation by diltiazem. Comparison with verapamil and nifedipine and inhibitory potencies of diltiazem metabolites. Circulation Research 52 (Suppl. I): 115-119 (1983).
Klein, H.O.; Ninio, R.; DiSegni, E.; David, D.; Lang, R.M. and Kaplinsky, E.: Improved left ventricular function at rest and handgrip exercise with nifedipine in a placebo-controlled study. (Abstract.) European Heart Journal (Suppl. 1): 9 (1984).
Klein, W.; Brandt, D.; Vrecko, K. and Härringer, H.: Role of calcium antagonists in the treatment of essential hypertension. Circulation Research 52: 174-181 (1983).
Kleinbloesem, C.H.; van Harten, J.; de Leede, L.G.J.; van Brummelen, P. and Breimer, D.D.: Nifedipine kinetics and dynamics during rectal infusion to steady state with an osmotic system. Clinical Pharmacology and Therapeutics 36: 396-401 (1984c).
Kleinbloesem, C.H.; van Brummelen, P.; Faber, H.; Danhof, M.; Vermeulen, N.P.E. and Breimer, D.D.: Variability in nifedipine pharmacokinetics and dynamics: A new oxidation polymorphism in man. Biochemical Pharmacology 33: 3721-3724 (1984d).
Kleinbloesem, C.H.; van Brummelen, P.; Sandberg, T.W.H. and Breimer, D.D.: Pharmacokinetics and haemodynamic interaction between nifedipine and propranolol. British Journal of Clinical Pharmacology 19: 537P (1985).
Kleinbloesem, C.H.; van Brummelen, P.; van de Linde, J.A.; Voogd, P.J. and Breimer, D.D.: Nifedipine: Kinetics and dynamics in healthy subjects. Clinical Pharmacology and Therapeutics 35: 742-749 (1984a).
Kleinbloesem, C.H.; van Harten, J.; van Brummelen, P. and Breimer, D.D.: Liquid chromatographic determination of nifedipine in plasma and of its main metabolite in urine. Journal of Chromatography 308: 209-216 (1984b).
Klugmann, S.; Salvi, A. and Camerini, F.: Haemodynamic effects of nifedipine in heart failure. British Heart Journal 43: 440-446 (1980).
Klütsch, V.R.; Schmidt, P. and Grosswendt, J.: Der Einfluss von Bay a 1040 auf die Nierenfunktion des Hypertonikers. Arzneimittel-Forschung 22: 377-380 (1972).
Kneussl, M.; Burghuber, O.; Harmuth, P.; Silberbauer, K.; Sinzinger, H. and Haber, P.: Nifedipine protects acetylcholine induced bronchoconstriction: The role of mediator release. American Review of Respiratory Disease 127 (Suppl. 2): 108 (1983).
Kober, G.; Schulz, W.; Bamberg, E. and Kaltenbach, M.: Cardiac and peripheral effects of nifedipine; in Lichtlen et al.: (Eds) International Adalat Panel Discussion: New Experimental and Clinical Results, pp. 86-93 (Excerpta Medica, Amsterdam 1979).
Koch, G.: Plasma renin activity, epinephrine and norepinephrine at rest and during exercise in young adults and boys. Scandinavian Journal of Clinical and Laboratory Investigation 37 (Suppl. 147): 107 (1977).
Koch, G.: Beta-receptor and calcium blockade in ischemic heart disease: Effects on systemic and pulmonary hemodynamics and on plasma catecholamines at rest and during exercise; 4th International Adalat Symposium, pp. 131-142 (1980).
Koide, T.; Kakihana, M.; Takabatake, Y.; Iizuka, M.; Uchida, Y.; et al.: Long-term clinical effect of calcium inhibitors in hypertrophic cardiomyopathy compared to the effect of Beta-blocking agents. A preliminary report with special reference to the beneficial effect of nifedipine on angina pectoris. Japanese Heart Journal 22: 87-102 (1981).
Kondo, S.; Kuchiki, A.; Yamamoto, K.; Akimoto, K.; Takahashi, K.; et al.: Identification of nifedipine metabolites and their determination by gas chromatography. Chemical and Pharmaceutical Bulletin 28: 1-7 (1980).
Kopf, G.S.; Riba, A. and Zito, R.: Intraoperative use of nifedipine for hemodynamic collapse due to coronary artery spasm following myocardial revascularization. Annals of Thoracic Surgery 34: 457-460 (1982).
Koppermann, G. and Kaukel, E.: Effect of nifedipine on the allergen-induced bronchoconstriction. Respiration 46 (Suppl. 1): 28 (1984).
Kramer, P.H.; Chatterjee, K.; Schwartz, A.; Swedberg, K.; Rouleau, J.-L.; et al.: Alterations in angina threshold with nifedipine during pacing induced angina. British Heart Journal 52: 308-313 (1984).
Krikler, D. and Rowland, E.: Effect of nifedipine as compared with verapamil on atrioventricular conduction; 4th International Adalat Symposium, pp. 241-244 (1980).
Kroneberg, G.: Pharmacology of nifedipine (Adalat); 1st International Nifedipine 'Adalat' Symposium, pp. 3-10 (1975a).
Kroneberg, G.: Pharmacology of nifedipine; 2nd International Adalat Symposium, pp. 12-19 (1975b).
Kroneberg, G. and Krebs, R.: Pharmacology of nifedipine; 4th International Adalat Symposium, pp. 14-24 (1980).
Kubo, K.; Shiraishi, K.; Muto, H.; Suzuki, T. and Sugino, N.: Treatment of hypertension in haemodialysis patients with nifedipine. Hypertension 5 (Suppl. II) 109-112 (1983).
Kuhlmann, J.: Effects of nifedipine and diltiazem on plasma levels and renal excretion of beta-acetyldigoxin. Clinical Pharmacology and Therapeutics 37: 150-156 (1985).
Kuhlmann, J. and Marcin, S.: Lack of significant effect of nifedipine and diltiazem on the pharmacokinetics of digitoxin. (Abstract No. 792.) II World Conference on Clinical Pharmacology and Therapeutics, Washington D.C. (31 July-5 August 1983).
Kuhlmann, J.; Marcin, S. and Frank, K.H.: Effects of nifedipine and diltiazem on the pharmacokinetics of digoxin. Naunyn-Schmiedeberg's Archives of Pharmacology 324 (Suppl.): R81 (1983).
Kuhlmann, J.; Marcin, S. and Frank, K.H.: Pharmakokinetik und kardiale Wirksamkeit von β-Acetyldigoxin und Digitoxin unter einer Kombinationstherapie mit Nifedipin. Klinische Wochenschrift 62: 451-457 (1984).
Kurnik, P.B.; Tiefenbrunn, A.J. and Ludbrook, P.A.: The dependence of the cardiac effects of nifedipine on the responses of the peripheral vascular system. Circulation 69: 963-972 (1984).
Kurosawa, N.; Morishima, S.; Owada, E.; Ito, K.; Ueda, K.; et al.: Determination of nifedipine in human plasma by gas chromatography equipped with flame thermionic detector (FTD). Yakugaku Zasshi 104: 775-779 (1984).
Kusano, E.; Asano, Y.; Takeda, K.; Matsumoto, Y.; Ebihara, A. and Hosoda, S.: Hypotensive effect of nifedipine in hypertensive patients with chronic renal failure. Arzneimittel-Forschung 32: 1575-1580 (1982).
Kusano, E.; Asano, Y.; Takeda, K.; Terao, N. and Hosoda, S.: Acute and chronic hypotensive effects of nifedipine and niludipine in hypertensive patients with chronic renal failure. Arzneimittel-Forschung 34: 624-629 (1984).
Kuwajima, I.; Ueda, K.; Kamata, C.; Matsushita, S.; Kuramoto, K.; et al.: A study on the effects of nifedipine in hypertensive crises and severe hypertension. Japanese Heart Journal 19: 455-467 (1978).
Lacché, A. and Basaglia, P.: Hypertensive emergencies: effects of therapy by nifedipine administered sublingually. Current Therapeutic Research 34: 879-887 (1983).
Lacché, A.; Feltrin, G.; D'Amico, A.; Zucchinetti, L. and Basaglia, P.: L'uso della nifedipina come farmaco anti-ipertensivo in pazienti in età geriatrica. Giornale di Gerontologia 29: 295-301 (1981).

Landmark, K.: Antihypertensive and metabolic effects of long term therapy with nifedipine slow-release tablets. Journal of Cardiovascular Pharmacology 7: 12-17 (1985).

Landmark, K.; Sire, S.; Thaulow, E.; Amlie, J.P. and Nitter-Hauge, S.: Acute influences of nifedipine, propranolol and the combined administration of the two drugs on haemodynamics in patients with hypertrophic obstructive cardiomyopathy; 5th International Adalat Symposium, pp. 81-90 (1983).

Lappe, R.W.; Saslow, B.A. and Wendt, R.L.: Effects of nifedipine on the hypotensive actions of α_2-agonists in conscious spontaneously hypertensive rats. Journal of Cardiovascular Pharmacology 6: S748-S752 (1984).

Latta, G.; Verheggen, R.; Rücker, W. and Schrör, K.: Inhibition of human platelet aggregation and thromboxane formation by calcium antagonists. Naunyn-Schmiedeberg's Archives of Pharmacology 324 (Suppl.): R49 (1983).

Lederballe Pedersen, O.: Calcium blockade in arterial hypertension: Review. Hypertension 5 (Suppl. II): 74-79 (1983).

Lederballe Pedersen, O.; Christensen, C.K.; Mikkelsen, E. and Ramsch, K.D.: Relationship between the antihypertensive effect and steady state plasma concentration of nifedipine given alone or in combination with a beta adrenoceptor blocking agent. European Journal of Clinical Pharmacology 18: 287-293 (1980a).

Lederballe Pedersen, O.; Christensen, N.J. and Rämsch, K.D.: Comparison of acute effects of nifedipine in normotensive and hypertensive man. Journal of Cardiovascular Pharmacology 2: 357-366 (1980b).

Lederballe Pedersen, O. and Mikkelsen, E.: Acute and chronic effects of nifedipine in arterial hypertension. European Journal of Clinical Pharmacology 14: 375-381 (1978).

Lederballe Pedersen, O.; Mikkelsen, E. and Andersson, K.-E.: Effects of extracellular calcium on potassium and noradrenaline induced contractions in the aorta of spontaneously hypertensive rats – increased sensitivity to nifedipine. Acta Pharmacologica et Toxicologica 43: 137-144 (1978).

Lederballe Pedersen, O.; Mikkelsen, E.; Christensen, N.J.; Kornerup, H.J. and Pedersen, E.B.: Effect of nifedipine on plasma renin, aldosterone and catecholamines in arterial hypertension. European Journal of Clinical Pharmacology 15: 235-240 (1979).

Lederman, D.; Lumerman, H.; Reuben, S. and Freedman, P.D.: Gingival hyperplasia associated with nifedipine therapy. Oral Surgery, Oral Medicine, Oral Pathology 57: 620-622 (1984).

Lee, T.H.; DiSesa, V.J.; Cohn, L.H.; Lilly, L.S. and Antman, E.M.: Correction of intraoperative diastolic myocardial dysfunction with nifedipine. Clinical Cardiology 6: 549-552 (1983).

Lehmann, H.-U. and Hochrein, H.: Differentialtherapie mit Calciumantagonisten. Deutsche Medizinische Wochenschrift 110: 674-680 (1985).

Leier, C.V.; Patrick, T.J.; Hermiller, J.; Dalpiaz Pacht, K.; Huss, P.; et al.: Nifedipine in congestive heart failure: Effects on resting and exercise hemodynamics and regional blood flow. American Heart Journal 108: 1461-1468 (1984).

Leier, C.V.; Patrick, T.J.; Hermiller, J.B.; Magorien, R.D. and Unverferth, D.V.: Regional hemodynamic effects of nifedipine in congestive heart failure (Abstract.) Circulation 68 (Suppl. III): 8 (1983).

Lejeune, Ph.; Boehme, K.; Schreiber, U.; Breitkopf, P.; Luther, P.; et al.: Hypertonie-Therapie: Wirkung der fixen Kombination von Nifedipin und Mefrusid (BAY O 8063). Münchener Medizinische Wochenschrift 126: 1393-1396 (1984).

Lejeune, Ph.; Gunselmann, W.; Hennies, L.; Hess, K.; Rittgerodt, K.; et al.: Effects of BAY 15240, a fixed combination of low dose nifedipine and acebutolol on hypertension: Comparison with standard dose nifedipine. European Journal of Clinical Pharmacology 28: 17-21 (1985).

Leon, M.B.; Rosing, D.R.; Bonow, R.O. and Epstein, S.E.: Combination therapy with calcium-channel blockers and beta blockers for chronic stable angina pectoris. American Journal of Cardiology 55: 69B-80B (1985).

Leonetti, G.; Cuspidi, C.; Sampieri, L.; Terzoli, L. and Zanchetti, A.: Comparison of cardiovascular, renal, and humoral effects of acute administration of two calcium channel blockers in normotensive and hypertensive subjects. Journal of Cardiovascular Pharmacology 4 (Suppl. 3): S319-S324 (1982).

Lesko, L.J.; Miller, A.K.; Yeager, R.L. and Chatterji, D.C.: Rapid GC method for quantitation of nifedipine in serum using electron capture detection. Journal of Chromatographic Science 21: 415-419 (1983).

Lette, J.; Gagnon, R.-M.; Lemire, J.G. and Morissette, M.: Rebound of vasospastic angina after cessation of long-term treatment with nifedipine. Canadian Medical Association Journal 130: 1169-1174 (1984).

Lever, A.M.L.; Corris, P.A. and Gibson, G.J.: Nifedipine enhances the bronchodilator effect of salbutamol. Thorax 39: 576-578 (1984).

Lewis, B.H.; Muller, J.E.; Rutherford, J.; Mudge, G.H. and Collins, J.J.: Nifedipine for coronary-artery spasm after revascularization. New England Journal of Medicine 306: 992-993 (1982).

Lewis, J.G.: Adverse reactions to calcium antagonists. Drugs 25: 196-222 (1983).

Lewy, R.I.; Wiener, L.; Walinsky, P.; Lefer, A.M.; Silver, M.J. and Smith, J.B.: Thromboxane release during pacing-induced angina pectoris: Possible vasoconstrictor influence on the coronary vasculature. Circulation 61: 1165-1171 (1980).

Lichtlen, P.R.; Engel, J.; Wolf, R. and Hundeshagen, H.: Effect of nifedipine on regional myocardial blood flow at rest and in pacing-induced ischemia. (Abstract.) Circulation 60 (Suppl. II): 249 (1979a).

Lichtlen, P.R.; Engel, J.G.; Wolf, R. and Pretschner, P.: Regional myocardial blood flow in patients with coronary artery disease after nifedipine; in Lichtlen et al. (Eds) International Adalat Panel Discussion: New Experimental and Clinical Results, pp. 69-85 (Excerpta Medica, Amsterdam 1979b).

Lichtlen, P.R.; Rafflenbeul, W.; Amende, R.; Simon, R. and Reil, G.: The influence of Ca^{2+}-entry blockers on hemodynamics and coronary blood flow, and its importance for the treatment of angina pectoris; in Godfraind et al. (Eds) Calcium Entry Blockers in Cardiovascular and Cerebral Dysfunction, pp. 161-179 (Martinus Nijhoff, Boston 1984).

Lindsey, G.; McCullough, R.G.; Seaman, J.; Hawkins, R.; Weil, J. and Steigerwald, J.: Nifedipine may be harmful in the treatment of Raynaud's phenomenon secondary to systemic sclerosis. (Abstract no. 27.) Arthritis and Rheumatism 28 (Suppl.): S18 (1985).

Linhart, J.: Effect of calcium blocking agents on peripheral circulation. European Heart Journal 2 (Suppl. A): 83 (1981).

Littler, W.A.; Watson, R.D.S.; Stallard, T.J. and McLeay, R.A.B.: The effect of nifedipine on arterial pressure and reflex cardiac control. Postgraduate Medical Journal 59 (Suppl. 2): 109-113 (1983).

Löfdahl, C.-G.; Svedmyr, K. and Svedmyr, N.: Effects of nifedipine or atenolol on ventilatory capacity and hemodynamics in asthmatic patients: Interaction with terbutaline. Current Therapeutic Research 36: 282-291 (1984).

Lombardi, C.; Spedini, C. and Govoni, S.: Effect of calcium entry blockade on ethanol-induced changes in bronchomotor tone. European Journal of Clinical Pharmacology 28: 221-222 (1985).

Lorell, B.H.: Use of calcium channel blockers in hypertrophic cardiomyopathy. American Journal of Medicine 78 (Suppl. 2B): 43-54 (1985).

Lorell, B.H.; Turi, Z. and Grossman, W.: Modification of left ventricular response to pacing tachycardia by nifedipine in patients with coronary artery disease. American Journal of Medicine 71: 667-675 (1981).

Lorentsen, E. and Landmark, K.: The acute effects of nifedipine

on calf and forefoot blood flow in patients with peripheral arterial insufficiency. Angiology 34: 46-52 (1983).
Losardo, A.A.; Klein, N.A.; Beer, N.; Strom, J.A.; Wexler, J.P.; et al.: Beneficial effects of sublingual nifedipine in patients with ischemic heart disease and depressed left ventricular function. Angiology 33: 811-817 (1982).
Love, S.J.; Yeh, J.; Kann, J.; Levitt, M.J. and Reitberg, D.P.: Effect of mode of administration on nifedipine pharmacokinetics (Abstract.) Clinical Pharmacology and Therapeutics 37: 209 (1985).
Ludbrook, P.A.; Tiefenbrunn, A.J.; Reed, F.R. and Sobel, B.E.: Acute hemodynamic responses to sublingual nifedipine: Dependence on left ventricular function. Circulation 65: 489-498 (1982).
Lunde, P. and Rasmussen, K.: Long-term beneficial effect of nifedipine in primary pulmonary hypertension. American Heart Journal 108: 415-416 (1984).
Lund-Johansen, P. and Omvik, P.: Haemodynamic effects of nifedipine in essential hypertension at rest and during exercise. Journal of Hypertension 1: 159-163 (1983).
Lydtin, H.; Lohmöller, G.; Lohmöller, R. and Walter, I.: Hemodynamic studies on nifedipine in man; 1st International Nifedipine 'Adalat' Symposium, pp. 97-106 (1975a).
Lydtin, H.; Lohmöller, G.; Lohmöller, R.; Schmitz, H. and Walter, I.: Hemodynamic studies on Adalat in healthy volunteers and patients; 2nd International Adalat Symposium, pp. 112-123 (1975b).
Macdonald, J.B.: Muscle cramps during treatment with nifedipine. British Medical Journal 285: 1744 (1982).
MacGregor, G.A.; Markandu, N.D.; Smith, S.J. and Sagnella, G.A.: Captopril: Contrasting effects of adding hydrochlorothiazide, propranolol, or nifedipine. Journal of Cardiovascular Pharmacology 7 (Suppl. 1): S82-S87 (1985).
MacGregor, G.A.; Rotellar, C.; Markandu, N.D.; Smith, S.J. and Sagnella, G.A.: Contrasting effects of nifedipine, captopril, and propranolol in normotensive and hypertensive subjects. Journal of Cardiovascular Pharmacology 4 (Suppl. 3): 358-362 (1982).
MacGregor, G.A.; Rotellar, C.; Markandu, N.D.; Smith, S.J. and Sagnella, G.A.: The acute response to nifedipine is related to pre-treatment blood pressure. Postgraduate Medical Journal 59 (Suppl. 2): 91-94 (1983).
Maeda, K.; Tanaka, C.; Tsukano, Y.; Minamikawa, H.; Komatsu, H.; et al.: Antihypertensive effects of the calcium antagonistic agent nifedipine. Arzneimittel-Forschung 32: 267-271 (1982).
Magometschnigg, D.: Acute hypotensive response to nifedipine. Hypertension 5 (Suppl. II): 80-84 (1983).
Magometschnigg, D. and Pichler, M.: Effective and safe treatment of hypertensive crisis with nifedipine. (Abstract.) American Journal of Cardiology 47: 469 (1981).
Magorien, R.D.; Leier, C.V.; Kolibash, A.J.; Magorien, D.J. and Unverferth, D.V.: Nifedipine improves resting and exercise coronary hemodynamics in congestive heart failure. (Abstract.) Clinical Research 31: 708A (1983).
Maigaard, S.; Forman, A.; Andersson, K.-E. and Ulmsten, U.: Comparison of the effects of nicardipine and nifedipine on isolated human myometrium. Gynaecologic and Obstetric Investigations 16: 354-366 (1983).
Majid, P.A. and De Jong, J.: Acute hemodynamic effects of nifedipine in patients with ischemic heart disease. Circulation 65: 1114-1118 (1982).
Malacoff, R.F.; Mudge Jr, G.H.; Holman, B.L.; Bifolck, L. and Cohn, P.F.: Beneficial effect of nifedipine on regional myocardial blood flow during the cold pressor test in patients with coronary artery disease (Abstract.) Clinical Research 29: 220A (1981).
Malacoff, R.F.; Lorell, B.H.; Mudge Jr, G.H.; Holman, B.L.; Idoine, J.; et al.: Beneficial effects of nifedipine on regional myocardial blood flow in patients with coronary artery disease. Circulation 65 (Suppl. I): 32-37 (1982).
Malaisse, W.J. and Boschero, A.C.: Calcium antagonists and islet function. XI. Effect of nifedipine. Hormone Research 8: 203-209 (1977).
Malaisse, W.J. and Sener, A.: Calcium-antagonists and islet function – XII. Comparison between nifedipine and chemically related drugs. Biochemical Pharmacology 30: 1039-1041 (1981).
Malamet, R.; Wise, R.A.; Ettinger, W.H. and Wigley, F.M.: Nifedipine in the treatment of Reynaud's phenomenom. Evidence for inhibition of platelet activation. American Journal of Medicine 78: 602-608 (1985).
Malik, S.; O'Reilly, J. and Sudlow, M.F.: Effects of sublingual nifedipine on inhaled histamine and methacholine-induced bronchoconstriction in atopic subjects. Thorax 37: 230 (1982).
Manga, P. and Vythilingum, S.: Unstable angina precipitated by nifedipine. South African Medical Journal 66: 144 (1984).
Mannhold, R.: Calcium antagonists: Basic chemical and pharmacological properties. Drugs of Today 20: 69-90 (1984).
Maroko, P.R.: Experimental infarction studies. Clinical and Investigative Medicine 3: 139-142 (1980).
Maseri, A.; Severi, S.; DeNes, M.; L'Abbate, A.; Chierchia, S.; et al.: Variant angina: One aspect of a continuous spectrum of vasospastic myocardial ischemia. American Journal of Cardiology 42: 1019-1035 (1978).
Masotti, G.; Poggesi, L.; Castellani, S.; Morettini, A.; Galanti, G. and Scarti, L.: A study of the antihypertensive effect and some pharmacodynamic aspects of nifedipine in medium-term treatment. International Journal of Clinical Pharmacology Research 4: 71-79 (1984).
Massie, B.M.; Hirsch, A.T.; Inouye, I.K. and Tubau, J.F.: Calcium channel blockers as antihypertensive agents. American Journal of Medicine 77: 135-142 (1984).
Matsumoto, S.; Takashi, I.; Toshikatsu, S.; Takahashi, M.; Su, K.; et al.: Hemodynamic effects of nifedipine in congestive heart failure. American Journal of Cardiology 46: 476-480 (1980).
McAllister Jr, R.G.: Clinical pharmacokinetics of calcium channel antagonists. Journal of Cardiovascular Pharmacology 4: 5340-5345 (1982).
McKenzie, W.B.; Lee, C.L. and Wilcken, D.E.L.: Acute and long term effects of nifedipine in patients with primary and secondary pulmonary hypertension. Australian and New Zealand Journal of Medicine 13: 423 (1983).
McLeay, R.A.B.; Stallard, T.J.; Watson, R.D.S. and Littler, W.A.: The effect of nifedipine on arterial pressure and reflex cardiac control. Circulation 67: 1084-1090 (1983).
McLeod, A.A.; Wise, J.R.; Daly, K. and Jewitt, D.E.: Nifedipine in primary and secondary pulmonary hypertension. (Abstract No. 678.) Circulation 64 (Suppl. IV): IV-180 (1981).
Medenwald, H.; Schlossmann, K. and Wünsche, C.: Strukturaufklang der renalen Ausscheidungsprodukte von 4-(2'-nitrophenyl)-2,6-dimethyl-1,4-dihydropyridin-3,5-dicarbonsäuredimethylester. Arzneimittel-Forschung 22: 53-56 (1972).
Michael, J.P.; Kennedy, T.P.; Fitzpatrick, S. and Rosenstein, B.J.: Nifedipine inhibits hypoxic pulmonary vasoconstriction during rest and exercise in patients with cystic fibrosis and cor pulmonale. American Review of Respiratory Disease 130: 516-519 (1984).
Middleton Jr, E.: Antiasthmatic drug therapy and calcium ions: Review of pathogenesis and the role of calcium. Journal of Pharmaceutical Sciences 69: 243-251 (1980).
Midtbø, K.; Hals, O. and van der Meer, J.: Verapamil compared with nifedipine in the treatment of essential hypertension. Journal of Cardiovascular Pharmacology 4 (Suppl. 3): 363-368 (1982).
Mielke Jr, C.H.: Comparative effects of aspirin and acetaminophen on hemostasis. Archives of Internal Medicine 141: 305-310 (1981).
Mikkelsen, E.; Andersson, K.E. and Lederballe Pedersen, O.: Verapamil and nifedipine inhibition of contractions induced by

potassium and noradrenaline in human mesenteric arteries and veins. Acta Pharmacologica et Toxicologica 44: 110-119 (1979).

Millar, J.A. and Reid, J.L.: Decreased vascular and adrenal responses to angiotensin II after administration of nifedipine; 5th International Adalat Symposium, pp. 122-132 (1983).

Millard, R.W.; Lathrop, D.A.; Grupp, G.; Ashraf, M.; Grupp, I.L. and Schwartz, A.: Differential cardiovascular effects of calcium channel blocking agents: Potential mechanisms. American Journal of Cardiology 49: 499-506 (1982).

Miller, D.D.; Théroux, P.; Waters, D.D. and Pelletier, G.B.: Action of nifedipine in ischemic heart disease. Canadian Family Physician 29: 703-708 (1983).

Mimran, A. and Ribstein, J.: Effect of chronic nifedipine in patients inadequately controlled by a converting enzyme inhibitor and a diuretic. Journal of Cardiovascular Pharmacology 7 (Suppl. 1): S92-S95 (1985).

Mitchell, L.B.; Schroeder, J.S. and Mason, J.W.: Comparative clinical electrophysiologic effects of diltiazem, verapamil and nifedipine: A review. American Journal of Cardiology 49: 629-635 (1982).

Miyazaki, K.; Kohri, N.; Arita, T.; Shimono, H.; Katoh, K.; et al.: High-performance liquid chromatographic determination of nifedipine in plasma. Journal of Chromatography 310: 219-222 (1984).

Moll, M.G.; Dominguez, J.M.; Obrador, D.; Oter, R. and Tomás, L.: Nifedipine (N) vs. propranolol (P) in unstable angina (A): A prospective randomized study. (Abstract No. 1247.) European Heart Journal 5 (Abstract Suppl. I): 238 (1984).

Mori, K.; Onoe, T.; Ohka, T. and Kanaya, H.: Hemodynamic effects of concomitant nitroglycerin ointment and nifedipine treatment in acute myocardial infarction. Japanese Heart Journal 23: 739-747 (1982).

Moriyama, K.; Matsuno, Y.; Nagase, H.; Nihei, T. and Morioka, S.: Long-term oral nifedipine therapy for refractory heart failure. (Abstract No. 2.) Japanese Journal of Medicine 22: 267 (1983).

Morse, J.R.: A comparison between nifedipine and isosorbide dinitrate when used adjunctively with propranolol. (Abstract No. 212.) Circulation 68 (Part II): III-53 (1983).

Moses, J.W.; Wertheimer, J.H.; Bodenheimer, M.M.; Banka, V.S.; Feldman, M. and Helfont, R.H.: Efficacy of nifedipine in rest angina refractory to propranolol and nitrates in patients with obstructive coronary artery disease. Annals of Internal Medicine 94: 425-429 (1981).

Moskowitz, R.M.; Piccini, P.A.; Nacarelli, G.U. and Zelis, R.: Nifedipine therapy for stable angina pectoris: Preliminary results of effects of angina frequency and treadmill exercise response. American Journal of Cardiology 44: 811-816 (1979).

Mostbeck A.; Partsch, H. and Peschl, L.: Extracardial effects of nifedipine: Measurements of liver blood flow in animals and humans and of peripheral circulation in the lower limbs; 1st International Nifedipine 'Adalat' Symposium, pp. 136-143 (1975a).

Mostbeck, A.; Partsch, H. and Peschi, L.: Extracardial effects of nifedipine (Adalat): Measurements of liver blood flow in animals and humans and of peripheral circulation in the lower limbs; 2nd International Adalat Symposium, pp. 303-310 (1975b).

Mostbeck, A.; Partsch, H. and Peschl, L.: Investigations on peripheral blood distribution; 3rd International Adalat Symposium, pp. 91-97 (1976).

Mueller, H.S. and Chahine, R.A.: Interim report of multicenter double-blind, placebo-controlled studies of nifedipine in chronic stable angina. American Journal of Medicine 71: 645-657 (1981).

Muiesan, G.; Agabiti-Rosei, E.; Castellano, M.; Alicandri, C.L.; Corea, L. et al.: Antihypertensive and humoral effects of verapamil and nifedipine in essential hypertension. Journal of Cardiovascular Pharmacology 4 (Suppl. 3): 325-329 (1982).

Müller, F.B.; Bolli, P.; Erne, P.; Kiowski, W. and Bühler, F.R.: Use of calcium antagonists as monotherapy in the management of hypertension. American Journal of Medicine 77: 11-15 (1984).

Muller, J.E.; Morrison, J.; Stone, P.H.; Rude, R.E.; Rosner, B. et al.: Nifedipine therapy for patients with threatened and acute myocardial infarction: A randomized double-blind, placebo-controlled comparison. Circulation 69: 740-747 (1984a).

Muller, J.E.; Turi, Z.G.; Pearle, D.L.; Schneider, J.F.; Serfas, D.H. et al.: Nifedipine and conventional therapy for unstable angina pectoris: A randomized, double-blind comparison. Circulation 69: 728-739 (1984b).

Murphy, M.B.; Brown, M.J.; Scriven, A.J.I.; Heavey, D.J. and Dollery, C.T.: Nifedipine and alpha adrenoceptor antagonism. Clinical Pharmacology and Therapeutics 36: 745-749 (1984).

Murphy, M.B.; Scriven, A.J.; Brown, M.J.; Causon, R. and Dollery, C.T.: The effects of nifedipine and hydralazine induced hypotension on sympathetic activity. European Journal of Clinical Pharmacology 23: 479-482 (1982).

Murphy, M.B.; Scriven, A.J.I. and Dollery, C.T.: Efficacy of nifedipine as a step 3 antihypertensive drug. Hypertension 5 (Suppl. II): 118-121 (1983a).

Murphy, M.B.; Scriven, A.J.I. and Dollery, C.T.: Role of nifedipine in treatment of hypertension. British Medical Journal 287: 257-259 (1983b).

Myers, A; Songeharsen, S.; Harisdangkul, V.; Raju, S. and Fredericks, R.: Nifedipine in the treatment of Raynaud's phenomenon. (Abstract No. D60) Arthritis and Rheumatism 27 (Suppl.): 585 (1984).

Mysliwiec, M.; Rydzewski, A. and Bulhak, W.: Calcium antagonist withdrawal syndrome. British Journal 286: 1898 (1983).

Naeije, R.; Mélot, C.; Mols, P. and Hallemans, R.: Effects of vasodilators on hypoxic pulmonary vasoconstriction in normal man. Chest 82: 404-410 (1982).

Nair, N.; Townley, R.G.; Againdra, B. and Nair, C.K.: Safety of nifedipine in subjects with bronchial asthma and COPD. Chest 86: 515-518 (1984).

Nakashima, T.; Inoki, M. and Nakanishi, Y.: Nifedipine serum concentration; effects upon blood pressure and heart rate in normotensive volunteers. European Journal of Drug Metabolism and Pharmacokinetics 9: 73-78 (1984).

Nasrallah, S.M.; Tommaso, C.L.; Singleton, R.T. and Backhaus, E.A.: Primary esophageal motor disorders: Clinical response to nifedipine. Southern Medical Journal 78: 312-315 (1985).

Nayler, W.G.: Cardioprotective effects of calcium ion antagonists in myocardial ischemia. Clinical and Investigative Medicine 3: 91-99 (1980).

Nayler, W.G.: Calcium and cell death. European Heart Journal 4 (Suppl. C): 33-41 (1983).

Nayler, W.G.; Ferrari, R. and Williams, A.: Protective effect of pretreatment with verapamil, nifedipine and propranolol on mitochondrial function in the ischemic and reperfused myocardium. American Journal of Cardiology 46: 242-248 (1980).

Nayler, W.G. and Grinwald, P.: Calcium entry blockers and myocardial function. Federation Proceedings 40: 2855-2861 (1981).

Nehring, J. and Camm, A.J.: Calcium antagonist withdrawal syndrome. British Medical Journal 286: 1057 (1983).

Nelson, G.I.C.; Silke, B.; Ahuja, R.C.; Hussain, M.; Forsyth, D. and Taylor, S.H.: The effect on left ventricular performance of nifedipine and metoprolol singly and together in exercise-induced angina pectoris. European Heart Journal 5: 67-79 (1984a).

Nelson, G.I.C.; Silke, B.; Ahuja, R.C.; Verma, S.P.; Hussain, M. and Taylor, S.H.: Hemodynamic effects of nifedipine during upright exercise in stable angina pectoris and either normal or severely impaired left ventricular function. American Journal of Cardiology 53: 451-455 (1984b).

Nicita-Mauro, V.; Ciraolo, O.; Barbera, N.; Buemi, M. and Ceruso, D.: La nifedipine nel trattamento dell 'ipertensione arteriosa nell' anziano. Considerazioni preliminari. Giornale di

Gerontologia 28: 357-364 (1980).
Nijsen-Karelse, M.; Dion, R.A.E. and Jambroes, G.: Nifedipine in cardiac operations. Journal of Thoracic and Cardiovascular Surgery 84: 145 (1982).
Nilsson, H.; Jonasson, T. and Ringqvist, I.: Treatment of digital vasospastic disease with the calcium-entry blocker nifedipine. Acta Medica Scandinavica 225: 135-139 (1984).
Nobile-Orazio, E. and Sterzi, R.: Cerebral ischaemia after nifedipine treatment. British Medical Journal 283: 948 (1981).
Norn, S.; Jensen, C. and Skov, P.S.: *In vivo* and *in vitro* inhibition of histamine release by calcium antagonists. European Journal of Respiratory Diseases 64 (Suppl. 128): 394-397 (1983).
Ochs, H.R.; Rämsch, K.-D.; Verburg-Ochs, B.; Greenblatt, D.J. and Gerloff, J.: Nifedipine: Kinetics and dynamics after single oral doses. Klinische Wochenschrift 62: 427-429 (1984).
Ocken, S.; Reinitz, E. and Strom, J.: Nifedipine treatment for pulmonary hypertension in a patient with systemic sclerosis. Arthritis and Rheumatism 26: 794-796 (1983).
Olivari, M.T.; Bartorelli, C.; Polese, A.; Fiorentini, C.; Moruzzi, P. and Guazzi, M.D.: Treatment of hypertension with nifedipine, a calcium antagonistic agent. Circulation 59: 1056-1062 (1979).
Olivari, M.-T.; Levine, T.B.; Weir, E.K. and Cohn, J.N.: Hemodynamic effects of nifedipine at rest and during exercise in primary pulmonary hypertension. Chest 86: 14-19 (1984).
Olson, G.W.; Logic, J.R. and Whitlow, P.L.: Comparative vasodilator responses to nifedipine, hydralazine and nitroprusside in patients with congestive heart failure. (Abstract.) Journal of the American College of Cardiology 3: 479 (1984).
Ono, H. and Kimura, M.: Effect of Ca^{2+}-antagonistic vasodilators, diltiazem, nifedipine, perhexiline and verapamil, on platelet aggregation *in vitro*. Arzneimittel-Forschung 31: 1131-1134 (1981).
Opie, L.H.; Jee, L. and White, D.: Antihypertensive effects of nifedipine combined with cardioselective beta-adrenergic receptor antagonism by atenolol. American Heart Journal 104: 606-612 (1982a).
Opie, L.H. and White, D.A.: Adverse interaction between nifedipine and β-blockade. British Medical Journal 281: 1462 (1980).
Opie, L.H.; White, D.; Lee, J. and Lubbe, W.F.: Alternatives to β-blockade in therapy of hypertension with angina pectoris: Role of nifedipine or labetalol. British Journal of Clinical Pharmacology 13 (Suppl. 1): 115-122 (1982b).
Packer, M.: Vasodilator and inotropic therapy for severe chronic heart failure: Passion and skepticism. Journal of the American College of Cardiology 2: 841-852 (1983).
Padeletti, L.; Franchi, F.; Brat, A.; Dabizzi, R.P. and Michelucci, A.: The cardiac electrophysiological effects of nifedipine. International Journal of Clinical Pharmacology and Biopharmacy 17: 290-293 (1979).
Parisi, A.F.; Strauss, W.E.; McIntyre, K.M. and Sasahara, A.A.: Considerations in evaluating new antianginal drugs. Circulation 65 (Suppl. I): 38-42 (1982).
Parratt, J.R. and Coker, S.J.: Cardioprotection with calcium antagonists by suppression of early ischaemia and reperfusion-induced arrhythmias. European Heart Journal 4 (Suppl. C): 49-54 (1983).
Parrillo, S.J. and Venditto, M.: Elevated theophylline blood levels from institution of nifedipine therapy. Annals of Emergency Medicine 13: 216-217 (1984).
Pasanisi, F. and Reid, J.L.: Plasma nifedipine levels and fall in blood pressure in a 53-year-old woman. European Journal of Clinical Pharmacology 25: 143-144 (1983).
Patakas, D.; Vlachoianni, E.; Tsara, V.; Louridas, G. and Argiropoulou, P.: Nifedipine in bronchial asthma. Journal of Allergy and Clinical Immunology 72: 269-273 (1983).
Patel, K.R.: Effect of nifedipine on bronchomotor tone and histamine reactivity in asthma. British Medical Journal 283: 796 (1981a).
Patel, K.R.: The effect of calcium antagonist, nifedipine, in exercise-induced asthma. Clinical Allergy 11: 429-432 (1981b).
Patel, K.R.: Calcium antagonists in exercise-induced asthma. British Medical Journal 282: 932-933 (1981c).
Patel, K.R. and Al-Shamma, M.: Effect of nifedipine on histamine reactivity in asthma. British Medical Journal 284: 1916 (1982).
Paulus, W.J.; Lorell, B.H.; Craig, W.E.; Wynne, J.; Murgo, J.P. and Grossman, W.: Comparison of the effects of nitroprusside and nifedipine on diastolic properties in patients with hypertrophic cardiomyopathy: Altered left ventricular loading or improved muscle inactivation? Journal of the American College of Cardiology 2: 879-886 (1983).
Payen, D.M.; Pinaud, M.L.J.; Lampron, N.; De Kersaint Gilly, A. and Nicolas, F.M.: Common carotid haemodynamic and metabolic effects of acutely administered nifedipine in human subarachnoid haemorrhage. Cardiovascular Research 18: 626-631 (1984).
Pedersen, K.E.; Dorph-Pedersen, A.; Hvidt, S.; Klitgaard, N.A.; Kjaer, K. and Nielsen-Kudsk, F.: Effect of nifedipine on digoxin kinetics in healthy subjects. Clinical Pharmacology and Therapeutics 32: 562-565 (1982).
Pepine, C.J.; Feldman, R.L.; Hill, J.A.; Conti, C.R.; Mehta, J. et al.: Clinical outcome after treatment of rest angina with calcium blockers: Comparative experience during the initial year of therapy with diltiazem, nifedipine, and verapamil. American Heart Journal 106: 1341-1347 (1983).
Perez, J.E.; Sobel, B.E. and Henry, P.D.: Effects of nifedipine, diltiazem, and nitroglycerin on regional myocardial shortening in dogs with coronary occlusion. (Abstract.) Circulation 60 (Suppl. II): 214 (1979).
Perez-Olea, J. and Quevedo, M.: Protective effect of nifedipine upon digitalis intoxication. Arzneimittel-Forschung 34: 1271-1274 (1984).
Petralito, A.; Lunetta, M.; Liuzzo, A.; Fiore, C.E. and Mangiafico, R.A.: Influenza della nifedipina sulla curva de carico di glucosio in sogetti normali e in sogetti con metabolismo glicidico alterato. Bollettino Della Societa Italiana Di Cardiologia 24: 184-186 (1979).
Pfeiffer, C.; Kremer, G.; Erbel, R. and Meyer, J.: Der akute Effekt einer intravenoesen Gabe von Nifedipin beim krisenhaften Blutdruckanstieg. (Abstract.) Zeitschrift für Kardiologie 72 (Suppl. 2): 66 (1983).
Pfisterer, M. and Burkart, F.: Comparative effects of nitroglycerin (NTG), nifedipine (NIF) and metoprolol (MET) on normal, ischemic and scar myocardial segments in man. American Journal of Cardiology 49: 942 (1982).
Pfisterer, M.; Glaus, L. and Burkart, F.: Comparative effects of nitroglycerin, nifedipine and metoprolol on regional left ventricular function in patients with one-vessel coronary disease. Circulation 67: 291-301 (1983).
Pfisterer, M.; Müller-Brand, J. and Burkart, F.: Combined acebutolol/nifedipine therapy in patients with chronic coronary artery disease: Additional improvement of ischaemic-induced left ventricular dysfunction. American Journal of Cardiology 49: 1259-1266 (1982).
Pietta, P.; Rava, A. and Biondi, P.: High-performance liquid chromatography of nifedipine, its metabolites, and photochemical products, Journal of Chromatography 210: 516-521 (1981).
Pinto, A.; Novo, S.; Davi, G.; Fazio, M.; Riolo, F. and Strano, A.: Evaluation of antianginal effects of nifedipine-acebutolol and isosorbide dinitrate-acebutolol associations, by bicycle ergometer test, in stable effort angina. (Abstract.) European Heart Journal 2 (Suppl. A): 196 (1981).
Pitlik, S.; Manor, R.S.; Lipshitz, I.; Perry, G. and Rosenfeld, J.: Transient retinal ischaemia reduced by nifedipine. British Medical Journal 287: 1845-1846 (1983).
Polese, A.; Fiorentini, C.; Olivari, M.I. and Guazzi, M.D.: Clinical

use of a calcium antagonist (nifedipine) in acute pulmonary edema. American Journal of Medicine 66: 825-830 (1979).
Prinzmetal, M.; Kennamer, R.; Merliss, R.; Wada, T. and Bor, N.: Angina pectoris. I. A variant form of angina pectoris. American Journal of Medicine 27: 375-388 (1959).
Raemsch, K.D. and Sommer, J.: Pharmacokinetics and metabolism of nifedipine. Hypertension 5: II-18-II-24 (1983).
Raffestin, B.; Boillot, J.; Derrieux, C.; Comoy, E. and Martre, H.: Exercise and the calcium-blocker, nifedipine, in normal subjects. (Abstract.) Scientific Meeting of the European Society for Clinical Investigation, Milan 17-19 April (1984).
Rahwan, R.G.: Mechanisms of action of membrane calcium channel blockers and intracellular calcium antagonists. Medicinal Research Reviews 3: 21-42 (1983).
Ramon, Y.; Behar, S.; Kishon, Y. and Engelberg, I.S.: Gingival hyperplasia caused by nifedipine – a preliminary report. International Journal of Cardiology 5: 195-204 (1984).
Ravens, K.G.: Effects of nifedipine on glucose-tolerance in man. 8th International Congress of Pharmacology, Tokyo 19-24 July, 1981. Abstract No. 1843, p. 776 (1981).
Redman, C.W.G.: Treatment of hypertension in pregnancy. Kidney International 18: 267-278 (1980).
Reitberg, D.P.; Love, S.J. and Zinny, M.: Effect of food on nifedipine pharmacokinetics. (Abstract.) Clinical Pharmacology and Therapeutics 37: 223 (1985).
Ren, J.-H.; Unverferth, D.V.; Magorien, R.D. and Leier, C.V.: Postural influences on the hemodynamic responses to vasodilating drugs in congestive heart failure. Archives of Internal Medicine 145: 641-644 (1985).
Resnick, L.M.; Sealey, J.E. and Laragh, J.H.; Calcium metabolism and the renin-aldosterone system determine the acute blood pressure response to calcium channel blockade. Circulation 66 (Suppl. 2): II-107 (1982).
Reves, J.G.; Barker, S. and Smith, L.R.: Significance of nifedipine plasma levels and hemodynamic changes during anesthesia induction. Anesthesiology 59: A41 (1983).
Rich, S.; Ganz, R. and Levy, P.S.: Comparative actions of hydralazine, nifedipine and amrinone in primary pulmonary hypertension. American Journal of Cardiology 52: 1104-1107 (1983).
Richter, J.E.; Dalton, C.B. and Castell, D.O.: Nifedipine: A potent inhibitor of esophageal contractions in normals and patients with the nutcracker esophagus. (Abstract.) Gastroenterology 86: 1219 (1984).
Rizzon, P.; Scrutinio, D.; DeToma, L.; Mangini, S.; Lagioia, R. et al.: Effects of nifedipine, isosorbide dinitrate, and acebutolol alone and in combination on exercise tolerance in patients with angina pectoris; 5th International Adalat Symposium, pp. 218-235 (1983).
Robinson, B.F.: The response of forearm resistance vessels to dilator agents in patients with primary hypertension: Use of nifedipine in long term therapy. Postgraduate Medical Journal 59 (Suppl. 2): 104-108 (1983).
Robinson, B.F.; Dobbs, R.J. and Kelsey, C.R.: Effects of nifedipine on resistance vessels, arteries and veins in man. British Journal of Clinical Pharmacology 10: 433-438 (1980).
Robson, R.H. and Vishwanath, M.C.: Nifedipine and beta-blockade as a cause of cardiac failure. British Medical Journal 284: 104 (1982).
Rodeheffer, R.J.; Rommer, J.A.; Wigley, F. and Smith, C.R.: Controlled double-blind trial of nifedipine in the treatment of Raynaud's phenomenon. New England Journal of Medicine 308: 880-883 (1983).
Rodger, C. and Stewart, A.: Side effects of nifedipine. British Medical Journal 1: 1619-1620 (1978).
Romano, M.; DeCaprio, L.; Chiariello, M.; Meccariello, P.; Scarfile, P. et al.: Nifedipine in stable angina. A double-blind study in normotensive and hypertensive patients. Current Therapeutic Research 30: 461-467 (1981).
Rosenkranz, H.; Schlossmann, K. and Scholtan, W.: Die Bindung von 4-(2'Nitrophenyl)-2,6-dimethyl-1,4-dihydropyridin-3,5-dicarbonsäuredimethyl ester (Nifedipine) sowie von anderen Koronar wirksamen Stoffen an die Eiweisskörper des Serums. Arzneimittel-Forschung 24: 455-466 (1974).
Rosenthal, J.: Antihypertensive effects of nifedipine, mefruside and a combination of both substances in patients with essential hypertension; 5th International Adalat Symposium, pp. 175-181 (1983).
Rosseel, M.T. and Bogaert, M.G.: Determination of nifedipine in human plasma by capillary gas chromatography with nitrogen detection. Journal of Chromatography 279: 675-680 (1983).
Rotmensch, H.H.; Roth, A.; Liron, M.; Rubinstein, A.; Gefel, A. and Livni, E.: Lymphocyte sensitisation in nifedipine-induced hepatitis. British Medical Journal 281: 976-977 (1980).
Rowland, E.; Evans, T. and Krikler, D.: Effect of nifedipine on atrioventricular conduction as compared with verapamil: Intracardiac electrophysiologic study. British Heart Journal 42: 124-127 (1979).
Rowland, E.; Razis, P.; Sugrue, D. and Krikler, D.M.: Acute and chronic haemodynamic and electrophysiological effects of nifedipine in patients receiving atenolol. British Heart Journal 50: 383-389 (1983).
Rozkovec, A.; Minty, K.; Stradling, J.; Shepherd, G.; MacDermot, J. et al.: Value of acute vasodilator studies in management of primary pulmonary hypertension. (Abstract No. 196.) Circulation 66: II-49 (1982).
Rubenfire, M.; Blevins, R.; Housholder, S. and Kerin, N.: The influence of calcium antagonists on the natural history of inoperable coronary artery disease. (Abstract.) Clinical Research 32: 201A (1984).
Rubin, L.J.; Nicod, P.; Hillis, L.D. and Firth, B.G.: Treatment of primary pulmonary hypertension with nifedipine. A hemodynamic and scintigraphic evaluation. Annals of Internal Medicine 99: 433-438 (1983).
Rubin, P.C.; McCabe, R. and Low, R.A.L.: Calcium channel blockade with nifedipine combined with atenolol in the management of severe pre-eclampsia. Clinical and Experimental Hypertension B3: 379 (1984).
Rud, T.; Andersson, K.-E. and Ulmsten, U.: Effects of nifedipine in women with unstable bladders. Urologia Internationalis 34: 421-429 (1979).
Ruddy, T.D.; Koilpillai, C.; Liu, P.P.; Mahon, W.A.; Henderson, M.A. et al.: Evaluation of chronic nifedipine therapy in nonobstructive hypertrophic cardiomyopathy. (Abstract No. 94.) Circulation 66 (Suppl. II): II-24 (1982).
Russi, E.W. and Ahmed, T.: Calcium and calcium antagonists in airway disease. A review. Chest 86: 475-482 (1984).
Saadjian, A.; Arnaud, A.; Philip-Jouet, F. and Torrésani, J.: Hemodynamic responses to nifedipine in chronic cor pulmonale. (Abstract.) European Heart Journal 5: 80 (1984).
Saeed, M.; Holtz, J.; Elsner, D. and Bassenge, E.: Attenuation of sympathetic vasoconstriction by nifedipine: The role of vascular α_2-adrenoceptors. European Journal of Pharmacology 94: 149-153 (1983).
Saito, D.; Haraoka, S.; Yoshida, H.; Kusachi, S.; Yasuhara, K. et al.: Primary pulmonary hypertension improved by long-term oral administration of nifedipine. American Heart Journal 105: 1041-1042 (1983).
Sandahl, B.; Ulmsten, U. and Andersson, K.-E.: Trial of the calcium antagonist nifedipine in the treatment of primary dysmenorrhoea. Archives of Gynecology 227: 147-151 (1979).
Sando, H.; Katagiri, H.; Okada, M.; Shoda, R.; Arai, Y. et al.: The effect of nifedipine and nicardipine on glucose tolerance, insulin and C-peptide. Diabetes 32: 66A (1983).
Santos, S.R.C.J.: Analysis of nifedipine in blood; in Turner, P. and Padgham, C. (Eds) World Conference on Clinical Pharmacology and Therapeutics. (Abstract No. 0575.) [Macmillan Publishers Ltd, London 1980].

Saris, S.D.; Lowenthal, D.T.; Falkner, B.; Broderman, S.; Bravo, E.V. and Stein, D.T.: Do antihypertensives and calcium-channel blockers blunt the catecholamine response to static exercise. Clinical Pharmacology and Therapeutics 35: 272 (1984).
Sarkozi, J.; Bookman, A.A.H.; Mahon, W.; Ramsay, C. and Keyston, E.C.: Nifedipine in the treatment of idiopathic Raynaud's syndrome (IRS). (Abstract No. 71.) Arthritis and Rheumatism 27: S27 (1984a).
Sarkozi, J.; McCarthy, D.D. and Lee, P.: The use of longterm nifedipine in a patient with Raynaud's syndrome secondary to mixed corrective tissue disease. Journal of Rheumatology II: 408-410 (1984b).
Sassano, P.; Kerihuel, J.C.; Banzet, O. and Carrol, P.: Nifedipine lowers blood pressure in long term therapy. (Abstract.) Presented at the Symposium on New Developments in Treatment of Cardiovascular Diseases with Nifedipine, Lisbon, 4-5 March (1983).
Sauza, J.; Kraus, A.; González-Amaro, R. and Alarcón-Segovia, D.: Effect of the calcium channel blocker nifedipine on Raynaud's phenomenon. A controlled double blind trial. Journal of Rheumatology II: 362-364 (1984).
Schanzenbächer, P.; Deeg, P.; Liebau, G. and Kochsiek, K.: Paradoxical angina after nifedipine: Angiographic documentation. American Journal of Cardiology 53: 345-346 (1984).
Schanzenbächer, P.; Göttfert, G.; Leibau, G. and Kochsiek, K.: Coronary hemodynamic and metabolic effects of nifedipine in patients with coronary artery disease treated with beta-blocking drugs. American Journal of Cardiology 55: 33-36 (1985).
Schanzenbächer, P.; Liebau, G.; Deeg, P. and Kochsiek, K.: Effect of intravenous and intracoronary nifedipine on coronary blood flow and myocardial oxygen consumption. American Journal of Cardiology 51: 712-717 (1983).
Schanzenbächer, P.; Schick, K.D. and Kochsiek, K.: Nifedipin bei hypertropher obstruktiver Kardiomyopathie. Deutsche Medizinische Wochenschrift 107: 1842-1846 (1982).
Schartl, M.; Dougherty, C. et al.: Hemodynamic effects of molsidomine, isosorbide dinitrate, and nifedipine at rest and during exercise. Am. Heart J. 109: 649-653 (1985).
Scheidt, S.: The role of calcium blockers in the treatment of chronic stable angina; in Flaim, S.F. and Zelis, R. (Eds) Calcium Blockers: Mechanisms of Action and Clinical Applications, pp. 231-244 (Urban and Schwarzenberg, Baltimore 1982).
Schick, E.C.; Liang, C.-S.; Heupler, F.A.; Kahl, F.R.; Kent, K.M. et al.: Randomized withdrawal from nifedipine: Placebo-controlled study in patients with coronary artery spasm. American Heart Journal 104: 690-697 (1982).
Schlossman, K.: Fluorometrische Bestimmung des 4-(2′-nitrophenyl)-2,6-dimethyl-1,4-dihydropyridin-3,5-dicarbonsauredimethylester und seinen Hauptmetaboliten. Arzneimittel-Forschung 22: 60-62 (1972).
Schlossman, K.; Medenwald, H. and Rosenkranz, H.: Investigations on the metabolism and protein binding of nifedipine; 2nd International Adalat Symposium, pp. 33-39 (1975).
Schmier, J.; Bruckner, U.B.; Mittman, U. and Wirth, R.H.: Intercoronary collaterals and intramyocardial blood distribution in dogs following nifedipine administration compared with controls; 3rd International Adalat Symposium, pp. 42-49 (1976).
Schreiner, G.; Erbel, R.; Henkel, B.; Pop, T. and Meyer, J.: Verbesserung der Ischaemietoleranz während transluminaler Angioplastie (PICA) durch antianginoese Substanzen. (Abstract.) Zeitschrift für Kardiologie 72 (Suppl. 2): 53 (1983).
Schroeder, J.S.: Treatment of coronary spasm with calcium blockers – variant and unstable angina; in Flaim and Zelis (Eds) Calcium Blockers. Mechanisms of Action and Clinical Applications, pp. 219-230 (Urban and Schwarzenberg, Baltimore-Munich 1982).
Schroeder, J.S.; Rosenthal, S.; Ginsburg, R. and Lamb, I.: Medical therapy of Prinzmetal's variant angina. Chest 78 (Suppl.): 231-233 (1980).
Schulte, K.-L.; Meyer-Sabellek, W.A.; Distler, A. and Gotzen, R.: Long-term treatment with diltiazem and nifedipine in essential hypertension. Journal of Hypertension 2: 93 (1984).
Schultz, H.; Kober, G.; Bamberg, E. and Kaltenbach, M.: Antianginoese Wirkung der Ca-Antagonisten Nifedipin bei intrakoronarer and intravenoeser Applikation. Zeitschrift für Kardiologie (Suppl. 5): 66 (1978).
Schultz, W.; Jost, S.; Kober, G. and Kaltenbach, M.: Relation of antianginal efficacy of nifedipine to degree of coronary arterial narrowing and to presence of coronary collateral vessels. American Journal of Cardiology 55: 26-32 (1985).
Schultz, W.; Kober, G.; Krauss, G. and Kaltenbach, M.: Influence of intracoronary and intravenous nifedipine on diameters of coronary vessels and stenoses; in Rafflenbeul et al. (Eds) Unstable Angina Pectoris, pp. 259-265 (Georg Thieme, Stuttgart 1981).
Schultz, W.; Wendt, T.; Kaltenbach, M. and Kober, G.: Active and passive changes in coronary artery diameters after vasodilatation; 5th International Adalat Symposium, pp. 309-321 (1983).
Schurtz, Cl.; Lesbre, J.P.; Kalisa, A.; Jarry, G. and Fardelonne, P.: Intérêt des inhibiteurs calciques dans l'angor d'effort stable. Diltiazem versus nifédipine. Annales de Cardiologie et d'Angéiologie 32: 337-341 (1983).
Schwartz, J.B. and Migliore, P.J.: Effect of nifedipine on serum digoxin concentration and renal digoxin clearance. Clinical Pharmacology and Therapeutics 36: 19-24 (1984).
Schwartz, J.B.; Raizner, A. and Akers, S.: The effect of nifedipine on serum digoxin concentrations in patients. American Heart Journal 107: 669-673 (1984a).
Schwartz, M.L.; Rotmensch, H.H.; Vlasses, P.H. and Ferguson, R.K.: Calcium blockers in smooth muscle disorders. Archives of Internal Medicine 144: 1425-1429 (1984b).
Scoble, J.E.; Uff, J.S. and Eastwood, J.B.: Nifedipine nephritis. (Correspondence.) Clinical Nephrology 21: 302 (1984).
Selwyn, A.P.; Welman, E.; Fox, K.; Horlock, P.; Pratt, T. and Klein, M.: The effects of nifedipine on acute experimental myocardial ischemia and infarction in dogs. Circulation Research 44: 16-23 (1979).
Serfas, D.; Shoback, D.M. and Lorell, B.H.: Phaeochromocytoma and hypertrophic cardiomyopathy: Apparent suppression of symptoms and noradrenaline secretion by calcium-channel blockade. Lancet 2: 711-713 (1983).
Serruys, P.W.; Booman, F.; Steward, R.; Michels, R.; Reiber, J.H.C. and Hugenholtz, P.G.: Unstable angina pectoris and coronary arterial vasomotion: Which role for nifedipine?: In Rafflenbeul et al. (Eds) Unstable Angina Pectoris: International Symposium, Hanover 1980, pp. 103-120 (Georg Thieme Verlag, Stuttgart-New York; Thieme-Stratton, New York 1981a).
Serruys, P.W.; Brower, R.W.; Katen, H.J.T.; Bom, A.H. and Hugenholtz, P.G.: Regional wall motion from radiopaque markers after intravenous and intracoronary injections of nifedipine. Circulation 63: 584-591 (1981b).
Serruys, P.W.; Hooghoudt, T.E.H.; Reiber, J.H.C.; Slager, C.; Brower, R.W. and Hugenholtz, P.G.: Influence of intracoronary nifedipine on left ventricular function, coronary vasomobility, and myocardial oxygen consumption. British Heart Journal 49: 427-441 (1983a).
Serruys, P.W.; Steward, R.; Booman, F.; van den Brand, M. and Reiber, J.H.C.: Effects of intracoronary nifedipine on coronary vasomobility and left ventricular hemodynamics. (Abstract.) Circulation 62 (Suppl. III): 86 (1980).
Serruys, P.W.; van den Brand, M.; Brower, R.W. and Hugenholtz, P.G.: Regional cardioplegia and cardioprotection during transluminal angioplasty, which role for nifedipine? European Heart Journal 4 (Suppl. C): 115-121 (1983b).
Shen, A.C. and Jennings, R.B.: Myocardial calcium and magnesium in acute ischemic injury. American Journal of Pathology 67: 417-440 (1972).

Sherman, L.G. and Liang, C.-S.: Nifedipine in chronic stable angina: A double-blind placebo-controlled crossover trial. American Journal of Cardiology 51: 706-711 (1983).

Sia, S.T.B.; MacDonald, P.S.; Triester, B.; Oliver, L.E.; Horowitz, J.D. and Goble, A.J.: Aggravation of myocardial ischaemia by nifedipine. Medical Journal of Australia 142: 48-50 (1985).

Silke, B.; Verma, S.P.; Nelson, G.I.C.; Ahuga, R.C.; Hussain, M. and Taylor, S.H.: The effects on left ventricular performance of nifedipine and verapamil in exercise-induced angina pectoris. British Journal of Clinical Pharmacology 17: 735-743 (1984).

Silver, P.J.; Dachiw, J. and Ambrose, J.M.: Effects of calcium antagonists and vasodilators on arterial myosin phosphorylation and actin-myosin interactions. Journal of Pharmacology and Experimental Therapeutics 230: 141-148 (1984).

Simonneau, G.; Escourrou, P.; Duroux, P. and Lockhart, A.: Inhibition of hypoxic pulmonary vasoconstriction by nifedipine. New England Journal of Medicine 304: 1582-1585 (1981).

Simonsen, S. and Nitter-Hauge, S.: Effect of nifedipine (Adalat) on coronary hemodynamics in patients with coronary arteriosclerotic disease. Acta Medica Scandinavica 204: 179-184 (1978).

Singh, B.N.; Ellrodt, G. and Nademanee, K.: Calcium antagonists: Cardiocirculatory effects and therapeutic applications; in Hurst, J.W. (Ed.) Clinical Essays on the Heart, Vol. 2, pp. 65-97 (McGraw-Hill, New York 1984).

Singh, B.N.; Hecht, H.S.; Nademanee, K. and Chew, C.Y.C.: Electrophysiological and hemodynamic actions of slow channel blocking compounds. Progress in Cardiovascular Diseases 25: 103-132 (1982).

Singh, B.N.; Nademanee, K. and Baky, S.H.: Calcium antagonists: Clinical use in the treatment of arrhythmias. Drugs 25: 125-153 (1983).

Singh, B.N. and Phil, D.: Pharmacological basis for the therapeutic applications of slow-channel blocking drugs. Angiology 33: 492-515 (1982).

Singlas, E.; Martre, H.; Taburet, A.-M.; Jacobs, C. and Sari, R.: Effet de l'hémodialyse sur les taux plasmatiques de nifédipine. Presse Médicale 13: 943-944 (1984).

Sirnes, P.A.; Overskeid, K.; Pedersen, T.R.; Bathen, J.; Drivenes, A. et al.: Evolution of infarct size during the early use of nifedipine in patients with acute myocardial infarction: the Norwegian nifedipine multicenter trial. Circulation 70: 638-644 (1984).

Sloan, P.J.M. and Beevers, D.G.: Nifedipine in combination therapy for resistant hypertension. Pharmatherapeutica 3: 349-353 (1983).

Snedden, W.; Fernandez, P.G.; Galway, B.A. and Kim, B.K.: Specific HPLC assay for serum nifedipine. Clinical and Investigative Medicine 7: 173-178 (1984a).

Snedden, W.; Fernandez, P.G. and Kim, B.K.: Specific assay for serum nifedipine with co-administered drugs in normo- and hypertensives. Clin. Pharmacol. and Therap. 35: 276 (1984b).

So, S.Y.; Lam, W.K. and Yu, D.Y.C.: Effect of calcium antagonists on allergen-induced asthma. Clinical Allergy 12: 595-600 (1982).

Sobel, B.E.: Calcium antagonists in cardiovascular therapeutics. Practical Cardiology 7: 1-8 (1981).

Sodeyama, O.; Ikeda, K.; Matsuda, I.; Fukunaga, A.F. and Bishay, E.G.: Nifedipine for control of post operative hypertension. Anesthesiology 59: A18 (1983).

Spital, A. and Scandling, J.D.: Nifedipine in continuous ambulatory peritoneal dialysis. Archives of International Medicine 143: 2025 (1983).

Spivack, C.; Ocker, S. and Frishman, W.H.: Calcium antagonists. Clinical use in the treatment of systemic hypertension. Drugs 25: 154-177 (1983).

Staffurth, J.S. and Emery, P.: Adverse interaction between nifedipine and beta-blockade. British Medical Journal 282: 225 (1981).

Stein, D.T.; Lowenthal, D.T.; Porter, R.S.; Falkner, B.; Bravo, E.L. and Hare, T.W.: Effects of nifedipine and verapamil on isometric and dynamic exercise in normal subjects. American Journal of Cardiololgy 54: 386-389 (1984).

Stern, Z.; Zylber-Katz, E. and Levy, M.: Nifedipine plasma concentration in patients treated for angina pectoris. International Journal of Clinical Pharmacology, Therapy and Toxicology 22: 198-203 (1984).

Stone, D.L.; Stephens, J.D. and Banim, S.O.: Comparative coronary haemodynamic effects of nifedipine and nitroglycerin. (Abstract.) Circulation (Suppl. III): 86 (1980a).

Stone, D.L.; Stephens, J.D. and Banim, S.O.: Coronary haemodynamic effects of nifedipine. Comparison with glyceryl trinitrate. British Heart Journal 49: 442-446 (1983a).

Stone, P.H.; Antman, E.M.; Muller, J.E. and Braunwald, E.: Calcium channel blocking agents in the treatment of cardiovascular disorders. Part II: hemodynamic effects and clinical applications. Annals of Internal Medicine 93: 886-904 (1980b).

Stone, P.H. and Muller, J.E.: Nifedipine therapy for recurrent ischemic pain following myocardial infarction. Clinical Cardiology 5: 223-230 (1982).

Stone, P.H.; Muller, J.E.; Turi, Z.G.; Geltman, E.; Jaffe, A.S. and Braunwald, E.: Efficacy of nifedipine therapy in patients with refractory angina pectoris: Significance of the presence of coronary vasospasm. American Heart Journal 106: 644-652 (1983b).

Stornello, M.; Di Rao, G.; Iachello, M.; Pisani, R.; Scapellato, L. et al.: Hemodynamic and humoral interactions between captopril and nifedipine. Hypertension 5 (Suppl. III): 154-156 (1983).

Strauer, B.E.; Atef Mahmoud, M.; Bayer, F.; Bohn, I. and Motz, U.: Reversal of left ventricular hypertrophy and improvement of cardiac function in man by nifedipine. European Heart Journal 5 (Suppl. F): 53-60 (1984).

Streifler, J.; Wittenberg, C. and Rosenfeld, J.B.: Effects of different single doses of nifedipine on blood pressure, renal function, plasma aldosterone and renin in hypertensive subjects; 5th International Adalat Symposium, pp. 164-174 (1983).

Strickland, W.G.; Blackmore, P.F. and Exton, J.H.: Nifedipine and alpha-adrenergic blockade. New England Journal of Medicine 307: 757-758 (1982).

Svedmyr, K.; Löfdahl, C.-G. and Svedmyr, N.: Nifedipine – a calcium channel blocker – in asthmatic patients. Interaction with terbutaline. Allergy 39: 17-22 (1984).

Taburet, A.M.; Singlas, E.; Colin, J.-N.; Benzet, O.; Thibonnier, M. and Corvol, P.: Pharmacokinetic studies of nifedipine tablet. Correlation with antihypertensive effects. Hypertension 5: II-29-II-33 (1983).

Taggart, E.J. and Zelis, R.: The role of calcium blockers in the treatment of other cardiovascular disorders; in Flaim, S.F. and Zelis, R. (Eds) Calcium blockers: Mechanisms of action and clinical application, pp. 265-281 (Urban and Schwarzenberg, Baltimore 1982).

Takahara, K.; Kuroiwa, A.; Matsushima, T.; Nakashima, Y. and Takasugi, M.: Effects of nifedipine on platelet function. American Heart Journal 109: 4-8 (1985).

Takekoshi, N.; Murakami, E.; Murakami, H.; Matsui, S.; Masuya, K. et al.: Treatment of severe hypertension and hypertensive emergency with nifedipine, a calcium antagonistic agent. Japanese Circulation Journal 45: 852-860 (1981).

Taylor, S.H.; Nelson, G.I.C.; Silke, B.; Verma, S.P.; Hussain, M. and Forsyth, D.: Comparative effects of labetalol and nifedipine in hypertensive complicating acute myocardial infarction. (Abstract No. A-571.) VII Asian-Pacific Congress of Cardiology, p. 154, November 27-December 2, 1983, Taiwan, Republic of China (1983)

Terry, R.W.: Nifedipine therapy in angina pectoris: Evaluation of safety and side effects. American Heart Journal 104: 681-689 (1982).

Théroux, P.; Taeymans, Y. and Waters, D.D.: Calcium antagonists. Clinical use in the treatment of angina. Drugs 25: 178-195 (1983).

Théroux, P.; Waters, D.D.; Debaisieux, J.C.; Szlachcic, J.; Micgala, H.F. and Bourassa, M.G.: Hemodynamic effects of calcium ion antagonists after acute myocardial infarction. Clinical and Investigative Medicine 3: 81-85 (1980).

Thibonnier, M.; Bonnet, F. and Corvol, P.: Antihypertensive effect of fractionated sublingual administration of nifedipine in moderate essential hypertension. European Journal of Clinical Pharmacology 17: 161-164 (1980).

Tiefenbrunn, A.J.; Sobel, B.E.; Gowda, S.; McKnight, R.C. and Ludbrook, P.A.: Nifedipine blockade of ergonovine-induced coronary arterial spasm: Angiographic documentation. American Journal of Cardiology 48: 184-187 (1981).

Timmermans, P.B.M.W.M.; de Jonge, A.; van Meel, J.C.A.; Mathy, M.-J. and van Zwieten, P.A.: Influence of nifedipine on functional responses *in vivo* initiated at α_2-adrenoceptors. Journal of Cardiovascular Pharmacology 5: 1-11 (1983a).

Timmermans, P.B.M.W.M.; Mathy, M.-J.; Wilffert, B.; Kalkman, H.O.; Thoolen, M.J.M.C. et al.: Differential effect of calcium entry blockers on α_1-adrenoceptor-mediated vasoconstriction *in vivo*. Naunyn-Schmiedeberg's Archives of Pharmacology 324: 239-245 (1983b).

Timmermans, P.B.M.W.M.; van Meel, J.C.A. and van Zwieten, P.A.: Calcium antagonists and -receptors. European Heart Journal 4 (Suppl. C): 11-17 (1983c).

Tirlapur, V.G. and Mir, M.A.: Cardiorespiratory effects of isosorbide dinitrate and nifedipine in combination with nadolol: A double-blind comparative study of beneficial and adverse antianginal drug interactions. American Journal of Cardiology 53: 487-492 (1984).

Toggart, E.J. and Zelis, R.: The role of calcium blockers in the treatment of other cardiovascular disorders; in Flaim and Zelis (Eds) Calcium Blockers: Mechanism of Action and Clinical Applications, pp. 265-283 (Urban and Schwarzenberg, Baltimore-Munich 1982).

Tolins, M.; Weir, K.; Chesler, E. and Pierpont, G.L.: 'Maximal' drug therapy is not necessarily optimal in chronic angina pectoris. Journal of the American College of Cardiology 3: 1051-1057 (1984).

Traube, M.; Hongo, M.; Magyar, L. and McCullum, R.W.: Effects of nifedipine in achalasia and in patients with high-amplitude peristaltic esophageal contractions. Journal of the American Medical Association 252: 1733-1736 (1984).

Traube, M.; Hongo, M.; McAllister Jr, R.G. and McCallum, R.W.: Correlation of plasma levels of nifedipine and cardiovascular effects after sublingual dosing in normal subjects. Journal of Clinical Pharmacology 25: 125-129 (1985).

Tsukiyama, H.; Otsuka, K. and Yamamoto, Y.: Effect on pindolol and nifedipine alone and in combination on haemodynamic parameters/variables in essential hypertension. Journal of International Medical Research 12: 154-162 (1984).

Tweddel, A.C.; Beattie, J.M.; Murray, R.G. and Hutton, I.: The combination of nifedipine and propranolol in the management of patients with angina pectoris. British Journal of Clinical Pharmacology 12: 229-233 (1981).

Ueda, K.; Kuwajima, I.; Itoh, H.; Kuramoto, K. and Murakami, M.: Nifedipine in the management of hypertension; in Lichtlen et al. (Eds) International Adalat Panel Discussion – New Experimental and Clinical Results, p. 105 (Excerpta Medica, Amsterdam 1978).

Ueda, K.; Kuwajima, I.; Murakami, M. and Yoshida, H.: The effect and safety of the long term antihypertensive therapy with nifedipine. Jananese Journal of Medicine 23: 324 (1984).

Ueda, K. and Murakami, M.: A controlled, comparative multicenter study on the clinical efficacy of nifedipine in the treatment of severe hypertension; 5th International Adalat Symposium, pp. 146-157 (1983).

Ulmsten, U.; Andersson, K.-E. and Forman, A.: Relaxing effects of nifedipine on the nonpregnant human uterus *in vitro* and *in vivo*. Obstetrics and Gynecology 52: 436-441 (1978).

Ulmsten, U.; Andersson, K.-E. and Wingerup, L.: Treatment of premature labor with the calcium antagonist nifedipine. Archives of Gynecology 229: 1-5 (1980).

Valdés, G.; Soto, M.E.; Croxatto, H.R.; Bellolio, T.; Corbalan, R. and Casanegra, P.: Effects of nifedipine during low, normal and high intakes of sodium in patients with essential hypertension. Clinical Science 63 (Suppl. 8): 447s-450s (1982).

Valdés, G.; Montero, J.; Tobar, M.; Chacon, C. and Croxatto, H.R.: Efecto inicial y cronico de nifedipina en pacientes hipertensos. Revista Médica de Chile 111: 1237-1240 (1983).

Van der Wall, E.E.; De Jong, J.P.; Eenige Van, M.J.; Scholtalbers, A.G. and Roos, J.P.: Long-acting effects of nifedipine on exercise tolerance in patients with stable angina pectoris. Current Therapeutic Research 34: 574-580 (1983).

Van Meel, J.C.A.; De Jonge, A.; Kalkman, H.O.; Wilffert, B.; Timmermans, P.B.M.W.M. and van Zwieten, P.A.: Organic and inorganic calcium antagonists reduce vasoconstriction *in vivo* mediated by postsynaptic α_2-adrenoceptors. Naunyn-Schmiedeberg's Archives of Pharmacology 316: 288-293 (1981).

Van Meel, J.C.A.; Timmermans, P.B.M.W.M. and van Zwieten, P.A.: Hypotensive activity of calcium entry blockers in rats. Relationship with depression of α_2-adrenoceptor-mediated vasopressor responses. European Journal of Pharmacology 92: 27-34 (1983a).

Van Meel, J.C.A.; Towart, R.; Kazda, S.; Timmermans, P.B.M.W.M. and van Zwieten, P.A.: Correlation between the inhibitory activities of calcium entry blockers on vascular smooth muscle constriction *in vitro* after k^+ depolarisation and *in vivo* after α_2-adrenoceptor stimulation. Naunyn-Schmiedeberg's Archives of Pharmacology 322: 34-37 (1983b).

Van Zwieten, P.A.; van Meel, J.C.A. and Timmermans, P.B.M.W.M.: Pharmacology of calcium entry blockers: Interaction with vascular alpha-adrenoceptors. Hypertension 5: II8-II17 (1983).

Vessby, V.; Abelin, J.; Finnson, M.; Hellsing, K. and Lithell, H.: Effects of nifedipine treatment on carbohydrate and lipoprotein metabolism. Current Therapeutic Research 33: 1075-1081 (1983).

Vey, G.; Wiese, K.H.; Schramm, A. and Walter, J.: Vergleichende Untersuchung zum Einfluss des Calciumantagonisten Nifedipin, der Beta-Rezeptorenblocker Acebutolol and Propranolol und der Kombination auf elektrophysiologische Parameter beim Menschen. Zeitschrift für Kardiologie 73: 101-105 (1984).

Vuori, I.; Kallio, V.; Hämäläinen, H. and Pietila, J.: Effects of nifedipine and glyceryltrinitrate on the ergometric performance of patients after myocardial infarction. Current Therapeutic Research 21: 435-448 (1977).

Van der Wall, E.E.; Tuinzing, D.B. and Hes, J.: Hyperplasie van de gingiva: een mogelijke bijwerking van nifedipine. Nederlands Tijdschrift voor Geneeskunde 128: 1954-1955 (1984)

Waller, D.G.; Nicholson, H.P. and Roath, S.: The acute effects of nifedipine on red cell deformability in angina pectoris. British Journal of Clinical Pharmacology 17: 133-138 (1984a).

Waller, D.G.; Renwick, A.G.; Gruchy, B.S. and George, C.F.: The first pass metabolism of nifedipine in man. British Journal of Clinical Pharmacology 18: 951-954 (1984b).

Walters, B.N.J. and Redman, C.W.G.: Treatment of severe pregnancy-associated hypertension with the calcium antagonist nifedipine. British Journal of Obstetrics and Gynaecology 91: 330-336 (1984).

Waters, D.D.; Miller, D.D.; Szlachcic, J.; Bouchard, A.; Méthé, M. et al.: Factors influencing the long-term prognosis of treated patients with variant angina. Circulation 68: 258-265 (1983).

Waters, D.D.; Szlachcic, J.; Théroux, P.; Dauwe, F. and Mizgala, H.F.: Ergonovine testing to detect spontaneous remissions of variant angina during long term treatment with calcium antagonist drugs. American Journal of Cardiology 47: 179-184 (1981a).

Waters, D.D.; Théroux, P.; Szlachcic, J. and Dauwe, F.: Provocative testing with ergonovine to assess the efficacy of treatment with nifedipine, diltiazem and verapamil in variant angina. American Journal of Cardiology 48: 123-130 (1981b).

Weiss, E.B. and Markowicz, J.: Inhibition of anaphylaxis in airways smooth muscle by the calcium channel drugs verapamil and nifedipine. American Review of Respiratory Disease 123 (Suppl. 4): 42 (1981).

Wertheimer, J.H.; Moses, J.W.; Banka, V.S.; Bodenheimer, M.M.; Watson, J.D.; et al.: Nifedipine for recurrent rest ischemia after recent myocardial infarction. (Abstract.) American Journal of Cardiology 49: 1024 (1982).

White, C.J.; Phillips, W.A.; Abrahams, L.; Watson, T.D. and Singleton, P.: Objective benefit of nifedipine in the treatment of Raynaud's phenomenon: A double-blind study. (Abstract No. 10.) Circulation 70 (Part II): II3 (1984).

Wiess, A.T.; Shefer, A.; Lewis, B.S.; Witt, H.; Halon, D.A. and Gotsman, M.S.: The effect of nifedipine on normal and ischemic left ventricular function during atrial pacing stress. Cardiology 71: 190-198 (1984).

Wilkins, M.R.; Woods, K.L.; Jack, D.B.; Kendall, M.J. and Laugher, S.J.: Separate and combined effects of nadolol and nifedipine on the cardiac response to exercise. European Journal of Clinical Pharmacology 28: 113-117 (1985).

Williams, D.O.; Barnes, P.J.; Vickers, H.P. and Rudolf, M.: Effect of nifedipine on bronchomotor tone and histamine reactivity in asthma. British Medical Journal 283: 348 (1981).

Winniford, M.D.; Fulton, K.L.; Corbett, J.R.; Croft, C.H. and Hillis, L.D.: Propranolol-verapamil versus propranolol – nifedipine in severe angina pectoris of effort: A randomized, double-blind crossover study. American Journal of Cardiology 55: 281-285 (1985).

Winniford, M.D.; Gabliani, G.; Johnson, S.M.; Mauritson, D.R.; Fulton, K.L. and Hillis, L.D.: Concomitant calcium antagonist plus isosorbide dinitrate therapy for markedly active variantangina. American Heart Journal 108: 1269-1273 (1984).

Winniford, M.D.; Johnson, S.M.; Mauritson, D.R. and Hillis, L.D.: Ergonovine provocation to assess efficacy of long-term therapy with calcium antagonists in Prinzmetal's variant angina. American Journal Cardiology 51: 684-688 (1983).

Winniford, M.D.; Johnson, S.M.; Mauritson, D.R.; Rellar, J.S.; Redish, G.A. et al.: Verapamil therapy for Prinzmetal's variant angina: Comparison with placebo and nifedipine. American Journal of Cardiology 50: 913-918 (1982a).

Winniford, M.D.; Markham Jr, R.V.; Firth, B.G.; Nicod, P. and Hillis, L.D.: Hemodynamic and electrophysiologic effects of verapamil and nifedipine in patients on propranolol. American Journal of Cardiology 50: 704-710 (1982b).

Winniford, M.D.; Willerson, J.T. and Hillis, L.D.: Calcium antagonists in the treatment of individuals with ischemic heart disease. Angiology 33: 522-539 (1982c).

Winston, E.L.; Pariser, K.M.; Miller, K.B.; Salem, D.N. and Creager, M.A.: Nifedipine as a therapeutic modality of Raynaud's phenomenon. Arthritis and Rheumatism 26: 1177-1180 (1983).

Wit, A.L. and Cranefield, P.: Effect of verapamil on the sinoatrial and atrioventricular nodes of the rabbit and the mechanisms by which it arrests re-entrant atrioventricular nodal tachycardia. Circulation Research 35: 413-425 (1974).

Woo, T.Y.; Wong, R.C.; Campbell, J.R.; Goldfarb, M.T.; Voorhees, J.J. and Callen, J.P.: Nifedipine in scleroderma ulcerations. International Journal of Dermatology 23: 678-680 (1984).

Yagil, Y.; Kobrin, I.; Leibel, B. and Ben-Ishay, D.: Ischemic ECG changes with initial nifedipine therapy of severe hypertension. (Correspondence.) American Heart Journal 103: 310-311 (1982).

Yagil, Y.; Kobrin, I.; Stessman, J.; Ghanem, J.; Leibel, B. and Ben-Ishay, D.: Effectiveness of combined nifedipine and propranolol treatment in hypertension. Hypertension 5 (Suppl. II): 113-117 (1983a)

Yagil, Y.; Kobrin, I.; Stessman, J.; Leibel, B. and Ben-Ishay, D.: Acute oral management of hypertension: Blood pressure response to prazosin and nifedipine. Israel Journal of Medical Sciences 19: 277-279 (1983b).

Yokoyama, S. and Kaburagi, T.: Clinical effects of intravenous nifedipine on renal function. Journal of Cardiovascular Pharmacology 5: 67-71 (1983).

Yokoyama, M.; Koizumi, T.; Fujitani, K.; Mizutani, T. and Fukazaki, H.: Adverse response to nifedipine in unstable angina pectoris. Chest 81: 646-648 (1982).

Yoshimura, M.; Takashina, R.; Shikuma, R.; Takahashi, H.; Takeda, K. et al.: Antihypertensive effect of nifedipine and its relationship to severity of hypertension Arzneimittel-Forschung 33: 254-257 (1983).

Young, K.D. and MacDonald, G.: Treatment of angina pectoris in general practice with a combination of nifedipine and betablocker. British Journal of Clinical Practice 36: 103-110 (1982).

Zacca, N.M.; Verani, M.S.; Chahine, R.A. and Miller, R.R.: Effect of nifedipine on exercise-induced left ventricular dysfunction and myocardial hypoperfusion in stable angina. American Journal of Cardiology 50: 689-695 (1982).

Zar, M.A. and Gooptu, D.: Effect of nifedipine on the contractile responses of human colonic muscle. British Journal of Clinical Pharmacology 16: 339-340 (1983).

Zipes, D.P., and Fischer, J.C.: Effects of agents which inibit the slow channel on sinus node automaticity and atrioventricular conduction in the dog. Circulation Research 34: 184-192 (1974).

Zylber-Katz, E.; Koren, G.; Granit, L. and Levy, M.: Bioavailability of nifedipine. A comparison between two preparations. Biopharmaceutics and Drug Disposition 5: 109-115 (1984a).

Zylber-Katz, E.; Koren, G. and Levy, M.: Pharmacokinetic study of digoxin and nifedipine coadministration. (Abstract.) Clinical Pharmacology and Therapeutics 35: 286 (1984b).

Authors' address: *Eugene M. Sorkin* and *Stephen P. Clissold*, ADIS Drug Information Services, P.O. Box 34-030, Birkenhead, Auckland 10 (New Zealand).

Drugs 30: 275-283 (1985)
0012-6667/85/0009-0275/$04.50/0

Vertigo
Current Concepts in Management

W.J. Oosterveld

Vestibular Department, Ear, Nose and Throat Clinic, Academisch Medisch Centrum, Meibergdreef, Amsterdam

Summary *Vertigo is not a disease, but a symptom. The management of vertigo requires more than the treatment of the symptom alone, as it concerns the whole physical and psychological condition of the patient. In addition to causal treatment, symptomatic treatment is needed in many cases. This specific treatment consists of vestibular exercises and drug therapy. The efficacy and use of the different drugs available are discussed.*

The treatment of vertigo differs from the usual management of diseases in medical practice in that vertigo is not a definite disease but a symptom. The term 'vertigo' is often loosely used both by patients and by clinicians and it is of great diagnostic importance to separate vertigo from mere unsteadiness. Vertigo is a disturbance in the orientation-detecting system of a subject. Orientation is the person's ability to determine his or her body position within the framework of gravity and acceleration to which it is submitted. Orientation is achieved by integrating information from 3 main sources: the vestibular organs, vision, and the proprioceptors in muscles and joints. The collected information is processed in the sensory integratory area in the reticular formation. The processing of information under normal conditions and circumstances happens subconsciously but when the information contains elements that are new to the individual or have an uncommon character, a condition is created under which the phenomenon of vertigo can be generated. Vertigo is always a symptom and never a disease. The symptom is sometimes very difficult for a patient to describe, and so an exact definition always lacks in some way.

A systematic approach in eliciting the patient's history ensures a broad assessment of each individual. A general approach is essential and should include attention to such aspects as the presence of signs and symptoms from the central nervous system and circulatory system, secondary effects of other diseases, and also from non-organic causes.

The most reliable way to commence an assessment is to take a full history, which should begin with obtaining a detailed account of the type of the vertigo. One should always keep in mind that vertigo can be caused by a lesion in any part of the vestibular system, and this includes the ear as well as the nervous system. Thus the origin of vertigo is not restricted just to the vestibular system, but rather it should be considered as part of a disturbed integration process that becomes conscious.

Vertigo is present in about 5% of all patients consulting the general practitioner. Among patients examined by an otorhinolaryngologist, the incidence rate is 10 to 15%. The reasons for this high prevalence are 2-fold: vertigo is a symptom which accompanies a large number of diseases, and more than 80 possible causes have been described (Oosterveld, 1983).

1. Assessment of the Type of Vertigo

Vertiginous complaints need a careful history, which can only be performed properly by using a specific questionnaire. Four main questions need to be answered:

1. *What does the patient mean regarding the complaint of vertigo?*
   a) spinning sensations, turning sensations
   b) lift sensations
   c) blurred vision
   d) fear of height
   e) unsteadiness
2. *What is the frequency and duration of the vertigo?*
   a) attacks lasting seconds, days or weeks
   b) one attack, slowly fading away over several weeks
   c) chronically present, sometimes changing its intensity
3. *What is the effect on the vertigo of:*
   a) head and body movements
   b) head and body position
   c) noise
   d) time of day
   e) eating habits
4. *Are there other signs and symptoms related or not related to the vertigo?*
   a) nausea or vomiting
   b) hearing impairment, diplacusis
   c) tinnitus
   d) neurological symptoms
   e) states of lowered consciousness
   f) headache.

The answers to these questions give a good insight into the extent of the patient's complaints.

2. Management Principles

The management of a definite disease is usually relatively easy to describe. However, as emphasised above, vertigo is not a disease, so it becomes the mangement of a symptom. The therapy of vertigo is primarily directed at eliminating the underlying cause, but in many cases the origin of the complaint in vertiginous patients does not become clear. Even with sophisticated examination methods the cause of the vertigo in about 50% of the cases will not become apparent. According to Wilmot (1980) it is almost impossible for a clinician to distinguish where dizziness, giddiness or lightheadedness stops and true vertigo begins.

The therapy of vertigo is, by definition, a symptomatic treatment. Although many different diseases have vertigo among their symptoms and signs, the therapy of vertigo does not differ extensively. A confusing factor is that in many patients, vertigo continuously changes its character as well as its intensity (Oosterveld, 1984). For good management of vertigo an excellent doctor-patient relationship is extremely important. In many cases the vertigo affects the happiness of the whole family. It is fundamental for any healing process that the patient feels the support and understanding of his or her doctor regarding the social consequences of the condition.

Two categories in the management of vertigo can be distinguished: causal treatment and symptomatic treatment, which includes support of the patient in his or her daily life and work environment. A general scheme for management of vertigo is shown in figure 1.

3. Causal Treatment

Causal treatment consists primarily of measures intended to correct factors which are responsible for the onset and continuation of the vertigo. When the cause of the vertigo is known, in some cases adequate therapy is available. Labyrinthitis, hypertension, hyperthyroidism, acoustic neuroma and diabetes mellitus are examples of this. On the other hand, even if the cause is known, no therapy of the vertigo is possible in many other cases, e.g. multiple sclerosis, cerebral atherosclerosis, cervical vertigo and post-traumatic vertigo.

4. Symptomatic Treatment

During an acute attack of vertigo the patient should be instructed to lie still in bed – sometimes, if he or she wishes, in a darkened room. Often the patient experiences an exacerbation of his or her complaints when head or body movements are made, and thus immobilisation is helpful to decrease the vertigo. An acute attack of vertigo lasts from minutes up to several days, sometimes even weeks. The central nervous system has a strong ability to compensate a unilateral labyrinthine function loss as well as other kinds of vestibular imbalances. However, this can take from several days up to several months; age plays an important role here.

Symptomatic treatment consists of adaptation methods, surgical treatment and drug therapy.

4.1 Adaptation Methods

It has been known for centuries that the phenomenon of motion sickness heals spontaneously when the initiating movement pattern is maintained. The physiological background of this adaptation is still not well understood. The central nervous system has the ability to recalibrate the relationship between vestibular, visual and proprioceptive inputs. The mechanism at work during motion sickness is strongly related to the adaptation phenomenon shown after a labyrinthine function loss and other vestibular diseases, and is vital for recovery.

Cooksey (1945) and Cawthorne (1945) described the practical application of head and body movements in the treatment of vertigo. These vestibular exercises induce a compensation mainly in vertigo due to peripheral vestibular disorders. In central vestibular lesions little or no benefit at all must be expected from an exercise programme. Norré and De Weerdt (1980a,b) reported good results in cases with one hypofunctional labyrinth.

Table I. Vestibular exercises

In bed

Eye movements: at first slow, then with increasing speed
- Gazing up and down
- Gazing from side to side
- Focusing on finger moving from 10 to 50cm away from the face

Head movements: at first slow, then with increasing speed, and at first with open eyes, then with closed eyes
- Bending forward and backward
- Turning from side to side

Sitting
- Similar eye and head movements as above
- Shoulder shrugging and circling
- Bending forward and picking up objects from floor

Standing
- Similar eye, head and body movements as above
- Changing from sitting to standing position; at first with eyes open, then with eyes closed
- Throwing small ball from hand to hand (above head level)
- Throwing small ball from hand to hand, passing under one knee
- Changing from sitting to standing position, turning around in between

Moving about
- Walking across room with eyes open and then closed
- Walking up and down slope with eyes open and then closed
- Walking up and down steps with eyes open and then closed
- Walking and throwing a small ball in the air and catching it
- Playing any ball game involving stooping, stretching and aiming

The Cawthorne-Cooksey vestibular training programme is designed to gradually retrain the eye, neck and body musculature to use visual and proprioceptive input to compensate for the lost vestibular information. The exercises can be carried out in 4 different positions: in bed, in the sitting position, in the standing position, and when walking around. The scheme adapted by Baloh (1983) is very practical. Very good results have been reported in cases of benign paroxysmal positional vertigo (Brandt and Daroff, 1980) [table I]. A schedule of 3 exercise sessions per day for at least

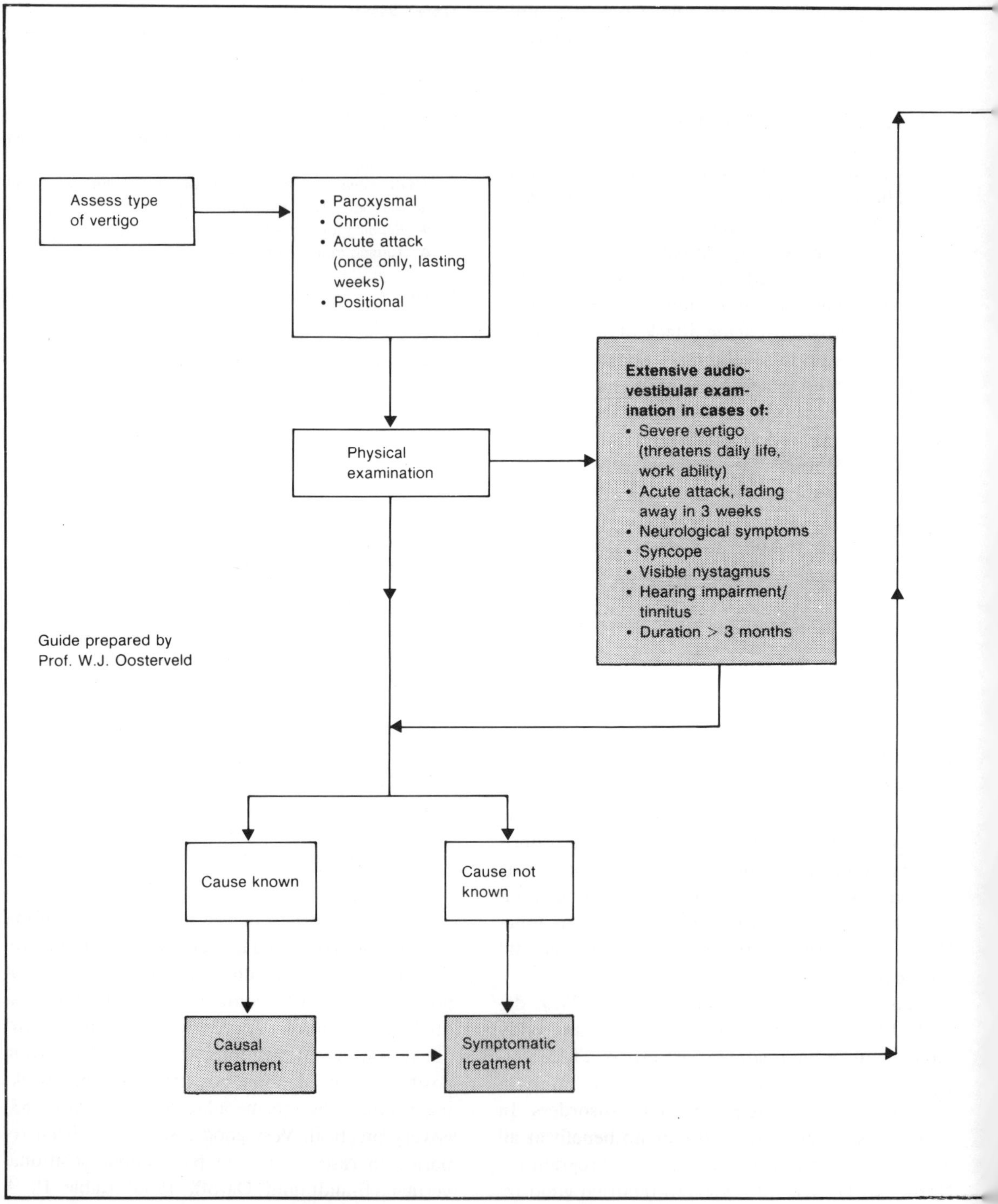

Fig. 1. Summary of the management of vertigo.

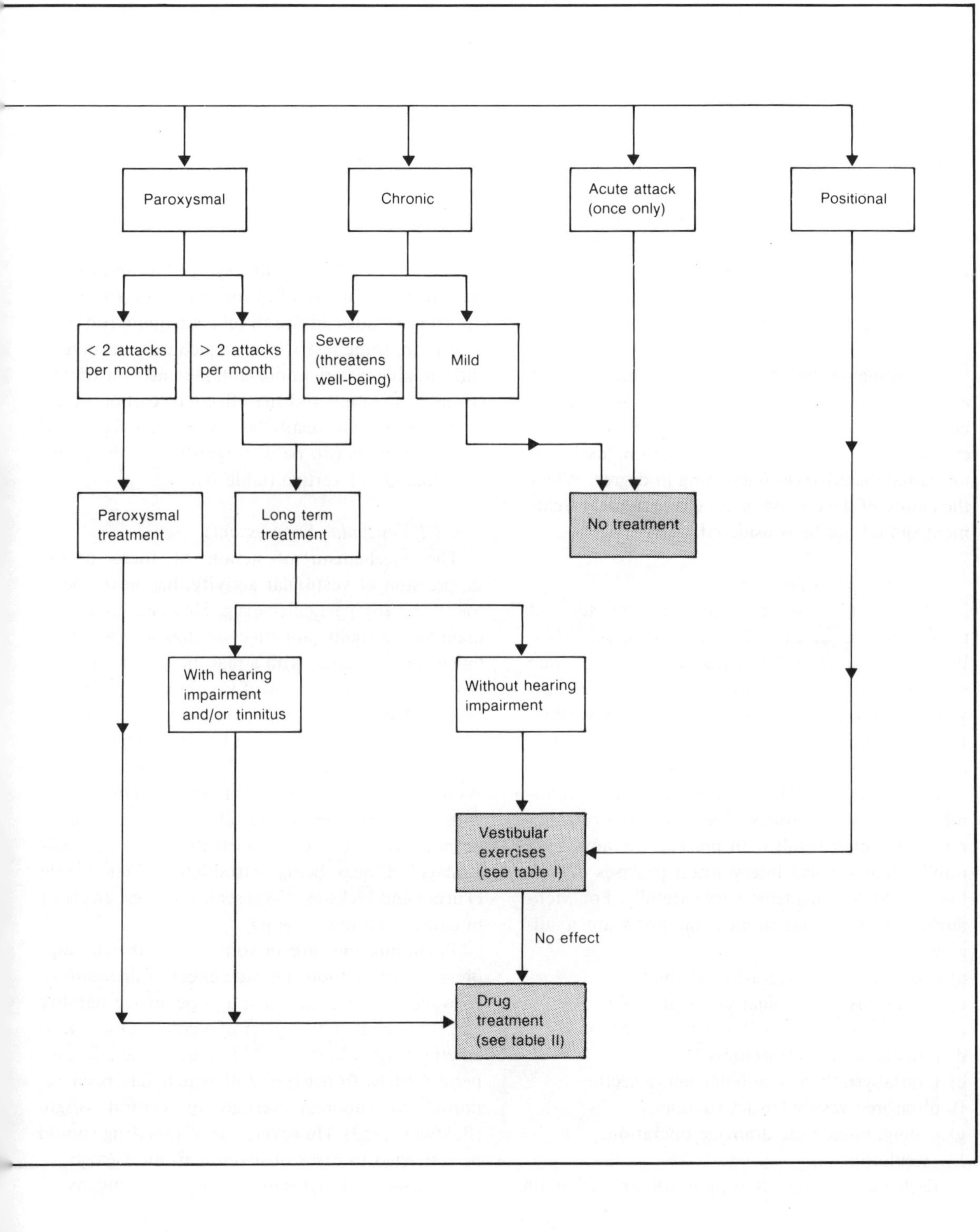
Paroxysmal
Chronic
Acute attack (once only)
Positional
< 2 attacks per month
> 2 attacks per month
Severe (threatens well-being)
Mild
Paroxysmal treatment
Long term treatment
No treatment
With hearing impairment and/or tinnitus
Without hearing impairment
Vestibular exercises (see table I)
No effect
Drug treatment (see table II)

5 minutes is recommended. The movements that cause vertigo must be especially practiced, since the more frequently vertigo is induced the more quickly compensation occurs (Cawthorne, 1945).

The purpose of the training programme should be explained to the patient and written instructions should be given. The training period must last from 1 to 3 months, with individual differences; younger people need less time than aged people. Returning to normal body activities and work situations should be encouraged.

4.2 Surgical Treatment

According to Baloh (1983), the rationale for ablative surgical treatment of vertigo is that the nervous system is better able to compensate for a complete unilateral vestibular function loss than for partial disturbances fluctuating in degree. When the nature of the disease is not clear, surgical treatment should *not* be considered.

4.2.1 Ménière's Disease

There is still a lot of discussion about surgical intervention in cases of Ménière's disease. When there is no functional hearing remaining on one side and hearing on the other side is normal, surgery can be considered in cases with severe vertigo. However, the results of this therapy in Ménière's disease are in many cases disappointing.

Bretlau et al. (1983) reported that surgical treatment in Ménière's disease does not produce a significantly better result than placebo therapy. This implies that surgical intervention in cases of vertigo should be considered very carefully. For Ménière's disease several surgical therapies are available:

a) endolymphatic subarachnoid shunt
b) middle fossa vestibular nerve section
c) retrolabyrinthine vestibular nerve section
d) transcanal labyrinthectomy
e) translabyrinthine vestibular nerve section
f) ultrasonic vestibular destruction
g) endolymphatic sac drainage operations
h) sacculotomy.

Each method has its supporters, and each its positive and negative aspects. A description of the various methods is beyond the scope of this article. Sometimes post-traumatic vertigo after head injuries can be treated by means of a vestibular nerve section (Sanna and Ylikosky, 1983). Gazek (1982) has reported benefit from singular neurectomy in cases of benign paroxysmal vertigo.

4.3 Drug Therapy

The relief of the patient's symptoms and his or her rehabilitation are of immediate concern to the clinician. Besides advice to take adequate rest and relaxation, some restriction on alcoholic beverages and smoking is very important; the vasoconstrictor effects of nicotine and the effects of carbon monoxide threaten the vestibular system. The following groups of drugs can be distinguished in the pharmacotherapy of vertigo (table II).

4.3.1 Vestibular Suppressants

The mechanism of action of these drugs, suppression of vestibular activity, has never been traced for any particular drug. However, many of them have a significant effect on dizziness and vertigo when compared with a placebo. Dix (1984) recently published a review of vestibular suppressant drugs. Among the antihistamines, cinnarizine (Towse, 1980) has proven to be an effective agent. Flunarizine (Holmes et al., 1984; Oosterveld, 1982; Wouters et al., 1983) is a derivative of cinnarizine with a stronger action, but also with some more pronounced side effects. These drugs have the advantage of also being vasodilators. Astemizole (Turner and Jackson, 1983) seems to exert an effect in cases of chronic vertigo.

Phenothiazines are in some cases able to suppress vertigo without the side effect of drowsiness. However, these drugs have a dependence liability and they enhance the effect of alcohol. Other antiemetic drugs which have been used include droperidol (dehydrobenzperidol) which has been reported to suppress vertigo of central origin (Baldwin, 1983). However, use of this drug should be restricted to cases of severe chronic vertigo.

Transdermal hyoscine, applied by means of

Table II. Drugs used in the treatment of vertigo (after Avery, 1980; Leonard and Lawrence, 1971; Rubin, 1973)

Class	Action	Drug	Dosage[a]
Vestibular suppressants			
Antihistamines (also anticholinergic and sedative effect)	Suppress vestibular end-organ receptors, inhibit activation of central cholinergic pathways	Astemizole	10mg 8-hourly
		Cinnarizine	25mg 4- to 6-hourly
		Cyclizine	50mg 4- to 6-hourly
		Dimenhydrinate	50mg 4- to 6-hourly
		Diphenidol[b]	50mg 4- to 6-hourly
		Flunarizine	10mg daily
		Meclozine	25-50mg daily
		Promethazine	25mg 12-hourly
		Diphenhydramine	100mg 6-hourly
Antiemetics			
Phenothiazines	Suppress action central vestibular nucleii and pathways	Prochlorperazine	10mg 4-hourly
		Thiethylperazine	6.5mg 8- to 24-hourly
Anticholinergics	Inhibit activation of central cholinergic pathways	Atropine sulphate	0.4mg im
		Hyoscine (scopolamine) hydrobromide	0.6mg 3-hourly
		Hyoscine	1.5mg 72-hourly (transdermally)
Vasodilators	Improve blood flow to labyrinth and brain stem	Betahistine	32-72mg daily
		Co-dergocrine (dihydroergotoxine)	1.5mg 6- to 8-hourly
		Papaverine	150mg 12-hourly
Diuretics	Decrease intralabyrinthine fluid pressure	Acetazolamide	250mg daily for 2 out of 3 days
		Hydrochlorothiazide	25mg 12-hourly
Psychotherapeutic drugs	Modify sensation of vertigo	Piracetam	400-800mg 8-hourly
		Chlordiazepoxide	10mg 8-hourly
		Diazepam	2-5mg 8-hourly
		Lorazepam	1mg 8-hourly
		Phenobarbitone	15-45mg 8-hourly
		Amitriptyline	25mg 8-hourly
		Nortriptyline	10mg 8-hourly
Corticosteroids	Suppress intralabyrinthine oedema due to viral infection	Methylprednisolone	40-80mg daily for 4-5 days, then 20mg daily for next 4 days
Miscellaneous		Acetyl-leucine	500mg 8-hourly

a Oral administration unless otherwise specified.
b Not an antihistamine.

stickers behind the auricle, seems to suppress motion sickness very well (Hornick et al., 1983). It can be expected that in cases of chronic vertigo of peripheral origin this method is able to give relief.

4.3.2 Diuretics

The use of diuretics is based on the assumption that vertigo is caused in some cases by endolymphatic hydrops. These drugs may be effective when given for a limited period (Klockhoff et al., 1974).

4.3.3 Vasodilators

Induction of vasodilatation improves the blood flow in the labyrinthine area. With this assumption, vasodilators are prescribed in vertigo with a peripheral labyrinthine origin.

Nicotinic acid was one of the first drugs used for this purpose (Stahle et al., 1981). Cyclandelate (Towse, 1980) and piracetam (Oosterveld, 1980) have been reported to be of benefit. Similarly, betahistine (Oosterveld, 1984) has also proven to be effective, especially when given in a high dosage (72 mg/day) for a prolonged period.

4.3.4 Psychotherapeutic Drugs

As would be expected in vertigo, tranquillisers are sometimes effective. Besides a general psychogenic effect, their muscle relaxant properties also play a role (McClure and Willett, 1980). Piracetam improves CNS function and suppresses vertigo in some patients, especially in the elderly (Oosterveld, 1980). Chlordiazepoxide, diazepam, lorazepam and phenobarbitone are useful when anxiety is a feature in the response to vertigo. When depression is the major response, amitriptyline and nortriptyline may be useful.

4.4 Treatment of Acute Attacks of Vertigo

In an acute attack of vertigo, especially when accompanied by vegetative symptoms, the oral route is not suitable for treatment. Rapid relief can be achieved by blocking the stellate ganglion with procaine. However, this method has some risks. As well as aggressive methods such as paracentesis, which in some cases immediately stops an attack, parenteral drug therapy can be employed but only when specialised medical care is available. Drugs which may be used parenterally include atropine sulphate 0.4mg intramuscularly, diazepam 10mg intravenously, and thiethylperazine 6.5mg intramuscularly.

In cases of paroxysmal vertigo, as in Ménière's disease, patients can use suppositories to suppress an attack. Especially when there are prodromes, it is worthwhile to try to cut off an attack at an early stage. Drugs which may be used for this purpose are prochlorperazine (25mg daily), domperidone (60mg 6- to 12-hourly) and thiethylperazine (6.5mg, 8- to 12-hourly).

5. Conclusion

Therapy of vertigo is needed in many cases. When the origin of the underlying disease is known, a causal treatment must be applied – if available. However, in many patients who complain of vertigo the cause remains obscure. In these cases, and also in cases where no causal treatment is available, antivertiginous therapy is desirable.

The treatment of peripheral and central vestibular vertigo does not differ greatly. Some drugs have a more central action, such as antiemetics and psychotherapeutic drugs, while others such as cinnarizine, flunarizine and acetyl leucine have a more peripheral action. Vasodilators work both centrally and in the labyrinths.

In practice, many patients suffering from vertigo are relieved by some kind of treatment. Vertigo not infrequently changes its character with regard to severity and vegetative signs and symptoms. This is not only the case in chronic or in paroxysmal vertigo, but also in vertigo of central as well as peripheral causes. Only when drug treatment fails, and the complaint threatens the patient's way of life seriously, should surgical intervention be considered.

References

Avery, G.S.: Drug Treatment. 2nd ed. (ADIS Press, Sydney, 1980).
Baldwin, R.L.: Droperidol in the treatment of vertigo. Southern Medical Journal 76: 1271-1272 (1983).

Baloh, R.W.: The dizzy patient. Symptomatic treatment of vertigo. Postgraduate Medicine 73: 5, 317-324 (1983).
Brandt, T. and Daroff, R.B.: Physical therapy for benign paroxysmal positional vertigo. Archives of Otolaryngology 106: 184-185 (1980).
Bretlau, P.; Thomsen, J.; Tos, M. and Johnsen, N.J.: Surgical management of Ménière's Disease, with special attention to endolymphatic sac surgery; in Oosterveld (Ed.) Ménière's Disease, A Comprehensive Study, pp. 109-127 (John Wiley & Sons, New York 1983).
Cawthorne, T.: Vestibular injuries. Proceedings of the Royal Society of Medicine 39: 270-273 (1945).
Cooksey, F.S.: Rehabilitation in vestibular injuries. Proceedings of the Royal Society of Medicine 39: 273-275 (1945).
Dix, M.R.: The clinical examination and pharmacological treatment of vertigo; in Dix Hood (Eds) Vertigo, pp. 37-55 (John Wiley & Sons, New York 1984).
Gacek, R.R.: Singular neurectomy update. Annals of Otology, Rhinology and Laryngology 91: 469-473 (1982).
Holmes, B.; Brogden, R.N.; Heel, R.C.; Speight, T.M. and Avery, G.S.: Flunarizine: A review of its pharmacodynamic and pharmacokinetic properties and therapeutic use. Drugs 27: 6-44 (1984).
Hornick, J.L.; Kohl, R.L.; Reschke, M.F.; Degioanni, J. and Cintron-Trevino, N.M.: Transdermal scopolamine in the prevention of motion sickness: Evaluation of the time course of efficacy. Aviation, Space and Environmental Medicine S4: 994-1000 (1983).
Klockhoff, I.; Lindblom, U. and Stahle, J.: Diuretic treatment of Ménlère's disease. Long term results with chlorthalidone. Archives of Otolaryngology 100: 262-265 (1974).
Leonard, J.R. and Lawrence, R.A.: Pharmacologic properties of antivertiginous drugs. Eye, Ear, Nose and Throat Monthly 50: 391-417 (1971).
McClure, J.A. and Willett, J.M.: Lorazepam and diazepam in the treatment of benign paroxysmal vertigo. Journal of Otolaryngology 9: 472-477 (1980).
Norré, M.E. and de Weerdt, W.: Treatment of vertigo based on habituation. 1. Physio-pathological basis. Journal of Laryngology and Otology 94: 689-696 (1980a).
Norré, M.E. and de Weerdt, W.: Treatment of vertigo based on habituation. 2. Technique and results of habituation training. Journal of Laryngology and Otology 94: 971-977 (1980b).
Oosterveld, W.J.: The efficacy of piracetam in vertigo. A double-blind study in patients with vertigo of central origin. Arzneimittel-Forschung 30: 1947-1949 (1980).
Oosterveld, W.J.: Flunarizine in vertigo. A double-blind placebo-controlled cross-over evaluation of a constant dose schedule. ORL – Journal for Oto-Rhino-Laryngology and its Related Specialities 44: 72-80 (1982).
Oosterveld, W.J.: The vertiginous syndrome. Advances in Oto-Rhino-Laryngology 29: 39-49 (1983).
Oosterveld, W.J.: Betahistine dihydrochloride in the treatment of vertigo of peripheral vestibular origin. Journal of Laryngology and Otology 98: 37-41 (1984).
Rubin, W.: Vestibular suppressant drugs. Archives of Otolaryngology 97: 135 (1973).
Sanna, M.; Ylikosky, J.: Vestibular neurectomy for dizziness after head trauma. ORL – Journal for Oto-Rhino-Laryngology and its Related Specialities 45: 216-225 (1983).
Stahle, J.; Lyttkens, L. and Larsson, B.: Some news on medical treatment in Ménière's disease: Use of urea and target seeking drugs; in Vosteen et al. (Eds) Ménière's Disease, pp. 199-208 (Thieme, Stuttgart 1981).
Towse, G.: Cinnarizine – a labyrinthine sedative. Journal of Laryngology and Otology 94: 1009-1015 (1980).
Turner, J.S. and Jackson, R.T.: Astemizole: Its use in patients with chronic vertigo and ENG signs. Laryngoscope 93: 898-902 (1983).
Wilmot, T.J.: The medical management of vertigo. Current Medical Research and Opinion 6: 43-49 (1980).
Wouters, L.; Amery, W. and Towse, G.: Flunarizine in the treatment of vertigo. Journal of Laryngology and Otology 97: 697-704 (1983).

Address for correspondence and reprints: Prof. Dr *W.J. Oosterveld*, Vestibular Department, Ear, Nose and Throat Clinic, Academisch Medisch Centrum, Meibergdreef 9, 1105 A2 Amsterdam (The Netherlands).

General Information

Publication data: Two volumes of *Drugs* are published annually. Each volume comprises six 96-page issues. The annual subscription price is US$320.00/Sw.F.750/Aust$390.00 including postage. *Drugs* is published by ADIS Press Limited, P.O. Box 34-030, Birkenhead, Auckland 10, New Zealand.

Editorial matter is prepared by our own professionally qualified editorial staff and by honorary specialist consultants from all fields of medicine. While great care has been taken in compiling and checking the information contained in *Drugs*, the publisher cannot accept responsibility or be in any way liable for errors or omissions. The inclusion or exclusion of any product does not mean that the publisher advocates or rejects its use either generally or in any particular field or fields.

Drug nomenclature: Approved names of the British Pharmacopoeia Commission are used throughout the text. When the Commission has not adopted a name for the drug under discussion, the United States Adopted Name (USAN – United States Pharmacopeial Convention Inc.) or the International Non-Proprietary Name (INN – WHO) is used. When available, all three names are given at the head of the 'Drug Evaluations' and 'Review Articles' sections, and elsewhere in the text as appropriate. Other synonyms (e.g. research code names of new drugs) are also given.

Manuscripts: Information on the preparation of manuscripts will be provided to authors.

Drugs 30: 285-312 (1985)
0012-6667/85/0010-0285/$14.00/0

Meptazinol
A Review of its Pharmacodynamic and Pharmacokinetic Properties and Therapeutic Efficacy

B. Holmes and *A. Ward*

ADIS Drug Information Services, Auckland

Various sections of the manuscript reviewed by: ***F. Camu,*** Department of Anaesthesiology, Academish Ziekenhuis Vrije Universiteit, Brussels, Belgium; ***M. Evans,*** Whitchurch Hospital, Cardiff, Wales; ***A. Hedges,*** Department of Clinical Pharmacology, St Bartholomew's Hospital Medical College, London, England; ***M.B.A. Jackson,*** Louise Margaret Maternity Wing, Cambridge Military Hospital, England; ***L. Lasagna,*** Tufts University, Sackler School of Graduate Biomedical Sciences, Boston, Massachusetts, USA; ***M. Levy,*** Clinical Pharmacology Unit, Hadassah University Hospital, Jerusalem, Israel; ***D.G. Moyes,*** University of Witwatersrand Medical School, Johannesburg, South Africa; ***N.J. Paymaster,*** Department of Anaesthetics, Clatherbridge Hospital, Bebington, England; ***M.T. Rosseel,*** J.F. and C. Heymans Institute, Voor Farmakodynamie en Terapie, Gent, Belgium; ***P.J. Slatterly,*** Department of Pharmacology and Clinical Pharmacology, School of Medicine, The University of Auckland, Auckland, New Zealand; ***G. Stacher,*** Psychophysiologisches Laboratorium, Universitätsklinik Wien, Vienna, Austria.

Contents

Summary 286
1. Pharmacodynamic Studies 288
1.1 Opioid-Like Agonist Activity 289
1.1.1 Antinociceptive Activity 289
1.1.2 Analgesic Activity in Animals 289
1.1.3 Analgesic Activity in Man 290
1.2 Opioid Antagonist Activity 291
1.3 Respiratory Effects 291
1.3.1 Studies in Healthy Volunteers 292
1.3.2 Studies in Patients with Postoperative Pain 292
1.3.3 Studies in Mothers and Neonates 292
1.3.4 Studies in Preoperative and Anaesthetised Patients 292
1.3.5 Studies in Other Patients 293
1.4 Haemodynamic Effects 293
1.5 Dependence Liability 293
1.5.1 Animal Studies 293
1.5.2 Human Studies 294
1.6 Mechanism of Action 294
2. Pharmacokinetic Studies 295
2.1 Absorption 295

2.1.1 Oral Administration 295
2.1.2 Intravenous Administration 296
2.1.3 Intramuscular Administration 296
2.1.4 Rectal Administration 297
2.2 Distribution 297
2.2.1 Plasma Protein Binding 297
2.3 Elimination 297
2.3.1 Metabolism 297
2.3.2 Excretion 297
2.4 Influence of Age on Pharmacokinetics 299
3. Therapeutic Trials 300
3.1 Open Studies 300
3.2 Controlled Studies 300
3.2.1 Comparisons with a Placebo 300
3.2.2 Comparisons with Morphine 300
3.2.3 Comparisons with Pentazocine 301
3.2.4 Comparisons with Pethidine (Meperidine) 301
3.2.5 Comparisons with Other Analgesics 306
3.3 Use in Premedication and Anaesthesia 306
3.4 Other Uses 306
4. Side Effects 306
5. Drug Interactions 308
6. Overdosage 308
7. Dosage and Administration 308
8. Place of Meptazinol in Therapy 309

Summary

Synopsis: *Meptazinol*[1] *is a new opioid-type analgesic with mixed agonist/antagonist properties. It may be given orally, intravenously or intramuscularly. In studies in patients with moderate to severe pain of various aetiologies, usually following surgery or in obstetrics, the characteristics of analgesia with meptazinol were comparable to those seen with equianalgesic doses of pentazocine, pethidine or a combination of dextropropoxyphene and paracetamol. Preoperative use and use as a component of anaesthesia require further investigation before conclusions may be drawn on its effectiveness in these areas. Onset of action, recorded in a few studies, was faster than that with the other analgesics but duration was shorter than that of morphine, buprenorphine and pentazocine. Only a small number of patients with chronic pain have received long term therapy with meptazinol; in such patients there was no need for increased doses as treatment progressed.*

Respiratory depression has only been observed in patients receiving meptazinol as a premedication or while undergoing anaesthesia. Similarly any haemodynamic changes have been limited to preoperative patients or patients undergoing anaesthesia. Like other agonist/antagonist analgesic drugs, the abuse potential of meptazinol seems relatively low, but only wider clinical use for longer periods can establish this with certainty. The most commonly reported side effects have been gastrointestinal in nature, and although the incidence of central nervous system side effects has been relatively low, drowsiness and dizziness have caused occasional problems. Thus, meptazinol is a relatively potent but safe addition to the analgesics available for treatment of the patient with moderate to severe pain.

Pharmacodynamic Studies: The opioid agonist activity of meptazinol has been demonstrated in standard animal tests, with a profile of activity characteristic of agonist/antagonist analgesic compounds. The analgesic action is believed in part to be due to

1 'Meptid' (Wyeth).

reaction of the drug with opioid receptors, and partly due to an effect on central cholinergic transmission. In analgesic potency assays in animals, meptazinol was estimated to be 2 to 5 times less potent than morphine and less potent than, or equipotent to, pentazocine. Studies in healthy subjects reported meptazinol 200mg to be significantly better than placebo but less effective than pentazocine 50mg in providing analgesia from experimentally induced pain. This result contrasts with those seen in patients.

The narcotic antagonist properties of meptazinol have been demonstrated in various animal models, including the appearance of withdrawal symptoms in morphine-dependent monkeys and exacerbation of the ongoing abstinence syndrome in those animals previously withdrawn for 12 to 14 hours.

Although animal studies revealed an antiarrhythmic effect for meptazinol, no clinically relevant haemodynamic changes have been recorded in healthy subjects or in patients receiving meptazinol for pain of various origins. During anaesthesia, however, meptazinol has resulted in significant alterations of blood pressure, cardiac output, mean arterial pressure, heart rate and rate/pressure product in some patients. Improved ventricular performance has also been reported in some patients.

The respiratory depressant activity of meptazinol has been looked at in healthy volunteers, pre- and postoperative patients, obstetric patients and neonates, and patients undergoing anaesthesia. Significant decreases in respiratory rate were seen only in those given premedication and in patients undergoing anaesthetic procedures.

Animal and human studies suggest that the abuse potential of meptazinol is relatively low. Withdrawal of meptazinol following long term administration in monkeys resulted in minimal abstinence signs. Injection of nalorphine in these animals produced very slight signs, while naloxone injection resulted in slightly more intense signs of withdrawal. Opioid-dependent patients on a methadone withdrawal programme did not suffer any typical withdrawal symptoms following administration of meptazinol.

Pharmacokinetic Studies: Only limited data are available on the pharmacokinetics of meptazinol in man. Oral administration in healthy subjects resulted in rapid absorption, with peak plasma concentrations being reached within 0.5 to 2 hours. However, as with other phenolic analgesics, bioavailability was low (8.69%) due to an extensive first-pass conjugation. No consistent accumulation was encountered following multiple dosing. Intramuscular administration produced peak plasma levels within 30 minutes, with 99% of steady-state concentrations being achieved before the third dose. Similarly, rectal administration resulted in peak levels which were considerably higher than after oral administration, within 30 minutes of dosing.

Animal studies have demonstrated high concentrations of meptazinol in the lung, spleen, liver and kidneys with some penetration into the brain, especially after intravenous administration. Values for apparent volume of distribution averaged 4.99 L/kg, which is similar to that for pethidine. Neonatal/maternal plasma concentration ratios have ranged from 0.57 to 0.96. A relatively low level of protein binding (27.1%) compared with butorphanol (80%) and buprenorphine (96%) was reported in young healthy subjects. Meptazinol is thought to be extensively metabolised with less than 5% of unchanged drug being recovered in the urine, the major metabolite being the glucuronide conjugate of the parent drug. Excretion was fairly rapid and took place chiefly via the urine with over 50% of the dose predominantly in the conjugated form being recovered in the first 9 hours. Elimination half-lives averaged 2 hours or less and plasma clearance values averaged 2.2 L/min. Age seemed to have little influence on the kinetics of meptazinol because, although the elimination half-lives in the elderly were extended (3.39h after a single dose and 4.97h after multiple doses), peak plasma concentrations after single and multiple doses were similar.

Therapeutic Trials: A number of open studies have reported meptazinol to be an effective analgesic when given orally (100 to 700mg daily), intravenously (100 to 200mg daily) or intramuscularly (100mg daily) in patients with moderate to severe pain from a variety of causes. Meptazinol given orally has proved to be significantly more effective than placebo in providing relief of pain in a limited number of patients with moderate to severe pain of different origin.

Meptazinol, usually given orally or intramuscularly, has been compared with morphine, pentazocine, pethidine (meperidine), buprenorphine, papaveretum, paracetamol (acetaminophen), a combination of dextropropoxyphene and paracetamol, and one of hyoscine-N-butylbromide and dipyrone. Generally, similar analgesic effects were evident for meptazinol and pethidine, pentazocine or the combination of dextropropoxyphene and paracetamol; in one or two studies a greater degree of analgesia was produced by meptazinol than pethidine or pentazocine. The single studies involving comparisons of meptazinol with papaveretum and paracetamol found no significant difference in the analgesia produced by the 2 drugs. Only buprenorphine has proven significantly more effective than meptazinol in provision of analgesia. The results of studies with morphine would suggest that meptazinol may be as effective in maintaining analgesia. Duration of effect of meptazinol was less than that of morphine, buprenorphine and, in 1 study, pentazocine, but equal to that of pethidine, and a combination of hyoscine butylbromide and dipyrone. However, onset of action (where recorded) showed meptazinol to be significantly faster than morphine, pentazocine and the hyoscine-N-butylbromide/dipyrone combination.

Meptazinol given intramuscularly in doses of 75 to 150mg has proved to be an effective obstetric analgesic and is without serious adverse effects on the neonate. The use of meptazinol in anaesthesia has not been adequately investigated. One trial reported an adequate response when combined with hyoscine as a premedication, whilst the other found an unacceptably high level of side effects when meptazinol was included in the anaesthetic technique.

Side Effects: The most common side effects associated with meptazinol administration are the gastrointestinal effects such as nausea and vomiting. Drowsiness and dizziness may also be a frequent problem, but the incidence of other central nervous system side effects has been comparatively low. Although a slightly higher incidence of adverse effects was seen during obstetric use, the condition of the majority of newborn babies was unaffected by the drug. Significant decreases in respiratory rate were seen only preoperatively and in anaesthetised patients, while no serious haemodynamic changes were reported following meptazinol administration.

Dosage and Administration: Meptazinol is available for oral and parenteral use. Recommended oral doses for adults are 200mg 3- to 6-hourly as required, with a usual dose of 200mg 4-hourly. Intramuscular doses of 75 to 100mg may be repeated every 2 to 4 hours if required. Slightly higher intramuscular doses (100 to 150mg) are used in obstetrics, calculated on a weight basis of approximately 2 mg/kg. Slow intravenous injections of 50 to 100mg may be repeated 2- to 4-hourly as required. The possibility of withdrawal symptoms precipitated by meptazinol should be looked for in patients who have previously taken opioids for long periods.

1. Pharmacodynamic Studies

Meptazinol is a centrally acting analgesic belonging to the hexahydroazepine series. The structural formula of meptazinol has some similarities to that of the opiates (fig. 1) and in many ways its action resembles that of the mixed opioid agonist/antagonist analgesics. However, studies both in animals and in man have revealed other properties which were not typical of this class of compound, in particular the low incidence of respiratory depression, constipation and miosis.

1.1 Opioid-Like Agonist Activity

1.1.1 Antinociceptive Activity

Opioid drugs with mixed agonist and antagonist properties exhibit marked activity in mouse writhing tests but tend to be inactive or to show only weak activity in rodent antinociceptive tests involving heat as the noxious stimulus. In contrast, opioid drugs with predominantly agonist activity consistently induce pronounced changes in nociceptive thresholds (Collier et al., 1968; O'Callaghan and Holtzmann, 1975; Tyers, 1980).

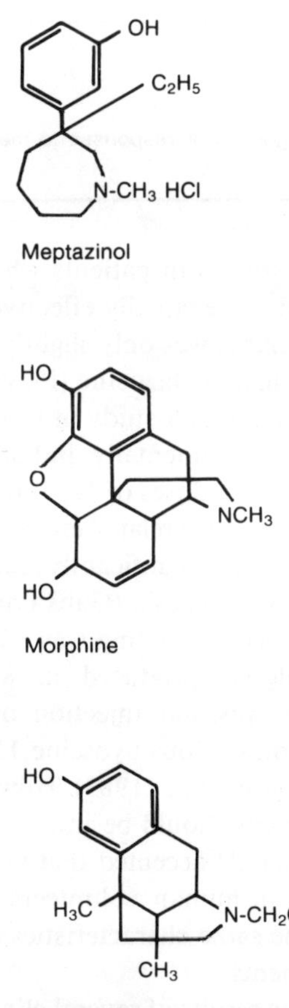

Fig. 1. Structural formulae of meptazinol, morphine and pentazocine.

In an attempt to establish that the antinociceptive activity of meptazinol depends on both opioid and cholinergic mechanisms, Bill et al. (1983) examined the antinociceptive responses to meptazinol, morphine and oxotremorine and the effects of pretreatment with naloxone or hyoscine on these responses in mice and rats (table I). Meptazinol behaved in a manner similar to that of established opioid partial agonists in the rat, but the amplitude of the responses to this agent in the mouse tail immersion and hot plate procedures was longer than that expected of a partial agonist. The responses to meptazinol were consistently partially antagonised by naloxone (requiring a higher dose of naloxone than that necessary to produce the same level of antagonism of morphine), but the action of hyoscine on responses to meptazinol differed substantially depending on the antinociceptive test and species studied. These observations led to the suggestion that meptazinol may affect a central cholinergic mechanism in addition to its effect on opioid receptors.

1.1.2 Analgesic Activity in Animals

In early animal studies, meptazinol was found to be at least as effective in producing analgesia than pentazocine, but less potent than morphine. For example, the ED_{50} of meptazinol against the acetylcholine-induced writhing response of mice was 0.9 mg/kg subcutaneously and 2.15 mg/kg orally. Morphine was slightly more potent by both routes of administration (0.7 mg/kg subcutaneously and 1.5 mg/kg orally), whereas pentazocine was approximately equipotent when given by the subcutaneous route, but 15 times less potent than meptazinol following oral administration (Collier et al., 1964). Meptazinol demonstrated approximately one-eighth the potency of morphine in the mouse heat-induced tail flick test, while buprenorphine produced a very similar dose/response curve after both oral and subcutaneous administration of morphine (unpublished data on file, Wyeth). Doses of drugs producing a 50% analgesic response (relative time taken for each rat to flick its tail from a radiant heat source) in the rat tail flick test conducted by Goode et al. (1979) were:

Table I. Inhibition of antinociceptive responses to subcutaneous analgesics by naloxone and hyoscine[a] given intraperitoneally in the mouse (n = 10 per treatment group) [after Bill et al., 1983]

Stimulus	Response	Analgesic agent	Dose (mg/kg)	Dose of antagonist (mg/kg) to reduce response by 50% (ID_{50})	
				naloxone	hyoscine
Tail immersion in hot water (50°C)	Distinct tail flick	Meptazinol	25	0.51	0.16
		Morphine	5	0.037	> 10
		Oxotremorine[b]	0.064	> 3	0.14
Hot plate (55°C)	Drumming or licking effect	Meptazinol	20	0.41	0.05[c]
		Morphine	6	0.11	> 2.5
		Oxotremorine	0.12	> 3	0.045
Injection of phenylbenzyl quinone (PBQ)	Number of abdominal writhes 5-15 min post PBQ	Meptazinol	8	0.24	> 2.5[d]
		Morphine	2	0.028	> 2.5[d]
		Oxotremorine	0.04	> 10	< 0.5

a Hyoscine; centrally acting anticholinergic drug.
b Oxotremorine; a centrally acting cholinergic drug with analgesic properties.
c Maximum inhibition was approximately 50%.
d Hyoscine alone caused significant reduction of writhing frequency but no sign of antagonism or responses to meptazinol or morphine at the dose shown.

meptazinol, 3.4 mg/kg; pentazocine, 10.9 mg/kg (by extrapolation); and morphine, 1 mg/kg. Assessment of pain perception in the rhesus monkey, using modifications of the leg shock method (Malis and Gluckman, 1974), reported a 50% increase in the intensity of the electrical stimulus that initiated lever pressing after intramuscular administration of meptazinol 6 mg/kg. Morphine and pentazocine induced changes of a similar magnitude at 3 and 15 mg/kg intramuscularly, respectively (unpublished data on file, Wyeth).

1.1.3 Analgesic Activity in Man

The results of a study by Stacher et al. (1983) in 24 healthy subjects showed that oral meptazinol (100, 200 and 400mg) produced dose-related effects on threshold and tolerance to electrically induced pain, and on threshold to thermally induced pain. Meptazinol 400mg was significantly more active than placebo and as active as pentazocine 50 and 100mg. Meptazinol 200mg was clearly more active than placebo, but significantly less effective than pentazocine 50mg, in increasing the threshold and tolerance to electrically induced pain. This result contrasts with studies in patients where the 2 dosages were found to be equally effective (Ward, 1981) or that meptazinol was only slightly (not significantly) weaker than pentazocine (Flavell-Matts and Ward, 1980). In another study in healthy subjects experiencing experimentally induced tooth pulp pain, meptazinol in doses of 50, 100, 150 and 200mg produced linear dose-related effects, but only the 200mg dose proved significantly better than placebo in producing analgesia (Gabka and Price, 1982). Intravenous naloxone 2mg was effective in reversing the analgesia produced in 8 healthy volunteers by intramuscular injection of meptazinol 100mg, but intravenous hyoscine 1.6mg was ineffective (Warrington et al., 1983). However, the results of these studies should be interpreted with caution as it is generally accepted that experimentally induced pain in human volunteers does not necessarily have the same characteristics as pathological pain in patients.

In a review of the results of several clinical trials meptazinol would appear to afford relief from moderate to severe pain of different aetiologies (see section 3). Meptazinol appears to produce pain relief in a dose-dependent manner over a range of 25 to 400mg (fig. 2; Paymaster 1976a; Stephens et al., 1978).

1.2 Opioid Antagonist Activity

Actions of meptazinol which have closely resembled those of the typical opioid antagonists include the appearance of withdrawal signs in morphine-dependent monkeys when given meptazinol 3 to 12 mg/kg, as well as an exacerbation of the ongoing abstinence syndrome in the animals withdrawn for 12 to 14 hours. Morphine-induced analgesia in the monkey was rapidly reversed by nalorphine (2 mg/kg intramuscularly), but that induced by meptazinol was not significantly modified by nalorphine. Similarly, the acute effects of a large dose (50 mg/kg subcutaneously) of morphine in rats, including depression of the corneal reflex, respiration and general locomotion and enhancement of muscle tone, were significantly reduced following the intravenous administration of meptazinol 6 mg/kg (Stephens et al., 1978).

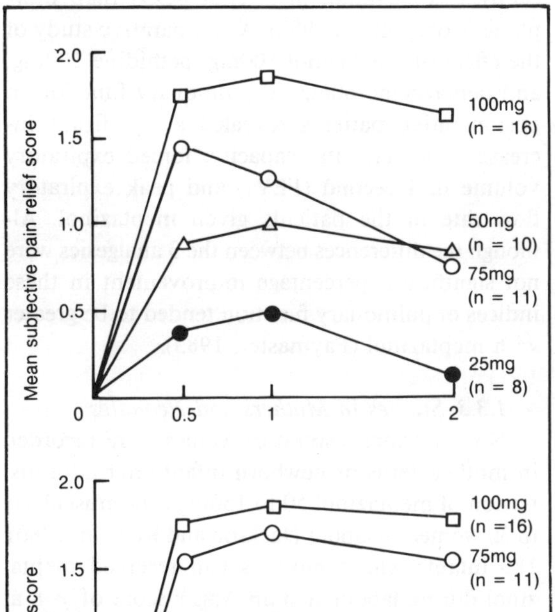

Fig. 2. Patient and investigator assessments of the intensity of pain on a 6-point scale postoperatively and at 0.5, 1.0 and 2.0h after the intramuscular administration of meptazinol. The pain relief score was calculated as the pretreatment pain score minus the post-treatment pain score (after Paymaster, 1976a).

Additional evidence suggesting that meptazinol has opioid-antagonist activity is afforded by its ability to inhibit naloxone binding *in vitro*. Pure opioid antagonists inhibit naloxone binding equally in the presence or absence of sodium ions, whereas opioid agonists are considerably more potent in the absence of sodium ions (Pert and Snyder, 1974). Most agonists have a sodium ratio (concentration required to inhibit naloxone binding in the presence of sodium ions to that in the absence of sodium ions) of >12, pure antagonists have a ratio of 1 and mixed agonist/antagonists a ratio intermediate between these two extremes (Snyder, 1977). The sodium ratio of meptazinol is 1.7, indicating that its effect on naloxone binding is largely unaffected by sodium ions (unpublished data on file, Wyeth).

1.3 Respiratory Effects

It has been proposed that the degree of respiratory depression induced by meptazinol in animal studies is limited by its opioid antagonist and chloruretic properties. Cowlrick and Shepperson (1985) found that the small but significant increase in arterial pCO_2 in rats induced by meptazinol (7.5 to 30 mg/kg) was attenuated by naloxone and enhanced by pretreatment with atropine. In addition, both (+) and (−) enantiomers increased pCO_2, but only the (−) enantiomer reduced the respiratory depressant effect of morphine.

The effect of meptazinol on respiration has been looked at in several groups of subjects – healthy volunteers, pre- and postoperative patients, obstetric patients, and neonates – but only in those patients receiving premedication or undergoing anaesthesia have significant respiratory depressant effects been seen.

1.3.1 Studies in Healthy Volunteers

No significant change in the ventilatory response to rebreathing carbon dioxide was observed after intramuscular injection of meptazinol (100 mg/70kg) or placebo in a double-blind crossover trial in 7 healthy volunteers. However, intramuscular administration of morphine (10 mg/70kg), pentazocine (60 mg/70kg) and diazepam (15 mg/70kg) depressed the slope of the ventilatory response (−30%, −31.6% and −50%, respectively). When breathing room air, end-tidal carbon dioxide tension increased significantly following all 3 analgesic drugs, but not after diazepam. The increase in end-tidal carbon dioxide tension when averaged over 3 hours after meptazinol (0.22 kPa) was significantly less than that following morphine (0.40 kPa) and pentazocine (0.59 kPa). To determine whether the ability of a patient with an abnormal respiratory load to maintain adequate ventilation was impaired, the effect of these analgesics on end-tidal carbon dioxide tension in healthy volunteers subjected to a severe inspiratory load of 8 kPa[1] was also studied. End-tidal carbon dioxide tension increased significantly with all 3 analgesics – meptazinol and morphine produced an increase of 0.51 kPa, and pentazocine produced an increase of 0.8 kPa (Jordan et al., 1979). These findings would indicate that meptazinol and morphine interfere with the regulatory processes involved in loaded inspiration, i.e. the reflex increase in neural activation, to a similar extent (Camu, personal communication).

In 8 healthy volunteers taking part in a double-blind study there was no significant alteration of respiratory rate after placebo or intramuscular administration of meptazinol 100mg (Warrington et al., 1983). Treatment of experimentally induced pain in 24 healthy volunteers with orally administered meptazinol 100 to 400mg did not significantly alter respiratory rates in these subjects (Stacher et al., 1983).

1.3.2 Studies in Patients with Postoperative Pain

Most studies involving the postoperative use of meptazinol in patients have reported no significant change in measurements of ventilation or blood gas tensions (Gibbs and Johnson, 1980; Paymaster, 1976a,b, 1977; Verschraegen et al., 1976; Verschraegen and Rolly, 1979). But in a double-blind study of intramuscular meptazinol 100mg and morphine 15mg in the relief of postoperative orthopaedic pain, both drugs caused a significant fall in respiratory rate, and meptazinol caused significantly less elevation of arterial pCO_2 than morphine (Cohen et al., 1983). A comparative study of the effect of meptazinol 100mg, pethidine 100mg, and pentazocine 60mg on pulmonary function in postoperative patients revealed a significant increase in forced vital capacity, forced expiratory volume in 1 second (FEV_1) and peak expiratory flow rate in the patients given meptazinol. Although the differences between the 3 analgesics were not significant, percentage improvement in these indices of pulmonary function tended to be greater with meptazinol (Paymaster, 1983).

1.3.3 Studies in Mothers and Neonates

No abnormal respiratory values were recorded in mother, fetus or newborn infant after administration of meptazinol 50 to 150mg intramuscularly to 30 women in labour (Jackson and Robson, 1980). 186 infants whose mothers had received meptazinol during labour had an Apgar score of ≥ 8 at 1 minute, which was a significantly greater value than the 172 infants whose mother had received pethidine. Incidence of apnoea and time to sustained regular respiration was shorter in the meptazinol-treated group, but not significantly so (Nicholas and Robson, 1982).

1.3.4 Studies in Preoperative and Anaesthetised Patients

Premedication of 51 patients with meptazinol 50 to 100mg in combination with intramuscular hyoscine 0.2 to 0.4mg resulted in a significant reduction in respiratory rate which was similar in extent to that produced by papaveretum 10 to 20mg plus hyoscine 0.2 to 0.4mg (Broadley et al., 1982).

Respiratory rate showed significant decreases in 2 studies using meptazinol (25 to 100mg) in anaesthetised patients (Slatterly et al., 1982, 1983). Slatterly et al. (1983) also reported a significantly increased end-tidal carbon dioxide concentration. Hardy (1983) reported a case of apnoea, 10 minutes after administration of intravenous meptazinol 100mg, which required manual ventilation. Spontaneous respiration returned with a decreased minute volume (11 to 4L) and halved respiratory rate (20 to 10/min).

1.3.5 Studies in Other Patients

No significant alterations of respiratory parameters were recorded in patients with myocardial infarction pain (Sonecha et al., 1983), pain following trauma (Copeland, 1983), or in patients receiving epidural meptazinol (30 to 90mg) for chronic pain (Budd et al., 1983).

1.4 Haemodynamic Effects

Animal studies have revealed an antiarrhythmic effect for meptazinol at doses which have little effect on other cardiovascular parameters (Fagbemi et al., 1983; Rashid, 1981; Rashid and Waterfall, 1979).

No clinically relevant changes in pulse or blood pressure have been found in studies involving healthy volunteers given doses of meptazinol ranging from 50 to 200mg (Davies et al., 1982; Gabka and Price, 1982; Warrington et al., 1983).

Similarly, no significant alterations of haemodynamic parameters such as heart rate, blood pressure, circulatory or ECG changes have been recorded in postoperative patients (Budd, 1983; Church, 1983; Gibbs and Johnson, 1980; Kingston, 1983; Moyes et al., 1979; Paymaster, 1976a,b, 1977, 1983; Pereira, 1980; Verschraegen and Rolly, 1979; Verschraegen et al., 1976), or in patients in pain from various other causes, such as renal failure (Oosterlinck and DeSy, 1975), myocardial infarction (Sonecha et al., 1983), trauma (Copeland, 1983) chronic pain treated with epidural meptazinol (Budd et al., 1983) and severe pain of various origins (Coutinho, 1980), apart from the occurrence of sinus bradycardia in 2 of the patients with myocardial infarction. Only Cohen et al. (1983) reported a significant decrease in heart rate after administration of intramuscular meptazinol 100mg to patients with postoperative orthopaedic pain. No adverse effects on blood pressure or pulse rates were found in mothers given meptazinol 100mg intramuscularly during labour (Nel et al., 1981).

Preoperative use of meptazinol has resulted in significant decreases (Broadley et al., 1982) as well as significant increases (Verschraegen et al., 1976) in blood pressure, while heart rate remained unchanged (Verschraegen et al., 1976). De Rosayro et al. (1981) reported an improved ventricular performance in 6 patients given meptazinol 1 mg/kg preoperatively, due to shortening of the pre-ejection period (PEP) and lengthening of the left ventricular ejection time (LVET) resulting in a reduction of the PEP/LVET ratio. In another study, cardiac output, mean arterial pressure, heart rate and the rate/pressure product all fell significantly in 9 anaesthetised patients given doses of meptazinol 2 to 4 mg/kg before surgery. Systemic and pulmonary vascular resistance remained stable, as did pulmonary capillary wedge pressure, mean pulmonary artery pressure and myocardial contractility. Meptazinol is thus thought to improve the myocardial oxygen demand/supply ratio by a negative chronotropic effect combined with an ability to decrease afterload (Camu and Rucquoi, 1983).

1.5 Dependence Liability

Agonist-antagonist analgesics like meptazinol produce a qualitatively different type of physical dependence than that seen with morphine-like agonists, with milder withdrawal symptoms and less drug-seeking behaviour (Errick and Heel, 1983).

1.5.1 Animal Studies

Animal studies have indicated a low dependence liability for meptazinol. It did not prevent withdrawal weight loss at doses equianalgesic to the maintenance dose of morphine in rats made dependent on morphine by 9 days of daily dosing via a subcutaneous implanted reservoir. The signs produced by meptazinol 15 mg/kg subcutaneously in this test were of a similar intensity to those induced by 10 mg/kg nalorphine (Goode and White, 1971; Stephens et al., 1978). In contrast, the administration of meptazinol to rats via a subcutaneous implanted reservoir for 9 days followed by abrupt cessation of the drug resulted in very mild withdrawal signs. Rats that had received 62 mg/kg/day morphine over the same period lost 16.3% of their bodyweight and voided, on average, 6.1g more faeces than control animals over the 7-hour period immediately following the withdrawal of morphine. However, rats receiving meptazinol 139 mg/kg/day lost only 3.4% of bodyweight and voided only 0.7g more faeces than controls during the same period after the drug was removed from the reservoir (Stephens et al., 1978).

The observation that meptazinol did not prevent the abstinence syndrome in morphine-dependent monkeys (see section 1.2) may be taken as indirect evidence of a lack of dependence liability. These animals exhibited typical withdrawal signs when given meptazinol, while 12 to 14 hours later the ongoing abstinence syndrome was only exacerbated by the administration of meptazinol. Minimal dependence liability was again demonstrated following long term dosing with meptazinol in the monkey. Rhesus monkeys were given meptazinol subcutaneously every 6 hours for 47 days; the doses on the first day were 8 mg/kg and thereafter 16 mg/kg. Abstinence signs were minimal (grade 0 or 1 compared with the maximum grade 8 after morphine) following abrupt withdrawal of the drug on day 48. Subcutaneous nalorphine 2 mg/kg produced similar very slight (grade 0-1) signs, while naloxone 2 mg/kg by the same route showed slightly more intense (grade 2) signs of withdrawal (Stephens et al., 1978).

1.5.2 Human Studies

In an investigation of the dependence potential of meptazinol injection was conducted in 8 opioid-dependent patients in a double-blind study. The subjects who were on a prolonged withdrawal regimen of methadone had no typical opioid withdrawal symptoms following intravenous administration of meptazinol 100mg. None of the patients reported pleasurable sensations following meptazinol injection, which, if anything, had a dysphoric effect (Evans et al., 1983). A very similar double-blind study by Keen and Owen (1985) in 8 opioid-dependent patients on methadone, who were given meptazinol 100mg intramuscularly, found that a variety of unpleasant psychological and physical effects were produced in the addicts and consequently was not liked by them.

1.6 Mechanism of Action

Meptazinol is a centrally acting analgesic with similar actions to the mixed opioid agonist/antagonist analgesics. For example, the analgesia it produces can be almost completely reversed by the opioid antagonist naloxone (although at higher doses than are needed to reverse the effects of 'pure' opioid agonists such as morphine). In addition, meptazinol reverses the signs of acute morphine overdosage in animals and it precipitates an abstinence syndrome in animals that are morphine dependent (Bill et al., 1983; Stephens et al., 1978).

However, although animal experiments have demonstrated that meptazinol has some opioid antagonist properties (Goode and White, 1971; Stephens et al., 1978), and the possibility that it acts as a mixed agonist/antagonist at opioid receptors cannot be ruled out, certain features of its pharmacology are not typical of the opioids. There is a relatively low incidence of such typical opioid properties as respiratory depression, constipation, and miosis, both in animal and in clinical studies, and receptor-binding studies utilising radioactive ligands have shown that meptazinol displays a greater affinity for μ_1-receptors than the other opioid receptors, but overall the affinity is comparatively low (Speigel and Pasternak, 1984) [table II]. However, high affinity binding sites have been identified, predominantly in the spinal cord and cortex – a distribution differing from that found with the opioids (Green, 1983). Similarly, in the electrically stimulated guinea-pig ileum and mouse vas deferens (preparations rich in opioid receptors) mep-

Table II. Comparison of the affinities of drugs for opioid receptors in the rat brain[a] (after Green, 1983)

Drug	Designation	μ_1-receptors	μ_2-receptors	δ-receptors	κ-receptors
Naloxone	Opioid antagonist	1	3	15	15
Pentazocine	Agonist-antagonist	19	14	90	120
Pethidine	Agonist-antagonist	1700	2100	2800	1800
Morphine	'Pure' agonist	3	6	20	400
Meptazinol	Agonist-antagonist	190	1800	20,000	100,000

a Concentrations (K_1 nmol) required to displace specific ligands from the individual receptor subtypes – the higher the figure the lower the affinity of the particular drug for that receptor.

tazinol injection gave results unlike those obtained with opioid agonists or mixed opioid agonist/antagonist (Stephens et al., 1978).

Certain cholinergic drugs such as oxotremorine are known to act centrally to produce analgesia in mice, and like these and other centrally acting analgesics, meptazinol injection is active in a test in which the tails of mice are subjected to a mild thermal stimulus and the response time is measured. It has been demonstrated that, unlike the actions of any opioid examined, the actions of meptazinol injection are antagonised by low doses of centrally acting anticholinergic drugs such as hyoscine, while anticholinergics such as atropine methylnitrate, which do not gain free access to the central nervous system when given peripherally, have a much smaller antagonist effect (Bill et al., 1983).

In conclusion, the possibility exists that meptazinol may act in part as a mixed agonist/antagonist at opioid receptors, but that a component of its analgesic action, in animals at least, is attributable to an effect on central cholinergic transmission. In this latter respect it differs from conventional analgesics.

2. Pharmacokinetic Studies

There is only limited information available on the pharmacokinetic properties of meptazinol in man.

2.1 Absorption

2.1.1 Oral Administration

Following oral administration of meptazinol 200mg to healthy subjects, peak plasma concentrations were achieved within 0.5 to 2 hours (fig. 3) [Franklin et al., 1976; Norbury et al., 1983; Stephens et al., 1978]. Peak plasma concentrations, however, showed considerable intersubject variability with levels ranging from 9.1 to 110 μg/L

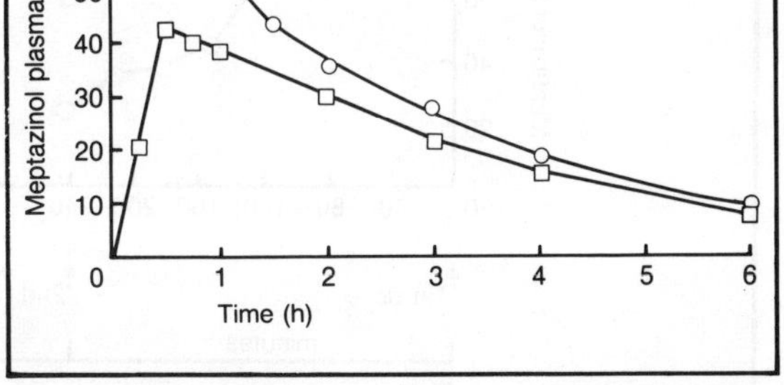

Fig. 3. Plasma concentration-time curves following administration of a single oral 200mg dose of meptazinol to 9 healthy volunteers (□) and a single intravenous dose of meptazinol 25mg in 5 healthy volunteers (○) [after Norbury et al., 1983].

(Norbury et al., 1983). As with other phenolic analgesics such as morphine (Brunck and Delle, 1974), pentazocine (Ehrnebo et al., 1978) and butorphanol (Caruso et al., 1979), meptazinol has demonstrated a low bioavailability (8.69%) due to an extensive first-pass conjugation. Norbury et al. (1983) also observed greater bioavailability during the initial rapid stages of absorption than when the maximum plasma concentrations were achieved, possibly due to saturation of the conjugating enzymes – a phenomenon previously observed in animal studies (Franklin, 1977). Multiple oral dosing with meptazinol (200mg 6-hourly for 3 days) did not lead to any consistent drug accumulation, with mean maximum plasma concentrations averaging 53.5 μg/L, compared with 55.4 μg/L after a single dose (Norbury et al., 1983).

2.1.2 Intravenous Administration

Changes of plasma concentration of meptazinol with time after a single intravenous dose of 25mg in healthy subjects following an initial rapid distribution phase are shown in figure 3 (Norbury et al., 1983). Rosseel et al. (1975) also observed an initial rapid distribution phase followed by a slower disposition phase following intravenous doses of 1 mg/kg in 4 healthy volunteers.

2.1.3 Intramuscular Administration

After intramuscular administration peak plasma concentrations were attained in less than 30 minutes in all of the 6 healthy subjects who received a 50mg dose (Davies et al., 1982). As can be seen from figure 4, and from the results of a study by Rosseel et al. (1976) where 4 healthy subjects received intramuscular doses of 60mg for 5 days, accumulation on repeated administration did not appear to be a problem, however the small but significantly higher pre-dose plasma level after the third and fourth injections cannot be ignored. 95%

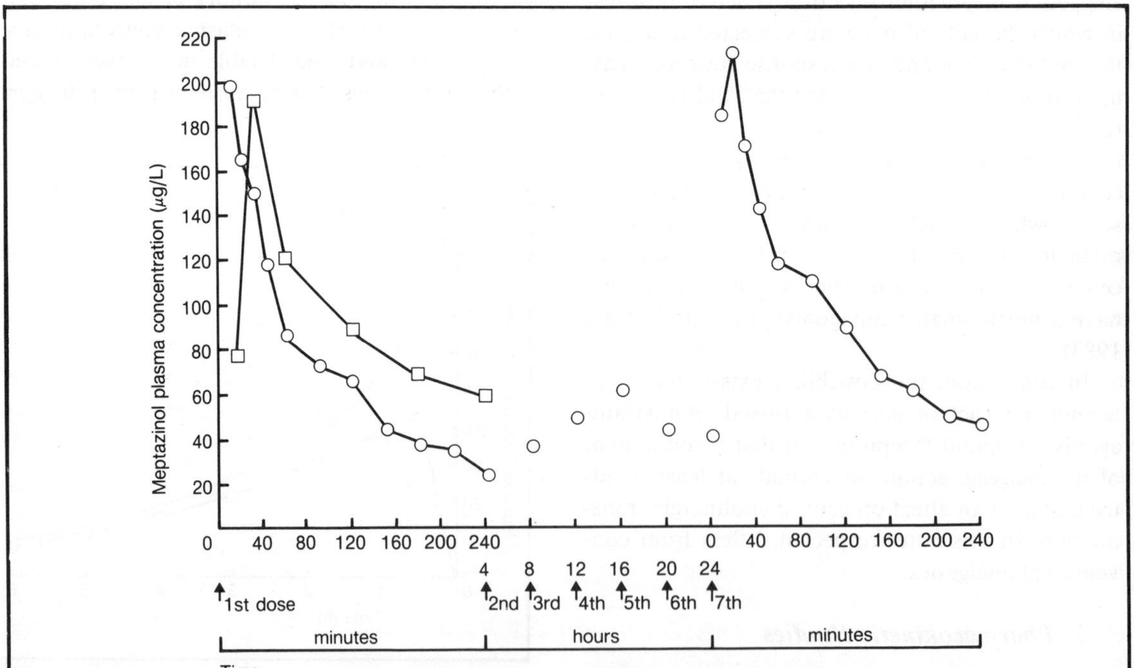

Fig. 4. Plasma concentration-time curve following administration of 7 intramuscular injections of meptazinol 50mg to 6 healthy volunteers (○) [after Davies et al., 1982] and after rectal administration of 50mg in 1 healthy volunteer (□) [after Franklin et al., 1977).

of the steady-state concentration was achieved before the second dose and 99% before the third dose (Davies et al., 1982).

2.1.4 Rectal Administration

In man, rectal administration of meptazinol both in healthy subjects and in elderly patients resulted in peak plasma concentrations of the drug within 30 minutes of dosing (Franklin et al., 1977; Rosseel et al., 1976) [fig. 4]. Urinary recovery of 65 to 99% of the administered dose suggested extensive absorption. Despite substantial interindividual variation in the observed maximum plasma concentrations (range 39 to 190 μg/L), they were considerably higher after rectal administration than those achieved following oral ingestion of the same dose (50mg) [Franklin et al., 1977]; this may be due to the lesser degree of first-pass phenomenon when the rectal route is used.

2.2 Distribution

Studies in animals have shown a tissue distribution pattern typical of a basic lipophilic drug, with relatively high concentrations being achieved in the highly perfused tissues such as the lung, spleen and liver (Franklin and Aldridge, 1976). High concentrations in the kidney may reflect extensive urinary excretion of the drug and metabolites. Concentrations in the brain reached 6 mg/kg an hour after intravenous administration of 8 mg/kg in monkeys, whereas brain concentration was only 0.3 mg/kg after oral administration of meptazinol 25 mg/kg.

The apparent volume of distribution after the intravenous administration of meptazinol 25mg in healthy subjects averaged 4.99 L/kg (Norbury et al., 1983), while values at steady-state following intravenous doses of 1 mg/kg and 3 mg/kg in healthy subjects and anaesthetised patients averaged 3.1 L/kg and 2.01 L/kg, respectively (Gepts et al., 1984; Rosseel et al., 1975). This value for apparent volume of distribution is similar to that for pethidine (4.36 L/kg) [Mather et al., 1974] and may indicate extensive penetration into extravascular tissues.

Neonatal/maternal plasma concentration ratios of 0.57 (Franklin et al., 1981; Jackson and Robson, 1983) and 0.96 (Jackson and Robson, 1980) have been reported for 13 women given intramuscular doses of meptazinol 100 to 150mg during labour and in 3 given 50 to 150mg intramuscularly, respectively.

2.2.1 Plasma Protein Binding

Plasma protein binding in healthy subjects, determined using ^{3}H-meptazinol, averaged 27.1% and did not vary significantly over the therapeutic range of 25 to 250 μg/L (Norbury et al., 1983). This is a low level of binding compared with 80% for butorphanol (Caruso et al., 1979) and 96% for buprenorphine (Heel et al., 1979). Plasma protein binding of meptazinol in elderly patients (Norbury et al., 1984) was reported to be slightly higher (33.8%) than that obtained in younger healthy subjects.

2.3 Elimination

2.3.1 Metabolism

Recovery of less than 5% of unchanged drug in the urine following oral and intravenous administration indicated extensive metabolism of meptazinol (Franklin et al., 1975, 1976). The major metabolite is thought to be the glucuronide conjugate of the parent drug. A minor metabolite amounting to 5 to 10% of the administered dose has been reported but not yet identified (Franklin et al., 1975). Conjugation of meptazinol is also thought to account for the major method of elimination of the drug in the neonate (Dowell et al., 1982).

2.3.2 Excretion

Elimination of both orally and intravenously administered drug from plasma took place in an apparently monoexponential fashion (Franklin et al., 1976; Norbury et al., 1983). Following intravenous doses of 25mg and 3 mg/kg, mean plasma clearance values were reported to be 132 L/h (Norbury et al., 1983) and 82.4 L/h (Gepts et al., 1984), respectively. Both studies indicated an intrinsically

Table III. Open studies on the use of oral, intramuscular (IM), intravenous (IV) and epidural (Ep) meptazinol in various pain states

Reference	Number of patients	Study population	Dose of meptazinol	Duration of therapy	Method of assessment	Results
Oral						
Paymaster (1976b)	51	Postoperative abdominal, vaginal, orthopaedic + plastic	50, 100, 250, 400, 500mg in a dose-ranging study	5 doses	Patient, + observer assessment of pain, level of consciousness, pulmonary function	50-100mg no analgesia; 250, 400, 500mg significant decrease in pain scores (1 to 4h)
Pearce and Robson (1980)	11	Moderate to severe pain	100mg	NA	Patient VAS alertness	Significant decrease in pain intensity after 30 minutes. No significant change in alertness
Price and Latham (1982a)	144	GP pts with chronic pain	200mg	12 mo	Patient VAS + GP assessment of pain severity, sleep impairment	Significant decrease in mean VAS scores from month 1-4
Wade and Ward (1981)	49	GP pts with chronic pain	550-710mg	NA	Patient VAS + observer VRS	Significant decrease in VAS from 2-72h
Intramuscular						
Copeland (1983)	19	Trauma	100mg	Single	Patient VAS + physician VRS, BP, pulse, RR, pupillary diameter	Effective analgesia
Coutinho (1980)	42	Severe and very severe urological pain, 19 postoperative, 22 renal colic, 1 testicular torsion	100mg	Single	Patient scoring, + comparison to pretreatment level of pain. Alertness, RR, pulse BP	Effective analgesia in 40 patients; duration 2-6h
Gibbs and Johnson (1980)	43	Postoperative abdominal	100mg	Mean 7 doses	Observer assessment of pain intensity	Provided satisfactory pain relief in the majority of cases
Nicholas (1983)	578	Women in labour	2 mg/kg	NA	Patient + observer VRS	Satisfactory to good in > 60% at 30 minutes. Effective analgesia in most pts at 1h. Effective analgesia in 72.6% at 90 minutes
Paymaster (1976a)	45	Postoperative abdominal	25, 50, 75 or 100mg sb	4 doses	Patient, + observer assessment of pain, level of consciousness, pulmonary function	Dose-related significant analgesia above 50mg, with a maximum effect after 1h and duration of 5h
Pereira (1980)	41	Postoperative orthopaedic	100mg	Single	NA	37 experienced an analgesic effect within 19 minutes

Verschraegen et al. (1976)	39	Postoperative abdominal surgery + lumbotomies	100mg	NA	Patient, nurse + anaesthetist completed pain scores	Effective analgesia, with an onset of 30 minutes and duration of 2h
Intravenous						
Sonecha et al. (1983)	17	Myocardial infarction	Titrated 100-200mg	24h	VAS, pulse, BP, RR, level of consciousness, pain intensity, 4-hourly	Effective analgesia in 15 of the 22 patients
Oosterlinck and DeSy (1975)	30	Acute renal colic	20-120mg	Single	NA	39 of 41 injections provided adequate analgesia
Epidural						
Budd et al. (1983)	23	Spinal or back pain	39-90mg	4 doses	VAS, pulse rate, BP, and respiration every 30 minutes	Effective analgesia achieved after 30mg in most cases, duration increased from 7.6h after the first dose to 11.8h after the fourth dose

Abbreviations: GP = general practitioner; sb = single blind; VAS = visual analogue scale; VRS = verbal rating scale; RR = respiratory rate; NA = not available; BP = blood pressure.

high hepatic clearance, approaching that of liver blood flow (21 ml/kg/min) with meptazinol clearance being a reflection of the delivery rate of the drug to the liver (Camu, personal communication).

Excretion of radioactivity following oral and intravenous administration of a mixture of [1-^{14}C]- and [7-^{3}H]-labelled meptazinol was rapid, irrespective of the dosage route. Urinary recovery was over 50% in the first 9 hours and more than 60% in the first 24 hours. Less than 10% was recovered in the faeces. Urinary recovery ranged from 65 to 90% following rectal administration of meptazinol 50 to 75mg (Franklin et al., 1977) and averaged 70% following intravenous doses of 1 mg/kg in healthy volunteers (Rosseel et al., 1975).

Elimination half-lives averaged 2 hours following intravenous (Franklin et al., 1976; Norbury et al., 1983) and rectal administration (Rosseel et al., 1975), while a slightly shorter value of 1.6 hours was recorded after intramuscular administration (Davies et al., 1982). During anaesthesia, the elimination half-life of intravenous meptazinol averaged 73 minutes (Gepts et al., 1984). A half-life for meptazinol in the newborn was reported to be similar to that in the adult, 3.4 hours (Jackson and Robson, 1983). This compares with the half-life for pethidine in the newborn of 22.7 hours (Caldwell et al., 1978).

2.4 Influence of Age on Pharmacokinetics

Oral administration of meptazinol 200mg to 10 elderly (> 70 years) patients resulted in peak drug concentrations of 41.3 μg/L at 0.5 to 3 hours after administration. Continued administration (13 consecutive 6-hourly doses) produced a higher value of 55.6 μg/L. Subsequent elimination proceeded with a half-life of 3.39 hours after a single dose and 4.97 hours following continuous dosing. Area under the plasma concentration-time curve (202 μg/L · h single, 481 μg/L · h multiple) and maximum plasma concentration values demonstrated no accumulation above the level expected from the single-dose results. Although this one study demonstrates an extended half-life for meptazinol in the elderly, peak plasma concentrations after single and multiple doses were similar to those of healthy adults, perhaps indicating that clearance remained largely unaltered (Norbury et al., 1983, 1984). In contrast, Levy (personal communication) believes that because the dosage interval used in this study was relatively long (maximum recommended for meptazinol) compared with the drug's normal half-life, a decreased renal clearance would not be easily detected from the results.

3. Therapeutic Trials

The subjective nature of pain, the difficulties in measuring pain relief, the variability of the placebo response and interpatient variation make studies on the therapeutic efficacy of analgesic drugs difficult to conduct. The correct design of the trial can minimise most of these problems through such measures as a double-blind design, random allocation of the treatments, the inclusion of a placebo control, and evaluation of the assessments of both observers and patients. Meptazinol has demonstrated analgesic properties in open studies, while a few double-blind placebo-controlled studies, one of which was crossover in design, all reported meptazinol as providing significantly more analgesia than placebo, using the patients', and in 2 trials, also the physicians' assessments to evaluate therapy. More extensive double-blind comparative trials which generally used a random allocation of treatments, and a few with a crossover design, were conducted. Patient and investigator assessments were more common in these trials, with only a few relying just on the patients' scoring.

3.1 Open Studies

Several open studies have shown meptazinol to be an effective analgesic when given orally, intravenously, intramuscularly or epidurally to patients with pain from a variety of causes (table III). Dose-ranging studies revealed a significant dose-related analgesia after intramuscular injection of meptazinol 25 to 100mg in patients following abdominal surgery.

In 51 postoperative patients, oral doses of meptazinol 250, 400 and 500mg (but not 50 or 100mg) produced significant decreases in pain scores 1 hour after administration (Paymaster, 1976a,b). A general trend of reduced dose with time was evident (from 730mg in the first month declining to 430mg during long term therapy) in patients with pain arising from 30 different aetiologies – most commonly musculoskeletal (29%) and osteoarthritic (20%) [Price and Latham, 1982a].

Epidural use of meptazinol in doses of 30 to 90mg effectively lowered visual analogue scale pain scores in 23 patients with spinal or back pain (Budd et al., 1983). The good analgesic success rate (60 to 70%) of meptazinol in an initial open study in women in labour, together with the rapid onset of action and lack of effect on the newborn infant, has led to further comparative studies, and may indicate a potential use for meptazinol in this area (see section 3.2.4).

3.2 Controlled Studies

3.2.1 Comparisons with a Placebo

Oral meptazinol has proved significantly more effective than placebo in providing analgesia in patients with pain from a variety of causes (table IV). In terms of pain relief, the placebo response has been assessed at between 20 and 40% (Cooper, 1980; Murray, 1964; Schindel, 1978). Overall though, meptazinol proved to be more efficacious than placebo, producing significantly more analgesia in patients with chronic pain after 4 to 8 and 11 to 14 days of therapy. However, in patients with acute pain, the difference in visual analogue scale scores was not significant.

This study also revealed a sex-dependent difference in pain response, with males obtaining significantly more pain relief than females (Price and Latham, 1982c). Meptazinol produced effective analgesia on 12 of the 14 occasions it was given intravenously for the relief of renal colic, whereas placebo was effective in only 1 of 8 injections (Oosterlinck and DeSy, 1975).

3.2.2 Comparisons with Morphine

Only 3 studies are so far available which com-

Table IV. Double-blind placebo-controlled studies of oral and intravenous (IV) meptazinol in patients with pain of various origins

Reference	Study population	Number of patients	Route of administration	Dose of meptazinol	Method of assessment	Result
Goldstuck and Ward (1983)	IUD insertion	29M 30P	Oral	100mg	NA	M > P
Hedges et al. (1977)	Hysterectomy	35M	Oral	400mg	Patient assessment	M > P
Parker and Langrick (1982)	Acute 40, chronic 22 Acute 32, chronic 35 GP pts	63M 68P	Oral	200mg 4-6 hrly for 14 days	Patient VAS daily + physician assessment at day 1 and 14	M > P
Price and Latham (1982c)	Acute 82, chronic 101 Acute 94, chronic 89	183M 183P	Oral	200mg 4-hrly	Patient VAS daily + physician assessment	M > P[a]
Oosterlinck and DeSy (1975)	Renal colic (15 episodes)	11M	IV	> 50-120mg	NA	M > P

a Placebo response of 20 to 40% reported. Difference in VAS scores for acute pain is much less than both acute and chronic scores, also males experienced significantly more pain relief.

Abbreviations: M = meptazinol; P = placebo; GP = general practitioner; NA = not available; Pt = patient; VAS = visual analogue scale; > = significantly better than.

pared meptazinol with morphine. In a double-blind study in 92 patients suffering traumatic injury of various types, intramuscular meptazinol 100mg provided a faster onset of analgesia and an equivalent or greater degree of analgesia than morphine 10 or 15mg. Blood pressure was not affected by meptazinol but fell significantly with morphine 15mg in the first 2 hours. Sedation was also more common with morphine but gastrointestinal effects and dizziness occurred more frequently with meptazinol (Westcombe and Price, 1985) [table V]. A significant improvement in mean pain scores in both the meptazinol and morphine treatment groups was seen in a study in patients with severe postoperative pain by Cohen et al. (1983). At 30 minutes the mean pain score improvement was significantly greater in the meptazinol group, but from 2 hours onwards pain relief became better in the morphine group, reaching a significant level after 6 hours. The overall linear analogue assessment of the patients at 24 hours was significantly better in the morphine (74.8) group than the meptazinol group (62). Similarly, the 24-hour observer assessment of the overall quality of treatment, taking into account side effects as well as analgesia, was significantly in favour of morphine (73) over meptazinol (61). Meptazinol was also found to be less effective than morphine in the relief of pain and duration of analgesia in a multicomparative study of postoperative analgesics by Harmer et al. (1983).

3.2.3 Comparisons with Pentazocine

In terms of degree of pain relief, meptazinol has been found to be better than (Griffiths and Thomas, 1985; Pearce and Robson, 1980; Verschraegen and Rolly, 1979) or equipotent to (Flavell-Matts and Ward, 1980; Paymaster, 1977; Staquet, 1978; Ward, 1981) pentazocine when given both by the intramuscular and oral route to patients with pain of various origins (table V). Onset of action with meptazinol has generally been faster than with pentazocine (Paymaster, 1977; Pearce and Robson, 1980; Verschraegen and Rolly, 1979), but duration of action appeared shorter in one study (Verschraegen and Rolly, 1979).

3.2.4 Comparisons with Pethidine (Meperidine)

As a Postoperative Analgesic

Meotazinol was found to be as effective as peth-

Table V. Comparative studies of intravenous (IV), intramuscular (IM), epidural (Ep) or oral (O) meptazinol (M) and morphine (m), pethidine (Pd), buprenorphine (B) and pentazocine (Pz)

Reference	No. of patients and diagnosis	Drug and dosage	Study design	Method of evaluation	Analgesic effect: pain relief	Analgesic effect: onset	Analgesic effect: duration	Side effects	Withdrawals
Comparison with morphine									
Cohen et al. (1983)	35M, 28m po orthopaedic	M 100 IM od, max 800 in 24h m 15 IM od, max 120 in 24h	random db	Pt and observer LAS plus observer assessment	M = m (LAS) m > M (24h)[a]	M < m	M > m	M = m (CV) M < m (R) M > m (GI)	5 patients (M) – 4 inadequate analgesia
Westcombe and Price (1985)	31M, 61m, Traumatic injury	M 100 m 10 to 15 } IM	random db	Pt and observer VAS and VRS	M > m	M < m	M = m	M < m (CV) M > m (GI)	
Comparison with morphine, pethidine and buprenorphine									
Harmer et al. (1983)	10B, 9M, 10m, 10Pd po cholecystectomy	B 0.15 M 50 m 5 Pd 50 } IM od[b]	db	Pt LAS at 24h plus observer assessment	B > m > M > Pd		B > m > M > Pd	B = M = m = Pd (nausea & drowsiness) Pd > B,M,m (dizziness)	1 patient (M) – inadequate analgesia
Comparison with pentazocine									
Flavell-Matts and Ward (1980)	60 chronic RA or OA moderate to severe pain	M 200 Pz 50 } O	db xover	Pt assessment	M = Pz			Pz > M nausea, vomiting and dizziness	3 patients (Pz) – side effects
Griffiths and Thomas (1985)	30M, 30Pz, 30P dental pain	M 200 Pz 50 P – } O	random db	Pt VAS and VRS	M > Pz > P	M < Pz	M > Pz		6 patients (Pz) 3 patients (M) 20 patients (P)
Pearce and Robson (1980)	30 elderly with moderate to severe pain	M 100 Pz 25 P – } O	random db xover	VAS for pain and mental confusion	M > Pz > P	M < Pz < P	M = Pz > P[d]	Pz > M > P (mental confusion)	
Staquet (1978)	*Trial I* 16 cancer patients	M 75 Pz 60 P – } IM	random xover	Pt scoring	M = Pz > P			M100 > Pz > M75 > P	3 patients (M) – severe side effects
	Trial II 9 cancer patients	M 100 Pz 60 P – } IM			M = Pz > P				

Verschraegen and Rolly (1979)	16M, 12Pz, 16P po lumbotomy for kidney disease	M 100 Pz 60 P –	IM	db	Pt and observer assessments	M > Pz > P	M < Pz < P	Pz > M > P	M = Pz = P (CV) M = Pz > P (R)[c]	
Ward (1981)	52M, 53Pz, chronic back pain	M 200 Pz 50	O	db random	Pt pain index[e] and global assessment	M = Pz			Pz > M	4 patients (M): and 9 (Pz) – side effects
Comparison with pentazocine and pethidine										
Paymaster (1977)	25M, 25Pz, 25Pd po orthopaedic[f] abdominal	M 100 Pz 60 Pd 100	IM[g]	db random	Pt and observer scoring	M = Pz = Pd			M = Pz = Pd	
Comparisons with pethidine										
Church (1983)	30 po abdominal	M 0.45 mg/kg/h Pd 0.3 mg/kg/h	cont. infusion	random	Pt VAS	M = Pd			Pd > M (R)	
Hedges et al. (1980)	24 × 3 po abdominal hysterectomy	M 60-100 Pd 100	IM	db	Pt scoring and observer assessment	M = Pd		M = Pd	M = Pd	
Jackson and Robson (1980)	163M 81Pd women in labour	< 60kg M 100-150 Pd 100-150	IM	sb	Pt scoring at 1h Apgar scores[h]	M > Pd		M = Pd		
Nel et al. (1981)	30M, 30Pd women in labour	M 100 Pd 100	IM	db random	Pt VAS for 2h observer assessments Apgar scores	M = Pd			M = Pd	
Nicholas and Robson (1982)	186M 172Pd women in labour	< 50kg M 75-150 Pd 75-150	Ep	db random	Pt verbal rating plus observer assessment Apgar scores	M > Pd[j]		M = Pd	M = Pd	
Slatterly et al. (1981)	20 po upper abdominal	M 24.1 mg/kg/24h Pd 9.94 mg/kg/24h	IV	db random assessment 2-4h	Pt LAS at 24h plus observer after	M = Pd			M > Pd (nausea) M = Pd (other)	1 patient (M) – inadequate analgesia

(see next page for footnotes)

a 24-hour assessment, taking into account observer and patient assessments.
b Cardiff Palliator, used to provide on-demand analgesia.
c A marked pCo_2 decrease following placebo.
d At 3 and 4 hours the pain relief afforded by meptazinol and pentazocine did not differ significantly.
e Pain index was calculated for the 4-day treatment period and included the daily pain assessment as well as the presence or absence of stiffness or discomfort.
f Pain relief in the orthopaedic group was significantly greater with both meptazinol and pentazocine.
g Median time of administration of second analgesic for meptazinol was 3.5 hours; pethidine 4.8 hours and pentazocine 6 hours; not a significant difference.
h Apgar score, an assessment of the condition of the newly born 1 or more minutes after birth. A score of 0, 1 or 2 is given in each of 5 variables: heart rate, respiratory effect, muscle tone, colour, and reflex irritability. Maximum score of 10.
j Pain relief assessments at 45 and 60 minutes were significantly greater in the meptazinol group, but after 90 and 120 minutes pain relief was the same in both groups.

Abbreviations: po = postoperative, od = on demand; Pt = patient; LAS = linear analogue scale; CV = cardiovascular; R = respiratory; GI = gastrointestinal; GP = general practitioner; P = placebo; VAS = visual analogue scale; RA = rheumatoid arthritis; OA = osteoarthritis; VRS = visual rating scale.

idine given either intravenously or intramuscularly in achieving pain relief in postoperative patients (table V). In the study by Slatterly et al. (1981) mean analogue pain scores after intravenous meptazinol and pethidine were almost identical at 43.1 and 42.7, respectively. However the meptazinol : pethidine consumption ratios ranged from 4.5 : 1 to 1.6 : 1 at varying times after surgery with a mean of 2.4 : 1 over 24 hours, which would seem to suggest that meptazinol was less potent than pethidine. Similarly, an average of 28 demands for meptazinol analgesia in 24 hours was recorded in a study of postoperative patients compared with an average of 20 demands in 24 hours with pethidine (Harmer et al., 1983). Although Hedges et al. (1980) found no significant difference in the pain relief produced by 3 different doses of intramuscular meptazinol (60, 75 and 100mg) and that produced by pethidine 100mg intramuscularly, patient preference for pethidine 100mg over meptazinol 60mg was significant.

As an Obstetric Analgesic

Pain relief produced by meptazinol 75 to 150mg intramuscularly in women in labour has proved to be significantly greater than that with pethidine 75 to 150mg, when assessed 1 hour after administration (Jackson and Robson, 1980; Nicholas and Robson, 1982). After 90 and 120 minutes this distinction was lost and pain relief was the same in both groups (Nel et al., 1981; Nicholas and Robson, 1982). Duration of action was similar for both drugs (Jackson and Robson, 1980; Nicholas and Robson, 1982). Most of the assessments of newborn infants, which generally involved an Apgar scoring system, as well as incidence of apnoea and clinical examination, did not reveal significant differences between the 2 drugs (Jackson and Robson, 1980, 1983; Nel et al., 1981). In a double-blind trial of 100 mothers who had received intramuscular meptazinol or pethidine 1.8 mg/kg, there was significantly more neonatal activity following meptazinol as judged by crying and movement, and the number of babies considered fit for discharge by the sixth day was also significantly greater in the meptazinol group. Weight loss and incidence of

Table VI. Comparative studies of intravenous (IV), intramuscular (IM) or oral meptazinol (M) and other drugs

Reference	No. of patients and diagnosis	Drug/dosage (mg)		Study design	Method of evaluation	Analgesic effect			Side effects
						relief of pain	onset	duration	
Moyes et al. (1979)	50 po hysterectomy	M 100 Pv 20	IM	db random	Pt and observer scoring	M = Pv			M = Pv
Oosterlinck and DeSy (1976)	20M, 20H acute renal colic	M 60 H 20	IV	db	Pt and observer assessments	M > H	M < H	M = H	M > H (dizziness) M = H (nausea and vomiting)
Price and Latham (1982b)	65M, 71D acute or chronic pain presenting to GP	M 200 D 2 tabs	0 3- to 6-hly 14 days	db random	Pt VAS, physician assessment	M = D			D > M
Videman et al. (1984)	34M 34Df acute low back pain	M 200 Df 250	0 qid	db random	Pt and observer assessment	M = Df			M = Df
Wade and Ward (1982a)	83 acute or chronic musculoskeletal pain presenting to GP	M 200 Pa 1g P	0 3- to 6-hly 72h	db	Pt and physician assessments of pain	M = Pa > P			M = Pa = P
Wade and Ward (1982b)	38M, 40D acute or chronic pain presenting to GP	M 200 D 2 tabs	0 3- to 6-hly for 72h	db random	Pt and physician pain assessments using VAS	M = D			D > M

Abbreviations: O = oral; P = placebo; db = double-blind; Pv = papaveretum; H = hyoscine-N-butylbromide 20mg and dipyrone 20mg; VAS = visual analogue scale; D = dextropropoxyphene 32.5mg and paracetamol 325mg; GP = general practitioner; Df = diflunisal; qid = 4 times daily.

neonatal jaundice was also lower in the meptazinol group, but not significantly so (Jackson and Robson, 1983).

3.2.5 Comparisons with Other Analgesics

Intramuscular buprenorphine 0.15mg was reported to give significantly more pain relief for a longer period than intramuscular morphine 5mg, meptazinol 50mg, and pethidine 50mg in a trial involving postoperative cholecystectomy patients (table VI; Harmer et al., 1983).

Meptazinol 200mg orally was found to be as effective as 2 tablets containing a combination of dextropropoxyphene (propoxyphene) and paracetamol in relieving pain in patients with acute or chronic pain presenting to their general practitioner. The incidence of side effects was lower with meptazinol in both studies (table VI; Price and Latham, 1982b; Wade and Ward, 1982b]. In treating patients presenting to their general practitioner with acute or chronic musculoskeletal pain, meptazinol 200mg administered orally was as effective as paracetamol 1g orally, both of which proved to be significantly better than placebo (Wade and Ward, 1982a).

Patients with acute renal colic obtained greater pain relief from a single intravenous dose of meptazinol 60mg than from an injection of a combination of hyoscine butylbromide 20mg and dipyrone 2.5g. Onset of action was faster with meptazinol, with 18 of 20 patients experiencing some pain relief within 5 minutes, compared with 10 of 20 patients after a combination of hyoscine butylbromide and dipyrone. Dizziness was a frequent problem with meptazinol, occurring in 13 patients, but nausea and vomiting were reported almost equally after both treatments (Oosterlinck and DeSy, 1976).

Comparable relief of pain following hysterectomy was achieved by meptazinol 100mg and papaveretum 20mg given intramuscularly to 50 women (Moyes et al., 1979). Despite the absence of anti-inflammatory properties, meptazinol produced a similar rate of clinical efficacy and side effect profile to diflunisal in outpatients with acute lumbago (Videman et al., 1984).

3.3 Use in Premedication and Anaesthesia

Broadley et al. (1982) compared a mixture of meptazinol (mean dose 81.5mg) and hyoscine (mean dose 0.33mg) with a papaveretum (mean dose 15.9mg) and hyoscine (mean dose 0.32mg) combination, as surgical premedications in a randomised double-blind trial involving 101 patients. Small but significant reductions in blood pressure and respiratory rate were noted in both groups. After both treatments most patients were calm and relaxed and there was no difference between the groups in sedation score, extent of salivary secretion or postoperative analgesic requirements. Antiemetics were administered to 13 patients receiving meptazinol and 18 receiving papaveretum. The incidence of side effects was similar: 25% and 28% given meptazinol and papaveretum, respectively.

In contrast, Verschraegen et al. (1976) using meptazinol (1.6 mg/kg intravenously) in 22 surgical patients found an unacceptably high incidence of side effects such as heavy perspiration, salivation, lacrimation and vomiting in 45% of cases.

3.4 Other Uses

The potentially fatal Jarisch-Herxheimer reaction, which can often follow antibiotic (generally tetracycline) treatment of spirochaetal diseases, was unaffected by naloxone 30 to 40mg intravenously, but was diminished by meptazinol 300 to 500mg intravenously. Compared with naloxone and placebo, meptazinol reduced the clinical severity of the reaction, significantly delayed and shortened its chill phase, delayed the rise in temperature, and reduced peak temperature and changes in pulse and respiratory rates and leucocyte count (Teklu et al., 1983).

4. Side Effects

The effects of meptazinol on the respiratory and cardiovascular system in patients has already been discussed (see sections 1.3 and 1.4). Meptazinol therapy has generally resulted in an incidence of

Table VII. Side effects reported in 592 postoperative patients treated with meptazinol (after Robson, 1983) [data taken from submissions to the Committee on Safety of Medicines]

	No. patients reporting	Incidence (%)
Vomiting	55	9.3
Nausea	45	7.6
Sleepy/drowsy	33	5.6
Dizzy	22	3.7
Sweating	16	2.7
Euphoria	6	1.0
Restless/jumpy	3	0.5
Dry mouth	2	0.3
Retching	2	0.3
Headache	2	0.3
Hypoventilation	1	0.2
Faintness	1	0.2
Blurred vision	1	0.2
Heartburn	1	0.2
Dysphoria	1	0.2
Numb feeling in limbs	1	0.2
Cramp in legs	1	0.2
Felt heart stopping	1	0.2
Pain at injection site	1	0.2

side effects similar to the other analgesic in comparative studies, but a lower incidence than pentazocine or a combination of dextropropoxyphene and paracetamol. The only exception was in the study by Staquet (1978) who found that an intramuscular dose of meptazinol 100mg produced a higher incidence of side effects (75%) than pentazocine 60mg (44%) or meptazinol 75mg (24%).

A summary of all side effects reported in 592 patients treated with meptazinol for postoperative pain is shown in table VII. The incidence of central nervous system side effects excluding drowsiness is comparatively low: of 1225 patients who received parenteral meptazinol in various indications, 0.65% experienced euphoria, 0.2% restlessness, 0.2% hallucinations, 0.1% dysphoria and 0.1% amnesia [Robson, 1983]. In a long term (1- to 12-month) study of oral meptazinol in 144 patients with chronic pain, complaints were primarily concerned with the gastrointestinal tract: 6.9% of patients reported nausea, 1.4% vomiting, 2.1% dyspepsia, 2.1% indigestion, 0.7% abdominal pain, 0.7% constipation, and 0.7% diarrhoea. No major central nervous system effects were reported, although 2.75% of patients complained of feeling giddy/dizzy (Price and Latham, 1982a).

Jackson (1983) analysed the side effects in 3 obstetric clinical trials which involved 597 patients, 293 having received meptazinol and 304 pethidine. A similar spectrum of side effects was observed, except that the incidence of drowsiness was significantly less in the meptazinol group of patients. Obstetric use of meptazinol, as with pethidine, tended to produce a higher incidence of side effects, with 28% of patients in the meptazinol group and 35% in the pethidine group reporting a similar spectrum of adverse effects. Nicholas and Robson (1982), who conducted the largest double-blind comparison of meptazinol and pethidine in obstetrics, reported an incidence of maternal side effects shown in figure 5. Meptazinol 2 mg/kg intramuscularly did not adversely affect Apgar scores, duration of initial apnoea, time to sustained regular respiration and method of resuscitation in neonates whose mothers received the drug during labour (table VIII). Similarly, the number of neonates showing abnormalities in terms of behav-

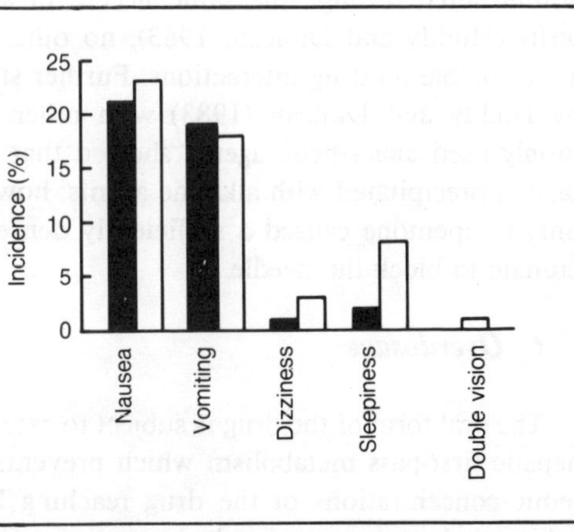

Fig. 5. Maternal side effects following parenteral administration of meptazinol (■) and pethidine (□) to 186 and 172 women in labour (after Robson, 1983).

Table VIII. Relationship of interval between meptazinol administration during labour, and delivery, with neonatal status. The results are expressed as percentage of neonates in each group (after Nicholas, 1983)

Status	Interval between injection and delivery (min)			
	≤ 35 (n = 76)	36-90 (n = 158)	91-180 (n = 300)	> 180 (n = 53)
With Apgar ≥ 8 at 1 min	76	84	82	79
at 5 min	100	98	99	100
With duration of initial apnoea < 1 min	84	99	93	92
Taking < 2 min to sustained regular respiration	84	99	95	96
Requiring only airway clearance and oxygen for resuscitation	88	96	92	91

ioural assessments (muscle tone, irritability/lethargy, feeding, jaundice and vomiting) within the first 24 hours of life were minimal (Nicholas, 1983).

5. *Drug Interactions*

Apart from preliminary *in vitro* evidence of meptazinol modifying the actions of neuromuscular blocking agents such as suxamethonium (succinylcholine) and tubocurarine (Strahan and Pleuvry, 1984), the *in vivo* potentiation of the antinociceptive response to meptazinol in mice by ibuprofen (Stephens, 1984), and a report of precipitation between meptazinol and thiopentone when administered through the same needle in a butterfly (Huddy and Duncan, 1983), no other data are available on drug interactions. Further studies by Huddy and Duncan (1983) with other commonly used anaesthetic agents showed that meptazinol precipitated with alkaline agents; however, only thiopentone caused a sufficiently dense precipitate to block the needle.

6. *Overdosage*

The oral form of the drug is subject to extensive hepatic first-pass metabolism which prevents systemic concentrations of the drug reaching levels achieved by parenteral administration. Consequently, overdoses are less likely than with the injections, but the recommended treatment includes gastric lavage, supportive therapy, and naloxone for respiratory depression if required. In the case of parenteral overdosage, normal resuscitative procedures should be used, and if necessary naloxone administered to reverse any respiratory depression.

7. *Dosage and Administration*

Meptazinol can be given orally, intravenously, or intramuscularly. Recommended oral doses for adults are 200mg 3- to 6-hourly as required for pain, with a usual dose of 200mg every 4 hours.

The dose by intramuscular injection should range between 75 and 100mg, and can be repeated every 2 to 4 hours as required. A slightly higher dose of 100 to 150mg is recommended in obstetric pain and should be calculated on a weight basis of approximately 2 mg/kg.

Intravenous doses of between 50 and 100mg should be given by slow intravenous injection which may be repeated 2- to 4-hourly as required. If vomiting occurs a suitable antiemetic is advised.

Meptazinol has not been evaluated for use in children and caution should be observed in treating patients with hepatic or renal insufficiency. Although clinical studies have indicated absence of clinically significant respiratory depression, caution is also indicated in patients with already severely compromised respiratory function. Safety for use in myocardial infarction has not been established. Administration of meptazinol to patients already receiving large doses of opioid drugs should be carefully undertaken until the response is established, since its antagonist activity could conceivably precipitate abstinence in this situation.

Use in pregnancy is limited to provision of analgesia during labour unless considered essential by the physician.

8. Place of Meptazinol in Therapy

Meptazinol appears to be an effective and potent analgesic when given by the oral, intravenous or intramuscular route. It possesses both opioid-like agonist and antagonist properties, and has been effectively used in moderate to severe postoperative and obstetric pain, as well as in pain of various other aetiologies.

In postoperative pain or pain from malignancies, meptazinol has in one study been judged significantly less effective than buprenorphine, and in an overall assessment less effective than morphine. Meptazinol and pethidine produced equal levels of analgesia, although sometimes a higher consumption of meptazinol was required to achieve this. Other studies found meptazinol as effective as pentazocine and papaveretum, but more effective than placebo, and in one study pentazocine.

Obstetric use of meptazinol has resulted in at least equal or more effective relief of pain during labour than pethidine. The condition of the majority of newborn babies following administration of meptazinol to the mother during labour was at least as good as, and in some cases better than, those whose mothers received pethidine.

Patients presenting to their general practitioner with acute or chronic pain, in many cases due to osteoarthritis or rheumatoid arthritis, have reported a greater degree of pain relief with meptazinol than with placebo, but judged pentazocine, paracetamol and a combination of dextropropoxyphene and paracetamol as giving similar amounts of relief. Data on its use preoperatively or in anaesthesia are too limited to comment on its potential in this area. Its duration of effect was shorter than that of morphine and buprenorphine but was similar to that of pentazocine, pethidine and a combination of hyoscine-N-butylbromide and dipyrone in patients with pain of various origins. In some patients its significantly shorter onset of action, however, could be considered an advantage over morphine and pentazocine.

A limited number of patients with chronic pain, treated for relatively long periods with meptazinol, did not show any signs of developing tolerance, a common drawback of the opioid analgesics. The abuse potential of meptazinol would appear to be very low compared with other opioid analgesics, but only much wider clinical experience will confirm this.

Respiratory depression and haemodynamic changes have not proven to be a problem with meptazinol therapy, being seen only in a small number of patients who have received the drug preoperatively or during anaesthesia. Side effects have been limited to those associated with the gastrointestinal system together with some drowsiness and dizziness, although generally the incidence of central nervous system adverse effects was relatively low.

In conclusion, meptazinol would seem to offer a safe, yet effective, alternative to some of the opioid analgesics in the treatment of pain states with a number of different aetiologies.

References

Bill, D.J.; Hartley, J.E.; Stephens, R.J. and Thompson, A.M.: The antinociceptive activity of meptazinol depends on both opiate and cholinergic mechanisms. British Journal of Pharmacology 79: 191-199 (1983).

Broadley, J.; Wilson, T. and Robson, F.: The use of meptazinol as premedication for surgical patients. Journal of International Medical Research 10: 225-228 (1982).

Brunck, S.F. and Delle, M.S.: Morphine metabolism in man. Clinical Pharmacology and Therapeutics 16: 51-57 (1974).

Budd, K.; Brown, P.M. and Robson, P.J.: The treatment of chronic pain by the use of meptazinol administered into the epidural space. Postgraduate Medical Journal 59: 68-71 (1983).

Caldwell, J.; Wakile, L.A.; Notarianni, L.J.; Smith, R.L.; Correy, G.J. et al.: Maternal and neonatal disposition of pethidine in childbirth – a study using quantitative gas chromatography-mass spectrometry. Life Sciences 22: 589-596 (1978).

Camu, F. and Rucquoi, M.: Cardiac and circulatory effects of high-dose meptazinol in anaesthetized patients. Postgraduate Medical Journal 59 (Suppl. 1): 60-63 (1983).

Caruso, F.S.; Pircio, A.W.; Maddisso, H.; Smyth, R.D. and Potcher, I.J.: Butorphanol. Pharmacol. Biochem. Prop. Drug Subst. 2: 19-57 (1979).

Church, J.J.: Continuous infusion of meptazinol and pethidine in the relief of post-operative pain. Postgraduate Medical Journal 59: 41-46 (1983).
Cohen, D.G.; Major, E.; Jothilingham, S.; Clark, G. and Coutinho, P.: Meptazinol in the treatment of severe post-operative pain. A comparison with morphine. Postgraduate Medical Journal 59: 35-40 (1983).
Collier, H.O.J.; Dinneen, L.C.; Johnson, C.A. and Schneider, C.: The abdominal constriction response and its suppression by analgesic drugs in the mouse. British Journal of Pharmacology 32: 295-310 (1968).
Collier, H.O.; Hammond, A.R.; Horwood-Barrett, S. and Schneider, C.: Rapid induction by acetylcholine, bradykinin and potassium of a nociceptive response in mice and its selective antagonism by aspirin. Nature 204: 1316-1318 (1964).
Cooper, S.A.: Double-blind comparison of zomepirac sodium, propoxyphene/acetaminophen and placebo in the treatment of oral surgical pain. Current Therapeutic Research 28: 630-638 (1980).
Copeland, S.A.: Preliminary evaluation of the use of meptazinol in trauma. Postgraduate Medical Journal 59: 64-66 (1983).
Coutinho, A.: Clinical evaluation of a new opium-antagonist analgesic – meptazinol. Journal of British Urology 6: 156-162 (1980).
Cowlrick, I.S. and Shepperson, N.B.: The effects of a new opioid analgesic, meptazinol, on the respiration of the conscious rat. British Journal of Pharmacology 85: 206 (1985).
Davies, G.; Sinclair, A.J.; Warrington, S.J.; Franklin, R.; Frost, T. et al.: Pharmacokinetics of meptazinol in man following repeated intramuscular administration. European Journal of Clinical Pharmacology 23: 535-538 (1982).
de Rosayro, M.; Healy, T.E.J. and Morris, G.K.: Meptazinol and morphine compared: A study using systolic time intervals. Pharmatherapeutica 2: 523-527 (1981).
Dowell, P.S.; Pierce, D.M.; Franklin, R.A.; Robson, P.J. and Jackson, M.B.A.: Routes of meptazinol conjugation in the neonate. British Journal of Clinical Pharmacology 14: 748-750 (1982).
Ehrnebo, M.; Boréus, L.O. and Lönroth, U.: Bioavailability and first pass metabolism of oral pentazocine in man. Clinical Pharmacology and Therapeutics 22: 883-892 (1978).
Errick, J.K. and Heel, R.C.: Nalbuphine: A preliminary review of its pharmacological properties and therapeutic efficacy. Drugs 26: 191-211 (1983).
Evans, M.; Robson, P.J.; Chadd, M.A.; Evans, C.M. and Fry, D.M.: Administration of meptazinol to opiate-dependent patients. Postgraduate Medical Journal 59: 78-84 (1983).
Fagbemi, O.; Kane, K.A.; Lepran, I.; Parratt, J.R. and Szekerès, L.: Antiarrhythmic actions of meptazinol, a partial agonist at opiate receptors, in acute myocardial ischaemia. British Journal of Pharmacology 78: 455-460 (1983).
Flavell-Matts, S.G. and Ward, P.J.: A double blind comparison of meptazinol versus pentazocine in chronic rheumatoid and osteoarthritis. British Journal of Clinical Practice 34: 286-289 (1980).
Franklin, R.A.: The influence of gastric emptying on plasma concentrations of the analgesic meptazinol. British Journal of Pharmacology 59: 565-569 (1977).
Franklin, R.A. and Aldridge, A.: Pharmacokinetics and metabolism of the new analgesic meptazinol in rats and patas monkeys. Xenobiotica 6: 499-508 (1976).
Franklin, R.A.; Aldridge, A. and de B. White, C.: Preliminary metabolic studies on the new analgesic meptazinol. British Journal of Clinical Pharmacology 2: 472-473 (1975).
Franklin, R.A.; Aldridge, A. and de B. White, C.: Studies on the metabolism of meptazinol, a new analgesic drug. British Journal of Clinical Pharmacology 3: 497-502 (1976).
Franklin, R.A.; Frost, T.; Robson, P.J. and Jackson, M.B.A.: Preliminary studies on the disposition of meptazinol in the neonate. British Journal of Clinical Pharmacology 12: 88-90 (1981).
Franklin, R.A.; Southgate, P.J. and Coleman, A.J.: Studies on the absorption and disposition of meptazinol following rectal administration. British Journal of Clinical Pharmacology 4: 163-167 (1977).
Gabka, J. and Price, R.K.J.: Tooth pulp stimulation: A method of determining the analgesic efficacy of meptazinol in man. British Journal of Clinical Pharmacology 14: 104-106 (1982).
Gepts, E.; Sonck, W.; Rucquoi, M.; Vercruysse, A. and Camu, F.: Disposition of meptazinol (mep), an agonist antagonist analgesic, in man. IUPHAR 9th International Congress of Pharmacology, Abstract No. 1766P, London (1984).
Gibbs, J.M. and Johnson, H.D.: A trial of meptazinol for the relief of pain after abdominal surgery. Anaesthesia and Intensive Care 8: 441-444 (1980).
Goldstuck, N.D. and Ward, P.J.: Treatment of pain following IUD insertion with meptazinol – a new centrally acting analgesic. Contraceptive Delivery Systems 4: 33-37 (1983).
Goode, P.G.: An implanted reservoir of morphine solution for rapid induction of physical dependence in rats. British Journal of Pharmacology 41: 558-566 (1971).
Goode, P.G.; Rhodes, K.F. and Waterfall, J.F.: The analgesic and respiratory effects of meptazinol, morphine, and pentazocine in the rat. Journal of Pharmacy and Pharmacology 31: 793-795 (1979).
Goode, P.G. and White, A.C.: Some properties of Wy 22811, a new analgesic compound. British Journal of Pharmacology 43: 462-463P (1971).
Green, D.: Current concepts concerning the mode of action of meptazinol as an analgesic. Postgraduate Medical Journal 59 (Suppl. 1): 9-12 (1983).
Griffiths, M.J. and Thomas, T.A.: A comparison of the analgesic effects of meptazinol and pentazocine following removal of impacted third molars. British Dental Journal 158: 19-21 (1985).
Hardy, P.A.J.: Meptazinol and respiratory depression. Lancet 2: 576 (1983).
Harmer, M.; Slatterly, P.J.; Rosen, M. and Vickers, M.D.: Intramuscular on demand analgesia: Double blind controlled trial of pethidine, buprenorphine, morphine and meptazinol. British Medical Journal 286: 680-682 (1983).
Hardy, P.A.J.: Meptazinol and Respiratory Depression. Lancet 2: 576 (1983).
Hedges, A.; Turner, P. and Wadsworth, J.: A double-blind comparison of meptazinol with pethidine in post-operative pain. British Journal of Anaesthesia 52: 295-298 (1980).
Hedges, A.; Rose, J.; Leighton, M. and Turner, P.: A double-blind comparison of meptazinol with placebo in post-operative pain. Journal of Clinical Pharmacology 17: 125-127 (1977).
Heel, R.C.; Brogden, R.N.; Speight, T.M. and Avery, G.S.: Buprenorphine: A review of its pharmacological properties and therapeutic efficacy. Drugs 17: 81-110 (1979).
Huddy, N.C. and Duncan, J.J.: Precipitation between meptazinol and thiopentone. Anaesthesia 38: 601-602 (1983).
Jackson, M.B.A.: Obstetric Analgesia. Proceedings of a Symposium on Current Advances on the Control of Acute and Chronic Pain. John Radcliffe Hospital, Oxford (1983).
Jackson, M.B.A. and Robson, P.J.: Preliminary experience of the use of meptazinol as an obstetric analgesic. British Journal of Obstetrics and Gynaecology 87: 296-301 (1980).
Jackson, M.B.A. and Robson, P.J.: Preliminary clinical and pharmacokinetic experiences in the newborn when meptazinol is compared with pethidine as an obstetric analgesic. Postgraduate Medical Journal 59 (Suppl. 1): 47-51 (1983).
Jordan, C.; Lehare, J.R.; Robson, P.J. and Jones, J.G.: A comparison of the respiratory effects of meptazinol pentazocine and morphine. British Journal of Anaesthesia 51: 497-502 (1979).
Kingston, H.G.G.: Meptazinol used after open heart surgery. Postgraduate Medical Journal 59: 54-56 (1983).
Keen, M.R. and Owen, A.: Comparison of the effects of single

i.m. dose of meptazinol (100mg), methadone (20 and 40mg) and placebo in opiate addicts. Postgraduate Medical Journal 61 (Suppl. 2): 27-28 (1985).
Malis, J. and Gluckman, M.: in Braude et al. (Eds) Narcotic Antagonists (Raven Press, New York 1974).
Mather, L.E.; Tucker, G.T.; Pflug, A.E.; Lindop, M.J. and Wilkerson, C.: Meperidine kinetics in man. Clinical Pharmacology and Therapeutics 17: 21-30 (1974).
Moyes, D.G.; Miller, M.T. and Aldridge, N.J.: A comparison between meptazinol and omnopon in the relief of post-operative pain. South African Medical Journal 55: 865-866 (1979).
Murray, W.J.: Evaluation of aspirin in treatment of headache. Clinical Pharmacology and Therapeutics 5: 21-25 (1964).
Nel, C.P.; Bloch, B. and Rush, J.M.: A comparison of meptazinol and pethidine for pain relief during the first stage of labour. South African Medical Journal 59: 908-910 (1981).
Nicholas, A.D.G.: Routine use of meptazinol in labour. Postgraduate Medical Journal 59: 52 (1983).
Nicholas, A.D.G. and Robson, P.J.: Double-blind comparison of meptazinol and pethidine in labour. British Journal of Obstetrics and Gynaecology 89: 318-322 (1982).
Norbury, H.M.; Franklin, R.A. and Graham, D.F.: Pharmacokinetics of the new analgesic, meptazinol, after oral and intravenous administration to volunteers. European Journal of Clinical Pharmacology 25: 77-80 (1983).
Norbury, H.M.; Franklin, R.A.; Graham, D.F. and Sinha, B.: Pharmacokinetics of meptazinol after single and multiple oral administration to elderly patients. European Journal of Clinical Pharmacology 27: 223-226 (1984).
O'Callaghan, J.P. and Holtzmann, S.G.; Quantification of the analgesic activity of narcotic antagonists by a modified hot plate procedure. Journal of Pharmacology and Experimental Therapeutics 192: 497-505 (1975).
Oosterlinck, W. and DeSy, W.: Preliminary clinical experience with meptazinol, a new analgesic. Current Medical Research and Opinion 3: 187-191 (1975).
Oosterlinck, W. and DeSy, W.: A double-blind comparison between meptazinol (Wy 22811) and 'Buscopan' Compositum in renal colic. Current Medical Research and Opinion 3: 716-718 (1976).
Parker, C.E. and Langrick, A.F.: A double-blind comparison of meptazinol and placebo in patients with acute and chronic pain presenting to the general practitioner. Journal of International Medical Research 10: 408-413 (1982).
Paymaster, N.J.: Clinical evaluation of meptazinol a new analgesic in post-operative pain. British Journal of Anaesthesia 48: 599-605 (1976a).
Paymaster, N.J.: Clinical assessment of oral meptazinol in post-operative pain. Acta Anaesthesiologica Belgica 27: 159-170 (1976b).
Paymaster, N.J.: Analgesia after an operation: A controlled comparison of meptazinol, pentazocine and pethidine. British Journal of Anaesthesia 49: 1139-1146 (1977).
Paymaster, N.J.: Intramuscular meptazinol analgesia after surgery: A study of the dose-response effect and a controlled comparison with pentazocine and pethidine. Postgraduate Medical Journal 59 (Suppl. I): 25-31 (1983).
Pearce, V. and Robson, P.J.: Double-blind crossover trial of oral meptazinol, pentazocine and placebo in the treatment of pain in the elderly. Postgraduate Medical Journal 56: 474-477 (1980).
Pereira, E.S.: Clinical assessment of intramuscular meptazinol in post-operative pain. Revista Brasileira de Clinica e Terapêutica 9: 408-413 (1980).
Pert, C.B. and Snyder, S.H.: Opiate receptor binding of agonists and antagonists affected differentially by sodium. Molecular Pharmacology 10: 868-879 (1974).
Price, R.K.J. and Latham, A.N.: Long-term assessment of the efficacy and safety of oral meptazinol (200mg) in general practice. Current Therapeutic Research 31: 807-812 (1982a).
Price, R.K.J. and Latham, A.N.: Double-blind comparison of meptazinol (200mg) and dextropropoxyphene/paracetamol in a multicentre, general practice setting. Current Medical Research and Opinion 8: 54-60 (1982b).
Price, R.K.J. and Latham, A.N.: Pain type and sex dependent responses to a placebo controlled multicentre analgesic trial. Clinical Trials Journal 19: 107-115 (1982c).
Rashid, S. and Waterfall, J.F.: Cardiovascular actions of meptazinol in comparison with pentazocine and morphine. General Pharmacology 10: 459-464 (1979).
Rashid, S.: Effect of antidysrhythmic and analgesic drugs on haemodynamics and fibrillatory threshold. Journal of the Pakistan Medical Association 31: 141-145 (1981).
Robson, P.J.: Clinical review of parenteral meptazinol. Postgraduate Medical Journal 59 (Suppl. I): 85-92 (1983).
Rosseel, M.T.; Bogaert, M.G.; Verschraegen, R. and Staquet, M.: Plasma concentrations of meptazinol (Wy 22811) after different routes of administration in man. Pharmatherapeutica 1: 270-276 (1976).
Rosseel, M.T.; Bogaert, M.G.; Belpaire, F.M. and Oosterlinck, W.: Meptazinol (Wy 22811), a new analgesic: Preliminary pharmacokinetic data. Current Medical Research and Opinion 3: 181-186 (1975).
Schindel, L.: The placebo dilemma. European Journal of Clinical Pharmacology 13: 231-235 (1978).
Slatterly, P.J.; Harmer, M.; Rosen, M. and Vickers, M.: Comparison of the respiratory depressant effects of IV meptazinol and pethidine. British Journal of Anaesthesia 55: 245P (1983).
Slatterly, P.J.; Harmer, M.; Rosen, M. and Vickers, M.D.: Naloxone reversal of meptazinol induced respiratory depression. Anaesthesia 37: 1163-1166 (1982).
Slatterly, P.J.; Harmer, M.; Rosen, M. and Vickers, M.D.: Comparison of meptazinol and pethidine given IV on demand in the management of post operative pain. British Journal of Anaesthesia 53: 927-931 (1981).
Snyder, S.H.: The brain's own opiates. Chemical and Engineering News (Nov 28): 26-36 (1977).
Sonecha, T.; Abdel-Hadi, O.; Basterman, E.M.M. and Kidner, P.H.: Initial assessment of meptazinol in the treatment of pain in myocardial infarction/unstable angina. Postgraduate Medical Journal 59: 57-59 (1983).
Speigel, K. and Pasternak, G.W.: Meptazinol: A novel Mu-1 selective opioid analgesic. Journal of Pharmacology and Experimental Therapeutics 288: 414-419 (1984).
Stacher, G.; Steinringer, H.: Winklehner, S.; Mittelbach, G. and Schneider, C.: Effects of graded oral doses of meptazinol and pentazocine in comparison with placebo on experimentally induced pain in healthy humans. British Journal of Clinical Pharmacology 16: 149-156 (1983).
Staquet, M.: A double-blind comparison of meptazinol with pentazocine and placebo in cancer pain. Journal of Clinical Pharmacology 18: 76-79 (1978).
Strahan, K. and Pleuvry, B.J.: Interactions between meptazinol and neuromuscular blocking agents. British Journal of Anaesthesia 56: 1290P (1984).
Stephens, R.J.: Evidence for a pharmacokinetic interaction between ibuprofen and meptazinol in the mouse. Journal of Pharmacy and Pharmacology 36: 779-781 (1984).
Stephens, R.J.; Waterfall, J.F. and Franklin, R.A.: A review of the biological properties and metabolic disposition of the new analgesic agent, meptazinol. General Pharmacology 9: 73-78 (1978).
Teklu, B.; Habte-Michael, A.; Warrell, D.A.; White, N.J. and Wright, D.J.M.: Meptazinol diminishes the Jarisch-Herxheimer reaction of relapsing fever. Lancet 1: 835-839 (1983).
Tyers, M.B.: A classification of opiate receptors that mediate antinociception in animals. British Journal of Pharmacology 69: 503-512 (1980).
Verschraegen, R. and Rolly, G.: Double blind study of mepta-

zinol *versus* pentazocine and placebo in post operative pain treatment. Acta Anaesthesiologica Belgica 30: 255-264 (1979).
Verschraegen, R.; Rosseel, M.T.; Bogaert, M. and Rolly, G.: Meptazinol: IM use in post operative pain. Acta Anaesthesiologica Belgica 27 (Suppl.): 123-132 (1976).
Videman, T.; Heikkilä, J. and Partanen, T.: Double-blind parallel study of meptazinol versus diflunisal in the treatment of lumbago. Current Medical Research and Opinion 9: 246-252 (1984).
Wade, A.G. and Ward, P.J.: First impressions of the use of meptazinol in general practice. Journal of International Medical Research 9: 74-78 (1981).
Wade, A.G. and Ward, P.J.: A double-blind comparison of meptazinol *versus* distalgesic in acute or chronic pain presenting to the general practitioner. Journal of International Medical Research 10: 104-108 (1982b).
Wade, A.G. and Ward, P.J.: A double-blind comparison of meptazinol *versus* paracetamol and placebo in acute and chronic painful conditions presenting to the general practitioner. Current Medical Research and Opinion 8: 191-196 (1982a).
Ward, P.J.: Double-blind comparison of meptazinol *versus* pentazocine in patients with chronic backache. Current Therapeutic Research 30: 507-514 (1981).
Warrington, S.J.; Barclay, S.P.; Brown, Z. and Robson, P.J.: Reversibility of the analgesic effect of meptazinol in volunteers. Postgraduate Medical Journal 59 (Suppl. I) 13-18 (1983).
Westcombe, R.E. and Price, R.K.J.: Meptazinol in the casualty department: A comparison against morphine. Current Therapeutic Research 37: 969-979 (1985).

Authors' address: *Barbara Holmes,* ADIS Drug Information Services, Private Bag, Mairangi Bay, Auckland 10 (New Zealand).

Drugs 30: 313-332 (1985)
0012-6667/85/0010-0313/$10.00/0

Xipamide
A Review of its Pharmacodynamic and Pharmacokinetic Properties and Therapeutic Efficacy

B.N.C. Prichard and *R.N. Brogden*

ADIS Drug Information Services, Auckland

Various sections of the manuscript reviewed by: ***D.C. Brater,*** Health Science Center at Dallas, Dallas, Texas, USA; ***W. Flamenbaum,*** Division of Nephrology and Hypertension, Beth Israel Medical Center, New York, USA; ***R. Greger,*** Max Planck Institut für Biophysik, Frankfurt, West Germany; ***D. Hutcheon,*** University of Medicine and Dentistry, Newark, New Jersey, USA; ***M.J. Kendall,*** Department of Therapeutics and Clinical Pharmacology, Queen Elizabeth Hospital, Birmingham, England; ***W.P. Leary,*** University of Natal Medical School, Durban, South Africa; ***T. Morgan,*** Department of Physiology, University of Melbourne, Melbourne, Australia; ***E.B. Raftery,*** Northwick Park Hospital, Harrow, Middlesex, England; ***F.O. Simpson,*** Department of Medicine, Otago University, Dunedin, New Zealand.

Contents

Summary 314
1. Pharmacodynamic Studies 316
   1.1 Diuretic Effects 316
   1.2 Effects on Urine Characteristics and Electrolyte Excretion 317
      1.2.1 Effects on Urinary Sodium Excretion 317
      1.2.2 Effects on Urinary Potassium Excretion 318
      1.2.3 Excretion of Other Electrolytes 319
   1.3 Site of Action of Xipamide 319
2. Pharmacokinetic Studies 320
   2.1 Absorption and Distribution 320
   2.2 Metabolism and Elimination 320
      2.2.1 Half-Life 320
   2.3 Effect of Renal Insufficiency on Pharmacokinetics 321
3. Therapeutic Use 321
   3.1 Use in Hypertension 321
      3.1.1 Open Studies 321
      3.1.2 Controlled Trials 322
   3.2 Xipamide in the Treatment of Oedema 324
      3.2.1 Heart Failure 324
      3.2.2 Renal Disease 325
      3.2.3 Oedema Associated with Rheumatoid Arthritis 326
      3.2.4 Miscellaneous Oedematous Conditions 326
4. Side Effects 326
   4.1 Subjective Complaints 326
   4.2 Effect on Bodyweight 327

4.3 Effects on Serum Electrolyte, Blood Urea and Urate Levels 327
4.3.1 Potassium 327
4.3.2 Sodium and Chloride 328
4.3.3 Magnesium and Calcium 329
4.3.4 Blood Urea and Serum Urate 329
4.3.5 Other Metabolic and Hormonal Effects 329
5. Dosage and Administration 330
6. The Place of Xipamide in Therapy 330

Summary

Synopsis: *Xipamide*[1] *is a diuretic derived from salicylic acid and has a structural resemblance to chlorthalidone. Its pharmacodynamic profile shows a diuretic efficacy is similar to that of frusemide (furosemide) at doses up to 40mg, but the onset and duration of action are comparable to those of hydrochlorothiazide. Xipamide has been studied mostly in the treatment of mild to moderate essential hypertension, with few controlled studies of its use in oedematous states. The efficacy of xipamide 20 to 40mg once daily in patients with mild to moderate hypertension is comparable to that of bendrofluazide 5mg, bumetanide 1mg or hydrochlorothiazide 50mg when used alone in newly treated or previously treated patients. The addition of xipamide 20 to 40mg daily to regimens containing β-blockers, adrenergic neuron-blocking drugs and/or methyldopa has resulted in a further reduction in blood pressure. A few studies in oedematous states suggest that xipamide 40 to 80mg is comparable in efficacy to equal doses of frusemide, and that the side effects of hypokalaemia, hyperuricaemia and increased blood glucose in diabetics or latent diabetics are similar to those of other diuretics. Thus, xipamide is a suitable alternative to other diuretics in the treatment of mild to moderate hypertension and combines the efficacy of frusemide with a less abrupt action in the treatment of oedema.*

Pharmacodynamic Studies: Although structurally related to chlorthalidone, xipamide is not a thiazide. Diuresis produced by xipamide over a 24-hour period is equivalent to that of an equal dose of frusemide, but the onset and duration of action of xipamide resembles that of hydrochlorothiazide. The natriuretic effect of xipamide is dose related, with a progressive increase in 24-hour sodium excretion up to a dose of 40mg daily, although in one single-dose study in volunteers sodium excretion with xipamide 40mg daily was only marginally greater than that with 20mg daily. Unlike frusemide, xipamide does not result in a 'rebound' effect after initial natriuresis, but like frusemide it does produce diuresis in patients with marked renal insufficiency.

Urinary sodium/potassium ratios after oral xipamide 20 to 60mg were not significantly different from those after hydrochlorothiazide 50 and 100mg or frusemide 40mg. However, there is some evidence that the sodium/potassium ratio is more favourable with xipamide than with chlorthalidone. Xipamide 40mg, given as a single dose, did not exhibit a kaliuretic effect when creatinine clearance was below about 25 ml/min. Xipamide-induced potassium loss can be prevented by concomitant administration of the potassium-sparing diuretic triamterene, and a combination tablet containing xipamide and triamterene in a ratio of 1 : 3 has been developed for clinical use.

Studies in healthy subjects demonstrated that xipamide, like hydrochlorothiazide, decreases free water clearance and increases osmolar clearance during maximal water diuresis. Xipamide also behaved similarly to hydrochlorothiazide during maximal hydropenia, thus suggesting that its site of action is on the distal convoluted tubules. However, xipamide resembles frusemide in producing diuresis in renal failure and had an effect additive to that of hydrochlorothiazide in animals – suggesting a mechanism of action somewhat different to that of the thiazides.

1 'Diurexan' (E. Merk Ltd).

Pharmacokinetic Studies: Following oral administration of xipamide 20mg, maximum plasma concentrations of around 3 mg/L occur within 1 hour. As calculated by the area under the plasma concentration-time curve (AUC) after intravenous and oral administration, absolute bioavailability is 73%. Xipamide is conjugated with glucuronide and during the first 24 hours after administration 26% of a dose was excreted in the conjugated form and 40 to 55% unchanged. Urinary excretion of radioactivity was 88%, 96 hours after a single dose of ^{35}S-xipamide given orally or intravenously. Elimination half-life in healthy subjects has been reported to be between 5.8 and 8.2 hours after oral administration. In patients with renal impairment, half-life is prolonged. However, since extrarenal clearance remains constant with increasing renal failure and therefore becomes proportionally more important, it is unlikely that xipamide will accumulate to any marked degree in renal failure.

Therapeutic Use: Xipamide has most often been studied as an antihypertensive drug in patients with mild to moderate hypertension. Open studies, in which xipamide 10 to 20mg daily was generally administered alone, have suggested that it is an effective antihypertensive drug. At a daily dose of 40mg, or when given at individually titrated optimum dosage, xipamide was superior to placebo. In double-blind crossover trials the efficacy of xipamide 40mg daily was not significantly different from that of bendrofluazide 5mg, bumetanide 1mg or hydrochlorothiazide 50mg daily. In one study, xipamide 20mg was more effective than cyclopenthiazide 0.5mg daily after 6 weeks of treatment. Most of these studies, however, involved only small numbers of patients and were of short duration, thus requiring confirmation in larger and more prolonged comparative studies. Dose-determining studies found no significant difference in antihypertensive efficacy between xipamide 20 and 40mg, although response to the higher dose was more consistent. Similarly no difference between xipamide 10 and 20mg daily was found in a small study, although patient numbers may have been too small to detect any small differences in efficacy that may have existed between the dosages.

In patients with mild to moderate hypertension xipamide has been compared with placebo, indapamide and bendrofluazide when added to an existing regimen that did not control blood pressure adequately. The addition of either xipamide 20mg or indapamide 2.5mg daily to nadolol 160mg daily resulted in a significant decrease in blood pressure, although potassium loss was greater with xipamide than with indapamide. Similarly, the addition of xipamide 20 to 40mg to β-blockers, adrenergic neuron-blocking drugs and/or methyldopa produced a significant fall in blood pressure, although xipamide 20mg was no more effective than a further dose of bendrofluazide 5mg in patients already receiving a β-blocker with or without bendrofluazide 5mg daily.

Several studies in small numbers of patients have suggested that xipamide is effective in the treatment of congestive heart failure. In a double-blind study, xipamide 40mg was similar in efficacy to frusemide 25mg in patients receiving digoxin and a controlled sodium intake.

Preliminary studies suggest that xipamide is useful in alleviating oedema associated with renal failure and nephrotic syndrome, and appears to be of comparable efficacy to an equal dose of frusemide. Symptomatic improvement of premenstrual syndrome was comparable with xipamide 20mg and frusemide 40mg.

Side Effects: Xipamide has generally been well tolerated at dosages used to treat mild to moderate hypertension. The most frequently reported side effects include mild upper gastrointestinal symptoms, anorexia or nausea (incidence 2 to 4%), and tiredness and fatigue (3 to 8%). Dizziness (often postural) and vertigo have also occurred infrequently and were probably related to the extent of reduction in blood pressure. Xipamide, like the thiazide and 'loop' diuretics, causes net potassium loss, but this has varied according to the country of investigation. There have been occasional reports of considerable decreases in serum potassium to concentrations as low as 2.2 mmol/L and of symptomatic hypokalaemia. As might be expected, xipamide has caused small increases in average blood urea and serum urate concentrations in some studies, and occasional increases in blood glucose and of plasma lipids in diabetic patients.

Dosage and Administration: The usual dose of xipamide in the treatment of mild to moderate hypertension is 20mg daily given as a single dose in the morning. A dose of 40mg may be needed in more severe grades of hypertension. In combination with other antihypertensive drugs the initial dose of xipamide should not exceed 20mg daily. In the treatment of oedema the usual initial dose is 40mg daily which should subsequently be adjusted according to response. Supplementary potassium may be needed to avoid hypokalaemia during long term treatment of cardiac, hepatic or renal oedema.

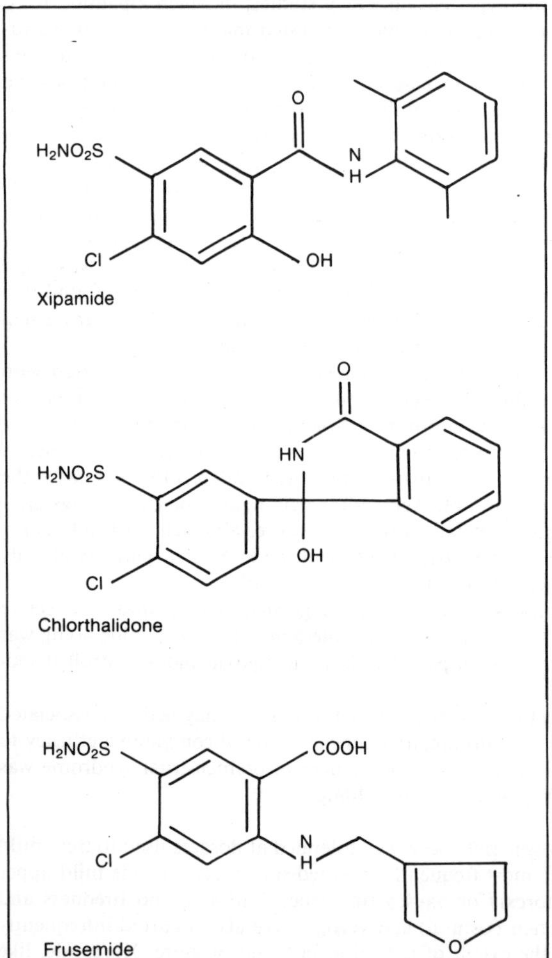

Fig. 1. Structural formulae of xipamide, chlorthalidone and frusemide (furosemide).

1. Pharmacodynamic Studies

Xipamide is a salicylic acid derivative with a structural resemblance to chlorthalidone (fig. 1) although xipamide is neither a thiazide nor a specific loop diuretic in its mechanism of action. Diuresis produced by xipamide over a 24-hour period is equivalent to that of frusemide (furosemide), but the time-course of the diuretic, natriuretic and kaliuretic effects of xipamide differs from that of frusemide, being similar to that of hydrochlorothiazide.

1.1 Diuretic Effects

In healthy patients xipamide produces a dose-related diuresis when administered orally at dosages of 5 to about 40mg (Hempelmann et al., 1975; Leary and Asmal, 1978a,b; Reyes and Leary, 1981a) [table I]. Peak diuretic activity of xipamide is similar to that of frusemide at doses up to 40mg, but doses higher than 40mg were not tested. Peak diuresis occurs about 3 to 4.5 hours after a single oral dose compared with 1.5 hours for frusemide and 1 hour for piretanide (Reyes and Leary, 1981b). Urine volume increases for at least 8 hours after a single dose but urinary excretion of sodium and chloride remain above baseline values for 12 to 24 hours. This is in contrast to findings with frusemide where the diuretic effect after oral administration is complete after 4 hours (Henness and Weng, 1979; Knauf and Mutschler, 1984; Reyes et al., 1980). The onset and duration of action of xipamide resemble those of hydrochlorothiazide

Table I. Increase in urinary volume and in urinary excretion of sodium and potassium over 24 hours relative to baseline in healthy subjects given single oral doses of xipamide (Xip), hydrochlorothiazide (H) or frusemide (F)

Reference	No. of subjects	Drug	Dose (mg)	Urine volume (ml)	Urinary sodium (mmol)	Urinary potassium (mmol)
Henness and Weng (1979)	10	Xip	10	982	148	15
		Xip	20	1520	306	12
		Xip	40	1509	320	14.5
		H	50	1045	222	6
		F	40	703	146	12
Leary and Asmal (1978a)	26	Xip	20	1039	209	17
		Xip	40	1430	264	32
		Xip	60	1276	233	37
		H	50	934	146	11
		H	100	1069	204	41
		F	40	1429	127	−7
Leary and Asmal (1978b)	12	Xip	5	632	94	15
		Xip	10	897	122	21
		H	50	787	113	13
Reyes and Leary (1981a)	26	Xip	5	635	67	7
		Xip	10	900	94	12
		Xip	20	1040	223	20
		Xip	40	1430	277	20
		Xip	60	1275	247	40

(Henness and Weng, 1979). The diuretic, natriuretic and chloruretic effects of xipamide 10mg are similar to those of hydrochlorothiazide 50mg (Henness and Weng, 1979; Leary and Asmal, 1978b). In healthy subjects, 84% of the 24-hour urine volume is excreted within 14 hours of frusemide 40mg, 74% after xipamide 40mg and 76% after hydrochlorothiazide 100mg (Leary and Asmal, 1978a; Leary et al., 1980). Intravenously administered xipamide causes a marked diuresis within minutes, with 80% more water excretion than control values during the first 15 minutes after xipamide 80mg (Schuetterle et al., 1969).

A study in patients with cardiac, renal or hepatic oedema indicated that xipamide 40mg daily and frusemide 40mg daily increased the mean urine output by 70 and 65%, respectively (Fischer and Lenhartz, 1970), although in another study in oedematous patients, equal doses of xipamide and frusemide increased urine volume by only 10 and 13%, respectively (Piyasena et al., 1975). In patients with congestive heart failure, xipamide 40mg daily produced diuresis similar to that with frusemide 25mg, both drugs producing their maximum effect after 3 days (Bonaduce et al., 1982).

1.2 Effects on Urine Characteristics and Electrolyte Excretion

1.2.1 Effects on Urinary Sodium Excretion

Early studies in normal volunteers have demonstrated a natriuretic effect with xipamide (Schuetterle et al., 1969). These results were confirmed by Hempelmann et al. (1975) who performed a dose-response study using oral doses from 0.035 mg/kg to 0.75 mg/kg. The increase in excretion of sodium rose rapidly (until xipamide dosage reached 0.125 mg/kg) to an excess excretion of 2.96 mmol/kg/24 hours. However, a more gradual increase in sodium excretion occurred at dosages of 0.25 to 0.75 mg/kg, with 3.57 mmol/kg/24 hours excess sodium being excreted after a dose of 0.75

mg/kg. In a study employing doses from 5 to 40mg, Knauf et al. (1980) stated that maximum natriuretic effect was obtained by 5mg; however, the actual data were not given in this report, only diagrams and levels of significance. Reyes and Leary (1981a) assessed xipamide 5, 10, 20, 40 and 60mg (previously reported in part; Leary and Asmal, 1978a,b), and observed a progressive increase in 24-hour sodium excretion up to a dose of 40mg daily. Further single-dose studies in volunteers revealed only marginally greater sodium excretion with xipamide 40mg compared with 20mg daily (Henness and Weng, 1979) [table I].

Comparative studies indicate that the initial natriuretic effects to frusemide is much greater than that of xipamide, hydrochlorothiazide or amiloride. However, the 24-hour natriuretic effect of xipamide 40mg is significantly greater than that of frusemide 40mg, and hydrochlorothiazide 50mg. However, the natriuretic effect of hydrochlorothiazide 100mg was not significantly different from that of xipamide 40mg (fig. 2; Knauf and Mutschler, 1984). Henness and Weng (1979) found xipamide 10mg was similar in effect to hydrochlorothiazide 50mg. Unlike frusemide, xipamide does not cause a 'rebound' effect after initial natriuresis (Knauf and Mutschler, 1984).

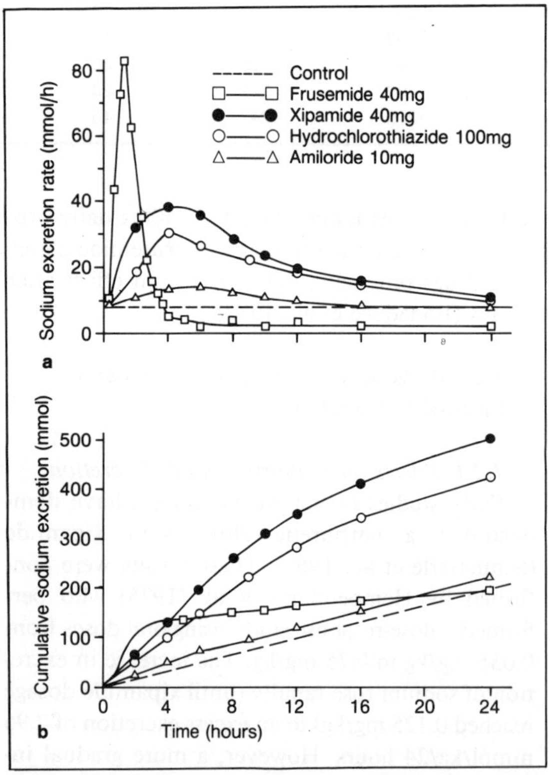

Fig. 2. Sodium excretion rate **(a)** and cumulative sodium excretion **(b)** following a single dose of different diuretics in comparison with the control period (after Knauf and Mutschler, 1984).

Single-dose studies in patients with renal insufficiency indicate that xipamide and frusemide may be of similar efficacy in such patients and that xipamide was effective even in patients with end-stage renal insufficiency (Knauf and Mutschler, 1984).

1.2.2 Effects on Urinary Potassium Excretion

Single doses of xipamide administered orally or intravenously have a lesser effect on potassium than on sodium excretion (table II). Up to a dosage of xipamide 40mg potassium excretion is about 1.5-fold greater than control values but this increases to 2-fold when the dosage is increased to 60mg (Reyes and Leary, 1981a).

In healthy volunteers the loss of potassium with xipamide for a given 24-hour excretion of sodium appears to be less than that with thiazides. Leary and Asmal (1978a) observed with xipamide 40mg a 3.1-fold increase in urinary sodium and a 1.7-fold increase in urinary potassium excretion per 24 hours. The corresponding figures for hydrochlorothiazide 100mg were 2.6- and 2.0-fold increases, respectively.

The effect of the dose of frusemide studied (40mg) was considerably less than xipamide in terms of sodium excretion (a 2.0-fold increase in 24 hours), with a 20% decrease in potassium excretion compared to control levels. However, urinary sodium/potassium ratios were not significantly different for xipamide 5mg or 10mg or hydrochlorothiazide 50mg (Leary and Asmal, 1978b), or for xipamide 20, 40 and 60mg, hydrochlorothiazide 50 and 100mg or frusemide 40mg (Lealy and Asmal, 1978a; Piyasena et al., 1975). Hempelmann et al. (1975) found xipamide 0.5 mg/kg produced greater 24-hour sodium excretion than chlorthali-

Table II. Urinary excretion of potassium and sodium following oral administration of xipamide, frusemide, hydrochlorothiazide or chlorthalidone to healthy subjects

Diuretic	Dose (mg)	Electrolyte excretion[a]		Plasma potassium change (mmol)	References[b]
		sodium	potassium		
Xipamide	10	1.8	1.2	−0.1	2
Xipamide	40	3.0-3.4	1.5-1.7	−0.26-0.32	1, 2, 3
Xipamide	60	3.2	2.0	−0.39	2
Frusemide	40	1.9	0.8	−0.26	1
Hydrochlorothiazide	50	2.1	1.2	−0.4	1
Hydrochlorothiazide	100	2.6	1.9	−0.48	1

a Change in electrolyte excretion relative to control values (1.0).
b *Reference key:* 1 Leary and Asmal (1978a); 2 Reyes and Leary (1981a); 3 Piyasena et al. (1975).

done, but the levels of potassium excretion were similar: 0.37 and 0.32 mmol/kg/24 hours, respectively. They also compared 0.5 mg/kg of xipamide and frusemide. The effect of xipamide on sodium excretion was greater than that of frusemide, as was the effect on urinary potassium excretion at 0.45 and 0.16 mmol/kg/24 hours, respectively.

Single-dose studies in patients with renal insufficiency indicated that xipamide 40mg did not exhibit a kaliuretic effect when the creatinine clearance was below about 25 ml/min (Knauf and Mutschler, 1984).

The undesirable electrolyte loss of the saliuretic loop and distal tubule diuretics can be largely counterbalanced by the administration of a potassium-sparing diuretic. Experiments in rats with the combination of xipamide and triamterene showed an additive effect on sodium excretion, whilst triamterene prevented the xipamide-induced potassium loss. The ratio of xipamide to triamterene dosage was between 1 : 1 and 1 : 1.5 (Armah et al., 1983; Hohenegger and Holzer, 1976). Triamterene has a similar half-life to xipamide in man, and the administration of the two drugs in combination did not alter the half-life of either drug (Diembeck et al., 1982). Subsequently, a combination tablet containing xipamide and triamterene in a ratio of 1 : 3 has been developed for clinical use.

1.2.3 Excretion of Other Electrolytes

Other than reports of the urinary excretion of sodium, chloride which parallels sodium, and potassium, there are few data on the effect of xipamide on other urinary electrolytes. Schuetterle et al. (1969) found that single doses of xipamide 80mg intravenously produced a 50% increase in calcium excretion ($p < 0.001$), with a non-significant 20% increase in urinary magnesium. Copper excretion also increased, but changes in zinc levels were not significant. Knauf and Mutschler (1984) also reported an increase in calcium and magnesium excretion after xipamide in normal volunteers and in patients with renal failure. Similar to their observations on potassium excretion, they also found a delayed loss of magnesium over the second and third day after xipamide. Indeed, Leary and Reyes (1984) reported significant loss of magnesium (25 to 45%), but which was not related to dose over a range of doses of 5 to 20mg of xipamide.

1.3 Site of Action of Xipamide

Xipamide produces a similar maximal diuresis to frusemide in animals (Leuschner, 1969) and also resembles frusemide in producing a diuretic effect in renal failure in man (Knauf and Mutschler, 1984). Also in common with the loop diuretics, xipamide apparently causes urinary loss of calcium (Knauf and Mutschler, 1984). However, the long term slight, but statistically significant, increase in serum calcium in hypertensive patients reported by Castro (1980) casts some doubt on the importance of these observations. As discussed by Knauf and Mutschler (1984), calcium reabsorption parallels sodium in the proximal nephron under various experimental conditions, the reabsorption of calcium due to thiazide diuretics occurring at the distal convoluted tubule. These investigators concluded that because of the effect of xipamide on calcium excretion, the effect of xipamide in renal failure, and structural similarities to frusemide (fig. 1), xipamide acts as a loop diuretic.

However, in accord with micropuncture studies in animals, the studies in man of Gold and Viljoen (1979), and the observations of Hempelmann (1975b) that xipamide and hydrochlorothiazide in rats have an additive effect, xipamide may act at the distal tubule but by a different mechanism to that which occurs with thiazides.

Xipamide, like hydrochlorothiazide, decreases free water clearance and increases osmolar clearance during maximal water diuresis in healthy subjects. Frusemide, however, surprisingly did not influence osmolar clearance or free water clearance under the same study conditions (Gold and Viljoen, 1979). During maximal hydropenia, induced by an infusion of vasopressin in saline, xipamide and hydrochlorothiazide also behaved similarly, increasing free water reabsorption in a linear relationship to osmolar clearance, whereas an increase in osmolar clearance with little effect on free water reabsorption was seen with frusemide. This evidence tends to support animal experiments which indicate that xipamide acts on the distal convoluted tubules. However, the atypical and rather fragmentary nature of some of the results which support these statements indicates that more studies are needed to clarify the site of action of xipamide, and also that current data should be interpreted with caution.

2. *Pharmacokinetic Studies*

2.1 Absorption and Distribution

Following oral administration of xipamide 20mg to 14 healthy volunteers, the drug appeared to be completely absorbed, with maximum plasma concentrations of about 3 mg/L occurring within 1 hour (Knauf and Mutschler, 1984). In an earlier study using ^{35}S-labelled xipamide, peak plasma radioactivity representing 13% of the dose per litre occurred 0.75 to 2 hours after oral administration of 42mg to 3 healthy volunteers (Hempelmann and Dieker, 1977).

A comparison of the area under the plasma concentration-time curve (AUC) after intravenous and oral administration of xipamide 20mg to healthy subjects indicated an absolute bioavailability of 73%. The volume of distribution of xipamide, as calculated from the total plasma clearance and elimination half-life, was 21L (Knauf and Mutschler, 1984).

2.2 Metabolism and Elimination

After oral and intravenous administration of xipamide 20mg in 14 healthy subjects, urinary recovery of unchanged drug (time period not stated) was 37 and 38%, respectively (Knauf and Mutschler, 1984). Urinary excretion of radioactivity 96 hours after administration of a single dose of ^{35}S-xipamide was 88% when given orally or intravenously (Hempelmann and Dieker, 1977). Radioactivity in the faeces over a period of 4 days accounted for about 3% of the administered dose. Xipamide is conjugated with glucuronide and during the first 24 hours 26% of the administered dose was excreted in the conjugated form and 40 to 55% unchanged (Hempelmann and Dieker, 1977; Knauf and Mutschler, 1984). Total plasma clearance of xipamide was calculated at 2.1 L/h, with renal clearance calculated to be 0.7 L/h (Knauf and Mutschler, 1984).

2.2.1 Half-Life

The mean plasma half-life of radioactivity after intravenous administration of ^{35}S-xipamide in 5 healthy subjects was 5 hours and after oral administration in 3 subjects values between 5.8 and 8.2 hours were obtained (Hempelmann and Dieker, 1977). Similar results were reported by Knauf and Mutschler (1984) who determined a terminal half-life of 7 hours, using a densitofluorimetric method of estimating xipamide (Sobel and Mutschler, 1980).

2.3 Effect of Renal Insufficiency on Pharmacokinetics

In 2 patients with renal failure, half-life was prolonged, most of the radioactivity was excreted in the faeces, and a higher proportion was conjugated (Hempelmann and Dieker, 1977). Knauf and Mutschler (1984) studied 14 patients with varying degrees of renal impairment down to a creatinine clearance of 3 ml/min. The elimination rate constant showed only a modest reduction with progressive renal impairment, with a plasma half-life calculated to be 9 hours in end-stage renal disease. The extrarenal clearance of xipamide (1.5 L/h) remains constant with increasing renal failure and therefore proportionally more important (Knauf and Mutschler, 1984). It is therefore not to be expected that xipamide will accumulate to any marked degree in renal failure.

3. Therapeutic Use

Although xipamide is an effective diuretic, it has been most widely evaluated for the treatment of hypertension rather than in the primary treatment of fluid retention. Most patients had mild to moderate essential hypertension and many had not previously been treated with antihypertensive drugs. Xipamide has been used alone in patients not previously treated for hypertension, in combination with a variety of other antihypertensive drugs, and has been substituted for other diuretics which were part of a treatment regimen. Most blinded studies have been of double-blind crossover design and have usually involved only small numbers of patients. Few studies have stated that blood pressure measurements were taken by the same observer under the same conditions at each clinic visit. Likewise, relatively few studies have used an observer bias-free sphygmomanometer or monitored patient compliance.

3.1 Use in Hypertension

3.1.1 Open Studies

Open studies in hypertension are not a reliable indication of the relative therapeutic efficacy of an antihypertensive, since a placebo response can occur in up to about 40% of patients with mild to moderate hypertension (Weber et al., 1977). Nevertheless, open studies, generally with xipamide alone, have suggested that it is an effective antihypertensive drug.

Earlier studies usually used a dosage of 40mg, as have also some more recent investigators (Acosta-Barrios et al., 1983; Ktenas and Aravanis, 1980), but after the demonstration in double-blind trials that 20mg gave similar effects to 40mg (Davies and Prichard, 1975; Weber et al., 1977), and then that 10mg was probably similar to 20mg (MacGregor et al., 1982), open studies have tended to use lower dosages. Several investigators used 20 and 40mg daily (Cruz and Cruz, 1980; Leary et al., 1978; Moreira et al., 1979). Studies with 20mg daily in the elderly have shown this dose was effective (Reyes et al., 1981).

In a longer term open study in 74 patients, Brochez et al. (1983) gave xipamide for an average of 10.4 months at dosages between 5 and 20mg (average 12.2mg). Blood pressures with placebo were 168/101mm Hg supine and 166/105 erect, and after xipamide were 146/87 and 145/91mm Hg, respectively. A double-blind phase (see section 3.1.2) gave less impressive results. Castro (1980) studied 22 patients for 2 years, adjusting the dosage according to the individual response. The dosage required to decrease standing diastolic blood pressure to $\leq$ 90mm Hg in mild hypertension and to $\leq$ 96mm Hg in moderate hypertension was 10mg in 2 patients and 20mg in 16 patients. Standing diastolic blood pressure was decreased to $\leq$ 100mm Hg by a dose of 40mg daily in 2 of 3 patients with initially severe hypertension ($\geq$ 120mm Hg diastolic).

Raftery et al. (1981) performed continuous intra-arterial monitoring of blood pressure before and after an average of 3 months' treatment with xipamide 20mg once daily in 18 patients (fig. 3), with full data being available in 13 patients. 11 patients attended for physiological testing. Supine blood pressures after resting for 30 minutes were 168/80mm Hg before xipamide and 138/64 after xipamide, whereas after 5 minutes of 60° tilt the figures were 174/90 and 140/74mm Hg, respectively. The effect of xipamide was significant on all of these values ($p < 0.01$). Systolic blood pressure after exercise was not significantly decreased by xipamide but the decrease in exercise diastolic pressure (112 to 102mm Hg) was significant.

In an open crossover study in 29 patients, Pasquel et al. (1981) randomly administered xipamide and hydrochlorothiazide. They titrated the dose of xipamide to control blood pressure, using 5mg in 17 patients, 10mg in 7 and 20mg in 5 patients. Hydrochlorothiazide was likewise titrated, 50mg being used in 18 patients, and 100mg in 3 patients. Each dose increment was given for 4 weeks. The two drugs were separated by a 4-week placebo washout period. The goals of treatment were reduction of supine diastolic blood pressure to ≤ 90mm Hg in mildly hypertensive patients and to ≤ 96mm Hg in moderate and severely affected patients. This was achieved in all patients during xipamide and in 72% of patients during treatment with hydrochlorothiazide. It is not clear why more patients were not given the 100mg dose of hydrochlorothiazide in view of the fact that only 72% were controlled on hydrochlorothiazide, although many physicians would hold the view that the larger doses of hydrochlorothiazide seldom give a greater fall of blood pressure.

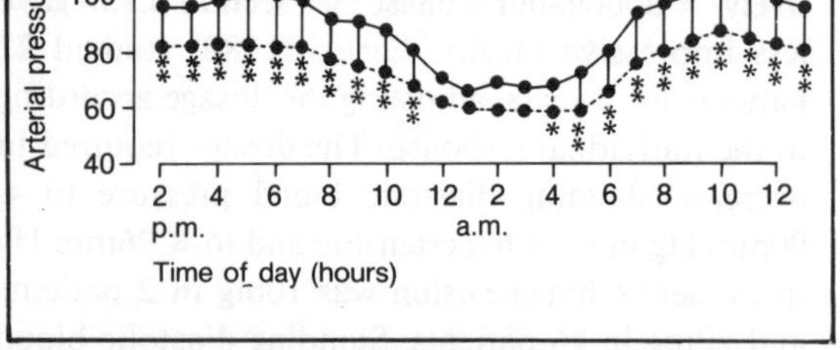

Fig. 3. Hourly records of intra-arterial blood pressure before (●——●) and during (●---●) treatment (mean 13 weeks) with xipamide 20mg daily in 13 patients with hypertension; * $p < 0.05$; ** $p < 0.01$ (after Raftery et al., 1981).

3.1.2 Controlled Trials

Comparisons with Placebo

A double-blind study in 47 patients found xipamide at individualised dosages to be superior to placebo (table III). Xipamide was substituted for existing treatment at a dosage found to be optimal during an earlier open phase of the study (Brochez et al., 1983). On the other hand, Harding et al. (1974) found no significant difference between the effects of xipamide 40mg daily and placebo when added to existing treatment in a small study with only 8 patients.

Dose-Determining Studies

Dose-response studies that have compared xipamide 20 and 40mg did not find any statistically significant difference between these doses when xipamide was given alone (Weber et al., 1977) or in combination with other drugs (Davies and Prichard, 1975), although in this small study the response to the 40mg dose was more consistent (table III). Similarly, there was no significant difference in antihypertensive efficacy between xipamide 10 and 20mg daily (MacGregor et al., 1982) or between doses of 5 and 10mg daily (Leary and Reyes, 1983), although in the latter study there was a tendency for Black patients to respond better to the 10mg dose while Caucasians responded similarly to each dose.

It seems probable, therefore, that 40mg of xipamide will only seldom be required in hypertension, 10 or 20mg will often be adequate, and sometimes 5mg (see section 5).

Table III. Summary of design and results of studies of the antihypertensive efficacy of xipamide compared with that of placebo and other diuretics in patients with mild to moderate hypertension

Reference	No. of patients[a]	Duration[b] (weeks)	Dosage (mg/day)	Added to existing therapy	Design[c]	Results (supine blood pressure, mm Hg)		
						baseline	xipamide	comparative treatment
Comparisons with placebo								
Brochez et al. (1983)	47	8	Adjusted to optimum	No	db, xo	169/101	146/87[d]	168/101
Harding et al. (1974)	8	8	Xip 40	Yes	sb, xo	133[e]	123[f]	132
Dose-finding studies								
Davies and Prichard (1975)	10	6	Xip 40	Yes	db, xo	Not stated	145/85[d]	162/93 (placebo)
			Xip 20			Not stated	147/89[d,g]	162/93
			Placebo					
Leary and Reyes (1983)	23	9	Xip 5	No	sb, xo	169/104	146/89[d]	
			Xip 10			170/103	147/87[d,g]	
Weber et al. (1977)	48	4	Xip 20	No	db, xo	Not stated	148/94[d]	159/97 (placebo)
			Xip 40			Not stated	145/90[d,g]	159/97
			Placebo					
Comparisons with other diuretics[i]								
Bonaduce et al. (1981)	40	6	Xip 40	No	db, xo	170/100[h]	152/88[d,g]	155/88[d]
			Ch 100					
Gabriel (1983)	24	12	Xip 40	No	?, xo	146/90	139/85[d,g]	
			Ben 5			146/90		146/88[f]
			Bum 1			146/90		145/87
Kumar et al. (1984)	17	4	Xip 40	Yes	db, xo	155/100[h] (placebo)	137/90[d,g]	150/100[f]
			Hyd 50					
	12	4	Xip 80	No	db, par	158/96 (placebo)	136/85[f,g]	142/88[f]
			Hyd 100					
MacGregor et al. (1982)	14	6	Xip 10	No	db, xo	181/115	158/104[d,g]	160/104[d]
			Xip 20				153/102[d,g]	
			Cyc 0.5					

a Number of patients who completed the trial.
b Duration of treatment with each active drug.
c db = double-blind; xo = crossover; sb = single-blind.
d Better than placebo or control.
e Mean blood pressure (1/3 systolic + diastolic).
f Not significantly different from control.
g No significant difference between active drugs.
h Figure extrapolated from graph.
i Ch = chlorthalidone; Ben = bendrofluazide; Bum = bumetanide; Hyd = hydrochlorothiazide; Cyc = cyclopenthiazide.

Comparisons with Other Diuretics

Xipamide 40mg daily has been compared with chlorthalidone 100mg, bendrofluazide 5mg, bumetanide 1mg and hydrochlorothiazide 50mg daily; xipamide 80mg was compared with hydrochlorothiazide 100mg, while lower doses of xipamide (10 and 20mg daily) were compared with cyclopenthiazide 0.5mg (table III). There is little indication of how these dosages were chosen, other than by their equivalent natriuretic effects.

Although no significant differences in mean supine blood pressure were noted between the drugs during treatment with xipamide or the other thiazides, MacGregor et al. (1982) reported that standing blood pressure was similar after 6 weeks' treatment with xipamide 10mg to that after the same period of treatment with cyclopenthiazide 0.5mg. Xipamide 20mg daily produced significantly greater decreases in blood pressure than either xipamide 10mg daily or cyclopenthiazide 0.5mg daily, but the higher dose was associated with significant hypokalaemia.

A tendency for a greater antihypertensive effect with xipamide 40mg than with chlorthalidone 100mg was noted by Bonaduce et al. (1981) who reported that the 20 patients given chlorthalidone first showed a further reduction in supine and standing blood pressure when crossed over to xipamide, but the 20 patients given xipamide first showed no further fall when chlorthalidone was substituted. However, in another crossover study of 6 weeks' duration, xipamide 20mg and chlorthalidone 50mg were not significantly different in efficacy (Dies and Heinz, 1978). A tendency for xipamide 40mg to be more effective than bendrofluazide 5mg and hydrochlorothiazide 50mg was noted by Gabriel (1983) and Kumar et al. (1984), respectively.

Xipamide in Combination with Other Drugs

Xipamide has been compared with placebo, indapamide and bendrofluazide when added to an existing regimen that did not provide a satisfactory decrease in blood pressure (table IV). In a well-designed study the addition of xipamide 20mg or indapamide 2.5mg daily to nadolol 160mg (2 × 80mg) daily resulted in a significant decrease in supine and standing blood pressure after 8 weeks' treatment. However, xipamide caused a greater reduction in serum potassium after 12 months of treatment than did indapamide (Dean et al., 1984). The addition of xipamide 20 to 40mg daily to existing regimens comprising β-blockers, adrenergic neuron-blocking drugs and/or methyldopa produced a significant decrease in supine and erect blood pressure in the study of Davies and Prichard (1975) and in erect blood pressure in the small study of Harding et al. (1974). In contrast, Ramsay and Freestone (1984) found xipamide 20mg no more effective than an additional 5mg of bendrofluazide in patients already receiving a β-blocker with or without bendrofluazide 5mg daily.

3.2 Xipamide in the Treatment of Oedema

3.2.1 Heart Failure

Several studies have indicated that xipamide is effective in heart failure. Thus, in open studies the fluid retention and symptoms of heart failure have been diminished by xipamide (Acosta-Barrios et al., 1983; Cox et al., 1981; Fischer and Lenhartz, 1970; Gold and Viljoen, 1978; Piyasena et al., 1975). In a 4-week open study in 8 elderly subjects with congestive heart failure, bodyweight fell from 54.7kg to 53.4kg (Cox et al., 1981). A further open study in 16 ambulant patients (average age 60 years; range 41 to 77 years) who had hypertension and heart failure reported that the administration of xipamide 40mg for 5 weeks resulted in a reduction in blood pressure from an average of 204/122 to 151/103mm Hg, and a clearing of the signs and symptoms of heart failure, dyspnoea, hepatojugular reflex and hepatomegaly. The only quantitative measurement quoted was that of ankle circumference which significantly decreased from 25.9cm before xipamide to 24.6cm after 1 week and to 24.2cm after 5 weeks of xipamide treatment.

There have been some comparative studies of xipamide with other diuretics. Bonaduce et al. (1982) performed a double-blind parallel group comparative study of 7 days' treatment with xip-

Table IV. Summary of design and results of therapeutic trials of xipamide used in combination with other antihypertensive drugs in patients whose blood pressure was not satisfactorily controlled with the basic regimen

Reference	No. of patients	'Basic' therapy[a]	Drug[b] dosage (mg/day)	Duration (weeks)	Design[c]	Results (average/mean blood pressure, mm Hg)		
						'basic'	xipamide	other drug
Davies and Prichard (1975)	10	Propranolol Bethanidine Methyldopa	Xip 20 Xip 40 Placebo	6	db, xo	162/93 (supine) 151/95 (erect)	147/89[d,e] (20mg) 145/85[d] (40mg) 133/85[d,e] (20mg) 129/85[d] (40mg)	
Dean et al. (1984)	19	Nadolol	Xip 20 Ind 2.5	8	db, xo	167/100 (supine) 165/101 (erect)	143/93[d,e] 147/97[d,e]	145/90[d,e] 146/95[d,e]
Harding et al. (1974)	8	Propranolol Guanethidine Debrisoquine Methyldopa	Xip 40 Placebo	4	db, xo	132[f] (supine) 117 (erect)	123 106[d]	
Heimsoth (1977)	23	Clonidine	Xip 80[g]	16	Open	174/119	158/104[d]	
Ramsay and Freestone (1984)	20	β-Blocker Bendrofluazide	Xip 20 Ben 5	6	sb, par	159/100 (supine) (erect)	161/101[e] 145/97	157/100[e] 148/100

a Therapy to which xipamide was added, consisting of one of these drugs or various combined regimens.
b Xip = xipamide; Ind = indapamide; Ben = bendrofluazide.
c db = double-blind; xo = crossover; par = parallel groups.
d Significantly superior to basic regimen.
e No significant difference between treatments added to the basic regimen.
f Mean blood pressure.
g Xipamide 40mg given for the first 2 weeks.

amide 40mg or frusemide 25mg in 30 patients with heart failure. All subjects received digoxin and a 40 mmol/day sodium diet throughout. It was found that the treatments were similar in their effect on bodyweight, and sodium and potassium excretion. Diagrams of the results are given, not actual figures, but no significant differences between drugs were reported. In an open study involving 19 patients with cardiac oedema, the substitution of xipamide 40mg for hydrochlorothiazide 50mg plus amiloride 5mg daily (7 patients), cyclopenthiazide 0.25mg plus 1 or 2 tablets (6 patients each) of slow-release potassium 0.6g daily resulted in the resolution of oedema in 6 patients, and its reduction in 7 patients. Bodyweight was reduced by an average of 1.4kg in 9 patients while there was no change in 7 and an increase of an average of 1.8kg in 3 patients (Wade, 1980). Viikari et al. (1979) briefly reported a study in 13 elderly patients; they suggested that xipamide 10mg was equivalent to chlorothiazide 250mg or frusemide 20 to 40mg. However, from the report it is not possible to draw any firm conclusions.

3.2.2 Renal Disease

Xipamide 20 to 40mg daily (average 32mg) given to 6 patients with renal insufficiency (creatinine 160 to 1000 μmol/L) and 3 with nephrotic syndrome ('heavy' proteinuria and a serum albumin less than 434 μmol/L for periods of up to 20 months) improved oedema in all patients (Thomas and Thomis, 1981). In the 6 patients with renal insufficiency, weight fell by 0.9kg after 1 month and 1.4kg by the time of the last reading, while in the 3 patients with nephrotic syndrome the corresponding decreases in bodyweight were 5.8kg and

7.0kg, respectively. In the group as a whole, blood pressure fell from 182/110mm Hg to 160/104 at 1 month and to 160/93 at the last reading. Serum sodium was reduced significantly from 140.3 mmol/L pre-xipamide to 136.7 mmol/L at the end of the study. Creatinine levels tended to decrease (by 37 μmol/L) but this change, and the slight reduction in serum potassium (0.24 mmol/L), was not statistically significant. In this study, a patient with a past history of gout had attacks after 6 and 17 months of xipamide treatment, while the only other possible side effect was transient nausea.

In a study of 11 patients with oedema, Gold and Viljoen (1978) included 8 patients with nephrotic syndrome. They gave xipamide 20mg daily for between 2 and 30 weeks and restricted fluid intake to 1 L/day. Seven of the 8 patients lost weight (on average 10.7kg), while it increased by 1.3kg in the remaining patient. There were no symptomatic side effects: however, in 1 patient serum potassium fell to 2.8 mmol/L but resolved spontaneously, rising to 4.1 mmol/L; 1 patient had symptomless hyperuricaemia, another an elevated blood sugar level.

In a short term non-blind study, xipamide 40mg and frusemide 40mg were compared in 15 patients with either proteinuria or elevated creatinine levels. Each drug was given for 7 days separated by a washout period of 3 days. Both drugs reduced oedema. In the 13 patients with complete data, 6 responded equally while 7 had a better response to xipamide. The overall reduction in bodyweight was 1.4kg on xipamide and 1.03kg on frusemide. The increase in 24-hour urinary sodium (83.1 mmol) on xipamide was significantly greater than the increase on frusemide (33.9 mmol/24 hours). While differences between the drugs were not significant, the greater natriuresis with xipamide was associated with an increase in urinary potassium, not seen with frusemide. Side effects on xipamide were minor (Mihindukulasuriya and Lee, 1982).

3.2.3 Oedema Associated with Rheumatoid Arthritis

Kalos et al. (1974) compared xipamide 40mg, frusemide 40mg and placebo given for 1 week in random order to 20 patients with oedema associated with rheumatoid arthritis. Ankle circumference decreased by 1.12cm during xipamide and by 1.13cm on frusemide. The weight reduction averaged 1.58kg with xipamide and 1.13kg with frusemide; this difference was significant ($p < 0.05$).

3.2.4 Miscellaneous Oedematous Conditions

There have been a few studies in which results of treatment of various forms of oedema have been grouped. Fischer and Lenhartz (1970) reported studies with 43 patients: 33 with cardiac, 7 with renal and 3 with hepatic oedema. Xipamide 40 or 80mg or frusemide 40mg were each given for 3 days in alternating order separated by 3 days free of diuretic. The various causes of oedema were grouped in the analysis of results; xipamide and frusemide overall were found to be similar in their effect. Piyasena et al. (1975) also studied a mixed group of patients with oedema, 3 with congestive cardiac failure, 3 with cirrhosis, and 1 each with cor pulmonale, nephrotic syndrome and malnutrition. They administered 80mg doses of xipamide and frusemide in 6 patients, and 40mg of each drug in the remaining 3 patients. Single doses of each drug were given on two occasions in random order with a drug-free day between each treatment. The 24-hour mean urine volume was 1769ml on xipamide and 1859ml on frusemide. Urinary excretion of sodium and potassium was similar with each drug, as was the sodium/potassium ratio. A patient with cirrhosis who had failed to respond to other diuretic therapy had a useful response to xipamide 20mg which was administered for 11 months. Weight reduction was between 2 and 6kg (Gold and Viljoen, 1978).

In a double-blind comparison in 40 women on xipamide 20mg and frusemide 40mg, each given for 5 days prior to menstruation, both drugs relieved symptoms of premenstrual syndrome – although xipamide appeared to be the more effective treatment (Khandelwal et al., 1982).

4. Side Effects

4.1 Subjective Complaints

A number of studies in hypertension involving

a total of 155 patients did not report any subjective side effects (Bonaduce et al., 1981; Heimsoth, 1977; Leary and Reyes, 1983; Leary et al., 1978; Pasquel et al., 1981; Raftery et al., 1981), and in those studies that did, interruption of treatment was seldom necessary.

Side effects reported most frequently included mild upper gastrointestinal symptoms, anorexia or nausea in 2 to 4% of patients (Brochez et al., 1983; Cruz and Cruz, 1980; Hammer and Dembowski, 1969), tiredness and fatigue in 3 to 8% (Brochez et al., 1983; Castro, 1980; Weber et al., 1977) and weakness, which occurred in 12% of patients in one study (Cruz and Cruz, 1980). However, some studies have not reported any such side effects. Other subjective effects that have been reported with some regularity were dizziness (often postural) and vertigo, although many studies have apparently not had any patients with this symptom (Dies and Heinz, 1978). These complaints were almost invariably reported as mild and did not necessitate withdrawal of xipamide. The incidence of such effects is probably largely, if not entirely, related to the extent of the reduction in blood pressure. Isolated cases have been reported in large series giving an incidence of about 1% (Brochez et al., 1983; Hammer and Dembowski, 1969), and individual patients have had symptoms of this nature in smaller series (MacGregor et al., 1982). However, others have found a higher incidence of up to 10% (Ktenas and Aravanis, 1980; Weber et al., 1977) or even more in one smaller double-blind study series where blood pressure was lowered to a greater degree than in many studies (Davies and Prichard, 1975). Patients in this latter study also received other antihypertensive drugs throughout, and dizziness, which was intermittent, occurred on placebo as well as on active treatment.

There have been occasional reports of other symptoms associated with xipamide administration: headache (MacGregor et al., 1982; Moreira et al., 1979), a case of leg cramps at night (Brochez et al., 1983), and paraesthesiae of the upper limbs (Hammer and Dembowski, 1969). Dry mouth, polyuria and nocturia were found in response to a questionnaire by Dies and Heinz (1978).

4.2 Effect on Bodyweight

Although a number of studies of xipamide in hypertension fail to mention its effect on bodyweight, most trials have reported an average weight loss of about 1kg (e.g. Brochez et al., 1983; Castro, 1980; Weber et al., 1977). An average weight loss of about 0.7kg has been reported by some investigators (Cruz and Cruz, 1980; Harding et al., 1974) while others have reported values of 1.5kg (MacGregor et al., 1982), 2kg (Ktenas and Aravanis, 1980; Pasquel et al., 1981) or 3kg (Hammer and Dembowski, 1969).

4.3 Effects on Serum Electrolyte, Blood Urea and Urate Levels

4.3.1 Potassium

As discussed in section 1.2.2, clinical pharmacological experiments indicate that for an equivalent loss of sodium, the potassium loss on xipamide and frusemide appears similar. There are some experiments that indicate that the selective loss of potassium relative to sodium is less with xipamide than with hydrochlorothiazide (Leary and Asmal, 1978b) or chlorthalidone (Hempelmann et al., 1975).

The most marked influence on potassium levels after the treatment of hypertension with xipamide appears to be geographical factors, presumably due to dietary differences (fig. 4). The average reduction in serum potassium has ranged from low levels of 0.1 to 0.3 mmol/L in studies conducted in Naples, Brazil and South Africa to higher levels of 0.7 to 1.2 mmol/L in the United Kingdom and Belgium. In one study in Germany, xipamide 20mg daily for 1.5 months was associated with a decrease in serum potassium of 0.1 mmol/L (Dies and Heinz, 1978), while in another German study using 80mg daily the average serum potassium level was reduced by 0.9 mmol/L over a 4-month period (Heimsoth, 1977).

Although average decreases in serum potassium are of interest, more important may be isolated greater responses. One of the 25 patients studied by Ktenas and Aravanis (1980) had a serum potassium of less than 2.5 mmol/L. Raftery et al. (1981), in their small series (n = 13) with an unusually large average reduction in potassium, reported 3 patients with serum potassium concentrations below 3.0 mmol/L, with 1 at 2.2 mmol/L. There are reports of symptomatic hypokalaemia with xipamide. Altmann and Hamblin (1982) reported a patient with ventricular fibrillation associated with a very low serum potassium concentration of 1.02 mmol/L after receiving xipamide 20mg daily. The patient responded to DC shock, and serum potassium subsequently returned to normal after vigorous replacement therapy. No evidence however, either way, is given to indicate whether this patient had primary hyperaldosteronism, and whether the patient was normokalaemic prior to xipamide. An unusual case was reported by Boulton and Hardisty (1982) in a 62-year-old patient with essential hypertension who had a long history of exercise-induced proximal muscle weakness, suggestive of hypokalaemic periodic paralysis. He had been treated for 6 weeks with xipamide 20mg daily, and prior to minor surgery had a serum potassium of 3.1 mmol/L. Postoperatively he developed severe muscle weakness with a serum potassium of 3.0 mmol/L. Xipamide was stopped, but then inadvertently restarted, and he experienced 4 episodes of post-exercise mild muscle weakness over 1 month, with a serum potassium of 3.4 mmol/L. Xipamide was again stopped and over 9 months' further observation no more attacks were reported and serum potassium had increased to 4.2 mmol/L.

4.3.2 Sodium and Chloride

Xipamide used in the treatment of hypertension may either not affect serum sodium or may produce a slight reduction. Most studies quoting the serum sodium levels either report no change (Harding et al., 1974; Heimsoth, 1977) or minimal

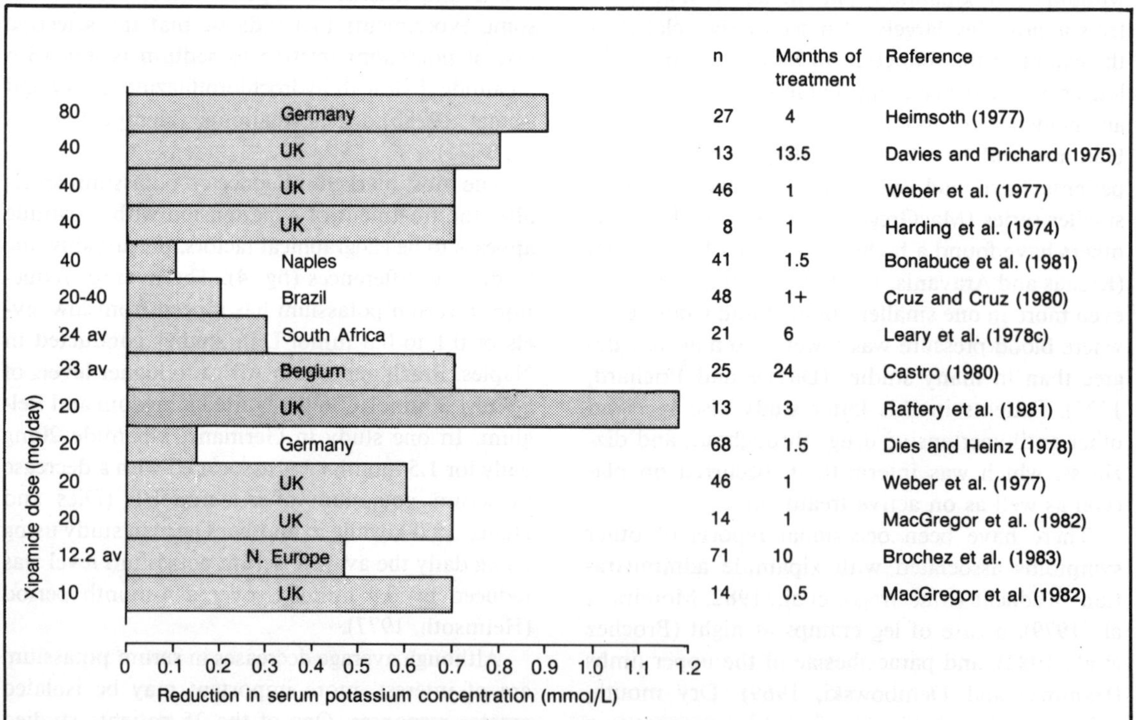

Fig. 4. Geographical variation in the reduction in serum potassium concentration during xipamide administration to patients.

insignificant falls of 1 to 2 mmol/L (Brochez et al., 1983; Cruz and Cruz, 1980; Dies and Heinz, 1978; Weber et al., 1977). Chloride levels also show slight statistically insignificant falls (Harding et al., 1974; Heimsoth, 1977; Weber et al., 1977), no change (Brochez et al., 1983), or minimal insignificant increases (Dies and Heinz, 1978).

4.3.3 Magnesium and Calcium

Recently it has become clear that diuretics lower serum magnesium concentration (Reyes and Leary, 1983; Sheehan and White, 1982), and in cardiac arrhythmias resistant to the correction of hypokalaemia this may be a causal factor (Dyckner and Wester, 1981; Reyes and Leary, 1981a). Leary and Reyes (1983) studied xipamide 5 and 10mg in 10 Caucasians and 13 Blacks. In the 8 patients treated with 5mg daily, magnesium levels showed a small fall from 0.80 to 0.74 mmol/L, within the normal range, after 8 weeks' treatment ($p = 0.05$). The effects of xipamide on serum calcium are mentioned in 2 reports: a significant increase (within normal range) by Castro (1980) after 2 years' treatment (actual figures are not given), but a slight but insignificant decrease by Dies and Heinz (1978) after 6 weeks' treatment.

4.3.4 Blood Urea and Serum Urate

As might be expected, xipamide causes a small increase in blood urea. The increases have been significant in some studies, e.g. increasing from 5.4 mmol/L to 6.4 mmol/L on 20mg and to 7.1 mmol/L on 40mg ($p < 0.01$ *vs* 20mg) in 46 patients treated by Weber et al. (1977); from 12.1 to 13.9 mmol/L, $p < 0.001$, in 72 patients (Brochez et al., 1983); and from 5.05 mmol/L to 6.5 mmol/L, $p < 0.01$, in 13 patients (Raftery et al., 1981). Other studies have recorded small increases which were both clinically and statistically insignificant (Cruz and Cruz, 1980; Dies and Heinz, 1978; Harding et al., 1974; MacGregor et al., 1982). When serum creatinine concentrations were reported, no significant changes occurred during xipamide therapy (Brochez et al., 1983; Cruz and Cruz, 1980; Dies and Heinz, 1978).

Xipamide causes small increases in serum urate concentrations which in some studies have reached statistical significance, ranging between 29 and 74.5 μmol/L (Brochez et al., 1983; Castro, 1980; Cruz and Cruz, 1980). In a double-blind trial conducted by Weber et al. (1977) mean serum urate concentration was 335 μmol/L on placebo, 406 μmol/L on xipamide 20mg and 414 μmol/L on xipamide 40mg. Other investigators have found either an insignificant increase in average values (Harding et al., 1974; Heimsoth, 1977; MacGregor et al., 1982) or no change (Dies and Heinz, 1978; Leary and Reyes, 1983). In a crossover comparison with hydrochlorothiazide, Pasquel et al. (1981) noted that serum urate was above 387 μmol/L in 6 patients during xipamide and in 12 during hydrochlorothiazide treatment.

4.3.6 Other Metabolic and Hormonal Effects

Many studies reported xipamide as having no effect on blood glucose levels (Cruz and Cruz, 1980; Hammer and Dembowski, 1969; Ktenas and Aravanis, 1980; Leary and Reyes, 1983; Leary et al., 1978; Moreira et al., 1979), even after 16 weeks' treatment with 80mg (Heimsoth, 1977), but did not state the actual values observed. Other investigators quote actual levels, reporting no change (Brochez et al., 1983) or only very small average increases (Dies and Heinz, 1978; MacGregor et al., 1982) in blood glucose during xipamide therapy. In contrast, there have been reports of larger increases in blood glucose in 6 latent diabetics (Heimsoth, 1977) or in diabetic patients, 7 receiving treatment with oral hypoglycaemic drugs, and 1 on diet (Castro, 1980). In these diabetic patients blood glucose averaged 6.5 mmol/L before xipamide therapy, and was increased to 8.5 mmol/L at 1 year, and to 8.6 mmol/L at 2 years of treatment.

Although serum cholesterol concentrations are generally elevated by diuretics, only a few studies have reported the effects of xipamide on this variable. Dies and Heinz (1978) found no change in average concentrations in 20 patients (6.7 mmol/L before and after therapy) while Brochez et al. (1983) noted an insignificant increase from 6.2 to 6.5 mmol/L in 56 patients. Significant increases were reported by Castro (1980) [no values given] and by Cruz and Cruz (1980) [from 5.43 to 6.25 mmol/L] while plasma lipids increased in 6 diabetics treated with xipamide 80mg for 3.5 months (Heimsoth, 1977).

Plasma renin activity was increased in one study from 0.92 ng/ml/h on placebo to 2.03 at 2 weeks and to 2.11 ng/ml/h after 4 weeks of treatment with xipamide 20mg daily (MacGregor et al., 1982). Elevation of renin by 'about 8-fold' and aldosterone 'about 2-fold' has also been reported in healthy volunteers and patients with renal insufficiency receiving xipamide (Knauf and Mutschler, 1984).

5. *Dosage and Administration*

In the treatment of mild to moderate hypertension the usual adult dose of xipamide is 20mg daily given as a single morning dose. A daily dose of 40mg may be required in more severe grades of hypertension. When used in combination with other antihypertensive drugs, the initial dose of xipamide should not exceed 20mg daily and lower doses may often be adequate.

In the treatment of oedema the usual dosage in the initial phase is 40mg given as a single dose in the morning. Subsequently, dosage may be reduced to 10 to 20mg daily if long term therapy is necessary. However, in severe refractory cases dosage may be increased to 80mg daily. Supplementary potassium or a potassium-sparing diuretic may be needed to avoid hypokalaemia during long term treatment of patients with cardiac, hepatic or renal oedema.

6. *The Place of Xipamide in Therapy*

Xipamide is a non-thiazide diuretic with a greater natriuretic effect than the thiazides and a less abrupt onset and longer duration of action than frusemide. There have been numerous studies of xipamide in hypertension but only relatively few studies in oedematous conditions. It is an effective antihypertensive drug; like most other diuretics, it causes potassium loss and appears to have other biochemical side effects similar to other diuretics.

There is evidence in man that xipamide, like the thiazides, acts on the distal tubule, but it also resembles frusemide in that it is an effective diuretic in patients with renal failure.

Xipamide appears to be a more effective diuretic than the thiazides and may cause a lesser potassium loss relative to sodium excretion than these drugs, but further comparative trials in adequate numbers of patients are needed to confirm these findings. It has yet to be determined whether xipamide will cause calcium retention, like the thiazides, or calcium loss like frusemide.

Thus, xipamide offers a suitable alternative to other diuretics in the treatment of patients with mild to moderate hypertension and in patients with oedema due to a variety of causes.

References

Acosta-Barrios, T.; Reyes, A.J.; Leary, W.P. and Van Der Byl, K.: Effects of xipamide in hypertensive patients with cardiac insufficiency: A clinical appraisal. Current Therapeutic Research 33: 855-859 (1983).

Altmann, P. and Hamblin, J.J.: Ventricular fibrillation induced by xipamide. British Medical Journal 284: 494 (1982).

Armah, B.; Dies, R. and Heinz, N.: Untersuchung der saluretischen und diuretischen Wirkung von Xipamid-Triamteren-Kombinationen in unterschiedlichen Dosisverhaltnissen an Ratten. Arzneimittal-Forschung 33 (I): 131-135 (1983).

Bonaduce, D.; Ferrara, N.; Petretta, M.; Canonico, V.; Romango, E. and Rengo, F.: Comparison of the antihypertensive activities of xipamide and chlorthalidone: A double-blind randomized crossover trial. Current Medical Research and Opinion 7: 247-252 (1981).

Bonaduce, D.; Ferrara, N.; Canonico, V.; Visciola, G.; Postiglione, M. et al.: Xipamide treatment in congestive heart failure: Double-blind trial with furosemide. Current Therapeutic Research 31: 293-301 (1982).

Boulton, A.J.M and Hardisty, C.A.: Hypokalaemic periodic paralysis precipitated by diuretic therapy and minor surgery. Postgraduate Medical Journal 58: 106-107 (1982).

Brochez, A.; Castro, M.; Odegaard, A. and Thomis, J.: Once daily administration of low-dose xipamide: A long-term study in mild to moderate hypertension. International Journal of Clinical Pharmacology, Therapy and Toxicology 21: 394-398 (1983).

Castro, M.: Xipamide ('Diurexan') in essential hypertension: A 24-month study. Current Medical Research and Opinion 6: 416-422 (1980).

Cox, J.R.; Shalaby, W.A.; Crabbe, S.J. and Richens, J.: The effect of xipamide on body fluids and electrolytes in elderly patients with congestive cardiac failure. Journal of Clinical Experimental Gerontology 3: 381-385 (1981).

Cruz, J. and Cruz, H.M.M.: Hypotensive action of a new diuretic: Xipamide. Revista Brasileira de Medicina 37: 526-534 (1980).

Davies, P.S. and Prichard, B.N.C.: A dose-response study of xipamide in hypertension used in combination with other antihypertensive drugs. Journal of International Medical Research 3: 389-394 (1975).

Dean, S.; Kendall, M.J.; Potter, S.; Thompson, M.H. and Jackson, D.A.: Nadolol in combination with indapamide and xipamide in resistant hypertensives. European Journal of Clinical Pharmacology 28: 39-33 (1984).

Diembeck, W.; Dies, R. and Heinz, N.: Pharmakokinetik von Xipamid und Triamteren bel gesunden Probanden. Arzneimittel-Forschung 32 (II): 1482-1484 (1982).

Dies, R. and Heinz, N.: Treatment of essential hypertension with xipamide and chlorthalidone. Klinikarzt 7: 571-576 (1978).

Dyckner, T. and Wester, P.O.: Relation between potassium, magnesium and cardiac arrhythmias. Acta Medica Scandinavica 647 (Suppl.): 163-169 (1981).

Fischer, R. and Lenhartz, A.: Experience with a new diuretic. Medizinische Welt 21 (N.F.): 270-273 (1970).

Gabriel, R.: Comparison of the hypotensive effects of bendrofluazide, bumetanide and xipamide. Current Medical Research and Opinion 8: 645-647 (1983).

Gold, C.H. and Viljoen, M.: Xipamide in the management of renal, hepatic and cardiac oedema. South African Medical Journal 54: 569-571 (1978).

Gold, C.H. and Viljoen, M.: Site of renal action of xipamide. Clinical Pharmacology and Therapeutics 25 (Part I): 522-527 (1979).

Hammer, O. and Dembowski, U.: Experience with a new saluretic in the treatment of essential hypertension. Medizinische Klinik 41: 1862-1864 (1969).

Harding, R.D.; Kalos, A.; Weber, J.C.P. and Dixon, A.St.J.: Treatment of hypertension with xipamid – a new diuretic. A double-blind controlled trial. Clinical Trials Journal (London) 11: 45-48 (1974).

Heimsoth, V.H.: Studies covering combined treatments with xipamide. International Journal of Clinical Pharmacology 15: 260-266 (1977).

Hempelmann, F.W.: The protein binding of xipamide (4-chloro-5-sulphamoyl-2′,6′-salicyloxylidide). Arzneimittel-Forschung 25: 258-259 (1975a).

Hempelmann, F.W.: The inhibition of carbonic anhydrase by xipamide (4-chloro-5-sulphamoyl-2′,6′-salicyloxylidide) in the modified Philpot test. Arzneimittel-Forschung 25: 259-260 (1975b).

Hempelmann, F.W. and Dieker, P.: Untersuchungen mit Xipamid (4-chlor-5-sulphamoyl-2′,6′-salicyloxylidid). Arzneimittel-Forschung 27 (2): 2143-2151 (1977).

Hempelmann, F.W.; Leuschner, F. and Liebenow, W.: The saluretic effect of xipamide (4-chloro-5-sulfamoyl-2′-6′-salicyl-oxylidide) in normal subjects. Arzneimittel-Forschung 25 (2): 252-255 (1975).

Henness, D.M. and Weng, T.S.: Single-dose evaluations of xipamide: A comparison study with furosemide and hydrochlorothiazide. Clinical Therapeutics 2: 277-286 (1979).

Hohenegger, M. and Holzer, F.: Effects of xipamide and triamterene – alone or in combination – on electrolyte excretion in the rat. International Journal of Clinical Pharmacology 13 (4): 298-303 (1976).

Kalos, A.; Dixon, A.St.J. and Weber, J.C.P.: Xipamid in the treatment of oedema in rheumatoid arthritis. Rheumatology and Rehabilitation 13: 81-87 (1974).

Khandelwal, S.; Khandelwal, P.D. and Narula, J.: A comparative study of Lasix and Xipamid in the management of premenstrual syndrome. Indian Medical Gazette 12: 368-369 (1982).

Knauf, H. and Mutschler, E.: Pharmacodynamics and pharmacokinetics of xipamide in patients with normal and impaired kidney function. Europ. J. Clin. Pharmacol. 26: 513-520 (1984).

Knauf, Von H.; Haase, W. and Mutschler, E.: Dosis-Wirkungs-Beziehungen von Xipamid bei gesunden Probanden. Arzneimittel-Forschung 30 (II): 1599-1607 (1980).

Ktenas, J.A. and Aravanis, C.: Antihypertensive action of a new compound, Xipamid. Current Therapeutic Research 28: 543-547 (1980).

Kumar, S.; Pandhi, P.; Wahi, P.L. and Sharma, P.L.: A randomized double-blind clinical trial of xipamide and hydrochlorothiazide in essential hypertension. International Journal of Clinical Pharmacology, Therapy and Toxicology 22: 549-551 (1984).

Leary, W.P. and Asmal, A.C.: Comparative effects of xipamide, furosemide and hydrochlorothiazide in healthy adults. Current Therapeutic Research 24: 662-672 (1978a).

Leary, W.P. and Asmal, A.C.: Xipamide: Diuretic effects of low dosage in healthy adults. Current Therapeutic Research 24: 656-661 (1978b).

Leary, W.P.; Asmal, A.C. and Reyes, A.J.: Time-courses of the diuretic, natriuretic and kaliuretic effects of xipamide. Current Therapeutic Research 27: 16-21 (1980).

Leary, W.P. and Reyes, A.J.: Effects of low doses of xipamide given as monotherapy in essential hypertension. Current Therapeutic Research 34: 888-899 (1983).

Leary, W.P. and Reyes, A.J.: Diuretic-induced magnesium losses. Drugs 28 (Suppl. 1): 182-187 (1984).

Leary, W.P.; Asmal, A.C.; Williams, P.C. and Herron, M.: Treatment of uncomplicated essential hypertension with xipamide. Current Therapeutic Research 24: 511-515 (1978).

Leuschner, F.: Chemie und Pharmakologie von 4-chlor-5-sulamyl-salicylsavre-2', 6'-dimethylanilid; in Kruck and Leppla (Eds) Klinische Pharmakologie der Diuretika, pp. 193-212 (Urban and Schwarzenberg, Munich 1969).

Liebenow, W. and Leuschner, F.: Struktur-Wirkungsbeziehungen beim Diuretikum Xipamid (4-chlor-5-sulfamoyl-2′,6′-salicyloxylidid). Arzneimittel-Forschung 25 (2): 240-244 (1975).

MacGregor, G.A.; Banks, R.A.; Markandu, N.D. and Roulston, J.: Xipamide and cyclopenthiazide in essential hypertension-comparative effects on blood pressure and plasma potassium. British Journal of Clinical Pharmacology 13: 859-863 (1982).

Mihindukulasuriya, J. and Lee, H.A.: Effect of xipamide in oedema of renal disease with varying degrees of renal insufficiency: A comparative trial with frusemide. Current Medical Research and Opinion 8: 208-214 (1982).

Moreira, J.; Chocair, P.R.; Coutinho, A.F. and Sabaga, E.: Treatment of arterial hypertension with a new diuretic – xipamide. A Folha Medica 78: 59-61 (1979).

Pasquel, R.; Wright Tribble, P. and Simon, A.: Hypotensive effects of xipamide in essential hypertension. Crossover comparison with hydrochlorothiazide. Journal of Clinical Pharmacology 21: 316-322 (1981).

Piyasena, K.H.G.; Havard, C.W.H. and Weber, J.C.P.: Xipamid, a potent new diuretic. Current Medical Research and Opinion 3: 121-125 (1975).

Raftery, E.B.; Melville, D.I.; Gould, B.A.; Mann, S. and Whittington, J.R.: A study of the antihypertensive action of xipamide using ambulatory intra-arterial monitoring. British Journal of Clinical Pharmacology 12: 381-385 (1981).

Ramsay, L.E. and Freestone, S.: Xipamide: No advantage over bendrofluazide in hypertension. British Journal of Clinical Pharmacology 18: 616-618 (1984).

Reyes, A.J. and Leary, W.P.: 24-hour urine volume, urinary electrolyte outputs and plasma potassium concentration as function of xipamide dose. Current Therapeutic Research 29: 120-125 (1981a).

Reyes, A.J. and Leary, W.P.: Antihypertensive diuretics: Difference from non-antihypertensive diuretics in time-course of excretory activity. Current Therapeutic Research 30: 217-226 (1981b).

Reyes, A.J. and Leary, W.P.: Magnesium deficiency provoked by diuretics. South African Medical Journal 63: 410-412 (1983).

Reyes, A.J.; Leary, W.P. and Asmal, A.C.: Urine volumes and flows after oral administration of xipamide, furosemide and hydrochlorothiazide to healthy adults. Current Therapeutic Research 28: 230-234 (1980).

Reyes, A.J.; Acosta-Barrios, T.N. and Leary, W.P.: The effects of

xipamide upon high blood pressure in geriatric hypertensives: A mathematical description. Current Therapeutic Research 30: 1089-1095 (1981).
Schuetterle, G.; Dieker, P. and Beckmann, D.: Relationship of the standard clearance and electrolyte excretion to zinc and copper after intravenous injection of 4-chloro-5-sulphamylsalicylic acid 2′,6′-dimethylanilide. Klinische Pharmakologie der Diuretika. Symposium in Travemunde, October, 1968, pp. 46-54 (Urban and Schwarzenberg, Munchen 1969).
Sheehan, J. and White, A.: Diuretic-associated hypomagnesaemia. British Medical Journal 285: 1157-1159 (1982).
Sobel, M. and Mutschler, E.: Fluorimetrische Bestimmung von Xipamid in biologischem Material mit einem neuen Fluoreszenzreagenz. Journal of Chromatography 183 (1): 124-130 (1980).
Strandhoy, J.W. and Gomoll, A.W.: Clearance and micropuncture studies of the diuretic xipamide in dogs. European Journal of Pharmacology 51: 173-176 (1979).
Thomas, H. and Thomis, J.A.: Preliminary experience with xipamide therapy in chronic renal failure and the nephrotic syndrome. Current Therapeutic Research 29 (2): 260-264 (1981).
Viikari, J.; Haataja, M. and Saarimaa, H.: Xipamide in cardiac insufficiency of geriatric patients. Current Therapeutic Research 26: 12-15 (1979).
Wade, A.G.: A patient compliance comparative study of three diuretics in the treatment of oedema. Journal of International Medical Research 8: 351-353 (1980).
Weber, J.C.P.; Bird, H.; Cosh, J.; Davies, P.S. et al.: Once daily treatment of mild to moderate hypertension with xipamid: A controlled study. British Journal of Clinical Pharmacology 4: 283-288 (1977).

Authors' address: *R.N. Brogden*, ADIS Drug Information Services, Private Bag, Mairangi Bay, Auckland 10 (New Zealand).

Review Article

Drugs 30: 333-354 (1985)
0012-6667/85/0010-0333/$11.00/0

Importance of Drug Enantiomers in Clinical Pharmacology

Kenneth Williams and *Edmund Lee*
Department of Clinical Pharmacology, St Vincent's Hospital, Darlinghurst, Sydney

Summary

The ordered asymmetry of biological macromolecules allows them to differentiate between the optical isomers of monomeric substrates. Optical isomers of drugs often have greatly different affinities at receptor sites, are metabolised at different rates, and have different affinities for tissue and protein binding sites. Despite this knowledge, many drugs are administered as their racemates. Manipulation of the enantiomeric ratio or the use of only one enantiomer of a drug may allow separation of toxicity and efficacy, and this may lead to a significant increase in therapeutic ratio and a more rational approach to therapeutics.

'All artificial bodies and all minerals have superposable images. Opposed to these are nearly all organic substances which play an important role in plant and animal life. These are asymmetric, and indeed have the kind of asymmetry in which the image is not superposable with the object.'

Louis Pasteur, 1860

All life as we know it is made up of ordered asymmetric macromolecular units. It is this ordered asymmetry which gives the macromolecules the necessary information to discriminate between the optical isomers of monomeric substrates such as amino acids and sugars. This ability to distinguish 'left'- from 'right'-handed molecules applies not only to endogenous substances, but extends to the recognition of 'left'- from 'right'-handed xenobiotics. Consequently, pharmacological activity often is associated predominantly with only one optical isomer of a drug.

The chemical synthesis of drugs generally leads to formation of both configurations at any given asymmetric centre. Mason (1984) has calculated that 82% of the synthetic chiral pharmaceuticals which appear in the 1980 edition of the US Pharmacopeial Dictionary of Drug Names are administered as their racemates, i.e. as equal mixtures of relatively 'active' and 'inactive' isomers. The 'inactive' form, however, may not be a passive component of the drug mixture. It may be an agonist, or an antagonist, or it may have actions at other receptors resulting in either unwanted side effects or contributing to overall drug efficacy. In addition, its metabolites may also be active or toxic. Furthermore, even as a totally inactive, passive component, it may place unnecessary burdens on the body's clearance mechanisms. On the other hand, advantage may be taken of differences in activity to tailor-make a drug with a specific ratio of the isomers to optimise some desired effect.

The problems and potential benefits of using drugs which are optically active have been largely neglected, because of the difficulties of separation of the isomeric forms both analytically and preparatively. This review does not discuss the analytical approaches which have allowed a study of the pharmacokinetics of these drugs (the interested reader should refer to articles by Lochmuller and Souter, 1975; Gil-Av, 1975; and Allenmark, 1984); rather it focuses on the clinical pharmacology and pharmacokinetics of racemic drugs commonly used in clinical practice, with occasional reference to experimental or infrequently prescribed drugs in order to make a general point. It is hoped that the review will increase awareness of the potential problems associated with administration of drugs as their racemates, and encourage interest in this growing area of clinical pharmacology.

1. Terminology

1.1 Optical Activity

A substance which rotates plane polarised light to the right is said to be *dextrorotatory* – symbolised by 'd' or (+). A substance which rotates polarised light to the left is said to be *levorotatory* – symbolised by 'l' or (−). Optical activity is not an independent variable. It is affected by sample concentration, temperature, light wavelength, solvent, and pH of aqueous solutions.

The necessary and sufficient condition for a molecule to show optical activity is that the molecule is not superimposable on its mirror image. Such a molecule is said to be *asymmetric* (or dissymmetric), and this asymmetry is generally conferred on the molecule by a carbon which has 4 different atoms or groups attached to it. (The word *chiral* is also used to describe asymmetry and a carbon atom may be described as a chiral carbon.) The pairs of non-superimposable mirror images are known variously as *optical isomers, optical antipodes* or *enantiomers.*

Changes in optical activity as a result of changing one or more of these variables is not the result of a change in the spatial orientation of the atoms in the molecule, i.e. its *configuration.* For example, by changing the pH of a solution of (+)-ibuprofen, not only can the magnitude of the rotation be altered but the direction can also be changed such that the solution becomes levorotatory, i.e. (−)-ibuprofen. This change in direction of rotation does *not* imply a change in configuration. The configuration can only be altered by the breaking and making of the atomic bonds. Consequently, optical rotation does not reveal anything about the configuration of a molecule. The signs d or (+) and l or (−) are useful only in the comparison of one enantiomer with its own mirror image. For some drugs, the configuration of the enantiomers is not known. Interenantiomer comparisons for a series of drug analogues must then be made using direction of rotation alone. Firm conclusions can only be made, however, when the absolute configuration has been determined.

1.2 Absolute Configuration

The *absolute configuration*, i.e. the actual orientation of the atoms in space, has been determined for many molecules by a combination of x-ray crystallography and known stereospecific synthetic transformations. The description of this orientation may then be made using the rules proposed by Cahn et al. (1956) and using the symbols 'R' (rectus) and 'S' (sinister). Given these symbols, the actual molecular configuration may be described. In this review, we have chosen to use R and S to describe drug enantiomers whose absolute configurations are known and (+) and (−) for those whose configurations have not been determined.

In the case of the amino acids (and sugars), the configuration is described by the symbols 'D' and 'L'. Again, although all the 'naturally' occurring amino acids are of the L-configuration, some are levorotatory and some are dextrorotatory. Furthermore, some L-amino acids when described according to the rules of Cahn et al. (1956) are R and some are S.

1.3 Stereospecific Index

The ratio of the activities of a pair of enantiomers is known as the *stereospecific index* and is dependent upon the optical purity of the enantiomers. This purity has not been adequately considered in some instances, as has been demonstrated for the enantiomers of chloroquine (Haberkorn et al., 1979) and benzhexol (Barlow et al., 1972), thus leading to underestimates of the respective stereospecific indices.

1.4 Racemisation

Thermodynamically, pure enantiomers are unstable. Thermodynamic equilibrium is attained when there is an equal mixture of the two enantiomers, i.e. a *racemate* [symbolised by (±); R,S- or d,l-]. The process whereby a pure enantiomer becomes a racemate is known as *racemisation.* This phenomenon, as it occurs for amino acids, has been applied to the dating of fossils, among other applications (Williams and Smith, 1977).

1.5 Diastereomers

Inversion at only 1 of the chiral carbons of a molecule with more than 1 centre of asymmetry results in a stereoisomer which is not a mirror image. Such a stereoisomer is known as a *diastereoisomer* or *diastereomer*, and this inversion is known as *epimerisation.* An example of a drug which undergoes spontaneous epimerisation in aqueous solution is the broad-spectrum oxalactam antibiotic latamoxef (moxalactam) [Miner et al., 1981; Wise et al., 1981]. Unlike enantiomers, diastereomers have different physical properties, such as melting points and solubilities.

1.6 Stereoselectivity

The terms '*stereoselective*' and '*stereospecific*' tend to be used interchangeably in the literature. This is hardly surprising as absolute stereospecificity of, for example, a receptor for one enantiomer is rarely observed, although the stereoselectivity may be 100-fold or more greater for the active enantiomer. Furthermore, the limits of experimental sensitivity may be the limiting factor in determining the activity of the less active enantiomer. For the purposes of this review, 'stereoselective' will be used unless no 'measurable' activity has been reported for one of the enantiomeric pairs.

2. *Pharmacodynamic Differences in Activities of Drug Enantiomers*

There is a large body of literature comparing the biological activities of a wide range of enantiomers of drugs using tissue perfusion studies and comparing effects in intact animals. These studies have demonstrated repeatedly the stereoselective nature of the interaction between drugs and cellular and tissue components, such as the uptake and storage of amines in adrenergic granules and brain synaptosomes. It is not within the scope of this review to cover this literature. The interested reader should refer to reviews by Ariens et al. (1983), Patil et al. (1970, 1975), Sastry (1973) and Smith (1984). Similarly, there is a large volume of literature which has shown that enzyme-catalysed reactions are stereoselective, and aspects of enzyme reaction stereoselectivity have been reviewed elsewhere (e.g. Rose, 1972).

The clinical application of this information is of great interest. In general, the basic known pharmacodynamic differences in activity between enantiomers have not been utilised to clinical advantage.

3. *Pharmacokinetic Differences in Behaviour of Drug Enantiomers*

Differences between the pharmacological activity of enantiomers may be of pharmacokinetic as well as of pharmacodynamic origin. Following administration of a drug as its racemate, concentration differences of the enantiomers at the receptors may be brought about by differential rates of absorption or by stereoselective presystemic extraction, metabolism, or protein or tissue binding.

3.1 Absorption

There is no difference between the lipid or aqueous solubilities of enantiomers. Since drug absorption generally is considered to be a passive process, it is not expected that there should be any stereoselectivity of drug absorption. For a drug which is actively transported across the intestinal mucosa, however, absorption may occur stereoselectively. Such a 'drug' is dopa whose L-enantiomer has been shown to be more rapidly absorbed than the D-enantiomer (Wade et al., 1973). Although D-dopa is not actively transported, it is still totally absorbed in man (Williams, unpublished data) by passive diffusion. This may be compared with methotrexate. Methotrexate, like dopa, is administered as the L-enantiomer and, like dopa, the L-enantiomer is absorbed actively. However, the oral availability of D-methotrexate has recently been shown to be only 2.5% of that for L-methotrexate following a 10mg dose. It appears that this is largely attributable to very poor passive absorption of D-methotrexate (Hendel and Brodthagen, 1984) and presumably the L-enantiomer is equally poorly absorbed by passive diffusion. The possible contribution of stereoselective first-pass metabolism and/or stereoselective metabolism by intestinal bacteria to the relative systemic availabilities of the enantiomers has not been investigated.

3.2 Presystemic Elimination

The asymmetric nature of enzymes results in differences in affinities between enantiomers for the reactive site, and thus the intrinsic free clearances for enantiomers often differ. First-pass extraction by both the liver and gut may result in differences in systemic availability for enantiomeric pairs of high extraction ratio drugs.

Significant stereoselective hepatic extraction has been demonstrated for metoprolol and this has been related to the oxidation phenotype (Lennard et al., 1983). Subjects in this study were phenotyped as

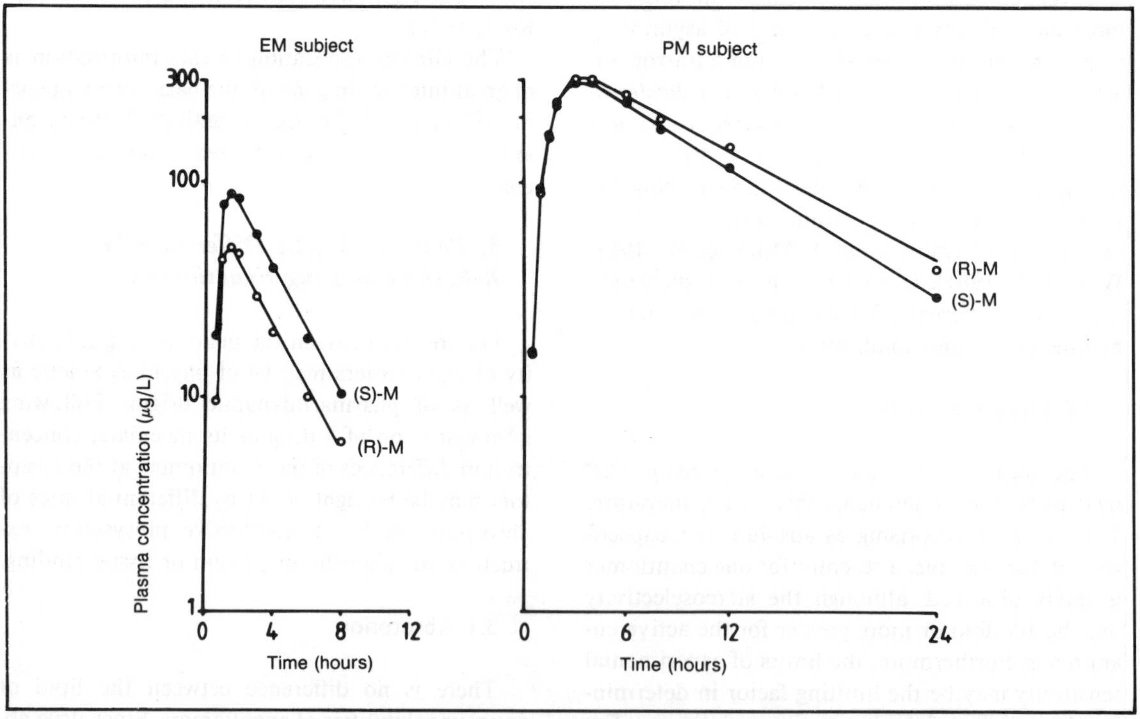

Fig. 1. Log plasma concentration-time curves for S-metoprolol (●) [(S)-M] and R-metoprolol (○) [(R)-M] after a dose of 200mg metoprolol orally to 1 extensive metaboliser (EM) and 1 poor metaboliser (PM) of debrisoquine (after Lennard et al., 1983; reproduced with permission of the authors and C.V. Mosby Co.).

extensive metabolisers (EM) or poor metabolisers (PM) of debrisoquine. In the EM group, metoprolol was a medium to high clearance drug and the systemic availability of the active S-enantiomer was approximately 1.4 times that of the inactive R-enantiomer. In the PM group, metoprolol was a low clearance drug, and the systemic availabilities of the enantiomers were apparently equal (fig. 1).

It has also been found that propranolol undergoes stereoselective presystemic clearance in dogs (Walle and Walle, 1979) and in man (Silber and Riegelman, 1980; Von Bahr et al., 1982a) [fig. 2]. However, contrary to these findings, Jackman et al. (1981) reported no difference between the extraction ratios of the propranolol enantiomers in man, although if their intravenous and oral data are considered separately there is evidence that intrinsic clearance of R(+)-propranolol exceeds that of the pharmacologically active S(−)-propranolol. *In vitro* studies using human liver microsomes have shown that oxidation of propranolol to 4-hydroxypropranolol and norpropranolol favours the R-enantiomer while glucuronidation is stereoselective for the S-enantiomer (Silber and Riegelman, 1980; Von Bahr et al., 1982b). It is not clear, however, whether stereoselective oxidation of R-propranolol fully accounts for the observed difference in presystemic elimination between the enantiomers. An additional consideration is that this difference in intrinsic clearance may be partly attributable to stereoselective differences in protein binding (Wilkinson and Shand, 1975). It has been reported that S-propranolol is more highly bound than R-propranolol to plasma proteins (Walle et al., 1983). Thus, the lower plasma free fraction of S-propranolol may also be a determinant of the greater area

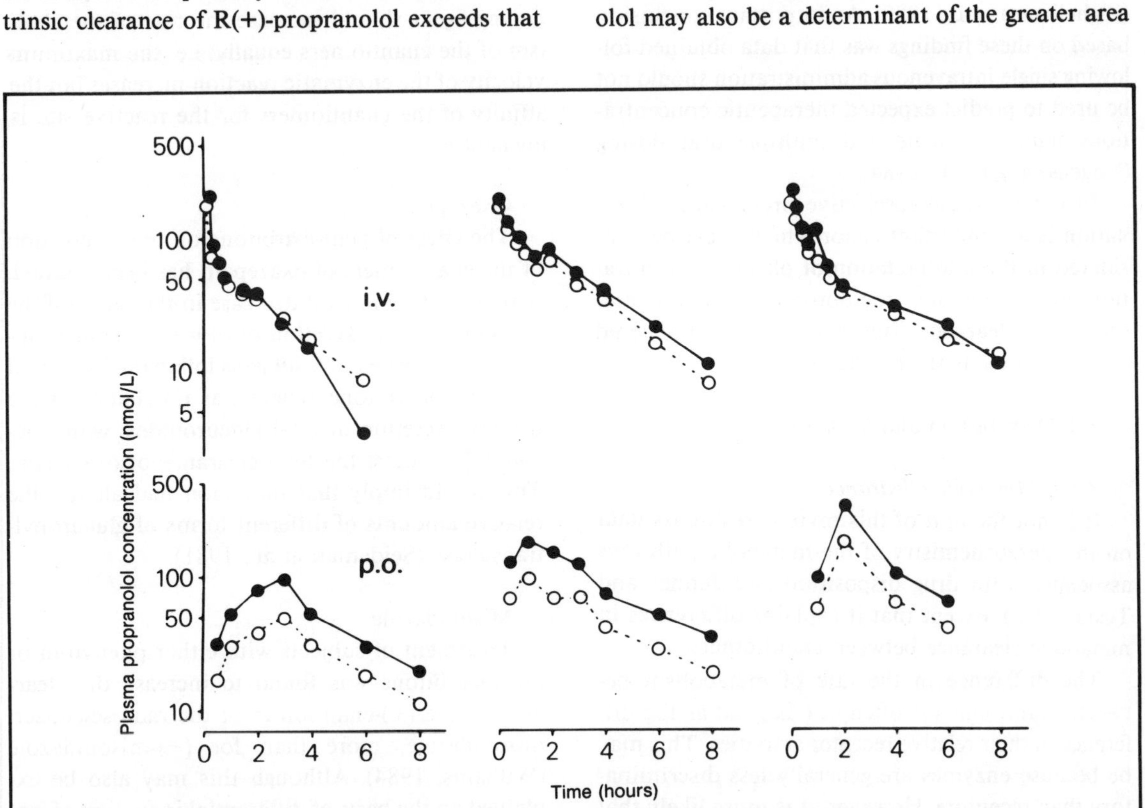

Fig. 2. Plasma concentrations of (+)- and (−)-propranolol obtained in 3 subjects after administration of racemic (±)-propranolol. A dose of 40mg propranolol was given orally (PO) and 5mg intravenously (IV); O---O = (+)-propranolol; ●—● = (−)-propranolol (after Von Bahr et al., 1982a; reproduced with permission of the authors and Blackwell Scientific Publications Ltd).

under the plasma concentration-time curve (AUC) observed for this enantiomer following oral administration.

The most recent and best documented example of stereoselective first-pass metabolism is that of verapamil (Vogelgesang et al., 1984). This study demonstrated that, consistent with their relative and very high plasma clearances and differences in plasma protein binding (Eichelbaum et al., 1984), the systemic availability of the more active (−)-enantiomer was 2 to 3 times smaller than for the (+)-enantiomer. The data explained the apparent paradox that when intravenous and oral doses of verapamil were titrated to give the same plasma concentration, there was a 2- to 3-fold difference in pharmacodynamic response with respect to the dromotropic effect on atrioventricular conduction (Eichelbaum et al., 1980). An important conclusion based on these findings was that data obtained following single intravenous administration should not be used to predict expected therapeutic concentrations following single and multiple oral dosing (Vogelgesang et al., 1984).

In our view, stereoselective presystemic elimination is an important factor which must be considered in the interpretation of plasma concentrations of propranolol, metoprolol, verapamil and other high clearance drugs which are administered and measured as their racemates.

3.3 Distribution and Clearance

3.3.1 Metabolic Clearance

It is not the aim of this review to discuss data on the stereochemistry of the metabolic pathways associated with drug disposition (see Jenner and Testa, 1973), except that it explains differences in metabolic clearance between enantiomers.

The difference in the rate of metabolism between enantiomers is often not as great as the difference in their relative receptor activities. This may be because enzymes are generally less discriminatory than receptors. However, it is more likely that this is because of the number of enzymatic steps involved in the metabolic clearance of a drug. Competing pathways may exhibit stereoselectivity in opposite directions for enantiomers, such as discussed above for propranolol. Additionally, any metabolic pathway may be catalysed by a number of isoenzymes, each of which may be highly stereoselective for an enantiomer. Finally, the stereoselectivity of enzymes (and receptors) will depend on the proximity of the asymmetric centre to the respective binding sites. Each of these factors may moderate any stereoselective difference in intrinsic free clearance. (The effects of tissue and protein binding on metabolic clearance are discussed in section 3.3.3.)

Evidence for stereoselective isoenzymes comes from studies of the effects of inducing agents on the clearance of enantiomers. It would be expected that if a pair of enantiomers were substrates for the same enzyme, then treatment with an enzyme-inducing agent should increase the rate of metabolism of the enantiomers equally; i.e. the maximum velocity of the enzymatic reaction increases but the affinity of the enantiomers for the reactive site is unchanged.

Oxazepam

The effect of pentobarbitone on the disposition of the enantiomers of oxazepam has been studied. A small but significant decrease in the ratios of the 24-hour urinary excretion of (+)- to (−)-glucuronides was observed in 6 subjects following treatment with pentobarbitone. There was no change in the urinary excretion of total glucuronides, which account for almost the total clearance of oxazepam. This would imply that induction had altered the relative amounts of different forms of glucuronyltransferase (Seideman et al., 1981).

Misonidazole

Treatment of subjects with either phenytoin or phenobarbitone was found to increase the clearance of the (+)-enantiomer of the radiosensitiser, misonidazole, more than for (−)-misonidazole (Williams, 1984). Although this may also be explained on the basis of differential induction of isoenzymes, it is likely that this effect was the result of differential induction of a metabolic pathway specific for the (+)-enantiomer.

2-Arylpropionic Acids

A novel stereospecific pathway is that associated with the metabolic clearance of the inactive R-enantiomers of the 2-arylpropionic acids. Interest in the stereochemistry of these non-steroidal anti-inflammatory drugs was aroused by observations that the differences in potency between the enantiomers of 2-arylpropionic acids in *in vitro* tests of anti-inflammatory activity were much greater than the differences in *in vivo* models. For instance, S(+)-ibuprofen is 160 times more potent than R(−)-ibuprofen in the inhibition of prostaglandin synthetase using bovine seminal vesicle preparations, while *in vivo*, using the acetylcholine writhing test in the mouse or pain threshold in the rat, S-ibuprofen has only 1.4 times the potency of its enantiomer (Adams et al., 1976). These observations together with data showing that urinary metabolites following administration of racemic drug were predominately dextrorotatory (Mills et al., 1973), led to the suggestion that there was an *in vivo* pathway for the stereospecific inversion of the inactive R-2-arylpropionic acids to their active S-enantiomers.

The relative *in vivo* and *in vitro* activities of the 2-arylpropionates have been summarised recently by Hutt and Caldwell (1984).

Data on the mechanism of this inversion (Nakamura et al., 1980) suggest that R-ibuprofen is stereospecifically activated by formation of its coenzyme A thioester, while S-ibuprofen does not appear to be a substrate for the ibuprofen CoA synthetase. R-ibuprofen-CoA is then racemised by ibuprofen-CoA racemase and following hydrolysis, R- and S-ibuprofen are released. Similarities of the mechanism with the *in vivo* racemisation of methylmalonic acid have led to our hypothesis that the enzyme responsible for racemisation of ibuprofen-CoA is methylmalonyl-CoA racemase (Lee et al., 1984).

The literature on the metabolic chiral inversion of 2-arylpropionic acids has been reviewed recently by Hutt and Caldwell (1983). The pharmacokinetics of this inversion and the disposition of the enantiomers in man have been poorly defined, partly because of the use of analytical methodology which was often non-discriminatory for the individual optical isomers.

The elimination of the enantiomers of 2-arylpropionic acids in man using stereospecific assays has been studied for benoxaprofen, carprofen, fenoprofen, indoprofen and ibuprofen. Bopp et al. (1979) demonstrated in 3 subjects that following administration of 400mg R(−)-benoxaprofen there was immediate appearance of S(+)-benoxaprofen whose concentrations exceeded that of the R-enantiomer from 48 hours onwards. It was inferred from these data that there was approximately a 50% inversion of R- to S-benoxaprofen, and Simmonds et al. (1980) estimated the half-life of inversion to be 108 hours in man.

Recently, we have characterised in detail the pharmacokinetics and extent of inversion of ibuprofen enantiomers in 4 volunteers following administration of racemic ibuprofen, R-ibuprofen and S-ibuprofen. Data was obtained by HPLC analysis of the diastereomeric S-2-octyl esters of ibuprofen (Lee et al., 1984). An estimated mean of 63 ± 6% of R-ibuprofen was inverted stereospecifically to S-ibuprofen (Lee et al., 1985) [fig. 3].

Data on the pharmacokinetics of the enantiomers of fenoprofen are of particular interest because of the apparent avidity of the inversion process (Rubin et al., 1985). However, in this study only racemic drug was administered, and consequently the relative clearances of the enantiomers and the fraction inverted is uncertain. This is an example of a drug for which total racemic drug concentrations are very similar to the concentration of active drug.

One 2-arylpropionic acid for which no inversion has been observed in man is indoprofen. No difference in either plasma or total urine concentrations of S-indoprofen was observed following administration of S-indoprofen (100mg) and R,S-indoprofen (200mg) to normal volunteers (Tamassia et al., 1984). Carprofen may also demonstrate little, if any, inversion (Stoltenborg et al., 1981).

All of the 2-arylpropionic acids, with the exception of naproxen, are administered as their racemates. It is likely that a factor contributing to the interindividual variability in response to many of

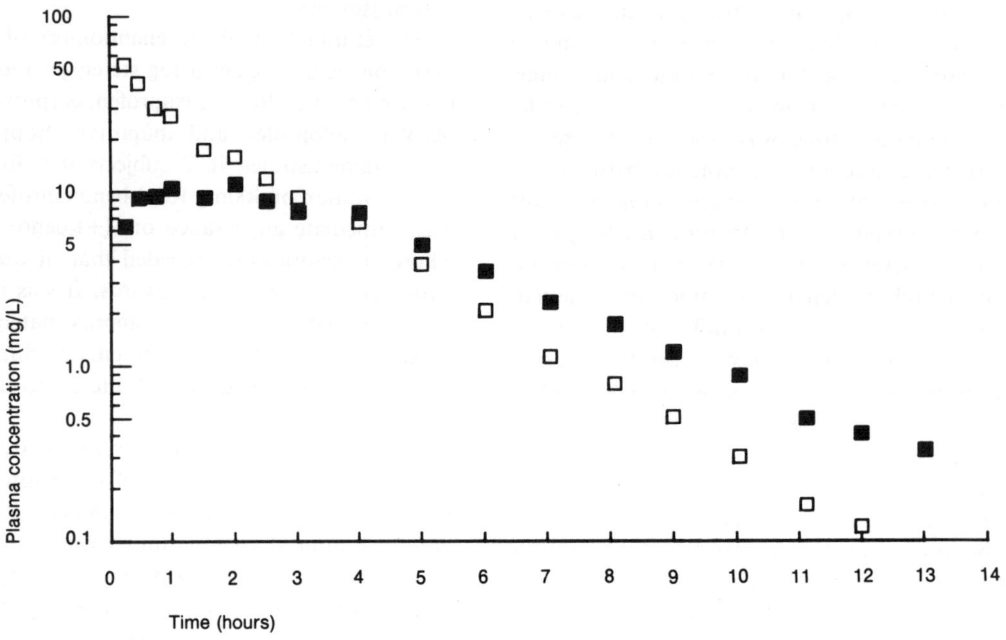

Fig. 3. The plasma concentration-time profile of R-ibuprofen (□), showing the formation and elimination of S-ibuprofen (■) in a single subject following oral administration of a solution of 400mg R-ibuprofen (after Lee et al., 1985).

these non-steroidal anti-inflammatory drugs is the variability in the extent of inversion of R- to S-enantiomer between individuals.

Coumarin Anticoagulants

The importance of knowing the clearances of the individual enantiomers of a drug for an understanding of the relative *in vivo* activities of those enantiomers is illustrated by the example of nicoumalone (acenocoumarol). Nicoumalone, along with the other coumarin anticoagulants warfarin and phenprocoumon, is administered as the racemate. For warfarin and phenprocoumon the S(−)-enantiomers are 2 to 5 times more potent than their R(+) counterparts. However, for nicoumalone the reverse activity has been reported, with R(+)-nicoumalone being several times more potent than the S(−)-enantiomer (Meinertz et al., 1978).

The reason for the reversal of the relative activities for the enantiomers of nicoumalone has been addressed by Godbillon et al. (1981). Data from this study revealed large differences between the pharmacokinetic parameters of the enantiomers. The ratios of the total body clearances of S- to R-nicoumalone were 10.0 and 13.7 in 2 subjects, while the ratios of the steady-state volumes of distribution were 1.9 and 1.4, respectively. These data demonstrate that the unpredicted greater anticoagulant activity of R-nicoumalone was due to its much lower plasma clearance.

3.3.2 Renal Clearance

The renal clearance of metoprolol has been found to be stereoselective for the inactive R-enantiomer (Lennard et al., 1983), and low clearance drugs such as warfarin with stereoselective differences in protein binding might also be expected to demonstrate stereoselective renal clearance. However, as renal excretion is only a minor route of elimination for metoprolol and warfarin, stereoselectivity of renal clearance will be unimportant clinically. Stereoselective renal clearance may occur for a drug which is actively secreted and/or reabsorbed. This may occur for both a high or a low renal clearance drug but there are no published data on this facet of renal function.

Stereoselectivity in filtration at the glomerulus will depend mainly on stereoselective differences in unbound (i.e. filterable) levels of the drug.

3.3.3 Distribution

The enantiomers of a drug may be distributed differently within the body as the result of differences in either tissue or protein binding.

Tissue Binding

Little is known about the stereoselectivity of tissue binding of enantiomers, but this factor may contribute to observed *in vivo* differences in enantiomer activity.

β-Adrenoceptor blockers: Stereoselective uptake by the heart has been demonstrated for S(−)-propranolol in rats (Kawashima et al., 1976) and this was suggested as the reason for the more rapid elimination of the R(+)-enantiomer in this species. The extravascular binding of S-propranolol is also greater than for R-propranolol in the dog (Bai et al., 1983). Similarly, a study of the tissue distribution of the enantiomers of timolol in the rat found that (−)-timolol was taken up much more avidly by the particulate fraction of heart, lung and brain than the (+)-enantiomer, which was bound only to nonspecific sites (Tocco et al., 1976). Evidence in this study suggested that the selectivity of binding was β-adrenoceptor related. In all cases, selective tissue binding should increase the elimination half-life of the more highly bound enantiomer and may contribute to differences in enantiomer concentrations at the relevant receptor.

2-Arylpropionic acids: A potential stereoselective pathway of tissue uptake is that relating to the disposition of the enantiomers of ibuprofen and other 2-arylpropionic acids. It has been reported that in rats treated long term with ibuprofen, there is a gradual accumulation of ibuprofen into fat (Adams et al., 1969). This is released very slowly (half-life approximately 6 days), while the corresponding plasma elimination half-life is about 2 hours. Furthermore, it has been demonstrated using rat liver and small intestine, that fenoprofen, ketoprofen and ibuprofen are incorporated into hybrid triglycerides (Caldwell and Marsh, 1983; Fears et al., 1978; Fears and Richards, 1981) presumably via formation of the CoA thioesters. As discussed above, this step is apparently stereospecific, in the case of ibuprofen, for the R-enantiomer; although S-ibuprofen CoA ester is formed via the racemase. It is likely that overall formation of hybrid triglycerides and uptake of 2-arylpropionic acids into fat will occur stereoselectively (Williams and Day, 1985). This is an interesting phenomenon although its clinical relevance is not known. It has been suggested that toxicity may be associated with formation of hybrid triglycerides as they may disrupt normal lipid metabolism and membrane function (Caldwell and Marsh, 1983).

Distribution into Saliva

The excretion of drugs into saliva may be considered a distributional or recycling phase of drug disposition, similar to the process of enterohepatic recycling. In general, it is believed that acidic drugs partition between saliva and plasma by passive diffusion in a manner that is dependent upon the pH of plasma and saliva, the pKa of the drug, and the unbound fraction of drug in plasma (Graham, 1982). However, this may not be true for basic drugs. In a recent study of the disposition of the enantiomers of tocainide it was found that the mean saliva to plasma ratio for the more active S(+)-enantiomer was 2.07, and 3.68 for the R(−)-enantiomer. These ratios were greater than predicted and showed that not only was there a stereoselective distribution of tocainide into saliva but that this occurred by a process of active secretion (Pillai et al., 1984). This finding highlights the problems associated with attempts to correlate plasma and salivary drug concentrations and again confirms the stereoselective nature of drug disposition.

Protein Binding

The binding sites on albumin and α_1-acid glycoproteins (αAGP) are generally considered to be non-stereoselective. However, the asymmetry of the plasma proteins results in a diastereomeric relationship between a pair of protein-drug enantiomer complexes, i.e. the dissociation constants for the binding of enantiomers will be expected to be different and it is only the magnitude of this difference which is in question.

The first stereoselective binding interaction described for human serum albumin (HSA) was with tryptophan (McMenamy and Oncley, 1958). L-Tryptophan was found to bind to a single site with an affinity of about 100 times that for D-tryptophan. Studies of the stereoselective binding of drug enantiomers to plasma proteins have been reviewed by Alebic-Kolbah et al. (1979) but this aspect of plasma protein binding has received little attention. The differences in affinity which have been described so far are not nearly so great for other drugs as for tryptophan. The exception to this is oxazepam hemisuccinate, whose (+)-enantiomer binds to a single site on human serum albumin with an affinity 40 times that for the (−)-enantiomer (Muller and Wollert, 1975a). Contrary to earlier understanding (Muller and Wollert, 1975b), recent data suggest that the tryptophan and benzodiazepine sites are 2 distinct stereoselective binding sites (Wanwimolruk, 1983).

Protein binding by αAGP is important for basic drugs and recent evidence shows that this binding is also stereoselective. αAGP has been shown to favour the binding of S-propranolol over R-propranolol (Albani et al., 1984; Bai et al., 1983; Walle et al., 1983), and S(+)-disopyramide over its (R(−)-enantiomer (Lima et al., 1984; Valdivieso et al., 1983). The stereoselective binding of αAGP and human serum albumin may not be in the same direction. While αAGP favoured the binding of S-propranolol, human serum albumin was found to favour the binding of R-propranolol (Walle et al., 1983).

Although differences in affinity between enantiomers for plasma proteins are not as great as for binding with receptors, differences in protein binding can be important. For drugs of *low intrinsic clearance*, the total body clearance is directly proportional to its free fraction (Wilkinson and Shand, 1975). For those drugs which are highly protein bound such as warfarin, phenprocoumon and ibuprofen, a small change in binding can result in a large change in drug clearance. The variability of the elimination of racemic warfarin in rats has been shown to be largely attributable to differences in protein binding between rats (Yacobi and Levy, 1975). Similarly, Yacobi et al. (1976) found a significant correlation between total body clearance and free fraction of warfarin in a study of 31 patients with cardiovascular disease.

It is reasonable to assume, therefore, that part of the intra- and interindividual variability in elimination between the enantiomers of drugs could be due to differences in protein binding of the enantiomers. The clinical significance of differential changes in protein binding of enantiomers is illustrated below (section 4.2).

Plasma protein binding may also affect the elimination rate of *high intrinsic clearance* drugs. The more highly bound enantiomer will have a shorter half-life (assuming equal intrinsic free clearances) as the result of a smaller volume of distribution (Evans et al., 1973). This shorter half-life will decrease the time to steady-state, while steady-state total concentrations will be the same for both enantiomers after intravenous administration. However, the more highly bound enantiomer will have a lower concentration of free drug available for interaction at the receptor or enzymatic binding site. In contrast, following oral administration, plasma concentrations are dependent on the intrinsic clearances of the enantiomers, which are in turn influenced by the extent that the enantiomers are bound to plasma proteins. In this case, even though total concentrations are different, the free plasma concentrations of the enantiomers will be similar.

The protein binding of drug enantiomers should be considered when estimating their relative potencies. Jahnchen et al. (1976) have reported that S-phenprocoumon is 1.6 to 2.6 times more active than R-phenprocoumon based on relative areas under the prothrombin complex activity-time curves and 1.5 to 2.3 times more potent when total plasma concentrations that elicited the same anticoagulant effect were compared. However, the difference in potency is even greater when corrected for unbound concentrations (Jahnchen et al., 1976), which were shown to be up to 2 times greater for the R-enantiomer (Brown et al., 1977; Jahnchen et al., 1976). A correction for protein binding thus gives an estimated potency ratio for S- to R-phenprocoumon of approximately 3.0 to 5.0. This value is similar to those reported for S- and R-warfarin of 3.8 (Breckenridge et al., 1974), 3.4 (O'Reilly, 1974) and 4.6 (Bjornsson et al., 1977). However, these warfarin potency ratios were also uncorrected for the R- to S- free fraction ratios which were found to range from 0.93 to 2.3 (Yacobi and Levy, 1977). Toon and Trager (1984) have recently reported a relative potency of S- to R-warfarin of 8 based on their estimations of free concentrations. There is evidence that potency ratios for warfarin enantiomers are dose and concentration dependent (Wingard et al., 1978).

It has been suggested that plasma protein binding of drugs might be used as an indicator of their relative activities at the receptors. This is an unlikely application. S-Warfarin is the more potent enantiomer and is more highly bound to human serum albumin (Sellers and Koch-Weser, 1975). In the case of propranolol, however, human serum albumin favours the less potent R-enantiomer, although overall plasma protein binding favours the active S-enantiomer (Walle et al., 1983).

4. Importance of Enantiomers in Drug Interactions

Administration of racemic drug allows for potential enantiomer-enantiomer interactions. One enantiomer may compete with the other for binding at plasma protein binding sites, the active sites of enzymes, or at receptors. Furthermore, drug interactions may occur stereoselectively such that a greater interaction may be observed with one enantiomer than with the other, i.e. drug-enantiomer interactions. In the assessment of drug interactions, determination of unbound enantiomer concentrations is preferred as these give more insight into the mechanism of such interactions.

4.1 Enantiomer-Enantiomer Interactions

The extraction ratio of propranolol in rats decreases with increasing dosage due to saturation of the enzyme and tissue binding sites (Shand et al., 1973). In such a situation it is likely that the presence of the inactive enantiomer will increase the availability of the active enantiomer, by competing with it for these binding sites.

Propoxyphene Enantiomers

Although there are no reports of such an interaction in man, Murphy et al. (1976) have observed this effect in rats for the enantiomers of propoxyphene. They observed that oral administration of (−)-propoxyphene significantly increased the plasma concentrations and enhanced the analgesic activity of (+)-propoxyphene due to a substantial increase in the systemic availability of (+)-propoxyphene.

Amphetamine Enantiomers

Competition at enzymatic binding sites may affect enantiomer clearance. R(−)-amphetamine when incubated alone with microsomes forms the hydroxylamine metabolite more rapidly than S(+)-amphetamine. However, when the racemate is incubated, it is the S-enantiomer which is preferentially oxidised. It is concluded that although S-amphetamine has the lower rate of metabolism, it has the higher affinity for the oxidative enzyme (Cho and Wright, 1978). Similar findings have been reported for the metabolism of the enantiomers of p-chloroamphetamine by rabbit liver microsomal preparations (Ames and Frank, 1982).

Methadone Enantiomers

There is some evidence that S(+)-methadone antagonises the respiratory depressant and miotic effects of R(−)-methadone (Olsen et al., 1977). Instead of the expected 2-fold difference in activity between R- and R,S-methadone, the observed potency ratio was 3.0 for respiratory depression and 2.7 for miosis. It is likely that there is competitive binding between the enantiomers for the receptors.

Propranolol Enantiomers

An interesting enantiomer-enantiomer interaction is that which occurs between the optical isomers of propranolol. The S-enantiomer has been shown to decrease cardiac output in man by 25%, and, liver blood flow in monkeys was decreased by 35%; the R-enantiomer was inactive in these studies (Nies et al., 1973a,b, 1976). Propranolol is a high clearance drug and consequently this stereospecific haemodynamic effect of S-propranolol is a significant factor affecting its own clearance as well as decreasing the clearance of the R-enantiomer when propranolol is administered as the racemate. In support of this conclusion, Nies et al. (1973b) found that R-propranolol had a higher clearance than S-propranolol in the monkey due to the absence of effect on liver blood flow, while Branch et al. (1973) showed that when flow was kept constant in perfused rat liver, the elimination of R- and R,S-propranolol were very similar.

Ibuprofen Enantiomers

Enantiomers may compete with each other for protein binding sites, although there are no studies which have demonstrated this potential interaction. Recently, we have observed that the clearance of R-ibuprofen in man is greater when administered as part of the racemate than when administered alone (Lee et al., 1985). The data also implied that the clearance of S-ibuprofen was similarly affected by administration of the isomers together. The explanation for this phenomenon may be either non-linearity of protein binding of the individual enantiomers or non-linearity of binding brought about by competition between R- and S-ibuprofen. We are presently examining the binding characteristics of the ibuprofen enantiomers to clarify this point.

4.2 Enantiomer-Drug Interactions

4.2.1 Stereoselective Interactions with Warfarin

Warfarin, more than any other drug used clinically as its racemate, has been investigated for a stereoselective basis for known or suspected drug interactions. The following discussion illustrates the importance of studying the enantiomeric disposition of drugs in suspected cases of drug-drug interactions.

Warfarin-Phenylbutazone Interaction

Interactions with the enantiomers of warfarin became of interest when it was demonstrated that the reported interaction between phenylbutazone and warfarin was stereoselective (Lewis et al., 1974; O'Reilly et al., 1980a). An increase in the clearance of R-warfarin with a concomitant decrease in the clearance of the more active S-enantiomer resulted in the original observation of an increased pharmacological response with no change in elimination half-life for the racemic drug. It was initially suggested that the mechanism of this interaction was one of protein binding displacement (Aggeler et al., 1967). However, this was subsequently discounted on theoretical grounds as it is now known that simple plasma protein displacement increases the free fraction of a low clearance drug but does not alter the free concentration, and hence the pharmacological effect is unperturbed. The explanation that phenylbutazone inhibits the metabolism of S-warfarin while inducing that of R-warfarin (Lewis et al., 1974; O'Reilly et al., 1980a; Serlin and Breckinridge, 1983), although possible, appears unlikely. Rather, the combination of protein displacement and metabolic inhibition is a more satisfactory hypothesis which finds support in the recent results of Toon and Trager (1983, 1984).

In an *in vitro* study of the protein binding of the enantiomers of warfarin, Toon and Trager (1983, 1984) reported that phenylbutazone and sulphinpyrazone stereoselectively displaced the R-enantiomer, although O'Reilly and Goulart (1981) were unable to find any effect with sulphinpyrazone. Banfield et al. (1983) found in a study of 3 volunteers that phenylbutazone caused displacement of warfarin from plasma protein binding sites, although this was not clearly stereoselective. Furthermore, they found a large decrease (78%) in un-

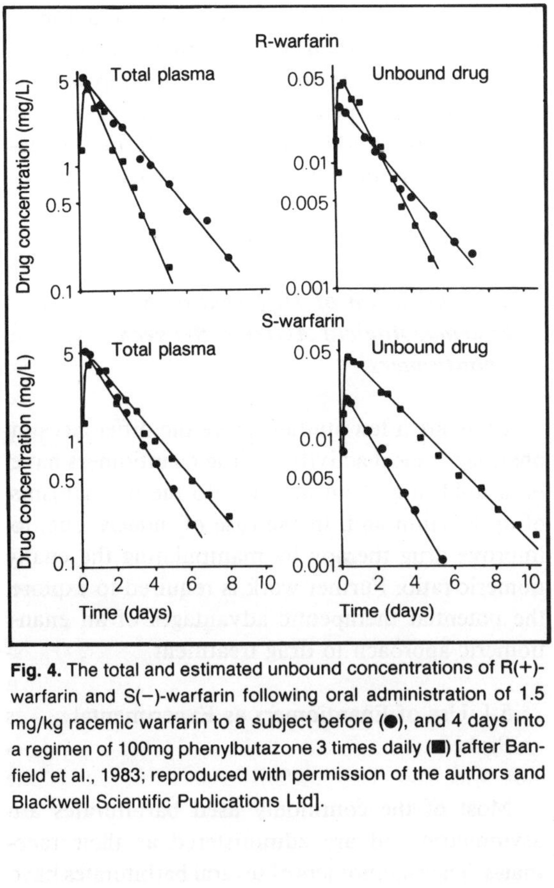

Fig. 4. The total and estimated unbound concentrations of R(+)-warfarin and S(−)-warfarin following oral administration of 1.5 mg/kg racemic warfarin to a subject before (●), and 4 days into a regimen of 100mg phenylbutazone 3 times daily (■) [after Banfield et al., 1983; reproduced with permission of the authors and Blackwell Scientific Publications Ltd].

bound clearance for S-warfarin while the observed decrease in unbound clearance for R-warfarin was much smaller (25%) [fig. 4]. The total body clearance for R-warfarin increased while that for S-warfarin decreased – as reported previously (Lewis et al., 1974). According to these data, the expected increase in total clearance for S-warfarin as the result of protein binding displacement is more than offset by the inhibitory effect of phenylbutazone on its metabolism. In the case of the R-enantiomer, the smaller inhibitory effect is not sufficient to overcome the opposing increase in clearance due to protein binding displacement, and the overall effect is an increase in total body clearance. The complex combination of these pharmacokinetic interactions is such that clearance of racemic drug appears unchanged. The effect on the more active S-enantiomer, however, results in the observed augmentation of response when phenylbutazone is taken concurrently with racemic warfarin.

Interactions of Warfarin with Other Drugs

Stereoselective interactions with warfarin leading to augmentation of the hypoprothrombinaemic response have also been described for metronidazole (O'Reilly, 1976), co-trimoxazole (O'Reilly and Motley, 1979; O'Reilly, 1980), sulphinpyrazone (Bailey and Reddy, 1980; Davis and Johns, 1978; Gallus and Birkett, 1980; O'Reilly, 1982a), clofibrate (Bjornsson et al., 1977; O'Reilly et al., 1972), disulfiram (O'Reilly, 1981) and tienilic acid (ticrynafen) [O'Reilly, 1982b] and quinalbarbitone (O'Reilly et al., 1980b).

Data relevant to the mechanism by which these drugs potentiate the hypoprothrombinaemic response to warfarin are summarised in table I. In general, it appears that drug interactions with warfarin have a pharmacokinetic rather than pharmacodynamic basis. Stereoselective inhibition of

Table I. Basis for drug interactions with warfarin enantiomers (i.e. R- and S-warfarin)

Drug	Pharmacokinetic mechanism				Pharmacodynamic potentiation	
	protein binding[a] displacement		enzyme inhibition			
	R	S	R	S	R	S
Phenylbutazone	R ≤ S		R < S		[b]	[b]
Sulphinpyrazone	R < S		R < S		[b]	[b]
Metronidazole	?[c]	?[c]	[b]	S	[b]	[b]
Co-trimoxazole	?[c]	?[c]	R < S		[b]	[b]
Clofibrate	R = S		?[c]	?[c]	R = S	
Disulfiram	[b]	[b]	[b]	[b]	[b]	S
Tienilic acid	[b]	[b]	[b]	S	[b]	[b]
Quinalbarbitone	?[c]	?[c]	R = S		[b]	[b]

a The unimportance of protein binding interactions on the hypoprothrombinaemic response is discussed in the text.
b No apparent effect.
c Data unavailable or uncertain.

the metabolism of the S-enantiomer is generally observed and this may also be associated with concurrent stereoselective displacement of S-warfarin from plasma protein binding sites, as discussed in detail above for phenylbutazone.

The data on the interaction of clofibrate with warfarin are difficult to assess. Veronich et al. (1979) reported that clofibrate increased the free fractions of both warfarin enantiomers equally *in vitro*, suggesting that the interaction occurred at secondary binding sites which are generally considered to be less or non-stereoselective. *In vivo*, Bjornsson et al. (1977) observed an increase in clearance and volume of distribution for R-warfarin in each of the 4 subjects investigated consistent with protein binding displacement. However, the effects on the pharmacokinetics of S-warfarin were variable. It was concluded that the interaction resulting in potentiation of hypoprothrombinaemia was pharmacodynamic, as simple protein binding displacement was not expected to increase free warfarin concentrations and hence to affect anticoagulation.

O'Reilly (1982a) has noted that these interactions generally do not have significant clinical consequences when patients begin treatment with both drugs, as simultaneous monitoring of the prothrombin time leads to stabilisation at a lower dose of warfarin than would otherwise be required in the absence of the second drug. The problem arises when these drugs are added to a stabilised regimen of warfarin as this may precipitate a haemorrhagic episode.

In all of the above interaction studies with warfarin, determination of the unbound clearances of the enantiomers of warfarin, as carried out by Banfield et al. (1983), would allow a clearer distinction to be made between the pharmacokinetic and pharmacodynamic contributions to these interactions.

4.2.2 Stereoselective Interactions with Other Drugs

Apart from interactions with warfarin, the study of stereoselective drug interactions has been almost totally ignored. Two exceptions have already been discussed. These are the effects of the induction of misonidazole metabolism by phenytoin and phenobarbitone, and the induction of oxazepam glucuronidation by pentobarbitone. The results of these studies together with the warfarin interactions demonstrate the need to investigate the enantiomeric disposition of drugs in suspected cases of drug-drug interactions.

5. Application of Differences in Pharmacological Activity Between Enantiomers

There are a few studies where the differences in pharmacological activity of drug enantiomers have been used to give an insight into the mechanisms of drug action and, in the case of indacrinone, to improve drug therapy by manipulating the enantiomeric ratio. Further work is required to explore the potential therapeutic advantages of an enantiomeric approach to drug treatment.

5.1 Use of Enantiomers as Experimental Probes

Most of the commonly used barbiturates are asymmetric and are administered as their racemates. The enantiomers of several barbiturates have been shown to have different intensities of activity (and even opposite activities), e.g. (−)-methylphenobarbitone is an anaesthetic while the (+)-enantiomer is inactive in this respect (Steen and Michenfelder, 1978). This difference in activity has been used to examine the mechanism of the protective effect of barbiturates in cerebral hypoxia. A study in mice demonstrated that (+)-methylphenobarbitone did not increase survival time, while the (−)-enantiomer significantly increased this time. It was concluded from these data that the protective effect of barbiturates is related to a stereospecific receptor that is the same for protection and anaesthesia. This assumes, however, that stereoselective metabolism of methylphenobarbitone enantiomers to phenobarbitone is not a significant consideration in the mechanism of action of this drug.

The β-blocking activity of S-propranolol is approximately 100 times greater than R-propranolol, while their membrane-stabilising and local anaesthetic activities are approximately equal (Barrett and Cullum, 1968). The differential activities of the propranolol enantiomers have been used to distinguish between the β-blocking and membrane-stabilising mechanisms of action of the racemic drug. The lack of β-activity of the R-enantiomer has been used to show that the effectiveness of propranolol in the suppression of essential tremor is due to the β-blocking effect of the S-enantiomer and not to its membrane-stabilising activity (Larsen and Teravainen, 1982). Conversely, the protective effect of propranolol in experimental myocardial, renal and cerebral tissue ischaemia was shown to be unrelated to β-activity, as R-propranolol was equally as effective as the racemate (Little et al., 1982). Finally, the differential effect of R- and S-propranolol on liver blood flow discussed earlier has been used to separate the effects of liver blood flow from the intrinsic clearance in studies of this high clearance drug (Nies et al., 1976).

5.2 Manipulation of the Enantiomeric Ratio

It has been pointed out that a racemic drug is in reality a fixed-ratio combination of 2 drugs (Ariens, 1984). This one-to-one combination may not be optimal even when there is some benefit in having both enantiomers present. This point is illustrated by data for the loop-acting diuretic indacrinone. Racemic indacrinone generally produces hyperuricaemia along with its desired diuretic action, although there may be transient uricosuric activity. The R(−)-enantiomer is the more potent natriuretic and the S(+)-enantiomer has a higher uricosuric/natriuretic potency ratio (Field et al., 1984; Irvin et al., 1980; Vlasses et al., 1981). However, the observed *in vivo* differences in activity may be largely attributable to stereoselective pharmacokinetic differences, as has been observed for the disposition of indacrinone in rhesus monkeys (Zacchei et al., 1982). On the basis of the relative difference in pharmacological activity of the enantiomers, Tobert et al. (1981) studied the dose-response relationship for the hypouricaemic and uricosuric activities of S-indacrinone in the presence of a fixed dose of R-indacrinone in normal volunteers. They showed that a R/S ratio of 10/40 (mg/mg) was isouricaemic while a ratio of 10/80 decreased plasma urate by 13%. More recently, Vlasses et al. (1984) reported that a 10/40 combination of the enantiomers had a significant hypouricaemic effect when compared with placebo-treated controls. Despite this conflict in findings, both studies support the conclusion that a ratio of S- to R-indacrinone of greater than 1 may lead to a significant increase in therapeutic index. It has been suggested that the diuretic profile may be further improved by the use of amiloride to give an isouricaemic, isokaluretic combination (Blaine et al., 1982).

These studies represent the first attempts to take advantage of differences in enantiomeric activities to optimise the therapeutic activity of a drug.

5.3 Use of One Enantiomer

In general, drugs of natural product origin are enantiomerically pure. However, there are some synthetic drugs which are resolved to give the active enantiomer. An example of such a drug is naproxen. The marketed drug, Naprosyn®, contains only the S(+)-enantiomer. The rationale for this resolution is not entirely clear, although the manufacturer's literature points to the possibility of undesirable side effects and the renal burden of clearing 'inactive' R(−)-naproxen (Feldman, 1976). However, as there is likely to be significant inversion of inactive R- to active S-naproxen (see section 3.3.1), and as naproxen has a very low renal clearance, the arguments for resolving the 2-arylpropionic acids to improve their clinical efficacy are not as clear as for other classes of racemic drugs.

Resolution of dopa for the treatment of Parkinson's disease was shown to be therapeutically advantageous. The use of D,L-dopa was associated with a significant incidence of granulocytopenia which was no longer a problem when only the L-enantiomer was used (Cotzias et al., 1969). Other catecholamines such as methyldopa and adrenaline (epinephrine) are also used as the active enantiomer alone.

Another drug used in an enantiomerically pure form is timolol. S(−)-Timolol is applied topically for the treatment of glaucoma but is not without some incidence of undesirable side effects due to β-adrenoceptor blockade. Recently, a study has demonstrated that R(+)-timolol, which has only 1/80 the activity of the S-enantiomer at extraocular receptors, also causes a significant decrease in intraocular pressure (Keates and Stone, 1984). The mechanism of this action is uncertain, but the data suggest that there is the potential for the use of this enantiomer for treating glaucoma without the risk of systemic side effects.

Basic pharmacological data on the differences in activity between enantiomers suggest that there are many other drugs for which an increase in therapeutic index might be obtained by using the appropriate enantiomer rather than the racemic drug. A discussion of some examples of drugs representative of major drug groups which potentially fall into this category follows.

5.3.1 Verapamil

The calcium antagonist activity of verapamil is attributable primarily to the (−)-enantiomer and it is also the (−)-enantiomer which leads to the greater reduction in myocardial oxygen consumption (Kaumann and Serur, 1975; Raschack, 1976; Saikawa and Arita, 1980; Satoh et al., 1980). The (+)-enantiomer has the greater sodium antagonist activity (Bayer et al., 1975) and, unlike (−)-verapamil, it has little negative chronotropic, dromotropic or inotropic effects in dogs at doses which double coronary blood flow (Satoh et al., 1980). The (+)-enantiomer also has been found to be responsible for the dromotropic effects of racemic verapamil on atrioventricular conduction in man (Echizen and Eichelbaum, 1984). Consequently, Satoh et al. (1980) suggested that (+)-verapamil may be a more desirable antianginal drug as it has less cardiodepressant action. The (+)-enantiomer also has a 2 to 3 times greater systemic availability than the (−)-enantiomer in man (Vogelgesang et al., 1984), as discussed previously.

5.3.2 Pentazocine

Clinical studies have compared the analgesic, respiratory and subjective effects of the enantiomers of pentazocine. Both analgesia and side effects reside in the (−)-enantiomer. The (+)-enantiomer has little if any analgesic activity but it does have some side effects, notably sedation and increased sweating (Berkowitz, 1974; Forrest et al., 1969). It has also been found (Bellville and Forrest, 1968) that subjects are more likely to be happy and relaxed with the (−)-enantiomer, while subjects are more likely to be sad and anxious with the (+)-enantiomer. The data support the view that use of the (−)-enantiomer alone may lead to a decrease in the incidence and/or severity of subjective side effects associated with the use of this strong analgesic.

5.3.3 Methadone

Methadone is a drug of variable availability (Meresaar et al., 1981) whose primary pharmacological activity resides in the R(−)-enantiomer, although the relatively inactive S(+)-enantiomer may undergo first-pass metabolism (Smits and Myers, 1974) to (−)-α-normethadol, which has greater opiate activity than R-methadone (Horng et al., 1976). The pharmacokinetics of the methadone enantiomers have been studied following both single-dose administration in volunteers (Olsen et al., 1977) and long term treatment of patients (Kreek et al., 1979; Nakamura et al., 1982). These data, together with studies of the kinetics of racemic methadone (Verebely et al., 1975), suggest that elimination may be altered between short and long term dosing. The half-life of R-methadone may be up to approximately twice that of the S-enantiomer.

Judson et al. (1976) found no advantage in using R-methadone over the racemic drug for the treatment of patients in long term methadone maintenence programmes, although Kreek et al. (1979) have suggested that use of R-methadone alone my be desirable in the following situations:

1. To facilitate attempts to correlate plasma concentrations with symptoms of narcotic abstinence

2. In severe liver disease, to reduce the metatolic load on the liver
3. To more readily predict the period of drug action
4. To take advantage of the slower elimination of R-methadone and minimise daily fluctuations in plasma concentrations.

These considerationo are also relevant to the general argument for the use of enantiomers rather than racemic drugs.

5.3.4 Opiates

The potential for separating the analgesic activity from the physical dependency activity of the opioid agonists is an interesting possibility which has received some attention. In particular, derivatives of the benzomorphan nucleus have been investigated (Ager et al., 1969; May and Takeda, 1970; Shiotani, 1979) with very favourable separation of morphine-like effects from physical dependence capacity in certain animal species. Further studies along these lines in man may prove clinically beneficial.

5.3.5 Cyclophosphamide

Similarly, data suggest that cyclophosphamide could be better employed if the (−)-enantiomer was used. Cyclophosphamide is an interesting molecule in that its dissymmetry is due to a chiral phosphorus atom rather than a chiral carbon atom. Cox et al. (1976) showed that (−)-cyclophosphamide was twice as effective as the (+)-enantiomer in killing tumour cells, but their LD_{50}s were equal. Consequently, the therapeutic index for (−)-cyclophosphamide was approximately 2 times higher than that for (+)-cyclophosphamide, and it was also 1.3 times greater than that for the racemate. Therefore the (−)-enantiomer may be a less toxic antitumour drug.

Similar stereoselective differences have been reported for the less effective antitumour drug 4-methylcyclophosphamide (Farmer et al., 1977).

5.3.6 Quinalbarbitone (secobarbitone)

The biggest disadvantage of the use of barbiturates as anticonvulsants is their potent sedative side effects. In general, the sedative and anticonvulsant effects of the racemic barbiturates are not independent. However, the enantiomers of the barbiturates have differing qualitative activities. For example, S(−)- and R(+)-quinalbarbitone demonstrate equipotent anticonvulsant activity, while the S(−)-enantiomer is more toxic and is a more potent anaesthetic (Ho and Harris, 1981). The data suggest that R(+)-quinalbarbitone could be investigated as an anticonvulsant in its own right.

5.3.7 Misonidazole

It is not in all situations that the asymmetric centre plays a role in the efficacy of a drug. In such circumstances, one enantiomer may contribute to drug toxicity more than the other. Misonidazole is a drug under clinical trial as a radiosensitising agent for the treatment of slow-growing solid tumours. The drug suffers from dose-related neurotoxic side effects which are best related to the area under the plasma concentration-time curve. Radiation therapy is given at the time of peak tumour misonidazole concentrations and, following this treatment, rapid elimination of the drug is desirable. The radiation interacts with the nitro substituent of the imidazole ring to produce free radicals which cause cytotoxic interactions with cellular DNA. The asymmetric centre of misonidazole resides in the aliphatic side chain and does not influence free radical formation, i.e. free radicals will be equally generated by both enantiomers. However, clearance of the drug is stereoselective (Williams, 1984) and may be influenced by enzyme-inducing agents (Williams et al., 1983; Workman, 1979). It is likely that the enantiomers have different degrees of neurotoxicity, as will their respective metabolites. There remains the potential to further refine use of this drug by carrying out clinical trials with each of its enantiomers.

5.3.8 Warfarin

It has been shown that the prothrombin complex activity of equieffective doses of the enantiomers of warfarin are not significantly different over a dosing interval despite their pharmacokinetic differences (Wingard and Levy, 1977). This may suggest that there is little advantage in using one enantiomer over either the racemate or the other enantiomer. But there is potential for avoiding drug interactions with racemic drugs like warfarin by selecting the enantiomer least involved in interactions with other drugs (O'Reilly, 1976).

With this in mind, Wingard et al. (1978) analysed previously published data on warfarin (O'Reilly, 1974) and found that the maintenance dose of S-warfarin, but not R-warfarin, required to produce the same degree of anticoagulation as the racemate can be predicted. Consequently, in the event of a known or suspected drug interaction, transition from racemate to S-warfarin can be made. Unfortunately, most drug interactions appear to occur stereoselectively with the S-enantiomer. However, this does not preclude the use of R-warfarin alone when initiating anticoagulant therapy.

The above discussion is illustrative of specific instances where use of only the one enantiomer of a drug may be clinically advantageous. There may be situations where use of the racemate is advantageous. It has been suggested, for example, that if one enantiomer is pharmacologically inactive and also inhibits metabolism of the active enantiomer, then the inactive enantiomer may be used to prolong drug action (Anders et al., 1973). However, no situations of this type have yet been demonstrated. In general, a more satisfactory approach to therapeutics would be to investigate each enantiomer for clinical efficacy. In the absence of pharmacological activity of one of the enantiomers, racemic drug should not be used unless it has been demonstrated that there is no toxicity associated with the 'inactive' enantiomer. Even in this situation it is preferable to use only the active enantiomer to decrease the burden placed on renal and/or metabolic clearance mechanisms. Furthermore, this approach will lessen the potential for drug-enantiomer interactions and enantiomer-enantiomer interactions, both of pharmacokinetic and pharmacodynamic origin.

6. Conclusions

Many drugs are administered as their racemates despite the pharmacokinetic, and often large pharmacodynamic, differences between the enantiomers. A non-stereoseleltive approach to the study of optically active drugs is often not only inaccurate, but may also be misleading. This review emphasises the importance of studying the activity and disposition of the individual enantiomers. It is hoped that through a better understanding of the stereoselective pharmacology of optically active drugs their clinical use may be improved.

References

Adams, S.S.; Bough, R.G.; Cliffe, E.E.; Lessel, B. and Mills, R.F.N.: Absorption, distribution and toxicity of ibuprofen. Toxicology and Applied Pharmacology 15: 310-330 (1969).

Adams, S.S.; Bresloff, P. and Mason, C.G.: Pharmacological differences between the optical isomers of ibuprofen: Evidence for metabolic inversion of the (−)-isomer. Journal of Pharmacy and Pharmacology 28: 256-257 (1976).

Ager, J.H.; Jacobson, A.E. and May, E.L.: Separation of morphine-like effects by optical resolution. Levo isomers as strong analgetics and narcotic antagonists. Journal of Medicinal Chemistry 12: 288-289 (1969).

Aggeler, P.M.; O'Reilly, R.A.; Leong, L. and Kowitz, P.E.: Potentiation of anticoagulant effect of warfarin by phenylbutazone. New England Journal of Medicine 276: 496-501 (1967).

Albani, F.; Riva, R.; Contin, M. and Baruzzi, A.: Stereoselective binding of propranolol enantiomers to human α_1-acid glycoprotein and human plasma. British Journal of Clinical Pharmacology 18: 244-246 (1984).

Alebic-Kolbah, T.; Rendic, S.; Fuks, Z.; Sunjic, V. and Kajfez, F.: Enantioselectivity in the binding of drugs to serum proteins. Acta Pharmaceutica Jugoslavica 29: 53-70 (1979).

Allenmark, S.: Recent advances in methods of direct optical resolution. Journal of Biochemical and Biophysical Methods 9: 1-25 (1984).

Ames, M.M. and Frank, S.K.: Stereochemical aspects of parachloramphetamine metabolism. Biochemical Pharmacology 31: 5-9 (1982).

Anders, M.W.; Cooper, M.J. and Takemori, A.E.: Kinetics of microsomal metabolism and binding of enantiomerically related substrates. Drug Metabolism and Disposition 1: 642-644 (1973).

Ariens, E.J.: Stereochemistry, a basis for sophisticated nonsense in pharmacokinetics and clinical pharmacology. European Journal of Clinical Pharmacology 26: 663-668 (1984).

Ariens, E.J.; Soudijn, W. and Timmermans, P.B. (Eds): Stereochemistry and Biological Activity of Drugs (Blackwell Scientific Publications, Oxford, London 1983).

Bai, S.A.; Walle, U.K.; Wilson, M.J. and Walle, T.: Stereoselective binding of the (−)-enantiomer of propranolol to plasma and extravascular binding sites in the dog. Drug Metabolism and Disposition 11: 394-395 (1983).

Bailey, R.R. and Reddy, J.: Potentiation of warfarin action by sulphinpyrazone. Lancet 1: 254 (1980).

Banfield, C.; O'Reilly, R.; Chan, E. and Rowland, M.: Phenylbutazone interaction in man: Further stereochemical and metabolic considerations. British Journal of Clinical Pharmacology 16: 669-675 (1983).

Barlow, R.B.; Franks, F.M. and Pearson, J.D.M.: The relation between biological activity and the degree of resolution of optical isomers. Journal of Pharmacy and Pharmacology 24: 753-761 (1972).

Barrett, A.M. and Cullum, V.A.: The biological properties of the optical isomers of propranolol and their effects on cardiac arrhythmias. British Journal of Pharmacology 34: 43-55 (1968).
Bayer, R.; Kalusche, D.; Kaufmann, R. and Mannhold, R.: Inotropic and electrophysiological actions of verapamil and D600 in mammalian myocardium. Naunyn-Schmiedeberg's Archives of Pharmacology 290: 81-97 (1975).
Bellville, J.W. and Forrest, W.H.: Respiratory and subjective effects of d- and l-pentazocine. Clinical Pharmacology and Therapeutics 9: 142-151 (1968).
Berkowitz, B.: Pharmacokinetics and neurochemical effects of pentazocine and its optical isomers; in Braude et al. (Eds) Narcotic Antagonists, Advances in Biochemical Psychopharmacology, Vol. 8, pp. 395-430 (Raven Press, New York 1974).
Bjornsson, T.D.; Meffin, P.J. and Blaschke, T.F.: Interaction of clofibrate with warfarin. I. Effect of clofibrate on the disposition of the optical enantiomorphs of warfarin. Journal of Pharmacokinetics and Biopharmaceutics 5: 495-505 (1977).
Blaine, E.H.; Fanelli, G.M.; Irvin, J.D.; Tobert, J.A. and Davies, R.O.: Enantiomers of indacrinone: A new approach to producing an isouricemic diuretic. Clinical and Experimental Hypertension – Theory and Practice A4: 161-176 (1982).
Bopp, R.J.; Nash, J.F.; Ridolfo, A.S. and Shepard, E.R.: Stereoselective inversion of R(−)-benoxaprofen to the S(+)-enantiomer in humans. Drug Metabolism and Disposition 7: 356-359 (1979).
Branch, R.A.; Nies, A.S. and Shand, D.G.: The disposition of propranolol. VIII. Drug Metabolism and Disposition 1: 687-690 (1973).
Breckenridge, A.; Orme, M.; Wesseling, H.; Lewis, R.J. and Gibbons, R.: Pharmacokinetics and pharmacodynamics of the enantiomers of warfarin in man. Clinical Pharmacology and Therapeutics 15: 424-430 (1974).
Brown, N.A.; Jahnchen, E.; Muller, W.E. and Wollert, U.: Optical studies on the mechanism of the interaction of the enantiomers of the anticoagulant drugs phenprocoumon and warfarin with human serum albumin. Molecular Pharmacology 13: 70-79 (1977).
Cahn, R.S.; Ingold, C.K. and Prelog, V.: The specification of asymmetric configuration in organic chemistry. Experientia 12: 81-124 (1956).
Caldwell, J. and Marsh, M.V.: Interrelationships between xenobiotic metabolism and lipid biosynthesis. Biochemical Pharmacology 32: 1667-1672 (1983).
Cho, A.K. and Wright, J.: Pathways of metabolism of amphetamine and related compounds. Life Sciences 22: 363-372 (1978).
Cotzias, G.C.; Papavasiliou, P.S. and Gellene, R.: Modification of Parkinsonism–chronic treatment with L-dopa. New England Journal of Medicine 280: 337-345 (1969).
Cox, P.J.; Farmer, P.B.; Jarman, M.; Jones, M.; Stec, W.J. and Kinas, R.: Observations on the differential metabolism and biological activity of the optical isomers of cyclophosphamide. Biochemical Pharmacology 25: 993-996 (1976).
Davis, J.E. and Johns, L.E.: Possible interaction of sulfinpyrazone with coumarins. New England Journal of Medicine 299: 955 (1978).
Echizen, H. and Eichelbaum, M.: Pharmacodynamics of verapamil isomers in man. Naunyn-Schmiedeberg's Archives of Pharmacology 325 (Suppl.): R86 (1984).
Eichelbaum, M.; Birkel, P.; Grube, E.; Gutgemann, U. and Somogyi, A.: Effects of verapamil on P-R-intervals in relation to verapamil plasma levels following single i.v. and oral administration and during chronic treatment. Klinische Wochenschrift 58: 919-925 (1980).
Eichelbaum, M.; Mikus, G. and Vogelgesang, B.: Pharmacokinetics of (+)-, (−)- and (±)-verapamil after intravenous administration. British Journal of Clinical Pharmacology 17: 453-458 (1984).
Evans, G.H.; Nies, A.S. and Shand, D.G.: The disposition of propranolol. III. Decreased half-life and volume of distribution as a result of plasma binding in man, monkey, dog and rat. Journal of Pharmacology and Experimental Therapeutics 186: 114-122 (1973).
Farmer, P.B.; Jarman, M.; Facchinetti, T.; Pankiewicz, K. and Stec, W.J.: The metabolism and antitumor activity of the enantiomers of cis- and trans-4-methylcyclophosphamide. Chemical and Biological Interactions 18: 47-57 (1977).
Fears, R.; Baggaley, K.H.; Alexander, R.; Morgan, B. and Hindley, R.M.: The participation of ethyl 4-benzyloxybenzoate (BRL 10894) and other aryl-substituted acids in glycerolipid metabolism. Journal of Lipid Research 19: 3-11 (1978).
Fears, R. and Richards, D.H.: Association between lipid-lowering activity of aryl-substituted carboxylic acids and formation of substituted glycerolipids in rats. Biochemical Society Transactions 9: 572-573 (1981).
Feldman, D.: Naprosyn (naproxen). Monograph and Clinical Practice Handbook (Syntex Laboratories Inc., Palo Alto 1976).
Field, M.J.; Fowler, N. and Giebisch, G.H.: Effects of enantiomers of indarinone (MK-196) on cation transport by the loop of Henle and distal tubule studied by microperfusion *in vivo*. Journal of Pharmacology and Experimental Therapeutics 230: 62-68 (1984).
Forrest, W.H.; Beer, E.G.; Bellville, J.W.; Ciliberti, B.J.; Miller, E.V. and Paddock, R.: Analgesic and other effects of the d- and l-isomers of pentazocine. Clinical Pharmacology and Therapeutics 10: 468-476 (1969).
Gallus, A. and Birkett, D.: Sulphinpyrazone and warfarin: A probable drug interaction. Lancet 1: 535-536 (1980).
Gil-Av, E.: Present status of enantiomeric analyses by gas chromatography. Journal of Molecular Evolution 6: 131-145 (1975).
Godbillon, J.; Richard, J.; Gerardin, A.; Meinertz, T.; Kasper, W. and Jahnchen, E.: Pharmacokinetics of the enantiomers of acenocoumarol in man. British Journal of Clinical Pharmacology 12: 621-629 (1981).
Graham, G.G.: Non-invasive chemical methods of estimating pharmacokinetic parameters. Pharmacology and Therapeutics 18: 333-349 (1982).
Haberkorn, A.; Kraft, H.P. and Blaschke, G.: Antimalarial activity in animals of the optical isomers of chloroquine diphosphate. Tropenmedizin Parasitologie 30: 308-312 (1979).
Hendel, J. and Brodthagen, H.: Enterohepatic cycling of methotrexate estimated by use of the D-isomer as a reference marker. European Journal of Clinical Pharmacology 26: 103-107 (1984).
Ho, I.K. and Harris, R.A.: Mechanism of action of barbiturates. Annual Review of Pharmacology and Toxicology 21: 83-111 (1981).
Horng, J.S.; Smits, S.E. and Wong, D.T.: The binding of the optical isomers of methadone, α-methadol, α-acetylmethadol and their N-demethylated derivatives to the opiate receptors of rat brain. Research Communications in Chemical Pathology and Pharmacology 14: 621-629 (1976).
Hutt, A.J. and Caldwell, J.: The metabolic chiral inversion of 2-arylpropionic acids. A novel route with pharmacological consequences. Journal of Pharmacy and Pharmacology 35: 693-704 (1983).
Hutt, A.J. and Caldwell, J.: The importance of stereochemistry in the clinical pharmacokinetics of the 2-arylpropionic acid nonsteroidal anti-inflammatory drugs. Clinical Pharmacokinetics 9: 371-373 (1984).
Irvin, J.D.; Vlasses, P.H.; Huber, P.B.; Feinberg, J.A.; Ferguson, R.K.; Scrogie, J.J. and Davies, R.O.: Different pharmacodynamic effects of the (+) and (−) enantiomers of indacrinone in man. Clinical Pharmacology and Therapeutics 27: 260 (1980).
Jackman, G.P.; McLean, A.J.; Lennings, G.L. and Bobik, A.: No stereoselective first-pass hepatic extraction of propranolol. Clinical Pharmacology and Therapeutics 30: 291-296 (1981).
Jahnchen, E.; Meinertz, T.; Gilfrich, H-J.; Groth, U. and Martini, A.: The enantiomers of phenprocoumon: Pharmacodynamic

and pharmacokinetic studies. Clinical Pharmacology and Therapeutics 20: 342-349 (1976).

Jenner, P. and Testa, B.: The influence of stereochemical factors on drug disposition. Drug Metabolism Reviews 2: 117-184 (1973).

Judson, B.A.; Horns, W.H. and Goldstein, A.: Side effects of levomethadone and racemic methadone in a maintenance program. Clinical Pharmacology and Therapeutics 20: 445-449 (1976).

Kaumann, A.J. and Serur, J.R.: Optical isomers of verapamil on canine heart. Naunyn-Schmiedeberg's Archives of Pharmacology 291: 347-358 (1975).

Kawashima, K.; Levy, A. and Spector, S.: Stereospecific radioimmunoassay for propranolol isomers. Journal of Pharmacology and Experimental Therapeutics 196: 517-523 (1976).

Keates, E.U. and Stone, M.D.: The effect of d-timolol on intraocular pressure in patients with ocular hypertension. American Journal of Ophthalmology 98: 73-78 (1984).

Kreek, M.J.; Hachey, D.L. and Klein, P.D.: Stereoselective disposition of methadone in man. Life Sciences 24: 925-932 (1979).

Larsen, T.A. and Teravainen, H.: Propranolol and essential tremor: Role of the membrane effect. Acta Neurologica Scandinavica 66: 289-294 (1982).

Lee, E.J.D.; Williams, K.M.; Graham, G.G.; Day, R.O. and Champion, G.D.: Liquid chromatographic determination and the plasma concentration profile of optical isomers of ibuprofen in humans. Journal of Pharmaceutical Sciences 73: 1542-1544 (1984).

Lee, E.J.D.; Williams, K.; Day, R.; Graham, G. and Champion, D.: Stereoselective disposition of ibuprofen enantiomers in man. British Journal of Clinical Pharmacology 19: 669-674 (1985).

Lennard, M.S.; Tucker, G.T.; Silas, J.H.; Freestone, S.; Ramsey, L.E. and Woods, H.F.: Differential stereoselective metabolism of metoprolol in extensive and poor debrisoquine metabolizers. Clinical Pharmacology and Therapeutics 34: 732-737 (1983).

Lewis, R.J.; Trager, W.F.; Chan, K.K.; Breckenridge, A.; Orme, M.; Roland, M. and Schary, W.: Warfarin. Stereochemical aspects of its metabolism and the interaction with phenylbutazone. Journal of Clinical Investigation 53: 1607-1617 (1974).

Lima, J.L.; Jungbluth, G.L.; Devine, T. and Robertson, L.W.: Stereoselective binding of disopyramide to human plasma protein. Life Sciences 35: 835-839 (1984).

Little, J.R.; Latchan, J.P.; Slugg, R.M.; Lesser, R.P. and Stowe, N.T.: Treatment of acute focal cerebral ischaemia with propranolol. Stroke 13: 302-307 (1982).

Lochmuller, C.H. and Souter, R.W.: Chromatographic resolution of enantiomers. Selective review. Journal of Chromatography 113: 283-302 (1975).

McMenamy, R.H. and Oncley, J.L.: The specific binding of L-tryptophan to serum albumin. Journal of Biological Chemistry 233: 1436-1447 (1958).

Mason, S.: The left hand of nature. New Scientist 1393: 10-14 (1984).

May, E.L. and Takeda, M.: Optical isomers of miscellaneous strong analgetics. Journal of Medicinal Chemistry 13: 805-807 (1970).

Meinertz, T.; Kasper, W.; Kahl, C. and Jahnchen, E.: Anticoagulant activity of the enantiomers of acenocoumarol. British Journal of Clinical Pharmacology 5: 187-188 (1978).

Meresaar, U.; Nilsson, M.I.; Holmstrand, J. and Anggard, E.: Single dose pharmacokinetics and bioavailability of methadone in man studied with a stable isotope method. European Journal of Clinical Pharmacology 20: 473-478 (1981).

Mills, R.F.N.; Adams, S.S.; Cliffe, E.E.; Dickinson, W. and Nicholson, J.S.: The metabolism of ibuprofen. Xenobiotica 3: 589-598 (1973).

Miner, D.J.; Coleman, D.L.; Shepard, A.M.M. and Hardin, T.C.: Determination of moxalactam in human body fluids by liquid chromatographic and microbiological methods. Antimicrobial Agents and Chemotherapy 20: 252-257 (1981).

Muller, W.E. and Wollert, U.: High stereospecificity of the benzodiazepine binding site on human serum albumin. Molecular Pharmacology 11: 52-60 (1975a).

Muller, W.E. and Wollert, U.: Benzodiazepines: Specific competitors for the binding of L-tryptophan to human albumin. Naunyn-Schmiedeberg's Archives of Pharmacology 288: 17-27 (1975b).

Murphy, P.J.; Nickander, R.C.; Bellamy, G.M. and Kurtz, W.L.: Effect of l-propoxyphene on plasma levels and analgesic activity of d-propoxyphene in the rat. Journal of Pharmacology and Experimental Therapeutics 199: 415-422 (1976).

Nakamura, K.; Hachey, D.L.; Kreek, M.J.; Irving, C.S. and Klein, P.D.: Quantitation of methadone enantiomers in humans using stable isotope-labelled $[^2H_3]$–$[^2H_5]$– and $[^2H_8]$ methadone. Journal of Pharmaceutical Sciences 71: 40-43 (1982).

Nakamura, Y.; Yamaguchi, T.; Takahashi, S.; Hashimoto, S.; Iwatani, K. and Nakagawa, Y.: Optical isomerization mechanism of R(−)-hydratropic acid derivatives. Proceedings of the 12th Symposium on Drug Metabolism and Action, Kanazawa, Japan (October, 1980).

Nies, A.S.; Evans, G.H. and Shand, D.G.: The hemodynamic effects of beta adrenergic blockade on the flow-dependent hepatic clearance of propranolol. Journal of Pharmacology and Experimental Therapeutics 184: 716-720 (1973a).

Nies, A.S.; Evans, G.H. and Shand, D.G.: Regional hemodynamic effects of beta adrenergic blockade with propranolol in the unanesthetized primate. American Heart Journal 85: 97-102 (1973b).

Nies, A.S.; Shand, D.G. and Wilkinson, G.R.: Altered hepatic blood flow and drug disposition. Clinical Pharmacokinetics 1: 135-155 (1976).

Olsen, G.D.; Wendel, H.A.; Livermore, J.D.; Leger, R.M.; Lynn, R.K. and Gerber, N.: Clinical effects and pharmacokinetics of racemic methadone and its optical isomers. Clinical Pharmacology and Therapeutics 21: 147-157 (1977).

O'Reilly, R.A.: Studies on the optical enantiomorphs of warfarin in man. Clinical Pharmacology and Therapeutics 16: 348-354 (1974).

O'Reilly, R.A.: The stereoselective interaction of warfarin and metronidazole in man. New England Journal of Medicine 295: 354-357 (1976).

O'Reilly, R.A.: Stereoselective interaction of trimethoprim-sulfamethoxazole with the separated enantiomorphs of racemic warfarin in man. New England Journal of Medicine 302: 33-35 (1980).

O'Reilly, R.A.: Dynamic interaction between disulfiram and separated enantiomorphs of racemic warfarin. Clinical Pharmacology and Therapeutics 29: 332-336 (1981).

O'Reilly, R.A.: Stereoselective interaction of sulphinpyrazone with racemic warfarin and its separated enantiomorphs in man. Circulation 65: 202-207 (1982a).

O'Reilly, R.A.: Ticrynafen-racemic warfarin interaction: Hepatotoxic or stereoselective? Clinical Pharmacology and Therapeutics 32: 356-361 (1982b).

O'Reilly, R.A. and Goulart, D.A.: Comparative interaction of sulfinpyrazone and phenylbutazone with racemic warfarin: Alteration *in vivo* of free fraction of plasma warfarin. Journal of Pharmacology and Experimental Therapeutics 219: 691-694 (1981).

O'Reilly, R.A. and Motley, C.H.: Racemic warfarin and trimethoprim-sulfamethoxazole interaction in humans. Annals of Internal Medicine 91: 34-36 (1979).

O'Reilly, R.A.; Sahud, M.A. and Robinson, A.J.: Studies on the interaction of warfarin and clofibrate in man. Thrombosis et Diathesis Haemorrhagica 27: 309-318 (1972).

O'Reilly, R.A.; Trager, W.F.; Motley, C.H. and Howald, W.: Stereoselective interaction of phenylbutazone with $[^{12}C/^{13}C]$ warfarin pseudoracemates in man. Journal of Clinical Investigations 65: 746-753 (1980a).

O'Reilly, R.A.; Trager, W.F.; Motley, C.H. and Howald, W.: Interaction of secobarbital with warfarin. Clinical Pharmacology and Therapeutics 28: 187-195 (1980b).

Pasteur, L.: Second lecture to the Chemical Society of Paris (1860); in Richardson (Ed.) The Foundations of Stereo Chemistry (American Book Company, New York 1901).

Patil, N.; LaPidus, J.B. and Tye, A.: Steric aspects of adrenergic drugs. Journal of Pharmaceutical Sciences 59: 1205-1233 (1970).

Patil, N.; Miller, D.D. and Trendelenberg, U.: Molecular geometry and adrenergic drug activity. Pharmacological Reviews 26: 323-392 (1975).

Pillai, G.K.; Axelson, J.E.; Kerr, C.R. and McErlane, K.M.: Stereospecific salivary excretion of tocainide enantiomers in man. Research Communications in Chemical Pathology and Pharmacology 43: 209-221 (1984).

Raschack, M.: Relationship of antiarrhythmic to inotropic activity and antiarrhythmic qualities of the optical isomers of verapamil. Naunyn-Schmiedeberg's Archives of Pharmacology 294: 285-291 (1976).

Rose, I.A.: Enzyme reaction stereospecificity: A critical review. CRC Critical Reviews in Biochemistry 1: 33-57 (1972).

Rubin, A.; Knadler, M.P.; Ho, P.P.K.; Bechtol, L.D. and Wolen, R.L.: Stereoselective inversion of R-fenoprofen to S-fenoprofen in humans. Journal of Pharmaceutical Sciences 74: 82-84 (1985).

Saikawa, T. and Arita, M.: Effects of verapamil and its optical isomers on repetitive slow responses induced by electrical depolarization in canine ventricular myocardium. Japan Heart Journal 21: 247-255 (1980).

Sastry, B.V.R.: Stereoisomerism and drug action in the nervous system. Annual Reviews of Pharmacology 13: 253-267 (1973).

Satoh, K.; Yanagisawa, T. and Taira, N.: Coronary vasodilator and cardiac effects of optical isomers of verapamil in the dog. Journal of Cardiovascular Pharmacology 2: 309-318 (1980).

Seideman, P.; Ericsson, O.; Groningsson, K. and von Bahr, C.: Effect of pentobarbital on the formation of diastereomeric glucoronides in man: Analysis by high performance liquid chromatography. Acta Pharmacologica et Toxicologica 49: 200-204 (1981).

Sellers, E.M. and Koch-Weser, J.: Interaction of warfarin stereoisomers with human albumin. Pharmacological Research Communications 7: 331-335 (1975).

Serlin, M.J. and Breckenridge, A.M.: Drug interactions with warfarin. Drugs 25: 610-620 (1983).

Shand, D.G.; Branch, R.A.; Evans, G.H.; Nies, A.S. and Wilkinson, G.R.: The disposition of propranolol. VII. Drug Metabolism and Disposition 1: 679-686 (1973).

Shiotani, S.: Optical resolution of some homobenzomorphan derivatives and their pharmacological properties. Journal of Medicinal Chemistry 22: 1558-1560 (1979).

Silber, B. and Riegelman, S.: Stereospecific assay for (−)- and (+)-propranolol in human and dog plasma. Journal of Pharmacology and Experimental Therapeutics 215: 643-648 (1980).

Simmonds, R.G.; Woodage, T.J.; Duff, S.M. and Green, J.N.: Stereospecific inversion of R(−)-benoxaprofen in rat and man. European Journal of Drug Metabolism and Pharmacokinetics 5: 169-172 (1980).

Smith, D.F. (Ed.): CRC Handbook of Stereoisomers: Drugs in Psychopharmacology (CRC Press Inc., Boca Raton, Florida 1984).

Smits, S.E. and Myers, M.B.: Some comparative effects of racemic methadone and its optical isomers in rodents. Research Communications in Chemical Pathology and Pharmacology 7: 651-662 (1974).

Steen, P.A. and Michenfelder, J.D.: Cerebral protection with barbiturates. Stroke 9: 140-142 (1978).

Stoltenborg, J.K.; Puglisi, C.V.; Rubio, F. and Vane, F.M.: High performance liquid chromatographic determination of stereoselective disposition of carprofen in humans. Journal of Pharmaceutical Sciences 70: 1207-1212 (1981).

Tamassia, V.; Jannuzzo, M.G.; Moro, E.; Stegnjaich, S.. and Groppi, W.: Pharmacokinetics of the enantiomers of indoprofen in man. International Journal of Clinical Pharmacology Research 4: 223-230 (1984).

Tobert, J.A.; Cirillo, V.J.; Hitzenberger, G.; James, I.; Pyror, J. et al.: Enhancement of uricosuric properties of indacrinone by manipulation of the enantiomeric ratio. Clinical Pharmacology and Therapeutics 29: 344-350 (1981).

Tocco, D.J.; Hooke, K.F.; Deluna, F.A. and Duncan, A.E.W.: Stereospecific binding of timolol, a beta-adrenergic blocking agent. Drug Metabolism and Disposition 4: 323-329 (1976).

Toon, S. and Trager, W.F.: Stereochemical aspects of drug-protein binding: The warfarin sulfinpyrazone interaction. 2nd World Conference on Clinical Pharmacology and Therapeutics, Washington DC (August, 1983).

Toon, S. and Trager, W.F.: Pharmacokinetic implications of stereoselective changes in plasma-protein binding: Warfarin-sulfinpyrazone. Journal of Pharmaceutical Sciences 73: 1671-1673 (1984).

Valdivieso, L.; Blaschke, T. and Giacomini, K.: Disopyramide enantiomers bind stereoselectively to human plasma protein. 2nd World Conference on Clinical Pharmacology and Therapeutics, Washington DC (August, 1983).

Verebely, K.; Volavka, J.; Mulé, S. and Resnick, R.: Methadone in man: Pharmacokinetic and excretion studies in acute and chronic treatment. Clinical Pharmacology and Therapeutics 18: 180-190 (1975).

Veronich, K.; White, G. and Kapoor, A.: Effects of phenylbutazone, tolbutamide and clofibric acid on binding of racemic warfarin and its enantiomers to human serum albumin. Journal of Pharmaceutical Sciences 68: 1515-1518 (1979).

Vlasses, P.H.; Irvin, J.D.; Huber, P.B.; Lee, R.B.; Ferguson, R.K. et al.: Pharmacology of enantiomers and (−) p-OH metabolite of indacrinone. Clinical Pharmacology and Therapeutics 29: 798-807 (1981).

Vlasses, P.H.; Rotmensch, H.H.; Swanson, B.N.; Irvin, J.D.; Johnson, C.L. and Ferguson, R.K.: Indacrinone: Natriuretic and uricosuric effects of various ratios of its enantiomers in healthy men. Pharmacotherapy 4: 272-283 (1984).

Vogelgesang, B.; Echizen, H.; Schmidt, E. and Eichelbaum, M.: Stereoselective first-pass metabolism of highly cleared drugs: Studies of the bioavailability of L- and D-verapamil examined with a stable isotope technique. British Journal of Clinical Pharmacology 18: 733-740 (1984).

Von Bahr, C.; Hermansson, J. and Tawara, K.: Plasma levels of (+) and (−)-propranolol and 4-hydroxypropranolol after administration of racemic (±)-propranolol in man. British Journal of Clinical Pharmacology 14: 79-82 (1982a).

Von Bahr, C.; Hermansson, J. and Lind, M.: Oxidation of (R)- and (S)-propranolol in human and dog liver microsomes. Species differences in stereoselectivity. Journal of Pharmacology and Experimental Therapeutics 222: 458-462 (1982b).

Wade, D.N.; Mearrick, P.T. and Morris, J.L.: Active transport of L-dopa in the intestine. Nature 242: 463-465 (1973).

Walle, T. and Walle, U.K.: Stereoselective oral bioavailability of (±)-propranolol in the dog. A GCMS study using a stable isotope technique. Research Communications in Chemical Pathology and Pharmacology 23: 453-464 (1979).

Walle, U.K.; Walle, T.; Bai, S.A. and Oranoff, L.S.: Stereoselective binding of propranolol to human plasma, α_1-acid glycoprotein and albumin. Clinical Pharmacology and Therapeutics 34: 718-722 (1983).

Wanwimolruk, S.: Protein binding of non-steroidal anti-inflammatory drugs: Basic and clinical aspects (Ph.D. Thesis, Flinders University of South Australia, 1983).

Wilkinson, G.R. and Shand, D.G.: A physiological approach to hepatic drug clearance. Clinical Pharmacology and Therapeutics 18: 377-390 (1975).

Williams, K.M.: Kinetics of misonidazole enantiomers. Clinical Pharmacology and Therapeutics 36: 817-823 (1984).
Williams, K.M. and Day, R.O.: Stereoselective disposition – basis for variability in response to NSAID's. Agents and Actions (Suppl.) (In press, 1985).
Williams, K.M. and Smith, G.G.: A critical evaluation of the application of amino acid racemization to geochronology and geothermometry. Origins of Life 8: 91-144 (1977).
Williams, K.; Begg, E.; Wade, D. and O'Shea, K.: Effects of phenytoin, phenobarbital and ascorbic acid on misonidazole elimination. Clinical Pharmacology and Therapeutics 33: 314-321 (1983).
Wingard, L.B. and Levy, G.: Comparative pharmacokinetics of coumarin anticoagulants. XXXVI: Predicted steady state patterns of prothrombin complex activity produced by equieffective doses of R(+)- and S(−)-warfarin in humans. Journal of Pharmaceutical Sciences 66: 1790-1791 (1977).
Wingard, L.B.; O'Reilly, R.A. and Levy, G.: Pharmacokinetics of warfarin enantiomers: A search for intrasubject correlations. Clinical Pharmacology and Therapeutics 23: 212-217 (1978).
Wise, R.; Wills, P.J. and Bedford, K.A.: Epimers of moxalactam: *In vitro* comparison of activity and stability. Antimicrobial Agents and Chemotherapy 20: 30-32 (1981).
Workman, P.: Effects of pretreatment with phenobarbitone and phenytoin on the pharmacokinetics and toxicity of misonidazole in mice. British Journal of Cancer 40: 335-353 (1979).
Yacobi, A. and Levy, G.: Comparative pharmacokinetics of coumarin anticoagulants. XIV: Relationship between protein binding, distribution and elimination kinetics of warfarin in rats. Journal of Pharmaceutical Sciences 64: 1660-1664 (1975).
Yacobi, A. and Levy, G.: Protein binding of warfarin enantiomers in serum of humans and rats. Journal of Pharmacokinetics and Biopharmaceutics 5: 123-131 (1977).
Yacobi, A.; Udall, J.A. and Levy, G.: Serum protein binding as a determinant of warfarin body clearance and anticoagulant effect. Clinical Pharmacology and Therapeutics 19: 552-558 (1976).
Zacchei, A.G.; Dobrinska, M.R.; Wishousky, T.I.; Kwan, K.C. and White, S.D.: Stereoselectivity in the disposition and metabolism of the uricosuric-diuretic agent, indacrinone, in rhesus monkeys. Drug Metabolism and Disposition 10: 20-27 (1982).

Address for correspondence and reprints: Dr *K. Williams*, Department of Clinical Pharmacology, St Vincent's Hospital, Darlinghurst, Sydney, NSW 2010 (Australia).

Review Article

Drugs 30: 355-367 (1985)
0012-6667/85/0010-0355/$06.50/0

Current Management of Hodgkin's Disease

Brent C. Behrens, Robert C. Young and *Vincent T. DeVita Jr*

Medicine Branch, Clinical Oncology Program, Division of Cancer Treatment, and Office of the Director, National Cancer Institute, Bethesda

Summary

The prognosis of patients with Hodgkin's disease has dramatically improved over the past few decades. Treatment with currently standard radiotherapy or combination chemotherapy programmes will result in durable complete remissions and probable cure in most patients. However, these programmes are intensive, technically demanding, and associated with a risk of certain acute side effects and long term complications which vary in nature and severity according to the specific therapy employed.

The outlook for the few patients who do not achieve complete remission with induction therapy, or for those who later relapse (especially after complete remissions induced by chemotherapy), is less optimistic. Current trials of innovative induction and salvage therapies may lead to improved treatment approaches for such patients.

Hodgkin's disease is a form of malignant lymphoma of unknown cause which accounts for approximately 1% of the new cases of cancer diagnosed annually in the US (Gutensohn and Cole, 1982). Four subtypes differing somewhat in natural history and response to therapy are distinguished by the Rye histopathological classification, according to features of the characteristic multinucleated Reed-Sternberg cells and the surrounding cells and connective tissue: (1) lymphocyte predominant; (2) nodular sclerosis; (3) mixed cellularity; and (4) lymphocyte depleted (Kaplan, 1980). The stage of Hodgkin's disease (table I), also influences prognosis as well as choice of therapy. The pathological stage represents the best estimates of disease extent, and is based on results of all diagnostic studies (DeVita and Hellman, 1982), including histopathological examination of specimens obtained at staging laparotomy (if performed) and biopsies of other tissues.

Table I. Stages of Hodgkin's disease: Ann Arbor classification (adapted from DeVita and Hellman, 1982)

Stage	Definition
I	Involvement of one lymph node region or localised involvement of one extralymphatic site (I_E)
II	Involvement of multiple lymph node regions on one side of the diaphragm, possibly accompanied by (II_E) localised involvement of one extralymphatic site
III	Involvement of lymph node regions on both sides of the diaphragm and possibly also the spleen (III_S); localised involvement of one extralymphatic site (III_E), or both (III_{SE})
IV	Diffuse or disseminated involvement of extralymphatic organ(s) with or without associated lymphatic involvement

N.B. The suffixes 'A' and 'B' denote the absence or presence, respectively, of constitutional symptoms (otherwise unexplained fever, night sweats or weight loss of more than 10% of bodyweight over the preceding 6 months).

Table II. Drug administration during one cycle of MOPP therapy

Drug	Full (100%) dose (mg/m^2)[a]	Route	Days[b]
Mustine (mechlorethamine; nitrogen mustard)	6	Intravenous	1 and 8
Vincristine ('Oncovin')	1.4	Intravenous	1 and 8
Procarbazine	100	Oral	1 through 14
Prednisone[c]	40	Oral	1 through 14

a Square metre of body surface area.
b Each cycle lasts 28 days.
c Cycle 1 and every subsequent third cycle only.

Dramatic advances in our understanding of Hodgkin's disease and its therapy have been made in the last several decades. Current treatment approaches, which offer a realistic expectation of complete remission and probable cure for most patients with this otherwise ultimately fatal malignancy (Kaplan, 1980), are the subject of this review.

1. Chemotherapy Regimens

1.1 MOPP Combination Chemotherapy

The MOPP regimen (mustine/vincristine/procarbazine/prednisone; see table II) will be examined in detail as it is effective and widely used, and because its success has strongly supported the philosophy of cancer treatment with combination chemotherapy programmes. The principles underlying the MOPP regimen have also been useful in the design of other programmes: use of several drugs selected from different pharmacological classes by consideration of their efficacy, potential cross-resistance and toxicity; use of these drugs at full dose and optimum schedule; use of treatment cycles incorporating periods without therapy to promote recovery of normal tissues; and use of intensive therapy for a flexible period in an attempt to induce complete remission, and then stopped completely if residual disease is not found at restaging (DeVita et al., 1980).

1.1.1 Optimum Dose Schedules

Each MOPP cycle lasts 28 days, with drugs given only during the first 14 days (table II); no therapy is given over the next 14 days, and the subsequent cycle is started on the following day. Drug doses after the first cycle are based on peripheral blood counts and a dose modification schedule (table III) because of the variable myelosuppression accompanying MOPP therapy. A new MOPP cycle may be postponed for up to 1 week in anticipation of further marrow recovery if less than 50% of the full mustine (mechlorethamine) and procarbazine doses are allowed by this schedule. Patients with documented bone marrow involvement are best treated with full drug doses, regardless of peripheral blood counts, although severe but transient cytopenias may result and necessitate support with blood products (Myers et al., 1974). Granulocytopenic patients require close observation for potential infectious complications and should receive broad spectrum antibiotics empirically when febrile, even if a specific infectious cause is not found (Pizzo et al., 1982). Vincristine dosage should also be modified (table III) if serious neurotoxicity develops.

Dose reductions or treatment delays for reasons other than severe, treatment-related myelosuppression or neurotoxicity decrease the effectiveness of therapy (Carde et al., 1983) and should be avoided.

1.1.2 Side Effects and their Management

Certain acute side effects may accompany MOPP chemotherapy. Mustine and vincristine are both potent vesicants and may cause serious ulcerations if extravasated. Nausea and vomiting usually occur on days 1 and 8 of each cycle, sometimes in anticipation of treatment, and antiemetics should be used routinely (Siegel and Longo, 1981). Nausea, vomiting and anorexia may also occur during the first half of each cycle as a side effect of procarbazine. Hair loss will develop in possibly 50% of all patients.

Paraesthesias and decreased deep tendon reflexes are common manifestations of vincristine neuropathy, but usually are at least partially reversible. Motor deficits, such as foot drop or adynamic ileus, are less frequent but much more serious, and mandate dose modification as they often improve slowly. Neurotoxicity is more common in the elderly and vincristine must be used cautiously in this age group. Procarbazine also infrequently causes paraesthesias as well as depression, drowziness and a maculopapular skin rash which usually resolves without drug discontinuation if prednisone is given in every cycle. Patients should avoid alcohol, tyramine-rich foods or monoamine oxidase inhibitor drugs, and potent hypnotic agents because of potential adverse drug interactions with procarbazine. These and other, less frequent, side effects of the drugs used in the MOPP regimen have been reviewed (Chabner and Myers, 1982).

1.1.3 Optimum Duration of Treatment

Patients should receive 2 cycles of MOPP therapy beyond the number required for maximum or complete clinical response, with a 6-cycle minimum. Approximately 25% of patients will require more than 6 cycles (Young and DeVita, 1979) and up to 11 cycles were required in the initial group of patients treated with MOPP (DeVita, 1981). Since treatment duration depends on tumour response, periodic patient assessment is essential. This variation in the rate of tumour response among patients may explain the superiority of flexible induction therapy over treatment of fixed or specific duration (Young and DeVita, 1979).

1.1.4 Restaging and Patient Evaluation Following Treatment

Restaging, including physical examination, abdominal (if lymphangiography was done) and chest radiographs, routine blood counts and chemistries, and *all* other tests or procedures (other than laparotomy) that demonstrated disease at any site before therapy should be performed 1 month after the last chemotherapy cycle. Some patients will need invasive studies. Lymphangiography should be repeated if initially abnormal and remaining contrast dye is insufficient for adequate evaluation. Extranodal sites initially involved, such as the liver or bone marrow, and any areas suspicious for residual disease should be biopsied. Meticulous restaging following therapy can reveal unsuspected disease in 12% of patients (Herman and Jones, 1978). Treatment must be resumed if residual disease is found, using a different approach (see section 4) if a maximum response to MOPP therapy was definitely obtained. Patients in complete remission documented by restaging do not benefit from further maintenance therapy (DeVita and Hellman, 1982).

Patients in complete remission after induction therapy require periodic evaluation for manifes-

Table III. Dose modification of MOPP therapy for myelosuppression and neurotoxicity

White blood cell count[a]	Platelet count[a]	Dosages[b,c]
⩾4000	⩾ 100,000	100% of all drugs
3000-3999	⩾ 100,000	100% prednisone and vincristine; 50% mustine and procarbazine
2000-2999	⩾ 50,000	100% prednisone and vincristine; 25% mustine and procarbazine
1000-1999	⩾ 50,000	100% prednisone; 50% vincristine; 25% mustine and procarbazine
< 1000	< 50,000	100% prednisone; no other drugs

Neurotoxicity	Vincristine dose[c]	Dose to be resumed if improvement occurs
None	100%	
Moderate paraesthesias (e.g. inability to button clothing)	50%	100%
Severe (e.g. difficulty with ambulation or adynamic ileus)	0%	50%

a Cells/mm^3 on day 1.
b The lowest drug dosages appropriate for the white blood count and platelet count should be used.
c Percentage of full dose specified in table II.

tations of both recurrent disease and potential chronic complications of therapy (see section 5). Patients who ultimately relapse after MOPP chemotherapy usually do so within 2 years, and rarely after 4 years following therapy (DeVita, 1981). As a result, we routinely evaluate patients every month for the first year, every 2 months for the second year, every 4 to 6 months for the third and fourth years, and yearly thereafter. Since relapses from chemotherapy-induced complete remission usually occur at sites involved initially, especially in patients with bulky disease or the nodular sclerosis subtype (Young et al., 1978), close observation of such sites is important and annual restaging may be useful during the first years of follow-up. Patient evaluation should include specific inquiries concerning possible symptoms of recurrent disease or chronic treatment complications, pertinent physical examination, routine blood counts and chemistries, and chest and possibly abdominal (for those with persistent lymphangiographic contrast dye) radiographs.

1.1.5 Results of MOPP Chemotherapy

Long term results of MOPP chemotherapy for advanced Hodgkin's disease are known. The overall complete response rate among 198 patients treated at the National Cancer Institute from 1964 to 1976 was 80.3% (DeVita et al., 1980), and similar rates have been reported from other institutions (reviewed in Coltman, 1980). The complete response rate varied among subgroups differing in sex, histopathological subtype, stage, extranodal involvement and constitutional symptoms, but only the latter reached statistical significance. The presence of systemic symptoms was also the most important determinant of the 5-year disease-free survival rate and of deaths related to Hodgkin's disease at both 5 and 10 years following treatment, although clinical stage and histopathological subtype were also significant prognostic factors. Overall, 68% of patients who achieved complete remission remained continually disease-free for 5 years, and 82% and 73% of the patients achieving complete remission survived more than 5 and 10 years, respectively.

Patients who did not achieve complete remission had a median survival of 11 months.

1.2 MOPP-Variant Combination Chemotherapy Regimens

Many alternative chemotherapy regimens for Hodgkin's disease are variants of the MOPP regimen (table IV) and are intended to improve efficacy, decrease toxicity, or both. The acute toxicity of MOPP chemotherapy is appreciable and exceeds that of some of the MOPP-variant regimens. For example, the MVPP regimen has less neurotoxicity than MOPP but comparable acute gastrointestinal and haematopoietic toxicity (Sutcliffe et al., 1978), and the ChlVPP regimen has even fewer acute adverse effects (Dady et al., 1982). The long term sequellae of treatment with these regimens are less well known than those following MOPP therapy (see section 5), and chronic toxicities are currently difficult to compare.

However, MOPP chemotherapy is tolerated by most patients and effectiveness is thus a more important consideration. It is difficult to precisely assess the relative therapeutic efficacy of MOPP and its variants, as studies have differed in important respects such as distribution of prognostic factors among patients. Nevertheless, there is no evidence to suggest that any MOPP-variant regimen is more effective than MOPP itself (Bonadonna and Santoro, 1982; Coltman, 1980). Complete response rates of approximately 60 to 80% have been obtained in previously untreated patients with the regimens listed in table IV, compared with about 70 to 100% with MOPP (Coltman, 1980), and 10-year follow-up data is available only for MOPP. In addition, direct comparisons in 8 prospective randomised clinical trials have shown no variant regimen to be more effective than MOPP (reviewed in Coltman, 1980).

1.3 Other Combination Chemotherapy Regimens

Chemotherapy programmes for Hodgkin's disease have also been based on the principles under-

Table IV. Selected MOPP-variant combination chemotherapy regimens

Regimen	Drugs [cycle duration in weeks]	Induction duration	Overall complete response rate (%)	Restaged?	Maintenance therapy?	Median disease-free survival (years)	References
BVCPP	BCNU, VB, C, PR, P [4]	Flexible	77	No	Yes	> 5	Glick et al. (1982)
		Fixed	68	No	Yes	> 4	Gams et al. (1982)
ChlVPP	Chlorambucil, VB, PR, P [6]	Flexible	74	No	No	> 5	Dady et al. (1982)
COPP	CCNU, VC, PR, P [4]	Fixed	65	No	Yes	> 4	Cooper et al. (1980)
CVPP	CCNU, VB, PR, P [4]	Fixed	69	No	Yes	> 4	Cooper et al. (1980)
CVPP	C, VB, PR, P [3]	Flexible	62	No	Yes	3	Diggs et al. (1977)
CVPP	C, VB, PR, P [6]	Fixed	74	No	Yes	> 7	Gibbs et al. (1981)
MOP-BAP	M, VC, PR, B, A, P [4]	Flexible	77	Yes	No	> 4	Jones et al. (1983)
MOPP-bleo	M, VC, PR, P, B [4]	Flexible	67	Yes	No	> 4	Jones et al. (1983)
Bleo-MOPP	B, M, VC, PR, P [4]	Fixed	58	No	No	5[a]	Glick et al. (1982)
MVPP	M, VB, PR, P [4]	Fixed	66	No	Yes	3	Cooper et al. (1980)
MVPP	M, VB, PR, P [6]	Fixed	69	Yes	Yes	> 5	Sutcliffe et al. (1978)

a Indeterminate as all responding patients subsequently received additional therapy.

Abbreviations: A = doxorubicin (adriamycin); B = bleomycin; BCNU = carmustine; C = cyclophosphamide; CCNU = lomustine; M = mustine (mechlorethamine; nitrogen mustard); P = prednisolone or prednisone; PR = procarbazine; VB = vinblastine; VC = vincristine.

lying MOPP chemotherapy rather than on the actual regimen itself. Interest in these programmes has been stimulated by the failure of any MOPP-variant regimen to be more effective than MOPP itself, and by the belief that use of drugs mostly different from those of the MOPP regimen might afford non-cross-resistant therapy effective against disease resistant to MOPP chemotherapy. Such alternative programmes are currently of special interest in salvage therapy (see section 4) and as components of alternating combination chemotherapy regimens (see sections 1.4 and 3). Although many such regimens have been developed (table V), available clinical data suggest that only the VABCD, ABDIC, ABVD and SCAB programmes are truly non-cross-resistant with MOPP if reasonable criteria (Longo et al., 1982) are applied. The ABVD and SCAB regimens have also been used in the initial therapy of advanced Hodgkin's disease. Chemotherapy with SCAB afforded a complete response rate in a small group of such patients similar to that reported for MOPP, but at the expense of substantial toxicity (Diggs et al., 1981). A prospective randomised clinical trial in patients with advanced disease also showed comparable complete response rates following 6 cycles of ABVD or MOPP chemotherapy (Bonadonna et al., 1982). However, other important aspects of therapeutic efficacy, such as response duration, cannot be assessed, as all responding patients subsequently received radiation therapy. The ABVD regimen as used in this study caused worse nausea and vomiting, comparable myelosuppression and less neurotoxicity than MOPP therapy. An appealing feature of this frequently used regimen is that it may be less carcinogenic and have less gonadal toxicity than MOPP chemotherapy (see section 5).

1.4 Alternating Non-Cross-Resistant Combination Chemotherapy Regimens

If the presence of drug-resistant tumour cells during treatment is related to the suboptimum response to chemotherapy of patients with advanced disease (especially those with large tumour burdens), then alternating administration of different and putatively non-cross-resistant combination chemotherapy regimens may be more effective than treatment with a single regimen alone (Bonadonna, 1982; Longo et al., 1982). This hypothesis led to a prospective randomised clinical trial in which patients with advanced disease treated with MOPP and ABVD alternating monthly did, in fact, have a significantly better complete response rate (92% *vs* 71%) and overall survival at 7 years (82% *vs* 61%) than those given a similar number of monthly cycles of MOPP alone (Bonadonna et al., 1984; Santoro et al., 1982a).

Treatment with alternating MOPP/ABVD cycles is a very promising new approach to induction therapy in such patients. Several other prospective randomised clinical trials are pertinent to this intriguing hypothesis. The National Cancer Institute of Italy is currently evaluating monthly combined abbreviated MOPP and ABVD cycles (Bonadonna, 1982), and the Cancer and Acute Leukemia Group B will study MOPP or ABVD therapy alone and alternating MOPP/ABVD therapy (Mayer, 1982). In addition, the National Cancer Institute is currently testing MOPP chemotherapy against alternating MOPP/SCAB therapy [Longo et al., 1982].

2. Radiation Therapy

In contrast to the systemic effects of chemotherapy, radiation therapy is effective only against disease exposed to the radiation beam. Radiation therapy of Hodgkin's disease is thus based on accurate pretreatment staging, individualisation of treatment volumes with specialised simulation and blocking techniques, and treatment of both known areas of disease and contiguous nodal regions. The latter requirement arises from the characteristic spread of Hodgkin's disease in an orderly but often clinically occult fashion, and can best be accomplished by irradiation of large fields with parallel opposed beams generated by a radiocobalt teletherapy unit or linear accelerator (Kaplan, 1980).

Table V. Combination chemotherapy regimens possibly non-cross-resistant with MOPP

Regimen	Drugs	Cycle duration (weeks)	Reference
ABDIC	A, B, DTIC, P, CCNU	4	Tannir et al. (1983)
ABVD	A, B, VB, DTIC	4	Santoro et al. (1982)
B-CAVe	B, CCNU, A, VB	6	Porzig et al. (1978)
B-DOPA	B, DTIC, VC, P, A	3	Lokich et al. (1976)
BVDS	B, VB, A, S	4	Vinciguerra et al. (1977)
CEP	CCNU, etoposide, prednimustine	4	Santoro et al. (1982b)
CVB	CCNU, VBL, B	4	Goldman and Dawson (1975)
SCAB	S, CCNU, A, B	4	Levi et al. (1977)
VABCD	VB, A, B, CCNU, DTIC	6	Einhorn et al. (1983)

Abbreviations: DTIC = dacarbazine; S = streptozotocin; others, see table IV.

2.1 Induction Schedules

Radiation therapy is generally given to a total dose of 3500 to 4400 rad, factionated into multiple daily doses of approximately 200 rad (Hoppe, 1980), although lower total doses are often used in combined modality therapy. Patients may receive either total lymphoid (total nodal) or subtotal lymphoid irradiation, depending on disease presentation and treatment philosophy. The former includes all major lymph node chains and often other lymphatic structures such as the spleen and Waldeyer's ring, and is given by sequential treatment of mantle and inverted Y fields. Subtotal lymphoid irradiation may be directed at only those areas known to harbour Hodgkin's disease (involved field therapy) or at both these areas and continuous nodal regions (extended field therapy).

Radiotherapy induction programmes generally involve irradiation of mantle and inverted Y or para-aortic fields. The mantle field includes all major lymph node regions above the diaphragm, while the inverted Y field includes such regions between the diaphragm and the femoral nodes, and may also include the spleen (if not removed at staging laparotomy) or the liver in patients at risk for occult hepatic involvement (Hoppe, 1980). Para-aortic or spade fields resemble a truncated inverted Y field.

2.2 Side Effects

A variety of acute side effects may occur during radiation therapy of Hodgkin's disease, especially during mantle irradiation (Hoppe, 1980; Kaplan, 1980; Kinsella et al., 1982; Thar and Million, 1980). Fortunately, most are transient and many are of minimal consequence. Anorexia is common and may be aggravated by altered sensations of taste and smell. Nutritional status may also decline because of nausea and vomiting, diarrhoea, and mucositis, possibly accompanied by difficulty or pain in swallowing, but the latter usually develops only near the end of treatment and the other problems are not common. Substantial weight loss during treatment is actually infrequent. Fatigue and an unusual lassitude, often worse on treatment days, may curtail normal activity in some. Dental evaluation (and necessary treatment, if possible) should be performed before mantle irradiation as such treatment may aggravate or cause dental problems, primarily due to resultant xerostomia, and osteoradionecrosis may complicate subsequent oral surgery.

Mantle irradiation also commonly causes minor skin reaction along the sides of the neck and axillary folds as well as temporary occipital area hair loss. Lhermitte's syndrome of transient radiation myelopathy occurs in 15 to 25% of patients but is not a harbinger of radiation myelitis. Affected patients experience a fleeting 'electrical shock' or tingling sensation running down the back and/or legs upon neck flexion which may occur over several months following therapy.

Leucocyte and platelet counts may decrease by as much as 50% during mantle irradiation and may decrease even further if another field is treated immediately afterwards. Thus, a rest period of 2 or more weeks is usually allowed between treatment of successive fields to promote recovery from bone marrow injury and other toxicities.

2.3 Results of Radiation Therapy

Radiation therapy offers effective treatment for most patients with early stage Hodgkin's disease. Ten-year survival rates for stage I-II patients of 83% (symptomatic patients) and 86% (asymptomatic) have been reported following total lymphoid irradiation (Hoppe, 1980). Extended field therapy afforded a 95% 10-year survival rate for asymptomatic stage I-II patients and an 8-year survival rate of 84% for stage IIB patients in another large series (Hellman and Mauch, 1982). Few patients in either series relapsed after 5 years following radiation therapy. Patients who continuously remain in complete remission for 5 years following initial radiotherapy may thus be cured.

Those patients who unfortunately do relapse can be effectively treated by chemotherapy (see section 4), and relapse-free survival rates are therefore lower than the above overall survival rates. Patients with stage IIIA disease do less well, with 10-year survival rates of only 63 to 67% following total lymphoid irradiation, and many patients require salvage therapy (Hellman and Mauch, 1982; Hoppe, 1980). Combination chemotherapy alone probably affords at least comparable survival rates in such patients and seems more effective in achieving permanent freedom from relapse (Crowther et al., 1984; Lister et al., 1983). Stage IIIA patients with infradiaphragmatic disease only in the upper abdomen (spleen or splenic, porta hepatis or coeliac lymph nodes only) may form a subset ('stage III_1 A') of patients with a better response to radiation therapy than those with lower abdominal disease ('Stage III_2 A') [Stein et al., 1980], although this has not been noted in all series (Hoppe, 1980). Radiation therapy alone is not commonly used for stage IIIB or IV Hodgkin's disease.

3. Combined Modality Therapy

Potential advantages of an induction programme combining irradiation and combination chemotherapy include increased effectiveness as well as decreased morbidity of staging and treatment for certain patients such as the very young and those with massive mediastinal involvement. Combined modality programmes were thus met initially with great enthusiasm. This has been tempered, however, by increasing recognition of the enhanced potential for treatment complications following such therapy (see section 5) and of the ability of combination chemotherapy regimens to induce durable second complete remissions, especially in those who relapse following radiation therapy (see section 4). Nevertheless, combined modality therapy may be reasonable for patients in certain poor-risk categories (Canellos et al., 1983).

3.1 Use in Common Presentations of Advanced Disease

Although relapses are more frequent following irradiation alone than after combined modality therapy of stage I and II disease, both retrospective (Hagemeister et al., 1982) and prospective (Hoppe et al., 1982; Nissen et al., 1982) studies have shown comparable survival rates with either method of treatment because of effective salvage therapy. Combined modality therapy is therefore generally not necessary in routine presentations of these stages. Combined modality therapy of advanced Hodgkin's disease, in contrast, is currently widely used. Uniformly high (80% or greater) complete response rates and impressive overall survival rates have been obtained by combining radiation therapy with various combination chemotherapy regimens, including MOPP (Bonadonna and Santoro, 1982; Rosenberg et al., 1978), ABVD (Bonadonna and Santoro, 1982), MVVPP (Farber et al., 1980), MOPP/ABDV(Strausetal.,1981a,b),MOPP/ABVD or CAD/MOPP/ABDV (Straus et al., 1984), and MOPP/CAVmP (Wagener et al., 1983). However, the patient follow-up reported for many programmes is short and several direct comparisons of single and combined modality treatment in prospective randomised clinical trials have shown comparable survival rates (Jones et al., 1982; Rosenberg et al., 1978). It is thus not clear that such programmes afford long term survival rates better than those with initial single modality therapy in common presentations of advanced disease.

3.2 Use in Patients with Massive Mediastinal Involvement

Presentations with massive mediastinal involvement need to be considered separately. Patients with a mediastinal mass whose largest diameter exceeds 30 to 35% of the maximum thoracic width have significantly higher relapse rates following radiotherapy than patients with lesser or no mediastinal involvement in some (Lee et al., 1980; Mauch et al., 1982) but not all (Prosnitz et al., 1980; Schomberg et al., 1984) series. Radiation therapy may be technically difficult in such patients and require special techniques and possibly higher total doses (Hoppe, 1980). Combined modality therapy has thus been used in these patients with the intent of decreasing relapse rates and treatment complications. However, radiation therapy can be both safe and effective in this setting (Prosnitz et al., 1980; Schomberg et al., 1984) and comparable survival following irradiation given alone or combined with MOPP chemotherapy has been shown in retrospective (Mauch et al., 1982) and prospective (Hoppe et al., 1982) studies. The role of combined modality therapy for these patients is thus incompletely defined, but may be best limited to those with disease preventing adequate shielding of the heart and lungs (Mauch et al., 1982) or those with an unchanged mass after the first 1500 rad of radiation therapy (Johnson et al., 1983).

4. Salvage Therapy

Additional 'salvage' therapy is required for those who do not obtain a complete response with primary therapy or who later relapse. Additional irradiation is generally not useful in patients initially treated with radiation therapy (Hoppe, 1980), but such patients respond to MOPP (DeVita et al., 1980) and several other combination chemotherapy regimens (Bonadonna and Santoro, 1982; Dady et al., 1982; Sutcliffe et al., 1978) at least as well as previously untreated patients. Salvage therapy after initial chemotherapy, however, is less successful. Radiation therapy is not commonly employed, but it may be useful in certain circumstances (Diehl et al., 1983). Retreatment with MOPP chemotherapy produces second complete responses in about 90% of patients who relapse from a complete remission which lasted more than 1 year, but in only about 30% of those who relapse sooner, with a median survival of approximately 5 years following induction of a second complete remission (Fisher et al., 1979).

Salvage therapy of patients with MOPP-resistant disease (progressive disease during therapy or early relapse) is less effective. The ABVD regimen had complete response rates in such patients of 55% (Papa et al., 1982) and 59% (Santoro et al., 1982c) in 2 studies is widely used, but much lower rates were reported in 4 other studies (reviewed in Longo et al., 1982), possibly because of differences among studies in patient characteristics and details of chemotherapy administration. Of interest is that MOPP therapy produced complete responses in only 25% of patients with ABVD-resistant disease (Santoro et al., 1982c). Other regimens with 25 to 60% complete response rates in salvage therapy (usually after MOPP failure) include ABDIC (Tannir et al., 1983), B-CAVe (Porzig et al., 1978), B-DOPA (Lokich et al., 1976), BVDS (Vinciguerra et al., 1977), CAD/MOPP/ABV (Straus et al., 1983), CEP and CEP/ABVD (Santoro et al., 1982b), CVB (Goldman and Dawson, 1975), MOPP/ABVD (Straus et al., 1981a,b), SCAB (Levi et al., 1977), and VABCD (Einhorn et al., 1983). However, second complete remissions in this setting are often brief and long term survival is not common. Single-agent therapy may be useful for palliative therapy of patients with truly refractory disease (Mead et al., 1982).

5. Treatment Complications

Complications of treatment and recurrent disease may have numerous manifestations, and both should be considered in the differential diagnosis of subsequent illnesses in patients with Hodgkin's disease. Recent reviews of the complications of therapy for Hodgkin's disease (Gams, 1980; Hoppe, 1980; Kaplan, 1980; Kinsella et al., 1982; Thar and Million, 1980) may be of assistance. Meticulous treatment planning and technique will minimise radiotherapy complications, but the thyroid gland cannot be adequately shielded during mantle irradiation and hypothyroidism will later develop in many patients. Thyroid-stimulating hormone level determinations should initially be performed 6-monthly, and patients with elevated levels should receive L-thyroxine (Schimpff et al., 1980). Patients treated with mantle irradiation and certain chemotherapy regimens are at increased risk for pulmonary complications, as drugs such as doxorubicin (adriamycin) and bleomycin may potentiate radiation injury and abrupt cessation of steroid therapy may precipitate radiation pneumonitis. Combined modality therapy may also potentiate haematopoietic toxicity as regeneration of irradiated marrow may not begin for years after therapy. Immunisation with pneumococcal vaccine may reduce the risk of fulminant bacterial sepsis (Levine et al., 1979).

5.1 Gonadal Toxicity

Chemotherapy causes primary ovarian failure in 25 to 50% of premenopausal women and premature menopause may occur in others (Horning et al., 1981; Schilsky et al., 1981; Whitehead et al., 1983). Most men treated with MOPP (DeVita, 1981) and MVPP (Chapman et al., 1981) and some of those treated with ABVD (Bonadonna and Santoro, 1982) become sterile. The National Cancer Institute is currently testing a lutenising-hormone-releasing-hormone (LHRH) analogue to determine if concomitant suppression of gonadal function reduces the testicular toxicity of MOPP therapy.

Radiation therapy often causes oligo- or azoospermia, but most men recover testicular function within 2 years following even total lymphoid irradiation (Thar and Million, 1980), and there seems to be no increased incidence of congenital anomalies in their offspring (Holmes and Holmes, 1978). Radiation therapy sparing the pelvis probably has little effect on ovarian function (Cunningham et al., 1982), and oophoropexy and special shielding may preserve ovarian function in some women even with total lymphoid irradiation (Horning et al., 1981).

Age during treatment with drugs or total lymphoid irradiation greatly influences subsequent ovarian function, with the least impairment noted in women younger than 25 years of age, and those who maintain normal or even irregular menses may have normal pregnancies, probably without increased risk of fetal wastage or congenital anomalies (Horning et al., 1981; Schilsky et al., 1981; Whitehead et al., 1983).

5.2 Secondary Malignancies

Therapy may also influence the development of secondary malignancies. Actuarial estimates of the cumulative probability of either preleukaemia or overt leukaemia are as high as 9.9% at 9 years following treatment (Pedersen-Bjergaard and Larsen, 1982). The chance of developing leukaemia is greater following chemotherapy than after radiation therapy, especially for older patients or those requiring additional salvage chemotherapy, and combined modality therapy may be associated with the greatest risk (Aisenberg, 1983; DeVita, 1981; Henry-Amar, 1983; Pedersen-Bjergaard and Larsen, 1982; Valagussa et al., 1980). Various solid tumours and non-Hodgkin's lymphomas may also occur after treatment, and again may be most frequent following combined modality therapy (Armitage et al., 1983; Krikorian et al., 1979; Nelson et al., 1981; Valagussa et al., 1980). The ABVD regimen, however, has been associated with secondary malignancies only in patients who also received radiotherapy (Amadori et al., 1983; Valagussa et al., 1980).

As apparent relapses of Hodgkin's disease may instead represent development of secondary malignancies, a tissue diagnosis should be secured whenever possible. Although these are certainly grave complications, it must be remembered that untreated Hodgkin's disease is uniformly fatal, and that secondary malignancies such as leukaemia are an uncommon cause of death in patients with Hodgkin's disease (Pedersen-Bjergaard and Larsen, 1982).

5. Current Treatment Recommendations

Many patients with Hodgkin's disease may be cured with currently standard treatment approaches. Although therapeutic decisions for a specific patient will be influenced by the medical resources available and by possible special circumstances (such as pregnancy, childhood, unusual disease presentation or intercurrent illness), the following general recommendations can be made for pathologically staged patients:

1. Those with stage I or IIA supradiaphragmatic disease without massive mediastinal involvement are best treated with extended field radiation therapy to mantle and para-aortic fields.

2. Patients with the infrequent infradiaphragmatic presentations of stages I or IIA disease should be treated with an inverted Y field except in cases of para-aortic disease, for which total lymphoid irradiation is indicated. Total lymphoid irradiation is also recommended in stage IIB and can be used

for stage IIIA disease, although combination chemotherapy alone probably affords at least comparable overall survival rates and may provide improved freedom from initial relapse.

3. Patients with stage I-IIA disease and massive mediastinal involvement can be reasonably treated with extended field radiotherapy alone, using special irradiation techniques or with combined modality therapy. Those with massive mediastinal involvement and more advanced disease require consideration on an individual basis. MOPP chemotherapy is advised for stage IIIB and IV patients.

4. Optimum therapy for certain presentations such as stage IIIA disease is not known, and suitable patients should be considered for entry into clinical trials.

Treatment approaches differing from the above general recommendations may thus be entirely reasonable and may eventually prove to be preferable. For example, combined modality therapy of certain advanced stage patients (such as those with bulky disease, the nodular sclerosis subtype, or stage III_2A disease) and alternating MOPP/ABVD chemotherapy of stage IV patients may become standard approaches if their apparent effectiveness is confirmed through further patient follow-up and additional clinical trials.

References

Aisenberg, A.C.: Acute non-lymphocytic leukemia after treatment of Hodgkin's disease. American Journal of Medicine 75: 449-454 (1983).

Amadori, S.; Papa, G.; Anselmo, A.P.; Fidani, P.; Mandelli, F. and Biagini, C.: Acute promyelocytic leukemia following ABVD (doxorubicin, bleomycin, vinblastine, and dacarbazine) and radiotherapy for Hodgkin's disease. Cancer Treatment Reports 67: 603-604 (1983).

Armitage, J.O.; Dick, F.R.; Goeken, J.A.; Foucar, K. and Gingrich, R.D.: Second lymphoid malignant neoplasms occurring in patients treated for Hodgkin's disease. Archives of Internal Medicine 143: 445-450 (1983).

Bonadonna, G.: Chemotherapy strategies to improve the control of Hodgkin's disease: The Richard and Linda Rosenthal Foundation Award Lecture. Cancer Research 42: 4309-4320 (1982).

Bonadonna, G. and Santoro, A.: ABVD chemotherapy in the treatment of Hodgkin's disease. Cancer Treatment Reviews 9: 21-35 (1982).

Bonadonna, G.; Viviani, S.; Bonfante, V.; Valagussa. P. and Santoro, A.: Alternating chemotherapy with MOPP/ABVD in Hodgkin's disease: updated results. Proceedings of the American Society of Clinical Oncology 3: 254 (1984).

Canellos, G.P.; Come, S.E. and Sharin, A.T.: Chemotherapy in the treatment of Hodgkin's disease. Seminars in Hematology 20: 1-24 (1983).

Carde, P.; MacKintosh, F.R. and Rosenberg, S.A.: A dose and time response analysis of the treatment of Hodgkin's disease with MOPP chemotherapy. Journal of Clinical Oncology 1: 146-153 (1983).

Chabner, B.A. and Myers, C.E.: Clinical pharmacology of cancer chemotherapy; in DeVita et al. (Eds) Cancer Principles and Practice of Oncology, pp. 156-197 (J.P. Lippincott, Philadelphia 1982).

Chapman, R.M.; Sutcliffe, S. and Malpas, J.S.: Male gonadal dysfuction in Hodgkin's disease. Journal of the American Medical Association 245: 1323-1328 (1981).

Coltman, Jr., C.A.: Chemotherapy of advanced Hodgkin's disease. Seminars in Oncology 7: 155-173 (1980).

Cooper, M.R.; Pajak, T.F.; Nissen, N.I.; Stutzman, L.; Brunner, K. et al.: A new effective four drug combination of CCNU [1-(2-chloroethy)-3-cyclohexyl-1-nitrosourea] (NSC-79038), vinblastine, prednisone and procarbazine for the treatment of advanced Hodgkin's disease. Cancer 46: 654-662 (1980).

Crowther, D.; Wagstaff, J.; Deakin, D.; Todd, I.; Wilkinson, P. et al.: A randomized study comparing chemotherapy alone with chemotherapy followed by radiotherapy in patients with pathologically staged IIIA Hodgkin's disease. Journal of Clinical Oncology 2: 892-897 (1984).

Cunningham, J.; Mauch, P.; Rosenthal, D.S. and Canellos, G.P.: Long-term complications of MOPP chemotherapy in patients with Hodgkin's disease. Cancer Treatment Reports 66: 1015-1022 (1982).

Dady, P.J.; McElwain, T.J.; Austin, D.E.; Barrett, A. and Peckham, M.J.: Five years' experience with ChlVPP: Effective low-toxicity combination chemotherapy for Hodgkin's disease. British Journal of Cancer 45: 851-859 (1982).

DeVita Jr, V.T.: The consequences of the chemotherapy of Hodgkin's disease: The 10th David A. Karnofsky Memorial Lecture. Cancer 47: 1-13 (1981).

DeVita Jr, V.T. and Hellman, S.: Hodgkin's disease and the non-Hodgkin's lymphomas; in DeVita et al. (Eds) Cancer Principles and Practice of Oncology, pp. 1331-1401 (J.P. Lippincott, Philadelphia, 1982).

DeVita Jr, V.T.; Simon, R.M.; Hubbard, S.M.; Young, R.C.: Berard, C.W. et al.: Curability of advanced Hodgkin's disease with chemotherapy. Annals of Internal Medicine 92: 587-595 (1980).

Diehl, L.E.; Perry, D.J.; Terebelo, H.; Baldwin, P.E.; Hurwitz, M.: Kimball, D.B. and Dorn, R.V.: Radiation as salvage therapy for patients with Hodgkin's disease relapsing after MOPP (mechlorethamine, vincristine, prednisone and procarbazine) chemotherapy. Cancer Treatment Reports 67: 827-829 (1983).

Diggs, C.H.; Wiernik, P.H.; Levi, J.A. and Kvols, L.K.: Cyclophosphamide, vinblastine, procarbazine and prednisone with CCNU and vinblastine maintenance for advanced Hodgkin's disease. Cancer 39: 1949-1954 (1977).

Diggs, C.H.; Wiernik, P.H. and Sutherland, J.C.: Treatment of advanced untreated Hodgkin's disease with SCAB – an alternative to MOPP. Cancer 47: 224-228 (1981).

Einhorn, L.H.; Williams, S.D.; Stevens, E.E.; Bond, W.H. and Chenoweth, L.: Treatment of MOPP-refractory Hodgkin's disease with vinblastine, doxorubicin, bleomycin, CCNU and dacarbazine. Cancer 51: 1348-1352 (1983).

Farber, L.R.; Prosnitz, L.R.; Cadman, E.C.; Lutes, R.; Bertino, J.R. and Fisher, D.B.: Curative potential of combined modality therapy for advanced Hodgkin's disease. Cancer 46: 1509-1517 (1980).

Fisher, R.I.; DeVita, Jr, V.T.; Hubbard, S.M.; Simon, R. and Young, R.C.: Prolonged disease-free survival in Hodgkin's disease with MOPP reduction after first relapse. Annals of Internal Medicine 90: 761-763 (1979).

Gams, R.A.: Complications of chemotherapy in the treatment of

Hodgkin's disease. Seminars in Oncology 7: 184-186 (1980).
Gams, R.A.; Durant, J.R. and Bartolucci, A.A.: Chemotherapy for advanced Hodgkin's disease: Conclusions from the Southeastern Cancer Study Group. Cancer Treatment Reports 66: 899-905 (1982).
Gibbs, G.E.; Peterson, B.A.; Kennedy, B.J.; Vosika, G. and Bloomfield, C.D.: Long-term survival of patients with Hodgkin's disease. Archives of Internal Medicine 141: 897-900 (1981).
Glick, J.H.; Barnes, J.M.; Bakemeier, R.F.; Prosnitz, C.R.; Bennett, J.M. et al.: Treatment of advanced Hodgkin's disease: 10 years experience in the Eastern Cooperative Oncology Group. Cancer Treatment Reports 66: 855-870 (1982).
Goldman, J.M. and Dawson, A.A.: Combination therapy for advanced resistant Hodgkin's disease. Lancet 2: 1224-1227 (1975).
Gutensohn, N. and Cole, P.: Epidemiology of Hodgkin's disease. Seminars in Oncology 7: 92-102 (1982).
Hagemeister, F.B.; Fuller, L.M.; Velasquez, W.S.; Sullivan, J.A.; North, L. et al.: Stage I and II Hodgkin's disease: Involved field radiotherapy versus extended-field radiotherapy versus involved-field radiotherapy followed by six cycles of MOPP. Cancer Treatment Reports 66: 789-798 (1982).
Hellman, S. and Mauch, P.: Role of radiation therapy in the treatment of Hodgkin's disease. Cancer Treatment Reports 66: 915-923 (1982).
Henry-Amar, M.: Second cancers after radiotherapy and chemotherapy for early stages of Hodgkin's disease. Journal of the National Cancer Institute 71: 911-916 (1983).
Herman, T.S. and Jones, S.E.: Systematic restaging in patients with Hodgkin's disease. Cancer 42: 1976-1982 (1978).
Holmes, G.E. and Holmes, F.F.: Pregnancy outcome of patients treated for Hodgkin's disease: A controlled study. Cancer 41: 1317-1322 (1978).
Hoppe, R.T.: Radiation therapy in the treatment of Hodgkin's disease. Seminars in Oncology 7: 144-154 (1980).
Hoppe, R.T.; Coleman, N.C.; Cox, R.S.; Rosenberg, S.A. and Kaplan, H.S.: The management of stage I-II Hodgkin's disease with irradiation alone or combined modality therapy: The stanford experience. Blood 59: 455-465 (1982).
Horning, S.J.; Hoppe, R.T.; Kaplan, H.S. and Rosenberg, S.A.: Female reproductive potential after treatment for Hodgkin's disease. New England Journal of Medicine 304: 1377-1382 (1981).
Johnson, D.W.; Hoppe, R.T.; Cox, R.S.; Rosenberg, S.A. and Kaplan, H.S.: Hodgkin's disease limited to intrathoracic sites. Cancer 52: 8-13 (1983).
Jones, S.E.; Coltman, Jr, C.A.; Grozea, P.N.; DePersio, E.J. and Dixon, D.O.: Conclusions from clinical trials of the Southwest Oncology Group. Cancer Treatment Reports 66: 847-853 (1982).
Jones, S.E.; Haut, A.; Weick, J.K.; Wilson, H.E.; Grozea, P. et al.: Comparison of adriamycin-containing chemotherapy (MOP-BAP) with MOPP-bleomycin in the management of advanced Hodgkin's disease. Cancer 51: 1339-1347 (1983).
Kaplan, H.S.: Hodgkin's Disease, 2nd ed. (Harvard University Press, Cambridge 1980).
Kinsella, T.J.; Fraass, B.A. and Glatstein, E.: Late effects of radiation therapy in the treatment of Hodgkin's disease. Cancer Treatment Reports 66: 991-1001 (1982).
Krikorian, J.G.; Burke, J.S.; Rosenberg, S.A. and Kaplan, H.S.: Occurrence of non-Hodgkin's lymphoma after therapy of Hodgkin's disease. New England Journal of Medicine 300: 452-458 (1979).
Lee, C.K.K.; Bloomfield, C.D.; Goldman, A.I. and Levitt, S.H.: Prognostic significance of mediastinal involvement in Hodgkin's disease treated with curative radiotherapy. Cancer 46: 2403-2409 (1980).
Levi, J.A.; Wiernik, P.H. and Diggs, C.H.: Combination chemotherapy of advanced previously treated Hodgkin's disease with streptozotocin, CCNU, adriamycin and bleomycin. Medical and Pediatric oncology 3: 33-40 (1977).
Levine, A.M.; Overturf, G.D.; Field, R.F.; Holdorf, D.; Paganini-Hill, A. and Feinstern, D.I.: Use and efficacy of pneumococcal vaccine in patients with Hodgkin's disease. Blood 54: 1171-1175 (1979).
Lister, T.A.; Dorreen, M.S.; Faux, M.; Jones, A.E. and Wrigley, P.F.M.: The treatment of stage IIIA Hodgkin's disease. Journal of Clinical Oncology 1: 745-749 (1983).
Lokich, J.; Frei, III, E.; Jaffe, N. and Tullis, J.: New multiple-agent chemotherapy (B-DOPA) for advanced Hodgkin's disease. Cancer 38: 667-671 (1976).
Longo, D.L.; Young, R.C. and DeVita, Jr, V.T.: Chemotherapy for Hodgkin's disease: The remaining challenges. Cancer Treatment Reports 66: 925-936 (1982).
Mauch, P.; Gorshein, D.; Cunningham, J. and Hellman, S.: Influence of mediastinal adenopathy on site and frequency of relapse in patients with Hodgkin's disease. Cancer Treatment Reports 66: 809-817 (1982).
Mayer, R.J.: Alternating drug combinations for advanced Hodgkin's disease. (Correspondence.) New England Journal of Medicine 307: 688 (1982).
Mead, G.M.; Harker, W.G.; Kushlan, P. and Rosenberg, S.A.: Single-agent palliative chemotherapy for end-stage Hodgkin's disease. Cancer 50: 829-835 (1982).
Myers, C.E.; Chabner, B.A.; DeVita, V.T. and Gralnick, H.R.: Bone marrow involvement in Hodgkin's disease: Pathology and response to MOPP chemotherapy. Blood 44: 197-204 (1974).
Nelson, D.F.; Cooper, S.; Weston, M.G. and Rubin, A.: Second malignant neoplasms in patients treated for Hodgkin's disease with radiotherapy or radiotherapy and chemotherapy. Cancer 48: 2386-2393 (1981).
Nissen, N.I. and Nordentoff, A.M.: Radiotherapy versus combined modality treatment of stage I and II Hodgkin's disease. Cancer Treatment Reports 66: 799-803 (1982).
Papa, G.; Mandelli, F.; Anselmo, A.D.; DeLuca, A.M.; Maurizienrici, R. et al.: Treatment of MOPP-resistant Hodgkin's disease with adriamycin, bleomycin, vinblastine and decarbazine (ABVD). European Journal of Cancer and Clinical Oncology 18: 803-806 (1982).
Pedersen-Bjergaard, J. and Larsen, S.O.: Evidence of acute non-lymphocytic leukemia, preleukemia and acute myeloproliferative syndrome up to 10 years after treatment of Hodgkin's disease. New England Journal of Medicine 307: 965-971 (1982).
Pizzo, P.A.; Robichaud, K.J.; Gill, F.A. and Witebsky, F.G.: Empiric antibiotic and antifungal therapy for cancer patients with prolonged fever and granulocytopenia. American Journal of Medicine 72: 101-111 (1982).
Porzig, K.L.; Portlock, C.S.; Robertson, A. and Rosenberg, S.A.: Treatment of advanced Hodgkin's disease with B-CAVe following MOPP failure. Cancer 41: 1670-1675 (1978).
Prosnitz, L.R.; Curtis, A.M.; Knowlton, A.H.; Peters, L.M. and Farber, L.R.: Supradiaphragmatic Hodgkin's disease: Significance of large mediastinal masses. International Journal of Radiation Oncology, Biology and Physics 6: 809-813 (1980).
Rosenberg, S.A.; Kaplan, H.S.; Glatstein, E.J. and Portlock, C.S.: Combined modality therapy of Hodgkin's disease. Cancer 42: 991-1000 (1978).
Santoro, A.; Bonadonna, G.; Bonfante, V. and Valagussa, P.: Alternating drug combinations in the treatment of advanced Hodgkin's disease. New England Journal of Medicine 306: 770-775 (1982a).
Santoro, A.; Bonfante, V. and Bonadonna, G.: Third-line chemotherapy with CCNU, etoposide and prednimustine in Hodgkin's disease (HD) resistant to MOPP and ABVD. Proceedings of the American Society of Clinical Oncology 1: 165 (1982b).
Santoro, A.; Bonfante, V. and Bonadonna, G.: Salvage chemotherapy with ABVD in MOPP resistant Hodgkin's disease. Annals of Internal Medicine 96: 139-143 (1982c).
Schilsky, R.L.; Sherins, R.J.; Hubbard, S.M.; Wesley, M.N.; Young, R.C. and DeVita, V.T.: Long-term follow-up of ovarian func-

tion in women treated with MOPP chemotherapy for Hodgkin's disease. American Journal of Medicine 71: 552-556 (1981).

Schimpff, S.C.; Diggs, C.H.; Wiswell, J.G.; Salvatore, P.C. and Wiernik, P.H.: Radiation-related thyroid dysfunction: Implications for the treatment of Hodgkin's disease. Annals of Internal Medicine 92: 91-98 (1980).

Schomberg, P.J.; Evans, R.G.; O'Connell, M.J.; White, W.L.; Banks, P.M.; Ilstrup, D.M. and Earle, J.D.: Prognostic significance of mediastinal mass in adult Hodgkin's disease. Cancer 53: 324-328 (1984).

Siegel, L.J. and Longo, D.L.: The control of chemotherapy-induced emesis. Annals of Internal Medicine 95: 352-359 (1981).

Stein, R.S.; Golomb, H.M.; Diggs, C.H.; Mauch, P.; Hellman, S. et al.: Anatomic substages of stage III-A Hodgkin's disease. Annals of Internal Medicine 92: 159-165 (1980).

Straus, D.J.; Lee B.J.; Koziner, B.; Nisce, L.Z.; Young, C.W. and Clarkson, B.D.: The treatment of advanced Hodgkin's disease. Blut 43: 119-124 (1981a).

Straus, D.J.; Myers, J.; Koziner, B.J. and Clarkson, B.D.: Combination chemotherapy for the treatment of Hodgkin's disease in relapse. Cancer Chemotherapy and Pharmacology 11: 80-85 (1983).

Straus, D.J.; Myers, J.; Lee, B. J.; Nisce, L.Z.; Koziner, B.J. et al.: Treatment of advanced Hodgkin's disease with chemotherapy and irradiation. American Journal of Medicine 76: 270-278 (1984).

Straus, D.J.; Passe, S.; Koziner, B.; Lee, III, B.J.; Young, C.W. and Clarkson, B.D.: Combination chemotherapy salvage of heavily pretreated patients with Hodgkin's disease: An analysis of prognostic factors in two chemotherapy trials and the literature. Cancer Treatment Reports 65: 207-211 (1981b).

Sutcliffe, S.B.; Wrigley, P.F.M.; Peto, J.; Lister, T.A.; Stansfeld, A.G. et al.: MVPP chemotherapy regimen for advanced Hodgkin's disease. British Medical Journal 1: 679-683 (1978).

Tannir, N.; Hagemeister, F.; Velasquez, W. and Cabanillas, F.: Long-term follow-up with ABDIC salvage chemotherapy of MOPP-resistant Hodgkin's disease. Journal of Clinical Oncology 1: 432-439 (1983).

Thar, T.L. and Million, R.R.: Complications of radiation treatment of Hodgkin's disease. Seminars in Oncology 7: 174-183 (1980).

Valagussa, P.; Santoro, A.; Kenda, R.; Fossati Bellani, F.; Franchi, F.; Banfi, A.; Rilke, F. and Bonadonna, G.: Second malignancies in Hodgkin's disease: A complication of certain forms of treatment. British Medical Journal 280: 216-219 (1980).

Vinciguerra, V.; Coleman, M.; Jarowski, C.I.; Degnon, T.J. and Silver, R.T.: A new combination chemotherapy for resistant Hodgkin's disease. Journal of the American Medical Association 237: 33-35 (1977).

Wagener, D.J.T.; Burgers, J.M.V.; Dekker, A.D.; Kazen, I.; van Peperzeel, H.A. et al.: Sequential non-cross-resistant chemotherapy regimens (MOPP and CAVmP) in Hodgkin's disease stage IIIB and IV. Cancer 52: 1558-1562 (1983).

Whitehead, E.; Shalet, S.M.; Blackledge, G.; Todd, I.; Crowther, D. and Beardwell, C.G.: The effect of combination chemotherapy on ovarian function in women treated for Hodgkin's disease. Cancer 52: 988-993 (1983).

Young, R.C.; Canellos, G.P.; Chabner, B.A.; Hubbard, S.M. and DeVita, Jr., V.T.: Patterns of relapse in advanced Hodgkin's disease treated with combination chemotherapy. Cancer 42: 1001-1007 (1978).

Young, R.C. and DeVita, Jr, V.T.: Chemotherapy of Hodgkin's disease. Clinics in Hematology 8: 625-644 (1979).

Address for correspondence and reprints: Dr *Brent C. Behrens*, Medicine Branch, Division of Cancer Treatment, National Cancer Institute, National Institutes of Health (Building 10, Room 12N226), Bethesda, MD 20205 (USA).

Drugs 30: 368-375 (1985)
0012-6667/85/0010-0368/$04.00/0

Warts
Fact and Fiction

F.E. Anderson
Tamworth

Warts were well known to the physicians of Greece and Rome and throughout history cures have been sought all over the world. Although warts are very common, their true incidence is difficult to determine because only those which cause concern present to the medical profession.

Warts are an infection of the skin or mucous membrane by a virus of the Papovavirus group. This group of viruses also causes papillomas in animals and includes the Shope virus of rabbits, the Polyoma virus of mice, the vacuolating virus of monkeys and a number of other viruses which cause papillomas in cattle, dogs, monkeys, goats, horses, sheep and pigs.

Investigation of viral proteins by restriction enzyme analysis, molecular hybridisation and immunofluorescence has demonstrated many types of wart virus and these have been named human papilloma virus (HPV). Table I shows the assocation between the clinical types of wart and human papilloma viruses. In humans the virus infects epidermal cells by direct inoculation with infected material. In experimental inoculation the incubation period averages 4 months. The viruses can be seen by electronmicroscopy in the nuclei of the upper layers of the stratum spinosum, but as the cells mature, viruses spill over from the nucleus to the cytoplasm and then can be found dispersed in the horny layer. As the wart ages, the quantity of virus present falls.

There is, of course, no specific treatment for warts. There is no doubt that many of the measures employed are relatively, and in many cases totally, ineffective. Sadly, several of these treatments are painful and some even scar the skin permanently. The great majority of warts are harmless and benign and their main importance to the patient is cosmetic. It is vitally important that the skin should not be damaged during the treatment of such minor problems and certainly it is sad when ordinary warts are treated under general anaesthesia.

The natural history of warts should always be remembered when a treatment regimen is being or-

Table I. Association between the clinical types of warts and human papilloma viruses (HPV) [after Bunney, 1982]

Virus types	Source of virus
HPV1	Palmoplantar warts
HPV2	Common warts
	Mosaic warts
	Some genital warts
	Some laryngeal papillomas
HPV3	Plane warts
HPV4	Some palmoplantar warts
HPV5	Epidermodysplasia verruciformis
HPV6	Anogenital warts
HPV7	Common warts (butcher)
HPV8	Epidermodysplasia verruciformis

ganised. One thousand institutionalised mentally defective children had all their warts recorded for a period of 2 years (Massing and Epstein, 1963). The overall incidence increased from 18 to 25% in 2 years, but two-thirds of the original lesions in 168 patients involuted during the 2-year period. It was interesting that new warts occurred 3 times more frequently in infected children than in uninfected children and it was concluded that there was a reservoir of warts in the community and that an individual reaction was an important prerequisite for infection. It was also considered that each colony of wart viruses probably had its own lifecycle.

New work, which has linked the wart virus and especially HPV6 to carcinoma of the cervix and occasionally to penile and anal carcinoma (Syrjanen, 1984), would suggest that there are some warts which should be treated energetically, but for the majority of warts gentle treatment is all that is required. Laryngeal papillomas are also occasionally premalignant.

1. Suggestion and Psychotherapy

There are probably more folk remedies for warts than for any other affliction of mankind. It is certainly widely believed that suggestion can cure warts and it is very difficult to invalidate the claims made for this modality of treatment. However, most investigations concerned with suggestion as treatment for warts have not taken the natural history into account and so it is difficult to know whether the suggestion has in fact been successful. It is also possible that many of the simple physical treatments given for warts may appear to be successful simply because the warts have resolved spontaneously. Cases have been described in which the cure by posthypnotic suggestion has deliberately been confined to one side of the body and it is difficult not to believe that the method has worked in these cases (Ullman, 1959).

Certainly, when treating warts one should always keep the possibility of spontaneous resolution in mind and it does seem worthwhile to use the power of suggestion as much as possible. It is remarkable how often resistant warts disappear quickly after referral to a dermatologist, possibly because the patient expects the expert to succeed. This may be attributable to suggestion.

Should the cure of a particular patient prove too difficult, perhaps the physician should resort to some historical remedies. Sir Francis Bacon had his warts cured by rubbing them with fat pork which was then hung out in the sun to melt fully, which took about 5 weeks – and by then the warts had gone. Warts also used to be rubbed with a green alder stick which was then buried in muck to rot. A Cornish vagrant charged for carrying warts out of the district by the simple expedient of writing their number inside his hat. One successful method was to rub the warts, without being observed, on the father of an illegitimate child. Even in modern times there are wart shrines in Tokyo, and recently a wart charmer appeared on British television.

2. Epidemiology

Epidemiological studies are confused by the long and variable incubation period but there seems no doubt that warts are transmitted by direct contact. For example, the infection can sometimes be inoculated from hands to feet or face and investigation has shown clearly that communal bathing and changing facilities are associated with an increase in the incidence of plantar warts. Occasionally warts may be transmitted by contaminated objects. It is very rare for hand warts to be passed to the anogenital region. These simple epidemiological facts should be remembered when warts are to be treated.

Anogenital warts (fig. 1) are firmly established as sexually transmitted. When they proliferate into large masses in this area they are called condylomata acuminata. Recently it has been shown that the wart virus is a precursor of carcinoma of the cervix (Syrjanen, 1984). An American authority reported that 60% of male partners of women with cancer or precancer of the cervix had wart infections of the penis. Australian pathologists have found what appears to be wart virus in 69.5% of 500 cases of cervical dysplasia. Although cancer of the vulva is rare there is evidence that the wart virus may be

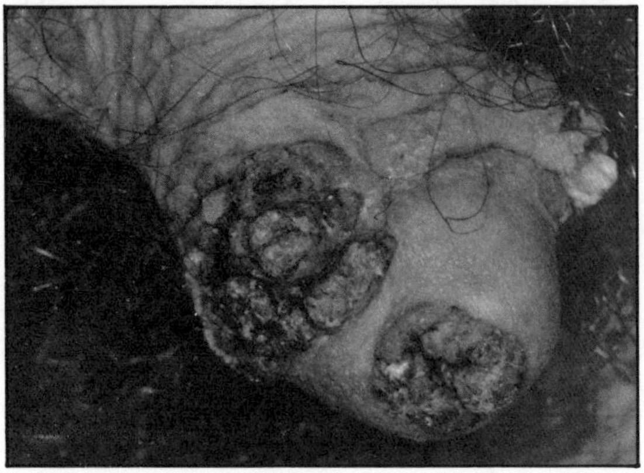

Fig. 1. Penile warts. (Photograph courtesy Dr H. Molloy.)

involved and from West Germany comes a report of a relationship between warts and cancer of the penis. In Sydney a blood test for the presence of wart virus has been developed, using the surface antigen of the virus. Blood samples from women with cervical carcinoma were positive for wart virus in 93% of cases; in those with anogenital warts the figure was 95%. The test may, in the future, be used to screen women for wart virus infection in the absence of obvious disease.

Thus, the fiction that warts are always harmless has been exploded but it is hoped that warts will not, in the future, generate all the fear and terror which surrounds the herpes simplex virus in the USA. Active treatment of warts in the anogenital area would obviously appear to be well justified.

2.1 Trauma

Trauma certainly plays a part in infection with the wart virus and if not prevented makes the cure much more difficult. The most obvious trauma associated with warts is nail biting and if the child or adult cannot be stopped from this habit it is almost impossible to effect a cure about the fingers and around the fingernails. Many plantar warts are on pressure points (fig. 2) and this must be considered in every patient suffering from this problem. Ill-fitting shoes, athletic injuries or minor orthopaedic foot problems may all aid the successful growth of the virus.

3. Immunology

In this era of organ transplantation with its accompanying induced immunosuppression, the importance of immune response in wart infections is very obvious. The incidence of warts is increased in patients with Hodgkin's disease and to a lesser extent in those with malignant lymphoma or chronic lymphatic leukaemia, but organ transplant patients suffer from extensive and prolonged problems. Reduction of cell-mediated immunity ap-

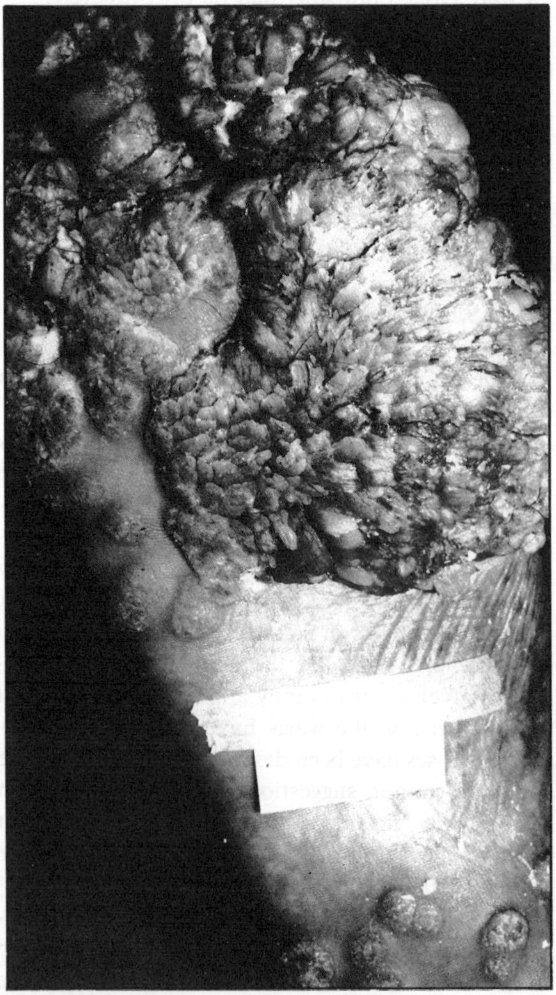

Fig. 2. Massive plantar warts. (Photograph courtesy Dr H. Molloy.)

pears to be the common problem. There is some evidence that cell-mediated immunity in children who have warts is less than that of a controlled group of children and that the diminution of the response of patients with persistent warts is proportionate to their duration (Morison, 1975b). An increased cell-mediated response can be demonstrated at or about the time of resolution of warts (Morison, 1974). The role of humoral antibodies is uncertain. The cure of warts is associated with a rise in the level of circulating immunoglobulin G and in patients with immunoglobulin M or low titres of immunoglobulin G the warts tend to persist (Pyrhonen and Johansson, 1975). However, reinfection or recurrence of warts can occur in the presence of circulating antibody.

Immunotherapy has been attemped in the treatment of warts. The patients were first sensitised to dinitrochlorbenzene by application of a 2% mixture in soft white paraffin. Sensitisation was proven by patch-testing and then a 0.1% dinitrochlorbenzene ointment was applied weekly to the warts in an attempt to enhance the local cell-mediated immunity. As so often happens in the treatment of warts there were early hopeful reports but this method of treatment has not stood the test of time.

Levamisole is an anthelmintic which is known to restore the capacity to develop cutaneous delayed hypersensitivity in anergic patients with cancer. Oral administration of levamisole has been tried in patients with very resistant warts in an attempt to enhance their cell-mediated immunity. However, again this has not been successful.

4. Treatment

4.1 Home Treatment

Numerous wart applications may be bought off the shelf and several others are prescribed by doctors. Most of these can be used at home and their effectiveness depends greatly on correct and sufficient application (table II). The patient should be carefully instructed in the method of applying medication and ideally should be given written instructions. Most remedies will take at least 12 weeks to effect a cure and the patient or the parents should have this explained to them. Periodic examination by the doctor, e.g. at 6-week intervals, should be arranged.

Table II. Example of written instructions to be given to the patient in the home treatment of warts (after Bunney, 1982)

Treat regularly every night – it may take 12 weeks for the warts to disappear

1. Wash the warts with hot soapy water and soak for 5 minutes
2. Dry with your own towel
3. Rub off old applications and dead wart material, with a pumice stone if necessary
4. Apply medicament as instructed:
   Paint: Apply a drop of paint to the centre of the wart with a pointed matchstick
   Paste: Rub the paste into the wart with a cotton wool bud
   Formalin solution: Pour the solution into a container and dip the wart into the solution, ensuring it does not rest on the base of the container. Soak for 10 minutes
5. If the warts are on the feet, cover with plaster

NB. If your warts become painful consult your doctor

Before application of the local preparation the warts should be soaked in hot soapy water for at least 5 minutes. Old applications or hard, dead material on top of the wart should be rubbed off with a pumice stone.

4.1.1 Salicylic Acid Paint (SLA)

The most useful application for most warts, except on the face or in the anogenital areas, is the so-called SLA made up as follows:

Salicylic acid	1 part
Lactic acid	1 part
Collodion	4 parts.

This should be applied with a pointed applicator before retiring to bed at night, e.g. a sharpened matchstick. On the hands the application does not need to be covered as the collodion hardens rapidly, but it is better to cover it on the sole of the foot in order to increase maceration of the thick skin, thus allowing the acids to penetrate. There is no contraindication to the application of this paint to periungual warts.

4.1.2 Upton's Paste

The following is the prescription for the old-fashioned Upton's paste:

Salicylic acid	7 parts
Trichloracetic acid	1 part
Glycerine as necessary to make thick paste.	

This is useful for resistant plantar warts or thick hand warts. A hole which is the same size as the wart is cut in a piece of sticking plaster which is applied to the skin so that the wart corresponds to the hole. The paste is applied and a further piece of plaster applied to seal the area. This is left on for 24 hours, the area is cleaned and washed, dead tissue is removed with the pumice stone and the paste is re-applied.

If the treatment causes pain the area should be rested until tenderness goes.

4.1.3 Formalin Preparations

Formalin preparations are well established in the treatment of plantar warts and are always the treatment of choice if there are multiple warts. It is usual to use a 3 to 10% aqueous solution of formalin, soaking the wart for 10 minutes each night having first rubbed away the dead tissue. The softer skin of the sole or the skin between the toes may become overdried and cracked by the formalin so must be carefully protected by the application of petroleum jelly.

The surface of the wart must not rest on the base of the container because the solution will not soak the wart. If there are few plantar warts a pledget of cotton wool may be soaked in the formalin solution and attached by plaster so that it stays in place overnight. The patient should be regularly reviewed.

4.1.4 Side Effects

Side effects of home treatment are not common. Overdrying of the skin or wart may lead to cracking and pain so that rest from treatment becomes necessary. Sensitisation to salicylic acid and more particularly to formalin must be considered a possibility.

4.2 Chemical Treatment by the Medical Practitioner

4.2.1 Podophyllin

Podophyllin is a complex resinous mixture containing podophyllotoxin which is known to inhibit mitoses and cause swelling and necrosis of cells. Originally used as a drastic purge, it can cause vomiting, lethargy, progressive stupor, neuropathy and eventually death. Being a strong antimitotic agent it is obviously hazardous in pregnancy. For all these reasons podophyllin should not be used as a home remedy.

Podophyllin is usually dissolved in spirit or compound tincture of benzoin to give a 2.5 to 20% solution. The treatment of anogenital warts depends greatly on the use of podophyllin and this will require weekly visits to the medical practitioner. A small quantity of 2.5% podophyllin in compound tincture of benzoin is applied carefully to the surface of the warts with a cotton wool bud. On subsequent weekly paintings stronger solutions can be used according to the degree of reaction from the previous painting. Some erythema and oedema are to be expected and this is followed by shrinkage and sloughing off of the warts. If the reaction is severe, analgesia may be necessary and cold compresses may help. The patient must be instructed to watch for recurrences so that these may be treated early. Podophyllin does not have any advantages in the treatment of warts in other body areas.

4.3 Cryotherapy

The freezing agents used are carbon dioxide snow which melts at −56.6°C and liquid nitrogen which vaporises at −195.8°C. Freezing is said not to affect the mature wart virus directly, but alternate freezing and thawing does so. The curative effect of freezing on warts depends on the destruction of host cells. Immune responses to wart virus develop in patients whose warts are cured by several freezing treatments, indicating stimulation of the immune system (Morison, 1975a).

Carbon dioxide snow can be made into a slush by adding a few drops of acetone and the slush may be applied to the wart on a cotton bud. Liquid nitrogen is much easier to use; a cotton bud made to correspond to the wart may be soaked in liquid nitrogen and then applied to the wart. Experience is of great help in knowing how long to apply the freezing agent. Usually the wart is frozen until a halo of about 1mm appears around the base, indicating that the full thickness has been frozen. Carbon dioxide slush takes about 3 times longer to freeze the wart than liquid nitrogen, which may take anything from 5 to 30 seconds.

Warts in any area may be treated by cryotherapy, which is now one of the most popular methods. Once-weekly attendances for freezing are advised. Blisters containing serous or bloodstained fluid may develop within a few hours and patients should be warned that this may occur and that there is no need to puncture the blister unless it is so large as to be a nuisance.

It is no longer thought to be necessary to freeze the wart severely enough to produce blisters intentionally. In the Edinburgh series discussed by Bunney (1982), an average of 3.7 treatments was required for cure.

4.4 Surgical Treatment

Patients often request surgical treatment in the mistaken belief that the warts will be cured immediately. Recurrence following surgical management is in fact higher than for other methods – around 30% (Vickers, 1961). In addition, the resultant scarring may be cosmetically unacceptable and on the fingertip or a weight-bearing area of the foot may be incapacitating. Other arguments against surgical treatment are postoperative pain, the need for anaesthesia and the possibility of secondary infection.

Excision of warts and repair by suturing should never be advised because recurrences are very frequent. The best surgical method is probably to inject the local anaesthetic and firmly curette out all the wart tissue. Occasionally the curettage is made easier by first frying the top of the wart with cautery. Once the wart has been curetted the bleeding may be very gently stopped using cautery. The best indication for curettage is probably the large single wart which has been present for a long time and which therefore does not contain copious quantities of virus. In expert hands periungual warts may be treated this way without nail damage, but follow-up of treatment and freezing of remnants is necessary. Similarly, anogenital warts may be cauterised and in some cases general anaesthesia is necessary.

4.5 Radiotherapy

There is no place for radiotherapy in the treatment of warts. Plantar warts were for many years treated by radiotherapy but it is now recognised that a safe dose is not sufficient to cure the lesion. A follow-up of 100 patients after approximately 11 years showed serious postirradiation damage in 7% and slight radiodermatitis in 31% (Faesster and Krebs, 1974). It is now unusual to use radiotherapy in benign lesions of the skin, and warts are certainly included in this category.

4.6 Alternative Treatments

The various methods of treatment outlined above will cure the majority of warts. There remains, however, a hard core of patients who have lesions which resist all ordinary attempts. Dinitrochlorbenzene and levamisole have already been mentioned but several other modalities are worth considering.

4.6.1 5-Fluorouracil

5-Fluorouracil is an antimetabolite which is used incorporated in a cream or a lotion for multiple superficial solar keratoses. It is irritating to skin and causes superficial ulceration. It has been used in wart treatment as a 5% cream and should be applied accurately to the wart each day with a cotton wool bud and covered with a waterproof plaster. It is not always successful and should be used only in exceptional circumstances and under supervision. Some authorities have claimed success using this agent in plane warts without covering.

4.6.2 Bleomycin

Bleomycin has been injected as a 0.1% solution into resistant plantar warts. In specialist practice this injection has also been made into large periungual warts. There is considerable pain afterwards but the success rate is high.

4.6.3 Retinoids

Retinoic acid has been used topically for warts with varying success. There have been reports of the oral use of the aromatic retinoid, etretinate, for severe recalcitrant warts. High doses are necessary and therefore side effects are severe, but this therapy could have a place in the future for serious problems.

4.6.4 Interferon

If this becomes more easily available it may be worthy of consideration for widespread lesions in allograft patients. Already some reports of success have been published and future investigations will be of interest.

4.6.5 Antiviral Drugs

Obviously drugs with a direct antiviral action would be ideal, but so far a satisfactory one has not been found. Idoxuridine has been used topically, dissolved in dimethylsulphoxide in concentrations as high as 40%, but was disappointing. However, 20% idoxuridine in a cream base under polythene occlusion gave promising results and will remove some recalcitrant warts.

Table III. Recommended treatments for warts, listed in order of choice

Plantar warts
1. Correct minor orthopaedic defects, ensure footwear is suitable and treat hyperhidrosis
2. Formalin solution
3. Salicylic acid paint
4. Upton's paste
5. Cryotherapy

Common warts
1. Cryotherapy
2. Salicylic acid paint
3. Upton's paste
4. Cauterisation (rarely)

Anogenital warts
1. Podophyllin paint
2. Curettage and cautery
3. Cryotherapy
4. If giant warts with recent enlargement in older patient, surgical excision and histological examination is necessary

Plane warts
1. Suggestion
2 Mild cryotherapy

5. Conclusion

The most common reason for patients or parents to seek treatment for warts is a cosmetic one. Children occasionally become very self-conscious about having warts, following taunting from their friends. Most warts can be cured painlessly and safely and the old dermatological maxim of 'primum non nocere' should always be remembered in these patients. Instruction sheets to help sufferers to understand more fully how treatment should be applied are valuable because attention to detail really pays dividends. The warning that a period of 12 weeks' treatment is to be expected also puts the process into better perspective. Immunosuppressed patients present special problems which have not been solved completely. Anogenital warts with their risk of future malignancy obviously require energetic management and these provide one of the very few instances where general anaesthesia is warranted.

References

Bunney, M.H.: Viral Warts: Their Biology and Treatment (Oxford University Press, New York 1982).

Faesster, R. and Krebs, A.: Long term re-examination of patients' plantar warts treated by Roentgen therapy. Dermatologica, Basel 148: 345-352 (1974).

Massing, A.M. and Epstein, W.L.: Natural history of warts: A two year study. Archives of Dermatology 87: 306-310 (1963).

Morison, W.L.: *In vitro* assay of cell-mediated immunity to human wart antigen. British Journal of Dermatology 90: 531-534 (1974).
Morison, W.L.: *In vitro* assay of immunity to wart virus. British Journal of Dermatology 93: 545-552 (1975a).
Morison, W.L.: Cell-mediated immune responses in patients with warts. British Journal of Dermatology 93: 553-556 (1975b).
Pyrhonen, S. and Johansson, E.: Regression of warts. An immunological study. Lancet 1: 592-596 (1975).
Syrjanen, K.J.: Current concepts of human papilloma virus infections in the genital tract and their relationship to intraepithelial neoplasia and squamous cell carcinoma. Obstetrical and Gynecological Survey 39: 252 (1984).
Ullman, M.: On the psyche and warts. I. Suggestion and warts: A review and comment. Psychosomatic Medicine 21: 473-488 (1959).
Vickers, C.F.: Treatment of plantar warts in children. British Medical Journal 2: 743-745 (1961).

Address for correspondence and reprints: Dr *F.E. Anderson,* P.O. Box 362, Tamworth, NSW 2340 (Australia).

Drugs 30: 377-381 (1985)
0012-6667/85/0011-0377/$02.50/0

Newer Non-Sedating Antihistamines
Will They Replace Older Agents?

Milan L. Brandon
Allergy Medical Group of San Diego, San Diego

There has been a resurgence of interest in antihistamines and their effects during the past decade since the development of terfenadine, astemizole, and other possibly non-sedating antihistamines such as mequitazine, BW825C (an analogue of hydroxyzine and meclozine which bears an acrylic acid chain ortho to the pyridine ring nitrogen atom of tripolidine), and UCB-P071 (a member of the cyclizine series of compounds). Further non-sedating antihistamines are also being evaluated, and among these is SK&F 93944; on the basis of extensive animal studies this compound is now being evaluated for the treatment of allergic rhinitis in humans at a dose of 100mg once or twice daily.

1. Differences in Activity Between Older and Newer Non-Sedating Antihistamines

Each of the above antihistamines is different in origin, chemical structure, and specificity of action and each is different in solubility and metabolic effects. However, they have in common the property of not readily penetrating the blood-brain barrier in usual therapeutic dosages. In contrast, most of the older antihistamines are highly lipid-soluble and thus readily cross the blood-brain barrier (Brandon and Weiner, 1982; Nicholson, 1983). The ideal pure H_1-antihistamine would have specificity for H_1-receptors without other effects, including no anticholinergic or α-adrenoceptor blocking activity. However, it is not clearly established that it must have a high affinity for peripheral H_1-receptors and not cross the blood-brain barrier to reach central H_1-receptors.

Due to diurnal differences in the rate of metabolism of some antihistamines, the duration of action and potency may differ depending on whether the drug is administered in the morning or evening. For example, a dose of 60mg terfenadine given at 7am may protect against allergic skin reactions for 24 hours, while a dose of 30mg given at 7pm may provide a similar degree of protection for the same period (Reinberg et al., 1978). Optimum therapy may therefore involve different doses given at different times of day for those antihistamines that do not protect for 24 hours with single daily doses and require twice daily administration.

Most antihistamines are not pure H_1-antagonists. On the contrary, they usually have multiple metabolic effects. Numerous biochemical processes and mediators are also involved in acute allergic reactions that involve release of histamine. However, the same nasal symptoms may be stimulated by mechanisms that do not involve allergy; vasomotor reactions, for example, are more common than allergic rhinitis. Pure H_1-antihistamines would thus be of no benefit in treating vasomotor reactions that do not involve the release of histamine. On the other hand, many of the older antihistamines have a broad spectrum of action, e.g. antihistaminic, anticholinergic, antiserotonergic, antibradykinin, sedative, and other properties. One would therefore expect such medications to be much more useful than the newer antihistamines in patients with mixed vasomotor, central allergic and other disturbances.

Once we fully appreciate the frequency and variety of non-allergic causes of upper and lower respiratory disorders and categorise them, pharmaceutical manufacturers may concentrate their efforts on development of more precise medications that act more specifically on each of the underlying disorders. In this way, appropriate specific therapy may be tailored to each patient, with optimum results.

2. Potential Adverse Effects of Older Antihistamines Avoided with the Newer Non-Sedating Agents

Antihistamines with anticholinergic activity may cause dryness of the mouth, blurred vision, dysuria or urinary retention, impotence, disordered coordination, increases in the pulse rate and other effects (Brandon and Weiner, 1980; Douglas, 1980). Promethazine and related compounds may exert both anticholinergic and α-adrenoceptor blocking activity (Douglas, 1980).

All antihistamines available before the advent of terfenadine and astemizole exhibit both anticholinergic and sedative properties, although these effects may vary greatly from one compound to another and also from one individual to another. Hence, the warning against activities that require mental alertness, such as driving a car, or operating other potentially dangerous machinery and appliances while taking H_1-blocking drugs.

There is evidence that some antihistamines may produce drowsiness by inhibiting histamine N-methyltransferase (Netter and Bodenschatz, 1967) and by blockade of central histaminergic (H_1) receptors (Uzan et al., 1979), but these studies must be interpreted with caution due to the complexity of action of the older antihistamines. Tolerance to their central effects may develop quickly (within a few days with some drugs) so that sedation is no longer troublesome (Nicholson, 1983). Many patients adapt well to the soporific sedative effect of the older antihistamines. They may in fact use them for their calming effect during the day and for insomnia at night, apparently leading to improved performance and coping with the stresses of daily life, including activities that require alertness. Patients may state that their attention span seems to be improved, and that they have less muscle tremor, tachycardia, and restlessness with medication in comparison to without medication. Consequently they may end up taking the drug for the sedating effects rather than the peripheral antihistaminic effects. Such patients often become upset and agitated when the medication is withdrawn and resort to similar over-the-counter antihistamines. The number of such individuals in the general population is probably much greater than might be expected.

The danger of dependence on over-the-counter antihistamines for their CNS effects also applies to other over-the-counter preparations in treatment of allergic and similar respiratory disorders. For example, ephedrine and other decongestants such as phenylpropanolamine may be taken primarily for their central stimulating, antidepressant and/or appetite suppressant effects rather than for their effects on the respiratory tract. These patients will continue to 'prefer' these drugs over the newer selective medications as they tend to lose sight of the original intent of their therapy. Of course, some will combine the new prescription antihistamine medications with their over-the-counter therapy, leading to various physiological and metabolic complications in addition to dependence on the CNS effects.

Evaluation of antihistamines is further complicated by the occurrence of paradoxical reactions in certain individuals. Although the older antihistamines generally cause sedation, they may occasionally cause nervousness, restlessness, and insomnia (Brandon and Weiner, 1980; Douglas, 1980). Thus, medications that spare the cerebral cortex are preferred in therapy.

Although the frequency of paradoxical reactions is not statistically significant, individually they may have life-threatening effects mentally and/or physically.

3. The Place of the Newer Non-Sedating Antihistamines in Clinical Practice

Blockade of H_1-receptors is of particular therapeutic value in the treatment of allergic seasonal and/or perennial allergic rhinitis, acute and chronic urticaria, and atopic dermatitis. Antihistamines used in clinical practice block the effects of histamine on smooth muscle and blood vessels released as a consequence of allergic stimuli by competitively binding to H_1-receptors (Douglas, 1980). Sodium cromoglycate (cromolyn sodium) is not an antihistamine; instead, one of its key effects is to act on mast cells to help prevent the release of histamine and other mediators (Brogden et al., 1974). Thus, an antihistamine may be used in conjunction with sodium cromoglycate to control symptoms that would otherwise result from any histamine that is released. Unfortunately, they cannot be combined in a single oral preparation because sodium cromoglycate is not absorbed from the gastrointestinal tract. Theoretically, however, they could be combined orally in the treatment of gastrointestinal food allergy and possibly certain other disorders involving mast cells in the enteric mucosa.

Pure H_1-antihistamines may often be only an adjunct or part of the treatment of allergic rhinitis and similar disorders. To help reduce side effects and achieve desired goals in therapy, a relatively pure non-sedating H_1-antihistamine may be used orally in combination with intranasal ipratropium or atropine solution to treat mixed allergic and vasomotor rhinitis.

Although many new modalities are available for the treatment of the allergic patient, antihistamines are still the first choice medication in therapy. In my view it is better to use a non-sedating antihistamine initially than to use decongestant or corticosteroid nasal sprays that can cause rhinitis medicamentosa, or in the case of corticosteroid sprays may interfere with normal fundamental defence mechanisms against viruses, fungi, and other infections, as well as causing atrophic changes and occasionally hoarseness or loss of voice, predisposing to petechial nasal bleeding, and affecting homeostatic mechanisms, such as normal responses to changes in temperature, humidity, barometric pressure, and organic and inorganic matter. Naturally, we should continue to follow allergy avoidance instructions and employ measures to stimulate normal immunity, such as appropriate allergy desensitisation injections in immunotherapy.

3.1 Terfenadine

It is of interest that some of the new non-sedating antihistamines, and in particular terfenadine, were developed as an offshoot of the search for drugs with improved selective central effects in the treatment of anxiety and depression. Many antidepressants and tranquillisers are powerful antihistamines. However, terfenadine is an exception in that it was found to have no central effects but retained antihistamine properties.

Along with astemizole, terfenadine may be regarded as the most specific H_1-receptor antagonist currently available. It does not readily cross the blood-brain barrier, in clinical dosage, but it binds to both peripheral and central H_1-receptors to a similar extent (Rose et al., 1982). Terfenadine has an elimination half-life of 16 to 23 hours and peak plasma concentrations are reached at 1 to 2 hours after a single oral dose. The drug is metabolised in the liver and its metabolites are excreted in the urine (primarily) and faeces (Sorkin and Heel, 1985).

Terfenadine does not cause CNS effects when administered in either high or low dosages (Brandon and Weiner, 1982). It has been thought that it may stimulate the CNS slightly (Nicholson, 1982), but there is no conclusive evidence in this regard. Similarly, there are no significant data to indicate that terfenadine causes sedation (Brandon and Weiner, 1982; Uzan and Le Fur, 1979).

Terfenadine has been evaluated and found effective as an H_1-receptor antagonist in reducing bronchial irritability, but it has no effect on histamine-induced permeability (Braude et al., 1984). Histamine increases lung capillary permeability by an H_2-receptor mechanism and bronchial reactivity by an H_1-receptor mechanism. The H_2-receptor antagonist cimetidine reduces the permeability response (Braude et al., 1984). Thus, the combined use of H_1- and H_2-receptor antagonists in the treatment of bronchial asthma may have some analogy to their combined use in the treatment of chronic urticaria and certain other disorders.

In addition to allergic rhinitis, terfenadine has also been demonstrated to be of value in exercise-induced asthma when given orally in a single dose of 120 or 180mg (Patel, 1984); a dose of 60mg was ineffective. It is suggested that terfenadine may act by competitive blockade of histamine at low concentrations and by a non-competitive blockade at higher concentrations (Hartley and Nogrady, 1980).

Terfenadine is also of value in the treatment of urticaria and dermographism. In a double-blind crossover study of 24 patients, the use of terfenadine in the treatment of chronic idiopathic urticaria was also reviewed (Cerio and Lessof, 1984). In each of the 3 studies, terfenadine was noted to be clinically effective without causing sedation or other side effects, and enabled discontinuance of corticosteroid therapy for the first time in some cases. In other studies, terfenadine has been shown to inhibit dermographic wealing and itch similar to histamine weal (Krause and Shuster, 1984). When the medication is discontinued, dermographism relapses toward its pretreatment state in 3 days, which confirms the long acting nature of terfenadine. The effect is sustained with continued therapy. In the treatment of this condition there is also some correlation between dosage and degree of therapeutic effect when comparing 60mg twice a day and 120mg 3 times daily, but this has not been established for allergic rhinitis.

In common with astemizole, terfenadine has no effect on itch as measured by nocturnal scratching or on induced dermographic wealing (Krause and Shuster, 1983). On the other hand, centrally acting sedative drugs, such as trimperazine or nitrazepam, may be effective antipruritics (Krause and Shuster, 1983). The new H_1-receptor antagonists may relieve itch of peripheral origin when it is due to histamine release, but may not relieve itch of central origin.

3.2 Astemizole

The available evidence indicates that astemizole penetrates the blood-brain barrier to only a small extent and acts primarily on H_1-receptors. In high dosages (not used clinically) it may have α-adrenocepor blocking and antiserotonergic effects.

Peak plasma concentrations of astemizole occur about 1 hour after administration, and the drug has an active metabolite with a half-life of about 104 hours, giving it a very long duration of action (Chapman and Rawlins, 1983). The recommended adult dose of 10mg suppresses skin weal and flare responses to histamine for several days. The usual dose is 10mg once daily, but doses as high as 20mg do not seem to adversely affect vision or performance (Nicholson and Stone, 1982). A number of studies have demonstrated the efficacy of astemizole in allergic rhinitis and beneficial effects have also been shown in chronic urticaria (Richards et al., 1984).

3.3 Mequitazine

Mequitazine does not readily cross the blood-brain barrier, and it does not cause sedation in the recommended dosage of 5mg twice daily (Uzan and LeFur, 1979). Plasma concentrations peak at about 6 hours after ingestion and the drug is cleared from the body about 38 hours after oral intake. Sedation apparently does not occur at the optimum recommended dose of 5mg twice a day. Lack of sedation is attributed to greater affinity for peripheral H_1-receptors than for central H_1-receptors (Uzan and LeFur, 1979).

Mequitazine has some anticholinergic activity and a dose of 10mg is associated with some central effects (Uzan and LeFur, 1979). Thus, the range between a potentially beneficial dose and one associated with side effects is small, which is not uncommonly seen with the older antihistamines.

4. Conclusion

Despite efforts to specifically identify the cause of symptoms in each patient with what seems to be allergic rhinitis, clinicians not infrequently prescribe a broad spectrum programme that includes avoidance measures, immunotherapy, antihistamines, decongestants, and possibly a choice of intranasal sodium cromoglycate or corticosteroid, oral corticosteroids and/or tranquillisers or antidepressants. The non-sedating antihistamines are a valuable tool, but we do have to appreciate their limitations, in that the amount of benefit to be obtained from them will depend on the role of histamine in each individual case. We must weigh carefully the possible factors involved in each case and prescribe medication accordingly. The new antihistamines should be employed along with other specific therapy and patients encouraged to avoid the potentially habit-forming older medications widely used in the treatment of allergic respiratory and other disorders.

Whenever possible, we should work with medications that spare the cerebral cortex and facilitate normal defence mechanisms, suppressing hyperreactive processes and facilitating hyporeactive processes. This is analogous to maintaining a satisfactory balance of receptors.

There is no doubt the new non-sedating antihistamines are a valuable adjunct in the therapy of the allergic patient. Although their non-sedating effect has been proven and provides a relative safety margin for these medications, this advantage is partly counterbalanced by their relatively narrow therapeutic range.

The new non-sedating antihistamines have been well accepted in those countries in which they are available, and the rise in their usage has been very rapid. They will lead to a better understanding of the role of histamine in allergic rhinitis and other disorders and to the development of agents that have a broader spectrum of action that is still non-sedating. The blood-brain barrier concept helps in appreciating the non-sedating role of these drugs, but compounds that do cross the blood-brain barrier and do not appear to cause sedation are also being evaluated. Thus, the old antihistamines are being replaced by the newer medications, initially on the basis of non-sedation, but possibly later on the basis of spectrum of action.

References

Brandon, M.L. and Weiner, M.: Clinical investigation of terfenadine, a new non-sedating antihistamine. Annals of Allergy 44: 71-75 (1980).

Brandon, M.L. and Weiner, M.: Clinical studies of terfenadine in seasonal allergic rhinitis. Arzneimittel-Forschung 32: 1204-1205 (1982).

Braude, S.; Coe, C.; Royston, D. and Barnes, P.J.: Histamine increases lung permeability by an H_2-receptor mechanism. Lancet 2: 372-374 (1984).

Brogden, R.N.; Speight, T.M. and Avery, G.S.: Sodium cromoglycate (cromolyn sodium): A review of its mode of action, pharmacology, therapeutic efficacy and use. Drugs 7: 164-282 (1974).

Cerio, R. and Lessof, M.H.: Treatment of chronic idiopathic urticaria with terfenadine. Clinical Allergy 14: 139-141 (1984).

Chapman, P.H. and Rawlins, M.D.: A randomized single blind study of astemizole and chlorpheniramine in normal volunteers. British Journal of Clinical Pharmacology 13: 593P (1983).

Douglas, W.: Histamine and 5-hydroxytryptamine (serotonin) and their antagonists; in Gilman et al. (Eds) The Pharmacological Basis of Therapeutics, 6th ed., pp. 609-646 (MacMillman, New York 1980).

Hartley, J.P.R. and Nogrady, S.G.: Effect of an inhaled antihistamine in exercise-induced asthma. Thorax 35: 675-679 (1980).

Krause, L. and Shuster, S.: Mechanism of action of antipruritic drugs. British Medical Journal 287: 1199-1200 (1983).

Krause, L.B. and Shuster, S.: The effect of terfenadine on dermographic wealing. British Journal of Dermatology 110: 73-79 (1984).

Netter, K.J. and Bodenschatz, K.: Inhibition of histamine-N-methyltransferase by some antihistamines. Biochemical Pharmacology 16: 1627-1631 (1967).

Nicholson, A.N.: Antihistaminic activity and central effects of terfenadine. A review of European studies. Arzneimittel-Forschung 32: 1191-1193 (1982).

Nicholson, A.N.: Antihistamines and sedation. Lancet 2: 211-212 (1983).

Nicholson, A.N. and Stone, B.M.: Performance studies with the H_1 receptor antagonists, astemizole and terfenadine. British Journal of Clinical Pharmacology 13: 199-202 (1982).

Patel, K.R.: Terfenadine in exercise induced asthma. British Medical Journal 288: 1496-1497 (1984).

Reinberg, A.; Levi, F.; Guillet, P.; Burke, J.T. and Nicolzi, A.: Chronopharmacological study of antihistamines in man with special reference to terfenadine. European Journal of Clinical Pharmacology 14: 242-252 (1978).

Richards, D.M.; Brogden, R.N.; Heel, R.C.; Speight, T.M. and Avery, G.S.: Astemizole: A review of its pharmacodynamic properties and therapeutic efficacy. Drug 28: 38-61 (1984).

Rose, C.; Quach, T.T.; Lorens, C. et al.: Relationship betwen occupation of cerebral H_1-receptors and sedative properties of antihistamines. Arzneimittel-Forschung 32: 1171-1173 (1982).

Sorkin, E.M. and Heel, R.C.: Terfenadine: A review of its pharmacodynamic properties and therapeutic efficacy. Drugs 29: 34-56 (1985).

Uzan, A. and LeFur, G.: Mequitazine et vigilance. Allergologica et Immunopathologia (Paris) 11: 27-30 (1979).

Uzan, A.; LeFur, G. and Malgouris, C.: Are antihistamines sedative via a blockade of brain H_1 receptors? Journal of Pharmacy and Pharmacology 32: 701-702 (1979).

Address for correspondence and reprints: Dr *Milan L. Brandon*, Allergy Medical Group of San Diego, 2800 Third Avenue, San Diego, CA 92103 (USA).

Drugs 30: 382-426 (1985)
0012-6667/85/0011-0382/$22.50/0

Cefotetan
A Review of its Antibacterial Activity, Pharmacokinetic Properties and Therapeutic Use

A. Ward and *D.M. Richards*

ADIS Drug Information Services, Auckland

Various sections of the manuscript reviewed by: ***G. Gialdroni Grassi,*** Cettedra di Chemoterapia, Universita di Pa[illegible] Pavia, Italy; ***P.O. Madsen,*** Urology Department, William S. Middleton Mem[illegible]s Hospital, Madison, Wisconsin, USA; ***S.W.B. Newsom,*** Department [illegible]pworth Hospital, Cambridge, England; ***P. Periti,*** Department [illegible]versity of Florence, Florence, Italy; ***R. Quintilliani,*** [illegible] Hartford Hospital, Hartford, Connecticut, USA; [illegible]gery, Brighton General Hospital, Brighton, England; [illegible]e, Tohuku University, Sendai, Japan; ***J.D. Williams,*** [illegible] London Hospital Medical College, London, Eng[illegible] Microbiology, Dudley Road Hospital, Birming[illegible]t of Communicable and Tropical Diseases, East [illegible]land.

[illegible]

Summary 383
1. Antibacterial Activity 386
1.1 *In vitro* Inhibitory Activity Against Aerobic Bacteria 387
1.1.1 Gram-Positive Bacteria 388
1.1.2 Gram-Negative Bacteria 388
1.2 *In Vitro* Inhibitory Activity Against Anaerobic Bacteria 395
1.3 Bactericidal Activity 395
1.4 Effect on Activity of Inoculum Size, Culture Media, pH and Serum 396
1.5 Antibiotic Synergy 396
1.6 β-Lactamase Resistance 399
1.7 Penetrability of Cefotetan 399
2. Nephrotoxicity 400
3. Pharmacokinetic Studies 400
3.1 Absorption and Plasma Concentrations 400
3.2 Distribution 401
3.3 Metabolism and Excretion 401
3.3.1 Half-Life 403
3.4 Effect of Disease States on Pharmacokinetics 404
4. Therapeutic Trials 405
4.1 Established Intra-Abdominal Infections 405
4.2 Surgical Prophylaxis 406
4.2.1 Appendicectomy 406

4.2.2 Colorectal Surgery 407
4.2.3 Biliary Tract Surgery 407
4.2.4 Other Surgical Operations 407
4.3 Obstetric and Gynaecological Infections 408
4.4 Use in Septicaemia and Immunologically Compromised Patients 408
4.5 Otorhinolaryngological Infections 409
4.6 Urinary Tract Infections 410
4.6.1 Studies in Adult Patients 411
4.7 Lower Respiratory Tract Infections 413
4.7.1 Studies in Adult Patients 413
4.7.2 Studies in Paediatric Patients 416
4.8 Skin and Soft Tissue Infections 417
4.9 Miscellaneous Therapeutic Use 417
5. Side Effects 418
5.1 Effects on Laboratory Values 418
6. Dosage and Administration 419
7. The Place of Cefotetan in Therapy 420

Summary

Synopsis: *Cefotetan*[1] *is a new semisynthetic cephamycin antibiotic administered intravenously or intramuscularly. It has a broad spectrum of activity against Gram-negative aerobic and most clinically important Gram-positive and anaerobic bacteria, and is generally more active against Gram-negative bacteria than the 'first and second generation' agents. Cefotetan is particularly active against* Enterobacteriaceae *but has little activity against* Pseudomonas aeruginosa.

An extended plasma elimination half-life of about 3.5 hours, and relatively high achievable serum and tissue levels, enables cefotetan to be administered on a twice daily basis in the treatment of mild to severe infections. Cefotetan has shown good clinical efficacy in intra-abdominal, obstetric and gynaecological infections, postoperative wound infections, and infections in immunocompromised patients – all of which are often complicated due to their polymicrobial nature or by the presence of anaerobic pathogens. A satisfactory clinical response is achieved in over 90% of paediatric patients with acute otorhinolaryngological infections, whereas in the treatment of chronic disease, as with other agents, the efficacy is dramatically reduced. Like other cephalosporins, cefotetan is effective in treating patients with complicated urinary tract infections and lower respiratory tract infections. Its efficacy in urinary tract infections is at least as good as cefoxitin, although in this and some other clinical areas its activity relative to that of other cephamycins and cephalosporins remains to be assessed.

Thus, with its convenient twice daily dosage schedule, cefotetan would appear to be a useful addition to a rapidly expanding group of antibacterial agents.

Antibacterial Activity: Cefotetan has a broad spectrum of *in vitro* antibacterial activity and is resistant to the activity of most β-lactamases. Like the 'third generation' cephalosporins and other cephamycins, cefotetan is active against a wide range of Gram-negative bacteria, with 90% of strains of *Escherichia coli, Klebsiella* species, *Proteus mirabilis* and *Proteus vulgaris* being inhibited at concentrations of less than 1 mg/L. Other Gram-negative rods (*Proteus, Providencia* and *Morganella* species, and *Haemophilus influenzae*), *Neisseria* species, *Salmonella* and *Shigella* species and *Yersinia enterocolitica* are susceptible at concentrations of less than 8 mg/L. The activity of cefotetan against *Serratia, Enterobacter* and *Citrobacter* species varied widely between studies ($MIC_{90} < 8$ to

1 'Apatef', 'Apacef', 'Cefotan', 'Yamatetan' (Yamanouchi, ICI).

$\geqslant$ 64 mg/L), but these species are consistently the least sensitive of the *Enterobacteriaceae* to cefotetan.

Unlike ceftazidime and some 'third generation' cephalosporins, cefotetan has little activity against *Pseudomonas aeruginosa* and other *Pseudomonas* or *Acinetobacter* species. Cefotetan displays modest activity (MIC_{90} = 2 to 16 mg/L) against most Gram-positive bacteria (streptococci and staphylococci) while enterococci, including *Streptococcus faecalis* and methicillin-resistant *Staphylococcus* species, show marked resistance.

Anaerobes, such as *Bacteroides, Clostridium* and *Fusobacterium* species, are usually more sensitive to cefotetan than other cephalosporins, although activity varies markedly between laboratories and species. 90% of isolates of *Clostridium perfringens, C. botulinum* and *B. urealyticus* are sensitive to cefotetan (MIC_{90} < 1 mg/L) whereas *B. thetaiotaomicron, B. ovatus, B. diastonis,* and *C. difficile* are markedly less sensitive. Cefotetan usually has modest activity against the clinically important *B. fragilis* and *B. asaccharolyticus* (MIC_{90} usually 8 to 32 mg/L).

In general, there is usually little difference between the minimum bactericidal concentrations (MBC) and minimum inhibitory concentrations (MIC) of cefotetan for most Gram-negative organisms, although there have been reports of 4-fold (or more) ratios of MBC_{90} : MIC_{90} for some species of *Salmonella, Klebsiella* and *Proteus.* The MIC_{90} of cefotetan for most strains tested is not greatly affected by increases in inoculum size up to 10^7 organisms per ml, by changes in pH down to 5.5 or by altering the growth medium (with the exception of the addition of 10% horse serum which caused 2- to 4-fold increases in the MIC of most bacteria).

Synergy between cefotetan and other antibacterial agents (including aminoglycosides, piperacillin and other cephalosporins) has been demonstrated in some isolates of Enterobacteriaceae that were poorly sensitive to cefotetan, with additive inhibition or no effects occurring in other strains.

Cefotetan has marked *in vitro* stability to most β-lactamases except those produced by *Pseudomonas aeruginosa* (type II) and certain uncommon isolates of *Bacteroides fragilis, Enterobacter cloacae, Serratia liquifaciens* and *Citrobacter freundii.* Marked direct β-lactamase inhibitory action has also been reported.

Pharmacokinetic Properties: Mean peak plasma concentrations of cefotetan (about 140 to 250 mg/L) are attained after a 1g intravenous bolus dose, and over a dosage range of 0.25 to 2g are almost linearly related with dose. Peak cefotetan concentrations of up to 270 and 90 mg/L are seen after 2g intravenous drip infusion (over 60 minutes) and intramuscular administration, respectively. Plasma concentrations were nearly 2-fold higher than those attained after latamoxef (moxalactam) administration at the same doses.

The volume of distribution after intravenous and intramuscular administration is usually between 8 and 13L in healthy adult volunteers. Concentrations of cefotetan likely to be active against susceptible organisms are achieved in a variety of tissues and body fluids, including female genital tissues, umbilical cord serum and amniotic fluid, gallbladder tissue and bile, prostatic tissue (but not prostatic fluid), palatine tonsillar tissue and maxillary sinus mucosa. In healthy subjects, protein binding is 78 to 91%. Breast milk concentrations are low and no accumulation has occurred with repeated doses. No metabolites of cefotetan have been detected in either plasma or urine. About three-quarters of a dose is excreted in the urine within 24 hours. Total plasma clearance has been recorded at 1.8 to 2.9 L/h, with renal clearance accounting for about 64 to 84%.

The plasma elimination half-life is between 2.8 and 4.2 hours after intravenous doses and between 3.4 and 4.4 hours after intramuscular doses. The plasma half-life is slightly shorter in paediatric patients but is considerably prolonged in patients with renal impairment (to over 10 hours). Increased renal dysfunction also leads to decreased urinary recovery of cefotetan.

Therapeutic Trials: The therapeutic efficacy of cefotetan 1 to 4g daily (usually given intravenously or intramuscularly every 12 hours) has been extensively documented in open and comparative trials in patients with intra-abdominal infections, obstetric and gynaecological infections, chronic, complicated urinary tract infection, lower respiratory tract infection, skin and soft tissue infection, or otorhinolaryngological disease. Cefotetan has also been used preoperatively (either alone or in combination with metronidazole) in the prevention of postoperative wound infection. However, there are only limited studies in important disease areas such as bacteraemia and septicaemia, gonorrhoea, meningitis and in immunocompromised patients.

Open and controlled studies of patients with intra-abdominal infections such as peritonitis (of various aetiology) report successful treatment in 82 to 100% of patients with cefotetan. Particularly impressive results have been achieved in peritonitis due to appendicitis or other diseases, where cefotetan therapy was an adjunct to surgery and drainage. In such patients cefotetan 1 to 2g twice daily has been at least as effective as cefmetazole 2g twice daily, latamoxef 2g 3 times daily or a combination of ampicillin, gentamicin and metronidazole.

Reductions in rates of postoperative infections have been seen with cefotetan in limited numbers of patients who have undergone appendicectomy (more effective than metronidazole), colorectal surgery (at least as effective as gentamicin plus metronidazole or tinidazole), biliary tract surgery (as effective as cefazolin), transurethral surgery (at least as effective as cefotaxime) and upper gastrointestinal tract surgery (more effective than cephazolin).

Obstetric and gynaecological infections are often caused by anaerobic bacteria. Therefore, although open studies in large numbers of women have shown a good or excellent clinical response to cefotetan (usually 1 to 4g daily) in over 80% of patients (some of whom were unresponsive to cefmetazole, piperacillin, dibekacin or benzylpenicillin), controlled studies are needed to assess the comparative efficacy of cefotetan with standard antibiotic therapy in anaerobic infections.

An overall clinical efficacy rate of 75 to 90% is seen in adults and children with acute otorhinolaryngological infections. Common causative organisms such as *Staphylococcus aureus*, streptococci, *Neisseria* species and *Haemophilus influenzae* are almost invariably eradicated, and treatment failures are usually only seen in acute exacerbations of chronic otitis media or in infections where *Pseudomonas aeruginosa, Acinetobacter* or *Corynebacteria* species are implicated.

In one study of immunocompromised patients with a variety of infections, high dose cefotetan (4 to 6 g/day) therapy produced a satisfactory clinical response in nearly 60% of patients, including patients with suspected sepsis. More studies are needed in these clinical fields. Cefotetan has been used successfully in a few patients requiring oral surgery (79 to 100%), in ophthalmological infections (78%), biliary diseases (80%), and septicaemia (92%).

In a large number of Japanese patients with urinary tract infections complicated by underlying urological abnormalities, treatment with cefotetan 1 to 2g daily for 5 days achieved a clinical success rate of about 60% and a bacteriological cure rate of 67 to 88%. Clinical success rates were greater in patients with infection due to a single organism than those with polymicrobial infection (65 *vs* 49%) and in those patients with no indwelling catheter compared to those with an indwelling catheter. However, in comparative studies conducted mostly in the United States and Europe successful treatment with cefotetan 1 to 2g twice daily occurred in 65 to 97% of patients, with this greater rate of response almost certainly being related to the fact that in Japan there are no strictly adhered to criteria for ensuring the *in vitro* sensitivity of the organism prior to treatment. Cefotetan was similar in clinical and bacteriological efficacy to cefmetazole 2g daily over a 5-day period; and cefotetan 2 to 4g daily was at least as effective as cefoxitin 3 to 12g daily administered for periods of 3 to 22 days. Eradication rates have exceeded 90% for most species of *Enterobacteriaceae* and *Staphylococcus,* whereas *Serratia, Pseudomonas* and *Acinetobacter* species, and particularly *Pseudomonas aeruginosa* and *Streptococcus faecalis* (eradication rates of 34 and 47%, respectively), were more resistant to cefotetan.

Cefotetan has produced a clinical 'success' rate of about 72% in open studies of patients with lower respiratory tract infections, and was somewhat more effective in patients with (non-mycoplasmal) pneumonia (79%) than in chronic pulmonary infections, lung abscess and pleural infections (65%). Bacteriological efficacy was assessed in over 300 Japanese patients: cefotetan eradicated over 90% of the common respiratory pathogens (*H. influenzae, K. pneumoniae* and *E. coli*), but was poorly active against *Pseudomonas* infections. Cefotetan was equally effective as cefmetazole in a large number of patients with a variety of respiratory tract infections.

In paediatric patients with community-acquired urinary tract and lower respiratory tract infections, cefotetan (usually 50 to 60 mg/kg/day) has shown a greater clinical (90 to 95%) efficacy than that seen in adults.

Side Effects: Cefotetan has generally been well tolerated by adults and children following intravenous or intramuscular administration. The most commonly reported clinical adverse effects are local reactions at the site of injection, particularly with intramuscular doses, hypersensitivity reactions, such as rash and fever, and gastrointestinal effects such as nausea, vomiting and diarrhoea. Low incidences of liver function test and haematological abnormalities have been recorded. Unlike many other cephalosporins, no clinical evidence of hypoprothrombinaemic bleeding problems or disulfiram-type reactions has been published.

Dosage and Administration: Cefotetan can be administered intravenously (either by bolus dose or drip infusion) or intramuscularly [with lignocaine (lidocaine) 0.5%]. The usual adult dosage is 0.5 to 1g 12-hourly, which may be increased in patients with very severe infections or immunocompromised patients to 4 to 6g daily. The recommended dose in paediatric patients is 40 to 60 mg/kg/day given 12-hourly, which may be increased to 100 mg/kg/day in serious infections.

1. Antibacterial Activity

Cefotetan is a new cephamycin antibiotic derived semisynthetically from oganomycin G produced by *Streptomyces oganonensis*. Structurally it is similar to cefoxitin and latamoxef (moxalactam), with a 7α-methoxy substitution of the cephalosporin structure (fig. 1). The modifications to its structure confer enhanced resistance to β-lactamases and a broad spectrum of activity, particularly against Gram-negative bacteria. The commercially available product exists as 2 epimers (R and S), although in weakly alkaline solutions a third tautomeric form is present. All 3 tautomers have equal antibacterial activity (Kees et al., 1984).

Cefotetan, although not technically a cephalosporin, is considered a 'third generation' cephalosporin in most currently available literature because of its spectrum of activity. It is generally more active than the 'first and second generation' cephalosporins against Gram-negative bacteria and has shown useful activity against anaerobic bacteria. However, the concept of cephalosporins in terms of 'generations' has recently been called into question, and a new method of classification has been proposed. This system divides the parenteral cephalosporins into 4 groups – those with high activity against Gram-positive bacteria (Group 1), Enterobacteriaceae (Group II), *Pseudomonas* and related species (Group III), or *Bacteroides* (Group IV) — and in this classification cefotetan falls into the Group IV category (Williams, 1985).

While the *in vitro* activity of an antibacterial agent can be assessed in many ways and it is difficult to determine which laboratory susceptibility tests will most accurately reflect the *in vivo* activity

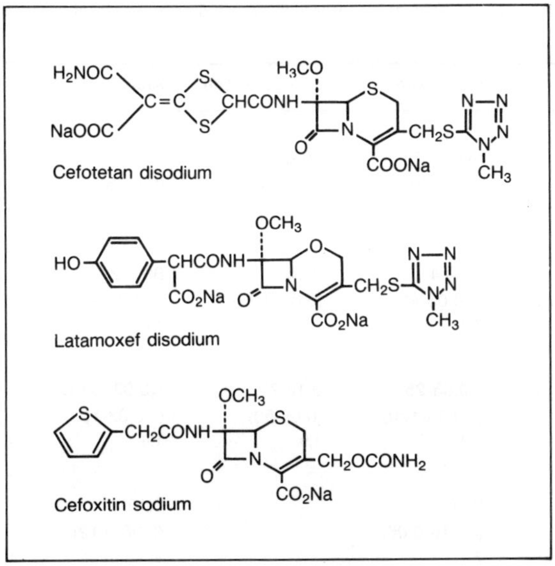

Fig. 1. Structural formulae of cefotetan disodium, latamoxef (moxalactam) disodium and cefoxitin sodium.

of a drug, the conclusions of this review are based largely on minimum concentrations inhibiting 90% of tested strains (MIC_{90}).

1.1 *In Vitro* Inhibitory Activity Against Aerobic Bacteria

In this review, bacterial isolates are considered to be 'susceptible' to cefotetan at a minimum inhibitory concentration (MIC) of ≤ 16 mg/L, and 'resistant' at an MIC ≥ 64 mg/L. In the intermediate MIC range of 17 to 63 mg/L, an organism will be considered 'moderately susceptible' and would usually only be inhibited by high doses which produce high antibiotic concentrations at the site of infection. The inhibitory activity of cefotetan *in vitro* has been extensively studied – including an attempt to collate the activity of cefotetan against more than 22,000 randomly collected clinical isolates obtained from 37 centres in Europe and North America (Hennessey, 1985). Studies reviewed here usually used a relatively large number of strains and an inoculum size of 10^4 to 10^6 colony-forming units.

Table I. Antibacterial activity of cefotetan and other antibacterial agents *in vitro* against Gram-positive aerobic bacteria (after Bauernfeind, 1983)

Organism	No. of isolates	MIC_{90} (mg/L)						
		cefotetan	latamoxef	cefoxitin	cefotaxime	cephalothin	cefamandole	penicillin G
Staph. aureus								
Penicillin-sensitive	25	7.5	7.5	3.3	1.85	0.23	0.19	0.045
Penicillin-resistant	83	7.5	7.5	3.4	2.5	0.40	0.80	9.5
Methicillin-resistant	9	135	> 256	> 256	220	52.0	17.5	54.0
Staph. epidermidis								
Penicillin-sensitive	13	7.9	7.3	1.7	1.5	0.16	0.20	0.03
Penicillin-resistant	19	42	64	8.5	11.5	0.44	0.77	3.20
Methicillin-resistant	18	56	68	12.5	11.5	0.79	1.80	8.50
Enterococci	100	> 64	> 128	> 128	> 128	32.0	46.0	1.25

Table II. Antibacterial activity *in vitro* of cefotetan and other antibacterial agents against streptococci, where 8 or more isolates were tested

Organism	Cefotetan	Latamoxef	Cefoxitin	Cefotaxime	Cefoperazone	Ampicillin
S. faecalis						
MIC_{90} range	16->256	>64->256	8->256	50->256	25-64	1
(overall range)	(1->256)	(>64->256)	(0.5->256)	(1->256)	(1.56-100)	(0.5-16)
References	1,2,5,6,9	1,6	1,2,6,9	5,6,9	1,6,9	1
S. pneumoniae						
MIC_{90} range	8-128	1-16	8	0.12-4	0.25	0.25-2
(overall range)	(0.12-256)	(0.25-16)	(0.12->256)	(<0.03-4)	(0.03-0.25)	(<0.03-4)
References	1,7,8	1,8	1	7,8	1	1,8
S. pyogenes						
MIC_{90} range	0.25-50	2	1-50	<0.03-25	0.12-25	<0.03-≤0.12
(overall range)	(0.25-100)	(0.5-2)	(0.19-100)	(<0.03-100)	(0.06-50)	(<0.03-1)
References	1,4,8,9,10	1	1,4,9	8,9	1,9	1,8
S. agalactiae						
MIC_{90} range	4-8	2	1-2	0.06		0.12
(overall range)	(4-16)	(1-4)	(0.5-2)	(0.016-0.06)		(0.06-0.12)
References	1,3,7	3	1,3	7		3

Reference Key: 1 Ayers et al. (1982); 2 Chattopadhyay and Teli (1982); 3 Clarke and Zemcov (1983); 4 Cocuzza et al. (1983); 5 Dette et al. (1983); 6 Grimm (1983); 7 Phillips et al. (1983); 8 Reeves et al. (1983); 9 Russo et al. (1983); 10 Wise et al. (1982).

1.1.1 Gram-Positive Bacteria

Cefotetan resembles latamoxef in its activity against Gram-positive bacteria, being moderately active against some species of Streptococci, and against penicillin-resistant but not methicillin-resistant *Staphylococcus aureus*. However, most other currently available cephalosporins, especially the older agents, are more active than cefotetan against this group in general.

The MIC_{90} of *S. aureus* isolates ranges from 8 to 16 mg/L in most studies (Ayers et al., 1982; Bauernfeind, 1983; Chattopadhyay and Teli, 1982; Clarke and Zemcov, 1983; Cocuzza et al., 1983; Daschner et al., 1982; Dette et al., 1983; Dublanchet, 1985; Grimm, 1983; Phillips et al., 1983; Wise et al., 1982). There is no reduction in activity of cefotetan against penicillin-resistant or β-lactamase-producing isolates of *S. aureus* (Bauernfeind, 1983; Dette et al., 1983; Grimm, 1983; Phillips et al., 1983), but there is diminished inhibition of methicillin-resistant strains of both *S. aureus* and *S. epidermidis* (MIC_{90} 32 to 135 mg/L) [table I; Ayers et al., 1982; Bauernfeind, 1983; Dublanchet, 1985; Phillips et al., 1983; Shah, 1983], and penicillin-resistant strains of *S. epidermidis* (MIC_{90} 42 mg/L; Bauernfeind, 1983).

Most strains of *Streptococcus pneumoniae, Strep. pyogenes,* and *Strep. agalactiae* are sensitive to cefotetan (MIC_{90} 2 to 8 mg/L) [table II], although occasionally laboratories have reported resistant isolates of *Strep. pneumoniae* (Phillips et al., 1983; Reeves et al., 1983; Russo et al., 1983). Isolates of enterococci are usually resistant to cefotetan (table I), including *Streptococcus faecalis* (table II; Hennessey, 1985). However, some strains of *Strep. faecalis* are moderately susceptible (Chattopadhyay and Teli, 1982; Russo et al., 1983). Resistance to cefotetan has also been reported in *Strep. bovis* (Ayers et al., 1982) and Group D streptococci (Clarke and Zemcov, 1983; Wise et al., 1982).

1.1.2 Gram-Negative Bacteria

Cefotetan exhibits a high degree of antibacterial activity against a wide spectrum of *Enterobacteri-*

aceae. Thus, cefotetan usually inhibits the growth of 90% of *Escherichia coli, Klebsiella* species, *Proteus mirabilis* and *P. vulgaris* at concentrations of ⩽ 1.0 mg/L. Against *Providencia* species, indole-positive and indole-negative *Proteus* species, *Morganella morganii, Neisseria* species and *Haemophilus influenzae*, cefotetan concentrations of 2 to 4 mg/L inhibit 90% of isolates. In contrast, many strains of *Enterobacter* species are resistant to cefotetan, and whilst most evidence suggests that *Serratia* species are moderately sensitive to cefotetan, resistant strains do occur. *Pseudomonas aeruginosa, Acinetobacter* and most other non-fermentative Gram-negative bacilli are essentially resistant to cefotetan.

Cefotetan concentrations of ⩽ 2 mg/L will usually inhibit 90% of *Salmonella* and *Shigella* species and *Yersinia enterocolitica*, giving it an activity similar to that of latamoxef and cefotaxime. In contrast, the latter 2 drugs are more active *in vitro* against *Citrobacter* species, many isolates of which are resistant to cefotetan. Only *C. diversus* shows any marked susceptibility to cefotetan.

Escherichia coli

Cefotetan is very active against *E. coli* with 90% of strains being inhibited by 0.13 to 1.0 mg/L, although in some studies the cefotetan MIC_{90} values have been somewhat higher (2.0 to 3.12 mg/L; Cocuzza et al., 1983; Russo et al., 1983; Wise et al., 1982). Generally cefotetan shows similar activity to latamoxef, ceftazidime and cefotaxime, and greater activity than cefoxitin and cefoperazone (table III), although in the 3 studies associated with a higher MIC_{90}, cefotetan showed greater activity than cefoxitin, ceftriaxone, cefazolin, cefoperazone, cefuroxime, gentamicin and piperacillin, equal activity to ceftazidime, but less potency than latamoxef (Cocuzza et al., 1983; Russo et al., 1983; Wise et al., 1982).

In one study, 6 β-lactamase-producing strains of *E. coli* were sensitive to cefotetan (Phillips et al., 1983). However, in another study, an MIC_{90} value of 3.78 mg/L for cefotetan was recorded in β-lactamase-producing strains of *E. coli*, compared with 0.45 mg/L in strains not producing β-lactamase, whereas the MIC_{90} value for cefotaxime only increased from 0.11 to 0.48 mg/L (Dette et al., 1983). Bauernfeind (1983) reported a 20-fold increase in potency against ampicillin-sensitive compared with ampicillin-resistant strains of *E. coli*. In contrast, the MIC_{90} of cefotetan in piperacillin-resistant isolates in one study did not increase whereas those of latamoxef, cefotaxime and cefoperazone did, although the sensitivities of these isolates were still in the susceptible range for all drugs (Grimm, 1983). Cefotetan was more active than cefotaxime, ceftriaxone, ceftazidime, cefoxitin, cefuroxime and cephradine against 42 gentamicin-resistant isolates of *E. coli* (Hart and Percival, 1983).

Klebsiella Species

Cefotetan is highly active against *Klebsiella* species (*K. pneumoniae, K. oxytoca* and *K. ozaenae*), with an overall range of activity of 0.02 to > 256 mg/L and an overall range of MIC_{90} values of 0.07

Table III. Antibacterial activity *in vitro* of cefotetan and other antibacterial agents against *Escherichia coli*, where 20 or more isolates were tested

Organism	Cefotetan	Latamoxef	Cefoxitin	Cefotaxime	Cefoperazone	Ceftazidime
E. coli						
MIC_{90} range	0.13-3.12	0.125-2	3.8->100	<0.12-8	0.5-32	0.125-2
Overall range	<0.03->128	0.03->128	0.125->256	<0.03-128	0.03->64	<0.03->128
References	1-14	1,2,5,7,11,13,14	1-5,7,10,12,14	2,5,6,7,10-14	1,5,7,12,13,14	5,11,13

Reference Key: 1 Ayers et al. (1982); 2 Bauernfeind (1983); 3 Chattopadhyay and Teli (1982); 4 Cocuzza et al. (1983); 5 Daschner et al. (1982); 6 Grimm (1983); 7 Morel et al. (1983); 8 Phillips et al. (1983); 9 Reeves et al. (1983); 10 Russo et al. (1983); 11 Shah (1983); 12 Wise et al. (1982).

to 4.0 mg/L. Cefotetan thus has a similar activity to latamoxef (MIC_{90} 0.12 to 4 mg/L) and cefotaxime (MIC_{90} 0.06 to 4 mg/L) [table IV]. *Klebsiella* isolates are very rarely resistant to cefotetan, even where multiple resistance to other antimicrobial agents is evident (see below).

At cefotetan concentrations of 8 to 16 mg/L, 99.5 to 100% of *Klebsiella* strains are usually inhibited (Ayers et al., 1982; Grimm, 1983; Shah, 1983). Only a slightly lower rate of inhibition is seen in piperacillin-resistant strains of *Klebsiella* (98%) at a concentration of 16 mg/L (Grimm, 1983; Periti et al., 1983). In a study of gentamicin-resistant isolates of *Klebsiellae* that were also resistant to tobramycin, streptomycin, spectinomycin, trimethoprim, tetracycline, chloramphenicol, cefazolin, cephaloridine and cefamandole, MIC_{90} values for cefotetan, cefotaxime, latamoxef and ceftriaxone (0.5 mg/L) were lower than those of cefoxitin or cefuroxime (4 mg/L) and netilmicin, cephalexin or cephradine (10 to 300 mg/L). Of the 8 isolates that were relatively insensitive to cefotetan, 7 were indole-positive strains of *K. oxytoca*. Both cefotetan and ceftazidime inhibited all strains of cefuroxime-resistant *Klebsiellae* species at concentrations of 0.5 to 1.0 mg/L (Hart and Percival, 1982). In a subsequent study 38 and 70 of 237 strains of *Klebsiellae* were resistant to cefoxitin and cefuroxime, respectively. Only a small number of these resistant isolates were also resistant to cefotetan (11% and 6%, respectively) or ceftazidime, whereas a significantly greater proportion were resistant to cefotaxime and ceftriaxone (Hart and Percival, 1983).

Enterobacter and *Serratia* Species

As with other cephalosporins and cephamycins, there is a very wide variation in the cefotetan susceptibility of *Enterobacter* and *Serratia* species between studies, with overall MIC_{90} values of 2 to 256 mg/L and 0.5 to 64 mg/L, respectively (table IV). These two genera (along with *Citrobacter* species) are consistently the least sensitive of the *Enterobacteriaceae* to cefotetan (Ayers et al., 1982; Bauernfeind, 1983; Clarke and Zemcov, 1983; Gialdroni Grassi et al., 1983; Grimm, 1983; Hart and Percival, 1983; Phillips et al., 1983; Shah, 1983; Wise et al., 1982). In most studies, cefotetan has an MIC_{90} value against *Enterobacter* species of $\geq$ 16 mg/L, with only the occasional laboratories reporting values lower than this (Cocuzza et al., 1983; Wise et al., 1982), although *E. agglomerans* (MIC_{90} 0.5 to 32 mg/L) may be more susceptible than other species (Ayers et al., 1982; Hennessey, 1985). Cefotetan is distinctly less active against cefuroxime-resistant than cefuroxime-sensitive isolates of *Enterobacter* species (Bauernfeind, 1983).

Cefotetan is moderately active against *Serratia* species and *S. marcescens*, with the MIC_{90} values for most studies falling within the range of 2 to 16 mg/L (Hennessey, 1985; table IV). Only occasionally have higher (Ayers et al., 1982; Reeves et al., 1983) or lower (Morel et al., 1983) values been reported. Cefotetan has greater activity against *Serratia* species and *S. marcescens* than cefoxitin, and usually has greater activity than cefoperazone against *Serratia* species, but less activity against *Enterobacter* species (Ayers et al., 1982; Daschner et al., 1982; Grimm, 1983; Russo et al., 1983; Shah, 1983). Cefotetan does not compare favourably with the newer cephalosporins and latamoxef against these species (table IV), and other antibacterial agents such as amikacin (Periti et al., 1983), gentamicin (Russo et al., 1983), netilmicin (Shah, 1983) and aztreonam (Clarke and Zemcov, 1983) also have considerably greater activity than cefotetan.

Proteus, Providencia and *Morganella* Species

Cefotetan is active *in vitro* against most strains of these closely related genera, with MIC_{90} values of 0.06 to 1.0 mg/L for *Proteus mirabilis*, 0.25 to 2.85 mg/L for *P. vulgaris*, 0.5 to 6.25 mg/L for indole-positive *Proteus* species, 0.5 to 12 mg/L for *Providencia stuartii*, 0.5 to 30 mg/L for *Providencia rettgeri* and 1 to 8 mg/L for *Morganella morganii* (table V; Hennessey, 1985). Cefotetan was equally effective against cefuroxime-sensitive and -resistant and cefamandole-sensitive and -resistant strains of *P. mirabilis* and *P. vulgaris* (Bauernfeind, 1983). In one study, all strains of *P. mirabilis, P. vulgaris* and *Prov. rettgeri*, and 95% of *M. morganii* were sensitive to cefotetan at concentrations $\leq$ 16 mg/L (Grimm, 1983), whereas in another study most

Table IV. Antibacterial activity *in vitro* of cefotetan and other antibacterial agents against *Klebsiellae, Enterobacter* and *Serratia* species, in studies where 15 or more isolates were tested

Organism	Cefotetan		Latamoxef	Cefoxitin	Cefotaxime	Ceftazidime	Ceftriaxone
	overall MIC range	MIC_{90} range	MIC_{90} range	MIC_{90} range	MIC_{90} range	MIC_{90} range	MIC_{90} range
Klebsiella pneumoniae	0.03-8.0	0.12-4.0	0.12-4.0	2.0-8.0	0.06-4.0	0.25-4.0	0.06
References	1,4,5,7,18,19		1,4,7,18,19	1,4,5,7,19	7,18	7,18,19	1
Klebsiella spp.	0.02->256	0.07-0.5	0.125-0.5	4.0-64	0.06-2.0	0.5-2.0	0.25-32
References	2,8-16		2,10,11,16	2,9-12,14,15	2,8-16	11,12,16	11,12,15
Enterobacter cloacae	0.12->256	2->160	0.25-50	>32->128	0.5-100	0.5-100	16
References	1,3,7,8,14		1,3,7	1,3,7,14	3,7,8,14	3,7	1
Enterobacter spp.	0.06->256	2->256	0.12-16	50->256	0.5-128	0.25->32	>25->32
References	2,4,5,6,9,10,12,13,16,17,19		2,5,10,16,19	2,4,5,6,9,10,12, 13,17,19	2,9,10,12,13,16,17	12,16,19	6,12
Serratia marcescens	0.12->32	3.2-32	2-6.25	64->256	3.12-8	3.12-8	
References	1,2,3,5,10,18		1,2,3,5,18	1,2,3,5,10	2,3,18	3,18	
Serratia spp.	0.25->128	0.5-64	8	16	<0.12-8	1	
References	8,13,14,16		16	13,14	8,13,14,16	16	

Key to references: 1 Ayers et al. (1982); 2 Bauernfeind (1983); 3 Campello et al. (1983); 4 Chattopadhyay and Teli (1982); 5 Clarke and Zemcov (1983); 6 Cocuzza et al. (1983); 7 Daschner et al. (1982); 8 Dette et al. (1983); 9 Dublanchet (1985); 10 Grimm (1983);[a] 11 Hart and Percival (1982);[b] 12 Hart and Percival (1983);[b] 13 Morel et al. (1983); 14 Phillips et al. (1983); 15 Ravizzola et al. (1983); 16 Reeves et al. (1983); 17 Russo et al. (1983); 18 Shah (1983); 19 Wise et al. (1982).

a Most isolates of *Klebsiella* and *Enterobacter* were piperacillin resistant.

b All isolates of *Klebsiella* were gentamicin resistant (and most multiresistant).

Table V. Antibacterial activity *in vitro* of cefotetan and other antibacterial agents against *Proteus, Providencia* and *Morganella* species in studies where 10 or more isolates were tested

Organism	Cefotetan		Latamoxef	Cefoxitin	Cefoperazone	Ceftazidime
	overall MIC range	MIC_{90} range	MIC_{90} range	MIC_{90} range	MIC_{90} range	MIC_{90} range
Proteus mirabilis	0.03-8.0	0.06-1.0	0.07-0.5	2.0-64	1.0-32	0.03-0.5
References	1-4,6,7,10,11,13		1,2,4,7,11,13	1-4,7,10,13	1,7	2,6,7,10,11
Proteus vulgaris	0.06-128	0.25-2.85	0.25-0.4	4.0-32	1.0	0.03-6.4
References	1,2,6,7,10		2,7	1,2,7,10	7	2,6,7,10
Indole-positive *Proteus*	0.06-16	0.5-6.25	0.25-0.5	4.0-25	4.0-128	<0.12-16
References	4,5,7,8,12,13		4,5,7,13	4,5,7,8,12,13	5,7,12	5,7,8,12
Indole-negative *Proteus*	<0.12-25	<0.12-3.12		2.0-25	6.25	<0.12-6.25
References	8,12			8,12	12	8,12
Providencia stuartii	0.03-64	0.5-12	0.06-4.0	4.0-40	32	0.5
References	1,2,4,9,10,13		1,2,4,13	1,2,4,10,13	1	10
Providencia rettgeri	0.06-32	0.25-30	0.11-0.5	16-64	4.0->64	0.06-4.0
References	1,2,6,7,10		1,2,7	1,2,7,10	1,7	6,7,10
Providencia spp.	0.03-32	0.125-8.0	0.06-2.0	4.0	4.0	0.06-5.0
References	6,7,11		7,11	7	7	6,7,11
Morganella morganii	0.125-32	1.0-8.0	0.25-0.5	16-32	8.0	0.5-5.2
References	1,6,7,9,10,11		1,7,11	1,7,10	7	1,6,7,10,11

Key to references: 1 Ayers et al. (1982); 2 Bauernfeind (1983); 3 Chattopadhyay and Teli (1982); 4 Clarke and Zemcov (1983); 5 Daschner et al. (1982); 6 Dette et al. (1983); 7 Grimm (1983); 8 Morel et al. (1983); 9 Periti et al. (1983); 10 Phillips et al. (1983); 11 Reeves et al. (1983); 12 Russo et al. (1983); 13 Wise et al. (1982).

strains of *Prov. rettgeri* were resistant to cefotetan, but sensitive to cefotaxime (Dette et al., 1983). Studies in a small number of isolates suggest that sensitivity of *Prov. alcalifaciens* and indole-negative *Proteus* species to cefotetan may be particularly high, with MIC_{90} values of 0.06 mg/L (Phillips et al., 1983) and < 0.12 mg/L (Morel et al., 1983) recorded, respectively.

Cefotetan is clearly more active *in vitro* against *Proteus, Providencia* and *Morganella* species than the 'second generation' cephalosporins, cefoxitin and cefoperazone (table V) and is also more active than gentamicin and piperacillin against *Providencia* species and *Proteus mirabilis*, but not indole-positive *Proteus* (Grimm, 1983; Periti et al., 1983; Wise et al., 1982). Cefotetan is equally active, in general, to cefotaxime against these genera, but somewhat less active than latamoxef, to which no strain has shown resistance in comparative studies with cefotetan (table V). Cefotetan has shown roughly equal *in vitro* activity to ceftazidime and ceftriaxone against *Proteus* species in some studies (Cocuzza et al., 1983; Daschner et al., 1982; Shah, 1983) but somewhat less activity in others (Ayers et al., 1982; Reeves et al., 1983; Wise et al., 1982).

Pseudomonas, Acinetobacter and Other Non-Fermentative Gram-Negative Bacilli

Pseudomonas species and other non-fermentative Gram-negative bacilli are essentially resistant to the 'first and second generation' cephalosporins, and demonstrate variable susceptibility to the newer cephamycins and cephalosporins.

Cefotetan shows very little *in vitro* activity against *P. aeruginosa* with all studies recording MIC_{90} values of over 32 mg/L (Ayers et al., 1982; Bauernfeind, 1983; Clarke and Zemcov, 1983; Cocuzza et al., 1983; Daschner et al., 1982; Dette et al., 1983; Grimm, 1983; Hart and Percival, 1983; Periti et al., 1983; Phillips et al., 1983; Reeves et al., 1983; Russo et al., 1983; Wise et al., 1982). Ceftazidime (MIC_{90} range of 2 to > 32 mg/L) was the most active of the cephalosporins tested (Daschner et al., 1982; Hart and Percival, 1983; Reeves et al., 1983; Wise et al., 1982), and aztreonam (MIC_{90} 8 mg/L), piperacillin (MIC_{90} 8 to 90 mg/L), amikacin (MIC_{90} 7.5 mg/L) and gentamicin (MIC_{90} 6.25 to 70 mg/L) also showed useful activity (Clarke and Zemcov, 1983; Grimm, 1983; Hart and Percival, 1983; Russo et al., 1983). Cefotetan has, however, shown some activity against other *Pseudomonas* species, with *Ps. stutzeri* and *Ps. acidovorans* and some strains of *Ps. cepacia* being most sensitive ($MIC_{90} \leq 8$ mg/L), but with *Ps. maltophila* (MIC_{90} 8 to 64 mg/L), *Ps. putida* and *Ps. thomasii* (MIC_{90} 32 to 128 mg/L) and *Ps. fluorescens* (MIC_{90} 64 to 512 mg/L) being resistant to cefotetan (Ayers et al., 1982; Daschner et al., 1982; Phillips et al., 1983).

In common with the structurally similar cefoxitin and latamoxef, the antibacterial activity of cefotetan against *Acinetobacter* species is poor (MIC_{90} > 32 to 256 mg/L) and does not compare favourably with cefotaxime (MIC_{90} 8 to > 32 mg/L) or ceftazidime (8 to 32 mg/L). However, in one study, remarkably low MIC_{90} values were obtained against *A. calcoaceticus* with cefotetan, cefoxitin and cefoperazone (0.78, 3.12 and 1.56 mg/L, respectively) compared with a much higher MIC_{90} value of 25 mg/L with cefotaxime (Russo et al., 1983). There does not appear to be any difference in the susceptibility of the *lwoffii* and *anitratus* subspecies of *A. calcoaceticus* (Ayers et al., 1982; Chattopadhyay and Teli, 1982; Daschner et al., 1982; Dublanchet, 1985; Hart and Percival, 1983; Morel et al., 1983; Phillips et al., 1983).

Other non-fermentative Gram-negative bacilli, such as *Alcaligenes, Achromobacter* and *Flavobacterium* species have also proven resistant to cefotetan *in vitro* (Ayers et al., 1982).

Haemophilus and *Neisseria* Species

Although data are somewhat limited, neither the presence of β-lactamase nor resistance to ampicillin appear to affect the *in vitro* activity of cefotetan against *H. influenzae* (Ayers et al., 1982; Clarke and Zemcov, 1983; Phillips et al., 1983; Wise et al., 1982). Most clinical isolates of this organism are inhibited by cefotetan 4 mg/L (MIC_{90} 1 to 4 mg/L) with an overall range of activity of 0.12 to 25 mg/L. Cefotetan possesses similar *in vitro* activity to cefoxitin, cefazolin and cefamandole, but ap-

Table VI. Antibacterial activity *in vitro* of cefotetan and other antibacterial agents against *Salmonella* and *Shigella* species

References	No. of isolates	Cefotetan overall MIC range	Cefotetan MIC_{90}	Latamoxef overall MIC range	Latamoxef MIC_{90}	Cefoxitin overall MIC range	Cefoxitin MIC_{90}	Cefotaxime overall MIC range	Cefotaxime MIC_{90}
Salmonella enteriditis									
Ayers et al. (1982)	13		≤0.12				4.0		
Chattopadhyay and Teli (1982)	42	0.125-2	1			2-8	8		
Clarke and Zemcov (1983)	6	0.03-0.5	0.5	0.03-1	1	1-4	4		
Salmonella spp.									
Cocuzza et al. (1983)	16	0.09-12.5	12.5			0.09-6.25	6.25		
Gialdroni Grassi et al. (1983)	30	0.05-3.2	1-6						
Grimm (1983)	20	0.031-0.06	0.063	0.031-0.125	0.063	1-2	2	0.031-0.125	0.063
Reeves et al. (1983)	9	0.06-0.12	0.12	0.06-0.12	0.12			0.06-0.5	0.5
Russo et al. (1983)	14	0.78-50	25			0.78-100	50	0.78-50	25
Shigella spp.									
Ayers et al. (1982)	16		0.5				4.0		
Clarke and Zemcov (1983)	10	0.06-12	0.06	0.03-0.12	0.12	2	2		
Grimm (1983)	20	0.063-4	0.125	0.063-0.5	0.125	2-64	4	0.016-1	0.063
Reeves et al. (1983)	9	0.06->128	>128	0.06-8	8			0.03-8	8

preciably less overall activity than latamoxef, cefuroxime, aztreonam, cefoperazone, ceftriaxone or ceftazidime against *H. influenzae*. However, the activity of cefotetan against ampicillin-resistant isolates may be similar to that of latamoxef and markedly better than cefazolin and cefamandole (Ayers et al., 1982; Hennessey, 1985).

Most isolates of *N. gonorrhoeae* are inhibited by cefotetan 4 mg/L (MIC_{90} 1 to 4 mg/L) with an overall range of activity of ≤ 0.008 to 8 mg/L (Ayers et al., 1982; Hennessey, 1985; Phillips et al., 1983; Reeves et al., 1983; Wise et al., 1982). Both β-lactamase-producing and non-producing, and penicillin-resistant strains of *N. gonorrhoeae* appear to be equally inhibited by cefotetan (Reeves et al., 1983). Cefotetan possesses similar *in vitro* activity to cefoxitin, cefazolin and cefamandole, but is less active than cefoperazone, latamoxef and ceftazidime, ceftriaxone and cefotaxime against *N. gonorrhoeae* (Ayers et al., 1982; Phillips et al., 1983; Reeves et al., 1983; Wise et al., 1982). *In vitro* activity of cefotetan against *N. meningitidis* (MIC_{90} 0.12 mg/L) is somewhat higher than that against *N. gonorrhoeae*, as was that of the other cephalosporins tested (Ayers et al., 1982; Hennessey, 1985).

Other Aerobic Gram-Negative Bacteria

Cefotetan is active *in vitro* against *Citrobacter* species (MIC_{90} 0.12 to 64 mg/L), *C. diversus* (MIC_{90} 0.12 mg/L) and *C. freundii* (MIC_{90} 1.0 to > 32 mg/L). Against *Citrobacter* species cefoxitin and cefamandole show markedly less activity than cefotetan, while latamoxef (MIC_{90} 0.12 to 0.5 mg/L), cefotaxime (0.25 to 50 mg/L) and ceftazidime show consistently greater *in vitro* activity (Ayers et al., 1982; Bauernfeind, 1983; Chattopadhyay and Teli, 1983; Dette et al., 1983; Grimm, 1983; Hart and Percival, 1983; Hennessey, 1985; Phillips et al., 1983; Reeves et al., 1983; Russo et al., 1983; Wise et al., 1982). In one study, the MIC_{90} value for cefotetan against *C. diversus* (0.12 mg/L) was lower than that of latamoxef (0.5 mg/L) [Ayers et al., 1982].

Cefotetan is very active against most strains of *Salmonella* and *Shigella* species with most studies reporting MIC_{90} values of 0.06 to 1.6 mg/L (table

VI; Hennessey, 1985). However, in one study, resistant strains were reported, which were moderately susceptible to latamoxef and cefotaxime (Reeves et al., 1983). Overall, the activity of cefotetan against *Salmonella* and *Shigella* is similar to that of latamoxef and cefotaxime (MIC_{90} 0.06 to 8 and 0.06 to 25 mg/L, respectively) and superior to that of cefoxitin (MIC_{90} 2 to 50 mg/L) [table VI].

Against *Yersinia enterocolitica* (128 isolates) a single study showed cefotetan (MIC_{90} 1 mg/L) to have greater activity than cefoperazone, piperacillin and cefoxitin (MIC_{90} 2 to 16 mg/L), but less activity than cefotaxime (MIC_{90} 0.06 mg/L) or latamoxef (MIC_{90} 0.25 mg/L). However, at the susceptibility 'breakpoint' of 16 mg/L, cefotetan, latamoxef, piperacillin and cefotaxime all inhibited 100% of strains (Grimm, 1983).

1.2 *In Vitro* Inhibitory Activity Against Anaerobic Bacteria

Cefotetan has modest *in vitro* activity against some clinically important Gram-negative anaerobes such as *Bacteroides fragilis, B. asaccharolyticus (B. melaninogenicus)* and *Fusobacterium* species and against most Gram-positive anaerobic bacilli, such as *Clostridium* species (table VII). However, the wide variation in sensitivity of anaerobes of the same genera (or even species) between laboratories suggests that local testing of isolates should be undertaken. Ascertaining the MIC_{90} value for cefotetan against *B. fragilis* is complicated in some studies by the lack of differentiation between *B. fragilis, B. ovatus, B. vulgatus, B. distasonis* and *B. thetaiotaomicron*, thus forming a *B. fragilis* 'group' of organisms. In studies which differentiated between these species, there are obvious differences in their susceptibility to cefotetan.

In general, cefotetan, cefoxitin and latamoxef are more active than the cephalosporins against most clinically important *Bacteroides* species, but less active than clindamycin, metronidazole and imipenem (N-formimidoyl thienamycin) [table VII]. Among the *B. fragilis* group, cefotetan is more active against the clinically important *B. fragilis* (MIC_{90} 8 to 32 mg/L), the rarely isolated *B. vulgatus* isolates (MIC_{90} 2 to 32 mg/L), and *B. asaccharolyticus* (MIC_{90} 0.5 to 64 mg/L) than against the less important *B. thetaiotaomicron, B. ovatus* or *B. distasonis* ($MIC_{90} \geqslant 32$ mg/L) [table VII; Hennessey, 1985, unpublished data on file, Stuart Pharmaceuticals]. Among other *Bacteroides* species, *B. uniformis, B. bivius, B. ruminicola* and *B. disiens* are sensitive to cefotetan (MIC_{90} 4 to 16 mg/L) and *B. ureolyticus* (MIC_{90} 0.06 to 1 mg/L) is highly sensitive (Phillips et al., 1983; Ruckdeschel, 1983; Werner, 1983). Somewhat higher MIC_{90} values were consistently reported for cefotetan against all *Bacteroides* species (MIC_{90} 64 to 256 mg/L) in one study where imipenem was particularly effective (Owens and Finegold, 1983).

The susceptibility of *Clostridium* species to cefotetan is also highly variable (MIC_{90} values range from 0.06 to 32 mg/L) [table VII; Hennessey, 1985], but *C. perfringens* and *C. botulinum* appear to be inhibited at far lower concentrations (MIC_{90} 0.06 to 1 mg/L) than does *C. difficile* (MIC_{90} 2 to 32 mg/L) [table VII]. Nevertheless, cefotetan seems to have greater activity than latamoxef, cefoxitin, ceftriaxone, ceftazidime or cefotaxime, but less activity than metronidazole or imipenem, against the latter organism (Kesado et al., 1982; Owens and Finegold, 1983).

Among anaerobic Gram-positive cocci, 90% of isolates of peptococci and peptostreptococci are inhibited by cefotetan 1 to 8 mg/L (Kesado et al., 1982; Owens and Finegold, 1983; Phillips et al., 1983). Cefotetan is usually active *in vitro* against *Fusobacterium* species (MIC_{90} 2 to 8 mg/L; Kesado et al., 1982; Phillips et al., 1983; Ruckdeschel, 1983), *Veillonella parvula* (MIC_{90} 2 mg/L; Kesado et al., 1982) and *Propionibacterium acnes* (MIC_{90} 0.5 mg/L; Owens and Finegold, 1983).

1.3 Bactericidal Activity

There is relatively little information available regarding the minimum bactericidal concentration (MBC) of cefotetan against Gram-positive or Gram-negative aerobic or anaerobic organisms. However, in general, there has been little difference between the MBC_{90} and MIC_{90} concentrations of cefotetan, with most values being identical or ≤ 2-fold higher for the MBC (Ayers et al., 1982; Cocuzza et al., 1983; Drugeon et al., 1985; Francisco and LeFrock, 1983; Gialdroni Grassi et al., 1983; Isono et al., 1982; Morel et al. 1983; Owens and Finegold, 1983; Phillips et al., 1983; Russo et al., 1983; Shah, 1983). Nevertheless, in some studies the MBC_{90}/MIC_{90} ratio has been increased to 4-fold for *Salmonella* species (Gialdroni Grassi et al., 1983), *Klebsiella* species (Morel et al., 1983) and *Staphylococcus aureus* (Shah, 1983) and even greater increases have been reported for indole-negative *Proteus* species, *Proteus vulgaris* and *Providencia rettgeri* (Gialdroni Grassi et al., 1983; Morel et al., 1983).

Killing curves for *Staphylococcus aureus, S. epidermidis, Escherichia coli, Klebsiella pneumoniae* and *Enterobacter aerogenes* show a rapid bactericidal activity at 2 to 4 times the MIC_{90} concentration. *Proteus vulgaris* regrows after exposure to these concentrations, as do other species, 24 hours after 1 to 2 times the MIC_{90} concentration – with the exceptions of *Enterobacter* species and *Proteus mirabilis,* which do not (Gialdroni Grassi et al., 1983; Shah, 1983).

1.4 Effect on Activity of Inoculum Size, Culture Media, pH and Serum

In most studies inoculum density over a range 10^3 to 10^7 organisms/ml appears to have little or no effect on the MIC_{90} of cefotetan against most isolates of Gram-negative and Gram-positive aerobic bacteria (Ayers et al., 1982; Clarke and Zemcov, 1983; Gialdroni Grassi et al., 1983; Morel et al., 1983; Russo et al., 1983; Wise et al., 1982) and anaerobic bacteria (Souza Dias et al., 1984). However, in one study, increasing the inoculum size from 5×10^3 to 5×10^5 organisms/ml clearly increased the concentration of cefotetan required to inhibit 90% of isolates of *E. coli* (β-lactamase-positive and -negative strains), *Klebsiella* species, *Enterobacter cloacae, Serratia* species, *Proteus mirabilis* and β-lactamase-positive and -negative *Staphylococcus aureus* isolates (Dette et al., 1983). Additionally, one genus (encompassing *Proteus, Providencia* and *Morganella* species) exhibited an 8-fold increase in MIC_{90} concentration over this inoculum range (Ayers et al., 1982), and a marked reduction in MIC_{90} of cefotetan was seen against *Staphylococcus aureus* and *S. epidermidis* at an inoculum size of 10^3 compared with 10^7 organisms/ml (Gialdroni Grassi et al., 1983).

The effect of the composition of growth medium on the *in vitro* antibacterial efficacy of cefotetan has been studied in several laboratories, the results from which suggest that the activity of cefotetan against Gram-negative bacilli was unaffected by using either Mueller-Hinton broth, Brain Heart Infusion extract broth, or 'Iso-Sensitest' broth and a number of other solid and liquid media (Gialdroni Grassi et al., 1983; Russo et al., 1983; Wise et al., 1982). However, the addition of 10% horse serum to Tryptic soy broth caused a 2- to 4-fold increase in MICs of all bacteria except *Klebsiella pneumoniae* where a 32-fold increase was seen (Gialdroni Grassi et al., 1983). Little or no change in activity was noted at different pH values in different solid and liquid media (Gialdroni Grassi et al., 1983; Yano et al., 1982), with only *Staphylococcus aureus* and *S. epidermidis* showing more susceptibility at pH values of 5.5 or lower (Gialdroni Grassi et al., 1983).

1.5 Antibiotic Synergy

There is only limited published information on the possibility of *in vitro* antibiotic synergy between cefotetan and aminoglycosides, cephalosporins or piperacillin. In the available studies, fractional inhibitory concentration (FIC) was assessed. Synergy was usually defined as an FIC ≤ 0.6 and addition as an FIC of 0.7 to 1.2. Results were based on both inhibitory activity and killing curves (Bauernfeind, 1983; Gialdroni Grassi et al., 1983; Just et al., 1984). When combined with aminoglycosides (gentamicin, netilmicin, amikacin, tobramycin) a synergistic effect was seen against 22% of Gram-negative isolates but only 2% of Gram-positive isolates. Additive inhibition was seen against 60 and 46% of Gram-negative and Gram-

Table VII. Antibacterial activity *in vitro* of cefotetan and other antibacterial agents against *Bacteroides* and *Clostridium* species

Organism	Cefotetan		Latamoxef MIC_{90} range	Cefoxitin MIC_{90} range	Cefotaxime MIC_{90} range	Clindamycin MIC_{90} range	Metronidazole MIC_{90} range	Imipenem MIC_{90} range
	overall MIC range	MIC_{90} range						
Bacteroides fragilis	0.12-256	4.0-128	2.0-85	8.0-128	16-128	0.25-4.0	0.03->64	0.25
References	1-12,14-20		4,5,9,10,12,14-17,19,20	1,2,4,5,8-10,16-20	5,7-10,15,16,17	2,5,9,12,14,16,17	2,9,12,14,15,17	9,11
B. thetaiotaomicron	2.0->256	>32-256	64-128	32-64	64-128	2.0->128	1.0-2.0	0.5
References	1,8,9,11,14,16-19		9,16,17,19	1,8,9,15,16,17	8,9,16,17	9,16	9,16	9,11
B. asaccharolyticus[a]	0.002-64	0.5-64	2.0-8.0	0.5-4.0	2.0	0.12-0.25	2.0	0.125
References	2,11,16,18		16,18	2,16,18	16	2,16	2,16	11
Other *Bacteroides* species	0.008-256	2.0->128	0.5-32	1.0-32	4.0-128	0.12->128	1.0-8.0	0.25-0.5
References	2,11,16-19		9,13,16,17	1,2,8,9,13,16,17	8,9,13,17	2,9,16	2,9,16	9,11
Clostridium perfringens	0.016-2.0	0.06-8.0	0.5-8.0	0.5-4.0	1.0-8.0	0.063-4.0	1.0-4.0	0.063
References	2,9,17-19		9,17,19	2,9,17,18,19	9,17	2,9,17	2,9,17	9
C. difficile	0.016-128	2.0-32	8.0-256	4.0-128	8.0-128	32->128	0.5-1.0	0.25-8.0
References	6,9,11,17,18		6,9,17	6,9,17	6,9,17	9	9	9,11
Other *Clostridium* species	0.03-256	0.25-8	1.0-80	1.0-64	2.0-8.0	0.063-4.0	0.5-2.0	0.125-1.0
References	2,9,11,15,17,19		9,15,17,19	2,9,17,19	9,15,17	2,9	2,9	9,11

a Also known as *B. melaninogenicus*.

Key to references: 1 Aldridge et al. (1984); 2 Ayers et al. (1982); 3 Chattopadhyay and Teli (1982); 4 Clarke and Zemcov (1983); 4 Dainelli et al. (1985); 6 Delmée et al. (1985); 7 Dette et al. (1983); 8 Dublanchet (1985); 9 Kesado et al. (1982); 10 Kesado et al. (1984); 11 Owens and Finegold (1983); 12 Periti et al. (1983); 13 Phillips et al. (1983); 14 Privivera et al. (1985); 15 Reeves et al. (1983); 16 Ruckdeschel (1983); 17 Souza Dias et al. (1984); 18 Watt and Brown (1985); 19 Werner (1983); 20 Wise et al. (1982).

positive isolates, respectively (Just et al., 1984). Synergy was seen against 50% of *Enterobacteriaceae* isolates that were previously poorly sensitive to cefotetan; against the remaining 50% of isolates the effects of the combination were usually additive (Bauernfeind, 1983; Gialdroni Grassi et al., 1983; Serra et al., 1985). Bauernfeind (1983) reported that in 3 of 8 strains against which synergy was exhibited the MIC for cefotetan remained above 16 mg/L, although the original MICs for these strains were ≥ 128 mg/L. Killing curves most often showed additive and negligible effects with combined therapy, although marked synergy occurred against *Enterobacter aerogenes* (Gialdroni Grassi et al., 1983). No synergy between cefotetan and amikacin against *Pseudomonas aeruginosa* was observed by Serra et al. (1985).

The combination of cefotetan with cefotaxime or piperacillin produced more examples of synergy against *Enterobacteriaceae* (43% and 33% of strains, respectively) than did combination with cefazolin or latamoxef (25% and 21%, respectively) [Gialdroni Grassi et al., 1983]. Combination of cefotetan with piperacillin or mezlocillin produced additive inhibition against 63%, and synergistic inhibition against 11%, of Gram-negative isolates (Just et al., 1984). No reduction of *in vitro* MIC values was seen in a variety of β-lactamase-producing isolates (mostly *Enterobacteriaceae*) when cefotetan and cefoxitin were combined with clavulanic acid (Moosdeen et al., 1983). Although no antagonism was noted between cefotetan and piperacillin, mezlocillin or aminoglycosides in one study (Just et al., 1984), in another study a combination of cefotetan and piperacillin was antagonistic in 25% of isolates (Barry et al., 1984).

1.6 β-Lactamase Resistance

Cefotetan has marked stability *in vitro* against a variety of β-lactamases produced by Gram-negative aerobic and anaerobic bacteria including the TEM type I β-lactamases (mainly cephalosporinases), type IV chromosomal broad spectrum β-lactamases, or by types Ia, IIIa, IIIb or IVc β-lactamases (Ayers et al., 1982; Bauernfeind, 1983; Chabbert and Derlot, 1983; Cocuzza et al., 1983; Hart and Percival, 1982; Jones and Wilson, 1983; Labia et al., 1983a,b; Moosdeen et al., 1983; Murata et al., 1981; Phillips et al., 1983; Ravizzola et al., 1983; Toda et al., 1981a,b; Wise et al., 1982). Like latamoxef, cefotetan shows some degree of hydrolysis by PSE II (*Pseudomonas aeruginosa*) β-lactamases (Ayers et al., 1982; Cocuzza et al., 1983; Jones and Wilson, 1983; Moosdeen et al., 1983), and has been inactivated by β-lactamases from occasional strains of *Enterobacter cloacae* (Bauernfeind, 1983; Chabbert and Derlot, 1983; Hennessey and Edwards, 1983; Jones and Wilson, 1983; Moosdeen et al., 1983; Ravizzola et al., 1983). Large increases in the MICs of *E. cloacae, Bacteroides fragilis, Serratia liquifaciens,* and *Citrobacter freundii* have also been reported, although evidence of inactivation by β-lactamases was not stated (Bauernfeind, 1983; Chabbert and Derlot, 1983).

Cefotetan also possesses direct β-lactamase inhibitory properties, in addition to its β-lactamase stability. Cefotetan, along with cefoxitin, latamoxef, cefotaxime, cefuroxime, ceftizoxime, cefmenoxime, cefmetazole and some semisynthetic penicillins inhibited the activity of cephalosporinases derived from *E. coli, Enterobacter cloacae, Citrobacter freundii, Serratia marcescens, Morganella morganii, Proteus rettgeri, Ps. aeruginosa* and *Bacteroides fragilis.* Cefotetan was less inhibitory against enzymes from *P. vulgaris,* and was ineffective against β-lactamase from *P. cepacia* and plasmid-mediated penicillinases type I and IV (Toda et al., 1981a,b). However, in another study the enzymes of *P. vulgaris* and OXA-1 type enzymes were rapidly inactivated, whereas cephalosporinases from *E. coli, M. morganii, E. cloacae* and *Ps. aeruginosa* were unaffected (Labia et al., 1983b).

1.7 Penetrability of Cefotetan

Penetrability studies have given conflicting evidence thus far. Surprisingly cefotetan had a far greater penetrability in 2 strains of *Pseudomonas aeruginosa* than cefoxitin, ceftizoxime, ceftazidime or cephaloridine, and a similar penetrability to these drugs with respect to *E. coli* strains in one study

(Cocuzza et al., 1983), although another showed poor penetrability into *Pseudomonas aeruginosa* (Suginaka et al., 1982).

2. Nephrotoxicity

Comparative studies after intravenous administration of cefotetan and other cephem antibiotics showed that, at single doses up to 2400 mg/kg, cefotetan along with cephalothin and cefazolin had markedly fewer renal effects than cephaloridine in rats (Imamura et al., 1982b) and markedly fewer renal effects than cefazolin after repeated doses up to 1200 mg/kg in rabbits (Suzuki et al., 1983). In 2 other studies in rats (one short term, the other over a 28-day period) cefotetan did not display any evidence of nephrotoxicity (Imamura, 1982b; Murgatroyd et al., 1985).

In healthy volunteers receiving cefotetan 2g twice daily for 3 days, there were no effects on proximal tubular enzyme activity, serum creatinine or creatinine clearance, although albumin and total protein levels in the urine were increased (Mondorf et al., 1985).

3. Pharmacokinetic Studies

The pharmacokinetic properties of cefotetan have been extensively studied in healthy subjects and in adult and paediatric patients after intramuscular injection and intravenous bolus or infusion. Serum concentrations have been determined by either microbiological assay or high pressure liquid chromatography, and occasionally by both methods. The influence of impaired renal function on the pharmacokinetics of cefotetan has also been studied.

3.1 Absorption and Plasma Concentrations

Immediately after an intravenous bolus dose of 1g to healthy adult volunteers mean peak plasma concentrations of cefotetan are about 140 to 250 mg/L (Naber et al., 1985a,b; Nakayama et al., 1981, 1982; Saito et al., 1982a,b) [table VIII]. A dose of 1 to 2g given by intravenous infusion over 60 minutes results in mean peak concentrations of about 70 to 270 mg/L (Nagasawa et al., 1982; Nakagawa et al., 1982a; Soejima et al., 1982). In dose-ranging studies in healthy volunteers, plasma concentrations increased almost linearly with dose after single intravenous administration of 0.25 to 2.0g (table VIII). Similarly, mean peak plasma concentrations after single intramuscular doses were also dose-related (23 to 91 mg/L) after cefotetan 0.5 to 2.0g, and were attained at 1.5 to 3 hours (Guibert et al., 1983; Yates et al., 1983b; fig. 2). Cefotetan is completely bioavailable after intramuscular administration (Guibert et al., 1983), and in one study there was no significant difference in the plasma concentrations and other pharmacokinetic parameters whether water or 0.5% lignocaine was used as the diluent for intramuscular doses (Yates et al., 1983b).

Mean steady-state plasma concentrations of 37.5 mg/L were attained 12 hours after the start of a continuous intravenous infusion (75.8 mg/hour) in healthy volunteers. The levels were attained much more quickly if an additional loading dose of cefotetan 0.5g was administered (Adam et al., 1983).

Mean peak plasma concentrations in children are usually comparable with those attained in adults

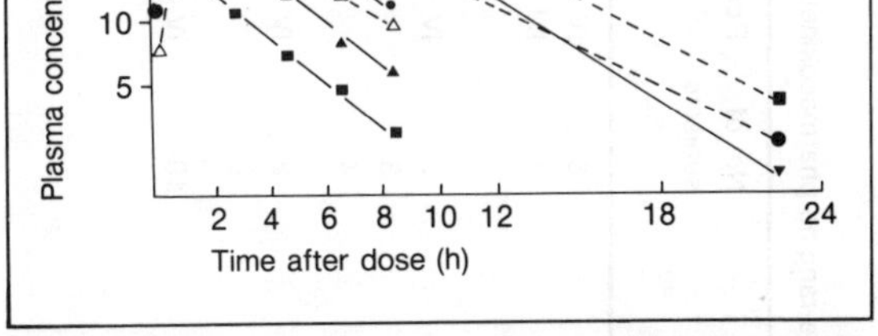

Fig. 2. Plasma concentrations of cefotetan (determined by HPLC) following single intravenous bolus doses of 0.25g (■——■), 0.5g (▲——▲), 1.0g (●——●) and 2.0g (▼——▼) and intramuscular doses of 0.5g (△---△), 1.0g (●---●) and 2.0g (■---■) [after Yates et al., 1983a,b].

Table VIII. Dose-ranging pharmacokinetic studies in healthy volunteers following single-dose parenteral administration of cefotetan

References	No. of subjects	Route	Dose (g)	C_{max} (mg/L)	T_{max} (min)	$t_{1/2\beta}$ (h)	Vd_{total} (L)	$Vd_{central}$ (L)	Total clearance (ml/min)	Renal clearance (ml/min)	% recovery in urine (h)	Assay techniques
Guibert et al. (1983)	6	IV	1.0	179	2	3.1	10.3	5.85	29.2 (plasma)		75 [24]	Bioassay
	6	IM	0.5	35	82	3.4-3.7	11.0				60 to 65 [24]	
			1.0	79	97		11.6					
Nakagawa et al. (1982a)	3	IV	0.5	132		3.11	8.9	3.9	37.3	29.7		HPLC
	3		1.0	253.2		3.40	8.0	3.9	30.7	23.5		Bioassay
	4		1.0	263.9		2.83	7.2	3.9	33.2			TLC
Stahl et al. (1985)	8	IV	1.0	229		3.8	10.4		30-32	20		Bioassay
	8		2.0	491		4.2	11.4					
Yates et al. (1983a)	10	IV	0.25	42	5	3.0	10.5		40.1		66 [18]	HPLC
			0.5	79		3.0	11.1		43.3		67 [18]	Bioassay
			1.0	142		3.5	13.0		45.5		70 [18]	
			2.0	237		3.6	14.8		49.0	31.3	66 [18]	
Yates et al. (1983b)	9	IM	0.5	23.3	180	3.4					66.5 [18]	HPLC
	8	IM	1.0	51.9	180	4.4					61 [18]	Bioassay
		IM	2.0	91.0	180	4.2						

Abbreviations: C_{max} = mean maximum plasma concentration; T_{max} = time to maximum plasma concentrations; $t_{1/2\beta}$ = plasma elimination half-life; Vd_{total} = total volume of distribution; $Vd_{central}$ = volume of distribution to the central compartment; HPLC = high performance liquid chromatography; TLC = thin-layer chromatography.

after intravenous bolus and infusion administration of comparable doses based on bodyweight; doses of 10 to 20 mg/kg produced peak concentrations of 55 to 216 mg/L (Aso et al., 1983; Fujii et al., 1983; Nishimura et al., 1983; Toyonaga et al., 1983). However, occasionally, somewhat lower plasma cefotetan concentrations have been observed (Iwai et al., 1983).

Three studies have compared the plasma concentrations of cefotetan with those after equal intravenous doses of other antibiotics. In healthy volunteers administered 1g doses, cefotetan peak plasma concentrations were 1.8-fold higher than those of latamoxef, 1.6-fold higher than cefotaxime and similar to cefazolin; at 2 hours onwards these differences were even more pronounced (Naber et al., 1985a,b; Nakagawa et al., 1982a; Nakayama et al., 1981).

Cefotetan plasma concentrations at 8 hours following single intravenous doses of 0.5 and 1.0g to healthy volunteers range from 7.6 to 9.1 mg/L, and from 13.5 to 16.3 mg/L, respectively (Koyama et al., 1982; Nakagawa et al., 1982a; Nakayama et al., 1981; Sawae et al., 1982; Tachibana et al., 1985), whereas serum concentrations of cefazolin and latamoxef 8 hours after 1g intravenous doses have fallen to 1.7 and 3.8 mg/L, respectively (Nakagawa et al., 1982a; Nakayama et al., 1981). Serum cefotetan concentrations of 10.5 mg/L were recorded 12 hours after 1g single intramuscular doses (Guibert et al., 1983), and 8 hours after 0.5g single intramuscular doses (Tachibana et al., 1985).

3.2 Distribution

The apparent volume of distribution in healthy adult volunteers administered a single intravenous bolus or intramuscular dose of cefotetan 0.5 to 1.0g is about 8 to 13L and is approximately equally divided between central and peripheral compartments (table VIII). A value of 14.8L was recorded after a 2g intravenous dose (Yates et al., 1983a).

Concentrations of cefotetan have been determined in a wide range of body tissues and fluids in man. Cefotetan concentrations likely to be inhibitory to susceptible bacteria were attained in most of these tissues and fluids. Indeed, concentrations high enough to inhibit even moderately susceptible bacteria (MIC_{90} 16 to 64 mg/L) were attained in wound secretions, stomach wall and mucosa, prostatic tissue, umbilical cord serum, intrapelvic organs, gallbladder tissue, bile and peritoneal fluid and palatine tonsillar tissue (table IX). Low cefotetan concentrations of 0.34 and 0.59 mg/L were measured in breast milk of puerperal women after 1g intravenous and intramuscular injections, with no accumulation of drug in milk after repeated doses (Cho et al., 1982; Novelli et al., 1983). Concentrations of cefotetan in non-traumatic joint effusion after 1g intramuscular doses were considered to be 'sufficient to inhibit many bacterial pathogens' (Bonadio et al., 1985).

Intravenous bolus doses (1g) have produced relatively high peak concentrations of cefotetan in prostatic tissue (38 mg/kg) in patients with prostatic hypertrophy, but not in the prostatic fluid (0.8 mg/L) of patients with prostatitis, where cefotetan produced less tissue penetration than cefoperazone, latamoxef, ceftizoxime or cefotaxime (Fujimura et al., 1982; Suzuki et al., 1981).

In 12 patients with cerebrovascular haemorrhage, administration of large intravenous doses of cefotetan (1g every hour for 12 hours or 2g every 3 hours for 24 hours) produced cerebrospinal fluid (CSF) cefotetan concentrations of 2.5 to 4.5 mg/L, respectively, and a CSF : plasma ratio of about 0.013 (Hirayama, 1985).

Protein binding of cefotetan in healthy subjects is 78 to 91% (Drumm et al., 1983; Gialdroni Grassi et al., 1983; Komiya et al., 1981; Tachibana et al., 1985; Wise et al., 1982; Yates et al., 1983a). Cefotetan is also bound to human liver ligandin (glutathione-S-transferase) to a much greater extent than cefazolin, chloramphenicol and gentamicin, which may explain the differences in the extent of biliary excretion of these drugs (Komatsu et al., 1981).

3.3 Metabolism and Excretion

A limited number of studies have been unable to identify metabolites of cefotetan in either plasma

Table IX. Concentrations of cefotetan in various body tissues and fluids after single-dose administration to patients

Tissue/body fluid	Type of patients	Doses (g)	Route(s) of administration	Peak tissue/ fluid concentration (mg/kg; mg/L)	Tissue/fluid : serum concentration ratio (%)	References
Peritoneal fluid	Abdominal infection patients	1.0-2.0	IV	48-80	85	Donovan et al. (1983) Wittke et al. (1985)
Wound secretions	Abdominal infection patients	2.0	IV	51	59	Wittke et al. (1985)
Stomach wall and mucosa	Abdominal infection patients	10	IV	19-30	9-13	Furuhata et al. (1985)
Prostatic tissue	Prostatic hypertrophy	1.0	IV	38		Fujimura et al. (1982)
Prostatic fluid	Prostatitis	1.0	IV	0.2-1.32	0.8	Suzuki et al. (1981, 1982d)
Umbilical cord serum	Pregnant women	0.5-1.0	IV	21-31.4	15.4-34	Seiga et al. (1982); Cho et al. (1982); Motomura et al. (1982); Takase et al. (1982)
Amniotic fluid	Pregnant women	0.5-1.0	IV	8.6-19.1	10.1-12.3	Seiga et al. (1982); Takase et al. (1982); Cho et al. (1982)
Breast milk	Puerperal women	1.0 1.0	IV IM	0.34 0.59	. . .[a]	Cho et al. (1982) Novelli et al. (1983)
Intrapelvic genital organs	Obstetric and gynaecology patients	1.0 2.0	IV IV	13.5-45 40-95	7.5-47	Cho et al. (1982) Daschner et al. (1985); Motomura et al. (1982);[b] Yasuda et al. (1983)
		1.0	Drip infusion	7.8-29.9	18-47	Cho et al. (1982); Nishino et al. (1982)[c]
Gallbladder tissue	Biliary tract infection	0.5-2.0	IM/IV	8-87.6	0.25	Furuhata et al. (1985); Owen et al. (1983a,b); Tanimura et al. (1982, 1985); Wittke et al. (1985)
Bile	Post-cholecystectomy	1.0	IV	171-408	>100	Fujimoto et al. (1982); Owen et al. (1983a,b)
	Biliary tract infections	1.0-2.0	IV	up to 1415	>100	Tanimura et al. (1982);[d] Wittke et al. (1985)
Palatine tonsils/ macillary sinus mucosa	Otorhinolaryngological patients	0.5-2.0	IV	5-20	12-35	Fujimaki et al. (1983); Iwasawa (1982); Sambe et al. (1982); Wada et al. (1982)
Cerebrospinal fluid	Children, meningitis	54-83 mg/kg	IV	1.1-4.8	0.8-3.6	Iwata et al. (1983)

Table IX. (Contd)

Tissue/body fluid	Type of patients	Doses (g)	Route(s) of administration	Peak tissue/ fluid concentration (mg/kg; mg/L)	Tissue/fluid : serum concentration ratio (%)	References
Sputum	Chronic bronchitis	0.5-1.0	IV		0.74-12	Matsumoto et al. (1982)
		0.5-1.0	Drip infusion	0.44-0.72		Nagasawa et al. (1982)
Suction blister fluid	Healthy volunteers	1.0	IM	12.5 mg/L	19.1	Periti et al. (1983)

a Ratio was 0.88% at 24 hours, 2.85% at 7 hours and 5% at 10 hours.
b Patients had uterine cancer.
c Various intrapelvic genital tissue concentrations (in descending order): portio > ovary > cervix > oviduct > endometrium > myometrium > uterine myoma.
d In patients with a T-tube, cefotetan biliary levels ≫ cefmetazole or cefazolin.

or urine of healthy subjects (Kuroda et al., 1982; Saito et al., 1982b). Cefotetan is excreted largely in the urine, with about 60 to 75% of a dose usually being recovered over a period of 18 to 24 hours after administration of single intravenous or intramuscular doses to healthy volunteers (table VIII). High cefotetan concentrations occur in urine of healthy subjects, and are highest during the first 3 hours after administration of intravenous 1.0g and intramuscular 0.5 and 1.0g doses (4513, 878 and 2354 mg/L), although significant amounts of drug are still excreted into the urine at 12 to 24 hours (43 to 77 mg/L). The half-life of urinary excretion is about 3 to 3.2 hours (Guibert et al., 1983; Nakayama et al., 1981; Yates et al., 1983a,b).

In man, cefotetan concentrations in bile of the common bile duct exceed plasma concentrations by up to 10-fold (Fujimoto et al., 1982; Owen et al., 1983a,b; Tanimura et al., 1982), whereas gallbladder bile concentrations depend on the functional state of the gallbladder. Cefotetan does not enter the biliary tree in patients with obstructive jaundice (Owen et al., 1983a,b).

Renal clearance of cefotetan after intravenous bolus or infusion is around 1.2 to 1.9 L/h and accounts for 64 to 84% of total plasma clearance (1.8 to 2.9 L/h) in healthy subjects (table VIII; Tachibana et al., 1985). Biliary excretion of cefotetan accounts for about 12% of intravenous dose in healthy volunteers (Lanzini et al., 1985).

Cefotetan exists in equilibrium with its tautomer in solution, which at neutral and acid pH strongly favours cefotetan. In man, the proportion of dose recovered as the tautomer has been recorded as 0.3 to 10%, and is not correlated with the state of renal function (Kuroda et al., 1982; Ohkawa et al., 1983; Nakayama et al., 1981; Saito et al., 1982b; Sawae et al., 1982; Tanimura et al., 1985).

3.3.1 Half-Life

In healthy adult subjects the mean elimination half-life of cefotetan has been recorded as 2.8 to 4.2 hours after intravenous administration of 0.5 to 2.0g when determined over a period of 8 to 24 hours (table VIII). After intramuscular administration of equal doses, the elimination half-life is 3.4 to 4.4 hours. The elimination half-life in the elderly may not be prolonged where renal function is good (Stahl et al., 1985); however, in patients with renal impairment the elimination half-life increases (section 3.4). In paediatric subjects a slightly shorter elimination half-life of 1.85 to 3.5 hours is commonly seen (Aso et al., 1983; Fujii et al., 1983; Iwai et al., 1983; Iwata et al., 1983), although in newborn infants with urinary tract infection a somewhat longer elimination half-life of 5.4 hours has been recorded (Serra et al., 1985).

In comparative studies in healthy volunteers the plasma cefotetan elimination half-life (2.8 to 3.4 hours) has been considerably longer than that of cefazolin (1.5 hours; Nakayama et al., 1982), latamoxef (1.9 hours; Nakayama et al., 1981) or cefotaxime (1.05 hours; Naber et al., 1985a,b).

3.4 Effect of Disease States on Pharmacokinetics

Several studies have recorded the influence of varying degrees of renal impairment on the disposition of cefotetan, using high performance liquid chromatography, thin layer chromatography and bioassay. There is a direct correlation between total body clearance and creatinine clearance and thus elimination of cefotetan will be delayed in patients with renal impairment (table X). A mild decrease in creatinine clearance (to around 60 to 100 ml/min) results in an increase in the mean elimination half-life to about 4.5 hours, and a creatinine clearance of around 30 ml/min will increase the half-life to at least twice the value in subjects with normal renal function. In patients with severe renal impairment (creatinine clearance less than 10 ml/min) this value will exceed 10 hours (Ohkawa et al., 1983; Wright et al., 1983) [fig. 3]. As might be expected, a decrease in renal function results in de-

Table X. Pharmacokinetic studies in patients with varying degrees of renal insufficiency following single-dose intravenous administration of cefotetan

References	No. of subjects	Creatinine clearance (ml/min/1.73m²)	Dose (g)	C_{max} (mg/L)	$t_{1/2\beta}$ (h)	AUC (mg/L · h)	Total clearance (ml/min)	Renal clearance (ml/min)	% recovery in urine [h]
Browning et al. (1985)	5	a	1.0		15.5 (7.9-31.7)		13.0		
Inamatsu et al. (1983)	8	40	0.5	104	7.64	659			
Ishito et al. (1983)	3	Healthy	0.5		3.0				77.0 [24]
	2	34-35			9.1				17.1 [24]
	2	7-15			15.3				22.8 [24]
Ohkawa et al. (1983)	8	Healthy	0.5	180	3.0	254	38.7	32.3	
	8	69-94			3.72	323.8	31.5	20.2	
	16	31-68			4.59	427.8	23.9	13.6	
	10	8-28			11.09	1171.0	10.1	3.3	
	7	0-7			13.11	1452.9	8.3	0.5	
Smith and LeFrock (1984)	4	>80	1.0	126	5.1				
	12	40-80		122	8.8				
	10	10-40		128	10.1				
Wright et al. (1983)	5	50-110	0.5		4.6				78.4 [24]
	3	15-50			7.0				65 [24]
	3	6-11			18.8				8 [24]
	4	0-5			35.1				4.9 [24]

a Patients undergoing continuous ambulatory peritoneal dialysis.

Abbreviations: C_{max} = mean maximum plasma concentrations; $t_{1/2\beta}$ = plasma elimination half-life; AUC = area under the plasma concentration-time curve.

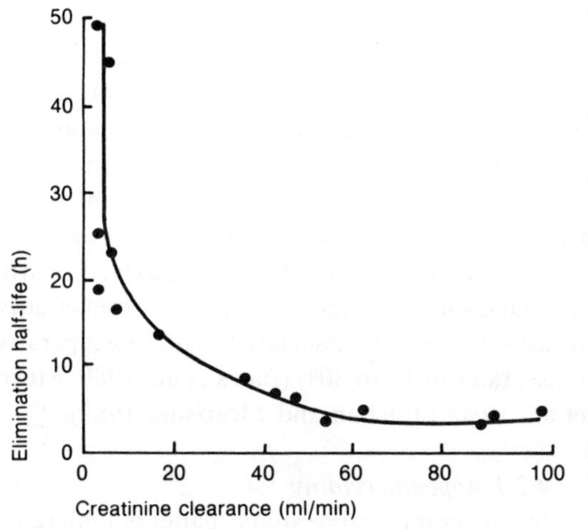

Fig. 3. The relationship between cefotetan elimination half-life and creatinine clearance in patients with varying degrees of renal impairment (after Wright et al., 1983).

creased renal clearance, total body clearance and urinary recovery of cefotetan (Ishino et al., 1982; Ishito et al., 1983; Ohkawa et al., 1983; Wright et al., 1983). The volume of distribution is not significantly altered in patients with severe renal impairment relative to that in healthy subjects (Ohkawa et al., 1983). In 5 patients undergoing chronic ambulatory peritoneal dialysis small amounts of cefotetan were excreted into the dialysate (5 to 9% of dose) [Browning et al., 1985].

4. Therapeutic Trials

Cefotetan has been used in the treatment of large numbers of patients with intra-abdominal, obstetric and gynaecological, skin and soft tissue infections, urinary tract and lower respiratory tract infections, and in patients requiring antibacterial prophylaxis prior to surgery. Many of the published studies have been conducted in Japan, but there is also a rapidly expanding amount of published literature of studies conducted in the United States and Europe drawn from the wealth of unpublished data available.

Generally, therapeutic use of cefotetan in the United States and Europe has been associated with higher success rates than that achieved in Japanese studies, probably due to the fact that in Japan there are no strictly adhered to criteria for ensuring the *in vitro* sensitivity of the organism prior to therapy. Thus, comparisons between these studies should be made with caution.

4.1 Established Intra-Abdominal Infections

Abdominal infections are often complicated by being polymicrobial in nature, and frequently involve both aerobes and anaerobes, the most important of which are *E. coli* and *Bacteroides fragilis*. Most of the patients treated with cefotetan for established infections suffered from peritonitis with an underlying diagnosis usually of perforated appendicitis, but also of sigmoid, jejunal, rectal or duodenal perforation, acute salpingitis, malignant lymphoma, or other diseases.

Impressive success rates of 88 to 100% have been recorded in 6 open studies following administration of cefotetan 1 to 2g twice daily for 4 to 15 days to a total of 105 patients with peritonitis due to appendicitis (almost all of whom also underwent appendicectomy and drainage), and to a smaller number of patients with peritonitis due to other diseases (some of whom also underwent gastrectomy or laparotomy and drainage) [Bax et al., 1985b; Fujimoto et al., 1982; Nakayama et al., 1982; Puleo et al., 1985; Yura et al., 1982; unpublished data on file, Stuart Pharmaceuticals].

Occasionally, higher doses of 2 to 6g daily have been used in such patients with similar results (Bax et al., 1985; Pfeiffer, 1985; Puleo et al., 1985). In patients with postoperative peritonitis, postoperative wound infection or abscess, the success rate with cefotetan was somewhat lower at about 65%, mostly without adjunct surgery (Fujimoto et al., 1982; Yura et al., 1982).

In a double-blind comparative study between cefotetan 2 g/day and cefmetazole 4 g/day in 150 patients with purulent peritonitis, there were no significant differences between the 2 drugs in the overall clinical success rates (82% *vs* 74%) or bacteriological cure rates (68% *vs* 74%), respectively. However, the success rate in those patients with severe peritonitis due to perforated duodenal and/or gastric ulcers treated with cefotetan (13/15) was greater than that with cefmetazole (19/27) [Tanimura et al., 1983].

In 3 other comparative studies in small numbers of patients with intra-abdominal infections (mostly peritonitis) intravenous cefotetan 2g twice daily has been compared with latamoxef 2g 3 times daily (data on file, ICI; Wilson et al., 1985) and with a combination of ampicillin 2 g/day, gentamicin 5 mg/kg/day and metronidazole 1.5 g/day (Haynes et al., 1985). In the latter study all patients were clinically cured, and in the former 2 studies 35 of 37 patients (95%) and 11 of 13 patients (85%) were cured with cefotetan and latamoxef, respectively. Excellent clinical success was achieved in these studies with all regimens, but cefotetan has the advantage of an easier dosing schedule.

Cefotetan has also been combined with piperacillin (2g twice daily and 4g 3 times daily, respectively) in patients with generalised peritonitis, and this combination compared with one of intravenous netilmicin 150mg and metronidazole 500mg, both 3 times daily. After a 5-day treatment period, 3 of 16 patients (19%) treated with the cefotetan-piperacillin combination still had a clinical infection (2 with serous wound discharge, 1 with chest infection) whereas 8 of 15 patients (53%) treated with the netilmicin-metronidazole regimen still had a clinical infection (5 with chest infections and 1 each with serous wound infection, subphrenic abscess or septicaemia and cardiorespiratory failure resulting in death) [Lindsay et al., 1985].

4.2 Surgical Prophylaxis

Before the introduction of prophylactic antibiotics to prevent postoperative infection, the sepsis rate following appendicectomy was estimated at 30% (Editorial, 1970), after cholecystectomy at 17 to 21% (Morran et al., 1978; Strachan et al., 1977) and after transurethral resection at up to 60% (Camey et al., 1983; Nielson et al., 1981). Postoperative wound infection poses difficulties for treatment because of the often polymicrobial nature of infection, or its association with anaerobic organisms. The literature in this field is also difficult to interpret because of wide regional variation in definitions of wound infection, stringency and duration of follow-up, risk factors within patient groups and surgical disciplines implemented. Metronidazole (either alone or combined with gentamicin) is commonly used as a prophylactic during intra-abdominal surgery, but such preventative measures are still associated with postoperative sepsis rates of 15 to 30% (Bates et al., 1980; Morris et al., 1980; Strachan and Morrison, 1982).

4.2.1 Appendicectomy

In one comparative study, patients undergoing appendicectomy received single intravenous doses of cefotetan 2g or metronidazole 0.5g (plus 1g rectally) immediately prior to surgery. In addition to prophylaxis, 18 patients received a 5-day course of postoperative therapy (11 received cefotetan 2g twice daily and 8 received metronidazole 1g rectally or 400mg orally 3 times daily). Of these, 2 of 47 patients (4.2%) receiving cefotetan and 8 of 41 patients (19.5%) receiving metronidazole developed postoperative wound infections. A further 23 patients received cefotetan 2g twice daily (n = 11) or metronidazole 400mg 3 times daily (n = 12) upon perioperative discovery of perforation or peritonitis, of whom 1 and 4 patients, respectively, developed wound infections (Buckels et al., 1985). In a similar trial in 54 patients who received single intravenous doses of cefotetan 2g or low dose metronidazole (0.5g) at induction of anaesthesia, postoperative wound infection occurred in 18.5 and 29.6%, respectively (Mitchell et al., 1983).

Taylor et al. (1985) studied the effect on postoperative sepsis rates of metronidazole 1g suppositories twice daily for 5 days before surgery, with or without the addition of intravenous cefotetan 1g on induction of anaesthesia, in 270 patients undergoing appendicectomy. Wound infection developed in 15% of patients receiving metronidazole alone, but in only 3% of those who received metronidazole plus cefotetan.

4.2.2 Colorectal Surgery

In patients undergoing colorectal surgery, cefotetan has been used to prevent postoperative wound sepsis in combination with metronidazole, and has been compared with combinations of gentamicin and either metronidazole or tinidazole.

Two studies in patients undergoing large bowel surgery show reduced postoperative wound infection rates when cefotetan is added to metronidazole. Hall et al. (1985) observed a 42% incidence of wound infection in 67 patients who received intravenous metronidazole 1g preoperatively, but in only 19% of 72 patients who received intravenous cefotetan 2g at induction of anaesthesia in addition to metronidazole. Similarly, in patients receiving intravenous metronidazole 0.5g preoperatively and 0.5g doses at 8 and 16 hours after surgery a wound infection rate of 32% was recorded, whereas a combination of intravenous cefotetan 2g and metronidazole 0.5g prior to induction of anaesthesia was associated with only a 9% incidence of postoperative sepsis (Lee et al., 1985).

Gray and Gray (1985) used either a regimen of intravenous cefotetan 2g preoperatively plus 2g intravenously at 12 hours after surgery, or gentamicin 120mg plus metronidazole 0.5g preoperatively followed by gentamicin 80mg and metronidazole 0.5g 3 times daily for 48 hours. These patients underwent colorectal surgery, and the high risk of infection with this operation was illustrated by the fact that only 3 of 57 patients were found to have clinically sterile swabs preoperatively. Postoperative wound infections occurred in 13.8% and 21.4% of patients, respectively, most of which — like the preoperative cultures — were due to *E. coli, B. fragilis* or *Strep. faecalis* (or combinations thereof). In the other study 86 patients (undergoing mainly appendicectomy, colorectal or upper gastrointestinal surgery) received intravenous cefotetan 2g at induction followed by further 2g doses at 12 and 24 hours after surgery, and 83 patients received gentamicin 120mg plus tinidazole 800mg at induction followed by gentamicin 80mg at 12 and 24 hours and tinidazole 800mg at 12 hours after surgery. At 6 weeks, wound infection occurred in 17 to 18% of both patient groups; however, the rate of wound sepsis in the minority of patients with sterile perioperative swabs was only 3.8% (Strachan et al., 1985). In both these studies some patients did receive additional antibiotics or an extended course of therapy.

4.2.3 Biliary Tract Surgery

In 2 studies of 74 and 199 patients, respectively, undergoing cholecystectomy for biliary tract disorders, comparisons between single intravenous preoperative doses of cefotetan 1g and cefazolin 1g were undertaken (Donovan et al., 1983; Royston et al., 1985). The lower postoperative wound infection rates of 8.1% *vs* 8.8% and 3.1% *vs* 10.4% for the two treatment groups reflects a lower incidence of bacteriologically positive perioperative swabs than seen in other abdominal surgery procedures. However, these rates represent 5-day follow-ups, whereas at 6 weeks significantly higher total sepsis rates of 13.5% and 14.7% were recorded (Donovan et al., 1983).

4.2.4 Other Surgical Operations

McGavigan and Stewart (1985) randomly assigned 100 patients undergoing elective gynaecological surgery to receive either no antibiotic prophylaxis or intravenous cefotetan 1g at induction of anaesthesia: postoperative infections occurred in 24% and 12%, respectively; additionally, postoperative urinary tract infections occurred in 14% and 4% (at 4 days), and 24% and 10% (at follow-up), respectively. In a smaller study in patients undergoing vaginal or abdominal hysterectomy, 5 of 20 patients (25%) receiving preoperative intravenous cefotetan 2g, and 3 of 10 patients (30%) receiving 3 doses of intravenous cefoxitin developed postoperative wound sepsis (Pastorek et al., 1985).

Prophylactic use of intravenous cefotetan 2g (99 patients) or gentamicin (95 patients) in patients undergoing prostatectomy was associated with 2 and 5% incidences of postoperative urinary tract infections, and 4 and 1% incidences of septicaemia, respectively (Leach, 1985).

In 69 patients undergoing major transurethral surgery, a single intravenous bolus dose of cefotetan 2g at induction was associated with asymptomatic and symptomatic bacteriuria rates of 6 and 36%, respectively, compared with rates of 43 and 57%, respectively, in patients receiving no prophylaxis (O'Boyle et al., 1983). Excellent results were seen in a comparative study of single-dose intramuscular cefotetan 2g *versus* cefotaxime (one 1g dose preoperatively and 2 doses postoperatively) in 101 patients: postoperative urinary tract infections occurred in 8 and 6%, respectively (Dorflinger et al., 1985).

In a total of 96 patients intravenous cefotetan 1g or cefazolin 1g were given as preoperative prophylaxis in elective upper gastrointestinal surgery. Cefotetan was associated with significantly fewer cases of postoperative wound sepsis than cefazolin (12.5 *vs* 25%, respectively) with no late infections manifest at 4- to 6-week follow-ups (Leaper et al., 1985).

4.3 Obstetric and Gynaecological Infections

Cefotetan has been used in open studies involving large numbers of women with obstetric and gynaecological infections of various aetiology. Results have been consistently good, with studies reporting good or excellent clinical responses in 80 to 100% of patients after receiving intravenous bolus, direct intravenous infusion or intramuscular cefotetan 1 to 6g daily for 5 to 27 days. The majority of these patients were treated for endometritis, parametritis, pelveoperitonitis, mastitis or adnexitis. Some of these infections were unresponsive to previous therapy with cefmetazole, cefuroxime, piperacillin, dibekacin or benzylpenicillin. Many patients had polymicrobial infections and in some the causative organisms were anaerobic bacteria or even *Streptococcus faecalis* (Cho et al., 1982; data on file, ICI; Motomura et al., 1982; Obata et al., 1983; Palumbo et al., 1985; Pastorek et al., 1985; Sweet, 1985; Takase et al., 1982; Yasuda et al., 1983).

In one particularly large open study of 225 patients with a variety of obstetric and gynaecological disorders, cefotetan 1 to 6g daily in divided doses given by intravenous infusion or bolus injection, or intramuscular injection produced an overall clinical and bacteriological response rate of 90% (table XI). Impressive results have also been reported in a study of cefotetan in anaerobic infections, including 82 women with gynaecological infections. Favourable results were seen in 96%, and clinical success occurred even when the organism was 'resistant' to cefotetan — MICs for *Bacteroides ovatus* and *B. thetaiotaomicron* were ≥ 64 mg/L (unpublished data on file, Stuart Pharmaceuticals).

Controlled, comparative studies are needed to establish the place of cefotetan therapy in this group of patients, particularly with regard to infections associated with anaerobic bacteria, where it appears to have particularly good potential.

4.4 Use in Septicaemia and Immunologically Compromised Patients

Experience with cefotetan in these patients is very limited at present. Bax et al. (1985a) reviewed 59 patients from the United States and Europe who were treated with cefotetan (usual dosage 2 to 3g intravenously twice daily for 7 to 8 days) for bacteriologically proven septicaemia associated with a number of underlying diseases (urinary tract infection in 20 patients; lower respiratory tract infection in 15; soft tissue infection in 8; intra-abdominal disease in 6; parotitis in 2; unknown causes in 8). 56 patients were clinically assessable, of whom 92% were cured of septicaemia and 79% cured of all infections. None of the organisms implicated in the septicaemia persisted. Of the 4 clinical 'failures', 3 had typhoid fever (although 5 other cases were cured) and 1 had right lower lobe pneumonia associated with *Streptococcus pneumoniae.* 12 patients had non-septicaemic infection which persisted: 4 urinary tract infections (3 associated with enterococci), 3 lower respiratory tract infections (2 associated with Gram-negative aerobes) and 5 other infections (included in analysis by Bax et al., 1985).

In an additional 40 patients with bacteriologically proven septicaemia secondary to other infections (mostly due to *Strep. pneumoniae* or *E. coli*) and 2 patients with primary bacterial septicaemia (*Staph. aureus* and *Strep. pneumoniae*), clinical

Table XI. Clinical results following administration of cefotetan 1 to 6g daily to 225 women with obstetric or gynaecological disorders (after Takase et al., 1982)

Diagnosis	No. of cases	Clinical response			Efficacy (%)
		excellent	good	poor	
Intrauterine infection					
Endometritis	20	6	14		100
Puerperal intrauterine infection	23	6	14	3	86.9
Other intrauterine infection	22	3	17	2	90.9
Sub-total	65	15	45	5	92.3
Intrapelvic infection					
Intrapelvic cellulitis	18	6	10	2	88.9
Parametritis	8	1	6	1	87.5
Pelvic peritonitis	22	4	16	2	90.9
Other intrapelvic	12	2	6	4	66.7
Sub-total	60	13	38	9	85.0
External genital infection	22		19	3	86.4
Adnexitis	55	19	31	5	90.9
Mastitis	8	4	3	1	87.5
Postoperative wound infection	8	1	7		100
Other infections	7	1	6		100
Total	225	53	150	22	203/225
(%)		(23.6)	(66.7)	(9.8)	(90.2)

signs and symptoms completely cleared and organisms were eradicated in all cases following treatment with cefotetan (data on file, ICI).

Cefotetan 4 to 6g daily was administered for 4 to 21 days to 66 patients with a variety of infections (including 48 patients with suspected sepsis), all of whom had underlying haematological disorders (mostly acute leukaemia) causing immunodeficiency. The overall clinical success rate was 57.6%, and that of patients with suspected sepsis was 56.3%. Of the 3 patients with bacteriologically confirmed sepsis only 1 was successfully treated with cefotetan, *Pseudomonas aeruginosa* being implicated in the other 2. Response to therapy was related to neutrophil count: 65% of patients with pretreatment count of 500 cells/mm^3 or more, 45% of patients with less than 500 cells/mm^3 and 28% of patients with less than 400 cells/mm^3 responded. In contrast, 5 of 7 patients with recovery of bone marrow to over 1000 cells/mm^3 responded well to cefofetan therapy, outlining the importance of neutrophils in treating infection (Shinohara et al., 1983).

4.5 Otorhinolaryngological Infections

Cefotetan has been used in a limited number of studies in otorhinolaryngological infections both in adults (Iwasawa, 1982; Sambe et al., 1982; Wada et al., 1982) and in children (Aoyama et al., 1983; Iwai et al., 1983).

Encouraging results were seen in adults, with between 75 and 90% of patients showing 'good' to 'excellent' clinical responses following cefotetan 1 to 2g daily, usually for 3 to 6 days. A number of common conditions such as acute tonsillitis, acute otitis media, and peritonsillar abscess almost invariably showed a good to excellent response. The majority of treatment failures wereseen in patients with acute exacerbations of chronic otitis media, where a success rate of only about 30% occurred despite often higher doses (2 to 4g daily) or treatment periods of up to 28 days. Other less common otorhinolaryngological conditions which have been successfully treated with cefotetan 1 to 2g daily for 3 to 6 days include frontal and maxillary sinusutis, cellulitus of the auricle and of epiglottitis, furuncle of ear, acute maxillary and epiglottic periostitis and acute pharyngitis (Iwasawa, 1982; Sambe et al., 1982; Wada et al., 1982).

The pathogens most commonly implicated in the above studies were *Staphylococcus aureus*, α- and β-haemolytic streptococci, *Neisseria* species and *Haemophilus influenzae,* which were nearly always eradicated by cefotetan. Those occasions where cefotetan therapy has been unsuccessful have been associated with less common organisms such as micrococcus, *Providencia inconstans,* corynebacterium (Iwasawa, 1982), *Pseudomonas aeruginosa* (Sambe et al., 1982), acinetobacteria (Wada et al., 1982) as well as resistant strains of *S. aureus* or streptococci.

In children with purulent tonsillitis, cefotetan has produced good to excellent clinical responses in all 4 patients treated at doses of 30 to 40 mg/kg daily for 3 to 4 days in one study (Aoyama et al., 1983) and in 8 of 9 such patients receiving 45 to 65 mg/kg daily for 2 to 6 days (Iwai et al., 1983).

4.6 Urinary Tract Infections

Experience with cefotetan has almost exclusively been in adult patients with chronic complicated urinary tract infections. Only a small number of patients with acute urinary tract infection have been studied, over 90% of whom responded to therapy with cefotetan 1.0 to 4.0g daily (Hara and Mashimo, 1981; Kumazawa et al., 1981; Martin, 1985; Romanelli et al., 1983). The majority of patients have been elderly (over 60 years old). The few paediatric patients treated with cefotetan 15 to 100 mg/kg/day in open trials also responded well (95% clinical efficacy) [Aoyama et al., 1983; Aso et al., 1983; Iwai et al., 1983; Nagamatsu et al., 1983; Nishimura et al., 1983; Serra et al., 1985; Toyonaga et al., 1983]. Published open studies have, with a few exceptions, been conducted in Japan, mainly under the auspices of the Urinary Tract Infection Group, who as stated previously, did not ensure the *in vitro* susceptibility of the organism to cefotetan prior to therapy. Thus, for the most part, the criteria for clinical and bacteriological efficacy and the protocol of administration of cefotetan were standardised. Unless otherwise stated, cefotetan was given by intravenous bolus or drip infusion at doses of 1.0 to 2.0g daily in single or divided doses for a period of 5 days, although the lack of follow-up would not detect the high relapse rates traditionally seen at 2 months in urinary tract infections. However, the majority of controlled studies have been conducted in the United States and Europe. Cefotetan has been compared with cefoxitin, cefmetazole and cefotaxime in published studies and with cefoxitin in unpublished studies.

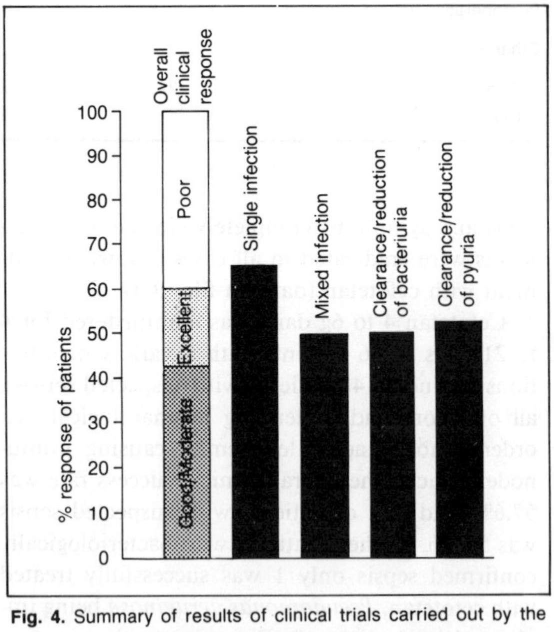

Fig. 4. Summary of results of clinical trials carried out by the Urinary Tract Infection Group (Japan) using intravenous (bolus or infusion) cefotetan 1 to 2 g/day for 5 days in chronic complicated urinary tract infection. *Studies included are:* Fujimura et al. (1982); Goto et al. (1982b); Hirano et al. (1982); Hirose et al. (1982); Ishino et al. (1982); Kamidono et al. (1983); Kumamoto et al. (1983); Kuroda et al. (1982); Matsuda et al. (1982); Mitsuhashi (1982); Nakamuta et al. (1982); Ohkawa et al. (1982); Saitou (1982); Suzuki et al. (1982d); Tsukada et al. (1982)

4.6.1 Studies in Adult Patients

Open Studies

Data from a large number of patients in open studies conducted in Japan suggest that the overall clinical 'success' rate is around 60% in patients with complicated urinary tract infection (fig. 4). A rather higher bacteriological cure rate is seen in these studies, with 66 to 88% of isolates being eradicated. In patients in whom a single pathogen was isolated a considerably higher clinical success rate is seen compared with patients infected with 2 or more pathogens (fig. 4; 64 *vs* 49%, respectively).

These studies also grouped patients according to whether they had an indwelling catheter, had undergone prostatectomy and whether the infection was situated in the upper or lower portion of the urinary tract (fig. 5). As a result, it was seen that patients with an indwelling catheter had a markedly lower than average rate of successful therapy (52.7 and 41.0%, with single or mixed infection, respectively) than other groups of patients. There was no apparent difference in the clinical efficacy of cefotetan in patients with upper or lower urinary tract infection. Differences in the overall clinical efficacy between studies may be explained by these factors; those with a high proportion of patients having indwelling catheters and/or mixed infections in the study showed the lowest success rate at the end of treatment (28%; Matsuda et al., 1982).

Intramuscular cefotetan 0.5mg once or twice daily for 5 days given to 24 elderly patients, mostly with uncomplicated urinary tract infections, produced an excellent clinical cure rate (96%; Stanbridge and Rash, 1985).

Among pathogens isolated from patients included in the Urinary Tract Infection Group studies, cefotetan eradicated over 90% of *Staphylococcus aureus* and *Staph. epidermidis,* and most *Enterobacteriaceae.* Considerably less activity was seen against *Serratia* species (78% eradicated), *Serratia marcescens* (81% eradicated), *Pseudomonas* species (68% eradicated) and *Acinetobacter* species (65% eradicated). *Pseudomonas aeruginosa* (34% eradicated) and *Streptococcus faecalis* (47% eradicated) proved quite resistant to cefotetan and were the organisms most commonly associated with reinfection (accounting for 56% of the total reinfections), with Streptococci, *Pseudomonas* species, *Acinetobacter* species, and *Enterobacteriaceae* accounting for most of the remaining reinfections. Yeast-like organisms were implicated in nearly 10% of reinfections (table XII).

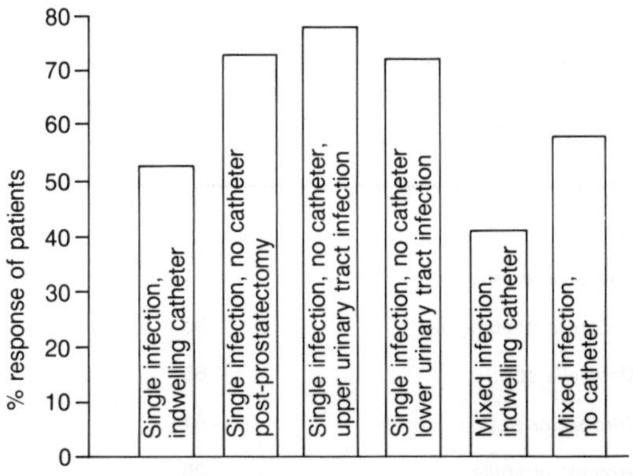

Fig. 5. Summary of percentage clinical success in various subgroups of patients from trials carried out by the Urinary Tract Infection Group (Japan) using intravenous (bolus or infusion) cefotetan 1 to 2 g/day for 5 days in chronic complicated urinary tract infection (refer to fig. 4 for further details).

Comparative Studies

In 4 published comparative studies in patients mostly with chronic complicated urinary tract infections, cefotetan has compared favourably with cefoxitin, cefotaxime and cefmetazole (table XIII). At doses of 1 to 2g twice daily, clinical and bacteriological cure rates have both been of the order of 65 to 87%. These bacteriological cure rates are almost identical to those seen in Japanese non-comparative studies, although the higher clinical success rates in those studies almost certainly reflect the high doses used. There is evidence of some improved clinical and bacteriological cure rates with cefotetan compared with cefoxitin 1 to 2g 3 times daily (Cox et al., 1983; Weissbach et al., 1985), cefmetazole (Kamidono et al., 1983), and cefotaxime

Table XII. Summary of bacteriological efficacy of cefotetan 1 to 2 g/day for 5 days against commonly isolated pathogens (more than 10 isolates) in studies undertaken by the Urinary Tract Infection Group (Japan) in patients with chronic complicated urinary tract infection

Organism	No. of strains	% eradication	No. of reappeared strains (% of total)	References
Escherichia coli	155	97.5	1 (0.4)	1-14
Enterobacter spp.	51	94	9 (3.3)	2-4, 6-8, 8-12, 14
Klebsiella pneumoniae	30	90	6 (2.2)	1-4, 6, 7, 9-14
Klebsiella spp.	65	95		5, 6, 8, 11, 12, 14
Citrobacter spp.	51	94		2, 3, 6-8, 11-14
Proteus mirabilis	26	100		3-5, 7, 9, 11, 12, 14
Proteus spp.	88	98[a]	2 (0.7)	1-4, 6-8, 10, 12-14
Morganella morganii	13	92		1, 7, 10, 11, 13, 14
Serratia marcescens	109	81	15 (5.4)	1-4, 6-9, 11-14
Serratia spp.	167	78		3, 5, 6, 8, 9, 12, 14
Pseudomonas aeruginosa	146	34	56 (20.3)	1-14
Pseudomonas spp.	76	68	21 (7.6)	1, 3-9, 12-14
Acinetobacter spp.	20	65	14 (5.1)	1, 6, 7, 9, 12
GNF[b]	16	87.5		2, 4, 6, 10, 14
Staphylococcus aureus	11	91		1, 3, 6, 7, 8, 13
Staphylococcus epidermidis	65	92	9 (3.3)	1-3, 5-12, 14
Streptococcus faecalis	193	47	99 (35.9)	1-14
GPC[c]	15	67		6, 13
GPB[d]	12	67		8
Yeast-like organisms			24 (8.7)	2, 3, 6, 10-14

a Indole-negative *Proteus* (100%), indole-positive *Proteus* (90%).
b Glucose non-fermenting Gram-negative rods.
c Gram-positive cocci.
d Other Gram-positive bacilli.
Key to references: 1 Fujimura et al. (1982); 2 Goto et al. (1982b); 3 Hirano et al. (1982); 4 Hirose et al. (1982); 5 Ishino et al. (1982); 6 Kamidono et al. (1983); 7 Kumamoto et al. (1983); 8 Kumazawa et al. (1981); 9 Kuroda et al. (1982); 10 Matsuda et al. (1982); 11 Mitsuhashi (1982); 12 Nakamuta et al. (1982); 13 Ohkawa et al. (1982); 14 Tsukada et al. (1982).

1g 3 times daily (Weissbach et al., 1985). When slightly lower doses of cefotaxime were used, similar relapse rates and a much lower rate of antibiotic resistance were seen (12.5% *vs* 35%) with cefotetan (Weissbach et al., 1985).

In 3 large (unpublished) controlled studies, cefotetan 1 to 4g daily and cefoxitin 9 to 12g daily were given to a total of 416 and 167 patients, respectively, and the duration of therapy was usually 5 to 10 days (mean 8 days) with both drugs. Over two-thirds of the patients had complicated urinary tract infections and the vast majority were community-acquired. The overall clinical success rates were excellent with both cefotetan (97%) and cefoxitin (96%) as was the bacteriological cure rate with cefotetan (93%). However, no data were given regarding follow-up rates of reinfection or superinfection in these studies (data on file, ICI).

4.7 Lower Respiratory Tract Infections

As was the case with urinary tract infections, clinical use of cefotetan in patients with lower respiratory tract infections has been primarily in open studies in small numbers of patients, conducted according to a common protocol by Japanese investigators (although the duration of treatment allocated to patients was not strictly adhered to and varied according to the clinical response of the patient). As pathogenic organisms were isolated from only a small proportion of patients, the bacteriological response to treatment was often inadequately assessed.

4.7.1 Studies in Adult Patients

A clinical response rate of about 71% was obtained in open studies of a large number of adult Japanese patients with respiratory tract infections. Most studies employed a dosage of 1 to 2g daily given as an intravenous bolus or drip infusion for periods of 7 to 21 days. In patients with pneumonia (excluding mycoplasma and interstitial pneumonias) the response rate was higher (about 80%) than in those with other diseases, such as lung abscess, bronchiectasis, chronic bronchitis, pleurisy or pyothorax (65%) [table XIV]. In a study by

Table XIII. Comparative studies of cefotetan and other cephalosporins in the treatment of urinary tract infections (UTI)

Reference	No. of patients	Dose (g)	Duration of therapy (days)	Clinical cure rate (%)	Bacteriological cure rate (%)	Reinfection rate (%)	Super-infection rate (%)
Cox et al. (1983)[a]	89	Cefotetan 1 to 2g bid	3 to 22	87	87		11
	40	Cefoxitin 1 to 2g tid		75	68		25
Hautmann et al. (on file, ICI)	69	Cefotetan 1 to 2g bid (mean 2.27 g/day)	4 to 22 (mean 10)	67	70	10	7.25
	68	Cefotaxime 1 to 2g tid (mean 3.74 g/day)		66	77	12	1.5
Kamidono et al. (1983)[b]	105	Cefotetan 0.5g bid	5	54	77		
	97	Cefotetan 1.0g bid		64	81		
	96	Cefmetazole 1g bid		52	81		
Weissbach et al. (1985)[c]	40	Cefotetan 1g bid	5	80	65	20	2.5
	20	Cefoxitin 2g tid		65	65	10	0
		Cefotaxime 1g tid		73	45	10	0
Unpublished data on file (ICI)[d]	416	Cefotetan 1 to 4 g/day	2 to 14 (mean 7.9)	97	93		
	167	Cefoxitin 3g tid or qid	2 to >22 (mean 8.1)	96			

a 93 patients had complicated UTI.
b 259 patients had complicated UTI.
c 47 patients had complicated UTI.
d Cumulative results from 3 studies; 414 patients had complicated UTI.

Table XIV. Clinical efficacy of cefotetan in Japanese open studies of adult patients (over 10) with lower respiratory tract infections

Reference	Patient diagnosis	No. of patients	Dose (g/day)	Duration (days)	Clinical response			Success rate (%)
					excellent	good	fair/poor	
Hayashi (1982)	Pneumonia (11) Other (2)	13	2	11-21	8	4	1	92.3
Hiraga et al. (1982)	Pneumonia (6) Chronic bronchitis (6) Other (6)	18	2	10-14	6	6	6	66.7
Kanzaki et al. (1982)	Pneumonia (7) Other (4)	11	1-4	4-14	3	4	4	63.6
Kato et al. (1982)	Pneumonia (18) Bronchitis (2) Mycoplasmal pneumonia (7)	27	1-2	6-19	0	15	12	55.5
Kaziki et al. (1982)	Pneumonia (3) Chronic bronchitis (7) Other (5)	15	1-2	6-19	9	4	2	86.7
Kobayashi et al. (1982)	Pneumonia (7) Chronic bronchitis (15)	22	2	6-15	14		8	63.6
Konishi et al. (1982)	Pneumonia/ bronchopneumonia (7) Bronchitis (4) Other (2)	13	1-4	5-31	3	7	3	76.9
Kurimura et al. (1982)	Bronchopneumonia (10) Mycoplasmal pneumonia (1) Bronchitis (1)	12	1-2	3-25	1	9	2	83.3
Matsumoto et al. (1982)	Pneumonia (1) Chronic bronchitis (8) Other (3)	12	1-2	4-14	2	8	2	83.3
Nagasawa et al. (1982)	Pneumonia (8) Chronic bronchitis (2) Mycoplasmal pneumonia (1) Other (4)	15	1-4	3-18	3	4	8	46.7
Nakagawa et al. (1982b)	Pneumonia (11) Mycoplasmal pneumonia (2) Other (3)	16	1-2	7-21	7	5	4	75.0
Oyama et al. (1982)	Pneumonia (21) Bronchitis (1)	22	1-2	4-17	4	12	8	72.7
Saito et al. (1982e)	Pneumonia (3) Bronchitis (8) Other (1)	12	1-2	6-78	1	9	2	83.3
Sekine et al. (1982)	Pneumonia (14) Other (23)	37	1-4	7-67	8	17	12	67.6
Soejima et al. (1982)	Pneumonia (9) Other (4)	13	1-2	7-21	0	9	4	69.3
Suzuki et al. (1982c)	Pneumonia (3) Chronic bronchitis (1) Other (14)	17	1-4	6-29	0	6	11	35.3

Table XIV. (Contd)

Reference	Patient diagnosis	No. of patients	Dose (g/day)	Duration (days)	Clinical response: excellent	good	fair/poor	Success rate (%)
Takebe et al. (1982)	Pneumonia (30) Bronchitis (6) Mycoplasmal pneumonia (2)	38	1-2	5-29	7	28	3	92.1
Watanabe et al. (1982a)	Pneumonia (5) Other (7)	12	2	4-22	3	6	3	75.0
Watanabe et al. (1982b)	Pneumonia (5) Other (6)	11			1	6	4	63.7
Totals		336			239		97	71.1

Hara and Mashimo (1981), the overall efficacy rate in 326 patients with lower respiratory tract infections was reported. An overall effective rate of 73% was reported, with effective rates of 78.3%, 59.3% and 50.0% seen in patients with pneumonia (including secondary and suppurative pulmonary diseases), chronic pulmonary infection (chronic bronchitis and bronchiectasis) and pleural infections, respectively. More impressive results have been recorded in open studies outside of Japan in a total of over 140 patients in whom infection was confirmed by the presence of purulent sputum, radiographic evidence and the isolation of pathogens. Cefotetan 2g every 12 hours for 4 to 17 days produced a satisfactory clinical response in 94, 93 and 85% of patients, respectively (unpublished data on file, ICI; Nolen, 1983; Petrie et al., 1985), and a satisfactory bacteriological response in 36 of 41 patients, respectively (Nolen, 1983).

In 2 comparative trials, intravenous doses of cefotetan 2 to 3g twice daily or latamoxef 1 to 2g 3 times daily were given to patients with acute lower respiratory tract infections. In the 2 larger studies (161 and 142 patients assessed) clinical cure or improvement was recorded in 94 and 97% with cefotetan, and 94 and 98% with latamoxef, respectively. Bacteriological cures occurred in over 90% of patients with both drugs (unpublished data on file, ICI; Nolen et al., 1985). In the other study all patients showed a satisfactory clinical response, with only 1 bacteriological failure (*Strep. pneumoniae*) in a patient treated with cefotetan (File et al., 1985).

In a double-blind comparative multicentre study, cefotetan 2g daily and cefmetazole 4g daily were administered to a total of 222 patients with extensive exclusion criteria employed. The overall clinical efficacy of both drugs was similar (73.4% and 71.6%, respectively), with cefotetan being more effective in patients with pneumonia (78.2%) than in chronic respiratory tract infection (65%), whereas cefmetazole was equally effective in both types of patient. There was a highly significant correlation between efficacy of cefotetan and the severity of disease seen in these patients, although the number with severe disease was very small. No significant differences between the drugs were seen with regard to their bacteriological efficacy (95.6 and 87.2%, respectively), their side effect profiles or the relief of symptoms (except cefotetan was superior in relieving fever and cefmetazole in relieving cough symptoms) [Nakagawa et al., 1983].

When bacteriological efficacy was assessed among 326 Japanese patients with lower respiratory tract infections, cefotetan demonstrated a high degree of efficacy against the most common respiratory pathogens [*H. influenzae* (92%), *K. pneumoniae* (93%) and *E. coli* (95%)], as well as against other Gram-negative bacteria, such as *P. mirabilis, E. cloacae, S. marcescens,* and Gram-positive

Table XV. Bacteriological results of cefotetan treatment of causative organisms in patients with lower respiratory tract infections (after Hara and Mashimo, 1981)

Organisms	No. of cases	Bacteriological effectiveness				Effective rate[a] (%)
		eliminated	decreased	replaced	unchanged	
Simple infection						
S. aureus	7	7				100
S. epidermidis	1	1				100
β-haemolytic streptococci	7	6		1		100.0
Strep. pneumoniae	14	9		2	3	78.6
Strep. faecalis	5	4			1	80.0
Other GPB[b]	3	3				100
Sub-total	37	30		3	4	89.2
E. coli	39	31	2	6		94.9
K. pneumoniae	30	23	1	5	1	93.3
K. oxytoca	2	1		1		50.0
Ps. aeruginosa	12	1	2	1	8	16.7
P. mirabilis	7	3		4		100
P. rettgeri	3	1		2		33.3
Enter. aerogenes	1	1				100
Enter. cloacae	5	4		1		100
Ser. marcescens	5	4		1		100
H. influenzae	48	39	3	5	1	91.7
Citrobacter spp.	1			1		0
Other GNB[c]	3	3				100
Sub-total	156	111	8	27	10	88.5
Bacteroides spp.	1				1	0
Total	194	141	8	30	15	88.1
Mixed infection						
Pseudomonas spp. + etc.	5	3			2	60.0
Serratia spp. + etc.	6	2	1	2	1	66.7
Proteus spp. + etc.	5	3	1	1		80.0
Klebsiella spp. + etc.	11	4	5	2		54.5
E. coli + etc.	2	2				100
Miscellaneous	9	7	1	1		88.9
Total	38	21	8	6	3	71.1
Grand total	232	162	16	36	18	85.3

a Effective rate = [(eliminated + replaced)/(eliminated + decreased + replaced + unchanged)].
b Gram-positive bacilli.
c Gram-negative bacilli.

staphylococci and streptococci. Bacteriological efficacy with cefotetan in mixed bacterial infection was somewhat reduced (71.1%) and was characteristically poor against infections caused by *Pseudomonas aeruginosa* (17%; table XV).

4.7.2 Studies in Paediatric Patients

The use of cefotetan in children with community-acquired lower respiratory tract infections [pneumonia, bronchopneumonia (with or without pyothorax) or acute bronchitis] has also been quite extensive in Japan, but limited entirely to open studies (table XVI). The overall clinical success rate was 90% in a series of small studies which followed a similar protocol for the assessment of effects following cefotetan doses of 20 to 108 mg/kg/day for

Table XVI. Clinical efficacy of cefotetan in Japanese open studies of paediatric patients with lower respiratory tract infections

Reference	Patient diagnosis	No. of patients	Dose (mg/kg/day)	Duration (days)	Clinical response			Success rate (%)
					excellent	good	fair/poor	
Aoyama et al. (1983)	Pneumonia/ bronchopneumonia[a]	23	20-100 (mean 58)	4-10	7	15	1[b]	96
Aso et al. (1983)	Pneumonia/ bronchopneumonia	13	60-85 (mean 70)	5-12	6	7	0	100
Iwai et al. (1983)	Bronchopneumonia	17[c]	40-98 (mean 62)	3-6	14	2	1	94
Meguro et al. (1983)	Pneumonia/ acute bronchitis	12	38-100 (mean 61)	2-6	7	2	3[d]	77
Nagamatsu et al. (1983)	Bronchitis/ bronchopneumonia/ pneumonia	16	38-93 (mean 50)	2-7	11	4	1[e]	94
Toyonaga et al. (1983)	Bronchopneumonia	14	25-104 (mean 63)	2-14	7	5	2[f]	86
Yanagisawa et al. (1983)	Bronchitis/ pneumonia	7	55-108 (mean 79)	2-12	5	0	2	72
Totals					57	33	10	90

a Excludes 5 cases of mycoplasmal pneumonia.
b Patient with pyothorax.
c Excludes 4 patients with mycoplasmal pneumonia.
d 2 cases with *Pseudomonas aeruginosa* infections.
e 1 case with *Pseudomonas aeruginosa* infection.
f 1 case had pleurisy.

2 to 14 days, and in a larger single study of 122 patients (details of the study design were unavailable; Fujii et al., 1983). Of those patients whose response to cefotetan was poor, 5 had either complicating factors, such as pyothorax or pleurisy, or had infections due to *Pseudomonas aeruginosa.*

4.8 Skin and Soft Tissue Infections

In 3 studies, a total of 110 patients requiring oral surgery for soft tissue infections — predominantly maxillary osteitis, cellulitis of the mouth floor and osteitis alveolaris — mostly due to infection with streptococci, other Gram-positive cocci and some anaerobes have been treated with cefotetan. Doses of 1 to 2g daily for 2 to 11 days produced overall subjective clinical success rates of 100%, 79% and 90%, respectively (Quayle et al., 1985; Takai et al., 1982; Yamada et al., 1982). In a further 30 patients with skin or soft tissue infections due exclusively to anaerobic bacteria, cefotetan 1 to 3g twice daily clinically cured all patients (Lee and Barry, 1985).

Cefotetan 1 to 2g twice daily for 5 to 10 days was also successfully used to treat 175 patients with a variety of skin and soft tissue infections in unpublished studies. Complete clinical clearing or significant improvement occurred in 98% of patients, and bacteriological cure in 80% of the 61 evaluable patients (data on file, ICI).

4.9 Miscellaneous Therapeutic Use

Cefotetan has been used in other types of in-

Table XVII. Cumulated side effect data following the use of cefotetan in North America, Europe and Japan

	N. America (1451 pts)	Europe (649 pts)	Japan (2798 pts)[a]
Phlebitis	5 (0.34%)	5 (0.78%)	
Local pain/ swelling	6 (0.41%)	30 (13.7%)[b]	2 (0.07%)
Other local reactions[c]	1 (0.07%)	7 (1.08%)	
Rash	9 (0.62%)	10 (1.54%)	32 (1.14%)
Itching/pruritus	3 (0.21%)		
Fever/chills	2 (0.14%)	1 (0.15%)	17 (0.61%)
Other hypersensitivity reactions[d]	4 (0.28%)	3 (0.46%)	1 (0.03%)
Diarrhoea	18 (1.24%)	4 (0.62%)	16 (0.57%)
Nausea	2 (0.14%)	8 (1.23%)	4 (0.14%)
Vomiting	1 (0.07%)	1 (0.15%)	2 (0.07%)
Abdominal pain		1 (0.15%)	1 (0.03%)
Other adverse effects[e]	7 (0.48%)	3 (0.46%)	14 (0.50%)
Total	58 (4.02%)	73 (11.2%)	89 (3.2%)

a Includes 310 children, 9 of whom had an adverse reaction.
b Percentage incidence in 219 patients receiving intramuscular cefotetan.
c Includes cellulitis, hypoaesthesia, stiffness, cramp.
d Includes urticaria, angioneurotic oedema, papular lesions, erythema, dermatitis.
e Includes candidal infection, monilial vaginitis, hypotensive symptoms, sore mouth/throat, fatigue, oedema, submandibular lymphadenopathy.

fection in small numbers of patients. In a series of 18 patients with a variety of ophthalmological infections in which *S. aureus, S. epidermidis* or unspecified Gram-negative or Gram-positive rods were the causative pathogens, cefotetan 1 to 2 g/ day for 2 to 10 days produced a clinical success rate of 78% (Ohishi and Nagai, 1982).

Cefotetan 2g daily was administered over a period of 3 to 16 days (average 8 days) to 36 patients with biliary diseases complicated by gallbladder, common bile duct or intrahepatic gallstones, pancreatic disease, or cardiac disease. 13 of 14 patients with cholecystitis, and 16 of 22 patients with cholangitis were successfully treated, which surprisingly included 5 of 6 patients who were infected or became superinfected with *Pseudomonas aeruginosa* or *Streptococcus faecalis* (Tanimura et al., 1982).

In 122 cases of bacteriologically confirmed acute gonorrhoea a single 500mg intramuscular dose of cefotetan produced a clinical and microbiological cure rate of 91% (Hunter et al., 1983).

Cefotetan 1 to 3g twice daily produced clinical and bacteriological cure in all 11 patients with bone or joint infections (osteomyelitis, septic bursitis, infected prosthesis), due to *Staph. aureus* (6), *K. pneumoniae* (1), *Strep. pyogenes* (1) and 3 of polymicrobial origin, in an open study (unpublished data on file, ICI).

5. Side Effects

Side effect data cumulated by the manufacturer on a total of 2798 patients from Japanese studies, 1451 patients from North American studies and 649 patients from European studies treated with cefotetan in open and comparative trials revealed overall clinical side effect incidences of 3.2%, 4.02% and 11.2%, respectively (table XVII). In European studies, the primary reason for a much higher incidence of side effects due to pain at the injection site is because of a disproportionate use of intramuscular cefotetan, mostly without the currently ommended dissolution in 0.5% lignocaine. Hypersensitivity reactions (such as rash and fever), gastrointestinal effects (such as nausea, vomiting and diarrhoea) and local reactions occurred most frequently.

Other adverse effects, such as hypotensive symptoms and general fatigue, only occurred very rarely (data on file, Yamanouchi).

5.1 Effects on Laboratory Values

The same manufacturer's analysis as that reported above determined the incidences of abnormalities of haematological and other laboratory parameters during cefotetan administration. The most commonly reported haematological abnormalities were changes in haemoglobin levels, eosinophilia,

Table XVIII. Abnormal biochemical and haematological changes during therapy with cefotetan

	Incidence (%)		
	Europe[a]	N. America[b]	Japan[b]
Haemoglobin	6.7		
White blood cell count	2.0		0.3
Polymorph count	0.6		
Eosinophilia	1.3	0.48	1.1
Platelet count	3.5	0.34	0.4
Prothrombin time	3.2	0.07	
Coombs' test positive	2.9	0.41	0.5
Neutropenia		0.07	0.1
Lymphocytosis			0.1
Bilirubin	1.2		0.2
AST (SGOT)	1.9	0.3	3.8
ALT (SGPT)	3.7	0.6	3.8
Gamma GT	1.6		
Urea	4.4		
Blood urea nitrogen	1.1		0.3
Creatinine	3.3		0.1
Alkaline phosphatase			0.8
Proteinaemia			0.1

a All changes regardless of patient's condition or administration of concomitant therapy.
b Changes reported as adverse reactions.

leucopenia, thrombocytopenia, and increased prothrombin time (table XVIII).

Unlike the structurally and bacteriologically similar compounds latamoxef and cefamandole, there has been no published evidence of hypoprothrombinaemic bleeding problems associated with therapy to date. The effects of cefotetan on haemostatic parameters, including platelet function, have been studied in patients, some of whom had renal impairment or hepatobiliary disease. There were no clinically significant effects on prothrombin time, thrombin time, platelet aggregation or other coagulation factors in most subjects. However, 1 malnourished patient showed clinical signs of vitamin K deficiency and 5 others with major complications unrelated to cefotetan therapy had abnormal prothrombin or bleeding times (Andrassy et al., 1985; Machin et al., 1985; Triger et al., 1985). Thus, it would seem that bleeding problems are unlikely to occur in most patients receiving cefotetan; nevertheless, if prothrombin levels fall or if patients are known to be vitamin K deficient, vitamin K supplements should be given at the start of treatment.

Liver function tests revealed low incidences of abnormal levels of serum ALT (alanine amino transferase; SGPT), serum AST (aspartate amino transferase; SGOT) and alkaline phosphatase. Abnormalities of blood urea nitrogen, Coombs test and serum creatinine were rare (table XVIII), and there was no evidence of abnormalities during urinalysis other than 1 case of raised urinary proteins (data on file, Yamanouchi).

6. Dosage and Administration

The type and severity of infection and the sensitivity of the causative organism largely determine the dosage, route and frequency of administration of cefotetan. The usual adult dosage is 2 to 4g daily given in divided doses every 12 hours either by intravenous bolus, intravenous drip infusion or by intramuscular injection (dissolved in 0.5% lignocaine). However, many studies have employed single daily parenteral doses, and in one direct comparison a regimen of cefotetan 2g once daily was as clinically and bacteriologically effective as cefotetan 1g twice daily in treatment of elderly patients with urinary tract infections (Fraschini and Gagliardi, 1985; Kumamoto et al., 1983).

For established intra-abdominal infections doses of 2g twice daily are recommended. The usual regimen for cefotetan when used as in surgical prophylaxis is 1 to 2g parenterally (usually given at premedication or induction of anaesthesia) followed by 1 or 2g 12 to 24 hours later. A single intramuscular dose of 0.5g is usually sufficient for treatment of gonorrhoea. In life-threatening infections and in immunocompromised patients, doses of 4 to 6g daily in divided doses may be necessary.

In children the recommended dosage of intravenous cefotetan is 40 to 60 mg/kg daily given 12-hourly, although doses in clinical trials have ranged from 15 to over 100 mg/kg daily.

In patients with impaired renal function (creatinine clearance 10 to 40 ml/min) the dosage should be decreased either by halving the dose or by doubling the dosing interval. In patients with a creatinine clearance of less than 10 ml/min a further halving of dose or doubling of dosing interval should be implemented.

Cefotetan is contraindicated in patients with a known hypersensitivity to cephalosporin and cephamycin antibiotics, and caution is advised in patients hypersensitive to penicillin due to the possibility of allergic cross-reactions. As with other broad spectrum antibiotics, prothrombin activity should be monitored, especially in patients with hepatic or renal impairment or a predisposition to haemorrhage. Concomitant ingestion of alcohol should be avoided due to potential disulfiram-type flushing reactions, although no examples of this reaction have been published.

7. The Place of Cefotetan in Therapy

A broad spectrum of *in vitro* antibacterial activity and high concentrations in most body tissues and fluids have been reflected in the clinical efficacy of cefotetan. An excellent success rate in the treatment of intra-abdominal, soft tissue and obstetric and gynaecological infections, and in the prophylaxis of postoperative wound sepsis has been achieved. These may be polymicrobial diseases (involving anaerobic and/or Gram-negative bacteria) and are often refractory to other cephalosporins.

Cefotetan has also been used successfully in large numbers of patients with chronic complicated urinary tract and lower respiratory tract infections. In smaller numbers of infected immunocompromised patients and patients with otorhinolaryngological infections, septicaemia, penicillin-resistant gonorrhoea, and bone and joint infections cefotetan has also shown clinical efficacy.

Unlike the aminoglycosides and some 'third generation' cephalosporins, cefotetan possesses little activity against *Pseudomonas aeruginosa* and is not recommended for use when this organism is the suspected pathogen. Cefotetan is not indicated in the treatment of bacterial meningitis.

Of practical importance it should be considered that, with the exception of ceftriaxone, cefotetan has the most prolonged plasma elimination half-life and half-life of urinary excretion of the currently available cephalosporins, thus enabling it to be given on a twice daily basis. To date, there has been no evidence (unlike the structurally similar compound latamoxef) of disulfiram-type reactions that may occur with some of the cephalosporins.

Thus, cefotetan offers a useful addition to a rapidly growing group of antibacterial agents used in the treatment of a variety of serious infections, and may prove particularly useful (due to its spectrum of antibacterial activity) in infections involving more than one organism or anaerobic bacteria.

References

Adam, H.K.; Houghton, H.L.; Yates, R.A.; Young J. and Donnelly, R.J.: Pharmacokinetics and tolerance of a 24-h infusion of cefotetan disodium (with and without loading dose) in normal Caucasian volunteers. Journal of Antimicrobial Chemotherapy 11 (Suppl. A): 193-199 (1983).

Aldridge, K.E.; Sanders, C.V.; Janney, A.; Faro, S. and Marier, R.L.: Comparison of the activities of penicillin G and new β-lactam antibiotics against clinical isolates of *Bacteroides* species. Antimicrobial Agents and Chemotherapy 410-413 (1984).

Andrassy, K.; Koderisch, J.; Bechtold, H. and Ritz, E.: Haemostasis during treatment with cefotetan; in Lode et al. (Eds). Cefotetan: A Long Acting Antibiotic, pp. 131-137 (Churchill Livingstone, Edinburgh 1985).

Aoyama, R.; Kakizaki, Y.; Ohnishi, A.; Izumi, Y.; Fujita, M. et al.: Basic and clinical studies on cefotetan in pediatric field. Japanese Journal of Antibiotics 36: 1191-1198 (1983).

Aso, K.; Nakashima, T.; Miyachi, Y.; Nishikawa, K.; Ogawa, A. et al.: Clinical evaluation of cefotetan in infants and children. Japanese Journal of Antibiotics 36: 1295-1300 (1983).

Ayers, L.W.; Jones, R.N.; Barry, A.L.; Thornsberry, C.; Fuchs, P.C. et al.: Cefotetan, a new cephamycin: Comparison of *in vitro* antimicrobial activity with other cephems, β-lactamase stability, and preliminary recommendations for disk diffusion testing. Antimicrobial Agents and Chemotherapy 22: 859-877 (1982).

Barry, A.L.; Packer, R.R. and Jones, R.N.: Unpredictable interactions between cefotetan and penicillins or amino-glycosides. Diagnostic Microbiology and Infectious Disease 2: 347-351 (1984).

Bates, T.; Touquet, V.L.; Tutton, M.K. et al.: Prophylactic metronidazole in appendicectomy: A controlled trial. British Journal of Surgery 67: 547-550 (1980).

Bauernfeind, A.: Cefotetan: Profile of *in-vitro* activity. Journal of Antimicrobial Chemotherapy 11 (Suppl. A): 19-29 (1983).

Bax, R.P.; Francis, A.J.; Kampfner, G.L. and Lesky, W.: Cefotetan monotherapy in septicaemia: A review of international studies; in Lode et al. (Eds) Cefotetan: A Long Acting Antibiotic, pp. 174-182 (Churchill Livingstone, Edinburgh 1985a).

Bax, R.P.; Kampfner, G.L.; Francis, A.J.; Lessman, F. and Walch, H.G.: Cefotetan monotherapy in intra-abdominal infections: A review of international studies; in Lode et al. (Eds) Cefotetan: A Long Acting Antibiotic, pp. 225-234 (Churchill Livingstone, Edinburgh 1985b).

Bonadio, M.; Giovannini, L.; Maccanti, O.; Bertelli, A.A.E.; Ciompi, M.L. and Bertelli, A.: Cefotetan concentration in non traumatic joint effusion. Proceedings of the 14th International Congress of Chemotherapy (Abstracts), p. 430 (Kyoto 1985).

Browning, M.; Chapman, S.; Cockshott, I.D.; White, L. and Yates, R.A.: Pharmacokinetics of cefotetan in patients requiring chronic ambulatory peritoneal dialysis; in Lode et al. (Eds) Cefotetan: A Long Acting Antibiotic, pp. 106-109 (Churchill Livingstone, Edinburgh 1985).

Buckels, J.A.C.; Brookstein, R.; Bonser, R.; Bullen, B.R. and Alexander-Williams, J.: A comparison of the prophylactic value of cefotetan and metronidazole in appendicectomy; in Lode et al. (Eds) Cefotetan: A Long Acting Antibiotic, pp. 274-278 (Churchill Livingstone, Edinburgh 1985).

Camey, N.; Botto, H.; Michon, J. and Le Duc, A.: The use of cefotaxime in prevention of intraoperative bacterial dissemination during urological endoscopic surgery; in Spitzy and Karrer (Eds) Proceedings of the 13th International Congress of Chemotherapy, Vienna, pp. 36-38 (1983).

Campello, C.; Stradoni, R. and Majori, L.: The *in-vitro* activity of cefotetan against *Serratia* spp. and *Enterobacter* spp. in comparison with other cephalosporins. Journal of Antimicrobial Chemotherapy 11 (Suppl. A): 87-93 (1983).

Chabbert, Y.A. and Derlot, E.: Comparative activity of cefotetan on *Escherichia coli* K12 possessing plasmid-mediated β-lactamases. Journal of Antimicrobial Chemotherapy II (Suppl. A): 159-167 (1983).

Chattopadhyay, B. and Teli, J.C.: Comparison of *in vitro* activity of cefotetan (ICI 156834), a new cephamycin derivative, with that of cefoxitin. Journal of Antimicrobial Chemotherapy 10: 151-154 (1982).

Cho, N.; Fukunaga, K. and Kunii, K.: Fundamental and clinical studies on cefotetan (YM 09330) in the field of obstetrics and gynecology. Chemotherapy 30: 832-842 (1982).

Clarke, A.M. and Zemcov, S.J.V.: Antibacterial activity of the cephamycin cefotetan: An *in-vitro* comparison with other β-lactam antibiotics. Journal of Antimicrobial Chemotherapy 11 (Suppl. A): 67-72 (1983).

Cocuzza, G.; Blandino, G. and Mattina, R.: Stability of cefotetan to Gram-negative β-lactamases. Journal of Antimicrobial Chemotherapy 11 (Suppl. A): 139-145 (1983).

Cox, C.E.; Childs, S.J. and Wells, W.G.: Comparative trial of cefotetan and cefoxitin in the treatment of urinary tract infection. Abstracts of the 23rd Interscience Conference on Antimicrobial Agents and Chemotherapy, p. 228, Miami Beach, Florida, October (1983).

Dainelli, B.; Magni, A.; Maragoni, F.; Gismondo, M.R. and Filadoro, F.: Cefotetan, a new cephamycin: *In-vitro* activity against *Bacteroides fragilis var. fragilis*; in Lode et al. (Eds) Cefotetan: A Long Acting Antibiotic, pp. 33-35 (Churchill Livingstone, Edinburgh 1985).

Daschner, F.D.; Goerke, C.; Bassler, M. and Just, M.: *In vitro* comparison of cefotetan with five other cephalosporins against nosocomial pathogens. Chemotherapy 28: 351-354 (1982).

Daschner, F.D.; Just, H-M.; Petersen, E.E.; Bassler, M. and Frank, U.: Penetration of cefotetan into the tissues of the female genital tract; in Lode et al. (Eds) Cefotetan: A Long Acting Antibiotic, pp. 110-112 (Churchill Livingstone, Edinburgh 1985).

Delmée, M.; Homel, M.; Janssens, M. and Wauters, G.: *In-vitro* activity of cefotetan and other cephalosporins against clinical isolates of *Clostridium difficile*; in Lode et al. (Eds) Cefotetan: A Long Acting Antibiotic, pp. 36-39 (Churchill Livingstone, Edinburgh 1985).

Dette, G.A.; Knothe, H. and Henckel, S.: Cefotetan: Antimicrobial activity *in vitro* compared with that of cefotaxime. Journal of Antimicrobial Chemotherapy 11 (Suppl. A): 11-17 (1983).

Donovan, I.A.; Wise, R.; Drumm, J. and Dent, J.: A comparison of cefotetan and cefazolin in prophylaxis against wound infection after cholecystectomy and the kinetics of cefotetan penetration into peritoneal fluid. Proceedings of the 13th International Congress of Chemotherapy, SS4.2/9 (part 25): 57-63 (1983).

Dorflinger, T.; Madsen, R.E. and Madsen, P.O.: A comparison of cefotetan and cefotaxime for prophylaxis in transurethral surgery; in Lode et al. (Eds) Cefotetan: A Long Acting Antibiotic, pp. 284-288 (Churchill Livingstone, Edinburgh 1985).

Drugeon, H.B.; Pirault, J.L.; Dubernat, H. and Courtieu, A.L.; Bactericidal activity of cefotetan and cefotaxime; in Lode et al. (Eds) Cefotetan: A Long Acting Antibiotic, pp. 57-62 (Churchill Livingstone, Edinburgh 1985).

Drumm, J.; Wise, R. and Donovan, L.A.: The effect of protein binding on the intraperitoneal penetration of β-lactam antibiotics. British Journal of Surgery 70: 297 (1983).

Dublanchet, A.: *In-vitro* evaluation of the antibacterial activity of cefotetan: Comparison with cefoxitin and cefotaxime; in Lode et al. (Eds) Cefotetan: A Long Acting Antibiotic, pp. 45-50 (Churchill Livingstone, Edinburgh 1985).

Editorial: Sepsis after appendicectomy. Lancet 1: 930-931 (1970).

File, T.M.; Tan, J.S.; Salstrom, S.J.; Johnson, L. and Douglas, G.: Cefotetan versus moxalactam in the treatment of acute bacterial lower respiratory tract infections. Proceedings of the 14th International Congress of Chemotherapy (Abstracts), p. 430 Kyoto (1985).

Francisco, M. and LeFrock, J.L.: Susceptibility of gentamicin resistant *Klebsiella pneumoniae* against cefotetan and other β-lactam antibiotics. Abstracts of the Annual Meeting of the American Society for Microbiology p. 6 (1983).

Fraschini, F. and Gagliardi, V.: Cefotetan in urinary tract infections: Comparison of two dosage schedules; in Lode et al. (Eds) Cefotetan: A Long Acting Antibiotic, pp. 162-166 (Churchill Livingstone, Edinburgh 1985).

Fujii, R.; Meguro, H.; Yoshioka, H.; Fujita, K.; Maruyama, S. et al.: Fundamental and clinical studies on cefotetan in pediatric field. Japanese Journal of Antibiotics 36: 1173-1184 (1983).

Fujimaki, Y.; Kawamura, S. and Sugita, R.: Studies on cefotetan in otorhinolaryngology. Japanese Journal of Antibiotics 36: 1317-1324 (1983).

Fujimoto, M.; Ueda, T.; Sakai, K.; Sawada, A.; Doi, S. et al.: A clinical trial on cefotetan (YM 09330) in the field of surgery. Chemotherapy 30: 817-826 (1982).

Fujimura, N.; Yuasa, M.; Yuasa, K.; Tanaka, K. and Kurokawa, K.: Fundamental and clinical studies on cefotetan (YM09330) in urological field. Chemotherapy 733-740 (1982).

Furuhata, H.; Iwai, S.; Takai, K.; Sato, T.; Matsushita, K. et al.: Cefotetan and cefmetazole concentrations in the tissue of patients at abdominal operations. Proceedings of the 14th International Congress of Chemotherapy (Abstracts) p. 194, Kyoto (1985).

Gialdroni Grassi, G.; Alesina, R.; Ferrara, A. and Peona, V.: *In vitro* antibacterial activity of cefotetan. Journal of Antimicrobial Chemotherapy 11 (Suppl. A): 45-48 (1983).

Goto, T.; Ohi, Y.; Kawabata, T.; Obata, M.; Okamoto, K. et al.: Fundamental and clinical studies on cefotetan (YM09330) in urinary tract infection. Chemotherapy 30: 753-769 (1982).

Gray, J.G. and Gray, J.: Prophylaxis of colorectal surgery: a comparison of cefotetan with gentamicin plus metronidazole. In Lode et al. (Eds) Cefotetan: A Long Acting Antibiotic, pp. 279-

283 (Churchill Livingstone, Edinburgh, 1985).

Grimm, H.: Susceptibility of bacterial pathogens to cefotetan judged by MIC and disc tests. Journal of Antimicrobial Chemotherapy 11 (Suppl. A): 37-43 (1983).

Guibert, J.; Kitzis, M.D.; Yuelin, C. and Acar, J.F.: Pharmacokinetics of single intravenous or intramuscular doses of cefotetan in normal human volunteers. Journal of Antimicrobial Chemotherapy 11 (Suppl. A): 201-206 (1983).

Hall, R.; Matheson, T.S.; Craven, J.L.; Lee, P.; Royston, C.S. and Edwards, M.H.: A multicentre comparative study of cefotetan + metronidazole *vs* metronidazole alone in the prophylaxis of wound infection in patients undergoing large bowel operations by a prospective randomised trial. Proceedings of the 14th International Congress of Chemotherapy (Abstracts) p. 317, Kyoto (1985).

Hara, K. and Mashimo, K.: Clinical study on YM09330 (cefotetan) in internal medicine; in Periti and Gialdroni Grassi (Eds) Current Chemotherapy and Immunotherapy, Vol. 1, pp. 436-439 (American Society for Microbiology, Washington 1981).

Hart, C.A. and Percival, A.: Resistance to cephalosporins among gentamicin-resistant klebsiellae. Journal of Antimicrobial Chemotherapy 9: 275-286 (1982).

Hart, C.A. and Percival, A.: Susceptibilities of gentamicin-resistant Gram-negative aerobic bacilli to cefotetan and other β-lactams. Journal of Antimicrobial Chemotherapy 11 (Suppl. A): 95-101 (1983).

Hautmann, R.E.; Hoffman-Fölkersamb, D.; Pranada, F. and Pusztai-Markos, Sz.: Comparative study of cefotetan and cefotaxime in the treatment of complicated urinary tract infections (unpublished data on file, ICI).

Hayashi, I.: Clinical studies on cefotetan (YM09330) in the treatment of respiratory tract infections. Chemotherapy 30: 362-368 (1982).

Hennessey, T.D.: Cefotetan: A compilation of susceptibility data of clinical isolates; in Lode et al. (Eds) Cefotetan: A Long Acting Antibiotic, pp. 14-22 (Churchill Livingstone, Edinburgh 1985).

Hennessey, T.D. and Edwards, J.R.: Antibacterial properties of cefotetan di-sodium, a cephamycin antibiotic. Drugs in Experimental Clinical Research 9: 115-123 (1983).

Hiraga, Y.; Kikuchi, K. and Nakahashi, M.: Clinical studies of cefotetan (YM09330) for respiratory tract infections. Chemotherapy 30: 323-331 (1982).

Hirano, M.; Ishito, N.; Miyata, K.; Kamata, H.; Takamoto, H. et al.: Fundamental and clinical studies on cefotetan (YM09330) in complicated urinary tract infections. Chemotherapy 30: 703-718 (1982).

Hirayama, A.: Clinical study on penetration of cefotetan into CSF. Proceedings of the 14th International Congress of Chemotherapy (Abstracts), p. 195, Kyoto (1985).

Hirose, T.; Sakai, S.; Nishio, A. and Kumamoto, Y.: Experimental and clinical studies on cefotetan (YM09330). Chemotherapy 30: 614-627 (1982).

Hunter, J.M.; Napier, I.R.; Roberts, J.E. and Lindsay, G.: An open evaluation of a single 500mg dose of cefotetan in the treatment of acute gonococcal infections. Proceedings of the 13th International Congress of Chemotherapy SS4.2/9 (Part 25): 37-41 (1983).

Imamura, K.; Sakai, T.; Yoshida, T.; Suzuki, H. and Shiobara, Y.: Nephrotoxicity of cefotetan (YM09330) in female rats. Chemotherapy 30: 258-266 (1982).

Inamatsu, T.; Urayama, K.; Noro, T. and Shimada, K.: Pharmacokinetics and clinical studies of cefotetan in aged patients. Proceedings of the 13th International Congress of Chemotherapy (SS4.2/9; Part 25): 5-10 (1983).

Ishino, T.; Masu, C.; Hatachi, K.; Fujii, M.; Nihira, H. et al.: Fundamental and clinical studies on cefotetan (YM09330) in the field of urology. Chemotherapy 30: 719-732 (1982).

Ishito, N.; Kumon, H.; Akazawa, N.; Miyata, K.; Okimune, M. et al.: Pharmacokinetics of antibiotics in patients with impaired renal function. Chemotherapy 32: 815-822 (1983).

Isono, M.; Yamada, N.; Watanabe, K. and Ueno, K.: Antibacterial activity of cefotetan (YM09330) against anaerobes. Chemotherapy 30: 51-64 (1982).

Iwai, N.; Sasaki, A.; Taneda, Y.; Mizoguchi, F. and Nakamura, H.: Fundamental and clinical evaluation of cefotetan in pediatric field. Japanese Journal of Antibiotics 36: 1279-1294 (1983).

Iwasawa, T.: Fundamental and clinical studies on cefotetan (YM09330) in the otorhinolaryngologic field. Chemotherapy 30: 883-901 (1982).

Iwata, S.; Iwasaki, Y.; Kanemitsu, T.; Tojo, M.; Jozaki, K. et al.: The basic and clinical studies on cefotetan in the pediatric field. Japanese Journal of Antibiotics 36: 1204-1218 (1983).

Jones, R.N. and Wilson, H.W.: Antimicrobial activity, β-lactamase stability and β-lactamase inhibition of cefotetan and other 7-α methoxy β-lactam antimicrobials. Diagnosis and Microbiology of Infectious Diseases 1: 71-83 (1983).

Just, H.-M.; Becker, C.; Bassler, M. and Daschner, F.D.: *In vitro* combination effect of cefotetan with four aminoglycosides, piperacillin and mezlocillin on Gram-positive and Gram-negative nosocomial bacteria. Chemotherapy 30: 387-391 (1984).

Kamidono, S.; Ishigami, J.; Arakawa, S.; Umezu, K.; Ohmori, H. and Ishito, N.: A double-blind comparative study of cefotetan and cefmetazole in complicated urinary tract infections. Japanese Journal of Antibiotics 36: 1325-1353 (1983).

Kanzaki, R.; Hayakawa, M.; Adachi, M.; Kawai, M.; Imataka, K. et al.: Experimental and clinical studies on cefotetan (YM09330). Chemotherapy 30: 374-379 (1982).

Kato, M.; Nagasaka, H.; Nanjo, K.; Takeuchi, T.; Kitaura, S. et al.: Clinical study of cefotetan (YM09330). Chemotherapy 30: 486-492 (1982).

Kaziki, A.; Takamoto, M. and Ishibashi, T.: Experience with cefotetan (YM09330) in respiratory tract infection and its serum concentration after continuous usage. Chemotherapy 30: 546-550 (1982).

Kees, F.; Grobecker, H. and Naber, K.G.: High performance liquid chromatographic analysis of cefotetan epimers in human plasma and urine. Journal of Chromatography 305: 363-371 (1984).

Kesado, T.; Watanabe, K.; Asahi, Y.; Isono, M. and Ueno, K.: Comparative antibacterial activities of 7α-methoxy cephalosporins and 7 β-methoxyiminoacetamido cephalosporins against *Bacteroides fragilis*. Antimicrobial Agents and Chemotherapy 25: 131-133 (1984)

Kesado, T.; Watanabe, K.; Asahi, Y.; Isono, M. and Ueno, K.: Susceptibilities of anaerobic bacteria to N-formimidoyl thienamycin (MK0787) and to other antibiotics. Antimicrobial Agents and Chemotherapy 21: 1016-1022 (1982).

Kobayashi, H.; Takamura, M.; Takeda, H. and Kawai, S.: Clinical evaluation of cefotetan (YM09330) in the field of respiratory tract infections. Chemotherapy 30: 455-459 (1982).

Komatsu, T.; Nishiya, H.; Iwata, K.; Watanabe, M. and Kunii, O.: Binding of antibiotics to human liver ligandin; in Periti and Gialdroni Grassi (Eds) Current Chemotherapy and Immunotherapy, Vol. 1, pp. 150-151 (American Society for Microbiology, Washington 1981).

Komiya, M.; Kikuchi, Y.; Tachibana, A. and Yano, K.: Pharmacokinetics of new broad-spectrum cephamycin, YM09330, parenterally administered to various experimental animals. Antimicroboal Agents and Chemotherapy 20: 176-183 (1981).

Konishi, K.; Nishioka, K.; Tanno, Y.; Sakamoto, M.; Satoh, S. and Takishima, T.: Clinical studies on cefotetan (YM09330). Chemotherapy 30: 342-345 (1982).

Koyama, M.; Nakagawa, K.; Komiya, M.; Kikuchi, Y.; Tachibana, A. and Yano, K.: Phase-1 clinical study on cefotetan

(YM09330). Chemotherapy 30: 150-162 (1982).

Kumamoto, Y.; Nishio, A.; Kuroda, K.; Tsuji, I.; Hunyu, T. et al.: Clinical effects of the comparative study between 2g once a day and 1g twice a day administration of cefotetan in complicated urinary tract infections. Chemotherapy 31: 851-875 (1983).

Kumazawa, J.; Momose, S. and Mashimo, K.: Clinical study on YM09330 (cefotetan) in urinary tract infection; in Periti and Gialdroni Grassi (Eds) Current Chemotherapy and Immunotherapy, Vol. 1, pp. 439-441 (American Society for Microbiology, Washington 1981).

Kurimura, O.; Sadamoto, K.; Sasaki, H.; Murai, T.; Nozaki, K. et al.: Antimicrobial activity and clinical effect of cefotetan (YM09330). Chemotherapy 30: 534-541 (1982).

Kuroda, Y.; Okada, H.; Harada, M.; Okada, Y.; Kamidono, J. and Ishigami, J.: Clinical application of cefotetan (YM09330) on urinary tract infections. Chemotherapy 30: 688-702 (1982).

Labia, R.; Morand, A.; Verchere-Beaur, C. and Doré, J.Ch.: Cefotetan and β-lactamases. An analysis of the affinity of cefotetan for β-lactamases. Journal of Antimicrobial Chemotherapy 11 (Suppl. A): 147-152 (1983a).

Labia, R.; Morand, A. and Peduzzi, J.: Cefotetan and β-lactamases. An unusual property: the inactivation of some β-lactamases by cefotetan. Journal of Antimicrobial Chemotherapy 11 (Suppl. A): 153-157 (1983b).

Lanzini, A.; Pigozzi, G.; Facchinetti, U.; Castellano, M.; Beschi, M. et al.: Biliary pharmacokinetic and gallbladder bile concentration of cefotetan in healthy volunteers. Proceedings of the 14th International Congress of Chemotherapy (Abstracts), p. 195, Kyoto (1985).

Leach, R.D.: Single dose perioperative prophylaxis during prostatectomy — A comparative study of gentamicin and cefotetan. Proceedings of the 14th International Congress of Chemotherapy (Abstracts), p. 312, Kyoto (1985).

Leaper, D.J.; Cooper, M.J. and Turner, A.: A comparative trial of cefotetan and cephazolin for wound sepsis prophylaxis during elective upper gastrointestinal surgery; in Lode et al. (Eds). Cefotetan: A Long Acting Antibiotic, pp. 263-268 (Churchill Livingstone, Edinburgh 1985).

Lee, J.C.H. and Barry, A.L.: Cefotetan in the treatment of anaerobic infections: Clinical efficacy and the comparison of clinical outcome with *in vitro* susceptibility of anaerobes. Proceedings of the 14th International Congress of Chemotherapy (Abstracts), p. 429, Kyoto (1985).

Lee, P.W.R.; Leighton, I. and Royston, C.M.S.: A single centre study of cefotetan plus metronidazole versus three dose metronidazole treatment in the prophylaxis of wound infection in patients undergoing large bowel surgery. Proceedings of the 14th International Congress of Chemotherapy (Abstracts), p. 317, Kyoto (1985).

Lindsay, G.; Taylor, E.W.; McLatchie, G. and Maccallum, J.R.: A prospective randomised study of cefotetan and piperacillin against netilmicin and metronidazole in the treatment of patients presenting with generalised peritonitis. Proceedings of the 14th International Congress of Chemotherapy (Abstracts), p. 311, Kyoto (1985).

Machin, S.J.; Bowcock, S.; Mackie, I.J.; Ho, D. and Pozniak, A.: Haemostatic parameters: Pilot study with cefotetan compared with other antibiotics; in Lode et al. (Eds) Cefotetan: A Long Acting Antibiotic, pp. 138-142 (Churchill Livingstone, Edinburgh 1985).

Martin, A.: Cefotetan in the treatment of elderly patients with acute infections; in Lode et al. (Eds) Cefotetan: A Long Acting Antibiotic, pp. 208-213 (Churchill Livingstone, Edinburgh 1985).

Matsuda, S.; Hasegawa, Y.; Kato, N.; Ban, Y.; Kawada, Y. and Nishiura, T.: Experimental and clinical studies on cefotetan (YM09330) in urinary tract infections. Chemotherapy 30: 678-687 (1982).

Matsumoto, K.; Noguchi, Y.; Taguchi, M.; Yoshida, T.; Yamamoto, M. et al.: Laboratory and clinical studies on cefotetan (YM09330). Chemotherapy 30: 595-605 (1982).

McGavigan, J. and Stewart, K.: Single dose prophylaxis with cefotetan in gynecological surgery. Proceedings of the 14th International Congress of Chemotherapy (Abstracts), p. 315, Kyoto (1985).

Meguro, H.; Ozawa, S-S.; Togo, T.; Kim, B.; Arimasu, O. et al.: Clinical evaluation of cefotetan therapy in children. Japanese Journal of Antibiotics 36: 1262-1270 (1983).

Mitchell, N.J.; Pollock, D.; Evans, D.S. and Jones, P.H.: A comparison of cefotetan with metronidazole as single dose therapy in preventing infection after colorectal surgery. Proceedings of the 13th International Congress of Chemotherapy SS4.2/9 (Part 34): 1-7 (1983).

Mitsuhashi, S-S.: Clinical studies of cefotetan (YM09330) in the treatment of chronic complicated urinary tract infections. Chemotherapy 30: 643-650 (1982).

Mondorf, A.W.; Klein, S. and Weise, M.: Evaluation of cefotetan in a volunteer study of kidney function; in Lode et al. (Eds) Cefotetan: A Long Acting Antibiotic, pp. 117-121 (Churchill Livingstone, Edinburgh 1985).

Moosdeen, F.; Maskell, J.; Philpott-Howard, I. and Williams, J.D.: Cefotetan activity against Gram-negative aerobes and anaerobes. Journal of Antimicrobial Chemotherapy 11 (Suppl. 4): 59-65 (1983).

Morel, C.; Vergnaud, M.; Langeard, M.M. and Dupuy, L.: Cefotetan: comparative study *in vitro* against 226 Gram-negative clinical isolates. Journal of Antimicrobial Chemotherapy 11 (Suppl. A): 31-36 (1983).

Morran, C.; McNaught, W. and McArdle, C.S.: Prophylactic cotrimoxazole in biliary surgery. British Medical Journal 2: 462-464 (1978).

Morris, W.T.; Innes, D.B.; Richardson, R.A. et al.: The prevention of post appendicectomy sepsis by metronidazole and cephazolin: A controlled double-blind trial. Australian and New Zealand Journal of Surgery 50: 429-433 (1980).

Motomura, R.; Teramoto, C.; Souda, Y.; Fujita, A.; Chiyoda, R. et al.: Fundamental and clinical study of cefotetan (YM09330) in the field of obstetrics and gynecology. Chemotherapy 30: 882-887 (1982).

Murata, T.; Minami, S.; Yasuda, K.; Iyobe, S.; Inoue, M. and Mitsuhashi, S.: Purification and properties of cephalosporinase from *Pseudomonas aeruginosa*. Journal of Antibiotics 34: 1164-1170 (1981).

Murgatroyd, L.B.; Goonetilleke, U.R.P.; Moseley, M.J.; Middleton, B.J. and Stewart, M.: Cefotetan, a new long-acting cephamycin antibiotic: An interaction study with gentamicin to examine the effects on the kidney; in Lode et al. (Eds) Cefotetan: A Long Acting Antibiotic, pp. 122-130 (Churchill Livingstone, Edinburgh 1985).

Naber, K.; Kees, F.; Meyer, G.P. and Grobecker, H.: *In vitro* activity, pharmacokinetics, safety and therapeutic efficacy of cefotetan in patients with complicated urinary tract infections. Proceedings of the 14th International Congress of Chemotherapy (Abstracts), p. 430, Kyoto (1985a).

Naber, K.; Kees, F.; Meyer, G.P.; Johnson, L.C.; Letzel, H. and Grobecker, H.: Comparative pharmacokinetic study of cefotetan and cefotaxime in healthy volunteers; in Lode et al. (Eds) Cefotetan: A Long Acting Antibiotic, pp. 88-97 (Churchill Livingstone, Edinburgh 1985b).

Nagamatsu, I.; Okuno, H.; Takase, A. and Tachibana, K.: Clinical experience with cefotetan in the infectious diseases of children. Japanese Journal of Antibiotics 36: 1199-1203 (1983).

Nagasawa, M.; Watanabe, K.; Tanaka, H.; Cho, K.; Ito, N. et al.: Laboratory and clinical studies on cefotetan (YM09330).

Chemotherapy 30: 564-594 (1982).
Nakagawa, K.; Watanabe, K.; Yaguchi, S.; Son, E.; Onodera, S. et al.: Double-blind clinical study of cefotetan and cefmetazole in treating respiratory infections. Japanese Journal of Antibiotics 36: 316-368 (1983).
Nakagawa, K.; Koyama, M.; Tachibana, A.; Komiya, M.; Kikuchi, Y. and Yano, K.: Pharmacokinetics of cefotetan (YM09330) in humans. Antimicrobial Agents and Chemotherapy 22: 935-941 (1982a).
Nakagawa, K.; Koyama, M.; Watanabe, K.; Kawaguchi, Y.; Nakazawa, H. and Yokozawa, M.: Clinical studies of cefotetan (YM09330). Chemotherapy 30: 422-441 (1982b).
Nakamuta, S.; Momose, S.; Kumazawa, J.; Sakamoto, K.; Ohshima, K. et al.: Clinical experience of cefotetan (YM09330) in chronic complicated urinary tract infections. Chemotherapy 30: 741-752 (1982).
Nakayama, I.; Akieda, Y.; Kawaguchi, H. and Ishiyama, S.: Comparative pharmacokinetic study of cefotetan (YM09330) and latamoxef; in Periti and Gialdroni Grassi (Eds) Current Chemotherapy and Immunotherapy, Vol. 1, pp. 433-435 (American Society for Microbiology, Washington 1981).
Nakayama, I.; Akieda, Y.; Tajima, K.; Kawamura, H.; Kawaguchi, H. and Ishiyama, S.: Antibacterial activity, absorption, excretion, metabolism, distribution in tissues and clinical use in surgical infections of a new cephamycin antibiotic, cefotetan (YM09330). Chemotherapy 30: 770-785 (1982).
Nielson, O.S.; Maigaard, S.; Frimodt-Moller, N. and Madsen, P.O.: Prophylactic antibiotics in transurethral prostatectomy. Journal of Urology 126: 60-62 (1981).
Nishimura, T.; Takashima, T.; Hiromatsu, K.; Tabuki, K. and Takagi, M.: Laboratory and clinical studies of cefotetan in the pediatric field. Japanese Journal of Antibiotics 36: 1301-1312 (1983).
Nishino, T.; Saito, M.; Obana, Y.; Ozaki, T.; Yoshizaki, M. and Tanino, T.: Bacteriological evaluation of cefotetan (YM09330) a new cephamycin antibiotic. Chemotherapy 30: 65-81 (1982).
Nolen, T.M.: Clinical evaluation of cefotetan in the treatment of lower respiratory tract infections. Abstracts of the 22nd Interscience Conference on Antimicrobial Agents and Chemotherapy, p. 228, Miami Beach, Florida (1983).
Nolen, T.M.; Phillips, H.L.; Hall, H.J.; Hutchison, J.M. and Whitman, B.H.: A comparison of the efficacy and safety of cefotetan with that of maxolactam in the treatment of hospitalised patients with acute lower respiratory tract infections. Proceedings of the 14th International Congress of Chemotherapy (Abstracts), p. 195, Kyoto (1985).
Novelli, A.; Mazzei, T.; Ciuffi, M.; Nicolletti, P.; Buzzoni, P. et al.: The penetration of intramuscular cefotetan disodium into human extra-vascular fluid and maternal milk secretion. Chemioterapia 2: 337-342 (1983).
Obata, I.; Imagawa, N.; Ochiai, K.; Koike, K. and Hachiya, S.: Clinical study on cefotetan in the field of obstetrics and gynecology. Japanese Journal of Antibiotics 36: 165-177 (1983).
O'Boyle, P.J.; Pether, J.V.S.; Smith, K.; Abel, P.; Kerle, D. and Chant, A.: Urinary tract infection: Prophylaxis with single dose cefotetan in transurethral surgery. Proceedings of the 13th International Congress on Chemotherapy SS 4.2/9 (part 34): 1-7 (1983).
Ohishi, M. and Nagai, S.: Fundamental and Clinical Studies of cefotetan (YM09330) in ophthalmology. Chemotherapy 30: 924-929 (1982).
Ohkawa, M.; Hirano, S.; Tokunaga, S.; Motoi, I.; Shoda, R. et al.: Pharmocokinetics of cefotetan (YM09330) in healthy volunteers and patients with renal insufficiency. Antimicrobial Agents and Chemotherapy 23: 31-35 (1983).
Ohkawa, M.; Motoi, I.; Shoda, R.; Ikeda, A.; Sugata, T. et al.: A clinical evaluation of cefotetan (YM09330) in chronic complicated urinary tract infections. Chemotherapy 30: 671-677 (1982).
Owen, A.W.M.; Manson, J.McK.; Yates, R.A.; Adshead, V.M.; Houghton, H.L. and Tweedle, H.L.: The pharmacokinetics of cefotetan excretion in the unobstructed biliary tree. Journal of Antimicrobial Chemotherapy 11 (Suppl. A): 217-221 (1983a).
Owen, A.W.M.; Rickards, D.; Yates, R.A.; Donnelly, R.J.; Adshead, V.M. et al.: The pharmacokinetics of the excretion of cefotetan into the biliary tree. Proceedings of the 13th International Congress of Chemotherapy (S.P. 4.2/9; Part 34): 8-17 (1983b).
Owens, W.E. and Finegold, S.M.: Comparative *in vitro* susceptibilities of anaerobic bacteria to cefmenoxime, cefotetan, and N-formidyl thienamycin. Antimicrobial Agents and Chemotherapy 23: 626-629 (1983).
Oyama, K.; Suzuki, K. and Shimizu, R.: Clinical study of cefotetan (YM09330). Chemotherapy 30: 478-485 (1982).
Palumbo, G.; Cianci, A.; Pafumi, C.; Russo, I.; Tempera, G. and Toscano, M.A.: Cefotetan in obstetric and gynaecological infections; in Lode et al. (Eds) Cefotetan: A Long Acting Antibiotic, pp. 149-151 (Churchill Livingstone, Edinburgh 1985).
Pastorek, J.; Faro, S.; Aldridge, K.; Cunningham, G. and McKenna, C.: Comparison of cefotetan with cefoxitin for gynecologic use: Prophylaxis and therapy. Proceedings of the 14th International Congress of Chemotherapy (Abstracts), p. 184, Kyoto (1985).
Periti, P.; Lamanna, S.; Nicoletti, P. and Orsi, A.: Comparative antimicrobial evaluation of cefotetan. Drugs and Experimental Clinical Research 9: 267-273 (1983).
Petrie, G.R.; Garnett, P.A.; Sandhu, P. and Choo-Kang, Y.F.J.: Clinical evaluation of cefotetan in the treatment of lower respiratory tract infections; in Lode et al. (Eds) Cefotetan: A Long Acting Antibiotic, pp. 214-217 (Churchill Livingstone, Edinburgh 1985).
Pfeiffer, M.: The efficacy and safety of cefotetan in the treatment of intra-abdominal infections; in Lode et al. (Eds) Cefotetan: A Long Acting Antibiotic, pp. 235-238 (Churchill Livingstone, Edinburgh 1985).
Phillips, I.; King, A.; Shannon, K. and Warren, C.: Cefotetan: *In vitro* antibacterial activity and susceptibility to β-lactamases. Journal of Antimicrobial Chemotherapy 11 (Suppl. A): 1-9 (1983).
Privitera, G.; Ortisi, G.; Vigo, B.; Rossi, R.; Setti, C. and Moroni, M.: *In vitro* activity of cefotetan, a new cephamycin against *Bacteroides fragilis*; in Lode et al. (Eds) Cefotetan: A Long Acting Antibiotic, pp. 28-32 (Churchill Livingstone, Edinburgh 1985).
Puleo, S.; Gismondo, M.R.; Sammartino, R.; Tempera, G. and Latteri, F.: Use of cefotetan in intra-abdominal and other surgical infections; in Lode et al. (Eds) Cefotetan. A Long Acting Antibiotic, pp. 239-241 (Churchill Livingstone, Edinburgh 1985).
Quayle, A.A.; Russell, C. and Hearn, B.: Cefotetan in the treatment of severe oro-facial infections of dental origin; in Lode et al. (Eds) Cefotetan: A Long Acting Antibiotic, pp. 218-224 (Churchill Livingstone, Edinburgh 1985).
Ravizzola, G.; Caruso, A.; Manca, N.; Savoldi, E. and Turano, A.: *In vitro* activity of cefotetan and other cephalosporins on *Klebsiella* and resistance to inactivating bacterial enzymes. Journal of Antimicrobial Chemotherapy 11 (Suppl. A): 133-138 (1983).
Reeves, D.S.; Bywater, M.J. and Holt, H.A.: Comparative activity *in vitro* of cefotetan, a new cephamycin antibiotic. Drugs in Experimental Clinical Research 9: 125-131 (1983).
Romanelli, G.; Agabiti-Rosei, E.; Muiesan, M.L.; Malerba, M.; Platto, L. and Muiesan, G.: Cefotetan in the treatment of nosocomial infections: A clinical review; in Lode et al. (Eds) Cefotetan. A Long Acting Antibiotic, pp. 192-197 (Churchill Livingstone, Edinburgh 1985).
Romanelli, G.; Ravizzola, G. and Turano, A.: Clinical effects of

cefotetan in urinary tract infections (UTI) in hospitalised patients. Proceedings of the 13th International Congress of Chemotherapy SS4-2/9 (Part 34): 85-90 (1983).

Royston, C.M.S.; Leighton, I. and Wale, R.J.: Prophylaxis in biliary surgery: a comparison of cefotetan and cephazolin; in Lode et al. (Eds) Cefotetan: A Long Acting Antibiotic, pp. 269-273 (Churchill Livingstone, Edinburgh 1985).

Ruckdeschel, G.: Activity *in vitro* of cefotetan against non-sporing anaerobes: A comparative study. Journal of Antimicrobial Chemotherapy 11 (Suppl. A): 117-124 (1983).

Russo, G.; Gismondo, M.R.; Toscano, M.A.; Speciale, A.M. and Nicoletti, G.: Comparative susceptibilities of organisms isolated in Sicily to cefotetan and other antibiotics. Journal of Antimicrobial Chemotherapy 11 (Suppl. A): 79-85 (1983).

Saito, T.; Koroku, T.; Yasuzuka, H.; Nakabayashi, T.; Yasuda, S. and Nagahama, F.: Studies on the clinical efficacy of cefotetan (YM09330) to lung infections. Chemotherapy 30: 317-322 (1982c).

Saito, A.; Shimada, J.; Oomori, M.; Siba, K.; Yamaji, T. et al.: Clinical studies on cefotetan (YM09330). Chemotherapy 30: 380-397 (1982a).

Saito, A.; Shinohara, M.; Tomizawa, M.; Sato, K.; Kikuchi, Y. and Tachibara, A.: Studies on cefotetan (YM09330). I. Pharmacokinetics in man. Chemotherapy 30: 163-173 (1982b).

Sambe, B.; Ueda, R.; Kobayashi, K.; Ito, Y. and Inafuku, M.: Fundamental and clinical study of cefotetan (YM09330) in otorhinolaryngology. Chemotherapy 30: 902-910 (1982).

Sawae, Y.; Okada, K.; Takemori, K. and Yokota, H.: Laboratory and clinical studies on cefotetan (YM09330). Chemotherapy 30: 551-563 (1982).

Seiga, K.; Minagawa, M.; Egawa, J.; Noma, M. and Sugiyama, Y.: Fundamental and clinical studies on cefotetan (YM09330). Chemotherapy 30: 843-868 (1982).

Sekine, O.; Usuda, Y.; Aoki, N.; Yuasa, Y.; Tsukada, Y. et al.: Clinical studies of cefotetan (YM09330). Chemotherapy 30: 466-477 (1982).

Serra, P.; Venditti, M.; Shinaia, M.; Micozzi, A.; Santini, C. and Martino, P.: Cefotetan and amikacin against Gram-negative bacilli: *In vitro* comparative study with other antibiotics and evaluation of their combined activity; in Lode et al. (Eds) Cefotetan: A Long Acting Antibiotic, pp. 71-73 (Churchill Livingstone, Edinburgh 1985).

Shah, P.M.: *In vitro* activity of cefotetan, other β-lactams, and netilmicin. Journal of Antimicrobial Chemotherapy 11 (Suppl. A): 73-78 (1983).

Shinohara, Y.; Matsubuchi, T.; Kawagoe, H.; Nagai, K.; Kanamuru, A. et al.: Cooperative studies on clinical effect of cefotetan for severe infections combined with hematological disorders. Japanese Journal of Antibiotics 36: 391-397 (1983).

Smith, B.R. and LeFrock, J.L.: Cefotetan pharmacokinetics in volunters with varying degrees of renal function. Drug Intelligence and Clinical Pharmacy 18: 491 (1984).

Soejima, R.; Matsushima, T.; Niki, Y.; Okimoto, J.; Kawanishi, M. and Nakahama, C.: Fundamental and clinical studies on cefotetan (YM09330). Chemotherapy 30: 524-533 (1982).

Souza Dias, M.B.; Jacobus, N.V.; Tally, F.P. and Gorbach, S.L.: Activity of cefotetan against anaerobic bacteria. Proceedings of the 24th Interscience Conference on Antimicrobial Agents and Chemotherapy, p. 316 (American Society for Microbiology, Washington 1984).

Stahl, J.P.; Croizé, J.; Bru, J.P.; Gaillat, J.; Tetelboum, R. et al.: The pharmacokinetics of cefotetan in the elderly; in Lode et al. (Eds) Cefotetan: A Long Acting Antibiotic, pp. 98-101 (Churchill Livingstone, Edinburgh 1985).

Stanbridge, T.N. and Rash, R.M.: Investigation of the effects of single daily doses of cefotetan in the treatment of urinary tract infections in the elderly; in Lode et al. (eds) Cefotetan: A Long Acting Antibiotic, pp. 170-172 (Churchill Livingstone, Edinburgh 1985).

Strachan, C.J.L. and Morrison, J.D.: Mezlocillin in abdominal surgery; in 249-254 (Eds) International Symposium on Acylureido Penicillins, Vol. III, pp. 153-155 (Excerpta Medica, London 1982).

Strachan, C.J.L.; Black, J. and Powis, S.J.A.: Prophylactic use of cephazolin against wound infection sepsis after cholecystectomy. British Medical Journal 1: 1254-1256 (1977).

Strachan, C.J.L.; Thom, B.T. and Tanner, A.G.: Contemporary use of antibiotics for the prevention of sepsis following abdominal surgery; in Lode et al. (Eds) Cefotetan: A Long Acting Antibiotic, pp. 255-260 (Churchill Livingstone, Edinburgh 1985).

Suginaka, H.; Takata, N. and Ogawa, M.: Mode of antibacterial action of cefotetan (YM09330) against *Escherichia coli* K12, *Pseudomonas aeruginosa* KM 338, and *Serratia marcescens* IFO 12648. Chemotherapy 30: 86-91 (1982).

Suzuki, H.; Imamura, K.; Yoshida, T.; Shibata, M.; Matsuzawa, T. et al.: Animal pharmacokinetics and toxicology of cefotetan — a new cephamycin antibiotic. Journal of Antimicrobial Chemotherapy 11: 179-183 (1983).

Suzuki, K.; Tachibana, A.; Nakata, K.; Okano, H.; Tanimoto, H. and Matsuoka, H.: Clinical study on cefotetan (YM09330) in the respiratory tract infection. Chemotherapy 30: 447-454 (1982a).

Suzuki, K.; Nagakubo, I.; Mitsui, H.; Ogawa, T.; Tamai, H. et al.: Clinical evaluation of cefotetan (YM09330) on urinary tract infections. Chemotherapy 30: 653-670 (1982b).

Suzuki, K.; Naide, Y.; Okada, K.; Ohkoshi, M. and Iki, Y.: Diffusion into human prostatic fluids of new cephem antibiotic drugs; in Periti and Gialdroni Grassi (Eds) Current Chemotherapy and Immunotherapy, Vol. 1, pp. 432-433 (American Society for Microbiology, Washington 1981).

Sweet, R.L.: Cefotetan in the treatment of obstetric and gynecologic infections: Results of non-comparative studies and a comparative study with moxalactam. Proceedings of the 14th International Congress of Chemotherapy (Abstracts), p. 86, Kyoto (1985).

Tachibana, A.; Kikuchi, Y.; Komiya, M. and Matsui, H.: Pharmacokinetics and excretion machanisms of cefotetan in humans. Proceedings of the 14th International Congress of Chemotherapy (Abstracts), p. 85, Kyoto (1985).

Takai, Y.; Mizuno, K.; Kuno, H.; Fujii, H.; Yamada, N. et al.: Clinical evaluation of cefotetan (YM09330) in acute infections in the field of oral surgery. Chemotherapy 30: 937-947 (1982).

Takase, Z.: Pharmacokinetics and clinical study of cefotetan in the field of obstetrics and gynaecology. Proceedings of the 13th International Congress on Chemotherapy SS 4.2/9 (Part 34): 55-60 (1983).

Takase, Z.; Fujiwara, M.; Kawamoto, Y.; Seto, M.; Shirafuji, H. and Uchida, M.: Laboratory and clinical studies of cefotetan (YM09330) in the field of obstetrics and gynaecology. Chemotherapy 30: 869-881 (1982).

Takebe, K.; Nakamura, T.; Sasaki, K.; Nakazono, M.; Kumasaka, Y. et al.: Clinical studies on cefotetan (YM09330). Chemotherapy 30: 332-341 (1982).

Tanimura, H.; Hikasa, Y.; Kobayashi, N.; Kato, H.; Sekiya, T. et al.: Comparative double-blind study of cefotetan and cefmetazole in patients with purulent peritonitis. Japanese Journal of Antibiotics 36: 369-390 (1983).

Tanimura, H.; Kobayashi, N.; Sato, T. and Saito, T.: Clinical effects of pharmacokinetics of cefotetan in patients with biliary tract infections. Proceedings of the 14th International Congress of Chemotherapy (Abstracts), p. 86, Kyoto (1985).

Tanimura, H.; Saito, T.; Sato,T.; Sekiya, T.; Kobayashi, N. et al.: Chemotherapy of biliary tract infection with special reference to biliary excretion, tissue concentration in gallbladder and clinical effects in patients treated with cefotetan (YM09330). Chemotherapy 30: 796-815 (1982).

Taylor, E.W.; Lindsay, G. and McGavigan, J.: A comparative study of metronidazole alone against metronidazole and cefotetan to prevent infection after appendicectomy. Proceedings of the 14th International Congress of Chemotherapy (Abstracts), p. 273, Kyoto (1985).

Toda, M.; Ikeuchi, T.; Tajima, M.; Inoue, M. and Mitsuhashi, S.: Comparative inhibition of β-lactamases by cephamycin antibiotics. Journal of Antibiotics 34: 114-117 (1981a).

Toda, M.; Inoue, M. and Mitsuhashi, S.: Properties of cephalosporinase from *Proteus morganii*. Journal of Antibiotics 34: 1469-1475 (1981b).

Toda, M.; Saito, T.; Inoue, M. and Mitsuhashi, S.: *In vitro* and *in vivo* antibacterial activity of cefotetan (YM09330). Chemotherapy 30: 1-17 (1982).

Toyonaga, Y.; Kurosu, Y.; Sugita, M.; Kita, A.; Yoshino, N. et al.: Experimental and clinical evaluation of cefotetan in the field of pediatric infection. Japanese Journal of Antibiotics 36: 1243-1261 (1983).

Triger, D.R.; Preston, F.E. and Malia, R.G.: Coagulation and platelet function in patients with impaired liver function receiving cefotetan; in Lode et al. (Eds) Cefotetan: A Long Acting Antibiotic, pp. 143-146 (Churchill Livingstone, Edinburgh 1985).

Tsukada, O.; Tominaga, T.; Niijima, T.; Nishimura, Y.; Nito, H. et al.: Clinical evaluation of cefotetan (YM09330) in complicated urinary tract infections. Chemotherapy 30: 628-638 (1982).

Wada, K.; Baba, S.; Hatano, T.; Murai, K.; Kinoshita, H. et al.: Laboratory and clinical studies of cefotetan (YM09330) in otorhinolaryngological field. Chemotherapy 30: 911-923 (1982).

Watanabe, A.; Aonuma, S.; Onuma, K.; Sasaki, M.; Oizumi, K. and Konno, K.: *In vitro* antimicrobial activity and clinical evaluation of therapeutic effects of cefotetan (YM09330) on respiratory tract infections. Chemotherapy 30: 346-361 (1982a).

Watanabe, K.; Hibino, J.; Shiina, K.; Izumi, A.; Mori, T. and Ikemoto, H.: Clinical studies on cefotetan (YM09330), a new semisynthetic cephamycin, in respiratory disease. Chemotherapy 30: 412-415 (1982b).

Watt, B. and Brown, V.: Anaerobes in clinical practice: significance and treatment; in Lode et al. (Eds) Cefotetan: A Long Acting Antibiotic, pp. 8-13 (Churchill Livingstone, Edinburgh 1985).

Weissbach, L.; Schlösser, R. and Herzög, F.A.: Cefotetan versus cefoxitin and cefotaxime in the treatment of urinary tract infections; in Lode et al. (Eds) Cefotetan: A Long Acting Antibiotic, pp. 152-161 (Churchill Livingstone, Edinburgh 1985).

Werner, H.: Inhibitory activity of cefotetan and other β-lactams against anaerobes. Journal of Antimicrobial Chemotherapy 11 (Suppl. A): 107-115 (1983).

Williams, J.D.: Classification of cephalosporins; in Williams (Ed.) The Cephalosporin Antibiotics, pp. 17-26 (ADIS Press, Auckland 1985).

Wilson, S.E.; Lewis, R.T. and Ton, G.T.: Comparative clinical evaluation of cefotetan with moxalactam in the treatment of hospitalised patients with serious intra-abdominal infections. Proceedings of the 14th International Congress of Chemotherapy (Abstracts), p. 86, Kyoto (1985).

Wise, R.; Andrews, J.M. and Hancox, J.: *In vitro* activity of cefotetan, a new cephamycin derivative, compared with that of other β-lactam compounds. Antimicrobial Agents and Chemotherapy 21: 486-491 (1982).

Wittke, R.R.; Adam, D. and Keemss, J.: Cefotetan in the treatment and prophylaxis of surgical infections: Pharmacokinetics in wound secretion, bile and tissues; in Lode et al. (Eds) Cefotetan: A Long Acting Antibiotic, pp. 255-262 (Churchill Livingstone, Edinburgh 1985).

Wright, N.; Wise, R. and Hegerty, A.: Cefotetan elimination in subjects with varying degrees of renal dysfunction. Journal of Antimicrobial Chemotherapy 1 (Suppl. A): 213-216 (1983).

Yamada, Y.; Sasaki, J. and Takeyasu, K.: Fundamental and clinical study on cefotetan (YM09330). Chemotherapy 30: 930-936 (1982).

Yanagisawa, K.; Hoshina, H. and Ichihashi, H.: Clinical study on cefotetan in pediatric field. Japanese Journal of Antibiotics 36: 1271-1278 (1983).

Yano, K.; Suzaki, K.; Saito, M.; Toda, M.; Naito, S. and Ohmi, Y.: Cefotetan, a new cephamycin antibiotic: *In vitro* and *in vivo* antibacterial activities. Japanese Journal of Antibiotics 35: 438-459 (1982).

Yasuda, J.; Yamamoto, T.; Itoh, M.; Honjo, H.; Okada, H. and Kanao, M.: Fundamental and clinical studies on cefotetan in obstetrics and gynecology. Japanese Journal of Antibiotics 36: 2455-2460 (1983).

Yates, R.A.; Adam, H.K.; Donnelly, R.J.; Houghton, H.L.; Chartesworth, E.A. and Lows, E.A.: Pharmacokinetics and tolerance of single intravenous doses of cefotetan disodium in male Caucasian volunteers. Journal of Antimicrobial Chemotherapy 11 (Suppl. A): 185-191 (1983a).

Yates, R.A.; Cockshott, I.D.; Houghton, H.L.; Wardleworth, A.; Adam, H.K. and Donnelly, R.J.: Pharmacokinetics and tolerance of single intramuscular doses of cefotetan in normal Caucasian volunteers. Journal of Antimicrobial Chemotherapy 11 (Suppl. A): 207-212 (1983b).

Yura, J.; Shinagawa, N.; Ishikawa, S.; Takaoka, T.; Hanai, T. et al.: Fundamental and clinical studies of cefotetan (YM09330) on the surgical field. Chemotherapy 30: 786-795 (1982).

Authors' address: *Alan Ward*, ADIS Drug Information Services, Centorian Drive, Private Bag, Mairangi Bay, Auckland 10 (New Zealand).

Review Article

Drugs 30: 427-443 (1985)
0012-6667/85/0011-0427/$08.50/0

Resistance to Loop Diuretics
Why it Happens and What to Do About It

D. Craig Brater

The University of Texas Health Science Center at Dallas, Departments of Pharmacology and Internal Medicine, Southwestern Medical School, Dallas

Summary

Resistance to loop diuretics is often encountered clinically. Studies in healthy subjects have shown that overall response to loop diuretics depends upon the interplay between the total amount of drug reaching the urine, the time course of its entry into urine and the pharmacodynamics of response to diuretic in the urine. The mechanism by which diuretic resistance occurs has been elucidated in several clinical conditions. Treatment with inhibitors of prostaglandin synthesis has no effect on diuretic appearance in urine but blunts response by blocking the increase in renal blood flow produced by loop diuretics. In the elderly and in patients with moderate renal insufficiency, the mechanism of resistance appears to be purely pharmacokinetic, involving altered access of diuretic into the urine. In contrast, patients with nephrotic syndrome and hepatic cirrhosis manifest a purely pharmacodynamic form of resistance: in nephrosis, diuretic may bind to protein in the urine; in cirrhosis the mechanism of resistance is unclear. Lastly, in patients with congestive heart failure, with intravenous administration, resistance represents a pharmacodynamic phenomenon. With oral administration, however, the time course but not the extent of absorption is altered; consequently, in this setting, both pharmacokinetic and pharmacodynamic changes may contribute to the subnormal response.

Strategies for overcoming resistance to loop diuretics in patients receiving NSAIDs or those with renal disease, hepatic cirrhosis or congestive heart failure include one or more of: increasing the dose size; administering frequent 'small' (but effective) doses; continuous intravenous infusion of the diuretic; or concomitant administration of another diuretic such as metolazone or hydrochlorothiazide.

Diuretic resistance is a common clinical problem. In the past, the focus has been on the physiological mechanisms of this phenomenon with little attention to possible pharmacological mechanisms. This review will emphasise pharmacological considerations, not to unduly de-emphasise the physiological considerations, but to offer a different perspective and demonstrate that ultimately the two approaches merge. Frusemide (furosemide) will be used as the prototype diuretic throughout this review, since more data are available with this drug and studies with other loop diuretics show similar results to those with frusemide.

1. The Role of Sodium Intake

The rationale for effecting diuresis in a patient is to create a net negative balance of sodium. Though simplistic, many clinicians often overlook the fact that accomplishing this goal depends not only on causing natriuresis but also on the magnitude of this effect relative to sodium intake. When a patient presents with florid congestive heart failure and large amounts of peripheral oedema, acute therapy often results in marked natriuresis with considerable weight loss while the patient is ingesting little or no sodium and receiving no sodium in intravenous preparations. That a net negative sodium balance ensues is obvious to clinician and patient alike.

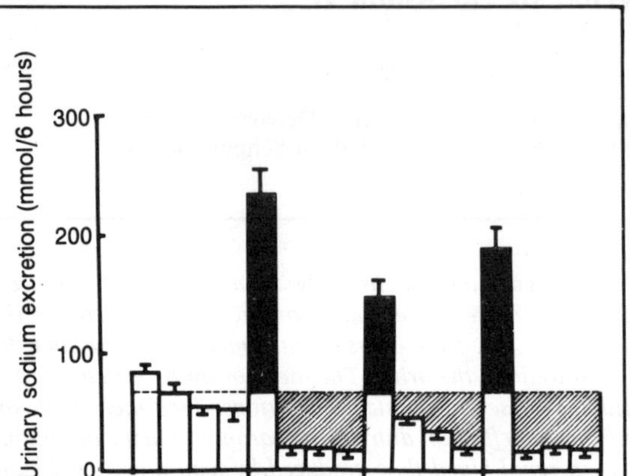

Fig. 1. Effects of frusemide on overall sodium balance during both high **(a)** and low **(b)** salt intakes; the horizontal dashed line represents intake. Columns above the line represent net loss of sodium while those below the line represent net gain. Columns represent urinary sodium excretion over 6 hours. With the high salt intake the net loss of sodium caused by frusemide (F) is matched by subsequent sodium retention. With low salt intake, sufficient sodium retention cannot occur to match losses and net negative sodium balance ensues (from Wilcox et al., 1983).

In contrast, many do not realise during institution of treatment in less dramatic settings, and with long term maintenance therapy with a diuretic, that sodium intake can easily offset the natriuretic effects of the diuretic. For example, a recent series of studies have assessed the impact of sodium intake on the ability to achieve a net negative sodium balance (Kelly et al., 1983; Wilcox et al., 1983). Six healthy volunteers received frusemide 40 mg/day for 3 days while on either a 20 or 270 mmol Na^+/day diet. During high salt intake, a negative sodium balance did not occur; the cumulative balance over the 3 days being 20 ± 63 mmol. In contrast, on the low sodium diet the cumulative balance was −146 ± 8 mmol, and in this phase of the study a significant decrease of approximately 1kg in weight occurred. During the phase with high sodium intake, frusemide caused a pronounced, short-lived natriuresis followed by avid sodium retention that matched that lost following the diuretic (fig. 1).

In essence then, although these studies were performed in healthy subjects, it would appear that a patient can easily ingest sufficient sodium to obviate the sodium loss caused by potent diuretics. Clinically, this could be partially overcome by administering the diuretic frequently and thereby lessening the opportunity for compensatory sodium retention to occur. Clearly, however, one must also be aware that a degree of sodium restriction may be necessary, the extent of which most likely will differ among patients. It is important to realise that this form of diuretic failure does not constitute diuretic resistance, for patients respond to the drug as expected. Rather, they have managed to simply overcome the effects of the diuretic by intake of sodium.

How does this compensatory sodium retention occur? During both high and low sodium intakes, plasma renin activity, and plasma angiotensin and aldosterone concentrations increase (Kelly et al., 1983; Wilcox et al., 1983). With a high intake of sodium, aldosterone-mediated sodium retention could conceivably account for this phenomenon.

However, treatment with captopril in sufficient doses to normalise aldosterone concentrations did not completely prevent the compensatory sodium retention. Volunteers ingesting 270 mmol Na^+/day treated with both frusemide and captopril had a neutral cumulative sodium balance of 42 ± 54 mmol (Kelly et al., 1983). Consequently, an intact renin-angiotensin-aldosterone system is not required for this compensation, and its mechanism remains unexplained.

Overall, the important clinical lesson from these data is that in patients who are not achieving a negative sodium balance the tendency is to focus on lack of response to the diuretics due to either pharmacological factors or because of the severity of the patients' disease. It is also important to be aware of the possible role of sodium intake in determining overall response to the diuretic.

2. *Determinants of Normal Response to a Loop Diuretic*

2.1 Importance of Urinary Concentrations of Frusemide

From *in vitro* and *in vivo* animal studies, it is clear that loop diuretics must reach the tubular lumen to be effective (Burg, 1976; Odlind, 1979a,b; Odlind and Beermann, 1980). These diuretics are all organic acids and are highly bound to serum proteins. As a consequence, they cannot reach the tubular lumen by glomerular filtration, for only a small fraction of the total drug in serum is free in the circulation and can be sieved through the glomerulus. These drugs reach the luminal compartment by being actively secreted from the blood into the urine via the organic acid transport pathway of the straight segment of the proximal tubule (Odlind, 1979a,b). To assess determinants of normal response to frusemide in man, it was important to determine whether observations in the basic laboratory could be extrapolated to man. Probenecid can be used to permute the relationship between concentrations of frusemide in blood and in urine and, thereby, as a tool to assess the importance of blood *versus* urinary frusemide concentrations in determining response. Pretreatment of healthy subjects with probenecid decreases both renal and non-renal clearance of frusemide by one-half, thereby greatly changing the relationship between blood and urinary frusemide concentrations (Chennavasin et al., 1979; Homeida et al., 1977; Honari et al., 1977). As shown in figure 2, this has no effect on the relationship between urinary frusemide concentration and response (Chennavasin et al., 1979). These data confirm the ability to extrapolate previous animal data to man, and that urinary frusemide concentration is the best correlate of response.

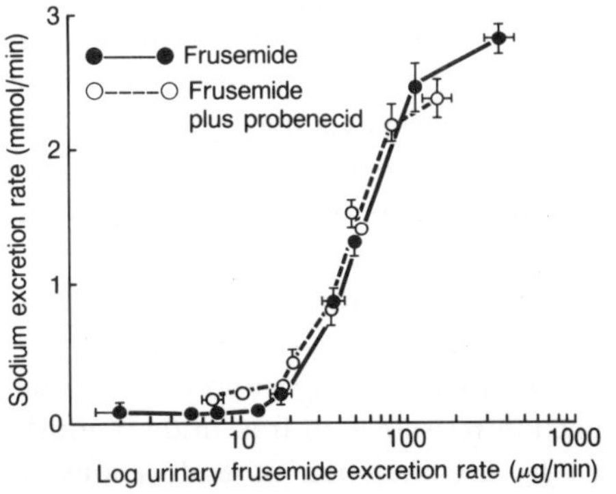

Fig. 2. Lack of effect of probenecid on the relationship between urinary frusemide excretion and response assessed as sodium excretion rate (from Chennavasin et al., 1979).

It is important to note the sigmoid nature of this relationship. It should be apparent that entry of drug into urine at a rate that never reaches the steep portion of the dose-response curve will result in no response even if substantial amounts of total drug reach the urine. This might occur, for example, with prolonged absorption where a constant ingress of small amounts of drug into the urine might never reach amounts sufficient to have an effect. In contrast, more rapid entry of the same total amount of drug might result in an effect. Another important aspect of the sigmoidal nature of the dose-response curve is that the upper plateau implies there is a point at which additional drug becomes superfluous. Hence, once the maximum is reached, more could be gained by giving multiple doses than by giving a larger single dose.

What determines access of frusemide and other organic acid diuretics to the urine? Since the sites of action are reached via the organic acid secretory pump at the proximal tubule, the presence of inhibitors of transport will affect access. Inhibitors include coadministered organic acids such as probenecid and accumulated endogenous organic acids of uraemia. As is discussed in greater detail subsequently, in patients with mild to moderate renal dysfunction resistance to frusemide is most likely caused by accumulation of endogenous organic acids which decrease access of frusemide to the site of action and thus alter response. This mechanism is in contrast to the changed response being a manifestation of decreased nephron mass (Rose et al., 1976a,b,c). The latter becomes predominant only with severe renal impairment.

Theoretically, decreases in protein binding of loop diuretics would allow more to be filtered at the glomerulus and thereby change the route of access to the site of action. In clinical conditions in which changed binding occurs – namely, azotaemia in which competitors to binding displace the drug, and in hypoalbuminaemic states of any cause in which the capacity for binding decreases – the increase in unbound drug is not quantitatively important relative to amounts entering the tubule via active secretion (Rane et al., 1978).

Access of the diuretic to the organic acid secretory site should also be determined by the amount of blood flowing to the proximal nephron. Hence, changes in renal blood flow might influence the amount of drug reaching the tubular lumen. However, the avidity of the transport system for loop diuretics appears to be so great that considerable decrements in renal blood flow must occur before access to the site of transport becomes limiting.

The most important determinant of how much drug reaches the urinary site of action, then, is the amount of drug circulating in blood. This, in turn, is a function of the bioavailability of the drug after an oral dose and its clearance; i.e. its pharmacokinetics. The pharmacokinetic characteristics of frusemide and their possible role in diuretic resistance are discussed subsequently as specific clinical conditions are considered. It is important to note, however, that the critically important determinant of diuretic response in man is a function of drug reaching the urinary site of action. Any change in serum concentrations of diuretic are only important to the extent that they affect concentrations in the urine.

Most clinicians would predict that the total amount of drug appearing in the urine would be a determinant of response, since larger doses result in increased diuresis. However, the time course of drug appearance in urine is also an important determinant.

2.2 Importance of the Time Course of Drug Delivery to the Site of Action

An unexpected finding in previous studies of frusemide was that pretreatment of healthy subjects with probenecid increased the overall natriuretic response from 262 ± 16 to 358 ± 11 mmol Na^+/8 hours ($p < 0.005$) [Brater, 1978]. Since 'dose-response' curves were identical (fig. 2), this effect did not occur, because of changed sensitivity of the nephron to frusemide. In addition, the total amount of frusemide delivered into the urine was unchanged; 19.7 ± 2.2 without probenecid *versus* 16.0 ± 1.4 mg/8 hours with probenecid pretreatment ($p = 0.252$). As a consequence, the only factor which could account for this difference in response between the 2 groups was a changed time course of delivery of frusemide into urine.

A similar phenomenon has been noted when comparing overall response to oral *versus* intravenous frusemide (Branch et al., 1977; Kaojarern et al., 1982). In our laboratory, 27 subjects who received frusemide intravenously had less than twice the natriuretic response of 21 subjects who received an oral dose (359 ± 43 *versus* 235 ± 25 mmol Na^+/24 hours, despite almost 3 times as much drug having reached the urine (21.2 ± 8 *versus* 7.9 ± 1.6 mg/24 hours) [Kaojarern et al., 1982]. As with the probenecid effect, there was a discrepancy between overall response relative to amounts of drug reaching the active site. Changed sensitivity could not account for the observation, for again 'dose-response' curves for the 2 formulations were superimposable. Consequently, as occurred with the probenecid studies, a difference in time course of delivery of drug into the urine was invoked to explain the results.

To probe the mechanism of this effect, we used the concept of the ratio of sodium to frusemide excretion to describe the efficiency of the diuretic (Kaojarern et al., 1982). This ratio has been used by others, although in a somewhat different context, to describe the influence of indomethacin on the response to frusemide in the dog (Data et al., 1978), and to describe the interaction between probenecid or spironolactone and frusemide in man (Homeida et al., 1977). Applying this efficiency approach to the actual dose-response curve of frusemide allowed mathematical derivation (by taking the first derivative of the Hill equation) of the determinants of maximum efficiency:

$$\text{Amount with Maximum Efficiency} = [c^b (b - 1)]^{1/b}$$

where b is the slope factor of the dose-response curve and c is the amount of drug causing half-maximal response (ED_{50}). This quantitative derivation allowed comparison between dosing regimens in terms of the relationship between the actual time course of delivery of drug to the active site and that amount with maximal efficiency.

The amount of urinary frusemide with maximum efficiency derived from the preceding equation (21.5 μg/min) was considerably less than the ED_{50} (69.8 μg/min) for frusemide. Therefore, the importance of the time course of delivery in determining overall response was the manner in which delivery of drug to its active site related to a value at the relatively low end of the steep portion of the dose-response curve. After oral administration, amounts of frusemide more persistently approached that amount with maximal efficiency, and overall natriuresis was greater relative to total amounts of drug delivery to the active site. Similarly, pretreatment with probenecid caused a counterclockwise shift in the time course curve with less overall deviation from the amount with maximum efficiency (Brater, 1983). For frusemide then, the influence on cumulative response of the time course of delivery of drug to the urinary site of action was more importantly related to the derived value with maximum efficiency than it was to the ED_{50}, although the former is only one-third the latter.

Table I. Determinants of response to frusemide

Pharmacokinetic determinants	
Total amount of drug reaching the urine	
	Dose
	Amount absorbed if given by mouth
	Capacity for active secretion at the proximal tubule
Time course of delivery of drug into the urine	
	Capacity for active secretion
Pharmacodynamic factors	
Concentration *versus* response curve	

An extrapolation of these data is that patients may respond better to a continuous infusion of frusemide than to bolus administration. How they respond will depend on the parameters of their dose-response curve which determine the maximally efficient amount of diuretic; namely, the slope factor and ED_{50} and the ability to attain a delivery rate of drug into the urine which reaches the steep portion of the dose-response curve in individual patients. This potential strategy will be discussed subsequently for patients refractory to large doses of diuretics.

In summary, the determinants of response to frusemide are as shown in table I. From a pharmacokinetic perspective, overall response is a function of the total amount of drug with access to the site of action – which will be determined by dose of drug, its quantitative absorption, and the capacity of the organic acid transport pump to deliver drug from blood into urine. In addition, overall response is determined by the time course of drug delivery to the site of action, a function of drug clearance which for organic acid diuretics is again a function of the organic acid transport pathway. From a pharmacodynamic perspective, overall response is also independently affected by the 'dose-response' curve.

Table II. Effect of NSAIDs on urinary frusemide excretion (40mg intravenous dose) [from Chennavasin et al., 1980; Brater et al., 1985]

Drug	Urinary frusemide excretion (mg)	
	frusemide alone	frusemide plus NSAID
Ibuprofen	21 ± 1	21 ± 1
Indomethacin	20 ± 2	19 ± 2
Naproxen	21 ± 1	24 ± 1
Sulindac	21 ± 1	20 ± 1

It is apparent from the data discussed above that response to diuretics is a function of the relationship between the pharmacokinetic and pharmacodynamic properties of the drug. Evaluation of either is, in itself, of only marginal value. In using these drugs – in assessing reasons for abnormal response, and in devising therapeutic strategies for overcoming resistance – one must consider all these determinants of response, which have only recently become more fully elucidated.

3. Clinical Conditions of Diuretic Resistance

3.1 Non-Steroidal Anti-Inflammatory Drugs

The effect of non-steroidal anti-inflammatory drugs (NSAIDs) to decrease the natriuretic response to loop diuretics is a good example of using a pharmacological approach to probe the mechanisms of diuretic resistance and also to provide insight into the physiological role of renal prostaglandins. Clinically, on the other hand, this drug interaction is of less importance, for its magnitude of effect is small.

Initial observations that treatment with indomethacin decreased the natriuretic response to frusemide lead to speculation that endogenous prostaglandins might be mediators (or at least modulators) of the effects of loop diuretics (Patak et al., 1975). A host of studies followed using a variety of methods, most of which arrived at the same conclusion (for review, see Anderson et al., 1976; Dunn and Hood, 1977; Dunn and Zambraski, 1980; Gerber et al., 1982; Lee et al., 1976; Levenson et al., 1982; Stokes and Kokko, 1980). During the early pursuit of this area of research, however, a key potential mechanism of the interaction was often overlooked; i.e. indomethacin and other NSAIDs are organic acids which could compete with loop diuretics for active transport into the lumen. Thereby, the NSAIDs could decrease access of frusemide and other loop diuretics to the site of action and thus decrease response. Any effect on prostaglandins could, in fact, merely represent an epiphenomenon.

Consequently, we and others have gathered data assessing potential pharmacological determinants of diuretic response in the setting of administration of NSAIDs. Importantly, the effect observed is not unique to indomethacin but occurs with several different NSAIDs (Brater et al., 1985; Chennavasin et al., 1980) [and presumably all have this capacity in sufficient doses] and with other loop diuretics. There appear to be minor quantitative differences in the effect but all NSAIDs are qualitatively similar. Table II shows the lack of effect of 4 different NSAIDs on total amounts of frusemide appearing in urine. These NSAIDs decreased response to frusemide by a range of 14% (naproxen) to 32% (ibuprofen). Thus, the interaction cannot be accounted for by a decrease in the amount of diuretic reaching the active site.

Competition of NSAIDs for secretion of frusemide might affect the time course of delivery of the diuretic into urine without changing the total amount. Figure 3 shows that ibuprofen, naproxen and sulindac do not affect the time course of drug delivery. Similar results have been shown with indomethacin (Chennavasin et al., 1980). Consequently, a pharmacokinetic interaction cannot explain the effect of NSAIDs on response to frusemide.

This interaction, then, must represent a pharmacodynamic one which can be confirmed by assessing the relationship between urinary frusemide

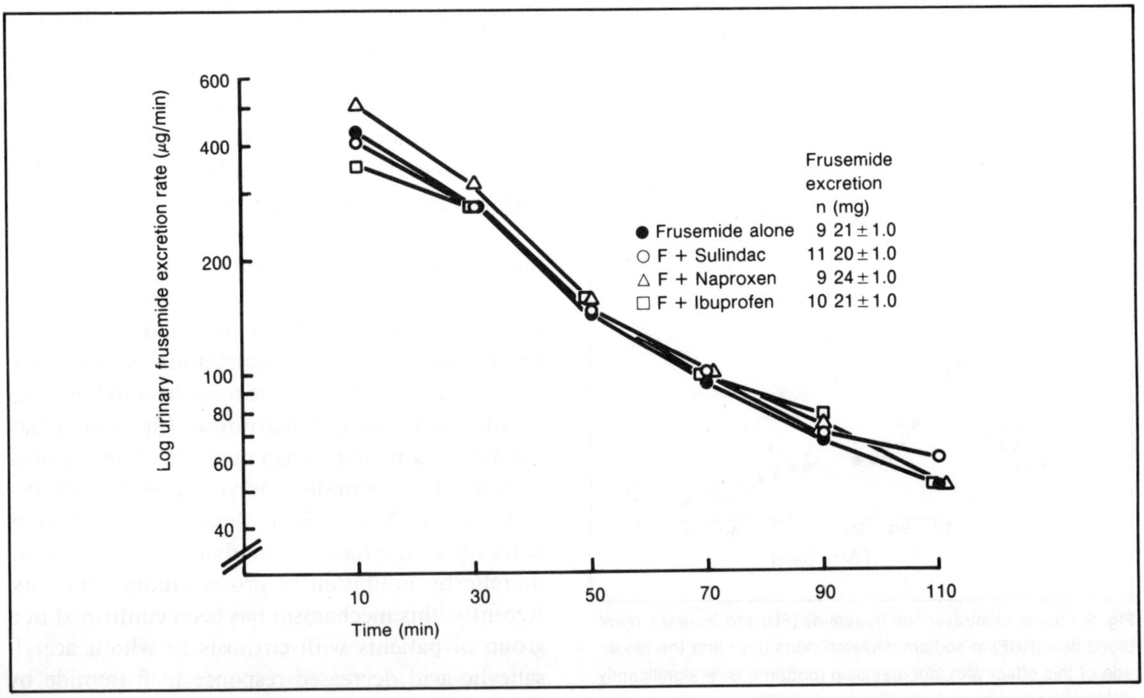

Fig. 3. Lack of effect of sulindac, naproxen or ibuprofen on total and time course of urinary excretion of frusemide (from Brater et al., 1985).

and sodium excretion; i.e. a 'dose'-response curve. This relationship is shown for indomethacin in figure 4. Similar results have been shown for ibuprofen, naproxen and sulindac, demonstrating that all of these NSAIDs have the same qualitative effect to blunt the response to frusemide (Brater et al., 1985; Chennavasin et al., 1980).

What is the mechanism of this pharmacodynamic interaction? Renal prostaglandins are known to play a potential role in renal haemodynamics and in tubular sodium homeostasis (for review, see Clive and Stoff, 1984; Dunn and Zambraski, 1980; Dunn, 1984; Garella and Matarese, 1984; Gerber et al., 1982; Levenson et al., 1982; McGiff and Wong, 1979). In turn, administration of loop diuretics causes increases in renal blood flow, and blocks tubular sodium reabsorption, both of which contribute to the overall natriuresis caused by these agents (Bourland et al., 1977; Burg, 1976; Dikshit et al., 1973; Kirkendall and Stein, 1968; Puschett

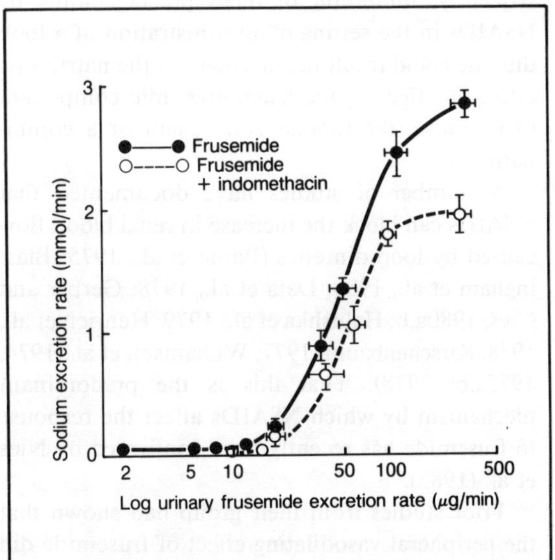

Fig. 4. Effect of indomethacin on the relationship between urinary frusemide and response (from Chennavasin et al., 1980).

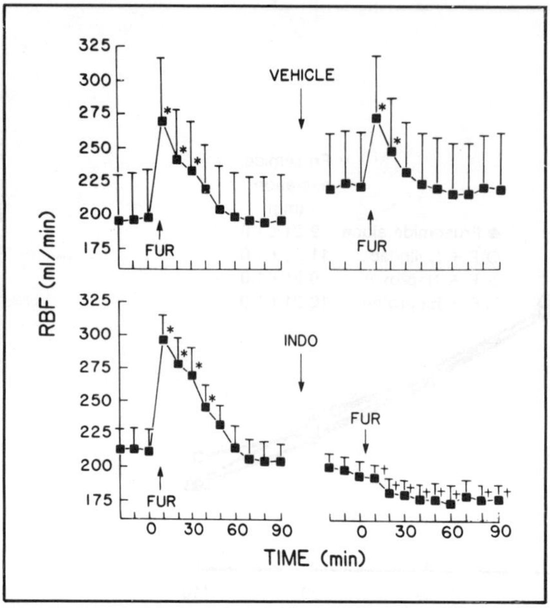

Fig. 5. Effects of intravenous frusemide (FUR) to increase renal blood flow (RBF) in sodium-depleted dogs (top) and the blockade of this effect with indomethacin (bottom); * = significantly different from control (from Nies et al., 1983).

and Goldberg, 1968; Tattersfield et al., 1974). Consequently, inhibition of renal prostaglandins by NSAIDs in the setting of administration of a loop diuretic could result in a decrease in the natriuretic effect by affecting the haemodynamic component of response, the tubular component or a combination.

A number of studies have documented that NSAIDs can block the increase in renal blood flow caused by loop diuretics (Bailie et al., 1975; Blasingham et al., 1980; Data et al., 1978; Gerber and Nies, 1980a,b; Halushka et al., 1979; Henrich et al., 1978; Kirschenbaum, 1977; Williamson et al., 1974, 1975a,b; 1978). That this is the predominant mechanism by which NSAIDs affect the response to frusemide has recently been confirmed by Nies et al. (1983).

Prior studies from their group had shown that the peripheral vasodilating effect of frusemide did not occur in sodium-replete subjects and that its occurrence in sodium-deprived subjects could be blocked by indomethacin (Gerber and Nies, 1980b). Hence, this haemodynamic effect was mediated by prostaglandins, and it could be suppressed physiologically by sodium repletion. This finding led to studies more specifically assessing renal haemodynamics (Nies et al., 1983). In sodium-depleted dogs, frusemide increased renal blood flow and as expected caused a striking natriuresis. Administration of indomethacin in this setting totally blocked the increment in renal blood flow (fig. 5) and decreased peak sodium excretion by 26%. In contrast, in sodium-replete dogs, frusemide did not increase renal blood flow, and administration of indomethacin had no effect on either renal haemodynamics or frusemide-induced natriuresis (fig. 6). Consequently, indomethacin had no effect on the tubular response to frusemide, implying that the mechanism of the NSAID-loop diuretic interaction is blockade of the renal haemodynamic effect of the diuretic by inhibition of prostaglandin synthesis. Recently, this mechanism has been confirmed in a group of patients with cirrhosis in whom acetylsalicylic acid decreased response to frusemide by blocking its renal haemodynamic effect (Planas et al., 1983).

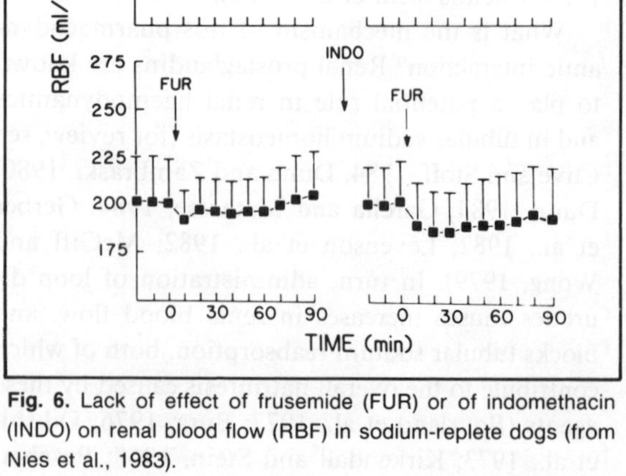

Fig. 6. Lack of effect of frusemide (FUR) or of indomethacin (INDO) on renal blood flow (RBF) in sodium-replete dogs (from Nies et al., 1983).

In summary, the NSAID-loop diuretic interaction is pharmacodynamic rather than pharmacokinetic in nature. Its mechanism is the blockade by the NSAID of increases in renal blood flow caused by the loop diuretic which in turn is mediated by diuretic-induced increases in prostaglandins.

3.2 Renal Disease

3.2.1 Renal Insufficiency

Patients with azotaemia often require large doses of loop diuretics to achieve a response. One might presume that diuretic resistance in these patients occurs solely because of decreased glomerular filtration of solute. However, as noted previously, a series of studies have suggested that a primary cause of diuretic resistance is decreased access of drug to the site of action (Rose et al., 1976a,b,c). As a consequence, large doses may be required to deliver enough diuretic into the tubular lumen to cause a response. This strategy is simply using principles of mass action. Two mechanisms exist by which secretion of frusemide might be reduced in azotaemia: (a) by decreased renal blood flow, less frusemide reaches secretory sites; and/or (b) accumulated endogenous organic acids block transport. The studies by Rose et al. (1976a,b,c) in dogs and in man showed the renal clearance of frusemide to be decreased in moderate uraemia, more so than that of tetra-ethylammonium (TEA) but similar to that of para-aminohippurate (PAH). The latter is an organic acid avidly secreted at the proximal nephron and subject to competition from endogenous organic acids of uraemia. On the other hand, TEA is an organic base that is also avidly secreted. Since accumulated acids do not compete for its secretion, it is a better index of renal blood flow in azotaemia than PAH. Since effects of uraemia on the renal clearance of frusemide were comparable to effects on clearance of PAH, and since both were diminished to a considerably greater extent than clearance of TEA, it is clear that a major limitation of access of frusemide into the urine is diminished secretion rather than decreased renal blood flow.

The effect of the decline in renal clearance of frusemide is to both decrease total amounts of drug reaching the urine and to delay the time course of its appearance (Andreasen et al., 1978; Beermann et al., 1977; Cutler et al., 1974; Rane et al., 1978). Presumably, the tubule responds normally to diuretic reaching the active site, although no data have been published to fully substantiate this hypothesis. That it is correct, however, is suggested by recent studies in the elderly.

The inexorable decline in renal function in the elderly results in decreased delivery of total amounts of frusemide into urine and to decreased response (Andreasen et al., 1983, 1984; Kerremans et al., 1983). Presumably this occurs by competition from endogenous organic acids as in patients with renal insufficiency of other causes, although no studies have addressed this question. In healthy elderly patients, the renal clearance of frusemide is approximately one-half that of young patients (Andreasen et al., 1983; Kerremans et al., 1983). These values are comparable to those of patients with mild to moderate renal insufficiency. Despite decreases in global renal function, these patients respond normally to amounts of frusemide reaching the urine when sufficient doses are administered to attain amounts on the steep portion of the dose-response curve (Andreasen et al., 1984; Kerremans et al., 1983) [fig. 7].

In summary, in patients with renal insufficiency the pharmacodynamics of response are normal when response is normalised for the decline in filtered sodium; i.e. expressed as fractional excretion. Decreased response appears to occur because of decreased delivery of drug to the site of action. Forcing sufficient amounts of drug into the urine will result in a natriuresis although the decreased filtration of sodium will limit the overall response that can be obtained. In patients requiring large doses of diuretics, the risk of ototoxicity might become limiting. In such cases, use of combination therapy using metolazone or hydrochlorothiazide may be effective by blocking sodium reabsorption at multiple tubule sites (Wollam et al., 1982).

3.2.2 Nephrotic Syndrome

Patients with nephrotic syndrome can require large doses of loop diuretics even if they have a

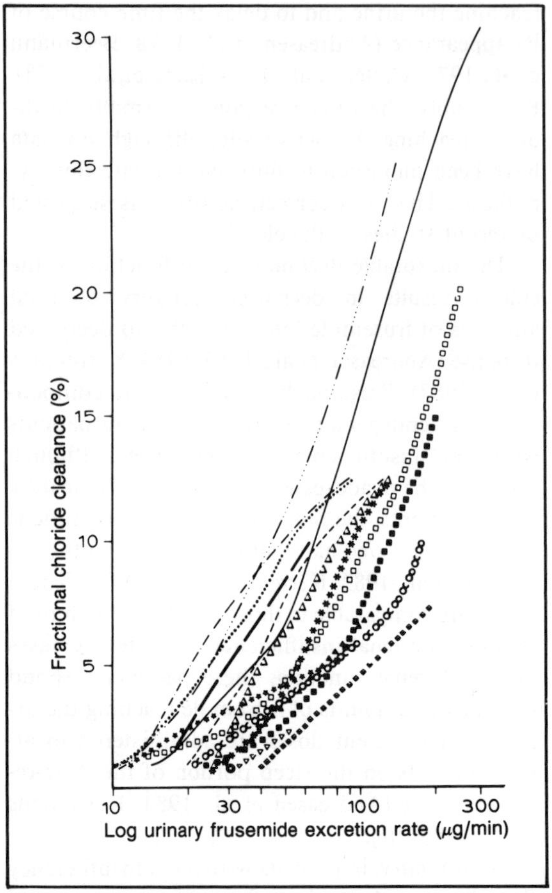

Fig. 7. Relationship between urinary frusemide excretion and fractional excretion of chloride. The solid line represents a young healthy subject (age 32 years); the remaining curves represent elderly subjects whose only abnormality is the decreased renal function of ageing (from Kerremans et al., 1983).

normal (or relatively normal) creatinine clearance. Since their glomerular filtration rate and renal blood flow are not affected, one would anticipate handling of frusemide to also be normal. Although some differences in pharmacokinetics occur due to decreased serum protein binding of the drug, both the total amount of diuretic delivered into the urine and its time course are identical to that in healthy subjects (Keller et al., 1982; Rane et al., 1978). Consequently, changes in pharmacokinetics of frusemide do not explain the resistance that occurs in this clinical setting. By exclusion then, there must be a decrease in the pharmacodynamics of response manifested by an altered 'dose'-response curve to frusemide.

A potential mechanism for this abnormal response to loop diuretics in nephrotic syndrome has been explored by Green and Mirkin (1980, 1981). They rendered rats nephrotic by pretreatment with puromycin aminonucleoside. 60 to 95% of the frusemide excreted into urine was bound to urinary protein, preventing the drug from interacting with its nephron site of action. This was reflected by a decrease in responsiveness to frusemide that was indirectly related to the amount of urinary protein. In other words, the greater the amount of protein in the urine, the greater the amount of diuretic bound, causing less frusemide to be available to exert a pharmacological effect. One would presume that response of the tubule would be normal if assessed relative to unbound or free amounts of frusemide in urine. However, this hypothesis has not yet been tested.

In summary, resistance to loop diuretics in patients with nephrotic syndrome and relatively normal renal function is pharmacodynamic in nature. The mechanism of this interaction may entail binding of the diuretic to urinary protein. If so, strategies may be developed in the future to cause endogenous displacement from protein binding. In the interim, several other approaches may prove fruitful. Administering large doses of frusemide would result in relatively more unbound drug in the urine causing greater effect. In addition, frequent administration of small doses could result in a cumulative natriuresis substantial enough to be beneficial. Importantly, each individual dose must be sufficient to elicit a response. This strategy uses the rationale discussed previously that a greater response will accrue if the steep portion of the dose-response curve is reached a number of times or if drug amounts that are maximally efficient are consistently maintained in urine, as opposed to increasing individual doses such that more time is spent at the upper plateau of the dose-response relationship. In the extreme this could be accomplished with a continuous intravenous infusion.

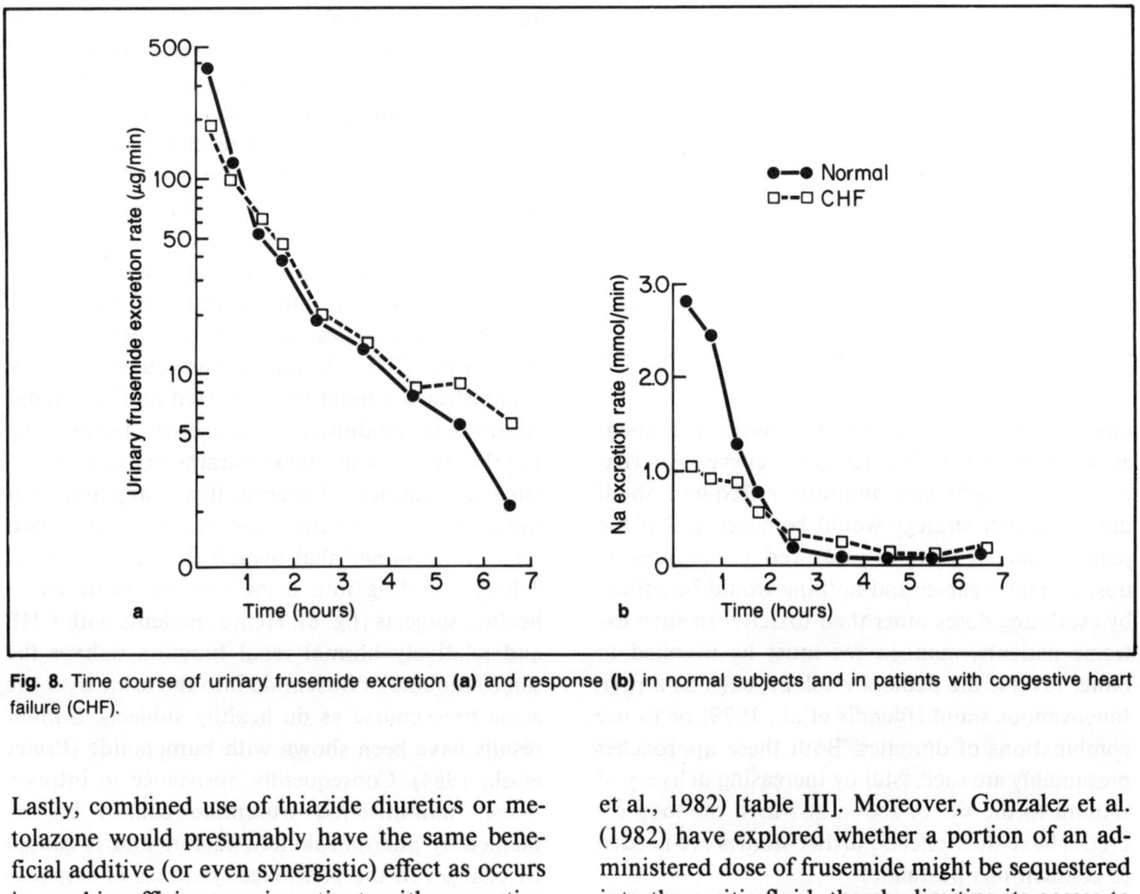

Fig. 8. Time course of urinary frusemide excretion **(a)** and response **(b)** in normal subjects and in patients with congestive heart failure (CHF).

Lastly, combined use of thiazide diuretics or metolazone would presumably have the same beneficial additive (or even synergistic) effect as occurs in renal insufficiency or in patients with congestive heart failure (see below).

3.3 Hepatic Cirrhosis

Although loop diuretics are infrequently administered to patients with cirrhotic liver disease, when they are used resistance to their effects is frequent. Minor differences in the pharmacokinetics of frusemide have been observed in this population of patients due to decreased serum protein binding. However, renal handling of the drug in such patients appears to be identical to that in healthy subjects, so that total amounts and the time course of entry of frusemide into urine are not different from normal and cannot explain the resistance that occurs (Allgulander et al., 1980; Gonzalez et al., 1982; Keller et al., 1981; Sawhney et al., 1981; Verbeeck et al., 1982) [table III]. Moreover, Gonzalez et al. (1982) have explored whether a portion of an administered dose of frusemide might be sequestered into the ascitic fluid, thereby limiting its access to the kidney. It appears that the diuretic can diffuse into the ascitic compartment, but at most this accounted for only 8% of an administered dose.

Consequently, similar to results in patients with nephrotic syndrome, pharmacokinetic mechanisms do not appear responsible for diuretic resistance in patients with cirrhosis, and a pharmacodynamic mechanism must account for the abnormal response. However, the nature of the mechanism is unclear. It presumably relates to the pathophysiology of sodium retention in this condition; namely, increased proximal tubular sodium reabsorption by unknown mechanisms and increased distal reabsorption caused by secondary hyperaldosteronism.

In view of the foregoing, what treatment strategies might prove successful? As discussed previ-

Table III. Renal clearance (ml/min) of frusemide in cirrhosis (mean ± SEM)

Healthy subjects	Patients with cirrhosis	References
95 ± 10	102 ± 16	Allgulander et al. (1980)
106 ± 12	103 ± 14	Sawhney et al. (1981)
126 ± 12	118 ± 11	Keller et al. (1981)
87 ± 8	66 ± 12	Verbeeck et al. (1982)

ously, large doses could result in more time spent at the top of the dose-response curve. Alternatively, one might also administer frequent small doses. Neither strategy would be successful if the patient had an extremely skewed or suppressed dose-response curve, and nothing would be gained by escalating doses other than toxicity. In such extreme patients, manoeuvres must be invoked to either reverse the pathophysiology, such as a peritoneovenous shunt (Blendis et al., 1979) or to use combinations of diuretics. Both these approaches presumably are successful by increasing delivery of sodium to the site of action at which the loop diuretics have their effect. Further studies are needed to confirm this postulate.

3.4 Congestive Heart Failure

Patients with congestive heart failure (CHF) probably represent the most common circumstance in which resistance to frusemide is encountered clinically. Many clinicians have presumed that considerable changes in the pharmacokinetics of loop diuretics would occur in such patients, particularly in absorption of drug from the gastrointestinal tract. Oedema of the gut, changed intestinal motility and perfusion, and a variety of other factors have been cited as potential causes of drug malabsorption in CHF (Benet et al., 1976; Benowitz and Meister, 1976). Recent data support some abnormalities of absorption, but their contribution to diuretic resistance remains unclear.

After intravenous administration of frusemide, the pharmacokinetics are relatively normal in patients with CHF. A study from our laboratory demonstrated a trend for decreased total and renal clearance of the diuretic (Brater et al., 1982) [table IV]. However, when these parameters were correlated to creatinine clearance, it was apparent that differences from normal were caused by decreased renal function and that overall the time course of delivery of drug into urine was the same as in healthy subjects (fig. 8). Hence, patients with CHF and relatively normal renal function deliver the same amounts of frusemide into the urine over the same time course as do healthy subjects. Similar results have been shown with bumetanide (Brater et al., 1984). Consequently, resistance to intravenously administered frusemide cannot be explained by pharmacokinetic factors and is caused by changes in the pharmacodynamics of response (Brater et al., 1982) [fig. 8]. The overall pattern of the dose-response curve in such patients is similar to that of patients with nephrotic syndrome and with cirrhosis. However, there is substantial variability among patients.

Some CHF patients have markedly suppressed, even flat, dose-response curves such that even very large amounts of diuretic in the urine elicit no re-

Table IV. Pharmacokinetics (mean ± SD) of frusemide in patients with congestive heart failure (CHF) [from Chennavasin et al., 1980]

	Half-life (min)	Volume of distribution (L/kg)	Clearance (ml/min/kg)	Renal clearance (ml/min/kg)
CHF (n = 16)	122 ± 64	0.20 ± 0.09	1.40 ± 1.24	0.56 ± 0.70
Healthy subjects (n = 8)	91 ± 27	0.35 ± 0.34	1.84 ± 1.02	1.05 ± 0.65

Table V. Time course of frusemide absorption (mean ± SEM) in decompensated *versus* compensated congestive heart failure (CHF) [from Vasko et al., 1985]

	Decompensated CHF	Compensated CHF
Time to peak (min)	242 ± 25	177 ± 21
Peak serum concentration (mg/L)	1.11 ± 0.24	1.57 ± 0.36

sponse. Such patients will not respond to large doses of diuretic administered singly or as frequent small doses. In this type of patient, a successful diuresis will occur only if the responsiveness of the tubule is improved – which might be achieved by alternative treatment of the primary disease such as afterload reduction. An additional potentially successful strategy which does not affect the tubule responsiveness to the loop diuretic is to use combination therapy. Clinically, this type of patient has a trivial or no response to a large parenteral dose of a loop diuretic. In fact, if a patient with CHF and relatively normal renal function does not respond to 400 to 500mg of intravenous frusemide or the equivalent of another loop diuretic, one can reliably presume that ancillary therapeutic strategies must be invoked.

On the other hand, many patients with CHF have suppressed dose-response curves but are sufficiently responsive to allow successful use of a loop diuretic. In these patients, strategies similar to those discussed in nephrotic syndrome (section 3.2.2) and cirrhosis (section 3.3) are useful.

As noted previously, many have assumed drugs to be malabsorbed in patients with CHF. However, we and others have shown that the same total amounts of frusemide are absorbed in patients with CHF as in healthy subjects; bioavailability in 25 healthy subjects was 38 ± 20% compared with 31 ± 12% in patients with CHF (Brater et al., 1982; Greither et al., 1979). Hence, an effect of CHF to diminish the total amount of drug absorbed cannot explain lack of response to orally administered frusemide in such patients.

Interestingly, however, it appears that the time course of drug absorption is affected by CHF, and that the magnitude of the effect is dependent upon the severity of the patient's disease. In patients with stable compensated CHF, absorption is delayed, so that the time at which peak amounts of either bumetanide or frusemide appear in the urine is prolonged 2-fold and the peak excretion rates of diuretic attained are approximately one-half those of healthy subjects (Brater et al., 1984). Moreover, if the time course of absorption of frusemide is assessed in the same patient while decompensated and again when compensated, the abnormalities noted above are more pronounced when the patient is in florid CHF (Vasko et al., 1985) [table V; fig. 9]. The delay in absorption and concomitant decreased peak concentrations of diuretic attained, albeit with normal total absorption of drug, could

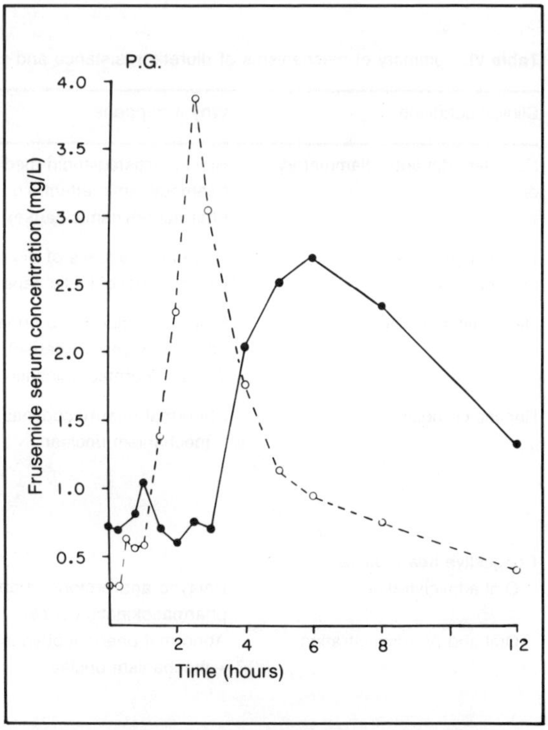

Fig. 9. Representative time course of frusemide serum concentration in a patient with congestive heart failure after oral administration of 160mg when in the decompensated state (●——●) and again when compensated (○——○) [from Vasko et al., 1985].

contribute to the diuretic resistance that occurs with oral administration in patients with CHF. Whether quantitatively this component is as important as the changed pharmacodynamics of response is unknown at present and is worthy of further study.

In summary, after intravenous administration to patients with CHF, resistance to loop diuretics is pharmacodynamic in nature. After oral administration, a pharmacokinetic component involving an altered time course of absorption of drug may also be contributory. To circumvent the latter component, the drug can be administered intravenously. However, if for some reason this were not possible, a large oral dose should eventually result in delayed attainment of amounts of drug in urine comparable to those after intravenous administration. Since peak concentrations are approximately one-half normal in this circumstance, and since the bioavailability of frusemide is approximately 40%, an oral dose 4 times larger than an effective intravenous dose would be necessary. Since bumetanide is 80% bioavailable, an oral dose twice the effective intravenous dose should suffice. This strategy would allow a peak concentration to be achieved comparable to that with intravenous administration. Hence, if an intravenous dose that causes a response is known, this extrapolation will provide an oral dose that should cause a response. It must be remembered, however, that the altered time course of absorption will also play a role. If the change causes more drug to stay at the steep portion of the dose-response curve for longer times, a greater overall response might occur relative to the intravenous dose. Whether this occurs should depend on the parameters of the individual's dose-response curve and on administering a dose sufficient that effective amounts of diuretic reach the urine.

Table VI. Summary of mechanisms of diuretic resistance and possible therapeutic strategies (IV = intravenous)

Clinical condition	Why it happens	What to do about it
Non-steroidal anti-inflammatory drugs	Blocks prostaglandin-mediated haemodynamic effect (i.e. pharmacodynamic cause)	More frequent doses
Renal insufficiency (including ageing)	Decreased access of diuretic to the urine (i.e. pharmacokinetic cause)	Larger doses. Combination therapy[a]
Nephrotic syndrome	Binding of diuretic to urinary protein (i.e. pharmacodynamic cause). ?Other pharmacodynamic causes	Larger doses. Frequent small doses or IV infusion. Combination therapy[a]
Hepatic cirrhosis	Abnormal pharmacodynamics of response – mechanism unclear	Larger doses. Frequent small doses. Alternative treatments of primary disease; e.g. peritoneovenous shunts. Combination therapy[a]
Congestive heart failure		
Oral administration	Delayed and prolonged absorption (i.e. pharmacokinetic cause)	IV administration
Oral and IV administration	Abnormal pharmacodynamics of response – mechanism unclear	Larger doses. Frequent small doses or IV infusion. Alternative treatments of primary disease; e.g. afterload reduction. Combination therapy[a]

a See text for further details.

In patients resistant to intravenous doses of loop diuretics, strategies similar to those suggested for cirrhosis can be attempted. A large dose can be given to extend the plateau of the dose-response curve. Alternatively, frequent administration of smaller effective doses could result in an overall beneficial cumulative effect. Theoretically, administering the dose as a continuous infusion over several hours should be more effective than giving the same dose as an intravenous bolus (presuming one gives an effective dose), and this approach could also be attempted (Kaojarern et al., 1982; Lawson et al., 1978). If these strategies prove unsuccessful, other treatments of the primary disease should be instituted if they have not been already. Improving cardiovascular haemodynamics by afterload reduction has been shown to increase the response to frusemide (Nomura et al., 1981).

A last manoeuvre that can be employed is to add other diuretics such as metolazone that decrease sodium reabsorption at nephron sites proximal to the site of action of the loop diuretics. Presumably by blocking solute reabsorption proximally, these diuretics allow delivery of sodium to the loop of Henle where the activity of the loop diuretics can then become manifest, often resulting in a synergistic rather than additive response (Epstein et al., 1977; Gunstone et al., 1971; Olesen, 1971; Olesen and Sigurd, 1971; Olesen et al., 1970; Oster et al., 1983; Ram and Reichgott, 1977; Sigurd and Olesen, 1978; Sigurd et al., 1975). If one invokes this strategy, it is important to realise that the effect may not occur quickly, since metolazone in particular is absorbed very slowly. Hence, if an effect is needed quickly, acetazolamide can be given intravenously followed by a loop diuretic (Rodicio and Hernando, 1977).

4. Conclusion

The different mechanisms for diuretic resistance require different therapeutic strategies. Table VI offers a summary of what is known to date, much of which has been learned recently by applying pharmacological approaches to this often vexing clinical problem. Many potentially fruitful avenues of research remain, the results of which should allow more rational, specific, and hopefully successful therapy.

References

Allgulander, C.; Beermann, B. and Sjogren, A.: Frusemide pharmacokinetics in patients with liver disease. Clinical Pharmacokinetics 5: 570-575 (1980).

Anderson, R.J.; Berl, T.; McDonald, K.M. and Schrier, R.W.: Prostaglandins: Effects on blood pressure, renal blood flow, sodium and water excretion. Kidney International 10: 205-215 (1976).

Andreasen, F.; Hansen, U.; Husted, S.E. and Jansen, J.A.: The pharmacokinetics of frusemide are influenced by age. British Journal of Clinical Pharmacology 16: 391-397 (1983).

Andreasen, F.; Hansen, U.; Husted, S.E.; Mogensen, C.E. and Pedersen, E.B.: The influence of age on renal and extrarenal effects of furosemide. British Journal of Clinical Pharmacology 18: 65-74 (1984).

Andreasen, F.; Hansen, H.E. and Mikkelsen, E.: Pharmacokinetics of furosemide in anephric patients and in normal subjects. European Journal of Clinical Pharmacology 13: 41-48 (1978).

Bailie, M.D.; Barbour, J.A. and Hook, J.B.: Effects of indomethacin on furosemide-induced changes in renal blood flow. Proceedings of the Society of Experimental Biology and Medicine 148: 1173-1176 (1975).

Bartha, J. and Hably, C.: Effect of indomethacin on extracellular space, sodium compartment and sodium excretion in saline loaded rats. Acta Physiologica Academiae Scintlarum Hungaricae 51: 335-342 (1978).

Beerman, B.; Dalen, E. and Lindstrom, B.: Elimination of furosemide in healthy subjects and in those with renal failure. Clinical Pharmacology and Therapeutics 22: 70-78 (1977)

Benet, L.Z.; Greither, A. and Meister, W.: Gastrointestinal absorption of drugs in patients with cardiac failure; in Benet et al. (Eds) The Effect of Disease States on Drug Pharmacokinetics, pp. 33-50 (American Pharmaceutical Association, Academy of Pharmaceutical Sciences, Washington, D.C. 1976).

Benowitz, N.L. and Meister, W.: Pharmacokinetics in patients with cardiac failure. Clinical Pharmacokinetics 1: 389-405 (1976).

Blasingham, M.C.; Shade, R.E.; Share, L. and Nasjletti, A.: The effect of meclofenamate on renal blood flow in the unanesthetized dogs: Relation to renal prostaglandins and sodium balance. Journal of Pharmacology and Experimental Therapeutics 214: 1-4 (1980).

Blendis, L.M.; Greig, P.D.; Langer, B.; Baigrie, R.S.; Ruse, J. and Taylor, B.R.: The renal and haemodynamic effects of the peritoneovenous shunt for intractable hepatic ascites. Gastroenterology 77: 250-257 (1979).

Bourland, W.A.; Day, D.K. and Williamson, H.E.: The role of the kidney in the early nondiuretic action of furosemide to reduce elevated left atrial pressure in the hypervolemic dog. Journal of Pharmacology and Experimental Therapeutics 202: 221-229 (1977).

Branch, R.A.; Roberts, C.J.C.; Homeida, M. and Levine, D.: Determinants of response to frusemide in normal subjects. British Journal of Clinical Pharmacology 4: 121-127 (1977).

Brater, D.C.: Pharmacodynamic considerations in the use of diuretics. Annual Review of Pharmacology and Toxicology 23: 45-62 (1983).

Brater, D.C.: Effects of probenecid on furosemide response. Clinical Pharmacology and Therapeutics 23: 259-265 (1978).

Brater, D.C.; Anderson, S.A.; Baird, B. and Campbell, W.B.: Effects of ibuprofen, naproxen, and sulindac on prostaglandins

in man. Kidney International 27: 66-73 (1985).
Brater, D.C.; Day, B.; Burdette, A. and Anderson, S.: Bumetanide and furosemide in heart failure. Kidney International 26: 183-189 (1984).
Brater, D.C.; Seiwell, R.; Anderson, S.; Burdette, A.; Dehmer, G.J. and Chennavasin, P.: Absorption and disposition of furosemide in congestive heart failure. Kidney International 22: 171-176 (1982).
Burg, M.B.: Tubular chloride transport and the mode of action of some diuretics. Kidney International 9: 189-197 (1976).
Chennavasin, P.; Seiwell, R. and Brater, D.C.: Pharmacokinetic-dynamic analysis of the indomethacin-furosemide interaction in man. Journal of Pharmacology and Experimental Therapeutics 215: 77-81 (1980).
Chennavasin, P.; Seiwell, R.; Brater, D.C. and Liang, W.M.M.: Pharmacodynamic analysis of the furosemide-probenecid interaction in man. Kidney International 16: 187-195 (1979).
Clive, D.M. and Stoff, J.S.: Renal syndromes associated with nonsteroidal anti-inflammatory drugs. New England Journal of Medicine 310: 563-572 (1984).
Cutler, R.E.; Forrey, A.W.; Christopher, T.G. and Kimpel, B.M.: Pharmacokinetics of furosemide in normal subjects and functionally anephric patients. Clinical Pharmacology and Therapeutics 15: 588-596 (1974).
Data, J.L.; Rane, A.; Gerkens, J.; Wilkinson, G.R.; Nies, A.S. and Branch, R.A.: The influence of indomethacin on the pharmacokinetics, diuretic response and hemodynamics of furosemide in the dog. Journal of Pharmacology and Experimental Therapeutics 206: 431-438 (1978).
Dikshit, K.; Vyden, J.K.; Forrester, J.S.; Chatterjee, K.; Prakash, R. and Swan, H.J.C.: Renal and extrarenal hemodynamic effects of furosemide in congestive heart failure after acute myocardial infarction. New England Journal of Medicine 288: 1087-1090 (1973).
Dunn, M.J.: Nonsteroidal anti-inflammatory drugs and renal function. Annual Reviews of Medicine 35: 411-428 (1984).
Dunn, M.J. and Hood, V.L.: Prostaglandins and the kidney. American Journal of Physiology 233: F169-F184 (1977).
Dunn, M.J. and Zambraski, E.D.: Renal effects of drugs that inhibit prostaglandin synthesis. Kidney International 18: 609-622 (1980).
Garella, S. and Matarese, R.A.: Renal effects of prostaglandins and clinical adverse effects of nonsteroidal anti-inflammatory agents. Medicine 63: 165-181 (1984).
Epstein, M.; Lepp, B.A.; Hoffman, D.S. and Levinson, R.: Potentiation of furosemide by metolazone in refractory edema. Current Therapeutic Research 21: 656-667 (1977).
Fuller, R.; Hoppel, C. and Ingalls, S.T.: Furosemide kinetics in patients with hepatic cirrhosis with ascites. Clinical Pharmacology and Therapeutics 30: 461-467 (1981).
Gerber, J.G. and Nies, A.S.: Furosemide-induced renal vasodilation: The role of the release of arachidonic acid. Advances in Prostaglandin Thromboxane Research 7: 1079-1082 (1980a).
Gerber, J.G. and Nies, A.S.: Furosemide-induced vasodilation: Importance of the state of hydration and filtration. Kidney International 18: 454-459 (1980b).
Gerber, J.G.; Anderson, R.J.; Schrier, R.W. and Nies, A.S.: Prostaglandins and the regulation of renal circulation and function; in J.A. Oates (Ed.) Prostaglandins and the Cardiovascular System, pp. 227-254 (New York 1982).
Gonzalez, G.; Arancibia, A.; Rivas, M.I.; Caro, P. and Antezana, C.: Pharmacokinetics of furosemide in patients with hepatic cirrhosis. European Journal of Clinical Pharmacology 22: 315-320 (1982).
Green, T.P. and Mirkin, B.L.: Furosemide disposition in normal and proteinuric rats: Urinary drug-protein binding as a determinant of drug excretion. Journal of Pharmacology and Experimental Therapeutics 218: 122-127 (1981).
Green, T.P. and Mirkin, B.L.: Resistance of proteinuric rats to furosemide: Urinary drug protein binding as a determinant of drug effect. Life Sciences 26: 623-630 (1980).
Greither, A.; Goldman, S.; Edelen, J.S.; Benet, L.Z. and Cohn, K.: Pharmacokinetics of furosemide in patients with congestive heart failure. Pharmacology 19: 121-131 (1979).
Gunstone, R.F.; Wing, A.J.; Shani, H.G.P.; Njemo, D. and Sabuka, E.M.W.: Clinical experience with metolazone in fifty-two African patients: Synergy with frusemide. Postgraduate Medical Journal 47: 789-793 (1971).
Halushka, P.V.; Margolius, H.; Allen, H. and Conradi, E.C.: Urinary excretion of prostaglandin E like material and kallikrein: Effects of furosemide. Prostaglandins 18: 359-368 (1979).
Hendrich, W.L.; Anderson, R.J.; Berns, A.S.; McDonald, K.M.; Paulsen, P.J. et al.: The role of renal nerves and prostaglandins in control of renal hemodynamics and plasma renin activity during hypotensive hemorrhage in the dog. Journal of Clinical Investigation 61: 744-750 (1978).
Homeida, M.; Roberts, C. and Branch, R.A.: Influence of probenecid and spironolactone on furosemide kinetics and dynamics in man. Clinical Pharmacology and Therapeutics 22: 402-409 (1977).
Honari, J.; Blair, A. and Cutler, R.: Effects of probenecid on furosemide kinetics and natriuresis in man. Clinical Pharmacology and Therapeutics 22: 395-401 (1977).
Kaojarern, S.; Day, B. and Brater, D.C.: The time course of delivery of furosemide into urine is an independent determinant of overall response. Kidney International 22: 69-74 (1982).
Keller, E.; Hoppe-Seyler, G.; Mumm, R. and Schollmeyer, P.: Influence of hepatic cirrhosis and end-stage renal disease on pharmacokinetics and pharmacodynamics of furosemide. European Journal of Clinical Pharmacology 20: 27-33 (1981).
Keller, E.; Hoppe-Seyler, G. and Schollmeyer, P.: Disposition and diuretic effect of furosemide in the nephrotic syndrome. Clinical Pharmacology and Therapeutics 32: 442-449 (1982).
Kelly, R.A.; Wilcox, C.S.; Mitch, W.E.; Meyer, T.W.; Souney, P.F. et al.: Response of the kidney to furosemide. II. Effect of captopril on sodium balance. Kidney International 24: 233-239 (1983).
Kerremans, A.L.M.; Tan, Y.; van Baars, H.; van Ginneken, C.A.M. and Gribnau, F.W.J.: Furosemide kinetics and dynamics in aged patients. Clinical Pharmacology and Therapeutics 34: 181-189 (1983).
Kirkendall, W.M. and Stein, J.H.: Clinical pharmacology of furosemide and ethacrynic acid. American Journal of Cardiology 22: 162-167 (1968).
Kirschenbaum, M.A.: The effect of prostaglandin inhibition on the natriuresis of drug-induced renal vasodilatation. Prostaglandins 13: 1103-1112 (1977).
Lawson, D.H.; Gray, J.M.B.; Henry, D.A. and Tilstone, W.J.: Continuous infusion of frusemide in refractory oedema. British Medical Journal 2: 476 (1978).
Lee, J.B.; Patak, R.V. and Mookerjee, B.K.: Renal prostaglandins and the regulation of blood pressure and sodium and water homeostasis. American Journal of Medicine 60: 798-816 (1976).
Levenson, D.J.; Simmons, C.E. and Brenner, B.M.: Arachidonic acid metabolism, prostaglandins and the kidney. American Journal of Medicine 72: 354-374 (1982).
McGiff, J.C. and Wong, P.Y.-K.: Compartmentalization of prostaglandins and prostacyclin within the kidney: Implications for renal function. Federation Proceedings 38: 89-93 (1979).
Nies, A.S.; Gal, J.; Fadul, S. and Gerber, J.G.: Indomethacin-furosemide interaction: The importance of renal blood flow. Journal of Pharmacology and Experimental Therapeutics 226: 27-32 (1983).
Nomura, A.; Yasuda, H.; Minami, M.; Akimoto, T.; Miyazaki, K. and Arita, T.: Effect of furosemide in congestive heart failure. Clinical Pharmacology and Therapeutics 30: 177-182 (1981).
Odlind, B.: Relation between renal tubular secretion and effects

of five loop diuretics. Journal of Pharmacology and Experimental Therapeutics 211: 238-244 (1979a).
Odlind, B.: Relationship between tubular secretion of furosemide and its saluretic effect. Journal of Pharmacology and Experimental Therapeutics 208: 515-521 (1979b).
Odlind, B. and Beermann, B.: Renal tubular secretion and effects of furosemide. Clinical Pharmacology and Therapeutics 27: 784-790 (1980).
Olesen, K.H.: The natriuretic effect addition of quinethazone and furosemide in congestive heart failure. Acta Medica Scandinavica 190: 229-232 (1971).
Olesen, K.H. and Sigurd, B.: The supra-additive natriuretic effect addition of quinethazone or bendroflumethazide during long-term treatment with furosemide and spironolactone. Acta Medica Scandinavica 190: 233-240 (1971).
Olesen, K.H.; Dupont, B. and Flensted-Jensen, E.: The combined diuretic action of quinethazone and furosemide in congestive heart failure. Acta Medica Scandinavica 187: 33-40 (1970).
Oster, J.R.; Epstein, M. and Smoller, S.: Combined therapy with thiazide-type and loop diuretic agents for resistant sodium retention. Annals of Internal Medicine 99: 405-406 (1983).
Patak, R.V.; Mookerjee, B.K.; Bentzel, C.J.; Hysert, P.E.; Babej, M. and Lee, J.B.: Antagonism of the effects of furosemide by indomethacin in normal and hypertensive men. Prostaglandins 10: 649-659 (1975).
Planas, R.; Arroyo, V.; Rimola, A.; Perez-Ayuso, R.M. and Rodes, J.: Acetylsalicylic acid suppresses the renal hemodynamic effect and reduces the diuretic action of furosemide in cirrhosis with ascites. Gastroenterology 84: 247-252 (1983).
Puschett, J.B. and Goldberg, M.: The acute effects of furosemide on acid and electrolyte excretion in man. Journal of Laboratory and Clinical Medicine 71: 666-677 (1968).
Ram, C.V.S. and Reichgott, M.J.: Treatment of loop-diuretic resistant edema by the addition of metolazone. Current Therapeutic Research 22: 686-691 (1977).
Rane, A.; Villeneuve, J.P.; Stone, W.J.; Nies, A.S.; Wilkinson, G.R. and Branch, R.A.: Plasma binding and disposition of furosemide in the nephrotic syndrome and in uremia. Clinical Pharmacology and Therapeutics 24: 199-207 (1978).
Rodicio, J.L. and Harnando, L.: Effects and interactions of furosemide and acetazolamide on tubular function in rat kidney. Revista Española de Fisiologia 33: 113-118 (1977).
Rose, H.J.; O'Malley, K. and Pruitt, A.W.: Depression of renal clearance of furosemide in man by azotemia. Clinical Pharmacology and Therapeutics 21: 141-146 (1976a).
Rose, H.J.; Pruitt, A.W.; Dayton, P.G. and McNay, J.L.: Relationship of urinary furosemide excretion rate to natriuretic effect in experimental azotemia. Journal of Pharmacology and Experimental Therapeutics 199: 490-497 (1976b).
Rose, H.J.; Pruitt, A.W. and McNay, J.L.: Effect of experimental azotemia on renal clearance of furosemide in the dog. Journal of Pharmacology and Experimental Therapeutics 196: 238-247 (1976c).
Sawhney, V.K.; Gregory, P.B.; Swezey, S.E. and Blaschke, T.F.: Furosemide disposition in cirrhotic patients. Gastroenterology 81: 1012-1016 (1981).
Sigurd, B. and Olesen, K.H.: Comparative natriuretic and diuretic efficacy of theophylline ethylenediamine and of bendroflumethiazide during long-term treatment with the potent diuretic bumetanide. Acta Medica Scandinavica 203: 113-119 (1978).
Sigurd, B.; Olesen, K.H. and Wennevold, A.: The supra-additive natriuretic effect addition of bendroflumethiazide and bumetanide in congestive heart failure. Permutation trial tests in patients in long-term treatment with bumetanide. American Heart Journal 89: 163-170 (1975).
Stokes, J.B. and Kokko, J.P.: Renal tubular sites of action of prostaglandins on salt transport; in Prostaglandins in Cardiovascular and Renal Function, pp. 425-442 (Spectrum Publications, 1980).
Tattersfield, A.E.; McNicol, M.W. and Sillett, R.W.: Haemodynamic effects of intravenous frusemide in patients with myocardial infarction and left ventricular failure. Clinical Science and Molecular Medicine 46: 253-264 (1974).
Vasko, M.R.; Cartwright, D.B.; Knochel, J.P.; Nixon, J.B. and Brater, D.C.: Furosemide absorption altered in decompensated congestive heart failure. Annals of Internal Medicine 102: 314-318 (1985).
Verbeeck, R.K.; Patwardhan, R.V.; Villeneuve, J.-P.; Wilkinson, G..R and Branch, R.A.: Furosemide disposition in cirrhosis. Clinical Pharmacology and Therapeutics 31: 719-725 (1982).
Wilcox, C.S.; Mitch, W.E.; Kelly, R.A.; Skorecki, K.; Meyer, T.W. et al.: Response of the kidney to furosemide. I. Effects of salt intake and renal compensation. Journal of Laboratory and Clinical Medicine 102: 450-458 (1983).
Williamson, H.E.; Bourland, W.A.; Marchand, G.R.; Farley, D.B. and VanOrden, D.E.: Furosemide induced release of prostaglandin E to increase renal blood flow. Proceedings for the Society of Experimental and Biological Medicine 150: 104-106 (1975a).
Williamson, H.E.; Bourland, W.A. and Marchand, G.R.: Inhibition of ethacrynic acid induced increase in renal blood flow by indomethacin. Prostaglandins 25: 297-301 (1974).
Williamson, H.E.; Bourland, W.A. and Marchand, G.R.: Inhibition of furosemide induced increase in renal blood flow by indomethacin. Proceedings of the Society of Experimental and Biological Medicine 148: 164-167 (1975b).
Williamson, H.E.; Gaffney, G.R.; Bourland, W.A.; Farley, D.B. and VanOrden, D.E.: Phenylbutazone-induced decrease in renal blood flow. Journal of Pharmacology and Experimental Therapeutics 204: 130-134 (1978).
Wollam, G.L.; Tarazi, R.C.; Bravo, E.L. and Dustan, H.P.: Diuretic potency of combined hydrochlorothiazide and furosemide therapy in patients with azotemia. American Journal of Medicine 72: 929-938 (1982).

Address for correspondence and reprints: Dr *D. Craig Brater*, The University of Texas Health Science Center at Dallas, Departments of Pharmacology and Internal Medicine, Southwestern Medical School, 5323 Harry Hines Boulevard, Dallas, TX 75235 (USA).

Drugs 30: 444-460 (1985)
0012-6667/85/0011-0444/$08.50/0

Risk of Haemorrhage Associated with Long Term Anticoagulant Therapy

Mark N. Levine, Gary Raskob and *Jack Hirsh*

Departments of Medicine, and Clinical Epidemiology and Biostatistics, McMaster University and Ontario Cancer Foundation Hamilton Clinic, Hamilton

Summary

This literature review was conducted to determine: (a) the rate of bleeding (major, minor and fatal) during long term oral anticoagulant therapy (greater than 4 weeks) in various disorders (ischaemic cerebrovascular disease, prosthetic cardiac valves, chronic atrial fibrillation, ischaemic heart disease and venous thrombosis); and (b) the clinical and laboratory risk factors which predispose such patients to bleeding. Using strictly defined methodological criteria, 167 studies were evaluated and classified into 1 of 5 categories based on the strength of the study design, with level I (randomised trials) representing studies which provided the most reliable information and level V (case series) the least reliable.

The risk of bleeding was substantial, and was most marked in patients with ischaemic cerebrovascular disease (29%), ischaemic heart disease (19%) and venous thromboembolism (23%). Major bleeding in venous thrombosis and cerebrovascular disease was frequently associated with an underlying risk factor. In venous thromboembolism these coexisting conditions (cancer, recent surgery and paraplegia) were also predisposing factors for thrombosis. In cerebrovascular disease major bleeding was almost always intracerebral, possibly because of associated hypertension or the cerebrovascular disease per se. *We were unable to determine whether bleeding events were concentrated soon after commencing anticoagulant therapy. Haemorrhagic episodes frequently occurred when the prothrombin time (or thrombotest) was within the targeted therapeutic range, but the relationship between bleeding and the level of anticoagulant therapy was properly evaluated in only 1 study (in venous thrombosis) which demonstrated that the risk of bleeding was reduced by using a less intense anticoagulant regimen.*

In conclusion, the risk of bleeding during oral anticoagulant therapy is substantial. Our analysis was limited by the lack of concise reporting of clinical and laboratory information and we would suggest that future clinical studies report these in greater detail.

1. Study Objectives

The main complication of anticoagulation therapy is bleeding. We have conducted a literature review of long term anticoagulant therapy to determine the rate of bleeding in patients with various clinical disorders and risk factors which predispose to bleeding. Long term therapy was defined as treatment with anticoagulants for greater than 4 weeks. The analysis was performed in patients with: ischaemic cerebrovascular disease (completed stroke, stroke-in-evolution, and transient ischaemic attacks); prosthetic cardiac valves; chronic atrial fibrillation with and without associated rheumatic valvular disease; ischaemic heart disease (angina, myocardial infarction); and venous thromboembolic disease.

Each report was reviewed seeking the following information:

1. Description of the cohort of patients being treated, including age, sex, indication for anticoagulant therapy, and duration of anticoagulant therapy (patient-years of exposure)
2. Evidence that bias was avoided by having a concurrent randomised placebo-treated control group
3. A clear description of the criteria used for assessing bleeding and evaluating the severity of bleeding
4. Evidence that a sufficient number of patients were treated to provide acceptable confidence limits for the reported rate of bleeding; for example, if the observed rate of bleeding is 15%, then 50 patients should be followed to achieve 95% confidence limits of ± 5%
5. The defined therapeutic range used for anticoagulant control and the type of thromboplastin used (whether human, rabbit or bovine in origin)
6. The results of the prothrombin time (PT) immediately before the haemorrhagic episode in patients who bled as well as the results of the prothrombin time obtained at regular intervals throughout the period of treatment in patients who both did and did not bleed
7. The interval between commencing anticoagulant therapy and the occurrence of bleeding, in addition to the number of patients exposed to anticoagulant therapy at each reported time of bleeding
8. A description of coexisting diseases and concomitant therapy, as hypertension, malignancy, ulcer disease and other drug therapy both in patients who bled and in those who did not bleed.

We were not able to achieve all of our objectives because the aim of most of the published reports was to evaluate the efficacy of anticoagulant therapy and not its safety. Hence, the information we were seeking was not always present. We also encountered difficulty in comparing the relationship between the intensity of anticoagulant therapy and the incidence of bleeding because of lack of information on the methods for monitoring anticoagulant therapy. Nevertheless, it was possible to obtain valid estimates of bleeding rates for each of the disorders of interest, and for some of the disorders we were able to determine the contribution of specific risk factors for both the occurrence of bleeding and its severity. Very few studies reported their success in maintaining patients within the stated therapeutic range, an important limitation of the analysis.

2. *Methods*

We analysed the results for each of the clinical indications separately. Potentially useful articles were identified through a computerised literature search and through relevant review articles. The reports were classified into 1 of 5 categories based on the strength of the study design; level I representing studies which provided the most reliable information and level V the least reliable:

1. *Level I:* randomised controlled trials with sufficient patient numbers (arbitrarily set at greater than 50) to provide a reliable index of bleeding, or in which a clinically and statistically important difference in bleeding was detected.

2. *Level II:* randomised controlled trials which either contained too few patients to provide a reliable index of the rate of bleeding or in which the method used to assess bleeding was not adequately described.

3. *Level III:* non-randomised prospective cohort studies between patients who did and did not receive anticoagulants, followed over the same time period.

4. *Level IV:* prospective cohort studies without a no-treatment control group.

5. *Level V:* non-randomised retrospective studies (case series), with or without historical control.

Case reports were not included in our analysis since they do not provide a valid estimate of bleeding rates or risk factors.

The major analysis for each of the indications was derived from studies in the highest category.

For example, there were a number of Level I studies available for ischaemic cerebrovascular disease, myocardial infarction and venous thromboembolism, whereas only Level IV studies were available for patients with prosthetic cardiac valves and only Level V studies for atrial fibrillation.

The definition of major and minor bleeding differed between studies. For the purposes of our review we classified episodes of haemorrhage as major if they were intracranial or retroperitoneal, or if they led directly to death, hospitalisation or transfusion. All other bleeding episodes (including some gastrointestinal bleeds, and most cases of epistaxis, haematuria, ecchymosis, and haemoptysis) were classified as being minor.

The control of oral anticoagulant therapy is based on the prothrombin time (PT) test, or less commonly the thrombotest (TT). The PT result can be expressed as time (in seconds), as a ratio (patient time in seconds over control time in seconds), as an index (which is control time over patient time multiplied by 100), or as a percentage of the value for normal control plasma using a saline dilution curve. The thromboplastins used to perform the PT are derived from either human brain, rabbit brain, or a mixture of rabbit brain and rabbit lung. The thromboplastin used in the TT is derived from bovine brain. The PT obtained on the plasma of patients treated with oral anticoagulants is influenced by the source of the thromboplastin. In general, human brain thromboplastins are more sensitive to deficiencies in the vitamin K-dependent clotting factors than the commercially available rabbit brain thromboplastins, although it is possible to prepare rabbit brain thromboplastins of approximately similar sensitivities to human brain thromboplastin. For the purpose of comparison between studies, we converted the reported test results for monitoring anticoagulant therapy into the International Normalized Ratio (INR).[1] In so doing we have made the following assumptions which are likely to be approximately, but not completely, correct:

1. That thromboplastins derived from human brain are approximately equivalent to the thromboplastin standard used in establishing the International Normalized Ratio

2. That thromboplastins derived from the commercially available rabbit brain or rabbit brain and lung thromboplastins are approximately equivalent to each other in their sensitivity to the anticoagulant effects of vitamin K antagonists. This assumption is supported by the observations of Bailey et al. (1971) [the relationship between the various rabbit brain thromboplastins used in the studies and the thromboplastin used to establish the International Normalized Ratio is shown in figure 1]

3. That the relationship between the thrombotest and the International Normalized Ratio is as shown in figure 1

4. That, unless otherwise stated, studies performed in the United Kingdom used human brain thromboplastin, studies performed in the United States have used rabbit brain or rabbit brain and lung thromboplastin, and studies in Scandinavia used bovine brain thromboplastin. The source of thromboplastin was stated explicitly in all studies reviewed from Scandinavia and the United Kingdom and the thromboplastins were reported to be bovine and human brain, respectively. The source of thromboplastin was also stated for the studies with the highest levels of evidence, i.e. Levels I and II for ischaemic cerebrovascular disease and ischaemic heart disease, Level IV for prosthetic heart valves and Level I for venous thrombosis, in over 85% of the reports; and

5. In the 2 studies where the prothrombin-proconvertin test (P&P) was used (Bjerkelund, 1963; Harvald et al., 1962) the P&P test result (expressed as percentage) was equivalent to the TT percentage (Owren, 1959).

1 The International Normalized Ratio (INR) is defined as the prothrombin time ratio results which would be obtained if the WHO primary international reference thromboplastin (IRP) were used to test the plasma sample. This is based on the determination of the International Sensitivity Index (ISI) of the thromboplastin used in the local laboratory. For a prothrombin time ratio using thromboplastin having an ISI value of 'c', the INR = (observed ratio)^c; thus, for thromboplastin with an ISI of 1.413, a ratio of 2.5 is equivalent to $(2.5)^{1.413} = 3.65$ with the IRP.

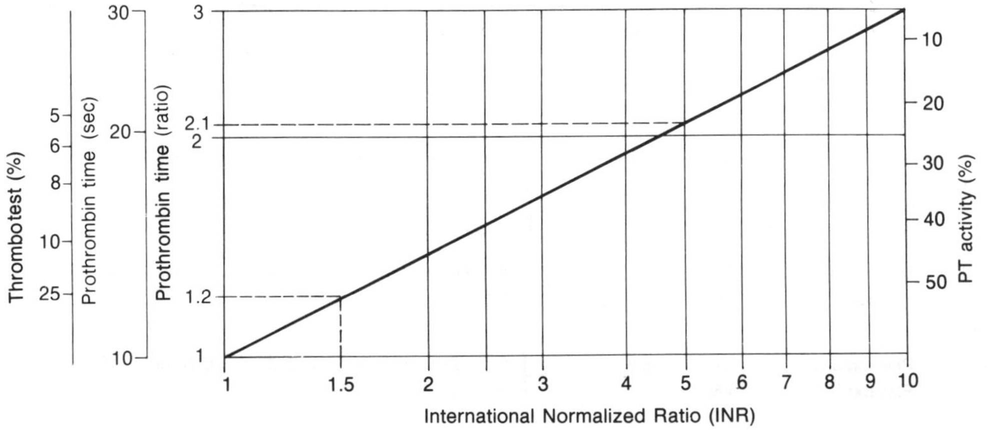

Fig. 1. Conversion of prothrombin time and thrombotest into an International Normalized Ratio (INR). See footnote, section 2 for further explanation.

3. *Results*

3.1 Ischaemic Cerebrovascular Disease

3.1.1 Level I Evidence

There were 6 studies which were classified as Level I (see table I). In only 3 of these was the duration of anticoagulant therapy clearly described (Baker, 1961; Enger and Boyesen, 1965; McDowell et al., 1963). In all 6 studies the rate of bleeding was greater in the treatment group than in the groups receiving no treatment or either low doses of anticoagulants or antiplatelet agents. The difference was statistically significant in 5 of the 6 studies and there was a strong trend in the sixth in which coumadin was compared with aspirin and dipyridamole (Olsson et al., 1980). The risk of bleeding was substantial, varying between 11.8 and 39.7%. The risk of major bleeding was also high, being 7% or more in 4 of the 6 studies (Baker, 1961; Baker et al., 1962; Enger and Boyesen, 1965; Fisher, 1961; Hill et al., 1960, 1962). Fatal haemorrhage occurred in more than 5% of patients in 4 studies (Baker, 1961; Baker et al., 1962; Enger and Boyesen, 1965; Fisher, 1961; Hill et al., 1960), and in more than 2% in the other 2 studies (McDowell et al., 1963; Olsson et al., 1980). The lowest bleeding rates were reported by Olsson et al. (1980). In this study, all patients were treated with anticoagulants for 2 months and were then randomised to either continue oral anticoagulants or to stop anticoagulants and receive antiplatelet agents. The low bleeding rates in this study might be explained by a selection bias since patients who bled before randomisation would not have been included in the analysis.

Our attempts to compare the targeted intensity of the anticoagulant effect and rate of bleeding between studies failed to reveal a clear relationship. For example, in the studies by Hill (1960, 1962) a therapeutic range of 2 to 2.5 times control with human brain thromboplastin (estimated INR 2 to 2.5) was used. This is likely to be equivalent to a PT of 1.2 to 1.4 times control using the presently available commercial rabbit brain thromboplastins; yet the rate of bleeding in Hill's study was greater than in the study reported by McDowell et al. (1963), in which the therapeutic range was 2 to 2.5 times control using rabbit brain thromboplas-

Table I. Studies analysed for incidence of bleeding in patients with ischaemic cerebrovascular disease (TIA, stroke, stroke-in-evolution). Randomised controlled trials (Level I), with >50 patients, in which bleeding episodes were described adequately [* $p < 0.001$]

References	Anticoagulant	No. of patients	Anticoagulant duration (patient-years)		Incidence of bleeding			Thromboplastin[c]	Targeted therapeutic range	INR equivalent
					total (%)	major (%)	fatal (%)[a]			
Baker (1961)	Warfarin/ dicoumarol	78	45.3	*	31 (39.7)	10 (12.8)	4 (5.1)	Rabbit	20%	5.6
	Untreated control	77			5 (6.5)	3 (3.9)	1 (1.3)			
Baker et al. (1962); Fisher (1961)	Dicoumarol	224	. . .[b]	*	88 (39.3)	18 (8.0)	12 (5.4)	Rabbit	15-25%	4.5-7.2
	Placebo	219			10 (4.6)	2 (0.9)	0			
Enger and Boyesen (1965)	Phenindione	52	96.8	*	10 (19.2)	4 (7.7)	3 (5.8)	Bovine	10-25%	1.5-2.1
	Placebo	48			0	0	0			
Hill et al. (1962)	Phenindione (high)	71	. . .[b]	*	15 (21.1)	5 (7.0)	5 (7.0)	Human	2-2.5×	2-2.5
	Phenindione (low)	71			1 (1.4)	1 (1.4)	0			
McDowell et al. (1963)	Warfarin	95	93.4	*	17 (17.9)	2 (2.1)	2 (2.1)	Rabbit	2-2.5×	4.4-7.5
	Untreated control	105			1 (1.0)	1 (1.0)	1 (1.0)			
Olsson et al. (1980)	Warfarin	68	. . .[b]		8 (11.8)	2 (2.9)	2 (2.9)	Bovine	7-15%	1.9-3.7
	Aspirin + dipyridamole	67			3 (4.5)	0	0			

a In anticoagulant groups, of 28 fatal bleeds 20 cerebral in origin.
b Long term anticoagulation, but duration uncertain.
c Test is prothrombin time when rabbit brain or human brain used, and thrombotest when bovine thromboplastin.

tin (estimated INR of 4.4 to 7.5). Similarly, Olsson et al. (1980) apparently used a more intense level of anticoagulation but reported a lower rate of bleeding than Enger (1965) [both used the thrombotest to monitor anticoagulant therapy].

Comparison of bleeding rates between studies has important limitations. However, our analysis shows that in patients with cerebrovascular disease the risk of haemorrhage, including major bleeding, was evident with relatively moderate anticoagulant therapy (INR of 2 to 2.5). In addition, there appears to be no clearcut relationship (or even a trend) between the intensity of the anticoagulant effect and the rate of bleeding.

As a group, patients with cerebrovascular disease have a high risk for bleeding. Hypertension was identified as a possible risk factor for cerebral bleeding (which was usually fatal) in 4 of the 6 studies (Baker, 1961; Baker et al., 1962; Enger and Boyesen, 1965; Hill et al., 1960). In 1 study 75% of the bleeders were hypertensive compared with 55% of the non-bleeders, which produces a relative risk of 2.4 (Baker et al., 1962).

The risk of bleeding appeared to be fairly evenly distributed throughout the duration of anticoagulant therapy, with no obvious clustering within the first few weeks or months.

Major bleeding in this group was dominated by cerebral haemorrhage. This raises the possibility that a proportion of patients in the studies reviewed (all performed before CT scanning was available) may have had a haemorrhagic stroke at presentation and the true risk of cerebral haemorrhage during anticoagulant therapy would be less if patients with haemorrhagic stroke had been excluded from analysis. However, this hypothesis is not supported by the reported bleeding rates in patients presenting with transient cerebral ischaemia (Baker, 1961; Baker et al., 1962; Fisher, 1961; Olsson et al., 1980), who showed a substantial risk of haemorrhage which was similar to that reported in patients with completed cerebral thrombosis. Therefore, within the limitations of available information we conclude that the high risk of bleeding in cerebrovascular disease is unlikely to be due to inappropriate treatment of cerebral haemorrhage, but is more likely to be related to a true risk of cerebral bleeding during anticoagulant therapy in patients with ischaemic cerebrovascular disease.

It was not possible to demonstrate a relationship between bleeding and the intensity of anticoagulant therapy. Although a number of studies documented major bleeding in association with excess hypocoagulability, major bleeding (including fatal bleeding) also occurred when the result of the PT or TT was within the targeted therapeutic range.

3.1.2 Ischaemic Cerebrovascular Disease – Level II Evidence

There were 6 randomised controlled trials in Level II (Baker et al., 1966; Buren and Ygge, 1981; Carter, 1961; Marshall and Shaw, 1959, 1960; Pearce et al., 1965; Wallace, 1964). In general, the incidence of bleeding was consistent with that found in Level I studies, although the range in incidences among studies was wider.

3.1.3 Ischaemic Cerebrovascular Disease – Level IV and V Evidence

Only a limited number of Level IV and V studies entered sufficient numbers of patients and described bleeding adequately to include in our analysis (Eriksson and Link, 1983; Olsson et al., 1976; Siekert et al., 1961; Terent and Andersson, 1980; Whisnant et al., 1978). The incidence of bleeding was high, ranging from 9 to 28%; major bleeding occurred in 4 to 9% of patients, and fatal bleeding in 4 to 9%. The most common cause of fatal bleeding was cerebral haemorrhage.

The time of the haemorrhagic event was equally distributed over the period of observation and bleeding was no more frequent in the first several months. In 2 of the studies some of the bleeders had hypertension (Siekert et al., 1961; Terent and Andersson, 1980), but the frequency of hypertension in the non-bleeders was not specified. Major bleeding was reported both in association with an excessive anticoagulant effect and with anticoagulant effects which were within the therapeutic range.

3.2 Prosthetic Heart Valves

3.2.1 Level IV Evidence

There were 4 Level IV studies of long term anticoagulant therapy in patients with prosthetic heart valves (table II). In all of these studies oral anticoagulant therapy alone was compared with a combination of oral anticoagulants and antiplatelet agents (Altman et al., 1976; Chesebro et al., 1983; Dale et al., 1977, 1980; Sullivan et al., 1971). Since none of these studies compared an oral anticoagulant with placebo or an antiplatelet agent alone, they were designated as Level IV studies (cohort) even though they were randomised trials. In 2 of the studies the duration of anticoagulant therapy was clearly documented (Altman et al., 1976; Chesebro et al., 1983). The frequency of bleeding varied between 1.2 and 10.7% in the patients treated with anticoagulant alone, and the frequency of major bleeding varied from 0 to 6.8%. Fatal bleeding did not occur in one study (Sullivan et al., 1971), but was as high as 4.1% in another (Dale et al., 1980) with most fatal bleeding being cerebral in origin.

The targeted therapeutic range was described in 2 of the 4 studies, with a desired intensity of anticoagulant therapy of INR 2.6 to 7.5 in one (Chesebro et al., 1983) and INR 2.0 to 2.2 in the second (Dale et al., 1977, 1980). The relationship between intensity of anticoagulant therapy and bleeding was not described in any of the studies. It is of interest that in 2 of the 4 studies there was a significantly greater frequency of bleeding when aspirin was added to coumadin, but not when dipyridamole was combined with coumadin (Chesebro et al., 1983; Sullivan et al., 1971). Most of the

Table II. Studies analysed for incidence of bleeding in patients with prosthetic heart valves. Randomised controlled trials (Level IV) [*p ≤ 0.05]

References	Anticoagulant	No. of patients	Anti-coagulant duration (patient-years)		Incidence of bleeding total (%)	major (%)	fatal (%)[a]	Thrombo-plastin	Targeted thera-peutic range	INR equivalent
Altman et al. (1976)	Acenocoumarin + aspirin (500mg)	57	121.8		7 (12.3)	1 (1.7)	1 (1.7)	Human	1.8-2.3×	1.8-2.3
	Acenocoumarin	65			7 (10.7)	1 (1.5)	1 (1.5)			
Chesebro et al. (1983)	Warfarin + aspirin (250mg bid)	170	166.7	*	23 (13.5)	20 (11.8)	3 (1.8)	Rabbit	1.5-2.5×	2.6-7.5
	Warfarin + dipyridamole (100mg qid)	180		*	7 (3.9)	4 (2.2)	0			
	Warfarin[b]	183			9 (4.9)	4 (2.2)	3 (1.6)			
Dale et al. (1977, 1980)	Warfarin + aspirin (500mg bid)	75	LTA[c]	*	15 (20.0)	12 (16)	1 (1.3)	Bovine	10-12%	2.0-2.2
	Warfarin	73			6 (8.2)	5 (6.8)	3 (4.1)			
Sullivan et al. (1971)	Warfarin + dipyridamole (400mg)	79	LTA[c]		3 (3.7)	2 (2.5)	2 (2.5)	Rabbit	–	–
	Warfarin	84			1 (1.2)	0	0			

a All fatal bleeds cerebral in origin.
b Non-randomised concurrent control.
c Reported to be on long term anticoagulants.

bleeding episodes during combined treatment with oral anticoagulants and aspirin were gastrointestinal in origin.

3.2.2 Prosthetic Heart Valves – Level V Evidence

Of the 53 descriptive studies[2] reviewed evaluating long term anticoagulant therapy in patients with prosthetic cardiac valves, only 28[2] mentioned bleeding complications. The reliability of the reported rates was low because there was no clear description of patient details, the duration of anticoagulant therapy was not described, and bleeding outcomes were not defined. The reported total incidence of bleeding ranged from 0 to 26%, and from 0 to 5% for fatal bleeding. Intracranial bleeding was the most common cause of fatal bleeding. Only 3 reports addressed the issue of time of bleeding and intensity of anticoagulant therapy. Thus, bleeding was equally distributed over the length of time that patients received treatment (Nunez et al., 1982); of 5 major bleeds only 2 were associated with a prolonged PT (2.5 and 3.6 times control, estimated INR 7.5 to >10) [Lieberman et al., 1978]; and of 15 major bleeds only 3 were associated with a PT of less than 10% (estimated INR 9) [Gonzalez-Lavin et al., 1978].

The study by Forfar (1979) provided some evidence for a relationship between bleeding and the intensity of anticoagulant therapy (see section 3.7). Although this study included patients with a variety of disorders, the majority of patients received anticoagulant therapy because they had prosthetic

2 Details provided on request from authors.

heart valves. Forfar reported an 8% risk of bleeding, with a 2% risk of major bleeding and a 0.4% risk of fatal bleeding. The probability of haemorrhage remained fairly constant throughout the duration of therapy. The intensity of anticoagulant treatment was mild by North American standards. A human brain thromboplastin ratio of 1.8 to 2.6 times control (INR 1.8 to 2.6) was used which is equivalent to a rabbit brain thromboplastin ratio of 1.2 to 1.5 times control.

In general, the rate of bleeding was lower in patients with prosthetic heart valves than in those with cerebrovascular disease.

3.3 Atrial Fibrillation - Level V Evidence

There are 7 studies, all Level V, describing bleeding in patients with atrial fibrillation. In only 2 studies was the frequency of bleeding adequately described, with rates of 7% and 36%, respectively (Fleming and Bailey, 1971; Foley et al., 1955).

3.4 Ischaemic Heart Disease

3.4.1 Level I Evidence

There were 7 studies which were classified as Level I (table III). In 5 of these, anticoagulant therapy was compared with placebo or control (Bjerkelund, 1957; Harvald et al., 1962; Loeliger et al., 1967; Meuwissen et al., 1969; Sixty-Plus Reinfarction Study Research Group, 1980), in the sixth anticoagulant was compared with aspirin (EPSIM Research Group, 1982), and in the seventh anticoagulant therapy was compared with aspirin and placebo (Breddin et al., 1980). The difference in total bleeding between the anticoagulant group and the control or aspirin groups was statistically significant in all of the studies. In 3 of the studies, patients were treated with anticoagulants for variable periods prior to randomisation (Loeliger et al., 1967; Meuwissen et al., 1969; Sixty-Plus Reinfarction Study Research Group, 1980). The risk of total bleeding was substantial, and varied between 3.8 and 36.5%. The incidence of major bleeding was variable; in 1 study there were no major bleeding episodes (Meuwissen et al., 1969), in 4 studies major bleeding episodes occurred in less than 5% of patients (Breddin et al., 1980; EPSIM Research Group, 1982; Loeliger et al., 1967; Sixty-Plus Reinfarction Study Research Group, 1980) and in 2 studies major bleeding occurred in greater than 10% of patients (Bjerkelund, 1957; Harvald et al., 1962). Fatal haemorrhages occurred less frequently than for stroke patients and those with prosthetic heart valves, the incidence ranging from nil in 3 studies (Breddin et al., 1980; Loeliger et al., 1967; Meuwissen et al., 1969), to 0.7 to 2.9% (Bjerkelund, 1957; EPSIM Research Group, 1982; Harvald et al., 1962; Sixty-Plus Reinfarction Study Research Group, 1980). When fatal bleeding occurred it was most commonly due to intracranial bleeding.

In none of these studies was the time of the bleeding event specified. Two of the studies (Breddin et al., 1980; EPSIM Research Group, 1982) included a group which received aspirin alone at a dose of 1.5g daily. In the EPSIM study there was significantly more bleeding in the anticoagulant group than the aspirin group, but there was significantly more gastritis and peptic ulcer disease in the aspirin group. In the second study by Breddin and colleagues no difference was detected in the incidence of bleeding between the anticoagulant and aspirin group. There were, however, more gastrointestinal ‘complaints’ in the aspirin group.

In 2 studies (Bjerkelund, 1957; Sixty-Plus Reinfarction Study Research Group, 1980) underlying risk factors for bleeding were described. In the Sixty-Plus study (1980, 1982), 4 patients with malignancies had bleeding episodes, and in the studies by Bjerkelund (1957, 1963) 2 patients bled from malignant lesions. In Bjerkelund's study, 4 of 5 incidents of cerebral bleeding occurred in hypertensive patients, 3 patients bled from duodenal ulcers, 2 had haematuria due to underlying urolithiasis, and 1 bled from an occult gastric carcinoma.

It is not possible from these reports to assess the relationship between bleeding and the intensity of anticoagulant therapy. Although a number of studies noted that major bleeding occurred when the PT was outside the targeted therapeutic range, bleeding often occurred with only moderately intense anticoagulant therapy.

Table III. Studies analysed for incidence of bleeding in patients with ischaemic heart disease (Level I) [* p < 0.01]

References	Anticoagulant	No. of patients	Anti-coagulant duration (patient-years)		Incidence of bleeding: total (%)	major (%)	fatal (%)[a]	Thrombo-plastin	Targeted thera-peutic range (%)	INR equivalent
Sixty-Plus Reinfarction Trial (1980, 1982)	Nicoumalone/ phenprocoumon	439	684.9	*	74 (17)	18 (4.1)	6 (1.4)	Bovine	5-10	2.2-5
	Placebo	439			6 (1.4)	1 (0.2)	1 (0.2)			
EPSIM Group (1982)	Nicoumalone (422) Fluindione (140) Ethylbiscoum-acetate (70) Phenindione (9) Tioclomarol (3)	652	LTA[b]	*	104 (16.0)	21 (3.2)	8 (1.2)	?	25-35	
	Aspirin (500mg tid)	651			35 (5.4)	5 (0.8)	4 (0.6)			
Breddin et al. (1980)	Phenprocoumon	320	LTA[b]		12 (3.8)	–	0	Bovine	5-12	2.0-5.0
	Aspirin (500mg tid)	317			9 (2.8)	–	0			
	Placebo	309			0		0			
Meuwissen et al. (1969)	Phenprocoumon	68	109.8	*	7 (10.3)	0	0	Bovine	5-15	1.9-5
	Placebo	70	122.9		0					
Loeliger et al. (1967)	Phenprocoumon	128	168.0	*	17 (13.3)	1 (0.8)	0	Bovine	5-13	2.0-5.0
	Placebo	122	138.0		7 (5.7)	1 (0.8)	1 (0.8)			
Bjerkelund (1957, 1963)	Dicoumarol	138	503.4	*	32 (23.2)	20 (14.5)	4 (2.9)	Human[c]	10-30	1.3-2.1
	Control	139			9 (6.5)	5 (3.6)	1 (0.7)			
Harvald et al. (1962)	Dicoumarol	145	362.5	*	53 (36.5)	28 (19.3)	1 (0.7)	Human[c]	10-25	1.5-2.1
	Placebo	170			8 (4.7)	0	0			

a All fatal haemorrhages cerebral in origin, except EPSIM study where not specified.
b Long term anticoagulants, but duration uncertain.
c Coagulation test used was P-P (prothrombin-proconvertin).

3.4.2 Ischaemic Heart Disease – Level II Evidence

There were 11 randomised controlled trials which we designated as Level II, mainly because of inadequate description of bleeding outcomes (Aspenstrom and Korsan-Bengsten, 1964; Boekhout-Mussert et al., 1981; Borchgrevink, 1960; Conrad et al., 1964; Ebert et al., 1969; Lygren, 1969; MacMillan et al., 1960; Medical Research Council, 1959, 1964; Moschos et al., 1964; Ritland and Lygren, 1969; Seaman et al., 1969; Veterans Cooperative Study, 1965; Wright et al., 1948, 1954). In these studies, the incidence of total bleeding ranged from 3 to 67%. The frequency of fatal bleeding ranged from 0.9 to 5.3%. Intracranial bleeding was the most common cause of fatal bleeding. In most studids the rate of bleeding was significantly greater in patients receiving anticoagulants than in the control group.

No inferences concerning the time of bleeding,

effect of coexisting conditions, or relationship of bleeding to intensity of anticoagulant therapy can be made. In a study by Moschos (1964), patients were randomised to 3 different intensities of warfarin therapy. The designated therapeutic PT ranges were 10 to 25% (INR 4.5 to 9) in the high dose group, 30 to 50% (INR 1.5 to 3.4) in the moderate dose group, and 60% (INR 1.2) in the low dose group. A significant difference in bleeding was detected when the high dose was compared to the moderate dosage group, but no significant difference was detected between the high dose and low dose groups. Unfortunately, bleeding was not well documented in the study; apparently, only a small number of bleeding episodes occurred, but the poor documentation of this aspect necessitates cautious interpretation of these findings.

3.4.3 Ischaemic Heart Disease – Level III and IV Evidence

There were 4 studies in Level III and 3 studies in Level IV (Feldman et al., 1952; Greisman and Marcus, 1948; Keyes et al., 1956; Manchester, 1957, 1964; Pollard et al., 1962; Rashkoff et al., 1951; Suzman et al., 1955). The incidence of total bleeding for the Level III studies ranged from 4.9 to 14.6% and for the Level IV studies from 4 to 37.3%. Major and minor bleeding were not often distinguished. It was not possible from these studies to assess the underlying risk factors for bleeding and to assess the relationship between bleeding and the level of anticoagulant therapy.

3.5 Venous Thromboembolism – Level I Evidence

There were 4 Level I studies that evaluated bleeding during anticoagulant therapy in patients with venous thromboembolism (Bynum and Wilson, 1979; Hull et al., 1979, 1982a,b) [see table IV]. In all of these studies, warfarin which was monitored to maintain the PT (rabbit brain) at approximately twice control (INR ≈4.5) was compared with a less intensely anticoagulated group. In 2 of the studies, the less intense treatment consisted of a fixed low dose of heparin (5000 units subcutaneously twice daily; Bynum and Wilson, 1979; Hull et al., 1979), while in the third it was adjusted dose subcutaneous heparin (Hull et al., 1982a), and in the fourth it was a less intense warfarin regimen which was monitored to maintain the standardised human brain prothrombin time at approximately

Table IV. Venous thromboembolism. Randomised controlled trials (Level I) [* $p < 0.01$]

Reference	Anticoagulant	No. of patients	Anticoagulant duration (months)		Incidence of bleeding: total (%)	Incidence of bleeding: major (%)[a]	Thromboplastin	Targeted therapeutic range	INR equivalent
Bynum and Wilson (1979)	Heparin (low dose SC)	24	6	*	1 (4.2)	0	Rabbit	1.5-2×	2.6-4.4
	Warfarin	24			9 (37.5)	4 (16.7)			
Hull et al. (1979)	Warfarin	33	3	*	7 (21.2)	4 (12.1)	Rabbit	1.5-2×	2.6-4.4
	Heparin (low dose SC)	35			0	0			
Hull et al. (1982)	Warfarin	53	3	*	9 (17.0)	3 (5.7)	Rabbit	1.5-2×	2.6-4.4
	Heparin (adjusted SC)	53			1 (1.9)	0			
Hull et al. (1982)	Warfarin	49	3	*	11 (22.4)	2 (4.1)	Rabbit	1.5-2×	2.6-4.5
	Warfarin (less intense)	47			2 (4.3)	2 (4.3)	Human	2×	2

a No fatal haemorrhages.

Table V. Pooled data showing incidence of haemorrhage during long term anticoagulant therapy

Indication	No. of patients	Incidence of bleeding			
		total (%)	minor (%)	major (%)	fatal (%)
Ischaemic cerebrovascular (Level I evidence)	588	169 (28.7)	128 (21.8)	41 (7.0)	28 (4.8)
Prosthetic heart valves (Level IV evidence)	405	23 (5.7)	13 (3.2)	10 (2.4)	7 (1.7)
Atrial fibrillation (Level V evidence)	302	46 (15.2)	43 (14.2)	3 (0.01)	1 (0.003)
Ischaemic heart disease (Level I evidence)	1890	299 (19.1)	199 (10.5)	88 (4.7)	19 (1.0)
Venous thromboembolism (Level I evidence)	159	36 (22.6)	23 (14.4)	13 (8.1)	0

2 times control (INR ≈2) [which is approximately equivalent to 1.3 times control using a rabbit brain thromboplastin; Hull et al., 1982b]. In all 4 studies total bleeding was significantly greater in the more intensely anticoagulated group. Bleeding during warfarin therapy, monitored by rabbit brain thromboplastin to maintain the prothrombin time at 1.5 to twice control (INR 2.5 to 4.3), varied between 17.0 and 37.5%, and major bleeding varied between 4.1 and 16.7%. There were no fatal episodes of bleeding. Thus, warfarin therapy in doses conventionally used in North America and elsewhere for 3 to 6 months in patients with venous thrombosis is associated with a substantial risk of bleeding.

The 3 studies carried out by Hull and associates were performed sequentially and with a similar protocol, and thus provided an opportunity to combine results to examine the risk factors associated with bleeding during warfarin therapy (Hull et al., 1979, 1982a,b). There were 135 patients treated with more intense warfarin therapy over a 3-year period. Bleeding occurred in a total of 27 patients, with major bleeding in 9 patients (6.7%). Each of these major haemorrhagic episodes was associated with an underlying predisposing cause. Two patients with major thigh haematomas were paraplegic and bled following trauma to an affected limb. In 1 patient, haemarthrosis occurred 1 week after knee surgery, and 3 episodes of gastrointestinal bleeding occurred in association with occult carcinoma of the colon (1 patient) or unsuspected duodenal ulcers (2 patients). Three major bleeding episodes occurred in patients who had undergone recent surgery. Two of these 9 major haemorrhagic episodes occurred with the PT more than 4 times control (INR >10) and 2 with the PT excessively prolonged but less than 3 times control (INR <10). 18 of the 135 patients had minor bleeding episodes; 2 were associated with trauma while in the remainder there was no obvious underlying cause. Of these 18 minor bleeding episodes, 9 occurred within the therapeutic range of 1.5 to 2 times control (INR 2.6 to 4.4), 6 with the PT 2 to 3 times control (INR 4.4 to 10), and 3 with the PT greater than 3 times control (INR >10). Thus, all of the major bleeding episodes were associated with underlying risk factors, some of which are also risk factors for venous thrombosis (i.e. hip surgery, malignancy and paraplegia).

3.6 Comparison Between Indications

The incidence of bleeding during long term anticoagulant therapy is substantial. Using pooled data, the incidence of total bleeding ranged from

5.7 to 28.7%, that of major bleeding from 1.4 to 8.1% and that of fatal bleeding from 0 to 4.8% (see table V).

There were differences in the incidence of bleeding among the 5 subgroups studied. The highest incidence was seen in patients with cerebrovascular disease and venous thromboembolism. Bleeding for most studies was expressed in terms of absolute rates; i.e. the proportion of patients who bled. It was possible to calculate bleeding per 100 patient-years of therapy for a number of studies, which provided information on exposure time (see table VI).

In ischaemic cerebrovascular disease total bleeding rates ranged from 10 to 68 per 100 patient-years, major bleeding rates ranged from 2 to 22 per 100 patient-years, and fatal bleeding from 2 to 9 per 100 patient-years. In prosthetic heart valves major bleeding was less, and in two studies was 0.8 per 100 patient-years. In myocardial infarction bleeding rates were substantial; total bleeding rates ranged between 6.4 and 14.6 per 100 patient-years, major bleeding from 0 to 7.7 per 100 patient-years, and fatal bleeding from 0 to 1.0 per 100 patient-years.

3.7 Relationship Between Intensity of Anticoagulant Therapy and Haemorrhage

It was possible to seek a relationship between intensity of anticoagulant therapy and risk of bleeding from only 3 of the studies (Forfar, 1979; Hull et al., 1982b; Moschos et al., 1964). Hull et al. (1982b) showed a strong relationship in venous thrombosis, with the incidence of bleeding in patients randomised to receive a less intense warfarin regimen (targeted INR 2.0) being significantly less (4% *vs* 22%) than in those receiving more intense therapy (targeted INR 2.5 to 4.5). All 13 patients in this study who bled did so when the Manchester Comparative Time (which is identical to the INR) was prolonged to more than 3 times the control value.

In Forfar's cohort study (1979) the targeted therapeutic range was a PT of 1.8 to 2.6 (INR 1.8 to 2.6) times control using human brain throm-

Table VI. Bleeding rates during long term anticoagulant therapy

Reference	No. of patients	Total exposure time (patient-years)	Number of bleeding episodes per 100 patient-years of anticoagulant therapy[a]		
			total	major	fatal
Patients with cerebrovascular disease					
Baker (1961)	78	45.3	68.0	22.0	9.0
Enger and Boyesen (1965)	52	96.8	10.0	4.0	3.0
McDowell et al. (1963)	95	93.4	18.0	2.0	2.0
Patients with heart valves					
Altman et al. (1976)	57	121.8	6.0	0.8	0.8
Chesebro et al. (1983)	183	166.7	1.8	0.8	0.6
Forfar (1979)	509	99.9	3.4	0.7	0.2
Patients with myocardial infarction					
Bjerkelund (1963)	119	418.3	7.6	4.8	1.0
Harvald et al. (1962)	145	362.5	14.6	7.7	0.2
Loeliger et al. (1967)	128	168.0	10.0	0.6	0
Meuwissen et al. (1969)	68	109.8	6.4	0	0
Sixty Plus (1982)	439	684.8	10.8	2.6	0.9

a A bleeding rate of 10 per 100 patient-years indicates that 10 bleeding episodes occur if 100 patients are followed for 1 year, or that the risk of bleeding for any individual patient is 10% per year.

boplastin. In 23 of 24 episodes of life-threatening haemorrhage, the PT was prolonged beyond the therapeutic range. In contrast the PT was prolonged beyond the therapeutic range on only 1 of 27 occasions of less serious haemorrhage – a relative risk of 40 in favour of a prolonged PT producing severe life-threatening haemorrhage. A PT ratio greater than 3.4 to 1 was recorded overall in 2.5% of patients who did not bleed; an observation which supports an association between intensity of anticoagulant effect and excess bleeding.

Finally, Moschos et al. (1964) randomised patients with ischaemic heart disease to 3 different intensities of warfarin therapy, with targeted therapeutic ranges for PT expressed in INR of 5 to 10 (high dose), 1.6 to 3.8 (moderate dose) and 1.2 (low dose). Although bleeding episodes were not well documented, the highest bleeding rate occurred in the high dose group, which is suggestive of a relationship between intensity of anticoagulation and bleeding.

The PT (or TT) was recorded at the time of the bleeding episode in a number of studies. Inter-study comparisons of the relationship between intensity of the anticoagulant effect and bleeding were not possible because the targeted therapeutic ranges varied among studies. Of 25 major haemorrhagic episodes in patients treated with anticoagulants for cerebrovascular disease, 18 occurred at a PT (or TT) above the desired therapeutic range, while 12 episodes occurred within a therapeutic range equivalent to 1.5 to 2 times control using rabbit brain thromboplastin (INR 2.6 to 4.4), a range which is commonly used in North America. In the 2 studies of patients with prosthetic heart valves where information on level of intensity of the anticoagulant effect was available (Chesebro et al., 1983; Dale et al., 1977, 1980), 9 of 15 haemorrhagic episodes occurred when PT was beyond the desired range. Similarly, of 113 bleeding events in patients treated with anticoagulants for ischaemic heart disease, 37 occurred at a PT (TT) above the therapeutic range. Finally, in venous thrombosis, 14 bleeding episodes occurred at a level of coagulation within the defined therapeutic range (INR 2.6 to 4.4).

Recently Furie et al. (1984) reported on alternative methods for monitoring oral anticoagulant control. Plasma and serum samples were assayed for PT, native prothrombin antigen, and abnormal prothrombin antigen in 133 patients receiving warfarin in an attempt to identify a value which discriminated between patients who bled and those who did not. 11 of 13 bleeding episodes occurred with the PT (rabbit brain) greater than 2 times control (INR 4.4). A native prothrombin antigen level of less than 12 μg/L was strongly predictive of bleeding; it correctly identified all 13 patients in whom bleeding occurred (sensitivity 100%). The prothrombin antigen, however, was less than 12 μg/L in many patients who did not bleed (positive predictive value of only 12%). Thus, although the negative predictive value of the prothrombin antigen was very high, it had poor positive predictive value. These encouraging results should be evaluated prospectively in future studies to determine the clinical usefulness of this test.

4. Discussion

The objective of our study was to review the literature to determine: (a) the rates of bleeding occurring during long term anticoagulant therapy; (b) the clinical risk factors responsible for bleeding; (c) the time of the bleeding in relationship to commencing anticoagulant therapy; and (d) the relationship between bleeding and the intensity of the anticoagulant effect (usually measured as the prothrombin time).

4.1 The Rate of Bleeding During Long Term Anticoagulant Therapy

A number of criteria should be met to reliably assess the rate of bleeding during anticoagulant therapy. Patient characteristics should be clearly defined, the duration of anticoagulant therapy including patient-years of exposure should be described, the nature and severity of bleeding should be defined clearly, and a sufficient number of patients should be treated to provide acceptable confidence limits for the rates of bleeding. In addition the targeted therapeutic range and the proportion of patients who achieved the desired range and the distribution of results within the range should be described.

Reliable estimates of bleeding rates were obtained for ischaemic cerebrovascular disease, ischaemic heart disease, prosthetic heart valves, and venous thromboembolism. The frequency of bleeding was expressed in terms of absolute rates (the proportion of patients who bled) and where possible as the annual incidence of bleeding. However, it was not possible to calculate the annual incidence of bleeding from most of the reports because they did not provide information on the total time of patient exposure to anticoagulant therapy. The risk of bleeding was substantial whether expressed as an absolute rate (percentage) or as the incidence of bleeding per 100 patient-years of exposure. Bleeding occurred most frequently in patients with ischaemic cerebrovascular disease, ischaemic heart disease, and venous thromboembolism. Major bleeding was most prominent in patients with ischaemic cerebrovascular disease and venous thromboembolism, possibly due to a higher prevalence of underlying risk factors in these conditions.

4.2 Clinical Risk Factors Responsible for Bleeding

To reliably assess the association of bleeding with clinical risk factors, knowledge of coexisting conditions and the patient's age and sex is required for all patients who bled and who did not bleed. From this information, relative risks can be calculated. It was possible to calculate relative risk ratios for only one risk factor, hypertension, in patients with ischaemic cerebrovascular disease. Hypertension increased the relative risk of bleeding in this group by more than 2-fold. Major bleeding was almost always intracerebral, possibly because of associated hypertension or the cerebrovascular disease *per se.* There was also strong evidence for an association of major bleeding with clinical risk factors in patients with venous thrombosis. Three of the documented risk factors in venous thromboembolism (cancer, recent surgery and paraplegia) are also predisposing factors for venous thrombosis.

From the reports of anticoagulant therapy in patients with prosthetic cardiac valves there was a greater frequency of bleeding when aspirin was added to warfarin but not when dipyridamole was combined with anticoagulant. A relationship between bleeding and age was sought, but could not be detected because the reports lacked the necessary information.

4.3 Time of the Bleeding Episode

To determine the relationship between bleeding onset and the time of commencing anticoagulant therapy, knowledge of both the time of the bleeding event and the number of patients at risk at that time is necessary. Although the time of bleeding was documented in a number of reports, information on the number of patients at risk at the time of bleeding was not available. Therefore, it was not possible to determine whether bleeding events were concentrated soon after commencing anticoagulant therapy.

4.4 Intensity of Anticoagulant Therapy

To reliably assess the relationship between the intensity of anticoagulant therapy and bleeding the following information is required: (a) a clear definition of the therapeutic range and of the thromboplastin used; and (b) the laboratory test (prothrombin time; PT) results in all patients who bled and who did not bleed. It was possible to seek a relationship between intensity of anticoagulant therapy and risk of bleeding from only 3 studies (Forfar, 1979; Hull et al., 1982b; Moschos et al., 1969). The relationship between bleeding and the level of anticoagulant therapy was most clearly demonstrated in the study by Hull et al. (1982b). This report, in patients with proximal vein thrombosis, demonstrated that the risk of bleeding was markedly reduced by using a less intense anticoagulant regimen monitored to maintain the PT (human brain thromboplastin) at 2 times control

(INR = 2), which is equivalent to a rabbit brain thromboplastin of 1.2 to 1.3 times control. Although the PT (or thrombotest) was recorded at the time of bleeding in a number of studies it was not possible to determine the clinical relevance of the result because appropriate information on patients who did not bleed was not available.

5. Therapeutic Implications

There is a strong association between major bleeding episodes during long term anticoagulant therapy and underlying risk factors. It would appear that the risk of bleeding is increased by increasing the intensity of the anticoagulant effect; there is evidence from 1 randomised study in patients with venous thrombosis that the risk of bleeding can be reduced without loss of efficacy by reducing the intensity of anticoagulant therapy. However, it is clear that a substantial incidence of bleeding occurs in all the indications examined even when the PT is within a therapeutic range equivalent to 1.5 to 2 times control using a rabbit brain thromboplastin (INR 2.6 to 4.4). This risk should be considered when evaluating whether or not to initiate (or continue) long term anticoagulant treatment.

References

Altman, R.; Boullon, F.; Rouvier, J.; Raca, R.; de la Fuente, L. and Favaloro, R.: Aspirin and prophylaxis of thromboembolic complications in patients with substitute heart valves. Journal of Thoracic and Cardiovascular Surgery 72: 127-129 (1976).

Aspenstrom, G. and Korsan-Bengsten, K.: A double-blind study of dicumarol prophylaxis in coronary heart disease. Acta Medica Scandinavica 176: 563-575 (1964).

Bailey, E.L.; Harper, T.A. and Pinkerton, P.H.: The 'therapeutic range' of the one-stage prothrombin time in the control of anticoagulant therapy: The effect of different thromboplastin preparations. Canadian Medical Association Journal 105: 1041-1043 (1971).

Baker, R.N.: An evaluation of anticoagulant therapy in the treatment of cerebrovascular disease: Report of the Veterans Administration cooperative study of atherosclerosis. Neurology 11: 132-138 (1961).

Baker, R.N.; Broward, J.A.; Fang, H.C.; Fisher, C.M.; Groch, S.N. et al.: Anticoagulant therapy in cerebral infarction: report on cooperative study. Neurology 12: 823-835 (1962).

Baker, R.N.; Schwartz, W.S.; Rose, A.S.: Transient ischemic strokes: A report of a study of anticoagulant therapy. Neurology 16: 841-847 (1966).

Bjerkelund, C.J.: The effect of long-term treatment with dicumarol in myocardial infarction. Acta Medica Scandinavica 158 (Suppl. I): 1-212 (1957).

Bjerkelund, C.J.: Therapeutic level in long-term anticoagulant therapy after myocardial infarction: Its relation to recurrent infarction and sudden death. American Journal of Cardiology 11: 158-163 (1963).

Boekhout-Mussert, M.; Van der Kolk-Schaap, P.J.; Hermans, J. and Loeliger, E.A.: Prospective double-blind clinical trial of bovine, human and rabbit thromboplastins in monitoring long-term oral anticoagulation. American Journal of Clinical Pathology 75: 297-303 (1981).

Borchgrevink, C.: Long-term anticoagulant therapy in angina pectoris and myocardial infarction: A clinical trial between intense and moderate treatment. Acta Medica Scandinavica (Suppl.) 359: 10-50 (1960).

Borchgrevink, C.: Long-term anticoagulant therapy in angina pectoris: A follow-up study. Lancet 1: 44-451 (1962).

Breddin, K.; Loew, D.; Lechner, K.; Uberla, K. and Walter, E.: Secondary prevention of myocardial infarction: A comparison of acetylsalicylic acid, placebo and phenprocoumon. Haemostasis 9: 325-344 (1980).

Buren, A. and Ygge, J.: Treatment program and comparison between anticoagulants and platelet aggregation inhibitors after transient ischemic attack. Stroke 12: 578-580 (1981).

Bynum, L.J. and Wilson, J.E.: Low-dose heparin therapy in the long-term management of venous thromboembolism. American Journal of Medicine 67: 553-556 (1979).

Carter, A.B.: Use of anticoagulants in patients with progressive cerebral infarction. Neurology 11: 601-609 (1961).

Chesebro, J.H.; Fuster, V.; Elveback, L.R.; McGoon, D.C.; Pluth, J.R. et al.: Trial of combined warfarin plus dipyridamole or aspirin therapy in prosthetic heart valve replacement: Danger of aspirin compared with dipyridamole. American Journal of Cardiology 51: 1537-1541 (1983).

Conrad, L.L.; Kyriacopoulos, J.D.; Wiggins, C.W. and Honick, G.L.: Prevention of recurrences of myocardial infarction: a double-blind study of the effectiveness of long-term oral anticoagulant therapy. Archives of Internal Medicine 114: 348-358 (1964).

Dale, J.; Myhre, E. and Loew, D.: Bleeding during acetylsalicylic acid and anticoagulant therapy in patients with reduced platelet reactivity after aortic valve replacement. American Heart Journal 99: 746-751 (1980).

Dale, J.; Myhre, E.; Storstein, O.; Stormorken, H. and Efskind, L.: Prevention of arterial thromboembolism with acetylsalicylic acid: A controlled study in patients with aortic ball valves. American Heart Journal 94: 101-111 (1977).

Ebert, R.V.; Borden, C.W.; Hipp, H.R.; Holzman, D.; Lyon, A.F. and Schnapper, H.: Long-term anticoagulant therapy after myocardial infarction. Journal of the American Medical Association 207: 2263-2267 (1969).

Enger, E. and Boyesen, S.: Long-term anticoagulant therapy in patients with cerebral infarction. Acta Medica Scandinavica 178 (Suppl. 438): 7-55 (1965).

Eriksson, S.E. and Link, H.: Evaluation of anticoagulants in patients with cerebral infarction with slight to moderate neurological deficit. Acta Neurologica Scandinavica 68: 96-106 (1983).

EPSIM Research Group: A controlled comparison of aspirin and oral anticoagulants in prevention of death after myocardial infarction. New England Journal of Medicine 307: 701-708 (1982).

Feldman, L.; O'Connor, W.R.; Friedman, I.A. and Fischer, J.W.: Anticoagulant therapy in acute myocardial infarction. American Heart Journal 44: 112-118 (1952).

Fisher, C.M.: Anticoagulant therapy in cerebral thrombosis and cerebral embolism. Neurology 11: 119-131 (1961).

Fleming, H.A. and Bailey, S.M.: Mitral valve disease, systemic embolism and anticoagulants. Postgraduate Medical Journal 47: 599-604 (1971).

Foley, W.T.; McDevitt, E.; Symons, C. and Wright, I.S.: Further experience with long-term anticoagulant therapy. Archives of Internal Medicine 95: 497-502 (1955).

Forfar, J.C.: A 7-year analysis of hemorrhage in patients on long-term anticoagulant treatment. British Heart Journal 42: 128-132 (1979).

Furie, B.; Liebman, H.A.; Blanchard, R.A.; Coleman, M.S.; Kruger, S.F. and Furie, B.C.: Comparison of the native prothrombin antigen and the prothrombin time for monitoring oral anticoagulant therapy. Blood 64: 445-451 (1984).

Gonzalez-Lavin, L.; Tandon, A.P.; Chi, S.; Blair, T.C.; McFadden, P.M. et al.: The risk of thromboembolism and hemorrhage following mitral valve replacement: A comparative analysis between the porcine xenograft valve and Ionescu-Shiley bovine pericardial valve. Journal of Thoracic and Cardiovascular Surgery 87: 340-351 (1978).

Greisman, H. and Marcus, R.M.: Acute myocardial infarction: detailed study of dicumarol therapy in seventy-five consecutive cases. American Heart Journal 36: 600-609 (1948).

Harvald, B.; Hilden, T. and Lund, E.: Long-term anticoagulant therapy after myocardial infarction. Lancet 2: 626-630 (1962).

Hill, A.B.; Marshall, J. and Shaw, D.A.: A controlled clinical trial of long-term anticoagulant therapy in cerebrovascular disease. Quarterly Journal of Medicine 29: 597-609 (1960).

Hill, A.B.; Marshall, J. and Shaw, D.A.: Cerebrovascular disease: Trial of long-term anticoagulant therapy. British Medical Journal 53: 1003-1006 (1962).

Hull, R.; Delmore, T.; Carter, C.; Hirsh, J.; Genton, E. et al.: Adjusted subcutaneous heparin versus warfarin sodium in the long-term treatment of venous thrombosis. New England Journal of Medicine 306: 189-194 (1982a).

Hull, R.; Delmore, T. and Genton, E.: Warfarin sodium versus low-dose heparin in the long-term treatment of venous thromboembolism. New England Journal of Medicine 301: 855-858 (1979).

Hull, R.; Hirsh, J.; Jay, R.; Carter, C.; England, C. et al.: Different intensities of oral anticoagulant therapy in the treatment of proximal-vein thrombosis. New England Journal of Medicine 307: 1676-1681 (1982b).

Keyes, J.W.; Drake, E.H. and Smith, F.J.: Survival rates after acute myocardial infarction with long-term anticoagulant therapy. Circulation 14: 254-259 (1956).

Lieberman, A.; Hass, W.K.; Pinto, R.; Isom, W.O.; Kupersmith, M. et al.: Intracranial hemorrhage and infarction in anticoagulated patients with prosthetic heart valves. Stroke 9: 18-24 (1978).

Loeliger, E.A.; Hensen, A.; Kroes, F.; van Dijk, L.M.; Fekes, N. et al.: A double-blind trial of long-term anticoagulant treatment after myocardial infarction. Acta Medica Scandinavica 182: 549-566 (1967).

MacMillan, R.L.; Brown, K.W.G. and Watt, D.L.: Long-term anticoagulant therapy after myocardial infarction. Canadian Medical Association Journal 83: 567-570 (1960).

Manchester, B.: The value of continuous (1 to 10 years) long-term anticoagulant therapy. Annals of Internal Medicine 47: 1202-1209 (1957).

Manchester, B.: Continuous anticoagulant therapy following myocardial infarction. Angiology 25: 19-26 (1964).

Marshall, J. and Shaw, D.A.: Anticoagulant therapy in cerebrovascular disease. Proceedings of the Royal Society of Medicine 52: 547-549 (1959).

Marshall, J. and Shaw, D.A.: Anticoagulant therapy in acute cerebrovascular accidents: A controlled trial. Lancet 1: 995-998 (1960).

McDowell, F.; McDevitt, E. and Wright, I.S.: Anticoagulant therapy: Five years experience with the patient with an established cerebrovascular accident. Archives of Neurology 8: 209-214 (1963).

Medical Research Council: An assessment of long-term anticoagulant administration after cardiac infarction. British Medical Journal 2: 803-810 (1959).

Medical Research Council: An assessment of long-term anticoagulant administration after cardiac infarction. British Medical Journal 2: 837-843 (1964).

Meuwissen, O.; Vervoorn, A.C.; Cohen, O.; Jordan, F.L.J. and Nelemans, F.A.: Double blind trial of long-term anticoagulant treatment after myocardial infarction. Acta Medica Scandinavica 186: 361-368 (1969).

Moschos, C.B.; Wong, P.C.Y. and Sise, H.S.: Controlled study of the effective level of long-term anticoagulation. Journal of the American Medical Association 190: 799-805 (1964).

Nunez, L.; Aguado, M.; Celemin, D.; Iglesias, A. and Larrea, J.L.: Aspirin or coumadin as the drug of choice for valve replacement with porcine bioprosthesis. Annals of Thoracic Surgery 33: 354-358 (1982).

Olsson, J.E.; Brechter, C.; Backlund, H.; Krook, H.; Muller, R. et al.: Anticoagulant *vs* antiplatelet therapy as prophylactic against cerebral infarction in transient ischemic attacks. Stroke 11: 4-9 (1980).

Olsson, J.E.; Muller, R. and Berneli, S.: Long-term anticoagulant therapy for TIAs and minor strokes with minimum residuum. Stroke 7: 444-451 (1976).

Owren, P.A.: Thrombotest. A new method for controlling anticoagulant therapy. Lancet 1: 754-758 (1959).

Pearce, J.M.S.; Gubbay, S.S. and Walton, J.N.: Long-term anticoagulant therapy in transient cerebral ischemic attacks. Lancet 1: 6-9 (1965).

Pollard, J.W.; Hamilton, M.J.; Christensen, N.A. and Achor, R.W.P.: Problems associated with long-term anticoagulant therapy: Observations in 139 cases. Circulation 25: 311-317 (1962).

Rashkoff, R.A.; Schaefer, L.E.; Magida, M.G. and Levy, H.: Evaluation of dicumarol therapy in 287 cases of acute myocardial infarction. Journal of Mt Sinai Hospital 18: 350-357 (1951).

Ritland, S. and Lygren, T.: Comparison of efficacy of 3 and 12 months' anticoagulant therapy after myocardial infarction: A controlled clinical trial. Lancet 1: 122-124 (1969).

Seaman, A.J.; Griswold, H.E.; Reaume, R.B. and Ritzmann, L.: Long-term anticoagulant prophylaxis after myocardial infarction: Final report. New England Journal of Medicine 281: 115-119 (1969).

Siekert, R.G.; Millikan, C.H. and Whisnant, J.P.: Anticoagulant therapy in intermittent cerebrovascular insufficiency: Follow-up data. Journal of American Medical Association 176: 19-22 (1961).

Sixty-Plus Reinfarction Study Research Group: A double-blind trial to assess long-term anticoagulant therapy in elderly patients after myocardial infarction. Lancet 2: 989-994 (1980).

Sixty-Plus Reinfarction Study Research Group: Risks of long-term oral anticoagulant therapy in elderly patients after myocardial infarction. Lancet 1: 64-68 (1982).

Sullivan, J.M.; Harken, D.E. and Gorlin, R.: Pharmacologic control of thromboembolic complications of cardiac-valve replacement. New England Journal of Medicine 284: 1391-1394 (1971).

Suzman, M.M.; Ruskin, H.D. and Goldberg, B.: An evaluation of the effect of continuous long-term anticoagulant therapy on the prognosis of myocardial infarction: A report of 82 cases. Circulation 12: 338-352 (1955).

Terent, A. and Andersson, B.: The outcome of patients with transient ischemic attacks and stroke treated with anticoagulants. Acta Medica Scandinavica 208: 359-365 (1980).

Veterans Cooperative Study: Long-term anticoagulant therapy after myocardial infarction: A study of 747 patients in 15 hospitals. Journal of the American Medical Association 193: 929-934 (1965).

Wallace, D.C.: Cerebral vascular disease in relation to long-term

anticoagulant therapy. Journal of Chronic Diseases 17: 527-537 (1964).
Whisnant, J.P.; Cartilidge, M.B. and Elveback, L.R.: Carotid and vertebral-basilar transient ischemic attacks: Effect of anticoagulants, hypertension, and cardiac disorders on survival and stroke occurrence – a population study. Annals of Neurology 3: 107-115 (1978).
Wright, I.S.; Beck, D.F. and Marple, C.D.: Myocardial infarction and its treatment with anticoagulants: Summary of findings in 1031 cases. Lancet 1: 92-95 (1954).
Wright, I.S.; Marple, C.D. and Beck, D.F.: Report on the committee for the evaluation of anticoagulants in the treatment of coronary thrombosis with myocardial infarction. American Heart Journal 36: 801-815 (1948).

Address for correspondence and reprints: Dr *Mark Levine,* Room 3H7, McMaster University Medical Centre, 1200 Main Street West, Hamilton, Ontario L8N EZ5 (Canada).

Drugs 30: 461-468 (1985)
0012-6667/85/0011-0461/$04.00/0

Current Management of Leg Ulcers

Terence J. Ryan
Department of Dermatology, Slade Hospital, Oxford

Summary *Leg ulceration is a common disease which in developed countries is age-related and a consequence of venous hypertension. Therapy should be founded on elevation of the leg and on exercise. Drug therapy is aimed at promoting granulation tissue and epithelialisation. However, the ulcer bed and surrounding skin is vulnerable and the clinician's first objective is to do no harm. The choice of a drug should therefore take into account its possible side effects.*

Pharmaceutical preparations for the treatment of ulcers of the leg, whether administered orally or applied topically will not be effective unless the causes of the ulcer are eliminated. Some preparations may actually cause harm to the especially vulnerable tissues associated with ulceration. Therefore, much should be done *before* prescribing, and the choice of a drug should take into account its possible side effects.

Leg ulcers have many causes, but in Western countries gravitational congestion or venous hypertension is the most significant cause. In countries where sitting on the ground is common and malnutrition not rare, venous disease is not so great a problem, but injury, infection, blood diseases and nutritional deficiencies play a greater role. These should not be forgotten even in the West, because the population of elderly people who suffer from leg ulcers are often subject to minor injuries of the leg, and healing may be impaired due to vitamin or protein deficiency.

This article will concentrate on the healing of leg ulcers from all causes and will assume that rarer eliminatable causes such as infections (e.g. deep mycoses) or blood diseases (e.g. sickle cell anaemia) have not been overlooked as a primary cause.

1. Pathophysiological Considerations

The blood supply of the skin of the lower leg has to adapt to the problems inherent in an upright stance, a position resulting in dependency of the leg which is adopted most of the day from childhood. To prevent the rise in capillary pressure which is due to gravitational accumulation of blood, there is reflex arteriolar vasoconstriction to the skin of the lower leg as the limb is lowered below the level of the heart. As well, there is always a factor of increased peripheral resistance in the arterial tree of the lower leg; by the age of 80 years, some 2% of persons suffer from arterial insufficiency. So far, the management of leg ulcers has not resulted in any research as to whether protection from vasoconstriction, either by elevation or by drugs, might be beneficial in the prophylaxis or cure of ulceration. However, it is well known that 30 to 40% of elderly persons with leg ulcers also have peripheral arterial disease with narrowing of arterial vessels to the leg, and surgical intervention to the artery is sometimes required.

The venous contribution to ulceration is an integral part of its aetiology. Absent venous valves, destruction by previous thrombosis, the opening up of communications between the deep and superficial venous systems, and reflux down the long saphenous vein from the iliac or femoral vein are well known causes, but their relative importance and the indications for surgical intervention are still the subject of debate.

The diagnosis of arterial disease should precede measures for managing venous disease. It should include the taking of the blood pressure in the lower leg. If this is less than 60% of that in the arm the chances of healing an ulcer are much diminished. Measuring the blood pressure in the lower leg is facilitated by an ultrasound stethoscope (Flowscope®, Hayashi Denki Co., Kawasaki, Japan).

2. Importance of Exercise and Elevation in Management

There is no debate, however, that to protect the microvascular system of the skin of the lower leg, the veins into which the skin capillaries drain must be emptied. This can be done either by exercise or by elevation. To facilitate the effect of exercise, support bandages or stockings are usually used. However, some patients cannot raise their legs, and others cannot wear stockings or cannot walk. No pharmaceutical preparation used in the management of leg ulcers has a chance to effect a cure without attention to the basic requirements of elevation or support bandaging and exercise.

It is unclear whether elevation with enforced bed rest merely increases the immobility and muscle atrophy and decreases the range of movements of the joints. Good management includes ankle exercises and preservation of muscle tone, even when resting. Elevation is not effective unless it is above the level of the heart. At night there should be slight elevation of up to 9 inches (by placing 2 blocks under the end of the bed); any higher, while sleeping, and it is impossible to maintain and the patient slips to the end of the bed. During the day (for instance, while watching television) it may be necessary to either lie on the floor or bring in a couch from the guest room into the living room. This is emphasised because so many people reserve their most useful furniture for a room in which they spend little time.

The habit of raising the legs is like 'weight watching' in the obese or giving up smoking – it requires zeal and reward. The weight watchers chart which can be used as a marking sheet for awards can be supplemented by a 'legs up' chart which records the exact amount of time the legs have been elevated.

If all this is done in every case, drugs used to supplement treatment may have some effect. Without elevation or exercise the drugs will not work, whatever their purpose.

3. Drug Treatment

Drug treatment can be divided into topical and systemic therapy. Topical therapy is used to control bacterial infection, promote granulation tissue, soothe the skin, relieve pain and remove slough or debris. These signs and symptoms are features of most leg ulcers, but at different times in their life history any one may be the most important. Because no two ulcers are identical and vary from week to week, it is difficult to perform a controlled clinical trial; thus data on most topical regimens are poorly documented. Documentation should include the size of the ulcer at any stage and the endpoint of healing. The latter is difficult to judge, but the former can be estimated using a planimeter and recording the ulcer edge on a cellophane sheet placed over the ulcer. The surface area can be plotted logarithmically and hence the healing rate can be read at a glance from the slope of the line.

3.1 Potential Problems in the Use of Topical Preparations

It is not certain from any study of topical drug therapy that its effect on the healing rate is highly significant. There are numerous studies which show some good effects and many observations (often unpublished) which show some harm. For this reason the wise clinician, realising that something has to be placed over or on an ulcer, will choose an agent which will do no harm.

Irritation of the surrounding skin is common and medicament allergy is not rare. Often the underlying, microvascular disease of congested leaking capillaries gives rise to gravitational eczema on which is superimposed variably pathogenic bacterial flora. It is important to recognise this eczematous response, to exclude infection, and distinguish it from medicament allergy. Gravitational eczema results from insufficient elevation or immobility and is usually accompanied by oedema. A low grade 'cellulitis' is indistinguishable from the inflammatory state due to leakage of protein and fibrin deposition known as liposclerosis, leading to end-stage fibrosis and hardening of the skin.

Very few drugs used topically are entirely bland. Many will damage granulation tissue or eczematous skin, and some bases are wetting and some are drying. The principle of a wet dressing is to soften debris and to keep it softened; however, if exposed to the air a wet dressing quickly dries. Dryness is good for a weeping area but it causes loss of suppleness and the stratum corneum may then crack. Dry skin may be moisturised by ointments and to some extent by creams, but these are quickly absorbed through eczematous skin. Pastes such as Lassar's paste are a mixture of zinc oxide, starch and salicyclic acid in an ointment base. The latter is absorbed leaving behind a cake of powder which can damage the skin. Because of all these difficulties, choosing the right agent at the right time is not easy and one may expect damage from agents used throughout the life of an ulcer simply because there is bound to be at least one stage at which the agent is unsuitable, i.e. too wetting or too drying, too toxic to granulation tissue, or too irritant to eczematous skin. There are some agents, such as corticosteroid creams, which are decongestant, antipruritic, anti-inflammatory and quickly control eczema. However, they also cause reabsorption of healthy granulation tissue and diminish resistance to infection and prevent wound contraction. A clean 'punched out' ulcer is the consequence.

3.2 The Problem of Infection: When is Specific Treatment Necessary?

Infection is one of the most puzzling problems in leg ulcer management simply because there is no certain way to distinguish between pathogens and non-pathogens. It is also not known how important aerobic *versus* anaerobic organisms may be. Thus, it is not certain that treatment for an organism identified by a bacteriology swab report is necessary. It is naive to think that an ulcer can be made sterile for more than a brief period without risking irritation, allergy or the emergence of resistant organisms. It is wise, however, to take swabs for bacteriological examination and treat appropriately (according to sensitivity patterns) certain infections such as those due to β-haemolytic streptococci type A and pathology such as cellulitis. It may also be wise to 'clean up' an ulcer prior to skin grafting.

It is generally believed that β-haemolytic streptococci group A warrant the prescription of a systemic antibiotic and that 'heavy' bacterial contamination of the ulcer bed is harmful. The latter can be reduced by irrigation or frequent wet dressings.

3.3 Removal of Slough

Healing requires a bed of granulation tissue and this is never compatible with slough or dead tissue. Surgical debridement is the quickest way to obtain clearance of slough, but medical debridement by soaking away debris is a slower and less damaging alternative. Agents which dissolve slough include protealytic enzymes such as chymotrypsin, collagenase and streptokinase/streptodornase, preparations such as 'Aserbine' (malic acid/benzoic acid/salicyclic acid), wetting agents, and occlusive preparations which allow natural exudate to collect and debride. Some agents, such as dextranomer ('Debrisan'), are designed to remove all exudate away from granulating surfaces. Others such as 'Granuflex' do just as well by retaining the exudate in excessive amounts.

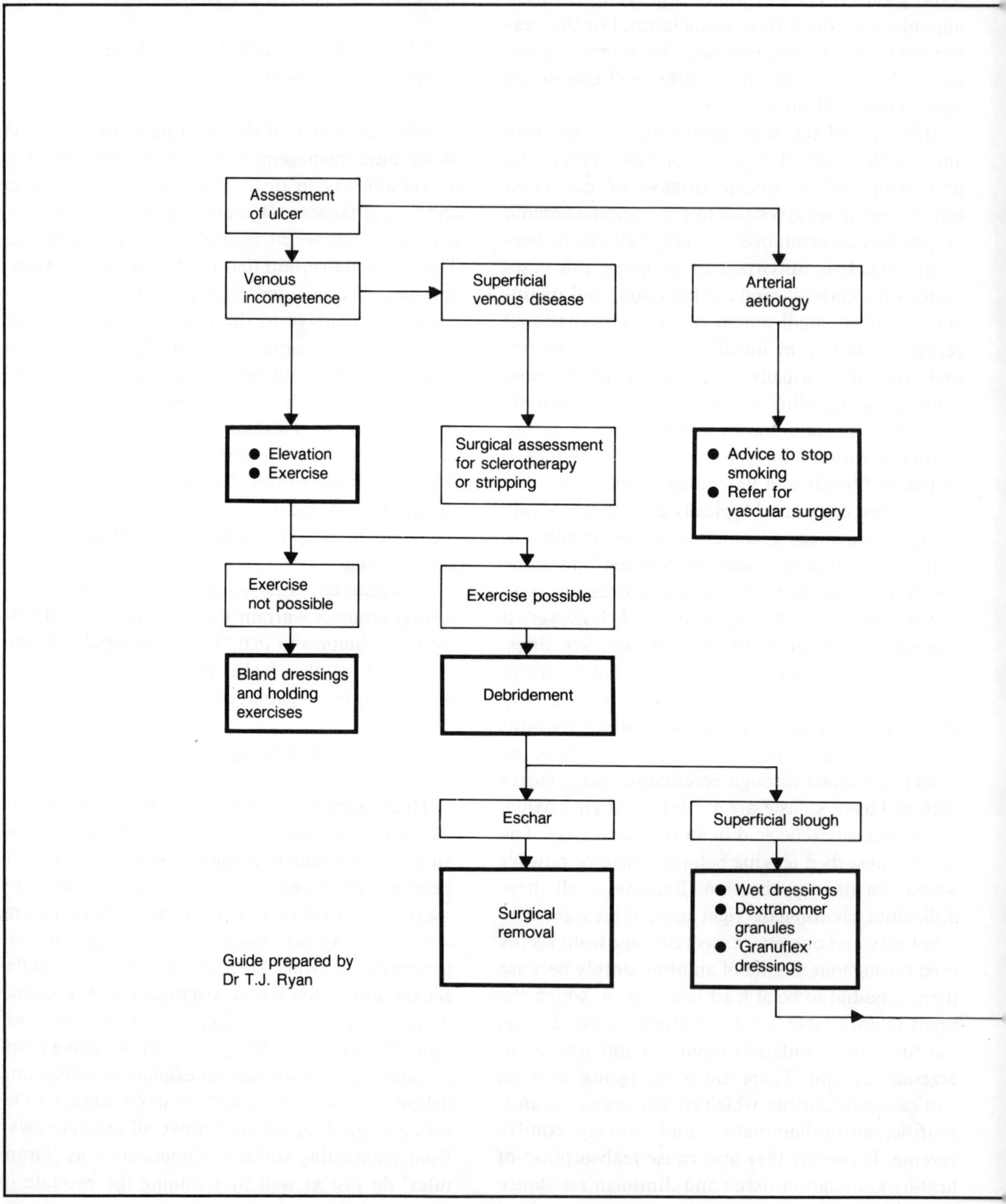

Fig. 1. Management plan for treatment of leg ulcers.

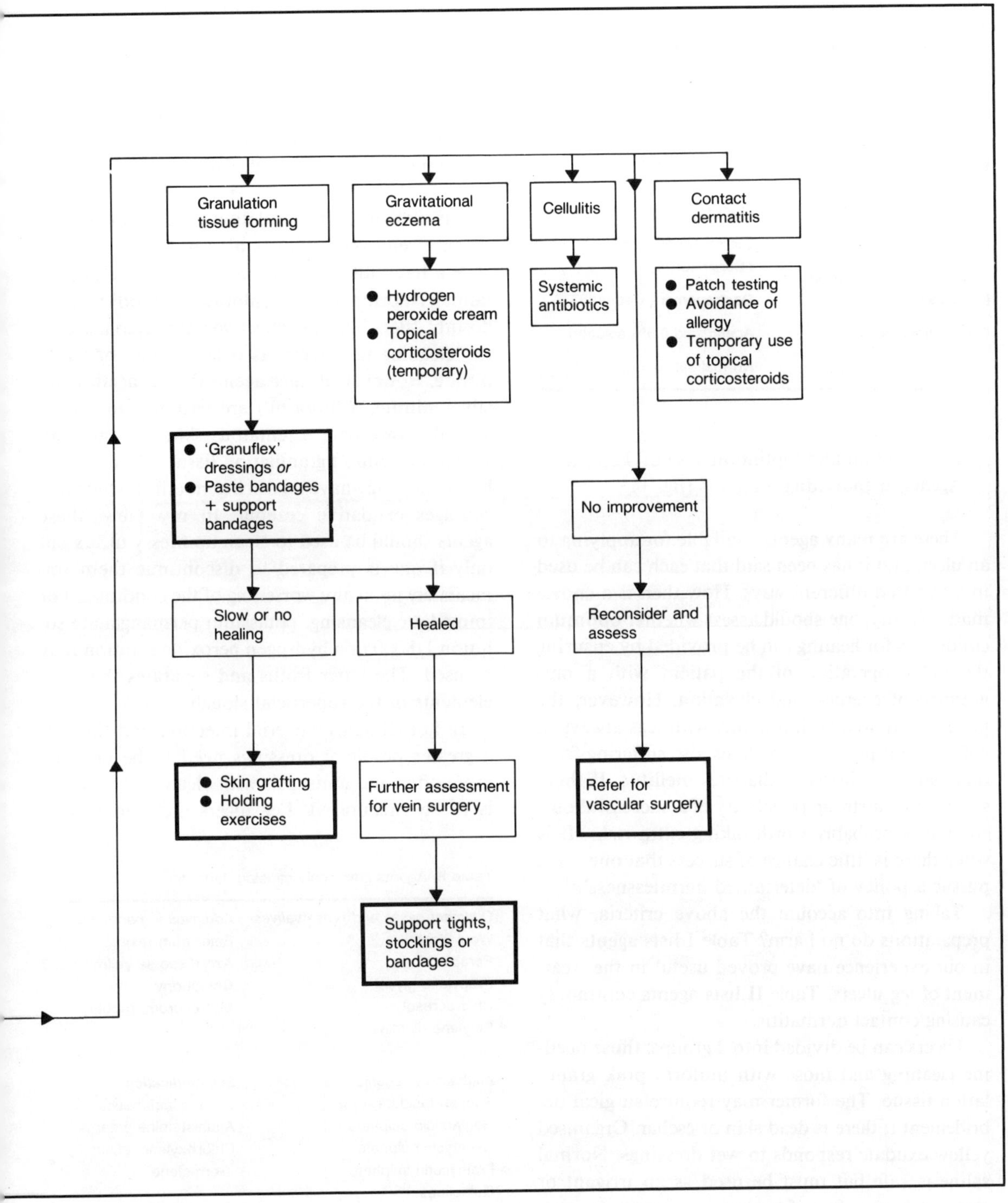
Granulation tissue forming
Gravitational eczema
Cellulitis
Contact dermatitis
● Hydrogen peroxide cream
● Topical corticosteroids (temporary)
Systemic antibiotics
● Patch testing
● Avoidance of allergy
● Temporary use of topical corticosteroids
● 'Granuflex' dressings or
● Paste bandages + support bandages
No improvement
Slow or no healing
Healed
Reconsider and assess
● Skin grafting
● Holding exercises
Further assessment for vein surgery
Refer for vascular surgery
Support tights, stockings or bandages

Table I. Some topical preparations which have proved useful in the treatment of leg ulcers

Eusol	Silver nitrate 0.5% solution
Gentian violet 1% paint	Potassium permanganate
Hydrogen peroxide solution	Hydrogen peroxide 1.5% cream ('Hioxyl')
Brilliant green/lactic acid ('Variclene')	Cadexomer iodine ('Iodosorb')
Sodium hypochlorite ('Chlorasol')	Starch copolymer ('Scherisorb')
Streptokinase/streptodornase ('Varidase')	Dextranomer ('Debrisan')
Pseudomonic acid	Acetic acid 0.5% solution
	Normal saline

3.4 Selection and Optimum Use of Topical Agents in Individual Patients (fig. 1)

There are many agents available for applying to an ulcer, and it has been said that each can be used in a hundred different ways. How then is a choice made? Firstly, one should assess whether optimum conditions for healing can be provided by ensuring the full cooperation of the patient with a programme of exercise and elevation. However, the patient may well be immobile, with legs always in a dependent position – perhaps also suffering from rheumatoid arthritis or diabetes mellitus. If there seems to be a strong possibility of a successful outcome it is probably worth taking extra risks. It is when there is little chance of success that one must pursue a policy of 'determined harmlessness'.

Taking into account the above criteria, what preparations do no harm? Table I lists agents that in our experience have proved useful in the treatment of leg ulcers. Table II lists agents commonly causing contact dermatitis.

Ulcers can be divided into 2 groups: those needing cleaning and those with uniform pink granulation tissue. The former may require surgical debridement if there is dead skin or eschar. Organised yellow exudate responds to wet dressings. Normal saline is safe but must be used as an irrigant or changed fairly often if bacteria are to be discouraged. Eusol, 0.5% acetic acid solution, and 0.5% silver nitrate solution are other wet dressings which inhibit bacterial growth up to a point. These preparations may be used 4-hourly. Some drying and adherence with their use may discourage bacteria, and removal of adherent dressings is one way of removing superficial slough. However, for the second class of ulcer with granulation tissue, these agents may depress granulation tissue, and any adherence removes seedlings of epithelium.

We have found halogenated preparations containing chlorine (Eusol, 'Chlorasol') or iodides ('Iodosorb', 'Betadine') are effective antibacterial agents for 'cleaning up' ulcers, as is acetic acid or silver nitrate. However, all such agents (Eusol, acetic acid, silver nitrate, 'Chlorasol') are irritants and occasionally exacerbate eczematous skin and they can sometimes inhibit granulation tissue. On the other hand, they may have an astringent effect which discourages exudative eczema. In my view, these agents should be used to clean up messy ulcers but only if one is prepared to discontinue them immediately upon any worsening of the condition. For immediate cleansing, potassium permanganate solution 1/8000 or a hydrogen peroxide solution may be used. The latter froths and separates the solid elements in the superficial slough.

In hot climates bacterial infection and flies are a greater problem; dressings need to be changed more often and antisepsis with cleaning of the legs is to be encouraged. Leg ulcers are a long term

Table II. Agents commonly causing dermatitis

Ointment bases and preservatives	*Additives in bandages*
Wool alcohols	Ester gum resin
Parabens	Azo disperse yellow No. 3
Propylene glycol	Colophony
Chlorocresol	Mbt thiurum (rubber)
Ethylene diamine	
Antibacterial agents	*Self-medication*
Sodium fusidate	Local anaesthetics
Gentamicin sulphate	Antihistamine creams
Neomycin sulphate	Chloroxylenol ('Dettol')
Framycetin sulphate	'Germolene'
Quinolines	

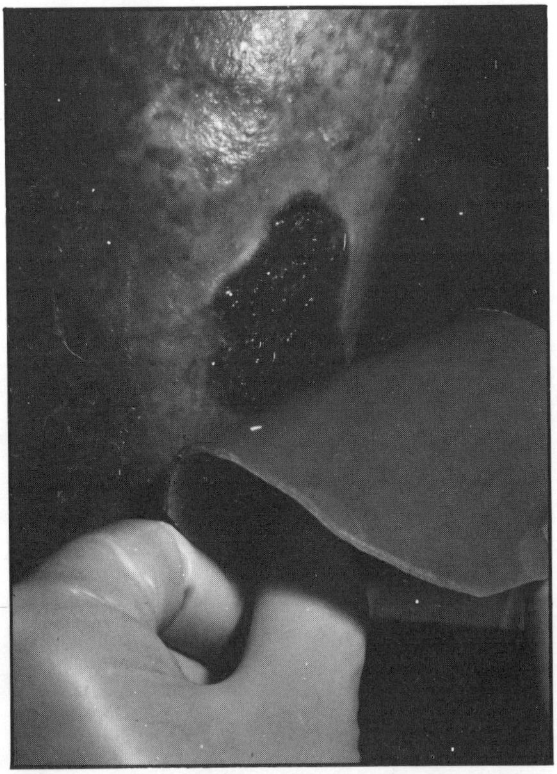

Fig. 2. The use of 'Granuflex' as an adhesive occlusive dressing over an ulcer.

problem and a policy of no bathing is an unhygienic rule which should be broken. 1% gentian violet paint or brilliant green (currently available in a cream form as 'Variclene') are other useful antiseptics which may retain some activity in the presence of exudate under a bandage.

In recent years a 1.5% hydrogen peroxide cream preparation ('Hioxyl') has proved to be a very useful addition to the therapeutic armamentarium. As it is a cream, twice daily application is necessary to maintain adequate moisturisation. Oxygen is slowly released from the bland base. So far, because it contains no potential allergenic agents, it has proved free of side effects. It is particularly soothing to eczematous skin surrounding an ulcer.

Our standard therapy for the management of leg ulcers in a population which for several reasons, such as lack of transport, can only be seen at the most twice weekly, are paste bandages with an overlying elastic support bandage (e.g. 'Lestreflex'). These are applied as a reasonably cosmetic sleeve rather than as a firm compression. The paste bandages used (Hardie et al., 1982) vary from the minimally irritant zinc paste and calamine bandage ('Calaband') to zinc paste bandages containing clioquinol ('Quinaband') used for antisepsis, or those containing coal tar or ichthammol ('Ichthopaste') which are used for pruritic lichen simplex or drying gravitational eczema.

Dextranomer granules or other polysaccharides produced as a powder or formulated in a jelly are recommended for cleaning ulcers. However, these are expensive preparations still needing further evaluation for their exact indications for any particular stage of ulceration and healing. Our own studies of healing rates using a wide range of agents have resulted in clear evidence of improved healing rates using 'Granuflex' applied for 3 days at a time. This results in dissolution of slough and stimulates granulation tissue. It is an adhesive dressing (fig. 2) which, like stoma adhesive, protects the surrounding skin. It may potentially encourage growth of anaerobic organisms since it is impermeable to oxygen, but the granulation tissue that develops in response to the dressing may preclude this and we have found no ill effects. All occlusive dressings such as 'Granuflex', 'Opsite' and 'Coretheum' relieve pain perhaps more effectively than any other class of therapeutic agent.

4. Other Considerations in Management

Two further aspects of leg ulceration deserve consideration. One is the current theory that fibrin deposition interferes with oxygenation (Burnand and Browse, 1982) and that removal of fibrin is therefore to be encouraged. Drugs such as stanozolol which promote fibrinolysis are currently undergoing trials (Burnand et al., 1980) and have been recommended for some of the sclerosis of the deep dermis often associated with leg ulcers. There is as yet no evidence that such drugs promote healing of ulcers. However, perhaps the most important problem of all in the healing of leg ulcers is the recurrence rate. More research needs to be done on how to produce effective support stockings which can be used by the elderly even when they are blind and/or arthritic.

References

Burnand, K.G. and Browse, N.L.: The postphlebitic leg and venous ulceration; in Recent Advances in Surgery, II, pp. 225-246 (Churchill Livingstone, Edinburgh 1982).

Burnand, K.; Clemenson, G.; Morland, M.; Jarrett, P.E.M. and Browse, N.L.: Venous lipodermatosclerosis treatment by fibrinolytic enhancement and elastic compression. British Medical Journal 280: 7-11 (1980).

Hardie, R.A.; Benton, E.C. and Hunter, J.A.A.: Adverse reactions to paste bandages. Clinical and Experimental Dermatology 7: 133-142 (1982).

Lookingbill, D.P.; Miller, S.H. and Knowles, R.C.: Bacteriology of chronic ulcers. Archives of Dermatology 114: 1765-1768 (1978).

Peachey, R.D.G.: Leg ulcers; in Rook, A. (Ed) Recent Advances in Dermatology (Churchill Livingstone, Edinburgh 1977).

Ryan, T.J.: The Management of Leg Ulcers (Oxford University Press, Oxford 1983).

Ryan, T.J.: An environment for healing. Royal Society of Medicine Symposium No. 88 (Oxford University Press, Oxford 1985).

Ryan, T.J. and Wilkinson D.S.: Diseases of veins and arteries; in Rood et al. (Eds) Textbook of Dermatology, 4th ed. (Blackwell Scientific Publications, in press 1985).

Teh, B.T.: Why do skin grafts fail? Plastic and Reconstructive Surgery 63: 323 (1979).

Address for correspondence and reprints: Dr *T.J. Ryan*, John Radcliffe Hospital, Headington, Oxford OX3 9DU (England).

Leading Article

Drugs 30: 469-474 (1985)
0012-6667/85/0012-0469/$03.00/0

How Dangerous Are Diuretics?

Edward D. Freis and *Vasilios Papademetriou*
Veterans Administration and Georgetown University Medical Center, Washington

Two major concerns that have been raised against the use of diuretics are: (a) diuretic-induced hypokalaemia may predispose to dangerous arrhythmias including sudden death (Kolata, 1982); and (b) long term diuretic use may cause an increase in serum cholesterol and thus an increased risk of arteriosclerosis, including coronary artery disease (Grimm et al., 1981).

Diuretics have provided the basic regimen for treating hypertension for many years and have served as the primary treatment in most of the controlled trials demonstrating the effectiveness of treatment. Although most physicians still believe that treatment for hypertension usually should begin with a thiazide diuretic, others are apt to try alternative regimens. This is due primarily to an increased concern with the potential risks of diuretic-induced hypokalaemia. These concerns resulted initially in a dramatic increase in the administration of potassium supplements or potassium-sparing diuretics, the cost of which in the USA totalled $250 million in 1981 alone (Harrington et al., 1982). Recently, because of fear of toxicity some physicians, especially in Scandinavia, have reduced the doses of hydrochlorothiazide to as low as 6.25 or 12.5 mg/day (e.g. Andrew et al., 1983; Berglund and Anderson, 1976).

Diuretics are the only known antihypertensive agents which lower blood pressure by reducing salt, water and extracellular fluid volume (Freis, 1976). Recent controlled trials indicate that when given as the sole treatment thiazide diuretics control blood pressure in approximately half of the patients treated (Veterans Administration Cooperative Study Group, 1982a,b,c, 1983), and in 85% of those given a diuretic plus a step-two drug (Editorial, 1977; Freis, 1976). Because they are effective, and certainly the least expensive of the antihypertensive agents, the validity of the charges against them needs to be carefully examined.

1. Diuretics and Hypokalaemia

1.1 Relationship Between Dose, Volume Depletion and the Antihypertensive Effects of Diuretics

There is a close association between volume reduction and the antihypertensive response to the diuretics. It has been known for many years that diuretics cause a moderate reduction in extracellular fluid volume and plasma volume, approximating 10 to 15% (Dustan et al., 1959; Wilson and Freis, 1959). This effect, although moderate, appears to play a major role in the reduction of blood pressure (Dustan et al., 1959; Freis, 1976). Volume loss occurs during the first 3 or 4 days of continuous treatment with diuretics after which no further volume depletion occurs (Freis, 1976; Papademetriou et al., 1984a). The net reductions in fluid volume are reflected in loss of bodyweight which approximates 1 to 2kg (Papademetriou et al., 1984a; Wilson and Freis, 1959). With respect to hydrochlorothiazide, doses of 50 mg/day were required to produce weight loss in most patients whereas lower doses of 25 or 12.5mg did not result in significant weight loss (McGregor et al., 1983). Thus, in many patients, doses smaller than 50 mg/day would not be sufficient to lower volume effectively and probably blood pressure as well.

The antihypertensive effectiveness of long term drug therapy is often difficult to assess. Because of spontaneous decreases in blood pressure such studies need to be carefully controlled. Following repeated visits to the clinic, blood pressure often reverts back to normal levels without any drug treatment (Carey et al., 1976; Management Committee Australian Therapeutic Trial in Mild Hypertension, 1982), and without proper controls it may be impossible to differentiate spontaneous and drug-induced reductions in blood pressure.

A few studies have suggested that when low doses of hydrochlorothiazide are given with a β-blocker the dose-response curve becomes flat after 6.25 or 12.5 mg/day of hydrochlorothiazide (Andrew et al., 1983; Berglund and Anderson, 1976). However, it is difficult to judge the effectiveness of one drug when it is combined with another, especially when there is no control evaluation of either drug used alone (Andrew et al., 1983).

On the other hand there is considerable evidence to indicate that the antihypertensive response to hydrochlorothiazide alone does not become flat at low levels but rather continues to increase to quite high doses of the diuretic. For example, in the Veterans Administration Cooperative Study, propranolol alone was compared with hydrochlorothiazide alone in patients with mild hypertension. Doses of hydrochlorothiazide were titrated as needed from 25mg twice daily to 50mg twice daily and finally to 100mg twice daily until the diastolic blood pressure was controlled to <90mm Hg (Veterans Administration Cooperative Study Group, 1982a,b). Of the patients controlled on hydrochlorothiazide alone, 50% attained the goal diastolic pressure with the 25mg twice daily dose. However, 30% required the 50mg twice daily dose and 20% needed 100mg of the diuretic twice daily before their diastolic blood pressure fell to <90mm Hg. These doses are far in excess of the 6.25 or 25mg recommended by others.

Studies other than the Veterans Administration trial have found that the dose-response curve of hydrochlorothiazide also does not remain flat after small doses, and that doses as high as 100 mg/day are required in many patients (Anderson et al., 1984; Henning et al., 1980). It would appear from these results that different patients vary in their responsiveness to the diuretics and that while small doses are satisfactory in some patients they are inadequate in others. As with most antihypertensive agents, the optimal dose of a diuretic is probably best found by individual titration.

1.2 Diuretic-Induced Hypokalaemia and Ventricular Arrhythmias

Reluctance to employ standard doses of diuretics in treating patients with uncomplicated essential hypertension derives primarily from the possibility that diuretic-induced hypokalaemia may predispose to the development of life-threatening or even fatal ventricular arrhythmias (Kolata, 1982; Multiple Risk Factor Intervention Group, 1982).

Contrary to popular opinion, diuretic-induced hypokalaemia is not associated with a major loss of total body potassium. The hypokalaemia is limited almost exclusively to the extracellular compartment. Review of various studies indicates that during continuous thiazide treatment, losses of body potassium approximate only a biologically unimportant 5 to 7% of the total body content (Kassirer and Harrington, 1977). These small losses are in contrast to changes in extracellular potassium, which is reduced by about 20%. Because potassium concentrations within the cells are much greater than in extracellular fluid, large changes in extracellular potassium may exert only a small influence on total body potassium. The large difference between extra- and intracellular potassium levels is maintained by sodium-potassium metabolic pump activity (Haddy and Pamnami, 1984).

Whether selective extracellular hypokalaemia without significant change in intracellular potassium, such as occurs with diuretic-induced hypokalaemia, predisposes to increased risk of ventricular arrhythmias is not known. Although adequate studies in experimental animals have not been performed (Harrington et al., 1982), the electrophysiological changes associated with selective extracellular hypokalaemia point towards a decreased rather than increased incidence of cardiac arrhythmias. According to the Nernst equation (Dyckner and Wester, 1979; Papademetriou, 1983) an increase in the intracellular/extracellular ratio which occurs in diuretic-induced hypokalaemia causes hyperpolarisation of the cell membrane. This raises the depolarisation threshold of the myocardium resulting in decreased rather than increased susceptibility of the heart to the development of arrhythmias. Hyperpolarisation of the cell membrane, however, may also raise conduction velocity which under special circumstances such as ischaemia, heart blocks or myocardial scars may either promote or retard re-entry phenomena. Regardless of these theoretical considerations, an increase in the ratio of intracellular/extracellular potassium of the type associated with thiazide diuretics has not been reported to produce life-threatening arrhythmias.

Diuretic-induced hypokalaemia may have differing physiological or pathological effects depending on the presence or absence of heart disease. For example, in the presence of congestive heart failure there may be a reduction in the intracellular concentration of potassium (Editorial, 1977). Localised changes in potassium may occur such as in acute myocardial infarction where high concentrations of potassium have been measured in the ischaemic zone (Hydegger et al., 1984). The elevated concentrations of potassium are thought to be the result of leakage of potassium from the injured cells. The role of whether diuretic-induced hypokalaemia in these special situations has not yet been clarified. This article, however, is not concerned with these forms of heart disease, but rather with the great majority of hypertensive patients who do not have overt heart disease and whose intracellular potassium content is apparently normal.

1.3 Hypokalaemia and Frequency of Ventricular Arrhythmias

The most practical and direct way of determining whether diuretic-induced hypokalaemia produces disturbances in cardiac rhythm is to carry out electrocardiographic monitoring. Using 48-hour continuous ambulatory monitoring, no association between hypokalaemia and the incidence of ventricular arrhythmias was found by Papademetriou et al. (1984b). Continuous electrocardiographic monitoring was carried out in patients with mild hypertension prior to any therapy and following hydrochlorothiazide treatment for 4 weeks. Patients were separated into those who developed hypokalaemia with thiazide therapy and those in whom serum potassium concentrations remained within the normal range. Following thiazide therapy no change was noted in either the frequency or severity of the arrhythmias in the patients who became hypokalaemic or those who remained normokalaemic. Other investigators using continuous electrocardiographic monitoring have confirmed the above findings (Leif et al., 1984; Madias et al., 1984). Further, in patients with overt hypokalaemia on long term diuretic therapy, administration of potassium supplements and potassium-sparing diuretics in amounts sufficient to raise serum potassium levels to normal had no effect on ventricular arrhythmias (Papademetriou et al., 1983).

A previous study by Holland et al. (1981) using electrocardiographic monitoring indicated that hypokalaemia secondary to the thiazides did increase the frequency and severity of ventricular arrhythmias. The difference between Holland's results and the more recent studies probably can be explained by differences in methodology. Holland excluded all patients who exhibited 6 or more ventricular premature beats/hour during the control period prior to thiazide administration. However, because of the great day-to-day spontaneous fluctuation in ectopic activity (Michelson and Morgenroth, 1980) the chances of these selected patients showing greater ectopic activity on the second (hypokalaemic) monitoring would be greatly enhanced simply by chance alone. Other investigators who did not select their patients on this basis found no increase in arrhythmias associated with the development of hypokalaemia (Leif et al., 1984; Madias et al., 1984; Papademetriou et al., 1984b).

Another previous study found an association between hypokalaemia and exercise-induced premature ventricular beats (Hollifield and Staton, 1981). The results are difficult to interpret, however, for a number of reasons: (a) the correlations were based on only 2- to 5-minute monitoring of arrhythmias which may be insufficient to distinguish chance occurrence of ectopic beats from those due to hypokalaemia; (b) the clinical significance of exercise-induced premature beats and their prognostic value is essentially unknown; and (c) the reproducibility of this method of assessing arrhythmias is very poor. This work has not been repeated and remains unconfirmed.

Additional concern with respect to diuretic-induced hypokalaemia has been generated by the recent observation that catecholamines which increase entry of potassium into cells may further aggravate the hypokalaemia resulting from treatment with thiazides (Struthers et al., 1983). However, these studies have not demonstrated that the hypokalaemia resulting from the combined effects of the diuretic and catecholamines has any effect on ventricular ectopic activity or that it increases either the frequency or severity of ventricular arrhythmias. As a result of catecholamine excess, potassium moves mostly into skeletal muscle cells with only minimal changes in potassium content of myocardial cells. The catecholamine-induced changes increase the ratio of intra- to extracellular potassium and theoretically at least should make the ventricle less rather than more susceptible to development of arrhythmias. Although catecholamines are known to increase ventricular arrhythmias they probably do so by other mechanisms than reduction in extracellular potassium.

1.4 Evidence from Clinical Trials

Most of the concern regarding the possible relationship between thiazide-induced hypokalaemia and sudden death has been generated by the results of the Multiple Risk Factor Intervention Trial (MRFIT) [Kolata, 1982; Multiple Risk Factor Intervention Trial, 1982]. It was suggested that data from MRFIT implicated thiazide diuretics as the cause for an increase in cardiac deaths in a subgroup of patients with minor electrocardiographic abnormalities. However, there are several problems with the interpretation of these data. The study was not designed to determine the relationship of cardiac deaths with respect to treatment with thiazide diuretics. The relationship between thiazide diuretics and sudden death was found after a retrospective search for correlations between many variables. This kind of retrospective procedure often leads to positive correlations by chance alone. Therefore, evidence so derived must be confirmed by independent studies. The results of other studies, however, have not been confirmatory.

Available data from similar trials such as The Hypertension Detection and Follow-up Program (HDFP) failed to confirm the findings of MRFIT. Thus, in HDFP no subgroup correlations were found between thiazide treatment and cardiovascular deaths (The Hypertension Detection and Follow-up Program, 1984). The HDFP investigators concluded that their results offered no support for the hypothesis raised in MRFIT that diuretics increase the mortality rates of patients with resting ECG abnormalities. The recently published morbidity-mortality results of the Medical Research Council Working Party (MRC Trial, 1985) indicated no significant differences between the effects of bendrofluazide in the prevention of all-cause mortality compared with propranolol ($p = 0.24$ and 0.71, respectively; cigarette smokers and non-smokers combined). Furthermore, in none of the studies (including MRFIT) has there been any correlation between diuretic dosage, serum potassium levels and deaths due to heart disease (Medical Research Council Working Party on Mild to Moderate Hypertension, 1983; MRFIT Trial, 1985).

The Medical Research Council Working Party on Mild to Moderate Hypertension (1983) reported 2 substudies with electrocardiographic monitoring. In one study without pretreatment baseline monitoring an increased incidence of ventricular ectopy occurred in hypertensive patients during long term treatment with thiazides compared to a group receiving only placebos. In this subgroup, however, there was no correlation between arrhythmias and serum potassium level, although there was a weak correlation with serum uric acid concentration. A second trial, better controlled, failed to confirm the first in that there was no increase in arrhythmias during treatment with thiazide diuretics for a period of 8 to 10 weeks.

The available evidence, therefore, fails to support the view that in patients without heart disease diuretic-induced hypokalaemia causes increased ventricular arrhythmias. But, because of the undue concern that has been generated, potassium replacement therapy has become widespread (Harrington et al., 1982), which if overdone could become potentially dangerous (Lawson, 1974).

2. *Diuretics and Serum Cholesterol*

Serum cholesterol usually increases slightly when thiazide diuretics are administered (Grimm et al., 1981). Some investigators have expressed concern that the elevation, even though slight, would over a period of many years aggravate and accelerate the development of coronary heart disease (Grimm et al., 1981). This fear would have some justification if it could be shown that the elevation of serum cholesterol is indeed persistent. The available evidence, however, indicates that it is not.

Three studies have shown that expected initial increases in serum cholesterol levels were followed later by reduction to or below the pretreatment levels. One of these trials was carried out in a Veterans Administration cooperative study in which 343 patients with mild hypertension received hydrochlorothiazide and no other drugs or dietary treatment (Veterans Administration Cooperative Study, 1982b). Plasma cholesterol rose during the first 3 months of treatment but at 12 months the cholesterol level fell to below baseline. Similarly, Alcazar et al. (1982) also found that plasma cholesterol only rose initially, and after 3 months returned toward the pretreatment baseline, remaining there for the next several years of observation. Data taken from the HDFP also indicated that the short term rise in plasma cholesterol was followed by a long term return to baseline (Williams et al., 1983). These observations are further supported by other studies which made only long term observations on changes in plasma cholesterol. When serum cholesterol levels were measured 1 or 2 years after beginning treatment they were not elevated in 2 studies (Amery et al., 1982; Kannel et al., 1977), but were elevated in 1 (Goldman et al., 1980).

Thus, elevated serum cholesterol concentration is not a risk during long term treatment with diuretics because the almost unanimous experience has been that elevation is not persistent after 6 months or 1 year of treatment.

3. *Summary and Conclusions*

The proposal that thiazide diuretics may increase cardiovascular risk receives no support from recent data. Current evidence does not indicate that diuretic-induced hypokalaemia is associated with increased ventricular arrhythmias. This evidence includes continuous electrocardiographic monitoring – which is the most sensitive technique for quantitating cardiac arrhythmias. In contrast to earlier reports, more recent studies found no evidence for increased arrhythmias during the period of hypokalaemia, or for decreased arrhythmic activity after correction of hypokalaemia. Similarly, studies claiming increased sudden death in patients on diuretic treatment have not been substantiated by the results of other large-scale trials.

Elevation of serum cholesterol concentrations with thiazide appears to be a short term phenomenon since most studies indicate the elevation reverts to baseline during long term treatment.

Thiazide diuretics remain as one of our most effective antihypertensive agents. Fears of their increasing the incidence of ventricular arrhythmias due to hypokalaemia, or constituting a risk factor for atherosclerosis by elevating serum cholesterol concentrations, appear largely unsubstantiated.

References

Alcazar, J.; Ruilope, L.; Ladron de Guevara, P.; Navarro, A.; Sang, J. et al.: Interrelationship between uric acid, cholesterol and triglycerides in essential hypertension (Meeting Abstract No. 8), Proceedings of Ninth Meeting, International Society on Hypertension, Mexico City, Feb 20-21 (1982).

Amery, A.; Birkenhager, C.; Bulpitt, D. et al.: Influence of antihypertensive therapy on serum cholesterol in elderly hypertensive patients. Acta Cardiologica 27: 235-244 (1982).

Anderson, P.O.; Henning, H.A.; Hagman, A. and Henning, R.: Potassium sparing by amiloride during thiazide therapy in hypertension. Clin. Pharmacol. Ther. 36: 197-200 (1984).

Andrew, L.; Weiner, L.; Svensson, A. and Hansson, L.: Enalapril with either a 'very low' or 'low' dose of hydrochlorothiazide is equally effective in essential hypertension. A double-blind trial in 100 hypertensive patients. Journal of Hypertension (Suppl. 2): 384-486 (1983).

Berglund, G. and Anderson, O.: Low doses of hydrochlorothiazide in hypertension: Antihypertensive and metabolic effects. European Journal of Clinical Pharmacology 10: 177-182 (1976).

Carey, R.M.; Reid, R.A.; Ayers, C.R.; Lynch, S.; McLain III, W.L. and Darracott Jr, V.E.: The Charlottsville blood pressure survey. Value of repeated blood pressure measurements. Journal of the American Medical Association 236: 847-851 (1976).

Dustan, H.P.; Cunning, G.R.; Corcoran, A.C. and Page, I.H.: A mechanism of chlorothiazide enhanced effectiveness of antihypertensive ganglioplegic drugs. Circulation 19: 360 (1959).

Dyckner, T. and Wester, P.O.: Ventricular extrasystoles and intracellular electrolytes in hypokalemic patients before and after potassium and magnesium infusion in patients on diuretic treatment. American Heart Journal 97: 12-18 (1979).

Editorial: Potassium in heart failure. Brit. Med. J. 1: 469 (1977).

Freis, E.D.: Salt, volume and the prevention of hypertension. Circulation 53: 589-595 (1976).

Goldman, A.I.; Steele, B.W.; Schnaper, H.W.; Fitz, A.E.; Frohlich, E.D. and Perry, H.M.: Sodium lipoprotein levels during chlorthalidone therapy. A Veterans Administration National Lung and Blood Institute Cooperative Study Group on Antihypertensive Therapy. Mild Hypertension. Journal of the American Medical Association 244: 1691-1695 (1980).

Grimm Jr, R.H.; Leon, A.S.; Hunninghake, D.B.; Leng, K.; Hannon, P. et al.: Effects of thiazide diuretics on plasma lipids and liproprotein in mildly hypertensive patients. A double blind controlled trial. Ann. Int. Med. 94: 11 (1981).

Haddy, F.J. and Pamnami, M.B.: The vascular Na^+-K^+ pump in low renin hypertension. J. Cardiov. Pharmacol. 6: 561 (1984).

Harrington, J.I.; Isner, J.M. and Kassirer, J.P.: Our national obsession with potassium. Amer. J. Med. 73: 155-159 (1982).

Henning, R.; Karlsberg, B.E.; Odar-Cederlöf, I.; Anderson, P.O.; Luis, L.E. et al.: Timolol and hydrochlorothiazide-amiloride in primary hypertension. Clin. Pharmacol. Ther. 28: 707 (1980).

Holland, O.B.; Nixon, J.V. and Kuhnert, I.: Diuretic-induced ventricular ectopic activity. Amer. J. Med. 770: 762 (1981).

Hollifield, J.W. and Slaton, P.E.: Thiazide diuretics, hypokalemia and cardiac arrhythmias. Acta Med. Scand. 647: 67-73 (1981).

Hydegger, C.; Anderson, G.; Hill, J. and Dennis, S.: Extracellular K^+ gradient across an ischemic boundary. Journal of the American College of Cardiology 3: 587 (1984).

The Hypertension Detection and Follow-up Program Cooperative Research Group: The effect of antihypertensive drug treatment on mortality in the presence of resting electrocardiographic abnormalities at baseline: The HDFP experience. Circulation 70: 996-1003 (1984).

Kannel, W.H.; Gordon, T. and McGee, D.: Diuretics and serum cholesterol. Lancet 1: 1362-1363 (1977).

Kassirer, J.P. and Harrington, J.T.: Diuretics and potassium metabolism: A reassessment of the need, effectiveness and safety of potassium therapy. Kidney International 11: 505-515 (1977).

Kolata, G.: Heart study produces a surprise result. Science 218: 31-32 (1982).

Lawson, D.H.: Adverse reactions to potassium chloride. Quarterly Journal of Medicine 43: 433-440 (1974).

Leif, P.D.; Beligon, I.; Mates, J. and Bank, N.: Diuretic-induced hypokalemia does not cause ventricular ectopy in uncomplicated essential hypertension. Kidney Internat. 25: 203 (1984).

Madias, J.E.; Madias, N.E. and Gavras, H.P.: Nonarrhythmogenicity of diuretic-induced hypokalemia. Archives of Internal Medicine 144: 2171-2176 (1984).

Management Committee of the Australian Therapeutic Trial in Mild Hypertension. Untreated mild hypertension. Lancet 1: 185-191 (1982).

McGregor, G.A.; Banks, R.A.; Markender, N.D.; Bayliss, J. and Roulston, J.: Lack of effect of beta-blocker in flat dose response to thiazide in hypertension: Efficacy of low dose thiazide combined with beta-blocker. Brit. Med. J. 286: 1535 (1983).

Medical Research Council Working Party on Mild to Moderate Hypertension: Ventricular extrasystoles during thiazide treatment: Substudy on MRC mild hypertension trial. British Medical Journal 287: 1249-1253 (1983).

Medical Research Council Working Party: MRC trial of treatment of mild hypertension: Principal results. British Medical Journal 291: 97 (1985).

Michelson, E.L. and Morganroth, J.: Spontaneous variability of complex ventricular arrhythmias detected by long-term electrocardiographic recording. Circulation 61: 690-695 (1980).

Multiple Risk Factor Intervention Trial Research Group: Multiple Risk Factor Intervention trial. Risk factor changes and mortality results. J. Amer. Med. Assoc. 248: 1465 (1982).

Multiple Risk Factor Intervention Trial Research Group: Baseline rest electrocardiographic abnormalities, antihypertensive treatment and mortality in the Multiple Risk Factor Intervention Trial. American Journal of Cardiology 55: 1-5 (1985).

Papademetriou, V.; Fletcher, R.; Khatri, I.M. and Freis, E.D.: Diuretic-induced hypokalemia in uncomplicated systemic hypertension: Effect of plasma potassium correction on cardiac arrhythmias. Amer. J. Cardiol. 52: 1017-1022 (1983).

Papademetriou, V.; Price, M.; Johnson, E.; Smith, M. and Freis, E.D.: Early changes in plasma and urinary potassium in diuretic-treated patients with systemic hypertension. American Journal of Cardiology 54: 1015-1019 (1984a).

Papademetriou, V.; Price, M.B.; Notargiacomo, A.; Fletcher, R.D. and Freis, E.D.: Effects of thiazide therapy on ventricular arrhythmias in patients with uncomplicated systemic hypertension. Amer. Fed. Clin. Res. 32: 2-337A (1984b).

Struthers, A.D.; Whitesmith, R. and Reid, J.L.: Prior thiazide diuretic treatment increases adrenaline-induced hypokalaemia. Lancet 1: 1358-1361 (1983).

Veterans Administration Cooperative Study Group on Antihypertensive Agents: Comparison of propranolol and hydrochlorothiazide for the initial treatment of hypertension. I. Results of short-term titration with emphasis on racial differences in response. J. Amer. Med. Assoc. 248: 1996-2003 (1982a).

V.A. Study Group: II. Results of long-term therapy. Journal of the American Medical Association 248: 2004-2011 (1982b).

Veterans Administration Cooperative Study Group on Antihypertensive Agents: Efficacy of nadolol alone and combined with bendroflumethiazide and hydralazine for systemic hypertension. Amer. J. Card. 52: 1230-1337 (1983).

Veterans Administration Cooperative Study Group on Antihypertensive Agents: Captopril: Evaluation of low doses, twice-daily doses and the addition of diuretic for the treatment of mild to moderate hypertension. Clin. Sci. 63: 4435 (1982c).

Williams, W.R.; Borhani, H.D.; Schnaper, H.W. et al.: The relationship between diuretics and serum cholesterol in HDFP participants. J. Amer. Coll. Card. 1: 623 (1983).

Wilson, I.M. and Freis, E.D.: Relationship between plasma and extracellular fluid volume depletion and the antihypertensive effect of chlorothiazide. Circulation 20: 1028 (1959).

Address for correspondence and reprints: Dr *Edward D. Freis*, Hypertension Research, VA Medical Center, Washington, D.C. 20422 (USA).

Leading Article

Drugs 30: 475-481 (1985)
0012-6667/85/0012-0475/$03.50/0

Therapeutic Use of Respiratory Stimulants
An Overview of Newer Developments

Barbara M. Galko and *Anthony S. Rebuck*
Division of Respiratory Medicine, Toronto Western Hospital, Toronto

Many drugs have been noted to stimulate ventilation in man, but because of their high incidence of unacceptable side effects few have found a place in clinical practice. Categories of potentially useful therapeutic agents include the methylxanthines, narcotic antagonists, progestagens, carbonic anhydrase inhibitors and the piperazine derivative, almitrene. Analeptics comprise an additional category, but have a small and unpredictable margin of safety between doses stimulating respiration and those producing stimulation of other brain centres. They have no clinical role in the management of poisoning from any sedative-hypnotic drug and, at best, serve as temporary measures in the management of chronic obstructive pulmonary disease. These drugs will therefore not be discussed further.

The recent interest in near-miss sudden infant death syndrome (SIDS) patients, and in the sleep apnoeas, has given new impetus to research in respiratory stimulants. These agents have long been useful in the therapy of chronic respiratory insufficiency, primary alveolar hypoventilation and narcotic and sedative overdose, but there is no universal agreement as to their clinical role. The objective of this article is to review briefly currently available respiratory stimulants, and to examine trends in current research that might point to the physiological properties required of the ideal agent.

1. Methylxanthines

The mechanisms of action of xanthines include competitive inhibition of the cyclic nucleotide phosphodiesterase (Butcher and Sutherland, 1962), the translocation of intracellular calcium (Blinks et al., 1972), and blockade of receptors for adenosine (Kakiuchi et al., 1969). The most widely used xanthine derivative is theophylline. For decades, this drug's major clinical role was that of a potent bronchodilator in the management of the asthmatic patient, and as an adjunct in the therapy of acute pulmonary oedema. Recently, interest has shifted to its properties of stimulating central respiratory neurons, enhancing the contractility of the diaphragm, and delaying fatigue in other respiratory muscles.

Evidence of stimulation of central respiratory neurons by xanthines has existed for some time. Thus Stroud et al. (1955) examined the effect of aminophylline and pethidine (meperidine) on the ventilatory response to CO_2. Aminophylline (6 mg/kg) produced sufficient respiratory stimulation to counter the respiratory depressant effects of 100mg of pethidine. More recently, studies in premature infants have demonstrated that oral or intravenous administration of aminophylline eliminates episodes of apnoea that last more than 20 seconds and markedly reduces those of shorter duration (Shannon et al., 1975).

Murciano et al. (1984) studied the effects of theophylline on diaphragmatic strength and fatigue in patients with severe chronic obstructive pulmonary disease. Maximal transdiaphragmatic pressure at functional residual capacity was increased by 16% after 7 days of administration of theophylline 13 mg/kg, this increase persisting after 30 days. Theophylline also suppressed diaphragmatic fatigue, as assessed by the high-low ratio of electrical activity of the diaphragm under conditions of resistive loaded breathing. Despite these findings, more recent work by Belman et al. (1985) question whether these changes were likely to improve long term ventilatory endurance. They measured maximal sustained ventilatory levels during prolonged isocapnoeic hyperpnoea as an index of ventilatory muscle function in 7 controls and 7 patients with chronic obstructive pulmonary disease, during intravenous infusion of saline and aminophylline in the usual therapeutic dose on 2 separate days. Although all subjects showed slightly higher sustained ventilatory levels during aminophylline infusion, the magnitude of the change was small and unlikely to have a significant clinical benefit in the setting of respiratory muscle fatigue.

Therapeutic Implications: Xanthine derivatives have been used since 1900 as therapy for reactive airways disease. Newly discovered actions of these drugs include dose-dependent improvement of diaphragmatic contractility, augmentation of ventilatory responses to hypoxia and an effect on breathing disturbances during sleep. While these newer roles of xanthines as respiratory stimulants are still evolving, they will continue to play an important role in the management of both acute and chronic airways obstruction. As respiratory muscle fatigue may tip the balance between success and failure during prolonged periods of weaning from mechanical ventilator support, and as most such patients benefit from maximal bronchodilatation, the addition of xanthines to the usual pharmacological regimen in such patients appears appropriate and justified.

2. Narcotic Antagonists

Narcotics, derived from the juice of the poppy *Papaver somniferum*, have been used medicinally since the third century BC. Though the problems of addiction and ventilatory depression have been noted for centuries, it was not until this century that compounds with opioid antagonist properties were studied. The narcotic antagonists have either pure antagonistic actions, such as naloxone (Foldes et al., 1969) or agonist-antagonist properties, such as nalorphine (Martin, 1967). As naloxone lacks any agonist properties, it has become the agent of choice for the reversal of ventilatory depression secondary to narcotic abuse, and has been shown to reverse narcotic-induced postoperative respiratory depression, although repeated doses (or a continuous infusion) may be necessary due to its short duration of action.

Endogenous opioids (or endorphins) have been postulated to be involved in the responses to chronic pain (Terenius, 1978), neuroendocrine regulation (Davis, 1979), and, more recently, in the control of breathing. Naloxone stimulates the output of central respiratory neurons in anaesthetised and ventilated cats (Lawson et al., 1979) and in fetal sheep (Moss and Scarpelli, 1979). However, naloxone has no effect on ventilatory responses to hypoxia or hypercapnia in normal subjects (Fleetham et al., 1980), or in anaesthetised human subjects (Foldes et al., 1969). Similarly, the hypercapnia associated with pulmonary disease (Butland et al., 1981) or hypothalamic disturbance (Dunger et al. 1980) is not altered by the administration of naloxone. Santiago et al. (1981) studied 14 normocapnoeic patients with chronic obstructive pulmonary disease and 8 healthy controls, measuring ventilation, pulmonary function, ventilatory response to CO_2 and the ventilatory response to flow-resistive loading, before and after the administration of naloxone. Before naloxone, increased resistance to breathing enhanced respiratory effort in all controls but in only 7 of 14 patients. After naloxone, these patients augmented their ventilatory response to loaded breathing, a pattern similar to that observed in healthy controls. These findings suggest that the elaboration of endorphins in patients with chronic obstructive lung disease minimise the stress of their chronic airway obstruction. Restoration of respiratory drive by naloxone in decompensated patients may allow for conservative management with avoidance of mechanical ventilation, though the results of clinical trials on this aspect of narcotic antagonist therapy are still awaited.

Therapeutic Implications: While naloxone has an established place in the resuscitation of otherwise healthy patients with narcotic overdose, or for reversing effects of narcotics postoperatively, the therapeutic role of narcotic antagonists as ventilatory stimulants is less certain in chronic respiratory acidosis. Until this is further clarified, narcotic antagonists are providing a useful tool for studying mechanisms of neuroendocrine regulation of breathing in research laboratories.

3. Progestagens

The hyperventilation now recognised to occur during pregnancy was originally described simultaneously by 2 groups over 70 years ago (Hasselbalch, 1912, Leimdorfer et al., 1912), and was subsequently found to be caused by increased levels of endogenous progesterone (Doring and Loeschcke, 1947). Exogenous progesterone, when administered to normal human subjects, increases minute ventilation (Heerhaber et al., 1948, Lyons and Antonio, 1959) and it is this property that has led to its use as a therapeutic agent.

Both parenterally administered progesterone (100mg daily) and sublingually administered medroxyprogesterone acetate (20mg every 8 hours) have produced improvements in alveolar ventilation in Pickwickian patients – a syndrome characterised by obesity, hypercarbia, hypoxia and elevated pulmonary vascular resistance (Lyons and Huang, 1968; Sutton et al., 1975). Progesterone-induced increases in alveolar ventilation have also been reported in emphysematous patients in respiratory failure (Tyler, 1960).

These encouraging results prompted Orr et al. (1979) to study 7 morbidly obese patients with sleep-related upper airway obstruction who underwent physiological measurements during sleep, before and during progesterone treatment (200mg sublingually, 3 times daily). All subjects had severe daytime somnolence, and 5 of 7 had congestive heart failure. There was no significant difference in the incidence, mean duration or rate per minute of apnoeic episodes occurring before and with progesterone treatment. Both severe hypoxaemia and cardiac arrhythmias during sleep persisted with treatment. However, over the course of treatment with progesterone, all of the patients were clinically improved, with a reduction in heart failure, peripheral oedema and daytime somnolence. The awake values of PaO_2 rose from a mean of 48 to 64mm Hg ($p < 0.05$) during progesterone therapy, though the reduction in $PaCO_2$ from a mean of 39 to 34mm Hg was considered not to be clinically significant. When measured during sleep, these parameters were unchanged before and during treatment. Therefore, in this group of morbidly obese patients the mechanisms of improvement of hypoxaemia were likely related to increased glomerular filtration, diuresis, and improved cardiac function, whereas increased minute ventilation played a minor role.

Therapeutic Implications: Progesterone administration leads to increased ventilation in healthy subjects, and in patients with chronic hypoventilation of any cause. It may have beneficial effects in patients with sleep apnoea syndromes. However, despite apparent improvement in patient well-being and arterial blood gases drawn while awake, potentially serious nocturnal arterial oxygen desaturation may occur and arrhythmias may persist.

4. Acetazolamide

Mobilisation of oedema fluid and the production of a negative extracellular fluid balance can be achieved by many diuretics that act directly on the kidney. When mobilisation of oedema fluid is rapid, e.g. with drugs such as ethacrynic acid, metabolic alkalosis can result from contraction of extracellular fluid volume (Mudge, 1975). With long term therapy, the combined effects of negative chloride balance and hypokalaemia are also associated with metabolic alkalosis. In healthy subjects. diuretic-induced (or for that matter any metabolically induced) alkalosis is compensated to some extent by hypoventilation (Sabatini et al., 1977), clearly an undesirable response in patients with impaired ventilatory drive. The induction of diuresis in patients with chronic respiratory insufficiency is therefore undertaken with caution attendant upon the realistic concern that fluid balance might be improved at the expense of further impairment of respiratory failure. While acetazolamide has limited usefulness as a diuretic, its action as a noncompetitive inhibitor of carbonic anhydrase results in an increased concentration of the bicarbonate anion in urine and a reduction in urinary chloride (Mudge, 1975). Consequently the concentration of bicarbonate in the extracellular fluid decreases and metabolic acidosis results. It is this latter property of acetazolamide that has suggested its use as a therapeutic agent in patients with impaired central respiratory drive.

Acetazolamide produces chronic hyperventilation in awake, normal subjects (Galdston, 1955; Nadell, 1953) by increasing blood hydrogen ion concentration, which acts at both peripheral and medullary chemoreceptor sites (Lane et al., 1977, Lerche et al., 1960). It has been used to improve hypoventilation in both acute (Miller and Berne, 1977) and chronic (Bear et al., 1977) metabolic alkalosis in patients with chronic obstructive pulmonary disease and decreases apnoeic awakenings and arousals in patients with central sleep apnoea (White et al., 1982).

While acetazolamide appears to stimulate ventilation through its renal acid-base mechanism there is now evidence that, like other respiratory stimulants, it might also have a direct although nonspecific effect on respiratory neurons. Thus, Cain (1961) gave a 12-minute intravenous infusion of the drug and found that ventilation had increased markedly even before the infusion was completed. It appears therefore that part of the respiratory stimulant action of acetazolamide may be unrelated to acidosis produced by the kidney but explained by increased cerebral blood flow. Despite our limited understanding of its action, acetazolamide has found a therapeutic use in the prophylaxis of acute mountain sickness and to augment the ventilatory effects of hypoxia at high altitudes (Larson et al., 1982).

Therapeutic Implications: Acetazolamide may be given orally or as an intravenous bolus to promote a bicarbonate diuresis and metabolic acidosis. In addition to its newest area of use, preventing acute mountain sickness, it has an important clinical role in critically ill patients who have developed compensatory and drug-induced (steroids, diuretics) metabolic alkalosis during the course of their chronic hypercapnic ventilatory insufficiency. During the course of management of patients with acute exacerbations of chronic obstructive lung disease, when intensive therapy is being directed to avoidance of or weaning from mechanical ventilation, acetazolamide will promote a significant diuresis and in so doing will act as a respiratory stimulant by correcting the complicating alkalaemia.

5. Almitrene

Almitrene bismesilate is a piperazine derivative that specifically stimulates peripheral chemoreceptors. It is pharmacologically unrelated to central-acting agents and is reported to be free of their side effects. The most convincing experimental evidence that almitrene has no effect on the central nervous system comes from the work of Laubie and Diot (1972) who have shown that after carotid denervation the action of the drug is abolished and no effect can be observed when the drug is injected directly into the cisterna. Its pharmacological action lasts for at least 6 hours when administered intravenously and carbon-label isotope studies suggest a half-life of 35 hours (Laubie and Diot, 1972). When almitrene is administered orally in a dose of 5 mg/kg in awake healthy subjects (Guillerm and Radziszewski, 1974) both tidal volume and respiratory frequency increase, with ventilation returning to normal levels within 1 minute of administration of pure oxygen. When administered intravenously in a dose of 1 mg/kg, healthy subjects increase their minute ventilation by approximately 12%, oxygen suppressing the increase in ventilation within 20 to 40 seconds (Flandrois and Guérin, 1980).

Aside from its effects as a primary ventilatory stimulant, almitrene has been shown to improve arterial oxygen tension in patients with chronic obstructive pulmonary disease to a degree that cannot be fully explained on the basis of lowering of the arterial pCO_2 tension. It appears that the drug improves ventilation-perfusion mismatching as a result of redistribution of blood flow away from poorly ventilated areas (Sergysels et al., 1978; Tenaillon et al., 1980).

In addition to improvements in blood gases with almitrene, the evidence that the drug affects the distribution of pulmonary blood flow comprise increased pulmonary vascular resistance with minor changes in cardiac output (Naeije et al., 1981) and an improvement in perfusion lung scans with an increase in blood flow to previously underperfused upper lung fields (Rigaud et al., 1980). Continuous monitoring of regional ventilation-perfusion ratios by an inert gas method (Wagner et al., 1974) substantiated the finding of redistribution of perfusion towards zones with higher ventilation-perfusion ratios in patients with severe chronic obstructive lung disease (Castaing et al., 1981).

The reported changes in distribution of pulmonary blood flow and pulmonary vascular resistance clearly give rise to some concern that pulmonary hypertension might be caused or exacerbated by almitrene, but its significant effect on impaired peripheral chemoreceptor drive justifies extensive study in these compromised patients. In this context, Powles et al. (1983) administered almitrene intravenously to 11 patients with severe chronic airflow obstruction and hypoxaemia in a randomised double-blind study, finding a reduction in venous admixture and improvement in blood gases in some but not all patients. The acute effects in most patients were to improve arterial pO_2 and pCO_2 either by increasing ventilation or improving ventilation-perfusion relationships. Oral administration (100mg) in patients with a similar degree of impaired pulmonary function achieved a significant improvement of arterial oxygen saturation with no change in pulmonary artery pressure or minute ventilation (Melot et al., 1983). As ventilation-perfusion mismatching is more marked in patients with chronic obstructive pulmonary disease than in healthy subjects, almitrene causes less improvement in blood gas tensions with more noticeable changes in minute ventilation in healthy volunteers (Pariente, 1983).

Therapeutic Implications: Almitrene increases tidal volume and respiratory frequency while simultaneously improving ventilation/blood flow mismatching by its effect on pulmonary blood flow distribution. Its therapeutic use is established for the restoration of peripheral chemosensitivity in halothane anaesthetised subjects, and it appears worthy of more extensive evaluation in patients with chronic obstructive lung disease. The potential but unproven hazard of exacerbating pulmonary hypertension may be outweighed by its obvious advantages over other respiratory analeptic drugs.

6. Conclusion

The ideal respiratory stimulant, if it existed, would be used in the treatment of the underventilation that follows oxygen therapy. The ideal response would be an increase in ventilation, a fall in pCO_2 and an improvement in the level of consciousness. The agent would not increase oxygen consumption, pulmonary vascular resistance or restlessness. It would have a wide margin between therapeutic and toxic doses and its effect should be apparent within hours. Desirable side effects would include bronchodilatation and improved diaphragmatic contractility. While the agents described in this article have among them many of these properties, none could be described as the ideal agent.

Acknowledgement

We wish to thank Ms M.T. Berk for secretarial assistance in preparation of the manuscript.

References

Bear, R.; Goldstein, M.; Philipson, E.; Ho, M.; Hammeke, M. et al.: Effect of metabolic alkalosis on respiratory function in patients with chronic obstructive lung disease. Canadian Medical Association Journal 117: 900-903 (1979).

Belman, M.J.; Sieck, G.C. and Mazar, A.: Aminophylline and its influence on ventilatory endurance in humans. American Review of Respiratory Diseases 131: 226-229 (1985).

Blinks, J.R.; Olson, C.B.; Jewell, B.R. and Braveny, RP.: Influence of caffeine and other methylxanthines on mechanical properties of isolated mammalian heart muscle. Evidence for dual mechanism of action. Circulation Research 30: 367-392 (1972).

Butcher, R.W. and Sutherland, E.W.: Adenosine 3′,5′-phosphate in biological materials. Journal of Biological Chemistry 237: 1244-1250 (1962).

Butland, R.J.; Woodcock, A.A.; Gross, E.R. and Geddes, D.M.: Endogenous opioids (endorphins) and the control of breathing. New England Journal of Medicine 305: 1096 (1981).

Cain, S.A.: A ventilatory effect of carbonic anhydrase in man. Proceedings of the Society for Experimental Biology and Medicine 106: 770 (1961).

Castaing, Y.; Manier, G.; Varene, N. and Guenard, H.: Effets de l'almitrene orale sur la distribution continue des rapport $V_A/\dot{Q}$ dans les bronchopenumopathies chroniques obstructives. Bulletin Européen de Physiopathologie Respiratoire 17: 917-932 (1981).

Davis, G.C.: Studies of the role of endorphins in normal subjects and psychiatric patients; in Bunney Jr W.E. (Moderator) Basic and Clinical Studies of Endorphins. Annals of Internal Medicine 91: 246-248 (1979).

Doring, G.H. and Loeschcke, H.H.: Atmung und Saure-Basengleichgewigt in der Schwangerschaft. Pfluegers Archiv für die Gesampte Physiologie des Menschen und der Tiere 249: 437-451 (1947).

Dunger, D.B.; Leonard, J.V.; Wolfe, O.H. and Preece, M.A.: Effect of naloxone in a previously undescribed hypothalamic syndrome. Lancet 1: 1277-1281 (1980).

Flandrois, R. and Guérin, J.C.: Action de l'almitrene sur le controle chémoreflexe de la ventilation chez l'homme sain et l'insuffisant respiratoire chronique. Revue Française des Maladies Respiratoires 8: 561-567 (1980).

Fleetham, J.A.; Clarke, H.; Dhingra, S.; Chernick, V. and Anthonisen, N.R.: Endogenous opiates and chemical control of breathing in humans. American Review of Respiratory Disease 121: 1045-1059 (1980).

Foldes, F.F.; Duncalf, D. and Kuwabara, S.: The respiratory, circulatory and narcotic antagonistic effects of nalorphine, levallorphan and naloxone in anaesthetized subjects. Canadian Anaesthetists Society Journal 16: 151-162 (1969).

Galdston, M.: Respiratory and renal effects of a carbonic anhydrase inhibitor (Diamox) on acid-base balance in normal man and in patients with respiratory acidosis. American Journal of Medicine 19: 516-532 (1955).

Guillerm, R. and Radziszewski, E.: Effets ventilatoires chez l'homme sain d'un nouvel analeptique respiratoire, le S2620. Bulletin Européen de Physiopathologie Respiratoire 10: 776-791 (1974).

Hasselbalch, K.A.: Ein Beirag zur Respirationphysiologie der Graviditaet. Skandinavishes Archiv für Physiologie 27: 1-12 (1912).

Heerhaber, I.; Loeschcke, H.H. and Westphal, U.: Eine Wirkung des progesterons auf die Atmung. Pflugers Archiv für die Gesampte Physiologie des Menschen und der Tiere 250: 42-55 (1948).

Kakiuchi, S.; Rall, T.W. and McIlwain, H.: The effect of electrical stimulation upon the accumulation of adenosine 3′,5′-phosphate in isolated cerebral tissue. Journal of Neurochemistry 16: 485-491 (1969).

Lane, D.J.; Horwell, J.B. and Stretton, T.B.: The effect of dichlorphenamide on blood and cerebrospinal fluid acid-base state in chronic ventilatory failure. Clinical Science 39: 391-406 (1977).

Larson, E.B.; Roach, R.C.; Schoene, R.B. and Hornbein, T.F.: Acute mountain sickness and acetazolamide. Clinical efficacy and effect on ventilation. Journal of the American Medical Association 248: 328-332 (1982).

Laubie, M. and Diot, F.: A pharmacological study of the respiratory stimulant action of S2620. Journal of Pharmacology 3: 363-374 (1972).

Lawson, E.E.; Waldrop, T.G. and Eldridge, F.L.: Naloxone enhances respiratory output in cats. Journal of Applied Physiology: Respiratory Environmental and Exercise Physiology 47: 1105-1111 (1979).

Leimdorfer, A.; Novak, J. and Porges, O.: Ueber die Kohlensaurespannung des Blutes in der Graviditat. Zeitschrift für Klinische Medizin 75: 301 (1912).

Lerche, D.; Katsaros, B.; Lerche, G. and Loescheke, H.: Vergleich der Wirkung verschiedener acidosen (NH_4Cl, $CaCl_2$, Acetazolamid) auf die Lungenbeluftung beim Menschen. Pflugers Archiv für die Gesampte Physiologie des Menschen und der Tiere 270: 450-460 (1960).

Lyons, H.A. and Antonio, R.: The sensitivity of the respiratory center in pregnancy and after the administration of progesterone. Transactions of the Association of American Physicians 72: 173-180 (1959).

Lyons, H.A. and Huang, C.T.: Therapeutic use of progesterone in alveolar hypoventilation associated with obesity. American Journal of Medicine 44: 881-888 (1968).

Martin, W.R.: Opiod antagonists. Pharmacological Reviews 19: 463-521 (1967).

Melot, C.; Naeije, R.; Hallemans, R.; Mols, P. and Lejeune, P.: Beneficial effects of almitrene bismesylate on pulmonary gas exchange in COPD. European Journal of Respiratory Diseases 126 (Suppl.): 249-254 (1983).

Miller, P.D. and Berne, A.S.: Acute metabolic alkalosis perpetuating hypercarbia: A role for acetazolamide in chronic obstructive pulmonary disease. Journal of the American Medical Association 238: 2400-2401 (1977).

Moss, I.R. and Scarpelli, E.M.: Generation and regulation of breathing in utero: Fetal CO_2 response test. Journal of Applied Physiology: Respiratory Environmental and Exercise Physiology 47: 527-531 (1979).

Mudge, G.H.: Diuretics and other agents employed in the mobilization of edema fluid; in Goodman and Gilman (Eds) Pharmacological Basis of Therapeutics, 5th ed., pp. 817-721 (MacMillan, New York 1975).

Murciano, D.; Aubier, M.; Lecocguic, Y. and Pariente, R.: Effects of theophylline on diaphragmatic strength and fatigue in patients with chronic obstructive pulmonary disease. New England Journal of Medicine 311: 349-353 (1984).

Nadell, J.: The effects of carbonic anhydrase inhibitor '6063' on electrolytes and acid base balance in two normal subjects and two patients with respiratory acidosis. Journal of Clinical Investigation 32: 622-629 (1953).

Naeije, R.; Melot, C.; Mols, P.; Hallemans, R.; Naeije, N. et al.: Effects of almitrene in decompensated chronic respiratory insufficiency. Bulletin Européen de Physiopathologie Respiratoire 17: 153-161 (1981).

Orr, W.C.; Imes, N.K. and Martin, R.J.: Progesterone therapy in obese patients with sleep apnea. Archives of Internal Medicine 139: 109-111 (1979).

Pariente, R.: Clinical pharmacology of Almitrene Bismesylate. European Journal of Respiratory Diseases 126 (Suppl.): 271-274 (1983).

Powles, A.C.P.; Tuxen, D.V.; Mahood, C.B.; Pugsley, S.O. and

Campbell, E.J.M.: The effect of intravenously administered almitrene, a peripheral chemoreceptor agonist, on patients with chronic air-flow obstruction. American Review of Respiratory Disease 127: 284-289 (1983).

Rigaud, D.; Dubois, D.; Boutet, J.; Brambilla, C.; Verain, A. and Paramelle, B.: Effets de l'almitrene sur la distribution isotropique de la ventilation et de la perfusion regionales chez l'insuffisant respiratoire chronique. Revue Françise des Maladies Respiratoires 8: 605 (1980).

Sabatini, S.; Arruda, J.A.L. and Kurtzman, N.A.: Disorders of acid-base balance. Medical Clinics of North America 62: 1223-1255 (1977).

Santiago, T.V.; Remolina, C.; Scoles, V. and Edelman, N.H.: Endorphins and the control of breathing. Ability of naloxone to restore flow-resistive load compensation in chronic obstructive pulmonary disease. New England Journal of Medicine 304: 1190-1195 (1981).

Sergysels, R.; Etien, J.L.; Schandevyl, W. et al.: Functional evaluation of a new analeptic drug in patients with chronic hypoxemia and hypercapnia (preliminary study). Acta Tuberculosia a Pneumologica Belgica 69: 237-246 (1978).

Shannon, D.C.; Gotay, F.; Stein, I.M.; Rogers, M.C.; Todres, I.D. and Moylan, F.M.B.: Prevention of apnea and bradycardia in low-birthweight infants. Pediatrics 55: 589-594 (1975).

Stroud, M.W.; Lambertsen, C.J.; Ewing, R.; Lough, R.H.; Gould, R.A. and Schmidt, C.F.: Effects of aminophylline and meperidine alone and in combination on the respiratory response to carbon dioxide inhalation. Journal of Pharmacology and Experimental Therapeutics 114: 461-469 (1955).

Sutton, F.D.; Zwillich, C.W.; Creagh, C.E.; Pierson, D.J. and Weil, J.V.: Progesterone for outpatient treatment of Pickwickian syndrome. Annals of Internal Medicine 83: 476-479 (1975).

Tenaillon, A.; Labrouse, J.; Longchal, J.; Bahloul, F. and Lissac, J.: Effects of almitrene on blood gases in chronic obstructive lung disease (COPD) with acute respiratory failure (ARF). (Abstract.) Intensive Care Medicine 6: 64 (1980).

Terenius, L.: Endogenous peptides and analgesia. Annual Review of Pharmacology and Toxicology 18: 189-204 (1978).

Tyler, J.M.: The effect of progesterone on the respiration of patients with emphysema and hypercapnia. Journal of Clinical Investigation 39: 34-41 (1960).

Wagner, P.D.; Salzman, H.A. and West, J.B.: Measurement of continuous distributions of ventilation-perfusion ratio: theory. Journal of Applied Physiology: Respiratory Environmental and Exercise Physiology 36: 588 (1974).

White, D.P.; Zwillich, C.W.; Pickett, C.K.; Douglas, N.J.; Findley, L.J. and Weil, J.V.: Central sleep apnea. Improvement with acetazolamide therapy. Archives of Internal Medicine 142: 1816-1819 (1982).

Address for correspondence and reprints: Dr *A.S. Rebuck*, Division of Respiratory Medicine, Toronto Western Hospital, Department of Medicine, 399 Bathurst Street, Suite 204, Edith Cavell Wing, Toronto, Ontario M5T 258 (Canada).

Drugs 30: 482-513 (1985)
0012-6667/85/0012-0482/$16.00/0

Norfloxacin
A Review of Its Antibacterial Activity, Pharmacokinetic Properties and Therapeutic Use

B. Holmes, R.N. Brogden and *D.M. Richards*

ADIS Drug Information Services, Auckland

Various sections of the manuscript reviewed by: ***R.R. Bailey,*** Department of Nephrology, Christchurch Hospital, Christchurch, New Zealand; ***A.L. Barry,*** Clinical Microbiology Institute, Tualatin, Oregon, USA; ***A. Bauernfeind,*** Institute of Hygiene and Medical Microbiology, University of Munich, Munich, West Germany; ***M. Bologna,*** Department of Biological Sciences, Collemaggio, Aquila, Italy; ***A. Digranes,*** Department of Microbiology and Immunology, Haukeland Hospital, Bergen, Norway; ***H. Giamarellou,*** Department of Propedeutic Medicine, Laikon General Hospital, Athens, Greece; ***H.C. Neu,*** Division of Infectious Diseases, College of Physicians and Surgeons of Columbia University, New York, USA; ***S.W.B. Newsom,*** Hospital Infection Society, Papworth Hospital, Cambridge, England; ***S.R. Norrby,*** Department of Infectious Diseases, University of Umeä, Umeä, Sweden; ***D.S. Reeves,*** Division of Pathology, Southmead Hospital, Bristol, England; ***J. Shimada,*** Department of Medicine, Jikei University School of Medicine, Tokyo, Japan; ***R. Wise,*** Department of Medical Microbiology, Dudley Road Hospital, Birmingham, England.

Contents

Summary 483
1. Antimicrobial Activity *In Vitro* 486
1.1 *In Vitro* Inhibitory Activity Against Aerobic Bacteria 486
1.1.1 Gram-Negative Bacteria 486
1.1.2 Gram-Positive Bacteria 489
1.2 Activity Against Anaerobic Bacteria and Other Organisms 489
1.3 Antifungal Activity 491
1.4 Activity Against Organisms Resistant to Other Antibacterial Drugs 491
1.5 Effect on Activity of Media, pH and Inoculum Size 492
1.6 Bactericidal Activity 494
1.7 Mechanism of Action and Development of Resistance 494
2. Pharmacokinetics 496
2.1 Absorption and Serum Concentrations 496
2.2 Distribution 497
2.3 Elimination 498
2.3.1 Half-Life 500
2.4 Effect of Decreased Renal Function on Pharmacokinetics 500
2.5 Effect of Decreased Liver Function on Pharmacokinetics 500
3. Therapeutic Trials 501
3.1 Uncomplicated Acute Urinary Tract Infection 501
3.1.1 Open Studies 501

3.1.2 Comparative Studies 501
3.2 Chronic and/or Complicated Urinary Tract Infections 504
3.2.1 Open Studies 504
3.2.2 Comparative Studies 505
3.3 Gonococcal and Non-Gonococcal Urethritis 505
3.4 Gastroenteritis and Prophylaxis of Sepsis in Neutropenic Patients 505
3.5 Other Infections 506
4. Side Effects 507
5. Dosage and Administration 508
6. The Place of Norfloxacin in Therapy 508

Summary

Synopsis: *Norfloxacin*[1] *is one of the new 4-quinolone antibacterial agents. A fluorinated piperazinyl-substituted congener of nalidixic acid, it demonstrates a much wider* in vitro *antibacterial spectrum and greater potency than the parent compound. Its antibacterial activity against most Gram-negative pathogens is enhanced in comparison to nalidixic acid, but is similar to that of some of the other new 4-quinolones like enoxacin, and slightly less than that of ciprofloxacin. Unlike nalidixic acid, norfloxacin is also active against* Pseudomonas aeruginosa *and some Gram-positive organisms.*

In acute or uncomplicated urinary tract infections, norfloxacin has repeatedly been shown to be as effective as co-trimoxazole. Single studies have demonstrated a significantly better bacteriological cure rate with norfloxacin than with pipemidic acid, and similar cure rates with norfloxacin and both a nalidixic acid/sodium citrate mixture and amoxycillin. Similar results were found in a few studies comparing norfloxacin to pipemidic acid or amoxycillin in patients with chronic and/or complicated urinary tract infections. Norfloxacin is as effective as spectinomycin in gonorrhoea due to penicillin-resistant N. gonorrhoeae, *and cures bacterial gastroenteritis caused by several gastrointestinal pathogens.*

Norfloxacin appears to be well tolerated and may have a low propensity to select for bacterial resistance during clinical use, although the latter needs further confirmation.

Antibacterial Activity: Norfloxacin is structurally related to nalidixic acid, but it has a broader *in vitro* antibacterial spectrum and is generally more active. Most Gram-negative pathogens including *Escherichia coli* and *Klebsiella, Enterobacter, Proteus* and *Citrobacter* species are susceptible to norfloxacin, and are inhibited by concentrations of 2 mg/L or less, with the exception of some strains of *Acinetobacter, Providencia* and *Serratia* species which are slightly less sensitive [minimum inhibitory concentration for 90% of tested strains (MIC_{90}): < 1 to 32 mg/L]. 90% of *Pseudomonas aeruginosa* isolates are inhibited by norfloxacin 1 to 2 mg/L. Although several times more active than nalidixic acid and some other quinolone antibacterial agents such as cinoxacin and oxolinic acid against these pathogens, norfloxacin is usually of similar potency to enoxacin and generally less active than ciprofloxacin. *Haemophilus influenzae* demonstrates marked sensitivity to norfloxacin (MIC_{90}: < 2 mg/L), as do *Neisseria gonorrhoeae* and *meningitidis,* and a range of organisms which commonly occur as gastrointestinal pathogens, e.g. *Salmonella* and *Shigella* species (MIC_{90}: < 1 mg/L). Campylobacter species are inhibited by slightly higher concentrations (MIC_{90}: ≤ 4 mg/L).

Staphylococci, including *S. saprophyticus,* are susceptible to norfloxacin (MIC_{90}: 1 to 4 mg/L) but the streptococci, including enterococci, are more resistant (MIC_{90}: 2 to 16

1 'Barazan', 'Floxacin', 'Zoroxin' (Merck Sharp and Dohme); 'Baccidal Kyorin' (Kyorin); 'Baccidal Torii' (Torii Yakuhin); 'Sebercim' (ISF); 'Fulgram' (ABC).

mg/L). Most strains of anaerobic bacteria are only moderately sensitive to norfloxacin, while some are resistant. Although norfloxacin has no intrinsic antifungal activity there is some evidence of synergy with antifungal agents against *Candida* species.

Despite the fact that norfloxacin has been demonstrated to be significantly less active *in vitro* in urine than in diagnostic sensitivity test (DST) agar (MIC_{90} values increasing 16 to 64 times), the high concentrations of the drug achieved in urine following oral administration make this of doubtful clinical significance. However, a definite pH effect has been noted for norfloxacin, activity decreasing considerably with decreasing pH below 5.5. Optimum activity is thought to occur between pH 7.5 and 8. Generally, higher concentrations of norfloxacin are required to inhibit organisms in Mueller Hinton broth than in agar, but similar values have been found for Mueller Hinton agar and DST agar.

Increasing the inoculum size from 10^3 to 10^6 colony-forming units (cfu) has only minor effects on MIC and minimum bactericidal concentration (MBC) values for norfloxacin. At 10^7 cfu, half the tested strains require twice the concentration of norfloxacin for inhibition, while at 10^8 cfu there are 2- to 4-fold increases in MIC values. MBC values are only slightly higher than MIC values for most organisms, although some strains of *P. aeruginosa* and *Serratia marcescens* require 4- to 8-fold increases in norfloxacin concentration for a bactericidal effect.

Norfloxacin is thought to act by inhibiting the A subunit of the essential enzyme DNA gyrase in the bacterial cell. Resistance to norfloxacin has so far been slow to develop clinically and the agent shows good activity against many multiresistant strains of bacteria. Nevertheless, resistance to norfloxacin can be induced experimentally. Cross-resistance has been observed between norfloxacin and nalidixic acid as well as some of the newer nalidixic acid analogues (ciprofloxacin, enoxacin, cinoxacin and oxolinic acid) and, in a few instance, some β-lactam antibiotics.

Pharmacokinetic Properties: Following single oral doses of norfloxacin 400mg, mean maximum serum concentrations of 1.35 to 1.58 mg/L have been achieved within 1 to 2 hours. An approximately linear relationship between maximum serum concentration, area under the concentration-time curve and dose was lost at doses in excess of 800mg and there is some uncertainty about the disposition of higher doses. Thus, the fraction of the dose absorbed over the first 12-hour period was lower at higher doses in 1 study, while another study reported disproportionately high serum concentrations and areas under the concentration time curve (AUC) at doses above 800mg. There does not appear to be any significant accumulation on multiple dose administration in healthy subjects.

Bioavailability appears to be approximately 70% and absorption is only delayed slightly when norfloxacin is administered with food.

Information on the distribution of norfloxacin into various body tissues is limited, but concentrations higher than those in serum have been found in both common duct and gallbladder bile as well as in liver tissue. Extrapolation of volume of distribution data from animal studies to man suggests values of around 25 to 35L, but the volume of distribution may prove to be much higher.

Approximately 30% of an oral dose is excreted as unchanged norfloxacin in urine. Six metabolites, 1 or more of which are thought to be microbiologically active, have been found in urine but account for less than 10% of an administered dose. Renal clearance has varied from 16.32 to 17.76 L/h with doses ranging from 200 to 1600mg. The urinary recovery of norfloxacin is halved by the coadministration of probenecid, indicating the involvement of some active renal tubular secretion. The elimination half-life of norfloxacin in healthy subjects ranges from 3.5 to 6.5 hours.

Decreased liver function has no significant effect on norfloxacin pharmacokinetics. In renal failure the serum half-life of norfloxacin increases with decreasing creatinine clearance. Values of around 6.5 hours have been noted in patients with moderate failure, rising to 7.7 hours in greater degrees of failure, while in haemodialysed patients the half life is around 7.9 hours.

Therapeutic Trials: Norfloxacin has been primarily studied in acute, uncomplicated urinary tract infections (UTI), with a smaller number of studies in chronic and/or complicated UTI, gonococcal and non-gonococcal urethritis, gastroenteritis and other infections. In open trials in acute or uncomplicated UTI the bacteriological cure rate with norfloxacin 300 to 800mg daily (usually for 3 to 10 days) has been reported to be 82 to 100%. Several comparative studies using random allocation of treatments show norfloxacin 400 to 800mg daily to be at least as effective as co-trimoxazole 320/1600mg daily; follow-up at 4 to 6 weeks demonstrated a slightly higher incidence of relapse or reinfection in the patients treated with co-trimoxazole than in those treated with norfloxacin. Norfloxacin 800mg daily for 3 days has produced a higher bacteriological cure rate 2 to 4 days post-therapy than a nalidixic acid/sodium citrate mixture, the difference becoming significant after the late follow-up at 4 to 6 weeks. Similarly, norfloxacin 300mg daily for 3 days has proved significantly more effective in eliminating bacteriura than pipemidic acid 750mg daily. Norfloxacin 800mg daily for 7 days has also produced higher bacteriological cure rates than amoxycillin 750mg daily, 4 to 9 days after therapy, but the difference did not reach a statistically significant level in this study.

In open trials in chronic and/or complicated UTI, the bacteriological response rate with norfloxacin (usually 300 to 900mg for 3 to 10 days) varies from 15 to 92%. However, adequate follow-up information is absent from all but 2 of these studies. Cumulated data from several Japanese trials reveal a decreased rate of eradication of bacteriura for norfloxacin in patients with indwelling catheters or in whom a prostatectomy has been performed. In 2 comparative trials in chronic and/or complicated UTI norfloxacin 800mg daily for 5 days was significantly better than pipemidic acid 2000mg daily, and in a single study the same dosage of norfloxacin for 7 days was at least as effective as amoxycillin 750mg daily.

Various dosage regimens of norfloxacin have been assessed in gonococcal urethritis; bacteriological cure rates of 93 to 100% are reported. Also, two 600mg doses of the 4-quinolone have proved to be as effective as a single intramuscular dose of spectinomycin 2g in men with gonorrhoea due to penicillin-resistant *N. gonorrhoeae.* Norfloxacin is less effective in non-gonococcal urethritis, with bacteriological cure rates of only 43 to 83%.

Norfloxacin 800 and 1200mg daily for 5 days have been found to be as effective as co-trimoxazole 320/1600mg daily in the eradication of harmful bacteria (rates of 98, 100 and 95%, respectively) in patients with acute bacterial gastroenteritis.

Side Effects: In comparative studies the incidence of adverse effects with norfloxacin has been generally lower than that with co-trimoxazole but similar to that with pipemidic acid. The most frequently reported adverse reactions to norfloxacin are gastrointestinal disturbances, which occur in about 2 to 4% of patients. Central nervous system reactions are generally minimal but include lightheadedness, drowsiness, headache and dizziness.

Dosage and Administration: In the treatment of urinary tract infections, the usual adult dosage is 400mg twice daily continued for 7 to 10 days. Three-day therapy has been shown to be effective in women with uncomplicated acute cystitis. In the treatment of chronic, relapsing urinary tract infection, the dosage of norfloxacin is 400mg twice daily for up to 12 weeks; if adequate suppression is obtained within the first 4 weeks the dosage of norfloxacin may be reduced to 400mg daily.

In acute bacterial gastroenteritis the usual dosage is 400mg twice daily for 5 days.

In patients with renal failure, in whom creatinine clearance is less than 30 ml/min/ $1.73m^2$ the recommended dosage is 400mg daily.

In the prophylaxis of sepsis in profound neutropenia, the recommended dosage is 400mg 3 times daily for the duration of profound neutropenia. However, data for recommending treatment beyond 8 weeks are presently not available.

The safety and efficacy of norfloxacin in children have not been established.

Place in Therapy: If wider clinical use confirms the efficacy, the low incidence of side effects and the apparently low propensity of norfloxacin to induce resistance clinically, it may not only offer worthwhile advantages over the standard agents used to treat urinary tract infections (e.g. co-trimoxazole and amoxycillin, as well as nalidixic acid and some of its early analogues), but it may become a valuable prophylactic and therapeutic antibiotic in several other clinical situations.

1. Antimicrobial Activity In Vitro

Norfloxacin, a γ-pyridone β-carboxylic acid structurally related to nalidixic acid, is one of the first of the new 'quinolone' group of antibacterial drugs (fig. 1). *In vitro,* its antibacterial spectrum is wider than that of nalidixic acid and includes *Pseudomonas* species and some Gram-positive cocci. It has also demonstrated a greater potency than nalidixic acid against most pathogens, although this high activity is reduced in the urine. Like pipemidic acid it contains a piperazinyl ring which confers antipseudomonal activity, while the 6-fluorine atom is thought to contribute to the electron stability of the molecule and to its greater potency (Newsom, 1984).

1.1 *In Vitro* Inhibitory Activity Against Aerobic Bacteria

There are several methods to assess the *in vitro* activity of an antibiotic. The conclusions of this review are based on the minimum inhibitory concentration (MIC).

Since the literature on the antibacterial activity of norfloxacin is fairly extensive, generally only studies using larger numbers of strains (usually clinical isolates) and an inoculum of 10^4 to 10^6 colony-forming units (cfu) were assessed.

1.1.1 Gram-Negative Bacteria

Enterobacteriaceae

As can be seen from tables I and II, 90% of tested strains of most species of Enterobacteriaceae were inhibited (MIC_{90}) by concentrations of norfloxacin at or below 2 mg/L, with the exception of *Serratia* and *Providencia* species in some studies. In contrast, most species required a minimum nalidixic acid concentration of 4 mg/L to achieve inhibition of growth of 90% of tested strains. While the comparative activity of norfloxacin and other 4-quinolones varied with different species of Enterobacteriaceae (table II), in general norfloxacin was much more active (several-fold) than cinoxacin and pi-

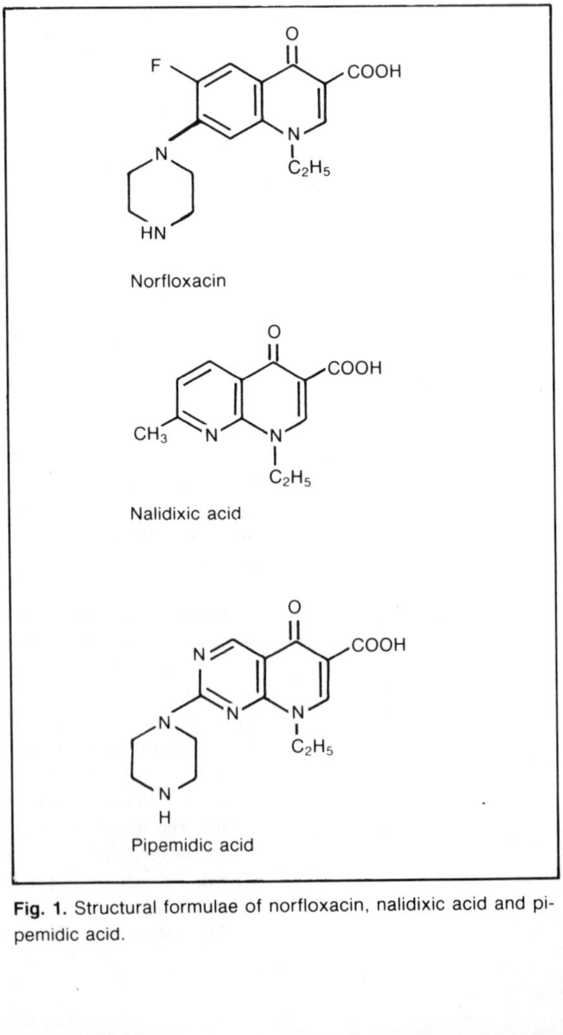

Fig. 1. Structural formulae of norfloxacin, nalidixic acid and pipemidic acid.

pemidic acid, similar in activity to enoxacin and slightly less active than ciprofloxacin. Norfloxacin was also more active than co-trimoxazole against Enterobacteriaceae.

Pseudomonas species

The results of a study of the *in vitro* activity of azlocillin, aminoglycosides and the 4-quinolones, norfloxacin and ciprofloxacin, against 100 epidemiologically diverse isolates of *P. aeruginosa* are shown in table III. The highest *in vitro* activity was clearly observed for ciprofloxacin, with 92% of the strains being inhibited by 0.25 mg/L. The activity of norfloxacin was 4 to 8 times lower than that of ciprofloxacin, but norfloxacin was inhibitory at lower concentrations than the aminoglycosides and azlocillin (Vangdal and Bergan, 1984a). These findings for norfloxacin are supported by the range of values obtained for MIC_{90} (1 to 2 mg/L) in other studies (Barry et al., 1984; Eliopoulos et al., 1984; King et al., 1984; Muytjens et al., 1983; Wise et al., 1983).

The minimum inhibitory concentration of norfloxacin against 90% of *Pseudomonas* species in these, and other studies has ranged from 0.5 to 16 mg/L (Barry et al., 1984; Digranes et al., 1984; Gadebusch et al., 1982; Husson et al., 1984; Jones and Barry, 1983; Khan et al., 1982; King et al., 1982; Muytjens et al., 1983; Nakamura et al., 1983; Neu and Labthavikul, 1982; Newsom et al., 1982; Norrby and Jonsson, 1983; Peddie, 1982; Reeves et al., 1984a; Wise et al., 1984a), although in 2 cases *P. maltophilia* has proved more resistant, with MIC_{90} values of 64 and > 128 mg/L (Jones and Barry, 1983; Corrado et al., 1983, respectively). In comparison, oxolinic acid was less active than norfloxacin against *Pseudomonas* species (MIC_{90}: 2 to 32 mg/L) [Barry et al., 1984; Jones and Barry, 1983; Vuye, 1983], and cinoxacin was even less active (MIC_{90}: 16 to > 512 mg/L) [Barry et al., 1984; Gadebusch et al., 1982; Jones and Barry, 1983; Norrby and Jonsson, 1983; Vuye, 1983]. Enoxacin, on the other hand, demonstrated a level of activity similar to that of norfloxacin (MIC_{90}: 2 to 6 mg/L) [Bauernfeind and Ullmann, 1984; Nakamura et al., 1983; Reeves et al., 1984a; Wise et al., 1984a].

Neisseria species

Both β-lactamase negative and β-lactamase positive strains of *N. gonorrhoeae* were inhibited by low concentrations of norfloxacin with MIC_{90} values of 0.015 to 0.03 mg/L and 0.06 mg/L, respectively (Khan et al., 1983; Peeters et al., 1984; Piffaretti et al., 1983). Other studies recording the activity of norfloxacin against *N. gonorrhoeae* support these findings (MIC_{90}: 0.016 to 0.06 mg/L) [Barry et al., 1984; Corrado et al., 1983; Gadebusch et al., 1982; King et al., 1982; Neu and Labthavikul, 1982; Newsom et al., 1982; Sweet et al., 1982]. Although not as active as ciprofloxacin and the newer cephalosporins, ceftriaxone and cefotaxime, against *N. gonorrhoeae* (MIC_{90}: 0.002 to 0.008 mg/L), norfloxacin demonstrated similar activity to the other quinolones, rosoxacin and ofloxacin (MIC_{90}: 0.008 to 0.06 mg/L) [Peeters et al., 1984].

Norfloxacin was also active in very low concentrations against *N. meningitidis* (MIC_{90} values < 0.05-$\leqslant 0.06$) [Barry et al., 1984; Neu and Labthavikul, 1982].

Other Gram-Negative Organisms

Acinetobacter species proved more resistant to norfloxacin with MIC_{90} values of 2 to 32 mg/L, as was true for nalidixic acid with MIC_{90} values of 4 to > 256 mg/L (Barry et al., 1984; Digranes et al., 1984; Gadebusch et al., 1982; Husson et al., 1984; Jones and Barry, 1983; King et al., 1982; Neu and Labthavikul, 1982; Newsom et al., 1982; Norrby and Jonsson, 1983). Norfloxacin and enoxacin (MIC_{90}: 2 to 12.5 mg/L) were similarly active against these species while ciprofloxacin was more active (MIC_{90}: 0.12 to 0.5 mg/L) and cinoxacin less active (MIC_{90}: $\geqslant$ 32 to 128 mg/L) [Barry et al., 1984; Bauernfeind and Ullmann, 1984; Gadebusch et al., 1982; Jones and Barry, 1983; Nakamura et al., 1983; Norrby and Jonsson, 1983].

Haemophilus influenzae, including β-lactamase producing strains, was very susceptible to norfloxacin with MIC_{90} ranging from $\leqslant$ 0.06 to 1.5 mg/L (table I; King et al., 1984; Nakamura et al., 1983; Wise et al., 1983, 1984a).

Norfloxacin also proved effective against a range of Gram-negative organisms which commonly oc-

Table I. *In vitro* activity of norfloxacin and nalidixic acid against Gram-negative organisms (medium used was Mueller-Hinton broth or agar and inoculum size ranged from 10^3 to 10^6 organisms/ml)

No. of strains	Norfloxacin		Nalidixic acid		References
	range of MIC	MIC_{90}[a]	range of MIC	MIC_{90}[a]	
E. coli					
542	0.025-2	0.19-0.5	0.39-128	4-8	2,6,8
204[b]	0.016-8	0.125	1-16	4	2
Klebsiella					
429 spp.	0.125-8	2	2-> 128	2-> 32	6,8
199 pneumoniae[b]	0.016-2	0.125	1-16	8	2
72 *oxytoca*	0.016-1	0.125	4-> 128	8	2
100 pneumoniae	≤ 0.025-1.56	0.19	0.78-100	12.5	9
Enterobacter					
436 *cloacae*	< 0.025-50	0.25-0.78	1-> 128	4-100	2,8,9
28 *aerogenes*	0.06-0.5	0.125-0.5	4-8	4-8	2,8
53 spp.	≤ 0.06-32	0.5	2-> 128	16	7
Proteus					
358 indole (+)	< 0.025-3.13	≤ 0.06-0.39	0.39-> 100	4-50	7-9
82 indole (−)		0.25		> 32	8
134 *mirabilis*	< 0.025-4	0.12-0.19	3.13-> 128	6-16	7,9
125 *mirabilis*[b]	0.016-0.5	0.063	1-16	4	2
70 *vulgaris*	0.016-0.25	0.063	1-16	4	2
Morganella					
40 *morganii*	0.016-2	0.063	1-64	4	2
Providencia					
36 spp.	< 0.03-2	0.12	0.5-≥ 64	≥ 64	4[c]
35 *rettgeri*	≤ 0.03-> 32	0.12-4	1-> 128	16-128	1,4
24 *rettgeri*[b]	0.016-1	0.25	1-16	16	2
Citrobacter					
254 *freundii*	≤ 0.025-100	0.125-3.13	0.39-> 128	8-> 100	2,7-9
8 *diversus*		0.5		16	8
Serratia					
171 *marcescens*	≤ 0.01-100	0.5-12.5	0.19-> 100	4-> 100	3,8,9
32 *marcescens*[b]	0.016-1	0.25	1-4	4	2

cur as gastrointestinal tract pathogens. Both *Salmonella* species and *Shigella* species were susceptible to norfloxacin, with MIC_{90} values of 0.05 to 0.25 mg/L and 0.06 to < 0.5 mg/L, respectively (Carlson et al., 1983; Diez-Enciso et al., 1984; Goossens et al., 1985; Kurimura et al., 1981; Neu and Labthavikul, 1982; Preblud et al., 1984; Shungu et al., 1983). *Yersinia enterocolitica* (MIC_{90}: 0.03 to 0.09 mg/L) [Carlson et al., 1983; Goossens et al., 1985; Shungu et al., 1983], *Aeromonas hydrophilia* (MIC_{90}: 0.05 and 0.125 mg/L), *Plesiomonas shigelloides* (MIC_{90}: ≤ 0.063 mg/L) [Carlson et al., 1983; Reinhardt and George, 1985], *Vibrio parahaemolyticus* (MIC_{90}: ≤ 0.05 and 0.06 mg/L) [Carlson et al., 1983; Shungu et al., 1983], and *Vibrio cholera* (MIC_{90}: 0.015 mg/L) [Shungu et al., 1983] were all easily inhibited by norfloxacin.

1.1.2 Gram-Positive Bacteria

In studies of the activity of norfloxacin against Gram-positive cocci, most staphylococcal strains, including *S. saprophyticus,* were susceptible to nor-

Table I. (contd)

No. of strains	Norfloxacin		Nalidixic acid		References
	range of MIC	MIC_{90}[a]	range of MIC	MIC_{90}[a]	
Acinetobacter					
31 *calcoaceticus*	0.5-32	16	1->256	>256	5
60 *calcoaceticus* variant *anitratus*	0.125-32	8	1-32	8	2
23 *calcoaceticus* variant *lwoffi*	0.25-4	4	2-32	4	2
48 spp.	0.78-50	6.25	3.13-100	25	9
Haemophilus influenzae					
40[d]	≤ 0.06-≤ 0.06	≤ 0.06	≤ 0.25-1	0.5	1[e]
40	≤ 0.05-3.13	0.125-1.56	0.25-25	12.5-32	9[f],3[g]

a MIC_{90} = minimum concentration to inhibit 90% of organisms (mg/L).
b Susceptible to nalidixic acid in concentrations < 16 mg/L.
c Medium PDM antibiotic sensitivity medium.
d Includes 20 β-lactamase producing strains.
e Mueller Hinton broth +3% blood + 25 mg/L nicotinamide dinucleotide.
f Brain heart infusion broth + horse serum (10 mg/L) + β nicotinamide adenine dinucleotide.
g Mueller-Hinton plus 10% lysed sheep blood.
References: 1 Barry et al. (1984); 2 Bauernfeind and Ullmann (1984); 3 Corrado et al. (1983); 4 Digranes et al. (1984); 5 Husson et al. (1984); 6 Khan et al. (1982); 7 Muytjens et al. (1983); 8 Newsom et al. (1982); 9 Sato et al. (1982).

floxacin 1 to 4 mg/L, while the streptococci, including enterococci, were more resistant, generally requiring concentrations of 2 to 16 mg/L to achieve 90% inhibition (table IV). By comparison, the studies in table IV which assessed nalidixic acid found very little activity against staphylococcal strains (MIC_{90}: 32 to > 128 mg/L) or against streptococci (MIC_{90}: > 32 to > 512 mg/L).

Staphylococci were generally less susceptible to inhibition by cinoxacin (MIC_{90}: > 32 to > 512 mg/L) [Barry et al., 1984; Gadebusch et al., 1982; Jones and Barry, 1983; Norrby and Jonsson, 1983; Vuye, 1983], cefotaxime (MIC_{90}: 2 to 32 mg/L) [Corrado et al., 1983; King et al., 1982] and oxolinic acid (MIC_{90}: 2 to 16 mg/L) [Barry et al., 1984; Jones and Barry, 1983; Vuye, 1983] than by norfloxacin, but were more susceptible to ciprofloxacin (MIC_{90}: 0.25 to 1 mg/L) [Barry et al., 1984; Eliopoulos et al., 1984; King et al., 1984; Muytjens et al., 1983; Reeves et al., 1984b; Wise et al., 1983]. The MIC_{90} for enoxacin against staphylococci (1 to 8 mg/L) was similar to that of norfloxacin (Bauernfeind and Ullmann, 1984; Chartrand et al., 1983; Nakamura et al., 1983; Reeves et al., 1984a; Wise et al., 1984a).

Norfloxacin was also considerably more active against streptococci than both cinoxacin (MIC_{90}: > 32 to > 512 mg/L) [Barry et al., 1984; Gadebusch et al., 1982; Jones and Barry, 1983; Norrby and Jonsson, 1983; Vuye, 1983] and oxolinic acid (MIC_{90}: 32 to > 128 mg/L) [Barry et al., 1984; Jones and Barry, 1983; Vuye, 1983], but the difference in potency between norfloxacin and enoxacin (MIC_{90}: 8 to 64 mg/L) was not as great (Bauernfeind and Ullmann, 1984; Nakamura et al., 1983; Reeves et al., 1984a; Wise et al., 1984a). As with staphylococci, ciprofloxacin was more potent than norfloxacin against streptococci (MIC_{90}: 0.5 to 8 mg/L) [Barry et al., 1984; Elipoulos et al., 1984; King et al., 1984; Muytjens et al., 1983; Reeves et al., 1984b].

1.2 Activity Against Anaerobic Bacteria and Other Organisms

Norfloxacin generally demonstrated poor activity against anaerobic bacteria, with most strains

Table II. Range of reported MIC_{90} values (mg/L) for norfloxacin against Enterobacteriaceae in comparative studies with other antibiotics. Most of the studies used larger numbers of strains (usually clinical isolates) and an inoculum of 10^4 to 10^6 colony-forming units

Bacterial species	Norfloxacin ( )[a]	Nalidixic acid (references)	Cinoxacin (references)	Pipemidic acid (references)	Oxolinic acid (references)	Ciprofloxacin (references)	Enoxacin (references)	Co-trimoxazole (references)	Other[b] (references)
Escherichia coli	0.05-1	4-32 (1,2,5,6,8-12,14,16-18,22)	4-32 (1,8,12,18,23)	4-16 (9,10,14,22)	0.5-4 (1,9,11,23)	≤ 0.06-0.015 (1,7,9,21,24)	0.125-1 (2,3,4,15, 20,24)	2-64 (6,8,11,12)	TMP: 1 (12) CTX: 0.2-0.3 (5,17)
Klebsiella spp.	0.25-2	2-64 (1,6,8,9,12, 14,16)		3-64 (9,10,14,22)	4-32 (1,9,11,23)	0.06-0.5 (1,14,20,24,25)	0.5-4 (20,24,25)	4-32 (1,6,8,11,12)	TMP: 1 (12) CTX: 0.06 (5)
K. pneumoniae	0.125-1	4-> 32 (2,5,11,18, 22,23)				≤ 0.06-0.25 (2,7,15,21)			
Enterobacter spp.	0.25-0.5	4-> 32 (1,6,12,14,18)				0.015-0.03 (15,20,21)	0.39-1 (15,20,21)		
E. cloacae	0.25-2	4-100 (2,5,8,11, 16,22)	8-> 32 (8,11,23)	12-64 (9,22)	0.25-2 (2,11,23)	≤ 0.06 (2,7)	0.25-2 (2,11,23)	0.5-128 (8,11)	CTX: 0.25-12.5 (5,17)
E. aerogenes	0.125-0.5					≤ 0.06 (2,7)	0.25 (2,7)		
Proteus spp.	0.063						0.25		
P. mirabilis	0.06-0.25	4-16 (1,5,6,8,11, 12,14)	4-64 (1,8,11,12, 18,23)	3-4 (14,22)	0.25 (1,11,23)	0.03-≤ 0.06 (7,15,20,21, 24,25)	0.25-0.78 (7,15,20,21, 24,25)	0.5-8 (6,8,11,12)	TMP: 32 (12) CTX: 0.06 (5)
P. vulgaris	≤ 0.06					0.125 (7)			
Proteus indole (+) 2-16[c]	0.12					0.06 (24)			
Morganella morganii	≤ 0.06					≤ 0.06 (7)			
Providencia rettgeri	0.5-≥ 16	16-> 128 (1,2,6,11,23)	128-> 128 (1,11,23)		0.5-16 (1,11,23)	1 (1)	0.5 (2)	> 16-≥ 128 (6,11)	
P. stuartii	0.12-4	16-> 128 (1,9,11,14, 16,17)	> 128 (1,11)	32-> 256 (9,14)	4-32 (1,9,11)	0.5-4 (14)	4 (2)	> 16 (11)	

Citrobacter spp.	0.06-1.56[c]	2-16[c] (1,2,8,11,12, 14,16,17,18)	4-16 (1,8,11,12, 18,23)	0.5-1 (1,11,23)	0.03-0.125 (1,14,15,20,21)	0.12-0.78 (15,20,21)
C. freundii	0.125-0.25				≤ 0.06 (2,7)	0.25 (2,7)
Serratia spp.	1-8				0.5-2 (20,21,24,25)	2-16 (20,21,24,25)
S. marcescens	0.125-12.5	2-> 152 (1,2,5,8,11,12, 16,17,22)	16-128 (1,8,11,12, 18,23)	0.25-4 (1,11,23)	0.125-2 (1,14)	0.25-16 (2,15)

a Results derived from all the references.

b TMP = trimethoprim; CTX = cefotaxime.

c Two studies reported higher values for norfloxacin (4 and 3.13 mg/L) with correspondingly higher levels for nalidixic acid (> 256 and > 100 mg/L) [Husson et al. (1984) and Sato et al. (1984), respectively].

References: 1 Barry et al. (1984); 2 Bauernfeind and Ullmann (1984); 3 Carlson et al. (1983); 4 Chartrand et al. (1983); 5 Corrado et al. (1983); 6 Digranes et al. (1984); 7 Eliopoulos et al. (1984); 8 Gadebusch et al. (1982); 9 Husson et al. (1984); 10 Ito et al. (1980); 11 Jones and Barry (1983); 12 Khan et al. (1982); 13 King et al. (1984); 14 Muytjens et al. (1983); 15 Nakamura et al. (1983); 16 Newsom et al. (1982); 17 Neu and Labthavikul (1982); 18 Norrby and Jonsson (1983); 19 Peddie (1982); 20 Reeves et al. (1984a); 21 Reeves et al. (1984b); 22 Sato et al. (1982); 23 Vuye (1983); 24 Wise et al. (1983); 25 Wise et al. (1984a).

only moderately sensitive and some resistant (table V). Results of the study by King et al. (1984) and those of other investigators (King et al., 1982; Reeves et al., 1984a,b; Sato et al., 1982; Wise et al., 1983, 1984a) indicated that both *Bacteroides* and *Clostridia* species are not susceptible to norfloxacin. The MIC_{90} for 23 strains of *Clostridium difficile* was 64 mg/L (Newsom et al., 1985).

Campylobacter (a Gram-negative microaerophilic organism), was inhibited by norfloxacin (MIC_{90}: 0.25 to 4 mg/L) [Carlson et al., 1983; Corrado et al., 1983; Diez-Enciso et al., 1984; Goossens et al., 1985; King et al., 1984; Larivière et al., 1984; Nakamura et al., 1983; Neu and Labthavikul, 1982; Shungu et al., 1983; Wang et al., 1984].

The MIC of norfloxacin for *Chlamydia trachomatis* was 8 mg/L (Heessen and Muytjens, 1984; van Roosbroeck et al., 1984).

1.3 Antifungal Activity

Norfloxacin has no intrinsic antifungal activity, but synergy has been observed between amphotericin B and norfloxacin against all tested strains of *Candida albicans* at concentrations of 2 and 32 mg/L, respectively (Vangdal and Bergan, 1984b). A similar study by Eng et al. (1982) resulted in a 2- to 32-fold reduction in the amphotericin B MIC for *C. albicans, Candida* species and *Cryptococcus* species in the presence of norfloxacin 1 to 12 mg/L. Synergy between norfloxacin and other antifungal agents such as ketaconazole, miconazole, fluocytosine and nystatin (8-fold reduction in the MIC_{90}) was also reported against *Candida* species by Walsh et al. (1983). Enhanced antifungal activity in the presence of norfloxacin is not explicable in terms of DNA gyrase activity (section 1.7) as the fungi are eukaryotes, but it could be explained by the inhibition of RNA activity and protein synthesis observed by Crumplin and Smith (1981).

1.4 Activity Against Organisms Resistant to Other Antibacterial Drugs

A few studies have been reported which specifically examined the activity of norfloxacan against

Table III. Cumulated frequency (%) of minimum inhibitory concentrations (MIC) of selected antibacterial drugs for 100 isolates of *Pseudomonas aeruginosa* tested on PDM antibiotic sensitivity medium after overnight growth at 37°C. Inocula size = 10^3 to 10^4 cfu (after Vangdal and Bergan, 1984a)

Antibiotic	MIC (mg/L)									
	< 0.25	0.25	0.5	1.0	2.0	4.0	8.0	16.0	32.0	> 32.0
Norfloxacin	15	15	54	87	92	96	99	100		
Ciprofloxacin	92	92	92	96	100					
Azlocillin	0	0	0	2	6	37	67	80	86	100
Gentamicin	0	0	0	2	2	35	78	91	97	100
Netilmicin	0	0	0	1	1	6	41	84	96	100
Tobramycin	0	1	17	79	85	96	97	100		

organisms showing varying degrees of antibiotic resistance. Multiresistant strains of *E. coli* were susceptible to norfloxacin ($MIC_{90} \leqslant 0.25$ mg/L) [Corigliano et al., 1984; Leigh and Osborne, 1982; Smith and Cherubin, 1983]. *K. pneumoniae* resistant to cefazolin and *S. marcescens* resistant to gentamicin (Corigliano et al., 1984), as well as multiresistant strains of both organisms (Smith and Cherubin, 1983), were inhibited by norfloxacin 2 and 4 mg/L, respectively. Multiresistant strains of *E. cloacae* were very susceptible to norfloxacin (MIC_{90} 0.08 and 0.11 mg/L: Yourassowsky et al., 1982; Leigh and Osborne, 1982, respectively). *P. aeruginosa* resistant to gentamicin (Corigliano et al., 1984; Forward et al., 1983; Ito et al., 1980), to both gentamicin and carbenicillin (Yourassowsky et al., 1982), or multiresistant strains (Leigh and Osborne, 1982; Martino et al., 1985; Smith and Cherubin, 1983) all showed norfloxacin MIC_{90} values of less than 8 mg/L. In one of these studies the combination of norfloxacin and imipenen was synergistic or partially synergistic in 37% of 54 multiresistant *P. aeruginosa* (Martino et al., 1985).

1.5 Effect on Activity of Media, pH and Inoculum Size

The activity of some of the antibiotics routinely used to treat urinary tract infections, in particular the aminoglycosides, is decreased in human urine. In contrast, the β-lactams have been found to be more active in urine than in broth or agar, except against *Proteus* species (Shah et al., 1976). The

Table IV. Antibacterial inhibitory activity of norfloxacin against Gram-positive organisms

Organisms	MIC_{90} (mg/L)	References
Staphylococcus aureus	1-4	2,5,7,9,10,12,13
S. aureus, MR	1-4	1,3,8
MS	0.5-2	
PS	2	8
S. epidermidis	0.5-3	3,4,7,12
S. saprophyticus	1-4	2,4,11,13
Streptococcus faecalis	2-8	1,3-13
S. pyogenes	8-32	1,5,12
S. agalactiae	4-8	1,8,13
S. pneumoniae	4-16	1,3,8
S. Gp ABCG	0.5-8	3,8,9

Abbreviations: MIC_{90} = minimum concentration inhibitory to 90% of tested strains; MR = methicillin-resistant; MS = methicillin-sensitive; PS = penicillin-sensitive.

References: 1 Barry et al. (1984); 2 Clarke et al. (1985); 3 Corrado et al. (1983); 4 Digranes et al. (1984); 5 Gadebusch et al. (1982); 6 Jones and Barry (1983); 7 Khan et al. (1982); 8 King et al. (1982); 9 Muytjens et al. (1983); 10 Newsom et al. (1982); 11 Norrby and Jonsson (1983); 12 Sato et al. (1982); 13 Vuye (1983).

MICs of norfloxacin determined simultaneously in diagnostic sensitivity test (DST) agar and in pooled human urine agar of pH 5.4 to 5.8 against the 4 most common urinary pathogens are shown in table VI. Norfloxacin was much less active in urine than in agar. Thus, MICs increased about 16-fold to a range of 1 to 32 mg/L for *E. coli* and *K. pneumoniae,* and by up to 64 times to 8 to 64 mg/L for *P. aeruginosa.* Although nalidixic acid, cinoxacin and pipemidic acid also showed a loss of activity when studied under the same conditions, in no instance was it as great as that with norfloxacin. The activity of norfloxacin against *E. coli* and *K. pneumoniae* in urine agar was only marginally better than that of nalidixic acid. However, since urine concentrations of norfloxacin have been reported to exceed 300 mg/L after a single oral dose of 400mg, it is unlikely that this loss of activity would become clinically relevant in uncomplicated urinary tract infections (Shah et al., 1983).

The reduction of activity in urine could be a pH effect. Thus, Lacey et al. (1984), who investigated the bactericidal effects of norfloxacin in urine, noted that the pH for optimum activity of norfloxacin in urine was 7.5 to 8.0, while Bauernfeind and Petermüller (1983a,b) observed the MIC of norfloxacin for *E. coli, S. aureus, S. epidermidis, Str. faecalis* and *P. mirabilis* at pH 5.8 (0.5 and 0.25 mg/L) to be 2 to 5 times that at pH 7.3. Similarly, the MIC of norfloxacin for 'nalidixic acid-sensitive' and '-resistant' strains of enterobacteria was about 8- to 16-fold higher at pH 5.5 than pH 7.2 using DST agar (Greenwood et al., 1984). Further support for a pH effect was provided by Newsom (1984) who found that the modal MIC of norfloxacin for 180 randomly selected strains of Enterobacteriaceae on agar was 0.06 mg/L at pH 7.2 compared with 8 mg/L at pH 6.

The magnesium (Mg^{++}) content of urine is much greater than that of nutrient broth or Mueller-Hinton media, even with Mg^{++} supplementation. Increases in the Mg^{++} concentration from 0.2 to 9 mmol/L have produced MIC increases of 2- to 8-fold in the quinolones, including norfloxacin. It is speculated that Mg^{++} interferes with the normal interaction of quinolones with DNA (Machka and Braveny, 1984; Neu, 1985; Ratcliffe and Smith, 1984).

Table V. Inhibitory activity of norfloxacin (NOR) against anaerobic bacteria compared with that of ciprofloxacin (CIP) [after King et al., 1984]. Medium used was diagnostic sensitivity test agar with 6% saponin lysed horse blood. Inoculum size = 10^4 cfu

Organism	No. of isolates	Antibiotic[a]	MIC_{90} (mg/L)
Bacteroides fragilis group	31	NOR	128
		CIP	16
Bacteroides melaningenicus and *oralis*	57	NOR	8
		CIP	256
Bacteroides ureolyticus	4	NOR	1
		CIP	0.12
Fusobacterium spp.	10	NOR	16
		CIP	2
Clostridium spp.	20	NOR	128
		CIP	16
Peptococcus spp.	44	NOR	8
		CIP	2
Peptostreptococcus spp.	21	NOR	4
		CIP	1
Eubacterium spp.	5	NOR	8
		CIP	2
Veillonella spp.	5	NOR	1
		CIP	0.12

a Nalidixic acid was ineffective against these anaerobes.

The minimum inhibitory concentrations of norfloxacin against usual inocula of a variety of bacterial species were about 4 to 8 times higher in Mueller-Hinton broth than in the corresponding agar. However, MIC values in Mueller-Hinton agar and DST were the same (Norrby and Jonsson, 1983; Shah et al., 1983).

Increasing the inoculum size from 10^3 to 10^7 cfu had only a minor effect on the MIC and minimum bactericidal concentration (MBC) of norfloxacin in Mueller-Hinton agar, although 11 of the 20 tested strains required 2-fold higher concentrations for inhibition of the larger inoculum (Neu and Labthav-

Table VI. Antibacterial activity of norfloxacin against 4 of the most common urinary pathogens in urine agar (pH 5.4 to 5.8) and diagnostic sensitivity test (DST) agar. Inocula size: 10^5 cfu (after Shah et al., 1983)

Organism (number of isolates)	Agar medium	Number of strains inhibited by an MIC (mg/L) of											
		≤ 0.06	0.12	0.25	0.5	1	2	4	8	16	32	64	≥ 128
Escherichia coli (97)	Urine					1	45	17	12	17	5		
	DST	65	17	11	2	1	1						
Enterobacter cloacae (68)	Urine		1	2	9	14	11	22	5	4			
	DST	41	12	12	2	1							
Klebsiella pneumoniae (87)	Urine				1	11	15	15	33	10	1	1	
	DST	26	33	20	2	3	1	2					
Pseudomonas aeruginosa (50)	Urine								2	15	9	21	3
	DST		7	12	6	10	7	5	1	1		1	

ikul, 1982). Similar effects were reported in Mueller-Hinton broth by Bauernfeind and Petermüller (1983a,b) and in DST agar by Shah et al. (1983). Increasing the inoculum size still further to 10^8 cfu resulted in 2- to 4-fold increases in MIC values for 37 enterobacteria studied by King et al. (1982). A 1000-fold increase (10^3 to 10^6 cfu) in inoculum size during MIC determinations by broth dilution for norfloxacin resulted in 8- to 16-fold increases in MIC values in 7 of 51 strains of a range of enterobacteria (Norrby and Jonsson, 1983). Sato et al. (1982) reported the MIC_{90} and MBC_{90} of norfloxacin for 50 strains of *E. coli, K. pneumoniae, P. aeruginosa,* and *S. aureus* to be either unchanged or doubled when the inoculum size was increased from 10^4 to 10^6 cfu.

1.6 Bactericidal Activity

In most cases MBCs were only slightly higher than the MICs for norfloxacin (King et al., 1982; Neu and Labthavikul, 1982; Norrby and Jonsson, 1983; Sato et al., 1982), although with certain organisms like *P. aeruginosa* and *S. marcescens* a 4- to 8-fold increase in concentration was required for a bactericidal effect (Neu and Labthavikul, 1982; Norrby and Jonsson, 1983; Sato et al., 1982).

1.7 Mechanism of Action and Development of Resistance

Norfloxacin has been shown to penetrate into bacterial cells much more readily than nalidixic acid. Investigations into the mechanism of action of norfloxacin upon susceptible strains of *E. coli* K12 suggest that the drug exerts a potent bactericidal effect resulting from the inhibition of the A subunit of the essential enzyme DNA gyrase (Crumplin et al., 1984). The critical imbalance in cellular metabolism resulting from the inhibition of DNA gyrase precipitates a sequence of cellular events which may lead to: (a) premature cell division; (b) delayed cell division; or (c) total failure of cell division leading to lysis of the cell. Reports by Hirai et al. (1982) that norfloxacin strongly inhibited DNA synthesis in *E. coli,* but only slightly inhibited ribonucleic acid and protein synthesis support these findings. An alternative theory, suggested by L.M. Fisher and colleagues, is that norfloxacin binds to specific sites on the DNA molecule which then prevents the binding of the DNA gyrase (S.W.B. Newsom, personal communication).

Clinical resistance of bacteria is usually obtained via plasmids mediating drug insusceptibility. The activity of the 4-quinolone antibacterials, however, is not decreased in the presence of plasmid. In fact, R-plasmids often increase bacterial sensitivity to 4-quinolone antibacterial agents. Additionally, these antibacterials often cause plasmid elimination from bacteria which harbour them (Crumplin and Smith, 1981) and can block the transfer of plasmids (Hooper et al., 1983).

Neu and Labthavikul (1982) did not find resistant colonies when subculturing *E. coli, Klebsiella* species and *Pseudomonas* species repeatedly in subinhibitory concentrations of norfloxacin, but later studies by Barry and Jones (1984), Bauernfeind et al. (1984a,b), Duckworth and Williams (1984) and Tenney et al. (1983) all succeeded in selecting resistant variants using similar methods. In the study by Tenney et al. (1983) *P. aeruginosa* which were inhibited only by concentrations of norfloxacin greater than 256 mg/L were rapidly selected by serial passage on agar with subinhibitory concentrations of the drug. However, despite a 512-fold increase in MIC to 16 mg/L, *E. coli* with MICs greater than the clinically achievable urine concentrations could not be selected.

Chin and Neu (1983) determined that the frequency of resistant variants for norfloxacin was generally $< 10^{-9}$ within different cultures. Consequently a very heavy inoculum would be needed to reliably select resistant cells within a population. Within a lighter inoculum random selection could require several passages before resistant cells were detected.

Greenwood et al. (1984) investigated the factors influencing the emergence of resistance to norfloxacin *in vitro* using a mechanical model simulating the hydrokinetic conditions that exist in the treatment of bacterial cystitis. In nalidixic acid-sensitive strains of *E. coli,* resistance to norfloxacin did not emerge even at the lowest dose, which achieved a peak concentration in the model of only 5 mg/L. In contrast, decreased norfloxacin susceptibility was selected for in a nalidixic acid-resistant strain of *E. coli* (but not in a nalidixic acid-resistant strain of *K. aerogenes)* tested in the model; since this decreased activity might be superimposed on reduced activity of norfloxacin in the acid conditions of infected urine, it is possible that norfloxacin may become subject to resistance problems.

Limited cross-resistance between norfloxacin and nalidixic acid was observed by Duckworth and Williams (1984) [table VII], but other studies have

Table VII. *In vitro* occurrence of cross-resistance between norfloxacin (NOR) and nalidixic acid demonstrated by 4 representative strains. Whether the resistant variants (RV) arose on norfloxacin plates or on nalidixic acid plates the MICs for the resistant variants were similar (after Duckworth and Williams, 1984)

Organism	Antibiotic on which RV isolated	Original MIC (mg/L)	New 'resistant' MIC (mg/L)	
			NA	NOR
K. pneumoniae	NA	1	64	2
	NOR	0.06	32	4
E. coli	NA	1	32	2
	NOR	0.06	8	2
Pseudomonas sp.	NA	4	256	2
	NOR	0.12	256	8
Citrobacter sp.	NA	2	> 256	1
	NOR	0.12	> 256	1

Table VIII. Pharmacokinetic variables after single oral doses of norfloxacin in healthy subjects

Number of subjects	Dose of norfloxacin (mg)	C_{max} (mg/L)	T_{max} (h)	$t_{½β}$ (h)	AUC_{0-24} (mg/L·h)	Urinary recovery (%) 0-24h; 0-48h	References
5	100	0.44	1	4-5		38; –	1
25	200	0.75-0.97	1-1.1	4-7.3	3.28	39; 24-30	1,3,6
37	400	1.36-1.58	1-1.5	3.5-7.4	4.1-6.26	27-33; 30	1,2,4,6,7
17	800	2.41-2.46	1-3	4-6.2	11.4	37; 30	1,6
14	1200	3.15	1.8	5.7	16.1	–; 30	6
18	1600	3.87-9.65	1.8-2	6-6.8	19.7	48; 30	1,6
5	2000	11.8	2.8		59.1	–; 30	5

Abbreviations: C_{max} = maximum serum concentration; T_{max} = time to maximum serum concentrations; $t_{½β}$ = elimination half-life; AUC = area under the serum concentration-time curve.
References: 1 Abiko et al. (1981); 2 Adhami et al. (1984); 3 Beerman et al. (1984); 4 Eandi et al. (1983); 5 Okada et al. 1981; 6 Swanson et al. (1983); 7 Wise et al. (1984b).

reported nearly complete cross-resistance between norfloxacin and nalidixic acid as well as several other 4-quinolones (ciprofloxacin, enoxacin, cinoxacin, ofloxacin and oxolinic acid) [Barry and Jones, 1984; Cullmann et al., 1985]. Jones and Barry (1983) demonstrated that Enterobacteriaceae with elevated MICs for cinoxacin, nalidixic acid or oxolinic acid also tended to be less susceptible to norfloxacin, and Fass (1983) observed a similar relationship for ciprofloxacin and norfloxacin. Traub (1985) reported incomplete cross-resistance of nalidixic acid- and pipemidic acid-resistant variants of *S. marcescens,* with ciprofloxacin, enoxacin and norfloxacin. In one of the few cases of resistance arising clinically, Sauerwein and Bauernfeind (1984) reported cross-resistance to several 4-quinolones in a strain of *P. aeruginosa* which became resistant to norfloxacin during therapy in a paraplegic patient (see section 3.2.1).

Cross-resistance between norfloxacin and antibiotics from other drug classes has been reported infrequently. Two ampicillin-resistant strains of *Enterobacter* species were cross-resistant to norfloxacin (Newsom et al., 1982). In a second study, 3 of 4 norfloxacin-selected resistant mutants of *K. pneumoniae* showed diminished susceptibility to both other quinolones and to β-lactam antibiotics [latamoxef (moxalactam), cefoxitin and cefotaxime; Sanders et al., 1984].

The mechanism(s) of resistance to norfloxacin are as yet unknown. An analogous mechanism to that which has been defined for nalidixic acid, i.e. a change in the configuration of bacterial DNA gyrase (Gellert et al., 1977) may in part explain the existence of cross-resistance (Husson et al., 1984). As the MICs and MBCs of norfloxacin are the same for many strains, the cryptic resistance associated with the β-lactams is unlikely to be a problem in treatment (Slack, 1984). The unusual pattern of cross-resistance reported by Sanders et al. (1984) between norfloxacin, other 4-quinolones and several cephalosporins (see above) was associated with changes in outer membrane proteins.

2. *Pharmacokinetics*

2.1 Absorption and Serum Concentrations

Several pharmacokinetic variables of norfloxacin are listed in table VIII. Following oral administration, maximum serum concentrations generally occur between 1 and 2 hours (table VIII; Okada et al., 1981; Shimada et al., 1981). Single oral doses of 400mg in healthy subjects resulted in mean maximum serum concentrations of 1.36 to 1.58 mg/L. Swanson et al. (1983) observed that, with rising doses, the mean maximum serum concentration (fig. 2), area under the serum concentration/time curve (AUC) from 0 to 12 hours, and the 0- to 12-hour urinary recovery of unmetabolised drug (see section 2.3) all became progressively lower relative to the amount of drug administered. For example, the AUC/dose ratio and maximum serum concentration/dose ratio for the 400mg dose of norfloxacin were significantly greater ($p < 0.01$) than for the 1600mg dose. This suggested that the fraction of the dose absorbed over the first 12-hour period was lower at the higher doses. However, by 48 hours the mean percentage recovery in urine was not substantially different for the various doses (range 27.4 to 31%), indicating that absorption may have only been delayed at the higher doses. In contrast, Abiko et al. (1981) found that 8 hours after administration, the concentration following the 1600mg dose was 6.5 times higher than that following the 800mg dose. A similar increase was noted for the serum AUC which was 12 mg/L • h in the 800mg group and about 60 mg/L • h in the 1600mg group.

In 3 healthy subjects administered norfloxacin 200mg 8-hourly for 7 days, there appeared to be little evidence of accumulation of the antibiotic, with no significant changes in the serum concentrations at 2 hours following the first, second and last dose (Abiko et al., 1981).

In a comparative study, Okada et al. (1981) found mean maximum serum concentrations of pipemidic acid (8 mg/L) to be about 2 to 3 times those of norfloxacin following administration of 500mg of each drug to healthy subjects. Similar results were reported by Ueda et al. (1981) who also noted that the peak concentrations of norfloxacin occurred somewhat later than those of pipemidic acid (0.5 to 1 hour).

Absorption is slightly delayed when norfloxacin is administered with food (unpublished data on file, Merck Sharp and Dohme). Given the pH dependency of the urinary solubility of norfloxacin (section 2.3), the effect of the concomitant administration of antacids on the absorption of the drug deserves study.

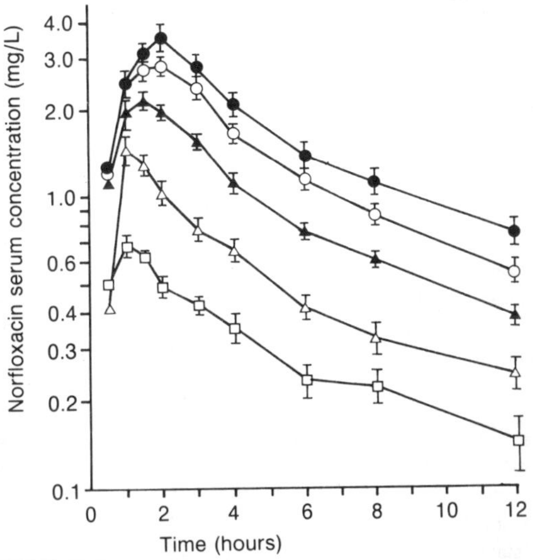

Fig. 2. Norfloxacin serum concentration-time curves in 14 healthy subjects following oral administration at weekly intervals of single doses: 200mg (□), 400mg (△), 800mg (▲), 1200mg (○), and 1600mg (●) [after Swanson et al., 1983].

Recovery of norfloxacin in faeces from 12 healthy volunteers given single oral 400mg doses averaged 28% over the ensuing 48 hours (Cofsky et al., 1984). As the drug is excreted in the bile to only a small extent (section 2.3), these results imply an oral bioavailability of approximately 70%.

2.2 Distribution

Since norfloxacin is not yet available in an intravenous form, accurate determination of the volume of distribution is impossible. However, animal studies would suggest that the distribution volume is very large (Shimada et al., 1983). Extrapolated to man, this would mean a distribution volume of 25 to 35L (Wise, 1984). However, it may prove to be much higher (R. Wise, personal communication).

Table IX. Concentration of norfloxacin in various tissue and tissue fluids following oral administration (after Norrby, 1983)

Tissue/fluid	Number of subjects	Dose of norfloxacin (mg)[a]	Sampling time (h after dose)	Norfloxacin concentration (mg/L or mg/kg)[b]	Reference
Sputum	4	200 q8h	1-6	< 0.05-0.16	5
Sputum	2	200 q8h	1-8	0.05-0.38	4
Palatine tonsilla	8	200	2	0.48-0.54	3
Maxillary sinus mucosa	4	200	2	0.3-0.38	3
Liver tissue	2	200	2	1.7-3.4	8
Gallbladder wall	2	200	2.5	< 0.2-0.48	8
Gallbladder bile	2	200	2	0.15-4.46	8
Common duct bile	2	200	2.5	0.41-4.2	8
Common duct bile	1	100	6	5.7	7
Bile	3	400	3-4	2.6-6	9
			6	1.4-2.5	9
Bile	1	100	3.6	3.16-5.68	11
Umbilical serum	14	200	0.13-10.5	< 0.05-0.38	10
Amniotic fluid	14	200	0.13-10.5	< 0.05-0.92	10
Breast milk	4	200	1-4	ND	10
Prostate	14	400[c]	3	0.75-3.3	6
Prostate	15	400[c]	3-4	0.29-2.5	2
Prostate	10	400[c]	2-6	< 0.25-4.65	1
Kidney	3	400[c]	2-6	3.9-16.2	1

a single dose unless indicated otherwise.
b ND = not detected (< 0.05 mg/L).
c 2 × 400mg doses given in the 12 hours before sampling.
References: 1 Bergeron et al. (1985); 2 Bologna et al. (1983a, 1985); 3 Iwasawa (1981); 4 Matsumuto et al. (1981); 5 Nakagawa et al. (1981); 6 Netto et al. (1984); 7 Ozaki et al. (1981); 8 Saito et al. (1981a); 9 Shimura et al. (1983); 10 Takase et al. (1981); 11 Yamamoto et al. (1981).

Information on the penetration of norfloxacin into different tissues is limited (table IX). Following oral administration of norfloxacin 200mg, concentrations in palatine tonsillar tissue, maxillary sinus mucosa, vaginal tissue, cervix tissue, salpinges, ovaries, renal cortex and the gallbladder wall were only slightly lower than serum concentrations (Fraschini et al., 1984; Iwasawa, 1981; Saito et al., 1981a). Concentrations higher than those in serum were found in both common duct and in gallbladder bile as well as in liver tissue and renal medulla (Fraschini et al., 1984; Ozaki et al., 1981; Saito et al., 1981a; Shimura et al., 1983; Yamamoto et al., 1981). Concentrations in sputum were relatively low (Matsumoto et al., 1981; Nakagawa et al., 1981). In amniotic fluid and umbilical serum, concentrations were lower than those in the mothers' serum, while no detectable concentration could be demonstrated in breast milk (Takase et al., 1981; unpublished data on file, Merck Sharp & Dohme). Norfloxacin penetrated into a mild inflammatory exudate induced by a cantharides impregnated plaster where the concentration was 1 mg/L after a 400mg dose, equivalent to approximately 67% of the peak serum concentration (Adhami et al., 1984).

Norfloxacin concentrations in urine are discussed in section 2.3.

Unpublished data from Merck Sharp & Dohme suggest a protein binding level of 14%.

2.3 Elimination

Although overall excretion of unchanged norfloxacin in urine appears to be approximately 30%, findings of studies have varied. The 24-hour urinary recovery in the study by Abiko et al. (1981)

ranged from 33 to 39% of the dose at doses of 100 to 800mg, but rose to 47.8% at the 1600mg dose (table VIII). However, Swanson et al. (1983) noted that the proportion of unchanged norfloxacin recovered in the urine over 0 to 12 hours became progressively lower relative to increased dose, although by 48 hours the mean urinary recovery did not alter substantially with dose (fig. 3). The variable urinary recovery with dose in this study may reflect a variation in absorption (section 2.1).

While the site of metabolism of norfloxacin is not yet known, 6 metabolites with modifications to the piperazine ring have been described for the drug, at least 1 of which has some microbiological activity. Urinary excretion of the metabolites of norfloxacin accounts for less than 10% of an administered dose (Adami et al., 1984; Ozaki et al., 1981; Wise et al., 1984b).

The renal clearance of norfloxacin was reported by Swanson et al. (1983) to vary from 16.32 to 17.76 L/h. Wise (1984), assuming a serum binding value of 14%, calculated a free renal clearance of 19.5 L/h. This fairly high value suggested that there was some active tubular secretion, a theory which was confirmed by the reduction in urinary recovery (from 28 to 14%) following probenecid administration (Shimada et al., 1983). However, the corresponding increase in terminal serum half-life was not significant, an inconsistency which has yet to be explained.

The concentration of norfloxacin attained in the urine varied with the volume of urine produced. A mean peak concentration of 478 mg/L was reported 1 to 2 hours following administration of single oral doses of 400mg to 14 healthy male volunteers (Swanson et al., 1983) and mean values of 180, 125 and 54 mg/L were reported 0 to 3 hours, 3 to 6 hours and 6 to 24 hours after administration of single 400mg oral doses to 6 healthy volunteers (Eandi et al., 1983).

The dependence of the urinary solubility of norfloxacin on pH and temperature is shown in figure 4. At 37°C norfloxacin was freely soluble (concentration < 40 g/L) at pH 5.5 or less, but at pH 7.5 solubility was at its lowest, peaking at 0.45 g/L at 25°C and 1.2 g/L at 37°C. Drug-related crystals were observed only at the highest (1200mg and 1600mg) doses of norfloxacin and only when urine pH values exceeded 7.0 (Swanson et al., 1983). On the other hand, Okada et al. (1981) administered 200mg to 5 healthy volunteers and failed to observe any crystal formation.

Quantitative biliary excretion of norfloxacin in 1 patient with choleductus cancer after a single oral dose of 100mg, amounted to 1.6% of the dose over 24 hours (Yamamoto et al., 1981). Similarly, low concentrations were found in the bile of patients

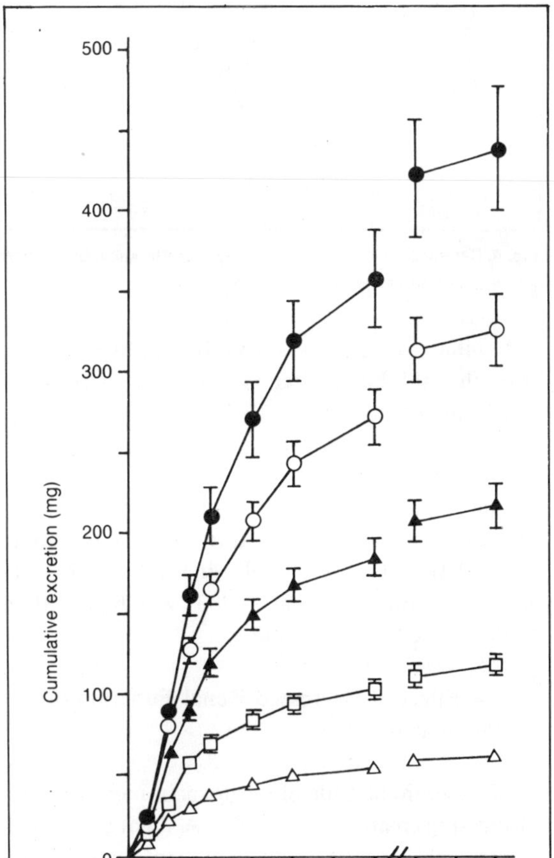

Fig. 3. Cumulative urinary excretion of unmetabolised norfloxacin in 14 healthy subjects following single oral doses of 200mg (△), 400mg (□), 800mg (▲), 1200mg (○) and 1600mg (●) [after Swanson et al., 1983].

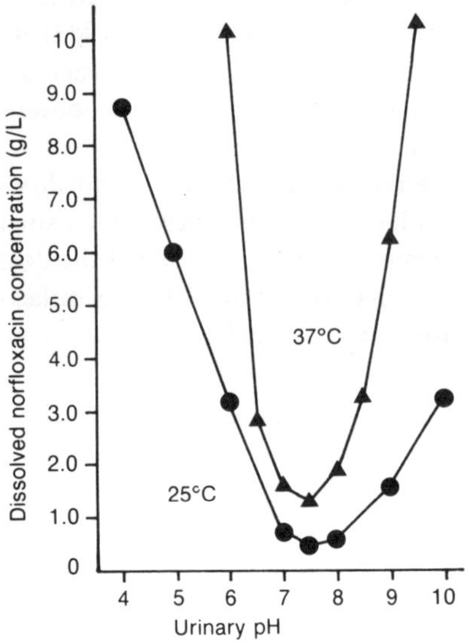

Fig. 4. Dependency of urinary solubility of norfloxacin on pH and temperature (after Swanson et al., 1983).

with biliary disease (table IX). It is unlikely, therefore, that the biliary tree is a significant route of norfloxacin elimination.

2.3.1 Half-Life

Mean elimination half-lives reported in various studies have generally ranged from 3.5 to 6.5 hours (table VIII). The serum elimination half-life reported by Swanson et al. (1983) was higher than that recorded in other studies.

2.4 Effect of Decreased Renal Function on Pharmacokinetics

The serum half-life of norfloxacin increases with decreasing creatinine clearance. A slight increase in serum half-life was found in patients with creatinine clearances of 30 to 80 ml/min/1.73m^2 (4.4 hours) and a greater increase occurred when creatinine clearance was between 10 and 29 ml/min/1.73m^2 (6.6 hours) compared with healthy volunteers (2.3 hours) [Fillastre et al., 1984]. In 3 patients with moderate impairment of renal function (creatinine clearance of 15-30 ml/min/1.73m^2), serum half-life was increased (mean 6.5 hours) compared with that in 6 normal volunteers (4.3 hours) following single oral doses of norfloxacin 400mg (Eandi et al., 1983). In this study there was also a slight decrease in the patients' urinary concentrations of the drug for the collection periods 0 to 3 hours (151 *vs* 180 mg/L in the healthy volunteers) and 3 to 6 hours (101 *vs* 125 mg/L). However, during the collection period 6 to 24 hours after administration, urinary concentrations were higher in the patients with moderately impaired renal function than in the healthy volunteers (62 *vs* 54 mg/L). The lengthening of half-life in patients with moderately impaired renal function was also associated with an increase in the serum AUC (Eandi et al., 1983; Hughes et al., 1984). With greater degrees of renal failure (creatinine clearances of below 10 ml/min/1.73m^2) serum half-life increased to 7.7 hours (Hughes et al., 1984; Fillastre et al., 1984). The mean half-life of norfloxacin was 7.9 hours in haemodialysed patients between dialysis sessions and was not influenced by haemodialysis (Fillastre et al., 1984).

Opinions as to whether dosage modifications are necessary in uraemic patients differ. Hughes et al. (1984) claim that modifications are essential when the glomerular filtration rate falls below 30 ml/min/1.73m^2, while Fillastre et al. (1984) feel that no alterations are necessary in patients with a creatinine clearance of 20 ml/min/1.73m^2 or more and that 400mg every 12 hours would be appropriate. They do, however, recommend either a doubling of the dosage interval or halving the dose in severe renal failure (creatinine clearance 2 to 10 ml/min/1.73m^2) [see also section 5].

2.5 Effect of Decreased Liver Function on Pharmacokinetics

Metabolism is a minor mechanism of elimination of norfloxacin (section 2.3). Thus, it is not surprising that neither the serum half-life nor the AUC were significantly different in patients with moderate impairment of liver function compared with healthy volunteers (Eandi et al., 1983).

3. Therapeutic Trials

Norfloxacin has been studied most extensively in the treatment of urinary tract infection. Many of the early therapeutic trials of norfloxacin are of Japanese origin. The Japanese studies have generally been open, non-comparative in design and have used a slightly lower dose range of norfloxacin (300 to 600mg daily) than that used in studies conducted in other countries (around 800mg daily). Brumfitt and Hamilton-Miller (1984) stress the importance of 'correct assessment' in the evaluation of a new antibiotic in urinary tract infection. They claim that the optimum time for the first follow-up assessment is 5 to 7 days after completion of treatment. This follow-up information is not available in most of the Japanese studies cited in this review, which made the data on relapse or reinfection more difficult to assemble and, due to the small number of patients who could be assessed in this way, less reliable. However, the definition of significant bacteriuria as based upon at least one bacterial count of 10^5/ml of urine from a midstream sample is generally apparent in both Japanese and non-Japanese studies. Several trials of norfloxacin in urinary tract infection have been of multicentre design, but in general practice patients such trials have the disadvantage of poorer quality of specimens and difficulties in persuading patients to return for long-term (6-week) follow-ups (Brumfitt and Hamilton-Miller, 1984). Several studies have compared norfloxacin with co-trimoxazole in urinary tract infection, but only a few have compared it with nalidixic acid, pipemidic acid and amoxycillin.

Norfloxacin has also been assessed in the treatment of other infections, in particular gonococcal and non-gonococcal urethritis and acute bacterial gastroenteritis. The drug is also indicated in the prophylaxis of sepsis in neutropenic patients.

3.1 Uncomplicated Acute Urinary Tract Infection

3.1.1 Open Studies

In open trials in the management of urinary tract infections (cystitis or pyelonephritis) described as 'simple', 'acute' or 'uncomplicated', norfloxacin in daily doses of 300 to 800mg for a usual duration of 3 to 7 days resulted in a bacteriological cure rate of 82 to 100% (Aoyama et al., 1981; Bailey et al., 1983a; Fujimura et al., 1981; Ganguli et al., 1985; Ishito et al., 1981; Kirby, 1984; Kiriyama et al., 1981; Kumamoto and Ishigami, 1983; Matsuoka et al., 1981; Nakamuta et al., 1981; Nishimura et al., 1980; Pantosti et al., 1984; Takebe et al., 1981; Tominaga et al., 1981; Unno and Yamamoto, 1981; Vogel et al., 1984). These response rates were defined as a sterile urine culture after a predetermined period of follow-up. However, only 5 of the above studies clearly stated when the follow-up was carried out (Bailey et al., 1983a; Ganguli et al., 1985; Kirby, 1984; Pantosti et al., 1984; Vogel et al., 1984). When interpreting the above cure rates one must take into account the fact that spontaneous remission occurs in about 50% of patients with dysuria and/or frequency with significant bacteriuria.

Reinfection occurred in 6% and relapse in 4% of patients after 2 weeks in the study by Vogel et al. (1984), while 1 patient was reinfected and 1 relapsed at 35 days in the study by Bailey et al. (1983a). Three patients were found by Kirby (1984) to have been reinfected by new organisms 2 to 4 weeks after starting therapy, while Pantosti et al. (1984) reported 1 reinfection after 4 weeks, and Ganguli et al. (1985) found 1 reinfection and 1 relapse by the final follow up at 5 weeks.

3.1.2 Comparative Studies

In urinary tract infections defined as acute, uncomplicated or both, norfloxacin has been compared with co-trimoxazole in several studies. Only single comparative studies have so far been reported for nalidixic acid, pipemidic acid and amoxycillin (table X). Most of these studies were open in design, but used a random allocation of treatments to 2 groups of patients.

The majority of studies which compared norfloxacin (400 to 800mg daily) with co-trimoxazole (160/800 to 320/1600mg daily), given in 2 divided doses for 7 to 10 days, found no statistically significant difference between bacteriological cure rates (range: norfloxacin 75 to 100%, co-trimoxazole 70

Table X. Summary of design, results and adverse effects of therapeutic trials comparing norfloxacin (NOR) with other antimicrobial agents in the treatment of uncomplicated and complicated or chronic urinary tract infection (UTI)

Reference	No. of patients (male/female; type of infection)	Study design	Dosage (mg/day)	Duration of treatment (days)	Follow-up	Bacteriological cure rate (%) [at end of follow-up]	Adverse effects (%)	No. pts. w/ reinfection or relapse/total no. assessed
Comparisons with co-trimoxazole (C)								
Bendall (1984)	27 (4M/23F; geriatric uncomplicated)	R	NOR 800 C 320/1600	10	5-9d 4-6wk	NOR 92 C 73	Nor 0 C 15	NOR 1/10 C 3/9
Bologna et al. (1983b)	20 (10M/10F; acute uncomplicated)	R	NOR 400 C 160/800	10	7d 30d	Nor 90 C 70	NOR 0 C 0	NOR 1/10 C 3/10
Giamarellou et al. (1983a)	61 (8M/53F; acute uncomplicated)	R	NOR 400 C 160/800	10	14d 6wk	NOR 92[a] C 96[b]	NOR C 3	NOR 2/26 C 1/26
Goldstein et al. (1985)	45 (M/F not stated; uncomplicated)	R	NOR 800 C 320/1600	7-10	5-9d 4-6wk	NOR 88 C 71	NOR 14 C 23	NOR 4/23 C 7/22
Guerra et al. (1983)	34 (1M/33F; acute uncomplicated)	R	NOR 800 C 320/1600	10	5-9d 4-6wk	NOR 95 C 100	NOR 47 C 60	NOR 3/19 C 1/15
Haase et al. (1984)	43 (0M/43F; acute uncomplicated)	R	NOR 800 C 320/1600	10	5-9d 4-6wk	NOR 95 C 90	NOR 13 C 14[c]	NOR 5/22 C 4/21
Newsom et al. (1983)	40 (1M/39F; not stated[d])	Not stated	NOR 800 C 320/1600	7	5-9d 6wk	NOR 75[e] C 75	NOR 15[f] C 40	NOR 2/20[e] C 3/20
Panichi et al. (1983)	38 (M/F not stated; uncomplicated[g])	Not stated	NOR 800 C 320/1600	10	5-9d 4wk	NOR 88 C 90	NOR 0 C 10	NOR 2/18 C 2/20
Sabbaj et al. (1985)	323 (82M/288F; uncomplicated)	R	NOR 800 C 320/1600	3-10	7d 4-6wk	NOR 97* C 90	NOR 6 C 14	NOR 9/101 C 15/125
Schaeffer and Sisney (1984)	39 (0M/39F; uncomplicated)	R	NOR 800 C 320/1600	10	7d 6wk	NOR 100 C 100	NOR 0 C 0	NOR 4/20 C 6/19

Watt et al. (1984)	103 (M/F not stated;[h] uncomplicated)	R	NOR 800 C 320/1600	7-10	5 to 9d 4-6wk	NOR 94 C 92.5	NOR 11.5* C 26.2	NOR 7/44 C 9/51
Comparison with nalidixic acid (NS)								
Reeves et al. (1984c)	110 (mainly women; uncomplicated)	R	NOR 800 NS[i] × 3	3	2-4d 4-6wk	NOR 96 NS 82	NOR 17 NS 26	
Comparisons with pipemidic acid (PI)								
Kamidono et al. (1982a)	197 (M/F not stated; acute uncomplicated)	db	NOR 300 PI 750	3	Not stated	NOR 91* PI 79	NOR 4.3 PI 2.7	
Kamidono et al. (1982b)	265 (M/F not stated; complicated)	db	NOR 800 PI 2000	5	Not stated	NOR 63* PI 48	NOR 1.2 PI 4.1	
Kumamoto and Ishigami (1983)	222 (complicated) 43 (complicated with indwelling catheter)	db	NOR 800 PI 2000	5	(on 5th day of therapy)	NOR 75[j] PI 62 NOR 52[k]* PI 41		
Comparisons with amoxycillin (AMX)								
Leigh et al. (1984)	40 (M/F not stated; geriatric complicated)	R	NOR 800 AMX 750	7	5-9d 4wk	NOR 95 AMX 75	NOR 0 AMX 0	NOR 0/20 AMX 3/20
Vogel et al. (1984)	91 (M/F not stated; uncomplicated)	R	NOR 800 AMX 750	7	4-9d 4-6wk	NOR 83 AMX 74	NOR 9 AMX 6	NOR 18% AMX 29%

a 7 patients lost to follow-up.
b 2 patients lost to follow-up.
c 2 patients with rash severe enough to warrant discontinuation of therapy.
d Presumably uncomplicated (general practice patients).
e Assuming 20 patients in each group.
f Candida infection was caused by co-trimoxazole in 4 patients and norfloxacin in 1 patient.
g 2 patients in the norfloxacin, and 1 in the co-trimoxazole group had upper UTI.
h Approximately equal distribution in 2 groups.
i NS = nalidixic acid 660mg plus sodium citrate 3.75g.
j 32% of norfloxacin and 25% of pipemidic acid patients had 'excellent' results.
k 24% of norfloxacin and 0% pipemidic acid patients had 'excellent' results.

Abbreviations: M = male; F = female; R = random allocation of treatment; db = double-blind; IM = intramuscular; d = day; wk = week; * = $p < 0.05$.

to 100%) [table X]. However, in the largest study norfloxacin produced bacteriological eradication in a significantly greater percentage of patients than co-trimoxazole (Sabbaj et al., 1985).

The immediate (2 to 4 days post-treatment) bacteriological outcome of 3 days' therapy with either norfloxacin 800mg or a nalidixic acid/sodium citrate mixture (1 sachet 3 times daily) was a higher cure rate for norfloxacin (96 *vs* 82%) which became significant (89 *vs* 67%; $p < 0.05$) at the later follow-up (4 to 6 weeks post-treatment). Among the bacteriuric patients, symptoms were recorded as having been 'improved' or 'cured' in a significantly greater proportion of patients on norfloxacin (64 and 36%) than on nalidixic acid (49 and 35%, respectively) [Reeves et al., 1984c].

A large double-blind study comparing 3 days of therapy in the treatment of acute simple cystitis revealed a significantly greater ($p < 0.03$) rate of elimination of bacteriuria in the patients treated with norfloxacin 300mg daily (91%) than in those treated with pipemidic acid 150mg daily (79.4%). Clinical efficacy was judged to be excellent in 80% and 68% of norfloxacin- and pipemidic acid-treated patients, respectively (Kamidono et al., 1982a).

The bacteriological efficacy 4 to 9 days after a 7-day course of norfloxacin 800mg daily was 83%, compared with 74% with amoxycillin 750mg daily. Four to 6 weeks after treatment bacteriological cure rates decreased to 63 and 48%, respectively. Neither difference was significant. Relapse of infection at 2 weeks was higher for amoxycillin (20%) than norfloxacin (9%), but rates of reinfection were the same at 9% each (Vogel et al., 1984).

3.2 Chronic and/or Complicated Urinary Tract Infections

3.2.1 Open Studies

As in uncomplicated urinary tract infection, studies of Japanese origin predominate the body of data on chronic/complicated urinary tract infection, with the results from only 4 non-Japanese studies published so far. Overall, in the Japanese studies, norfloxacin in doses of 300 to 800mg daily for 3 to 7 days has resulted in elimination of bacteriuria in 55% of patients (Ishito et al., 1981; Kiriyama et al., 1981; Maru, 1981; Matsuoka et al., 1981; Nakamuta et al., 1981; Nakatsu et al., 1981; Takada et al., 1981; Tominaga et al., 1981). However, these results should be interpreted with care because of the lack of follow-up information; bacteriological response in chronic and/or complicated urinary tract infection varies greatly according to when the patients are assessed. Clinical success rates for norfloxacin varied with the type of infection and underlying pathology (table XI). Clearly the presence of an indwelling catheter or the performance of a prostatectomy in a patient lowered the efficacy of norfloxacin, as has been noted with other antibiotics used in urinary tract infection.

Four non-Japanese open studies have evaluated the efficacy of norfloxacin in chronic and/or com-

Table XI. Overall clinical efficacy of norfloxacin 300 to 900mg daily for 3 to 7 days in open studies of patients with chronic and or complicated urinary tract infections (UTI) [data taken from Takada et al., 1981; Nakatsu et al., 1981; Fujimura et al., 1981; Ishito et al., 1981; Tominaga et al., 1981; Maru, 1981]

	Group	Total number of patients	Excellent (%)	Moderate (%)	Poor (%)
Single infection	Indwelling catheter	16	3 (19)	9 (56)	4 (25)
	Post prostatectomy	14	2 (14)	7 (50)	5 (36)
	Upper UTI	30	7 (22)	13 (43)	10 (33)
	Lower UTI	57	30 (53)	16 (28)	11 (19)
Mixed infection	Indwelling catheter	9	1 (11)	1 (11)	7 (77)
	No indwelling catheter	8	2 (25)	3 (37.5)	3 (37.5)

plicated urinary tract infection. Giamarellou et al. (1983b) evaluated norfloxacin 400mg daily for 10 days in 33 patients with recurrent urinary tract infections. All urine samples were sterile by the third day of therapy, but by the tenth day 2 of the 33 patients had experienced reinfection. Eradication of bacteria was maintained in 24 of the 26 and 22 of the 24 (92% each) patients evaluated at 2 and 6 weeks, respectively. 16 of the 19 (84%) courses of norfloxacin (800mg daily for 5 to 10 days) administered to 17 patients with complicated urinary tract infections resulted in eradication of the implicated *Pseudomonas* species (Leigh and Emmanuel, 1984). Bacterial eradication was reported in 85% of 20 patients with chronic relapsing prostatitis 30 days after a 10 day course of treatment with norfloxacin 800mg daily (Bologna et al., 1985). Sauerwein and Bauernfeind (1984) treated 52 paraplegics with recurrent urinary tract infection with norfloxacin in a total daily dosage of 400mg for 10 days. *Pseudomonas aeruginosa* was isolated from 53% of the patients prior to therapy and *Escherichia coli* was isolated from 18%, with Enterobacteriaceae and *Staphylococcus aureus* isolated from the others. 43% of the patients were symptom-free 7 days after therapy, 22% had a further infection with the same bacteria, 15% were infected with a new pathogen and in 20% of the patients the treatment was ineffective due to an increase in the MIC of the infecting bacteria. Indeed, 3 of 28 *P. aeruginosa* cultures showed an MIC increase after therapy, and 1 of the strains was cross-resistant to several other 4-quinolone antibiotics.

3.2.2 Comparative Studies

The results of 3 comparative studies, 1 with amoxycillin (Leigh et al., 1984) and 2 with pipemidic acid (Kamidono et al., 1982b; Kumamoto and Ishigami, 1983) in patients with complicated urinary tract infections are shown in table X. In the study by Leigh et al. (1984), failure of therapy occurred in only 1 patient on norfloxacin therapy but in 5 on amoxycillin therapy. Reinfection due to *Klebsiella* species, *Proteus* species or *P. aeruginosa* occurred in 3 of the amoxycillin-treated cases, but none of those treated with norfloxacin. Norfloxacin's ability to eliminate bacteriuria was significantly superior ($p < 0.04$) to that of pipemidic acid, while the overall clinical efficacy was classed as excellent in 30.5% and 21.2% of patients, respectively (Kamidono et al., 1982b). Similarly, in a double-blind trial of patients with complicated urinary tract infection with or without an indwelling catheter, norfloxacin had a higher rate of efficacy than did pipemidic acid in both patient groups, the difference reaching a statistically significant value in the patients with an indwelling catheter (Kumamoto and Ishigami, 1983).

3.3 Gonococcal and Non-Gonococcal Urethritis

Open studies of the efficacy of norfloxacin (300 to 600mg daily for 3 to 7 days) in a total of 55 patients with gonococcal urethritis reported bacteriological cure rates ranging from 93 to 100% (Ishigami et al., 1982; Nishimura et al., 1980; Saito, 1981). Additionally, in a comparative study, norfloxacin 1200mg administered to 59 men as 2 × 600mg oral doses 4 hours apart proved as effective as single doses of intramuscular spectinomycin 2g administered to 33 men; all patients in both treatment groups were infected with penicillin-resistant *Neisseria gonorrhoeae* and all patients were cured (Crider et al., 1984).

The norfloxacin response rate of 56 patients diagnosed as having non-gonococcal urethritis was much lower (43 to 83% bacteriological cure rate) [Ishigami et al., 1982; Nishimura et al., 1980; Saito, 1981] perhaps reflecting the lower level of activity of the drug against *Chlamydia trachomatis* (section 1.2).

3.4 Gastroenteritis and Prophylaxis of Sepsis in Neutropenic Patients

Norfloxacin is active against several pathogens commonly implicated in gastroenteritis, but demonstrates little activity against anaerobic organisms (section 1). Thus, the drug would be expected to be both clinically effective in gastroenteritis and to spare the normal faecal flora. Additionally, in neu-

Table XII. Bacteriological outcome of norfloxacin therapy in 159 patients with acute bacterial gastroenteritis with regard to the 15 infecting organisms (data on file, Merck Sharp and Dohme)

Organism	Norfloxacin 800mg		Norfloxacin 1200mg		Co-trimoxazole	
	eradicated	persisted	eradicated	persisted	eradicated	persisted
Aeromonas hydrophilia	6	0			4	0
Campylobacter spp.					1	0
Campylobacter fetus subsp. *jejuni*					1	1
E. coli (invasive)	–		1			
E. coli (enterotoxigenic)	15	1	19	0	9	1
Plesiomonas shigelloides	2		1		3	0
Salmonella spp.	4	0	2	0	7	1
Salmonella enteriditis					2	0
Shigella spp.					1	0
Shigella boydii	1	0			4	0
Shigella dysenteriae	1	0	3	0	2	0
Shigella flexneri	19	0	15	0	16	0
Shigella sonnei	5	0	4	0		
Vibrio cholerae			1	0		
Vibrio parahaemolyticus	3	0	3	0	2	0
Total[a]	56	1	49	0	52	3

a Includes 2 patients each infected with 2 pathogens.

tropenic patients the gastrointestinal tract frequently harbours norfloxacin-susceptible pathogens implicated in sepsis.

The clinical efficacy of norfloxacin in gastroenteritis has been assessed in a large multicentre trial conducted by 7 investigators in 7 countries. The efficacy of norfloxacin at 2 dose levels (800 and 1200mg daily) was compared with that of co-trimoxazole 320/1600mg daily for 5 days in 159 patients with acute bacterial gastroenteritis. Pathogenic bacteria were eradicated in 98% of patients treated with norfloxacin 800mg, 100% of patients treated with norfloxacin 1200mg and 95% of those treated with co-trimoxazole (table XII; unpublished data on file, Merck Sharp & Dohme).

Haase et al. (1984) studied the antimicrobial effects of norfloxacin and co-trimoxazole on periurethral and faecal microflora of patients being treated for urinary tract infection. The 2 drugs were of similar efficacy in eradicating the infecting organism from flora in the periurethra, but norfloxacin was significantly better than co-trimoxazole (93% *vs* 57% of patients, respectively) in the eradication of pathogens emanating from flora in the anal canal. It was also noted that the 3 urinary tract reinfections in the group of patients treated with co-trimoxazole appeared earlier than those in the norfloxacin group and were due to co-trimoxazole-resistant organisms, 2 of which were present in flora of the anal canal. This ability of norfloxacin to eradicate pathogens emanating from the faecal flora suggests a role for the drug in the prophylaxis of sepsis in neutropenic patients.

3.5 Other Infections

Japanese investigators have used norfloxacin in otorhinolaryngological and respiratory tract infections. Norfloxacin 600 to 800mg daily for 2 to 21 days was reported to produce 'excellent' to 'good' clinical results in 66 to 100% (mean of all studies 86%) of patients with acute otitis media, 33 to 91% (mean 55%) of patients with chronic otitis media, 100% of patients with chronic sinusitis and 67 to 100% (mean 82%) of patients with acute tonsillitis (Murai et al., 1981; Saito et al., 1981b; Sato et al., 1981; Sugita et al., 1981). One study used a higher dose of 1800 to 2400mg daily for 3 days (Kuriyama et al., 1981).

Administration of norfloxacin 300 to 800mg daily for periods of from 5 to 25 days produced 'excellent' to 'good' clinical results in 60 to 80% of patients with a variety of respiratory tract infections (Hayashi, 1981; Kabe et al., 1981), while a higher dose of 1800mg daily for 7 to 14 days achieved 'excellent' to 'good' clinical results in 74% of patients with chronic recrudescent bronchitis (Kobayashi et al., 1981). An important consideration in the treatment of respiratory tract infections is the poor *in vitro* activity of norfloxacin against *Streptococcus pneumoniae*; thus, it cannot be regarded as an alternative to other drugs active against pneumococci at concentrations readily achievable with usual dosages.

4. Side Effects

In the treatment of urinary tract infections, norfloxacin has been generally well tolerated. The overall incidence of adverse effects reported by the manufacturer in 1162 patients who received norfloxacin in a total daily dosage of 800mg was approximately 5% (table XIII). The incidence of abnormal laboratory values was low (0.01%). Increasing the dose of norfloxacin to 1200mg daily or considering neutropenic patients as a separate group did not seem to increase the overall incidence of drug-related side effects. However, Vogel et al. (1984), who treated 758 patients with norfloxacin for periods of 3 and 7 days, reported a higher overall incidence of 9%. Vogel's results are supported by data from comparative trials with co-trimoxazole, where the overall incidence of side effects was 9% with norfloxacin, and 18% with co-trimoxazole (table X). Norfloxacin also demonstrated a lower incidence of adverse effects than nalidixic acid (19 *vs* 26% overall, 5 *vs* 9% of moderate or greater severity; Reeves et al., 1984c), a similar incidence to pipemidic acid (2.7 *vs* 3.4%; Kamidono et al., 1982a,b) and in 1 study a slightly higher incidence than amoxycillin (9 *vs* 6%; Vogel et al., 1984).

Disorders of the gastrointestinal tract were the most commonly reported adverse effects with norfloxacin, occurring in 2 to 4% of patients, nausea and vomiting being the most frequent symptoms noted. Reactions such as lightheadedness and drowsiness were amongst the more commonly reported central nervous system effects. Generally these adverse effects were mild leading to with-

Table XIII. Adverse clinical effects reported by 1162 patients who received norfloxacin 400mg twice daily (data on file, Merck Sharp and Dohme)

Gastrointestinal (GI)		*Central nervous system*		*Dermatological*	
Abdominal pain	2	Anxiety	1	Erythema	2
Anorexia	1	Depression	1	Pruritus	2
Diarrhoea	1	Dizziness	6	Rash	3
Digestive system disorder	1	Euphoria	1		
		Hallucinations	1	*Other*	
Dyspepsia	4	Headache	4	Epiphora	1
Dysphagia	1	Insomnia	2	Taste perversion	2
GI cramps	1	Somnolence	1	Tinnitus	1
Nausea	13	Dry mouth	2	Vaginal swelling	1
Tongue enlargement	1			Tachycardia	1
				Total	57

drawal in only a small percentage of patients. Although the overall incidence of adverse effects in the Japanese studies was lower (3 to 4%), the effects were of a similar type and distribution. Of 2608 patients, 2 to 7% experienced gastrointestinal disturbances, nausea again being the most common (0.72%). 0.3% experienced dizziness and another 0.3% dermatological disorders.

Bailey et al. (1983b) reported tendinitis in 2 immunosuppressed men with poorly functioning renal transplants during long term treatment with norfloxacin. Symptoms resolved within 48 hours of discontinuing the antibiotic in 1 patient and in the other following a reduction in dosage.

Importantly, the photosensitivity associated with nalidixic acid therapy (Elmes, 1975) has not been reported with norfloxacin. In a comparative trial in acute urinary tract infection, 3 of 20 co-trimoxazole-treated patients experienced superinfection with *Candida, versus* only 1 of 20 norfloxacin-treated patients (Newsom, 1984). Also, in a comparative trial in women with recurrent uncomplicated urinary tract infection, no resistant strains of Enterobacteriaceae were cultured from the anus or vagina of the 20 women treated with norfloxacin 400mg 12-hourly either during or after therapy. In contrast, 3 of 15 patients with co-trimoxazole sensitive Enterobacteriaceae cultured from the anus developed resistant organisms and 2 patients had resistant organisms isolated from the vagina (Schaeffer and Sisney, 1985).

5. Dosage and Administration

In the treatment of urinary tract infections, the usual adult dosage is 400mg twice daily continued for 7 to 10 days. Three-day therapy has been shown to be effective in women with uncomplicated acute cystitis. In the treatment of chronic, relapsing urinary tract infection, the dosage of norfloxacin is 400mg twice daily for up to 12 weeks; if adequate suppression is obtained within the first 4 weeks the dose of norfloxacin may be reduced to 400mg daily.

In acute bacterial gastroenteritis the usual dosage is 400mg twice daily for 5 days.

In patients with renal failure, in whom creatinine clearance is less than 30 $ml/min/1.73m^2$ the recommended dosage is 400mg daily. In the prophylaxis of sepsis in profound neutropenia, the recommended dosage is 400mg 3 times daily for the duration of profound neutropenia. However, data for recommending treatment beyond 8 weeks are presently not available.

The safety and efficacy of norfloxacin in children have not been established.

6. The Place of Norfloxacin in Therapy

The broad spectrum of *in vitro* antibacterial activity of norfloxacin has been reflected in clinical efficacy comparable to that of co-trimoxazole in acute uncomplicated urinary tract infection. Also, initial comparative studies with pipemidic acid, nalidixic acid and amoxyxillin suggest that norfloxacin is more effective than the former and at least as effective as the latter 2 drugs in uncomplicated urinary tract infections. As occurs with other antibiotics, patients with chronic and/or complicated urinary tract infection were generally more resistant to norfloxacin therapy than were those with uncomplicated infection; initial comparative studies suggest that norfloxacin is superior to pipemidic acid in patients with indwelling catheters and similar in efficacy to amoxycillin in geriatric patients with complicated infections.

The high activity of norfloxacin against most important gastrointestinal pathogens but few anaerobes has allowed its effective use in bacterial gastroenteritis, while sparing the normal gastrointestinal flora. The wide spectrum of activity of the drug (again, sparing the normal faecal flora) is the basis of its being indicated in the prophylaxis of sepsis in neutropenic patients. Preliminary studies have demonstrated the efficacy of norfloxacin in the treatment of gonococcal urethritis and prostatitis, and the drug may eventually prove valuable in many types of infection.

Adverse effects associated with norfloxacin therapy have generally been mild, leading to withdrawals in less than 1% of patients.

Thus, if wider clinical use confirms the efficacy, the low incidence of side effects and the apparently low propensity of norfloxacin to induce resistance, it may not only offer worthwhile advantages over the standard agents used to treat urinary tract infections (e.g. co-trimoxazole and amoxycillin, as well as nalidixic acid and some of its early analogues) but it may become a valuable prophylactic and therapeutic antibiotic in other clinical situations.

References

Abiko, T.; Ishihama, A.; Ogawa, N.; Uchida, H.; Murayama, S.; Hirai, K. et al.: Phase I study on AM-715. Chemotherapy 29: 136-145 (1981).

Adhami, Z.N.; Wise, R.; Weston, D. and Crump, B.: The pharmacokinetics and tissue penetration of norfloxacin. Journal of Antimicrobial Chemotherapy 13: 87-92 (1984).

Aoyama, S.; Nakamura, H. and Hayashi, S.: Clinical study on AM-715 for the treatment of urinary tract infections. Chemotherapy (Tokyo) 29 (Suppl. 4): 669-672 (1981).

Bailey, R.R.; Kirk, J.A. and Peddie, B.A.: Norfloxacin-induced rheumatic disease. New Zealand Medical Journal 2: 590 (1983b).

Bailey, R.R.; Peddie, B.A. and Blake, E.: Norfloxacin for the treatment of uncomplicated urinary tract infections. New Zealand Medical Journal 96: 446 (1983a).

Barry, A.L. and Jones, R.N.: Cross-resistance among cinoxacin, ciprofloxacin, DJ-6783, enoxacin, nalidixic acid, norfloxacin and oxolinic acid after *in vitro* selection of resistant populations. Antimicrobial Agents and Chemotherapy 25: 775-777 (1984).

Barry, A.L.; Jones, R.N.; Thornsberry, C.; Ayers, L.W.; Gerlach, E.H. and Sommers, H.M.: Antibacterial activities of ciprofloxacin, norfloxacin, oxolinic acid, cinoxacin and nalidixic acid. Antimicrobial Agents and Chemotherapy 25: 633-637 (1984).

Bauernfeind, A.: Teichomycin and AM-715 activity on staphylococci and enterococci in comparison to other antibiotic agents. 21st Interscience Conference on Antimicrobial Agents and Chemotherapy, Chicago, Nov 4-6, 1981. Abstract No. 428 (1981).

Bauernfeind, A. and Petermüller, C.: Progress in chemotherapeutic heterocyclic carbonic acids. Drugs under Experimental and Clinical Research 9: 545-553 (1983a).

Bauernfeind, A. and Petermüller, C.: *In vitro* activity of ciprofloxacin, norfloxacin and nalidixic acid. European Journal of Clinical Microbiology 2: 111-115 (1983b).

Bauernfeind, A.; Petermüller, C. and Danninger, J.: Reduction of sensitivity to perfloxacin, ofloxacin, norfloxacin and ciprofloxacin in *Pseudomonas aeruginosa.* 24th Interscience Conference on Antimicrobial Agents and Chemotherapy, Washington D.C., Oct 8-10, 1984. Abstract No. 460 (1984a).

Bauernfeind, A.; Sauerwein, D.; Danninger, J. and Keding, M.: Reduktion der Empfindlichkeit von *Pseudomonas aeruginosa* gegen über neuen 4-chinolonen durch mutation *in vitro* und *in vivo.* Fortschritte der Antimikrobiellen und Antineoplastichen Chemotherapie 3-5: 521-529 (1984b).

Bauernfeind, A. and Ullmann, U.: *In vitro* activity of enoxacin, ofloxacin, norfloxacin, and nalidixic acid. Journal of Antimicrobial Chemotherapy 14 (Suppl. C): 33-37 (1984).

Beerman, D.; Wingender, W.; Zeiler, H.J.; Foerster, D.; Graefe, K.H. and Schacht, P.: Comparative pharmacokinetics of the new quinoline carboxylic acid antibiotics after oral administration in healthy volunteers. Journal of Clinical Pharmacology 24: 403 (1984).

Bergeron, M.G.; Thabet, M.; Roy, R.; Lessard, C. and Foucault, P.: Norfloxacin penetration into human renal and prostatic tissues. Antimicrobial Agents and Chemotherapy 28: 349-350 (1985).

Bendall, M.J.: A review of urinary tract infection in the elderly. Journal of Antimicrobial Chemotherapy 13 (Suppl. B): 69-78 (1984).

Bologna, M.; Vaggi, L.; Flammini, D.; Carlucci, G. and Forchetti, C.M.: Norfloxacin in prostatitis: correlation between HPLC tissue concentrations and clinical results. Drugs under Experimental and Clinical Research 11: 95-100 (1985).

Bologna, M.; Vaggi, L.; Forchetti, C.M. and Martini, E.: Bactericidal intra-prostatic concentrations of norfloxacin. Lancet 2: 280 (1983a).

Bologna, M.; Vaggi, L.; Martini, E. and Tomei, E.: Norfloxacin in the treatment of urinary tract infections. European Journal of Chemotherapy and Antibiotics 3: 41-46 (1983b).

Brumfitt, W. and Hamilton-Miller, J.M.T.: Review of the problem of urinary infection management and the evaluation of a potential new antibiotic. Journal of Antimicrobial Chemotherapy 13 (Suppl. B): 121-133 (1984).

Carlson, J.R.; Thornton, S.A.; DuPont, H.L.; West, A.H. and Mathewson, J.J.: Comparison of *in vitro* activities of ten antimicrobial agents against bacterial enteropathogens. Antimicrobial Agents and Chemotherapy 24: 509-513 (1983).

Chartrand, S.A.; Scribner, R.K.; Weber, A.H.; Welch, D.F. and Marks, M.I.: *In vitro* activity of Cl-919 (AT-2266), an oral antipseudomonal compound. Antimicrobial Agents and Chemotherapy 23: 658-663 (1983).

Chin, N.X. and Neu, H.C.: *In vitro* activity of enoxacin, a quinolone carboxylic acid, compared with those of norfloxacin, new β-lactams, aminoglycosides, and trimethoprim. Antimicrobial Agents and Chemotherapy 23: 754-763 (1983).

Clarke, A.M.; Zemcov, S.J.V. and Campbell, M.E.: *In vitro* activity of perfloxacin compared to enoxacin, norfloxacin, gentamicin and new β-lactams. Journal of Antimicrobial Chemotherapy 15: 39-44 (1985).

Cofsky, R.D.; DuBouchet, L. and Landesman, S.H.: Recovery of norfloxacin in feces after administration of a single oral dose to human volunteers. Antimicrobial Agents and Chemotherapy 26: 110-111 (1984).

Corigliano, B.E.; Appleman, M.D.; Heseltine, P.N.R. and Leedom, J.M.: Comparative *in vitro* activities of norfloxacin (MK-0366) and six commonly used antimicrobial agents against 199 urinary isolates showing various degrees of antibiotic resistance. Diagnostic Microbiology and Infectious Diseases 2: 101-106 (1984).

Corrado, M.L.; Cherubin, C.E. and Shulman, M.: The comparative activity of norfloxacin with other antimicrobial agents against Gram-positive and Gram-negative bacteria. Journal of Antimicrobial Chemotherapy 11: 369-376 (1983).

Crider, S.R.; Colby, S.D.; Miller, L.K.; Harrison, W.O.; Kerbs, S.B.J. and Berg, S.W.: Treatment of penicillin-resistant *Neisseria gonorrhoeae* with oral norfloxacin. New England Journal of Medicine 311: 137-140 (1984).

Crumplin, G.C.; Kenwright, M. and Hurst, T.: Investigations into the mechanism of action of the antibacterial agent norfloxacin. Journal of Antimicrobial Chemotherapy 13 (Suppl. B): 9-23 (1984).

Crumplin, G.C. and Smith, J.T.: Investigations into the mechanism of action of the antibacterial agent norfloxacin. Journal of Antimicrobial Chemotherapy 7: 379 (1981).

Cullmann, W.; Stieglitz, M.; Baars, B. and Opferkuch, W.: Comparative evaluation of recently developed quinolone compounds – with a note on the frequency of resistant mutants. Chemotherapy (Basel) 31: 19-28 (1985).

Diez-Enciso, M.; Mas-Jimenez, G.; Velasco-Cerrudo, A. and Gutierrez-Altes, A.: Comparison of the *in vitro* activity of ciprofloxacin (Bay 09867) and norfloxacin against gastrointestinal

tract pathogens. European Journal of Clinical Microbiology 3: 367 (1984).
Digranes, A.; Dibb, W.L. and Østervold, B.: Norfloxacin: *In vitro* activity compared with that of seven other antibacterial agents against urinary tract pathogens. Actá Pathologica, Microbiologica et Immunologica Scandinavica 92: 101-106 (1984).
Duckworth, G.J. and Williams, J.D.: Frequency of appearance of resistant variants to norfloxacin and nalidixic acid. Journal of Antimicrobial Chemotherapy 13 (Suppl. B): 33-38 (1984).
Eandi, M.; Viano, I.; DiNola, F.; Leone, L. and Genazzani, E.: Pharmacokinetics of norfloxacin in healthy volunteers and patients with renal and hepatic damage. European Journal of Clinical Microbiology 2: 253-259 (1983).
Eliopoulos, G.M.; Gardella, A. and Moellering Jr, R.C.: *In vitro* activity of ciprofloxacin, a new carboxyquinoline antimicrobial agent. Antimicrobial Agents and Chemotherapy 25: 331-335 (1984).
Elmes, P.C.: Antibacterial drugs used in miscellaneous infection. In Dukes, M.N.G. (Ed) Meyler's Side Effects of Drugs, Vol. 8, pp. 668-675 (Excerpta Medica, Amsterdam-Oxford American Elsevier Publishing Co., New York 1975).
Eng, R.H.K.; Smith, S.M.; Corrado, M.L. and Gadebusch, H.H.: Antifungal activity of norfloxacin (MK 0366) and amphotericin-B in combination. 22nd Interscience Conference on Antimicrobial Agents and Chemotherapy, Miami Beach, Oct 4-6, 1982. Abstract No. 479 (1982).
Fass, R.J.: *In vitro* activity of ciprofloxacin (Bay 09867). Antimicrobial Agents and Chemotherapy 24: 568-574 (1983).
Fillastre, J.P.; Hannedouche, Th.; Leroy, A. and Humbert, G.: Pharmacokinetics of norfloxacin in renal failure. Journal of Antimicrobial Chemotherapy 14: 439 (1984).
Forward, K.R.; Harding, G.K.M.; Gray, G.J.; Urias, B.A. and Ronald, A.R.: Comparative activities of norfloxacin and fifteen other antipseudomonal agents against gentamicin-susceptible and gentamicin-resistant *Pseudomonas aeruginosa* strains. Antimicrobial Agents and Chemotherapy 24: 602-604 (1983).
Fraschini, F.; Scaglione, F.; Proto, M.; Zanollo, A.; Gattei, G. et al.: Levels of norfloxacin in the tissue of the female genital apparatus and kidney. 4th Mediterranean Congress of Chemotherapy, Rhodes, Oct 19-25, 1984. Abstract No. 750 (1984).
Fujimura, N.; Yuasa, K.; Aga, Y. and Kurokawa, K.: Clinical efficacy of AM-715 on urinary tract and urogenital infection. Chemotherapy (Tokyo) 29 (Suppl. 4): 587-593 (1981).
Ganguli, L.A.; Keaney, M.G.L. and Gould, L.J.: Norfloxacin: a three-day course for the treatment of urinary tract infection. Drugs under Experimental and Clinical Research 13: 177-179 (1985).
Gadebusch, H.H.; Shungu, D.L.; Weinberg, E. and Chung, S.K.: Comparison of the antibacterial activity of norfloxacin (MK 0366, AM715), a new organic acid, with that of other orally absorbed chemotherapeutic agents. Infection 10: 41-44 (1982).
Gellert, M.; Mizuuchi, K.; O'Day, M.H.; Itoh, T. and Timizawa, J.: Nalidixic acid resistance: a second genetic character involved in DNA-gyrase activity. Proceedings of the National Academy of Science USA 74: 4772-4776 (1977).
Giamarellou, H.; Tsagarakis, J.; Petrikkos, G. and Daikos, G.K.: Norfloxacin *versus* cotrimoxazole in the treatment of lower urinary tract infections. European Journal of Clinical Microbiology 2: 266-269 (1983a).
Giamarellou, H.; Tsagarakis, J.; Seitanides, B. and Daikos, G.K.: Norfloxacin in the treatment of recurrent urinary tract infections. European Journal of Chemotherapy and Antibiotics 3: 27-30 (1983b).
Goldstein, E.J.C.; Alpert, M.L. and Ginsberg, B.P.: Norfloxacin *versus* trimethoprim-sulfamethoxazole in the therapy of uncomplicated, community-acquired urinary tract infections. Antimicrobial Agents and Chemotherapy 27: 422-423 (1985).
Goossens, H.; DeMol, P.; Coignau, H.; Levy, J.; Grados, O. et al.: Comparative *in vitro* activities of aztreonam, ciprofloxacin, norfloxacin, ofloxacin, HR810 (a new cephalosporin), RU28965 (a new macrolide) and other agents against enteropathogens. Antimicrobial Agents and Chemotherapy 27: 388-392 (1985).
Greenwood, D.; Osman, M.; Goodwin, J.; Cowlishaw, W.A. and Slack, R.: Norfloxacin: activity against urinary tract pathogens and factors influencing the emergence of resistance. Journal of Antimicrobial Chemotherapy 13: 315-323 (1984).
Guerra, J.G.; Falconi, E.; Palomino, J.C.; Benavente, L. and Antunez de Mayolo, E.: Clinical evaluation of norfloxacin *versus* cotrimoxazole in urinary tract infections. European Journal of Clinical Microbiology 2: 260-265 (1983).
Haase, D.A.; Harding, G.K.M.; Thomson, M.J.; Kennedy, J.K.; Urias, B.A. and Ronald, A.R.: Comparative trial of norfloxacin and trimethoprim-sulfamethoxazole in the treatment of women with localized acute, symptomatic urinary tract infections and antimicrobial effect on periurethral and fecal microflora. Antimicrobial Agents and Chemotherapy 26: 481-484 (1984).
Hayashi, I.: Clinical studies on AM-715 in the treatment of respiratory tract infections. Chemotherapy (Tokyo) 29 (Suppl. 4): 182-187 (1981).
Heessen, W.A. and Muytjens, H.L.: *In vitro* activities of ciprofloxacin, norfloxacin, pipemidic acid, cinoxacin and nalidixic acid against *Chlamydia trachomatis.* Antimicrobial Agents and Chemotherapy 25: 123-124 (1984).
Hirai, K.; Ito, A.; Suzue, S.; Irikura, T.; Inoue, M. and Mitsuhashi, S.: Mode of action of AM-715, a new nalidixic acid analog. Gunma Reports on Medical Sciences 19: 375-392 (1982).
Hooper, D.C.; Wolfson, J.S.; Tung, C. and Swartz, M.N.: Norfloxacin inhibits bacterial growth by antagonism of DNA gyrase and inhibits conjugal plasmid transfer. 23rd Interscience Conference on Antimicrobial Agents and Chemotherapy, Las Vegas Oct. 23-26, 1983. Abstract (1983).
Hughes, P.J.; Webb, D.B. and Asscher, A.W.: Pharmacokinetics of norfloxacin (MK366) in patients with impaired kidney function – some preliminary results. Journal of Antimicrobial Chemotherapy 13 (Suppl. B): 55-57 (1984).
Husson, M.O.; Izard, D. and Leclerc, H.: Comparative *in vitro* antibacterial activity of norfloxacin *versus* four other quinolone derivatives. Drugs under Experimental and Clinical Research 10: 315-319 (1984).
Ishigami, J.; Kamidono, S.; Matsumoto, O.; Arakawa, S.; Kataoku, N.; Saito, S. et al.: Efficacy of norfloxacin (AM-715) for the treatment of acute urethritis. Chemotherapy (Tokyo) 30: 1349-1360 (1982).
Ishito, N.; Okimure, M.; Miyata, K.; Takamoto, H.; Hirano, M.; Ohashi, T. et al.: A clinical study on AM-715 in urinary tract infections. Chemotherapy (Tokyo) 29 (Suppl. 4): 566-577 (1981).
Ito, A.; Hirai, K.; Inoue, M.; Koga, H.; Suzue, S. et al.: *In vitro* activity of AM-715, a new nalidixic acid analog. Antimicrobial Agents and Chemotherapy 17: 103-108 (1980).
Iwasawa, T.: Fundamental and clinical studies on AM-715 in the otorhinolaryngolic field. Chemotherapy (Tokyo) 29 (Suppl. 4): 714-729 (1981).
Jones, R.N. and Barry, A.L.: Norfloxacin (MK-0366, AM-715). *In vitro* activity and cross resistance with other organic acids including quality control limits for disk diffusion testing. Diagnostic Microbiology and Infectious Disease 1: 165-172 (1983).
Kabe, J.; Suehara, M.; Ishibashi, H. and Watanabe, T.: Clinical study of AM-715. Chemotherapy (Tokyo) 29 (Suppl. 4): 240-247 (1981).
Kamidono, S.; Tomioka, O.; Hikosaka, K.; Ishigami, J.; Niijima, T. et al.: A comparative double-blind study of norfloxacin (AM-715) and pipemidic acid in the treatment of acute simple cystitis. Chemotherapy (Tokyo) 30: 1159-1181 (1982a).
Kamidono, S.; Tomioka, O.; Hikosaka, K.; Ishigami, J.; Niijima, T. et al.: A comparative double-blind study of norfloxacin (AM-715) and pipemidic acid in the treatment of complicated urinary tract infection. Chemotherapy (Tokyo) 30: 1182-1211

(1982b).
Khan, M.Y.; Gruninger, R.P.; Nelson, S.M. and Klicker, R.E.: Comparative *in vitro* activity of norfloxacin (MK-0366) and ten other oral antimicrobial agents against urinary bacterial isolates. Antimicrobial Agents and Chemotherapy 5: 848-851 (1982).
Khan, M.Y.; Gruninger, R.P.; Nelson, S.M. and Simpson, M.L.: Comparative *in vitro* activity of Sch 29,482, a new oral penem, against *Neisseria gonorrhoeae.* Antimicrobial Agents and Chemotherapy 23: 481-482 (1983).
King, A.; Shannon, K. and Phillips, I.: The *in vitro* activity of ciprofloxacin compared with that of norfloxacin and nalidixic acid. Journal of Antimicrobial Chemotherapy 13: 325-331 (1984).
King, A.; Warren, C.; Shannon, K. and Phillips, I.: *In vitro* antibacterial activity of norfloxacin (MK-0366). Antibacterial Agents and Chemotherapy 21: 604-607 (1982).
Kirby, C.P.: Treatment of simple urinary tract infections in general practice with a 3 day course of norfloxacin. Journal of Antimicrobial Chemotherapy 13 (Suppl. B): 107-112 (1984).
Kiriyama, T.; Okada, K.; Okabe, T.; Okada, Y.; Nishibuchi, S. et al.: A phase II study of AM-715 on acute simple cystitis and complicated urinary tract infection. Chemotherapy (Tokyo) 29 (Suppl. 4): 531-545 (1981).
Kobayashi, H.; Takamura, M.; Takamura, K.; Kono, K. and Shimura, M.: A clinical study on AM-715 for the treatment of chronic respiratory tract infections. Chemotherapy (Tokyo) 29 (Suppl. 4): 248-254 (1981).
Kumamoto, Y. and Ishigami, J.: Clinical experience with norfloxacin in urinary tract infections. European Journal of Chemotherapy and Antibiotics 3: 31-39 (1983).
Kurimura, O.; Sadamoto, K.; Sasaki, H.; Murai, T.; Nozaki, K. et al.: Effects of AM-715 on typhoid fever and non-typhoidal salmonellosis. Chemotherapy (Tokyo) 29: 343-353 (1981).
Kuriyama, K.; Baba, K.; Okuzawa, Y.; Baba, Y.; Sato, K. and Furuuchi, I.: Clinical studies on AM-715 in the field of otorhinolaryngology. Chemotherapy (Tokyo) 29 (Suppl. 4): 730-737 (1981).
Lacey, R.W.; Lord, V.L. and Howson, G.L.: Bactericidal effects of norfloxacin towards bacteria in urine. Journal of Antimicrobial Chemotherapy 13 (Suppl. B): 49-54 (1984).
Lariviere, L.; Gaudreau, C. and Turgeon, F.: Antimicrobial susceptibilities of 163 strains of *Campylobacter jejuni.* Annals of the Royal College of Physicians and Surgeons of Canada 17: 333 (1984).
Leigh, D.A. and Emmanuel, F.X.S.: The treatment of *Pseudomonas aeruginosa* urinary tract infections with norfloxacin. Journal of Antimicrobial Chemotherapy 13 (Suppl. B): 85-88 (1984).
Leigh, D.A. and Osborne, M.: Comparative activity of MK 366, norfloxacin, cinoxacin and nalidixic acid against multiply resistant strains of Enterobacteriaciae and *Pseudomonas aeruginosa.* 22nd Interscience Conference on Antimicrobial Agents and Chemotherapy, Florida, Oct 4-6, 1982. Abstract No. 683 (1982).
Leigh, D.A.; Smith, E.C. and Marriner, J.: Comparative study using norfloxacin and amoxycillin in the treatment of complicated urinary tract infections in geriatric patients. Journal of Antimicrobial Chemotherapy 13 (Suppl. B): 79-83 (1984).
Machka, K. and Braveny, I.: Inhibitorische wirkung verschiedener factoren auf die activität von norfloxacin. Fortschritte der Antimikrobiellen und Antineoplastischen Chemotherapie 3-5: 557-562 (1984).
Martino, P.; Venditti, M.; Valente, B.; Brandimarte, C. and Serra, P.: N-formimidoyl-thienamycin and norfloxacin against multiple-resistant *Pseudomonas aeruginosa* strains: Combined *in vitro* activity and comparison with 14 other antibiotics. Drugs under Experimental and Clinical Research 11: 247-251 (1985).
Maru, A.: Clinical study on AM-715. Chemotherapy (Tokyo) 29 (Suppl. 4): 407-412 (1981).
Matsumuto, K.; Suziki, H.; Tsuchiahashi, K. et al.: Laboratory and clinical studies on AM-715 Chemotherapy (Tokyo) 29 (Suppl. 4): 370-379 (1981).
Matsuoka, K.; Eto, K.; Sakai, Y.; Yoshizumi, O. and Miyahara, S.: Clinical experience of AM-715 on urinary tract infection. Chemotherapy (Tokyo) 29 (Suppl. 4): 622-630 (1981).
Murai, K.; Baba, S.; Hondo, J.; Wada, K. and Hatano, K.: Laboratory and clinical studies on AM-715 in otorhinolaryngological field. Chemotherapy (Tokyo) 29 (Suppl. 4): 755-761 (1981).
Muytjens, H.L.; van der Ros-van de Repe, J. and van Veldhuizen, G.: Comparative activities of ciprofloxacin (Bay O 9867), norfloxacin, pipemidic acid, and nalidixic acid. Antimicrobial Agents and Chemotherapy 24: 302-304 (1983).
Nakagawa, K.; Watanabe, K. and Koyana, M.: Clinical study on AM-715. Chemotherapy (Tokyo) 29 (Suppl. 4): 220-234 (1981).
Nakamura, S.; Minami, A.; Katae, H.; Inoue, S.; Yamagishi, J. et al.: *In vitro* antibacterial properties of AT-2266, a new pyridone carboxylic acid. Antimicrobial Agents and Chemotherapy 23: 641-648 (1983).
Nakamuta, S.; Momose, S.; KumazawawJ.; Ishizawa, N.; Osada, S. and Nagatomo, K.: Clinical experience of AM-715 in urinary tract infection. Chemotherapy (Tokyo) 29 (Suppl. 4): 594-602 (1981).
Nakatsu, H.; Hatachi, K.; Fujii, M.; Nihira, H.; Masu, C. and Nakano, H.: Fundamental and clinical studies of AM-715 in complicated urinary tract infections. Chemotherapy (Tokyo) 29 (Suppl. 4): 578-586 (1981).
Netto Jr, N.R.; Palma, P.C.R.; Lemos, G.C.; Srulzon, G.B.; Cortado, P.L. and Fonseca, R.C.: Avaliação da concentração tecidual renal e prostática de norfloxacin. Revista Brasileira de Clinica e Terapeutica 13: 49-50 (1984).
Neu, H.C.: Effects of cations upon the activity of quinolone agents. In Shah, P.M. (Ed) Quinolone Bulletin: Reports on Gyrase Inhibitors. (m.i. publications, Frankfurt, 1985)
Neu, H.C. and Labthavikul, P.: *In vitro* activity of norfloxacin, a quinoline carboxylic acid, compared with that of β-lactams, aminoglycosides and trimethoprim. Antimicrobial Agents and Chemotherapy 22: 23-27 (1982).
Newsom, S.W.B.: The antimicrobial spectrum of norfloxacin. Journal of Antimicrobial Chemotherapy 13 (Suppl. B): 25-31 (1984).
Newsom, S.W.B.; Matthews, J.; Amphlett, M. and Warren, R.E.: Norfloxacin and the antibacterial γ pyridone β carboxylic acids. Journal of Antimicrobial Chemotherapy 10: 25-30 (1982).
Newsom, S.W.B.; Matthews, J. and Rampling, A.M.: Susceptibility of *Clostridium difficile* strains to new antibiotics: quinolones, efrotomycin, teicoplanin and imipenem. (Correspondence.) Journal of Antimicrobial Chemotherapy 15: 648-650 (1985).
Newsom, S.W.B.; Newsom, R.A. and Toase, D.: Norfloxacin *vs* cotrimoxazole for urinary tract infection in general practice. 23rd Interscience Conference on Antimicrobial Agents and Chemotherapy, Las Vegas, Oct. 24-26, 1983. Abstract No. 519 (1983).
Nishimura, Y.; Kishi, H.; Tsukada, O.; Tominga, T. and Niijima, T.: Clinical evaluation of AM-715 on urological infections. 20th Interscience Conference on Antimicrobial Agents and Chemotherapy, New Orleans, Sept. 22-24, 1980. Abstract No. 76 (1980).
Norrby, S.R.: Pharmacokinetics of norfloxacin: Clinical implications. European Journal of Chemotherapy and Antibiotics 3: 19-25 (1983).
Norrby, S.R. and Jonsson, M.: Antibacterial activity of norfloxacin. Antimicrobial Agents and Chemotherapy 23: 15-18 (1983).
Okada, K.; Ohkoshi, M.; Kawamura, N. and Murakami, Y.: Experimental and clinical studies on AM-715 in urological field. Chemotherapy (Tokyo) 29: 452-465 (1981).
Ozaki, T.; Uchida, H. and Irikura, T.: Studies on metabolism of

AM-715 in humans by high performance liquid chromatography. Chemotherapy (Tokyo) 29 (Suppl. 4): 128-135 (1981).
Panichi, G.; Pantosti, A. and Testore, G.P.; Norfloxacin (MK-0366) treatment of urinary tract infections in hospitalized patients. Journal of Antimicrobial Chemotherapy 11: 589-592 (1983).
Pantosti, A.; Guiliano, M.; Testore, G.P. and Panichi, G.: Microbiological and clinical study on a new chemotherapeutic agent for urinary tract infections: MK-0366. Drugs under Experimental and Clinical Research 10: 43-45 (1984).
Peddie, B.A.; Norfloxacin – a new oral antibacterial agent with anti-pseudomonal activity. New Zealand Medical Journal 95: 712 (1982).
Peeters, [illegible].; Van Dyck, E. and Piot, P.: *In vitro* activities of the spectinomycin analog U-6366 and four quinolone derivatives against *Neisseria gonorrhoeae*. Antimicrobial Agents and Chemotherapy 26: 608-609 (1984).
Piffaretti, J.C., Arini, A. and Peduzzi, R.: *In vitro* activity of norfloxacin against *Neisseria gonorrhoeae*. Chemotherapy (Basel) 29: 415-418 (1983).
Preblud, S.R.; Gill, C.J. and Campos, J.M.: Bactericidal activities of chloramphenicol and eleven other antibiotics against *Salmonella* spp. Antimicrobial Agents and Chemotherapy 25: 327-330 (1984).
Ratcliffe, N.T. and Smith, J.T.: Mechanism of reduced activity of 4-quinolone agents in urine. Fortschritte der Antimikrobiellen und Antineoplastichen Chemotherapie 3-5: 563-569 (1984).
Reeves, D.S.; Bywater, M.J. and Holt, H.A.: The activity of enoxacin against clinical bacterial isolates in comparison with that of five other agents, and factors affecting that activity. Journal of Antimicrobial Chemotherapy 14 (Suppl. C): 7-17 (1984a).
Reeves, D.S.; Bywater, M.J.; Holt, H.A. and White, L.O.: *In vitro* studies with ciprofloxacin, a new 4-quinolone compound. Journal of Antimicrobial Chemotherapy 13: 333-346 (1984b).
Reeves, D.S.; Lacey, R.W.; Mummery, R.V.; Mahendra, M.; Bint, A.J. and Newsom, S.W.B.: Treatment of acute urinary infection by norfloxacin or nalidixic acid/citrate: A multi-centre comparative study. Journal of Antimicrobial Chemotherapy 13 (Suppl. B): 99-105 (1984c).
Reinhardt, J.F. and George, W.L.: Comparative *in vitro* activities of selected antimicrobial agents against aeromonas species and *Plesiomonas shigelloides*. Antimicrobial Agents and Chemotherapy 27: 643-645 (1985).
van Roosbroeck, R.J.; Privinciael, D.R. and van Caekenberghe, D.L.: Activity of the newer quinolones against *Chlamydia trachomatis*. British Journal of Venereal Disease 60: 350 (1984).
Sabbaj, J.; Hoagland, V.L. and Shih, W.J.: Multiclinic comparative study of norfloxacin and trimethoprim-sulfamethoxazole for treatment of urinary tract infections. Antimicrobial Agents and Chemotherapy 27: 297-301 (1985).
Saito, T.: Clinical experience of AM-715. Chemotherapy (Tokyo) 29: 437-444 (1981).
Saito, S.; Fujii, K. and Miyake, H.: Clinical experience of AM-715 in otorhinolaryngological field. Chemotherapy (Tokyo) 29 (Suppl. 4): 745-749 (1981b).
Saito, T.; Yamada, Y. and Arai, T.: Studies on AM-715: Biliary excretion, tissue concentration of the liver and the gallbladder wall, and clinical evaluation in surgical field. Chemotherapy (Tokyo) 29: 631-638 (1981a).
Sanders, C.C.; Sanders Jr, W.E.; Goering, R.V. and Werner, V.: Selection of multiple antibiotic resistance by quinolones, β-lactams, and aminoglycosides with special reference to cross-resistance between unrelated drug classes. Antimicrobial Agents and Chemotherapy 26: 797-801 (1984).
Sato, K.; Ichikawa, T. and Yamada, Y.: Clinical experience of AM-715 in the otorhinolaryngological infections. Chemotherapy (Tokyo) 29 (Suppl. 4): 750-754 (1981).
Sato, K.; Matsuura, Y.; Inoue, M.; Une, T.; Osada, Y. et al.: *In vitro* and *in vivo* activity of DL 8280, a new oxazine derivative. Antimicrobial Agents and Chemotherapy 22: 548-553 (1982).
Sauerwein, D. and Bauernfeind, A.; Klinische Erfahrungen bei Behandlung von Harnwegsinfekten bei Querschnittgelämten mit Norfloxacin. Fortschritte der Antimikrobiellen und Antineoplastischen Chemotherapie 3-5: 759-764 (1984).
Schaeffer, A.J. and Sisney, G.A.: Comparison of norfloxacin and trimethoprim-sulfamethoxazole in the treatment of urinary tract infections. Journal of Urology 131: 204A (1984).
Schaeffer, A.J. and Sisney, G.A.: Efficacy of norfloxacin in urinary tract infections: biological effects on vaginal and fecal flora. Journal of Urology 133: 628-630 (1985).
Shah, P.M.; Ottrad, M. and Stille, E.: *In vitro* activity of norfloxacin in urine compared to that of cinoxacin, nalidixic acid and pipemidic acid. European Journal of Clinical Microbiology 2: 272-274 (1983).
Shah, P.M.; Schrinner, K.P.; Helm, E.B. and Stille, W.: Untersuchungen zur antibakteriellen Aktivität von Penicillin und Cephalosporinen in Urin. Arzneimittel Forschung 26: 1636-1638 (1976).
Shimada, K.; Inamatsu, T. and Urayama, K.: AM-715 therapy in complicated urinary tract infections. Chemotherapy (Tokyo) 29 (Suppl. 4): 255-258 (1981).
Shimada, J.; Yamaji, T.; Ueda, Y.; Uchida, H.; Kusajima, H. and Irikura, T.: Mechanism of renal excretion of AM-715, a new quinolone carboxylic acid derivative in rabbits, dogs and humans. Antimicrobial Agents and Chemotherapy 23: 1-7 (1983).
Shimura, H.; Yamamoto, H.; Igimi, H.; Arima, S.; Ohkuma, R. and Kuroda, Y.: Fundamental and clinical studies of norfloxacin (AM-715) in biliary tract infection. Chemotherapy (Tokyo) 31: 351-367 (1983).
Shungu, D.L.; Weinberg, E. and Gadebusch, H.H.: *In vitro* antibacterial activity of norfloxacin (MK-0366, AM-715) and other agents against gastrointestinal tract pathogens. Antimicrobial Agents and Chemotherapy 23: 86-90 (1983).
Slack, R.: Reviews of bacterial resistance – a challenge to the treatment of urinary infection. Journal of Antimicrobial Chemotherapy 13 (Suppl. B): 1-7 (1984).
Smith, S.M. and Cherubin, C.: Activity of norfloxacin (MK 0366) for 250 resistant clinical isolates. 83rd Annual Meeting of the American Society for Microbiology, New Orleans, March 6-11, 1983. Abstract No. A12 (1983).
Sugita, R.; Kawamura, S. and Fujimaki, Y.: Clinical experience of AM-715 in the otorhinolaryngological infections. Chemotherapy (Tokyo) 29 (Suppl. 4): 762-765 (1981).
Swanson, B.N.; Boppana, V.K.; Vlasses, P.H.; Rotmensch, H.H. and Ferguson, R.K.: Norfloxacin disposition after sequentially increasing oral doses. Antimicrobial Agents and Chemotherapy 23: 284-288 (1983).
Sweet, R.L.; Ohm-Smith, M.J. and Hadley, W.K.: Comparative *in vitro* activity of norfloxacin and selected antimicrobial agents against urinary tract pathogens and *Neisseria gonorrhoeae*. Journal of Antimicrobial Chemotherapy 10: 553-557 (1982).
Takada, K.; Sakakibara, T. and Ohbori, T.: Clinical experience of AM-715 on complicated urinary tract infections. Chemotherapy (Tokyo) 29 (Suppl. 4): 413-419 (1981).
Takahashi, H.; Kobayashi, Y. and Fujimori, I.: Clinical study on AM-715. Chemotherapy (Tokyo) 29 (Suppl. 4): 293-298 (1981).
Takase, Z.; Shirafuji, H. and Uchida, M.: Basic and clinical studies on AM-715 in the field of obstetrics and gynecology. Chemotherapy (Tokyo) 29 (Suppl. 4): 697-704 (1981).
Takebe, K.; Kumasaka, Y.; Nakahata, H.; Imamura, K.; Machida, K. et al.: Clinical studies on AM-715. Chemotherapy (Tokyo) 29: 157-171 (1981).
Tenney, J.H.; Maack, R.W. and Chippendale, G.R.: Rapid selection of organisms with increasing resistance on subinhibitory concentrations of norfloxacin in agar. Antimicrobial Agents and Chemotherapy 23: 188-189 (1983).

Tominaga, T.; Tsukada, O.; Kishi, H.; Kawabe, K.; Niijima, T. et al.: Antibacterial activity and clinical evaluation of AM-715 in the field of urology. Chemotherapy (Tokyo) 29 (Suppl. 4): 420-433 (1981).

Traub, W.H.: Incomplete cross-resistance of nalidixic and pipemidic acid-resistant variants of *Serratia marcescens* against ciprofloxacin, enoxacin and norfloxacin. Chemotherapy (Basel) 31: 34-39 (1985).

Ueda, Y.; Saito, A. and Shimada, J.: Clinical studies on AM-715. Chemotherapy 29 (Suppl. 4): 202-219 (1981).

Unno, R. and Yamamoto, Y.: Clinical experience of AM-715 in the urological field. Chemotherapy (Tokyo) 29: 466-474 (1981).

Vangdal, M. and Bergan, T.: *In vitro* activity of azlocillin, aminoglycosides and oxacins against *Pseudomonas aeruginosa*. Drugs under Experimental and Clinical Research 10: 433-436 (1984a).

Vangdal, M. and Bergan, T.: *In vitro* synergistic activity of norfloxacin and amphotericin-B against fungi. Drugs under Experimental and Clinical Research 10: 443-444 (1984b).

Vogel, R.; Deaney, N.B.; Round, E.M.; VandenBurg, M.J. and Currie, W.J.C.: Norfloxacin, amoxycillin, cotrimoxazole and nalidixic acid. Journal of Antimicrobial Chemotherapy 13 (Suppl. B): 113-120 (1984).

Vuye, A.: *In vitro* comparison of norfloxacin with nalidixic acid, cinoxacin and oxolinic acid. Arzneimittel-Forschung 33: 1623-1627 (1983).

Walsh, T.J.; Wharton, R.C.; Sprecher, S.; Moody, M.R. and Schimpff, S.C.: Augmentation of *in vitro* antifungal activity by norfloxacin. 23rd Interscience Conference on Antimicrobial Agents and Chemotherapy, Las Vegas, Oct. 24-26, 1983. Abstract No. 971 (1983).

Wang, W.-L.L.; BarthReller, L. and Blaser, M.J.: Comparison of antimicrobial susceptibility patterns of *Campylobacter jejuni* and *Campylobacter coli*. Antimicrobial Agents and Chemotherapy 26: 351-353 (1984).

Watt, B.; Chait, I.; Kelsey, M.C.; Newsom, S.W.B.; Newsom, R.A. et al.: Norfloxacin *versus* cotrimoxazole in the treatment of uncomplicated urinary tract infections – a multi-centre trial. Journal of Antimicrobial Chemotherapy 13 (Suppl. B): 89-94 (1984).

Wise, R.: Norfloxacin – a review of pharmacology and tissue penetration. Journal of Antimicrobial Chemotherapy 13 (Suppl. B): 59-64 (1984).

Wise, R.; Andrews, J.M. and Danks, G.: *In vitro* activity of enoxacin (CI-919), a new quinoline derivative, compared with that of other antimicrobial agents. Journal of Antimicrobial Chemotherapy 13: 237-244 (1984a).

Wise, R.; Andrews, J.M. and Edwards, L.J.: *In vitro* activity of Bay 09867, a new quinoline derivative, compared with those of other antimicrobial agents. Antimicrobial Agents and Chemotherapy 23: 559-564 (1983).

Wise, R.; Lockley, R.; Webberly, M. and Adhami, Z.N.: Pharmacokinetics and tissue penetration of enoxacin and norfloxacin. Journal of Antimicrobial Chemotherapy 14 (Suppl. C): 75-81 (1984b).

Yamamoto, Y.; Ihara, T. and Shimura, H.: Laboratory and clinical investigations of AM-715 in surgical field. Chemotherapy (Tokyo) 29 (Suppl. 4): 663-668 (1981).

Yourassowsky, E.; Van der Linden, M.P.; Lismot, M.J. and Crokaert, F.: Antibacterial activity of MK 0366 against multiresistant *Staphylococcus aureus, Pseudomonas aeruginosa, Enterobacter cloacae, Serratia marcescens* and *Haemophilus influenzae*. Current Therapeutic Research 32: 36-39 (1982).

Authors' address: *Barbara Holmes*, ADIS Drug Information Services, Private Bag, Mairangi Bay, Auckland 10 (New Zealand).

Drug Evaluation

Drugs 30: 514-538 (1985)
0012-6667/85/0012-0514/$12.50/0

Suprofen
A Review of Its Pharmacodynamic and Pharmacokinetic Properties, and Analgesic Efficacy

P.A. Todd and *R.C. Heel*

ADIS Drug Information Services, Auckland

Various sections of the manuscript reviewed by: ***H. Berry,*** Department of Rheumatology and Rehabilitation, King's College Hospital, London, England; ***S.A. Cooper,*** Stephen A. Cooper Associates Inc., Short Hills, New Jersey, USA; ***N. Fellmann,*** Rheumaklinik mit Physikalisch-Balneologischen Institut, Rheuma-Volksheilstätte, Leukerbad, Switzerland; ***F.D. Hart,*** Harley Street, London, England; ***A. Hedges,*** Department of Clinical Pharmacology, St. Bartholomew's Hospital, London, England; ***W.J. Honig,*** Nijmegen, The Netherlands.

Contents

Summary 515
1. Pharmacodynamic Properties 517
 1.1 Analgesic Activity 517
 1.2 Anti-Inflammatory Activity 518
 1.3 Antipyretic Activity 519
 1.4 Gastrointestinal Effects 520
 1.5 Effect on Prostaglandins 520
 1.6 Effects on the Endometrium 521
 1.7 Cardiovascular Effects 521
  1.7.1 Haematological Effects 521
  1.7.2 Haemodynamic Effects 522
 1.8 Other Effects 522
2. Pharmacokinetic Properties 522
 2.1 Absorption 522
 2.2 Distribution 523
 2.3 Elimination 523
3. Therapeutic Trials 523
 3.1 Studies in Acute Pain 524
  3.1.1 Comparisons with Placebo 524
  3.1.2 Comparisons with Diflunisal 524
  3.1.3 Comparisons with Aspirin and Aspirin/Codeine Combinations 528
  3.1.4 Comparisons with Codeine, Dextropropoxyphene, Dipyrone, Oxycodone, Pentazocine and Combinations 528
  3.1.5 Comparisons with Paracetamol, and in Combination with Paracetamol 530
  3.1.6 Comparisons with Other Non-Steroidal Anti-Inflammatory Drugs 530

3.2 Studies in Chronic Pain 530
3.2.1 Open Study 531
3.2.2 Comparisons with Aspirin 531
3.2.3 Comparisons with Dextropropoxyphene 531
3.2.4 Comparisons with Diclofenac, Ibuprofen, Indomethacin and Naproxen 531
3.3 Studies in Dysmenorrhoea 532
3.4 Studies in Fever 533
4. Side Effects 533
5. Effect on Laboratory Values 534
6. Drug Interactions 534
7. Overdosage 535
8. Dosage and Administration 535
9. The Place of Suprofen in Therapy 535

Summary

Synopsis: *Suprofen (sutoprofen)*[1] *is a non-steroidal anti-inflammatory analgesic, closely related structurally to drugs such as ibuprofen, ketoprofen and naproxen. In patients with acute pain, single oral doses of suprofen are at least as effective as: usual therapeutic doses of aspirin; codeine alone or combined with aspirin; dextropropoxyphene alone or in various combinations; oxycodone combined with aspirin; dipyrone; pentazocine; paracetamol (acetaminophen); diflunisal; ibuprofen; indomethacin; or mefenamic acid. In chronic pain due to osteoarthritis, suprofen is as effective as usual dosages of aspirin or dextropropoxyphene during long term therapy, and as effective as diclofenac, ibuprofen, indomethacin and naproxen during short term treatment. As with other non-steroidal anti-inflammatory drugs, gastrointestinal complaints are the most frequently reported side effects, although discontinuation due to gastrointestinal effects may be necessary less frequently with suprofen than with aspirin, dextropropoxyphene or combinations of the two.*

Suprofen appears to be a useful alternative to mild analgesics, analgesic combinations or the older more established non-steroidal anti-inflammatory drugs in the treatment of patients with acute or chronic pain. However, further definition of its efficacy and tolerability is required, especially in comparison with newer non-steroidal anti-inflammatory analgesics.

Pharmacodynamic Properties: *In vitro* studies show that suprofen, in common with aspirin and other non-steroidal anti-inflammatory drugs, is a potent inhibitor of prostaglandin synthesis. In standard animal models of analgesic activity, oral suprofen is similar in potency to ketoprofen, ibuprofen, diflunisal and sulindac, more potent than aspirin, paracetamol (acetaminophen) and codeine, and less potent than parenteral morphine. In a rat adjuvant arthritis flexion test, the analgesic activity of suprofen lasted about 4 hours with a rapid onset (0.5 hours). Suprofen is devoid of activity in animal tests specifically designed to detect narcotic-type analgesic activity. Suprofen is more potent as an analgesic than as an anti-inflammatory agent, and is generally equipotent to ibuprofen, indomethacin, ketoprofen and naproxen in animal models of acute and chronic inflammation. It is also similar in potency to these agents in reducing pyrogen-induced fever in animals. Because suprofen is more potent as an analgesic than as an anti-inflammatory agent, it has been developed as an analgesic and few anti-inflammatory studies have been conducted in man.

In a guinea-pig model of dysmenorrhoea, suprofen was more potent than aspirin, ibuprofen, indomethacin and naproxen in inhibiting arachidonic acid-induced uterine contractions.

1 'Supranol' (Cilag); 'Suprocil' (Cilag); 'Suprol' (Cilag, Ortho, McNeil).

The ulcerogenic activity of suprofen in animals is less than that of aspirin, ketoprofen and indomethacin when ulcerogenic dosages are related to dosages that effectively provide analgesia. In man, suprofen 800mg daily produces less faecal blood loss than aspirin 2600mg daily, although comparisons with other non-steroidal anti-inflammatory drugs have not been performed. As with other non-steroidal anti-inflammatory drugs, suprofen is a potent reversible inhibitor of platelet aggregation. Unlike aspirin, this inhibition is short lived.

Pharmacokinetic Properties: Suprofen is almost completely absorbed after oral administration and shows linear pharmacokinetics from dose-proportional bioavailability data, which fit a 2-compartment model. Following the oral administration of suprofen 200mg, maximum plasma concentrations are usually reached in about 1 hour, but this may vary between 0.25 and 2 hours in individual subjects. The peak plasma concentration after this dose ranges from 14.3 to 25.3 mg/L in healthy subjects. No accumulation occurs after repeated doses of suprofen 400mg every 6 hours. In common with other non-steroidal anti-inflammatory drugs, suprofen is extensively (99.4%) bound to human plasma proteins. There is minimal transfer of drug from maternal plasma to breast milk (about 0.015 to 0.03% of the usual adult dose). The elimination half-life of suprofen is short (1 to 3 hours). In man, 90% of the drug is excreted in urine following single-dose administration, and the principal urinary metabolite is a glucuronide conjugate. The influence of renal or hepatic insufficiency on the elimination of suprofen has not been studied.

Therapeutic Trials: Suprofen has been evaluated in many single-dose and a few short term studies in patients with acute pain due to headache, oral surgery, a variety of other surgical procedures, musculoskeletal disorders and primary dysmenorrhoea. Most of these studies were of a similar design and made reasonable attempts to overcome the inherent difficulties in evaluating analgesic drugs. In single-dose studies in patients with acute pain, suprofen 100 to 400mg usually proved more effective than aspirin 650mg. Suprofen 200 and 400mg proved as effective or superior to aspirin 650mg + codeine 60mg, aspirin 325mg + oxycodone 4.88mg, paracetamol 650mg, codeine 60mg, dipyrone 500mg, pentazocine 30mg, dextropropoxyphene hydrochloride 65mg, dextropropoxyphene napsylate 100mg + paracetamol 650mg, and dextropropoxyphene hydrochloride 65mg + aspirin 389mg + caffeine 32.4mg. The analgesic efficacy of suprofen was enhanced by the addition of paracetamol or codeine. Thus, a single dose of suprofen 100mg + paracetamol 650mg was clearly superior to suprofen 400mg or paracetamol 650mg alone. Single doses of suprofen 200 and 400mg provided equivalent analgesia to diflunisal 750mg. Diflunisal tended to show a longer duration of action but onset of analgesia tended to be faster with suprofen. Compared with other non-steroidal anti-inflammatory analgesics, single doses of suprofen 100 and 200mg were more effective than mefenamic acid 250mg, while suprofen 300mg daily was equivalent to indomethacin 75mg daily in patients with low back pain, and suprofen 800 and 1600mg daily was equivalent to ibuprofen 1600mg daily in primary dysmenorrhoea.

In patients with chronic pain due to osteoarthritis, suprofen 800 to 900mg daily proved at least as effective and was equally well tolerated as aspirin 2600 to 4000mg daily, dextropropoxyphene hydrochloride 260mg daily, ibuprofen 1600mg daily, indomethacin 150mg daily and naproxen 750mg daily. Suprofen 600mg daily was a more effective analgesic, with a faster onset, than diclofenac 150mg daily, and it was better tolerated.

Suprofen has not been compared with other newer non-steroidal anti-inflammatory analgesics, such as piroxicam, in patients with either acute or chronic pain.

Studies in adult and paediatric patients with fever also indicate that suprofen is an effective antipyretic agent. It appears at least as effective as standard agents, e.g. paracetamol, mefenamic acid, metamizol and aspirin.

Side Effects: Suprofen has been well tolerated in most patients to date. However, further data are required to determine clearly its side effect profile in patients receiving long term therapy, particularly when compared with other frequently used analgesics. The most frequent side effects are mild gastrointestinal complaints, followed by mild central nervous system effects and rash. In a summary of long term comparative studies, suprofen had a lower overall patient withdrawal rate because of side effects (17.7%) compared with aspirin, dextropropoxyphene and aspirin + dextropropoxyphene (23.9%). The respective withdrawal rates because of gastrointestinal problems were 10.9% and 17.2%.

Dosage: The recommended dosage of suprofen is 200mg 3 or 4 times daily for the treatment of mild or moderate pain. Suprofen is contraindicated in patients with active gastrointestinal ulceration or allergy to salicylates or other non-steroidal anti-inflammatory drugs. Caution or careful monitoring is required during administration in patients with impaired renal function, fluid retention, heart failure, hypertension, past history of gastrointestinal disease or coagulation disorders, and in patients receiving concomitant anticoagulant therapy.

1. Pharmacodynamic Properties

Suprofen (sutoprofen) is a non-steroidal, non-narcotic analgesic with anti-inflammatory and antipyretic activity. It is a propionic acid (phenylalkanoic acid) derivative (fig. 1), and during research was selected from a series of thienyl substituted benzene acetic acid derivatives as having the best separation of analgesic activity from gastrointestinal toxicity. *In vitro* and animal studies show that suprofen, in common with aspirin-like anti-inflammatory analgesics, is a tissue-selective inhibitor of prostaglandin (PG) synthesis.

1.1 Analgesic Activity

Suprofen was consistently more potent than aspirin, phenylbutazone and tolmetin, and generally comparable with ketoprofen, in the various animal models of analgesic efficacy shown in table I. Suprofen was usually similar in potency to indomethacin in analgesic efficacy but was less potent than indomethacin in the arachidonic acid-induced writhing test (Capetola et al., 1980) and in inhibiting adjuvant-induced arthritis in rats (Awouters et al., 1975a; Wong and Gardocki, 1983). The considerable potency differences between studies in the acetic acid-induced writhing tests in mice (Fujimura et al., 1982; Singh et al., 1983) and the adjuvant-induced arthritis tests in rats (Awouters et al., 1975a; Wong and Gardocki, 1983) are probably explained by different strains of test animals and other differences in experimental protocols.

In a rat adjuvant arthritis flexion test (Capetola et al., 1980), the analgesic activity of suprofen was evident at 0.5 hours, reached a peak at 2 hours, and was still statistically significant at 4 hours. Using the same model and comparing drug potencies at peak effect (Capetola et al., 1980), suprofen was equipotent to zomepirac, diflunisal, sulindac and ibuprofen, but was more potent than paracetamol [acetaminophen] (50 times) and codeine (5 times), and less potent than proquazone (1.56 times) and parenteral morphine (20 times). In the Randall-Selitto paw pressure test in rats (Capetola et al., 1980), oral suprofen was equipotent (weight-for-weight) to parenteral morphine, and 7, 142 and 238 times more potent than oral indomethacin, phenylbutazone and aspirin, respectively. Pain threshold in both normal and inflamed paws was raised by morphine (Capetola et al., 1980) and dextropropoxyphene (propoxyphene) [McGuire et al., 1978], whereas the other drugs raised the pain threshold in the inflamed paw alone. These findings together with the lack of analgesic effect of suprofen in the 'hot plate' and 'tail flick' tests in mice, and when administered intracerebroventricularly in adjuvant-induced arthritis in rats, and the inability of naloxone to block suprofen's analgesic activity, indicate that it is a peripherally acting analgesic (Capetola et al., 1980, 1981, 1983a,b).

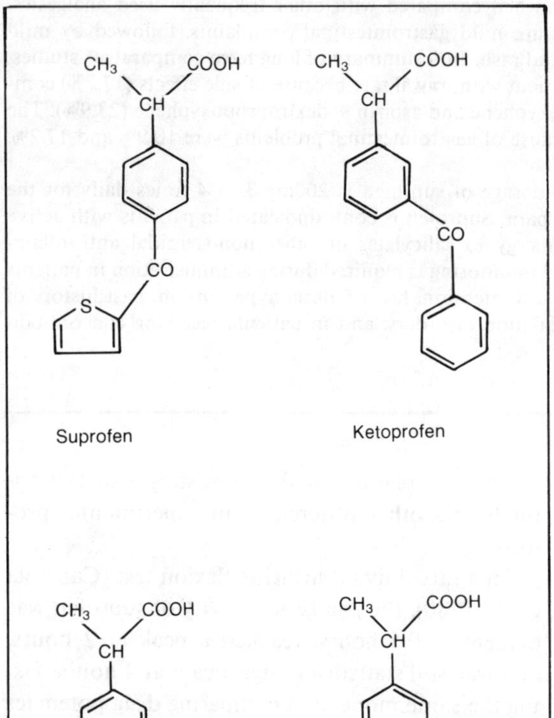

Fig. 1. Structural formulae of suprofen and other commonly used phenylalkanoic acid derivatives.

1.2 Anti-Inflammatory Activity

Suprofen appears more potent as an analgesic than as an anti-inflammatory agent in animal models (for review see Tolman et al., 1984) [table I], and the drug has therefore been developed primarily as an analgesic in man.

The analgesic and anti-inflammatory activities of suprofen can be separated in the rat adjuvant arthritic flexion test (Capetola et al., 1980): oral suprofen 10 mg/kg caused a statistically significant reduction in the number of vocalisations on flexion of the oedematous paw while there was no change in paw volume.

Comparison of oral ED_{50} values in an adjuvant-induced arthritis model of inflammation in rats showed that suprofen (24.8 mg/kg) was less potent than zomepirac (0.54 mg/kg), indomethacin (0.56 mg/kg), flufenamic acid (5.48 mg/kg), naproxen (14.5 mg/kg) and phenylbutazone (15.3 mg/kg), and more potent than fenoprofen (31.3 mg/kg), tolmetin (56.7 mg/kg), ibuprofen (136 mg/kg) and aspirin (452 mg/kg) [Wong and Gardocki, 1983; see also table I].

Oral suprofen was approximately equivalent to indomethacin and ketoprofen in reducing rat paw oedema induced by carrageenan, dextran, formalin and serotonin (5-hydroxytryptamine) [Fujimura et al., 1981] and by nystatin (Fujimura et al., 1982), but less potent than these drugs against mustard-induced paw oedema (Fujimura et al., 1982). However, suprofen tended to be more potent than indomethacin, ketoprofen or ibuprofen in reducing ultraviolet-induced erythema in guinea-pigs (Fujimura et al., 1981). Fujimura et al. (1981) also showed that the anti-inflammatory activity of suprofen is unaffected by adrenalectomy, indicating non-steroidal activity. Oral suprofen 5 to 40 mg/kg produced dose-dependent inhibition of granuloma tissue formation induced by the cotton pellet method in rats (Niemegeers et al., 1975d), and its potency was greater than that of ibuprofen, similar to ketoprofen, and less than that of indomethacin (Fujimura et al., 1982). Fujimura et al. (1982) concluded from their data that suprofen has a greater effect on the primary rather than the secondary stages of inflammation.

Suprofen 5% cream was as effective as triamcinolone acetonide 0.1% in the prevention of paw oedema induced by carrageenan. Suprofen 5% cream also inhibited the erythematous effect of arachidonic acid applied to the guinea-pig ear. This effect was enhanced by the addition of triamcinolone 0.1% (Capetola et al., 1981). In a placebo-controlled study in 8 human volunteers (Eaglstein

Table I. Analgesic, anti-inflammatory and antipyretic activity of suprofen compared with some other non-steroidal anti-inflammatory analgesics in animal models

Test (reference)	Oral ED_{50} (mg/kg)					
	suprofen	indomethacin	ketoprofen	tolmetin	aspirin	phenylbutazone
Analgesic activity						
Acetic acid-induced writhing in rats (1)	0.074	1.1	0.45	2.2	15.2	22.4
Acetic acid-induced writhing in mice (2)	53.7				100.0	67.6
Acetic acid-induced writhing in mice (3)	4.9	5.0	5.5			
Modified[a] Haffner's method in mice (3)	5.6	5.9	5.7			
Arachidonic acid-induced writhing in mice (4)	0.072	0.014			15.0	28.3
Phenylquinone-induced writhing in mice (2)	4.22				56.2	77.1
Sodium urate-induced arthritis in dogs (5)	0.64	2.47			>40.0	5.81
Anti-inflammatory activity						
Nystatin-induced oedema in rats (6)	2.7	6.2			38	34
Ultraviolet-induced erythema in guinea-pigs (7)	0.19	1.83	0.93	8.20		4.79
Ultraviolet-induced erythema in guinea-pigs (8)[b]	0.38	0.80	1.20		75.0	15.0
Adjuvant-induced arthritis in rats (9)	1.48	0.31		18.0	440	18.2
Adjuvant-induced arthritis in rats (10)	24.8	0.56	2.03	56.7	452	15.3
Antipyretic activity						
Yeast-induced pyresis in rats (11)	10.0	5.7		38	113	76
Yeast-induced pyresis in rats (12)	6.6	2.8			76.2	16.4

a In combination with morphine 2.0 mg/kg subcutaneously.
b Drugs administered intraperitoneally.
Reference key: 1 Niemegeers et al. (1975e); 2 Singh et al. (1983); 3 Fujimura et al. (1982); 4 Capetola et al. (1980); 5 Niemegeers and Janssen (1975); 6 Niemegeers et al. (1975a); 7 Awouters et al. (1975b); 8 Tsurumi and Fujimura (1983); 9 Awouters et al. (1975a); 10 Wong and Gardocki (1983); 11 Niemegeers et al. (1975b); 12 Vericat Cadesas et al. (1979).

et al., 1979), a combination of suprofen 5% and triamcinolone 0.1% cream applied after ultraviolet-B irradiation prevented subsequent erythema. This effect, lasting from 6 to 30 hours, was maximal when application of the cream was immediately after irradiation (5 minutes). The combination treatment was more effective than either agent alone, and suprofen was more effective than the steroid alone.

In a parallel, double-blind study in 207 patients with acute upper respiratory tract infection (Fujimori et al., 1983), suprofen 300 mg/day was more effective ($p < 0.05$) than aspirin 1500 mg/day in reducing the severity of sore throat, cough and pharyngeal redness after 3 days' treatment. Three patients receiving suprofen reported side effects compared with 7 on aspirin. Preliminary results from an ongoing parallel study (Stark et al., 1984) indicate that topical 0.5% suprofen tends to be more effective than placebo in preventing cystoid macular oedema following cataract surgery and lens implantation. All patients received standard treatment with neomycin and dexamethasone, and suprofen or placebo applied 4 times daily for 10 weeks started immediately before surgery. For the 16 patients so far completing treatment, 20% receiving suprofen developed cystoid macular oedema compared with 50% of those receiving placebo.

1.3 Antipyretic Activity

For the reference non-steroidal anti-inflammatory analgesics shown in table I, only indomethacin showed superior antipyretic activity to suprofen. At the fully effective antipyretic dose each of the reference agents produced transient hypothermia or in the case of indomethacin, protracted hypothermia, whereas suprofen did not produce hypothermia even at 4 times the fully effective antipyretic dose of 160 mg/kg (Niemegeers et al., 1975b). Suprofen was more effective than ibuprofen but less effective than ketoprofen and indomethacin (weight-for-weight) in reducing fever induced by lipopolysaccharide in rabbits or induced by yeast in rats (Fujimura et al., 1982).

1.4 Gastrointestinal Effects

Suprofen has been compared with a large number of other non-steroidal anti-inflammatory drugs for the prevention of endotoxin-induced diarrhoea in mice (Tsurumi and Fujimura, 1983) and castor oil-induced diarrhoea in rats (Awouters et al., 1978). Suprofen was more potent than indomethacin, ketoprofen, tolmetin, aspirin and phenylbutazone, and in both tests the ED_{50} values for the prevention of induced diarrhoea were closely related to the anti-inflammatory activity of the drugs. The authors therefore proposed that these tests could be used along with other standard tests for screening anti-inflammatory drugs.

The ulcerogenic activity of suprofen in rats has been investigated by several authors. Fujimura et al. (1981) showed that under normal physiological conditions the ulcerogenic dosage (UD_{50}) of suprofen (13 mg/kg) after repeated oral administration exceeded that of ketoprofen (2.2 mg/kg) and indomethacin (1.5 mg/kg). Niemegeers et al. (1975c) found the following UD_{50} values for single-dose oral administration under normal physiological conditions: aspirin (1190 mg/kg); suprofen (200 mg/kg); ketoprofen (46.0 mg/kg); and indomethacin (9.30 mg/kg). When these UD_{50} values are related to the analgesic ED_{50} values for these agents (Capetola et al., 1981) [see table I], then the therapeutic index (UD_{50}/ED_{50}) for suprofen (2703) exceeded that of indomethacin (78), ketoprofen (103) and aspirin (8.5). However, in cold stress-sensitised rats (Rainsford, 1977), suprofen was considered as having 'high' ulcerogenic activity, together with aspirin, ketoprofen and indomethacin, when compared with other non-steroidal anti-inflammatory agents. Rainsford (1978) also showed that suprofen inhibited ($p < 0.05$) gastrointestinal mucus glycoprotein production in rats as measured by ^{35}S incorporation *in vivo*. Other agents, e.g. diflunisal, naproxen and sulindac, caused no inhibition.

The ^{51}Cr-tagged erythrocyte method has been used to determine the effect of therapeutic doses of suprofen on faecal blood loss in man. In a 1-week double-blind crossover study (Arnold and Berger, 1983), aspirin 650mg 4 times daily caused more faecal blood loss than suprofen 200mg 4 times daily in 20 male volunteers (4.2 *vs* 1.8 ml/day, $p < 0.01$). In a 10-day double-blind parallel study in 30 male volunteers (Cohen and Smith, 1984), mean daily faecal blood loss on a combination of suprofen 200mg plus codeine 60mg 4 times daily was about half that with aspirin 325mg plus codeine 60mg 4 times daily (6.46 *vs* 3.58ml).

The gastrointestinal toxicity of suprofen has not been compared with that of the newer non-steroidal anti-inflammatory drugs, such as piroxicam, or the 'prodrugs' fenbufen and sulindac.

1.5 Effect on Prostaglandins

Suprofen is a potent inhibitor of prostaglandin biosynthesis, a mechanism by which many of its pharmacological effects are exerted (Capetola et al., 1981). It is a reversible inhibitor of cyclo-oxygenase, which catalyses the formation of cyclic endoperoxides (and eventually prostaglandins) from arachidonic acid (Ferreira et al., 1974; Vane, 1974).

Suprofen inhibits *in vitro* prostaglandin biosynthesis from bovine seminal vesicles (Capetola et al., 1980): ED_{50} values for suprofen, indomethacin, naproxen, ibuprofen and phenylbutazone were 1.82, 3.16, 14.42, 45.20 and 169.00 μmol/L, respectively. Basal PGE_2 production from rabbit renomedullary interstitial cells in tissue culture is also inhibited by suprofen (Zusman and Keiser, 1977): ED_{50} values for naproxen, ibuprofen, suprofen, indomethacin and aspirin were 0.04, 0.14, 1.5, 2.7 and 58 μmol/L, respectively. Suprofen inhibits the *in vitro* production of PGI_2 (prostacyclin) in rat aorta (Imai et al., 1982) and the *in vivo* production of prostaglandins in mouse small intestine (Borowska et al., 1981). Suprofen also inhibits arachidonic acid-induced malondialdehyde production from guinea-pig and cat platelets *in vitro* (Nevelsteen et al., 1984; Van Nueten et al., 1976), arachidonic acid hydroperoxide-induced contractions of guinea-pig ileum and rat fundic strips *in vitro* (Van Daele et al., 1975; Van Nueten et al., 1976), the peristaltic reflex of isolated guinea-pig ileum (Fontaine et al., 1977), arachidonic acid-induced bronchoconstriction in guinea-pigs *in vivo* (Rosenthale et al., 1981), arachidonic acid-induced writhing in mice *in vivo* (see section 1.1), and the lethal effect of arachidonic acid in rabbits (Fujimura et al., 1981; Imai et al., 1982).

When suprofen and indomethacin were compared in most of the aforementioned tests, they were in a similar potency range. However, suprofen 50 mg/L caused a 55% inhibition of arachidonic acid conversion into PGE_2 in rabbit heart or kidney *in vitro* while indomethacin 0.1 to 0.3 mg/L caused 100% inhibition (Capetola et al., 1980). These data, together with results showing that suprofen does not affect renal blood flow in dogs (section 1.7.2), suggest the tissue selective nature of prostaglandin inhibition by suprofen.

Topical suprofen 0.5% inhibited ($p < 0.05$) the release of PGE_2, $PGF_{2\alpha}$, PGI_2 and thromboxane B_2 from inflamed rabbit cornea, and appeared more effective than topical prednisolone 1% (Tong et al., 1984). Suprofen inhibited prostaglandin production by inflamed human gingival tissue *in vitro* only at concentrations greater than 10 mmol/L, which is much higher than for other tissues, indicating that suprofen is not selective for this tissue (Elattar and Lin, 1983).

Suprofen inhibited the mouse stretching response (Dubinsky and Schupsky, 1984) and guinea-pig uterine contractions (section 1.6) induced by arachidonic acid. This was taken as evidence of inhibition of prostaglandin biosynthesis via the cyclo-oxygenase pathway. However, at higher doses suprofen still blocks the stretching response and uterine contractions induced by endogenously applied PGE_2 and $PGF_{2\alpha}$, respectively. This suggests that suprofen may directly antagonise prostaglandin activity.

1.6 Effects on the Endometrium

There is evidence to suggest that prostaglandins play a role in the aetiology of primary dysmenorrhoea (Tolman et al., 1985). The role of kinins in dysmenorrhoea is unknown, but bradykinin induces uterine contractions and can potentiate the pain-producing action of prostaglandins (Capetola et al., 1981).

An *in vivo* guinea-pig model has been developed in which the effects of drugs on uterine contractions induced by prostaglandins, arachidonic acid and bradykinin can be studied (Carraher et al., 1981; Hahn et al., 1982). Oral pretreatment with prostaglandin synthetase inhibitors blocked the uterine response to arachidonic acid. The relative order of potency was suprofen (1) > indomethacin (0.65) > naproxen (0.52) > ibuprofen (0.43) > aspirin (0.31), and the maximal response to suprofen was greater ($p < 0.05$) than to each of the other agents. $PGF_{2\alpha}$ and bradykinin-induced contractions were also inhibited by suprofen. These data suggest that suprofen may be of use in the treatment of primary dysmenorrhoea.

1.7 Cardiovascular Effects

1.7.1 Haematological Effects

Like most other non-steroidal anti-inflammatory analgesics, suprofen is an inhibitor of induced platelet aggregation *in vitro* and *ex vivo* in diverse animal species (De Clerck et al., 1975a,b, 1976; Imai et al., 1982) and in man (De Clerck et al., 1975a). Suprofen dosing inhibits aggregation induced by arachidonic acid, collagen, thrombin and adrenaline (epinephrine). Only the secondary phase of ADP-induced aggregation is affected by suprofen. In general, suprofen is more potent than other non-steroidal anti-inflammatory analgesics (e.g. indomethacin, ketoprofen, ibuprofen). Oral single doses of suprofen as low as 0.31 mg/kg prolonged ($p < 0.05$) tail bleeding time in rats whereas whole blood clotting time was unaffected by doses up to 10 mg/

kg (De Clerck et al., 1975b). *In vivo* in man suprofen has been shown to have a mild inhibitory effect on haemostasis which is not of clinical significance. Return to normal occurs by 24 hours following administration (unpublished data on file, Ortho).

1.7.2 Haemodynamic Effects

Intravenous administration of suprofen 5 mg/kg had no effect on blood pressure, cardiac output or ECG in anaesthetised dogs (Capetola et al., 1981). Higher intravenous doses of suprofen 50 to 100 mg/kg (Fujimura et al., 1983) had no effect on heart rate or ECG in anaesthetised dogs and rabbits, although blood pressure and cardiac output were increased. Intravenous suprofen administration up to 10 mg/kg had no effect on renal blood flow in the anaesthetised dog whereas phenylbutazone 2 mg/kg caused a significant reduction ($p < 0.05$) [Capetola et al., 1980]. PGE_2 is capable of dilating renal vasculature, and some inhibitors of prostaglandin biosynthesis (e.g. phenylbutazone) can therefore reduce renal blood flow. Acute doses of suprofen 25 to 100 mg/kg caused a transient increase in renal blood flow in anaesthetised dogs but there was no effect on sodium, potassium or chloride excretion (Fujimura et al., 1983).

In man, the repeated intramuscular or intravenous administration of suprofen 200mg 3 times daily to healthy volunteers has no significant effect on heart rate or blood pressure (Michos et al., 1985a,b).

1.8 Other Effects

Suprofen inhibits secretion of lysosomal enzymes from guinea-pig neutrophils and phagocytosis by these cells *in vitro* (Smith, 1978). Ketoprofen was more active than suprofen, and sulindac was inactive. Lysosomal enzymes can mediate tissue injury, and their inhibition by suprofen may represent one mechanism, besides prostaglandin inhibition, by which the drug alleviates inflammation. Yokoya et al. (1984b) has shown that suprofen inhibits Type I (homologous passive cutaneous anaphylaxis in rats; histamine release from rat peritoneal mast cells; histamine and slow reacting substance of anaphylaxis release from guinea-pig lung tissue), Type II (Forssman cutaneous vasculitis in guinea-pigs) and Type III (Arthus reaction in guinea-pigs) allergic reactions. However, suprofen did not inhibit Type IV allergic reaction (delayed cutaneous hypersensitivity in guinea-pigs) or IgM or IgG antibody production in mice and rats.

2. Pharmacokinetic Properties

The pharmacokinetics of suprofen have been studied in animals and healthy subjects following single and repeated doses. The influence of disease on pharmacokinetics has not been studied in patients. High-performance liquid chromatography (HPLC) has been used to determine plasma suprofen concentrations (Alton and Patrick, 1978; Lagu et al., 1982; Müller et al., 1982).

2.1 Absorption

Following the parenteral and systemic administration of single and repeated therapeutic doses, the pharmacokinetics of suprofen are linear, with maximal plasma concentration and area under the plasma concentration time curve (AUC) being related to dosage (Abrams et al., 1983b; Zulliger and Fassolt, 1983, 1985). In healthy subjects the maximum plasma concentration is usually reached about 1 hour after oral administration but can vary between 0.25 and 2 hours in different subjects (Abrams et al., 1983a; Chaikin et al., 1983; Mori et al., 1985; Weintraub, 1978; Zulliger and Fassolt, 1983). Compared with oral administration, the maximum plasma concentration is reached more rapidly after intramuscular administration: about 20 to 30 minutes after 50 to 200mg (Michos et al., 1985b; Zulliger and Fassolt, 1983). However, total absorption is not significantly different after either route (corrected AUC 454.86 intramuscular *vs* 436.07 mg/L • h oral for 50mg).

The absolute bioavailability of suprofen 200mg taken as a capsule in healthy subjects is 92.2% compared with intravenous administration, indicating no significant first-pass effect (Zulliger and Fassolt, 1985). The maximum plasma concentration following oral and intramuscular administration of single and repeated doses of suprofen 200mg varies between mean values of 14.3 and 25.33 mg/L (Abrams et al., 1983a,b; Michos and Zulliger, 1985; Weintraub, 1978; Zulliger and Fassolt, 1983, 1985). On the basis of maximum and minimum plasma concentrations and AUC values, no accumulation occurs in healthy subjects after 6 to 7 days' treatment with oral suprofen 400mg every 6 hours (Abrams et al., 1983b), intramuscular suprofen 200mg 3 times daily (Michos et al., 1985b), or intravenous suprofen 200mg twice daily as a bolus or infusion (Zulliger et al., 1985).

Following administration of a single dose of suprofen 200mg as an oral solution or as 1 or 2 capsules (Weintraub, 1978), AUC values are similar – indicating equivalent physiological availability. Food and, to a lesser extent, milk cause a decrease in the maximum plasma concentration of suprofen and a slight decrease in AUC (Chaikin et al., 1982). This is consistent with data reported for other non-steroidal anti-inflammatory drugs. When suprofen 200 and 400mg is administered to elderly subjects, there is no trend to change the maximum plasma concentration or to prolong the elimination half-life. These results suggest that age does not alter the disposition of suprofen to any marked extent (unpublished data on file, Ortho).

2.2 Distribution

At times up to 24 hours after the oral or intravenous administration of ^{3}H-suprofen in mice and rats, the only organs to show concentrations similar to or greater than corresponding plasma samples are those involved with absorption, metabolism and excretion (gastrointestinal tract, liver and kidney) [Mori et al., 1984a,b; Yokoya et al., 1984a]. Mori et al. (1983a) showed that, following oral administration of ^{3}H-suprofen in rats, the drug crossed the placenta to a moderate extent. Also, in rats with carrageenan-induced oedema, the level of radioactivity in the inflamed paw reached about twice that of the non-inflamed paw.

Few data are available on the distribution of suprofen and its metabolites in man. The apparent volume of distribution after oral administration in healthy subjects is 11.9L (Zulliger and Fassolt, 1983). ^{3}H-Suprofen is extensively bound *in vitro* to human plasma protein (99.4%), principally to albumin (94.5%), independently of the drug concentration over the range 2.6 to 130 mg/L (Chaikin et al., 1980, 1983). There is minimal binding to human milk protein (10.4%). Based on simple passive diffusion, little transfer of suprofen from plasma to milk would be expected *in vivo*. This was confirmed in 6 nursing women administered a single oral dose of suprofen 200mg in whom the milk/plasma AUC ratio was 1.4% (Chaikin et al., 1983). Minimal suprofen ingestion (approximately 0.015 to 0.03% of the usual daily adult dose) would therefore be expected in a nursing infant whose mother is receiving suprofen.

2.3 Elimination

Few data are published on the metabolism and excretion of suprofen in man. In healthy subjects the elimination half-life is about 1 to 3 hours after single intravenous doses of 50 to 200mg, and plasma clearance is 5.72 to 7.62 L/h depending on dose and administration route (Zulliger and Fassolt, 1983, 1985). After a single dose of tritiated suprofen 200mg in man, about 90% of radioactivity is recovered in urine and 7% in faeces (Capetola et al., 1981). The major urinary metabolite is an acyl glucuronide of suprofen; other minor metabolites are formed by hydroxylation (Mori et al., 1985). Suprofen undergoes enterohepatic circulation and excretion into bile in rats (Mori et al., 1983b; Yokoya et al., 1984a), but it is not known if this occurs in man. The effects of renal or hepatic insufficiency on the metabolism and excretion of suprofen are not reported in the literature.

3. *Therapeutic Trials*

Methods employed in the clinical evaluation of analgesics, and problems encountered in these studies because of the complex nature and subjective variables of pain and pain relief, have been reviewed by Dundee (1980) and Littlejohns and Vere (1981).

The choice of a pain model requires careful consideration in any clinical evaluation of analgesics. The most sensitive assays of analgesic efficacy are single-dose studies in patients with acute pain, but multiple-dose studies in patients with acute or chronic pain provide information on the general clinical acceptability and safety of the analgesic. Some painful conditions (e.g. oral surgical pain, and episiotomy or meniscectomy pain) are particularly suitable models for analgesic efficacy studies, as the source of pain is understood, the duration of pain is fairly predictable, and a relatively homogeneous population of otherwise healthy subjects may be selected. Instances in which acute pain is likely to be more variable, but which represent important uses of analgesics, include headache, postsurgical pain, musculoskeletal pain and pain during dysmenorrhoea.

As there are substantial differences between acute and chronic pain, extrapolation of the results obtained from analgesic efficacy studies in patients with acute pain, in order to gain some indication of analgesic effectiveness in patients with chronic pain, is often unreliable. Psychological factors may considerably modify pain perception in patients experiencing chronic pain, and reaction to the pain may dominate the actual pain stimulus in some of these patients.

Suprofen is primarily indicated as an analgesic and has been studied in patients with acute pain (section 3.1), chronic pain (section 3.2) and dysmenorrhoea (section 3.3). Suprofen shows anti-inflammatory activity in animals but, because it is more potent as an analgesic, it has been developed as such and has been little studied in patients with inflammatory conditions (section 1.2). Suprofen is an effective antipyretic agent in man (see section 3.4).

3.1 Studies in Acute Pain

Suprofen has been compared with placebo (section 3.1.1) and a number of analgesics, analgesic combinations and non-steroidal anti-inflammatory drugs (tables II and III) in parallel double-blind studies in patients with acute pain. Most studies included a placebo control and used standard evaluation scales from which SPID (summed pain intensity difference) and TOTPAR (total pain relief) scores could be calculated. Single-dose studies were usually conducted within a clinic or hospital environment and used trained observers to try and minimise the effects of variability on assessments of pain perception. Multiple-dose studies were either of short duration or were only reported as abstracts. More published data are therefore required to determine the suitability of suprofen for longer term treatment.

3.1.1 Comparisons with Placebo

A single dose of suprofen 200mg has been compared with placebo in a double-blind parallel study in 77 patients with pain following tooth extraction (Ishibashi et al., 1982). Suprofen was superior ($p < 0.01$) to placebo for analgesic efficacy and overall clinical evaluation score. No side effects were reported with suprofen.

The majority of comparative studies reported in the remainder of this section on acute pain (section 3.1) were placebo controlled. Single doses of suprofen 100, 200 and 400mg were therefore compared with placebo in these studies. In general, all doses were superior to placebo, both statistically and clinically. A dose-related response was usually apparent, but not always (see Honig, 1983 and Mok et al., 1978) [table II and subsequent sections].

3.1.2 Comparisons with Diflunisal

Single doses of diflunisal 750mg and suprofen 200 or 400mg were approximately equipotent in relieving pain following meniscectomy (Honig, 1983). There was a tendency for suprofen 200mg to show better SPID and TOTPAR scores, as well as a faster onset of action, compared with the other treatments. Diflunisal tended to have a longer duration of action than suprofen. The incidence of side effects with either drug was not different to that seen with placebo.

Table II. Summary of randomised double-blind parallel studies comparing suprofen (S) with other analgesics in patients with acute pain

Reference	Population	Dosage (mg) and no. of patients[a]	Study design and dosage schedule[b]	Results				Comments
				SPID[c]	TOTPAR[c]	overall effects[d]	side effects	
Comparisons with diflunisal (DIF)								
Honig (1983)	Meniscectomy pain	S200 (32) S400 (32) DIF750 (32)	Single oral dose with 8h observation	S200 ⩾ DIF = S400	S ⩾ DIF	S = DIF	S = DIF	DIF ⩾ S for duration of analgesia
Comparisons with aspirin (ASA)								
Cooper et al. (1983)	Oral surgical pain	S200 (44) S400 (45) ASA650 (43)	Single oral dose with 6h observation	S > ASA	S > ASA	S > ASA	S = ASA	S > ASA for time to remedication
Markus and Gough (1980)	Oral surgical pain	S200 (46) ASA700 (47)	Every 6h orally as required for 6 days		S = ASA[e]		S ⩽ ASA	
Mok et al. (1978)	Undefined moderate pain	S100 (23) S200 (27) ASA650 (23)	Single oral dose with 6h observation	S ⩾ ASA	S ⩾ ASA		S = ASA (drowsiness)	
Silberman (1983)	Musculoskeletal pain	S200 (24) ASA650 (25)	Four times daily orally for 3 days	S > ASA	S > ASA	S ⩾ ASA	S ⩽ ASA	S > ASA for sleep and activity impairment
Comparisons with aspirin and aspirin/codeine (ASA + C) combinations								
Mehlisch (1985) [see also Frakes et al. (1984)]	Oral surgical pain	S200 (35) S400 (34) ASA650 (37) ASA650 + C60 (33)	Single oral dose with 6h observation	S400 > ASA and ASA + C	S400 > ASA and ASA + C; S200 > ASA	S400 > ASA and ASA + C	S = ASA and ASA + C	S400 > ASA and ASA + C for time to remedication
Sunshine et al. (1983)	Oral surgical pain	S200 (33) S400 (27) ASA650 (30) ASA650 + C60 (32)	Single oral dose with 4h observation	S = ASA and ASA + C	S = ASA and ASA + C	S = ASA and ASA + C	S = ASA + C ⩽ ASA	S ⩾ ASA and ASA + C for onset of analgesia
Vargha von Szeged and Michos (1983)	Neurological pain	S200 (40) S400 (39) ASA650 (37) ASA650 + C60 (40)	Single oral dose with 6h observation	S400 > S200 = ASA + C ⩾ ASA	S400 > S200 = ASA + C ⩾ ASA	S400 ⩾ S200 = ASA + C ⩾ ASA	S = ASA ⩽ ASA + C	

Continued on next page

Table II. Contd.

Reference	Population	Dosage (mg) and no. of patients[a]	Study design and dosage schedule[b]	Results				Comments
				SPID[c]	TOTPAR[c]	overall effects[d]	side effects	
Comparison with aspirin and aspirin/oxycodone (ASA + O) combinations								
Mehlisch et al. (1984)	Postsurgical pain (orthopaedic and general)	S200 S400 ASA650 ASA325 + O4.88[g] (206)[f]	Single oral dose with 6h observation	S ⩾ ASA and ASA + O	S ⩾ ASA and ASA + O	S ⩾ ASA and ASA + O	S = ASA and ASA + O	S ⩾ ASA and ASA + O for time to remedication. Abstract
Comparison with codeine (C), and in combination with codeine (S + C)								
Olson et al. (1984)	Postpartum pain	S100 S200 C30 S100 + C30 S200 + C30 S200 + C60 (392)[f]	Single oral dose with 4h observation	S+C ⩾ S and C	S+C ⩾ S and C			Abstract
Comparison with codeine (C) and dextropropoxyphene (D)								
Wagenberg et al. (1983)	Oral surgical pain	S200 C60 D65[h] (212)[f]	Single oral dose with 6h observation	S ⩾ C and D	S ⩾ C and D		S ⩽ C and D	Abstract
Comparison with DAC,[i] dextropropoxyphene/paracetamol (D + P) and aspirin/codeine (ASA + C) combinations								
Mehlisch and Eglsaer (1983)	Postsurgical pain (orthopaedic and general)	S200 DAC[j] D100[i] + P650 ASA650 + C60 (153)[f]	Single oral dose with 6h observation	S > all other treatments	S > all other treatments	S ⩾ all other treatments	S ⩽ all other treatments	Abstract
Comparison with dipyrone (DIP)								
Lorenzi et al. (1985)	Postsurgical pain (orthopaedic)	S200 (29) DIP500 (28)	Single oral dose with 6h observation	S ⩾ DIP	S ⩾ DIP		S = DIP	

Comparison with pentazocine (PEN)								
Bodner and Michos (1985) [see also Bodner 1985]	Postsurgical pain (general surgery)	S200 (29) PEN30 (29)	Single intramuscular dose with 6h observation[k]	S ≥ PEN	S ≥ PEN	S ≥ PEN	S = PEN	
Comparison with paracetamol (P), and in combination with paracetamol (S + P)								
Fassolt and Stocker (1983)	Postsurgical pain (general surgery)	S200 (32) S400 (28) P650 (29) S100 + P650 (29)	Single oral dose with 6h observation	S+P > S200; S+P ≥ S400 = P ≥ S200	S+P ≥ S400 ≥ P ≥ S200	S+P ≥ all other treatments	S = all other treatments	All treatments ≥ S200 for time to remedication

a Number of patients evaluated for efficacy in each group.
b All studies included a placebo control group, except Markus and Gough (1980).
c Summed pain intensity difference (SPID) and total pain relief scores (TOTPAR).
d Overall (global) effects as assessed by patient and investigators.
e Mean pain relief 1h after each dose.
f Total number of patients, including placebo.
g Oxycodone hydrochloride 4.5mg plus oxycodone terephthalate 0.38mg.
h Dextropropoxyphene hydrochloride.
i Dextropropoxyphene napsylate.
j DAC = dextropropoxyphene hydrochloride 65mg + aspirin 389mg + caffeine 32.4mg.
k Single-blind.

Symbols in all 'results' columns: > = statistically significant difference in favour of first drug; ≥ = tendency for first drug to be superior or statistical analysis not performed; ≤ = tendency for first drug to produce fewer and/or less severe side effects.

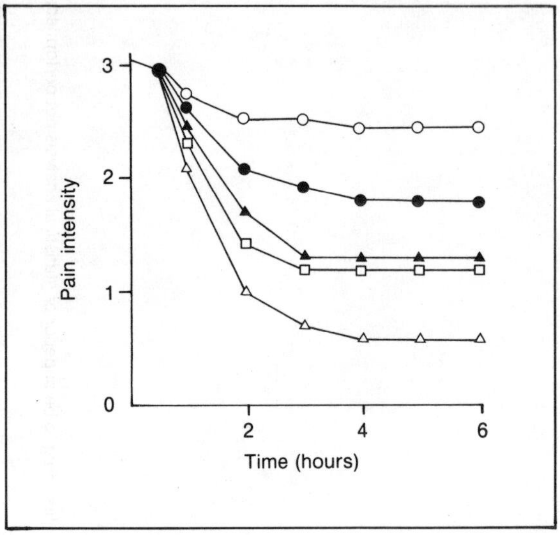

Fig. 2. Mean pain intensity scores (0 = no pain, 3 = severe pain) in 196 patients with neurological pain following a single dose of suprofen 200mg (□) and 400mg (△), aspirin 650mg (●), aspirin 650mg plus codeine 60mg (▲), and placebo (○) [after Vargha von Szeged and Michos, 1983].

3.1.3 Comparisons with Aspirin and Aspirin/Codeine Combinations

The analgesic efficacy of suprofen was generally superior to that of aspirin, in both single- and multiple-dose studies. Similarly, single doses of suprofen 400mg were usually superior to a combination of aspirin 650mg plus codeine 60mg, while suprofen 200mg showed similar analgesic efficacy to the aspirin combination (table II).

Suprofen 200mg and aspirin 700mg provided a similar degree of pain relief in patients with oral surgical pain (Markus and Gough, 1980). However, the patient groups in this study were not shown to be comparable for the degree of surgical trauma; and self-assessment of pain, while meant to be made 1 hour after each dose, was earlier on suprofen than on aspirin ($p < 0.001$). In another study in patients with pain following oral surgery, Sunshine et al. (1983) demonstrated a similar degree of analgesic efficacy following single-dose administration of suprofen 200 and 400mg, aspirin 650mg and a combination of aspirin 650mg plus codeine 60mg. Based on pain relief scores, Cooper et al. (1983) showed the duration of action of suprofen 400mg to be longer than that on 200mg in a single-dose study in patients with pain following periodontal surgery.

In patients with neurological pain (Vargha von Szeged and Michos, 1983), a single dose of suprofen 400mg was superior to 200mg, which in turn was approximately equivalent to aspirin 650mg combined with codeine 60mg and superior to aspirin 650mg (fig. 2).

A dose-related analgesic response to suprofen was not always apparent. Thus, Mok et al. (1978) noted a similar degree of analgesic efficacy with single doses of suprofen 100 and 200mg, and Sunshine et al. (1983) with suprofen 200 and 400mg.

Generally, suprofen did not cause more side effects than placebo, but central nervous system (CNS) and gastrointestinal symptoms were more frequent or more severe on aspirin and aspirin/codeine combinations.

3.1.4 Comparisons with Codeine, Dextropropoxyphene, Dipyrone, Oxycodone, Pentazocine and Combinations

Most of the studies reported in this section were reported as abstracts only, and lacked details of experimental protocol and results. Wagenberg et al. (1983) reported that a single dose of suprofen 200mg was 'substantially more effective' and produced fewer centrally mediated side effects than either dextropropoxyphene hydrochloride 65mg or codeine 60mg in patients with pain following periodontal surgery. A single dose of suprofen also gave statistically superior analgesia compared with 2 dextropropoxyphene combinations in patients with pain after general and orthopaedic surgery, and side effects were less severe and of shorter duration with suprofen (Mehlisch and Eglsaer, 1983). Mehlisch et al. (1984) noted that single doses of suprofen 200 and 400mg were 'consistently more effective' than a combination of aspirin 325mg and oxycodone (see table II) in patients with postsurgical pain. Olson et al. (1984) noted that the addition of codeine 30 or 60mg to single doses of suprofen 100 and 200mg appeared to increase the analgesic effect of suprofen in patients with postpartum pain. Bodner and

Table III. Summary of randomised double-blind parallel studies comparing suprofen (S) with other non-steroidal anti-inflammatory drugs in patients with acute pain

Reference	Population	Dosage (mg) and no. of patients[a]	Study design and dosage schedule[b]	Results: analgesic effect	Results: overall effect[c]	Results: side effects	Comments
Comparison with ibuprofen (IBU)							
Heffron et al. (1984)	Primary dysmenorrhoea	S200, S400, IBU400 (457)[d]	Four times daily as needed for up to 5 days	S400 ≥ S200 = IBU	S400 ≥ S200 = IBU	S = IBU	Abstract
Comparison with indomethacin (IM)							
Schichikawa et al. (1983)	Low back pain	S100 (81) IM25 (86)	Three times daily[e]		S = IM	S ≤ IM	
Comparison with indoprofen (IP)							
Honig and Michos (1984)	Meniscectomy pain	S200 intravenous (44) IP200 intravenous (43)	Single dose with 6h observation	S < IP	S = IP	S = IP	Abstract
Comparison with mefenamic acid (M)							
Pujalte et al. (1984)	Musculoskeletal pain	S100 (40) S200 (40) M250 (40)	Single dose with 4h observation	S > M	S > M	S = M	S ≥ M for time to remedication
Comparison with oxyphenbutazone (OX)							
Surace et al. (1982)	Pain (mainly back and post-traumatic)	S200 (30) OX100 (29)	Three times daily for up to 7 days	S = OX	S ≥ OX	S = OX	

a Number of patients evaluated for efficacy in each group.
b Studies by Heffron et al. (1984) and Honig and Michos (1984) included placebo control group.
c Overall (global) effect as assessed by patients and physicians.
d Total number of patients in all groups, including placebo group for Heffron et al. (1984).
e Duration not stated.

Symbols in all 'results' columns: > = statistically significant difference in favour of first drug; ≥ = tendency for first drug to be superior or statistical analysis not performed; < statistically significandifference in favour of second drug; ≤ = tendency for first drug to produce fewer and/or less severe side effects.

Michos (1985) showed that a single intramuscular dose of suprofen 200mg is an effective analgesic (determined from SPID and TOTPAR scores) compared with placebo in patients with moderate to severe pain following general surgery. A parallel group of patients receiving intramuscular pentazocine 30mg, a dose which might be considered therapeutically low, did not show results which were significantly different from placebo. Lorenzi et al. (1985) showed that a single oral dose of suprofen 200mg was marginally more effective than dipyrone 500mg in patients with acute pain following orthopaedic surgery.

3.1.5 Comparisons with Paracetamol, and in Combination with Paracetamol

In a single-dose study in patients with post-surgical pain, the analgesic efficacy of suprofen 400mg was similar to paracetamol (acetaminophen) 650mg, which tended to be better than suprofen 200mg (fig. 3). However, the most effective treatment was a combination of suprofen 100mg and paracetamol 650mg; the difference between this combination and suprofen was statistically significant. Results from animal experiments also show an additive analgesic effect when suprofen and paracetamol are combined (section 6), which may imply that this is a particularly suitable analgesic combination.

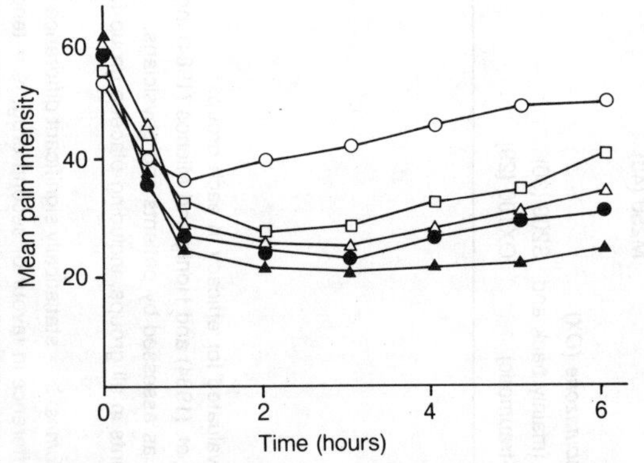

Fig. 3. Mean pain intensity scores on visual analogue scale (0 = no pain, 100 = unbearable pain) in patients with postsurgical pain following a single dose of suprofen 200mg (□) and 400mg (△), paracetamol 650mg (●), suprofen 100mg plus paracetamol 650mg (▲), and placebo (○) [after Fassolt and Stocker, 1983].

3.1.6 Comparisons with Other Non-Steroidal Anti-Inflammatory Drugs

The analgesic response to single doses of suprofen 100 and 200mg was approximately equivalent in patients with undefined musculoskeletal pain, and both doses were superior ($p < 0.05$) to a single dose of mefenamic acid 250mg as evaluated by SPID and TOTPAR scores. Schichikawa et al. (1983) found a similar global response to treatment with suprofen 100mg and indomethacin 25mg, each given 3 times daily, in 167 patients with low back pain. Side effects were reported by fewer patients with suprofen (7.6%) than with indomethacin (18.2%). In another repeated-dose study (Surace et al., 1982) in 59 patients with pain of diverse aetiology (low back pain, sciatica, and post-traumatic and postoperative pain), the reduction in pain compared with baseline after 7 days' treatment with suprofen 200mg and oxyphenbutazone 100mg, each given 3 times daily, was similar. Global assessments by the patients and physicians favoured suprofen. The number of side effects reported was similar on both treatments. This study was not placebo controlled.

Comparison of single intravenous doses of suprofen 200mg and indoprofen 400mg in 87 patients with postmeniscectomy pain showed no overall intergroup differences determined from the investigators' global evaluation of effectiveness, although SPID and TOTPAR scores significantly favoured indoprofen (Honig and Michos, 1984; unpublished data on file, Ortho).

3.2 Studies in Chronic Pain

There has been one open multiple-dose study of suprofen in patients with chronic pain, which was performed in a relatively small number of elderly patients studied for a short period (section 3.2.1).

In parallel double-blind multiple-dose studies, the analgesic efficacy of suprofen was similar to that with standard dosages of aspirin, dextropropoxyphene, ibuprofen, indomethacin and naproxen, but superior to that of diclofenac (table IV). These studies were either of short duration of performed in few patients or only reported as abstracts. More published data are therefore required to determine the role of suprofen in the treatment of chronic pain, especially with respect to long term efficacy and tolerability.

3.2.1 Open Study

The effects of suprofen 200mg every 4 hours as required (mean dosage 1050 mg/day) were examined in an open 4-week study in 19 patients of mean age 75.9 years with chronic pain, generally from osteoarthritis or rheumatoid arthritis (Denis and De Beer, 1983). All patients were receiving concomitant treatment for other disorders (e.g. diabetes, hypertension, bronchitis). No patients were withdrawn because of side effects, and all but 1 patient reported good tolerability. After 4 weeks 94% of patients had a moderate to very good reduction in pain severity, and 72% assessed their treatment with suprofen as better than their previous treatment.

3.2.2 Comparisons with Aspirin

Suprofen 200mg 4 times daily has been compared with aspirin 650 to 1000mg 4 times daily in several published (Bowers et al., 1984; Willkens, 1983; table IV) and unpublished (data on file, Ortho) double-blind parallel studies of 12 to 24 weeks' duration in patients suffering from chronic pain due to musculoskeletal disorders, osteoarthritis and rheumatoid arthritis. Relief of pain and inflammation, improvement in activity impairment, and global assessment scores were comparable with both drugs, as were the type and incidence of side effects. The clinical relevance of the study by Willkens (1983) was limited by the small number of patients completing the trial (8 in each group) and by the permitted use of supplementary analgesics (dextropropoxyphene or codeine), the consumption of which was not reported. These authors reported an increase ($p < 0.05$) in mean diastolic blood pressure for the group on suprofen (see section 4).

3.2.3 Comparisons with Dextropropoxyphene

Suprofen 200mg and dextropropoxyphene 65mg each given 4 times daily for 24 weeks produced similar analgesic responses and global assessment scores in a double-blind parallel study in 114 patients with chronic pain from osteoarthritis (Salzman and Brobyn, 1983) [table IV]. More patients were withdrawn because of side effects, primarily gastrointestinal complaints, on dextropropoxyphene (34%) than on suprofen (24%).

3.2.4 Comparisons with Diclofenac, Ibuprofen, Indomethacin and Naproxen

Suprofen has been compared with diclofenac, ibuprofen, indomethacin and naproxen in short term (1 to 2 weeks) double-blind parallel studies in patients with osteoarthritic pain (table IV).

Suprofen 200mg and diclofenac 50mg each given 3 times daily for 7 days were compared in 60 hospitalised women with acute exacerbation of osteoarthritic pain (Porzio, 1985). Suprofen proved clinically more effective and better tolerated than diclofenac. Not only was the degree of analgesia significantly greater with suprofen but it also had a faster onset of action. Global evaluation of efficacy by both patient and physician indicated a significantly better response with suprofen: 'very good or good' responses were recorded in all 30 suprofen patients compared with only 3 receiving diclofenac. Gastrointestinal side effects were reported by 15 patients receiving diclofenac compared with 4 of those receiving suprofen.

Suprofen 400mg and ibuprofen 400mg each given 4 times daily produced similar improvement of pain at rest, pain on motion, joint tenderness and joint mobility, and similar overall evaluations of efficacy and tolerability as assessed by both patients and investigators. There was a tendency for a more rapid analgesic effect with suprofen, and the improvement in pain on motion after 1 week compared with baseline was better ($p \leq 0.05$) with suprofen than with ibuprofen (Schuermans, 1983).

Table IV. Summary of randomised parallel double-blind studies comparing suprofen (S) with other analgesics in patients with osteoarthritis

References	Dosage (mg) and no. of patients[a]	Duration (weeks)	Results		
			analgesic effect	overall effect[b]	side effects[c]
Comparisons with aspirin (ASA)					
Bowers et al. (1984)	S200 qid ASA800 qid } (180)	24	S = ASA	S = ASA	S = ASA
Willkens (1983)	S200 qid (8) ASA650 qid (8)	12	S = ASA	S = ASA	S = ASA
Comparison with dextropropoxyphene (D)					
Salzman and Brobyn (1983)	S200 qid (48) D65 qid (51)	24	S = D	S = D	S ⩽ D
Comparison with diclofenac (DIC)					
Porzio (1985)	S200 bid (30) DIC50 tid (30)	1	S ⩾ DIC	S ⩾ DIC	S ⩽ DIC
Comparison with ibuprofen (IBU)					
Schuermans (1983)	S200 qid (21) IBU400 qid (21)	2	S = IBU	S = IBU	S = IBU
Comparison with indomethacin (IND)					
Hauzeur (1984, 1985)	S300 tid suppositories IND50 tid suppositories } (60)	1	S = IND	S = IND	S = IND
Comparison with naproxen (N)					
Fellmann et al. (1983)	S400 bid (39) N375 bid (40)	2	S = N	S ⩾ N	S = N

a Number of patients evaluated for efficacy in each group.
b ⩾ = tendency for first drug to be superior.
c ⩽ = tendency for first drug to produce fewer side effects.
Abbreviations: bid = twice daily; tid = 3 times daily; qid = 4 times daily.

In hospitalised patients with osteoarthritis, suprofen 300mg and indomethacin 50mg each administered as suppositories 3 times daily proved equipotent for the relief of pain and similar for tolerability. Local tolerability was considered good in 80% and 72% of patients on suprofen and indomethacin, respectively, when assessed by both the investigator and the patients (Hauzeur, 1984, 1985).

Suprofen 400mg twice daily relieved osteoarthritic pain as effectively as naproxen 375mg twice daily. Fair to very good global responses as assessed by the investigators were seen in 72% of patients receiving suprofen and in 60% of those on naproxen (Fellmann et al., 1983).

3.3 Studies in Dysmenorrhoea

Suprofen has been studied in over 900 women who suffer from primary dysmenorrhoea. For the most part, studies were double-blind, parallel or crossover, comparisons of suprofen with placebo, dextropropoxyphene plus paracetamol, or ibuprofen (Cooke et al., 1984, 1985; Heffron et al., 1984; unpublished data on file, Ortho). One open-label study (Deere et al., 1984) was conducted in which suprofen up to 800 mg/day was taken for 2 consecutive cycles. Over 80% of the women in this study experienced complete or moderate relief of menstrual symptoms during both cycles. Both the women and their physicians indicated a good or excellent response to suprofen in over 80% of the cycles treated. In the double-blind comparative studies, suprofen 200 to 400mg was shown to be statistically superior and clinically more acceptable than either the dextropropoxyphene combination or placebo. Suprofen 400mg was consistently better, though not statistically, than both suprofen 200mg and ibuprofen 400mg (Heffron et al., 1984).

3.4 Studies in Fever

In a dose-finding study (Weippl, 1985), paediatric patients with fever from respiratory tract infection were given a single dose of suprofen 1 to 10 mg/kg as a syrup. The optimal dose proved to be 5 mg/kg. This caused a peak reduction of rectal temperature of about 1.5°C after 3 hours, and the patients were maintained subfebrile for at least 4.5 hours. Higher doses did not produce any additional effect, and hypothermia was not seen.

The antipyretic effect of suprofen administered as capsules, syrup, drops and suppositories has been examined in a number of open studies and comparative trials against placebo and other standard antipyretic agents (Rizzo et al., 1983; Weippl, 1984; unpublished data on file, Ortho). These studies have involved several hundreds of adult and paediatric patients suffering from fever of diverse aetiologies (e.g. cancer, otitis media, respiratory tract infection). In most patients, effective fever control was achieved within 60 to 90 minutes, and they remained subfebrile with repeated doses. Suprofen showed a fast onset of antipyretic activity and was as effective as usual therapeutic doses of aspirin, paracetamol, mefenamic acid and metamizol.

4. Side Effects

Suprofen is well tolerated following single and repeated oral doses in patients with acute or chronic pain. Suprofen 200mg 3 times daily for 7 days administered systemically (intramuscularly and intravenously as a bolus or slow infusion) is also well tolerated both locally and systemically in healthy volunteers (Michos et al., 1985a,b; Zulliger et al., 1985). The most frequently occurring side effects are mild gastrointestinal disturbances (e.g. nausea, diarrhoea, constipation, gastralgia, heartburn, indigestion), mild CNS disturbances (e.g. headache, drowsiness, dizziness, somnolence) and skin rash (Denis and De Beer, 1983; Salzman and Brobyn, 1983; Schuermans, 1983; Silberman, 1983; Willkens, 1983). The incidence and nature of side effects in single-dose studies with suprofen is generally similar to that found with reference analgesics, and often with placebo. The clinical relevance of such 'side effects' must therefore be interpreted with caution as their relationshipo drug administration is often uncertain.

Suprofen produces less gastrointestinal bleeding than equipotent doses of aspirin in healthy volunteers (section 1.4). However, the incidence of gastrointestinal bleeding during suprofen administration relative to that of more established propionic acid derivatives (e.g. ibuprofen and naproxen) and newer agents (piroxicam) or prodrugs (fenbufen and sulindac) has not been determined. During long term administration of suprofen, gastrointestinal complaints remain the most frequently reported side effects (Salzman and Brobyn, 1983; Willkens, 1983), and peptic ulceration has been reported occasionally (Yeadon et al., 1983). In a 24-week study in patients with osteoarthritis, nausea and epigastric distress occurred in 3.7% and 7.4% of patients, respectively, receiving suprofen 200mg 4 times daily compared with 20% and 26.7% of patients, respectively, receiving dextropropoxyphene 65mg 4 times daily.

Other reactions infrequently associated with suprofen include single case reports of acute haemolytic anaemia (Tosato et al., 1985), and severe contact dermatitis following application of a topical suprofen cream (Dooms-Goossens et al., 1979). The latter patient was found to be cross-sensitive to ibuprofen, ketoprofen and naproxen. A very marked blood pressure elevation has been noted in

Table V. Frequency of withdrawals due to side effects in 1053 patients with osteoarthritis and musculoskeletal disorders receiving suprofen 200 to 400mg or reference drugs[a] 4 times daily in studies longer than 3 months (after Yeadon et al., 1983)

Side effect	Patients withdrawing because of side effects (%)	
	suprofen (n = 605)	reference drugs (n = 448)
Body as a whole	1.7	1.6
Cardiovascular/respiratory	1.7	1.3
Central nervous system	4.0	5.6
Cutaneous	3.6	1.6
Gastrointestinal	10.9	17.2
Genitourinary	0.8	0.4
Musculoskeletal	0.2	0.2
Special senses	0.8	2.9
Overall withdrawal[b]	17.7	23.9

a Aspirin 650 to 1000mg, dextropropoxyphene 65mg and a combination of dextropropoxyphene 65mg + aspirin 227mg + phenacetin 162mg + caffeine 32.4mg.
b Some patients withdrawn because of more than 1 side effect.

3 patients receiving suprofen (Willkens, 1983) but the authors did not discuss relationship to treatment, underlying disease or possible drug interaction.

In a summary of withdrawals due to side effects during long term double-blind trials (Yeadon et al., 1983), the overall withdrawal rate was lower on suprofen (17.7%) than with reference drugs (23.9%) [table V]. The withdrawal rate was similar with suprofen 200 and 400mg 4 times daily, and increased with age. Gastrointestinal complaints were the most frequent cause for withdrawal from suprofen (10.9%), but occurred at a lower rate than with the reference analgesics (17.2%).

5. *Effect on Laboratory Values*

Mild, clinically insignificant, leucopenia was reported in 8 of 605 patients receiving long term administration of suprofen. In addition, occasional elevations of serum bilirubin, alkaline phosphatase, lactate dehydrogenase, AST (SGOT) and ALT (SGPT) have been observed but without clinical symptoms or signs of liver disease. The uricosuric activity of suprofen causes a decrease in serum uric acid concentrations (Yeadon et al., 1983). Statistically significant reductions in haematocrit and haemoglobin, which are not clinically significant, have been noted during treatment with suprofen (Bowers et al., 1984; Denis and De Beer, 1983).

In a pharmacokinetic study in 45 healthy volunteers comparing diclofenac 25mg, suprofen 200mg and placebo administered intramuscularly 3 times daily for 7 days, diclofenac treatment had to be suspended after 4 days because of extreme increases in creatine phosphokinase. Creatine phosphokinase also increased with suprofen, but not to unacceptable levels. These enzyme elevations are probably attributable to tissue trauma from injection of the drugs since administration of the suprofen vehicle as placebo did not cause the enzyme elevation (Michos and Zulliger, 1985; Michos et al., 1985b; Zulliger, 1984).

6. *Drug Interactions*

At therapeutic concentrations suprofen does not displace warfarin and phenytoin from human albumin *in vitro* (Chaikin et al., 1980). De Clerck et al. (1975b) found that the anticoagulant effect of warfarin is only potentiated after repeated administration of very high doses of suprofen in rats (5 × 30 mg/kg). A crossover study conducted by Abrams et al. (1983a) in 24 healthy subjects given a single dose of suprofen 200mg alone and combined with liquid antacid (aluminium hydroxide 1.32g plus magnesium hydroxide 1.17g) showed that the antacid did not significantly alter the bioavailability of suprofen. Studies of the potential interaction of suprofen with other drugs after repeated administration in man have not been published.

The analgesic effects of suprofen and paracetamol potentiate each other when administered together in the rat adjuvant arthritic flexion test (Capetola et al., 1980). The analgesic effects of suprofen and paracetamol also appear to be additive in man, and this combination may therefore provide a useful analgesic combination. Codeine also adds to the analgesic effect of suprofen (sections 3.1.4 and 3.1.5).

7. *Overdosage*

There are few data on overdosage with suprofen. In a case report of a young woman who ingested suprofen 4g, the drug plasma concentration was 662 mg/L about 6 hours later (i.e. about 40 times the highest peak concentration with a single 200mg dose in healthy subjects). The patient remained fully conscious, and the authors concluded that suprofen is relatively non-toxic in overdosage (Freestone and Critchley, 1984).

8. *Dosage and Administration*

Suprofen is indicated in mild to moderate pain, such as musculoskeletal pain, episiotomy pain, postoperative pain following general surgery or dental procedures, headache, and pain associated with osteoarthritis, rheumatoid arthritis and dysmenorrhoea. The usual recommended dosage of suprofen is 200mg 3 or 4 times daily. Suprofen 400mg twice daily may provide an adequate dosage regimen (Fellmann et al., 1983). In acute pain, single doses of suprofen 400mg may provide a better analgesic response than lower doses.

As with other non-steroidal anti-inflammatory drugs, suprofen should be avoided in patients with active gastrointestinal ulcer or allergy to salicylates or other non-steroidal anti-inflammatory drugs. Suprofen should be used with caution in patients with impaired renal function, fluid retention, heart failure and hypertension, and those with a history of gastrointestinal ulceration. Close monitoring is required in patients with coagulation disorders and in patients receiving concomitant anticoagulants.

9. *The Place of Suprofen in Therapy*

Suprofen is an effective orally active analgesic for acute pain states of moderate intensity, including dysmenorrhoea. Single doses of suprofen provide equivalent or superior analgesia to therapeutic doses of other analgesics (e.g. aspirin, codeine, dextropropoxyphene, paracetamol, and their combinations). Suprofen is rapidly absorbed and therefore has a fast onset of action, but because of its short elimination half-life repeated doses may be required more frequently than with some other drugs, such as diflunisal. In chronic pain due to osteoarthritis or musculoskeletal disorders, suprofen appears as effective and as safe as aspirin, dextropropoxyphene, ibuprofen, indomethacin and naproxen. Its gastrointestinal tolerability may be superior to the former 2 drugs. In both acute and chronic pain, suprofen has not been compared with many other newer non-steroidal anti-inflammatory analgesics, such as piroxicam. In conclusion, suprofen appears to offer a suitable alternative to the older, more established simple analgesics and non-steroidal anti-inflammatory analgesics in the treatment of acute and chronic pain of moderate intensity.

References

Abrams, L.S.; Marriott, T.B. and Van Horn, A.: The effect of Maalox on the bioavailability of suprofen. (Abstract No. 69.) Clinical Research 31: 626A (1983a).

Abrams, L.S.; Marriott, T.B.; Chaikin, P.; Czerniecki, B.; Danna, R.P. and Friedmann, N.: Dose proportionality and multiple-dose pharmacokinetics of suprofen. (Abstract.) Clinical Research 31: 626A (1983b).

Alton, K.B. and Patrick, J.E.: High-performance liquid chromatographic assay for suprofen, a potent new analgesic, in plasma. Journal of Pharmaceutical Sciences 67: 985-987 (1978).

Arnold, J.D. and Berger, A.E.: Comparison of fecal blood loss after use of aspirin and suprofen. Pharmacology 27 (Suppl. 1): 14-22 (1983).

Awouters, F.; Niemegeers, C.J.E.; Lenaerts, F.M. and Janssen, P.A.J.: Delay of castor oil diarrhoea in rats: a new way to evaluate inhibitors of prostaglandin biosynthesis. Journal of Pharmacy and Pharmacology 30: 41-45 (1978).

Awouters, F.; Niemegeers, C.J.E.; Lenaerts, F.M. and Janssen, P.A.J.: The effects of suprofen in rats with Mycobacterium butyricum-induced arthritis. Arzneimittel-Forschung 25: 1526-1537 (1975a).

Awouters, F.; Niemegeers, C.J.E.; Lenaerts, P.M.H. and Janssen, P.A.J.: Suprofen, a potent antagonist of ultraviolet-erythema in guinea-pigs. Arzneimittel-Forschung 25: 1509-1511 (1975b).

Bodner, E.: Single-dose comparison of intramuscular suprofen, pentazocine, and placebo in patients with moderate-to-severe post-operative pain. Royal Society of Medicine International Congress and Symposium Series 90: 69-77 (1985).

Bodner, E. and Michos, N.: Clinically controlled comparative study of suprofen, pentazocine, and placebo. Arzneimittel-Forschung 35: 755-759 (1985).

Borowska, A.; Mackowiak, J. and Wisniewski, K.: Prostaglandins/PGs/ and peristalsis. Prostaglandins and Medicine 6: 13-16 (1981).

Bowers, D.E.; Honig, S.; Miller, J.L. and Gardner, M.C.: A long term double-blind evaluation of suprofen and aspirin in osteoarthritis. Poster presented at the 4th World Congress on Pain, Seattle (1984).

Capetola, R.J.; Argentieri, D.; Weintraub, H.S.; Chasin, M.; Doyle, P. et al.: Suprofen; in Goldberg (Ed.) Pharmacological and Biochemical Properties of Drug Substances Vol. 3, pp. 347-368 (American Pharmaceutical Association Academy of Pharmaceutical Sciences, Washington DC 1981).

Capetola, R.J.; McGuire, J.L. and Rosenthale, M.E.: Introduction to the pharmacology of suprofen. Pharmacology 27 (Suppl. 1): 1-13 (1983a).

Capetola, R.J.; Rosenthale, M.E.; Dubinsky, B. and McGuire, J.L.: Peripheral antialgesics: A review. Journal of Clinical Pharmacology 23: 545-556 (1983b).

Capetola, R.J.; Shriver, D.A. and Rosenthale, M.E.: Activity of a new non-narcotic analgesic, suprofen, on pathologic-induced pain in the rat. (Abstract No. 630.) Pharmacologist 20: 270 (1978).

Capetola, R.J.; Shriver, D.A. and Rosenthale, M.E.: Suprofen, a new peripheral analgesic. Journal of Pharmacology and Experimental Therapeutics 214: 16-23 (1980).

Carraher, R.P.; Hahn, D.W. and McGuire, J.L.: Pharmacological selectivity of suprofen, a new analgesic prostaglandin synthetase inhibitor. (Abstract No. 259.) Federation Proceedings 40: 280 (1981).

Chaikin, P.; Abrams, L.; McKenna, M. and Weintraub, H.: Suprofen protein binding studies *in vitro*. (Abstract No. 69.) Academy of Pharmaceutical Sciences (of the American Pharmaceutical Association), San Antonio, Texas, Nov 9-13 (1980).

Chaikin, P.; Marriott, T.B.; Simon, D. and Weintraub, H.S.: Comparative bioavailability of suprofen after coadministration with food or milk. (Abstract No. 88.) Academy of Pharmaceutical Sciences (of the American Pharmaceutical Association), San Diego, California, Nov 14-18 (1982).

Chaikin, P.; Chasin, M.; Kennedy, B. and Silverman, B.: Suprofen concentrations in human breast milk. Journal of Clinical Pharmacology 23: 385-390 (1983).

Cohen, A. and Smith, K.E.: Double-blind evaluation of safety and gastrointestinal blood loss following oral administration of suprofen plus codeine, aspirin plus codeine and placebo. (Abstract.) Journal of Clinical Pharmacology 14: 400-401 (1984).

Cooke, C.W.; Ellsworth, H.S. and Wentz, A.C.: Double-blind comparison of suprofen 200mg, suprofen 400mg, and placebo in the treatment of primary dysmenorrhoea. Royal Society of Medicine International Congress and Symposium Series 90: 1-10 (1985).

Cooke, C.W.; Ellsworth, H.S.; Wentz, A.C. and Czerniecki, B.: Efficacy and safety of two dosage regimens of suprofen in the treatment of primary dysmenorrhea. Poster presented at the 4th World Conference on Pain, Seattle (1984).

Cooper, S.A.; Wagenberg, B.; Eskow, R. and Zissu, J.: Double-blind evaluation of suprofen and aspirin in the treatment of periodontal pain. Pharmacology 27 (Suppl. 1): 23-30 (1983).

De Clerck, F.; Goossens, J. and Reneman, R.: Effects of anti-inflammatory, anticoagulant and vasoactive compounds on tail bleeding time, whole blood coagulation time and platelet retention by glass beads in rats. Thrombosis Research 8: 179-193 (1976).

De Clerck, F.; Vermylen, J. and Reneman, R.: Effects of suprofen, an inhibitor of prostaglandin biosynthesis, on platelet function, plasma coagulation and fibrinolysis I. *In vitro* experiments. Archives Internationales de Pharmacodynamie et de Therapie 216: 263-279 (1975a).

De Clerck, F.; Vermylen, J. and Reneman, R.: Effects of suprofen, an inhibitor of prostaglandin biosynthesis, on platelet function, plasma coagulation and fibrinolysis II. *In vivo* experiments. Archives Internationales de Pharmacodynamie et de Therapie 217: 68-79 (1975b).

Deere, J.L.; Howlett, R.J.; Jennings, C.L.; Kochell, R.L.; Newton, Z. and Purdon, T.F.: Suprofen in the treatment of primary dysmenorrhoea: Results of an open study. Advances in Therapy 1: 363-369 (1984).

Denis, F.R. and De Beer, J.M.M.: Clinical evaluation of suprofen in the treatment of elderly patients with pain of diverse etiology. Pharmacology 27 (Suppl. 1): 81-86 (1983).

Desjardins, P.J.; Wagenberg, B.; Eskow, R.; Reynolds, D.; Gallegos, O. and Kruger, G.: Analgesic efficacy of suprofen in two dental pain models. (Abstract No. A-25.) Clinical Pharmacology and Therapeutics 29: 240 (1981).

Dooms-Goossens, A.; Dooms, M.; Van Lint, L. and Degreef, H.: Skin sensitizing properties of arylalcanoic acids and their analogues. Contact Dermatitis 5: 324-328 (1979).

Dubinsky, B. and Schupsky, J.J.: Mechanism of action of suprofen, a new peripheral analgesic, as demonstrated by its effects on several nociceptive mediators. Prostaglandins 28: 241-252 (1984).

Dundee, J.W.: Clinical evaluation of mild analgesics. British Journal of Clinical Pharmacology 10 (Suppl.): 329S-334S (1980).

Eaglstein, W.H.; Ginsberg, L.D. and Mertz, P.M.: Ultraviolet irradiation-induced inflammation: Effects of steroid and non-steroid anti-inflammatory agents. Archives of Dermatology 115: 1421-1423 (1979).

Elattar, T.M.A. and Lin, H.S.: Effect of nonsteroidal anti-inflammatory agents on prostaglandins biosyntheses by human gingival tissue. (Abstract No. 270.) Journal of Dental Research 62: 679 (1983).

Fassolt, A. and Stocker, H.: Behandlung des postoperativen Wundschmerzes mit Suprofen. Arzneimittel-Forschung 33: 1327-1330 (1983).

Fellmann, N.; Stocker, H. and Reuteler, H.: Double-blind study of suprofen vs naproxen in the treatment of osteoarthritic pain. European Journal of Rheumatology and Inflammation 6: 216-221 (1983).

Ferreira, S.H.; Moncada, S. and Vane, J.R.: Prostaglandins and signs and symptoms of inflammation; in Robinson and Vane (Eds.) Prostaglandin Synthetase Inhibitors, pp. 175-187 (Raven Press, New York 1974).

Frakes, L.; Mehlisch, D.R. and Van Horn, A.W.: A double-blind evaluation of suprofen 200mg and 400mg, aspirin 650mg both alone and with codeine 60mg, and placebo in post-surgical dental pain. Poster presented at the 4th World Conference on Pain, Seattle (1984).

Fontaine, J.; Van Nueter, J.M. and Reuse, J.J.: Effects of prostaglandins on the peristaltic reflex of the guinea pig ileum. Archives Internationales de Pharmacodynamie et de Therapie 226: 341-343 (1977).

Freestone, S. and Critchley, J.A.J.H.: Self poisoning with sutoprofen. British Medical Journal 289: 470 (1984).

Fujimori, I.; Kono, M.; Sekita, T.; Takeda, Y.; Ogihara, K. et al.: A double-blind clinical evaluation of suprofen on acute upper respiratory infection comparing with aspirin. Journal of the Japanese Association for Infectious Diseases 57: 62-81 (1983).

Fujimura, H.; Nakayama, T.; Hiramatsu, Y.; Tamura, Y. and Maekawa, K.: General pharmacological studies of (±)-2-[p-(2-thenoyl)phenyl] propionic acid (suprofen). Pharmacometrics 26: 415-440 (1983).

Fujimura, H.; Tsurumi, K.; Hasegawa, J.; Yanagihara, M.; Hiramatsu, Y. and Maekawa, K.: Anti-inflammatory, analgesic and antipyretic activities of α-(p-thenoylphenyl) propionic acid. Folia Pharmacologica Japonica 79: 123-136 (1982).

Fujimura, H.; Tsurumi, K.; Nakayama, T.; Kokuba, S.; Hiramatsu, Y. and Tamura, Y.: Effect of α-(p-thenoylphenyl)-propionic acid (TN-762) on acute inflammatory reactions and prostaglandin biosynthesis. Folia Pharmacologica Japonica 77:

321-336 (1981).
Hahn, D.W.; Carraher, R. and McGuire, J.L.: Effects of suprofen and other prostaglandin synthetase inhibitors in a new animal model for myometrial hyperactivity. Prostaglandins 23: 1-16 (1982).
Hauzeur, J.P.: Comparison of effectiveness and tolerability of suprofen 300mg suppositories with indomethacin 50mg suppositories in osteoarthritis pain. Poster presented at the 4th World Congress on Pain, Seattle (1984).
Hauzeur, J.P.: Double-blind comparison of suprofen suppositories and indomethacin suppositories in patients with pain due to osteoarthritis. Royal Society of Medicine International Congress and Symposium Series 90: 61-68 (1985).
Heffron, W.; Gordon, S.; May, J.; Mehlisch, D.; Gravelee, L. et al.: A double-blind evaluation of two dosage regimens of suprofen and ibuprofen in primary dysmenorrhea. Poster presented at the 4th World Conference on Pain, Seattle (1984).
Honig, W.J.: Clinical comparison of the analgesic efficacy of suprofen, diflunisal and placebo in the treatment of pain after meniscectomy. Pharmacology 27 (Suppl. 1): 74-80 (1983).
Honig, W.J. and Michos, N.: Comparison of suprofen and indoprofen after intravenous injection in pain following meniscectomy. Poster presented at the 4th World Conference on Pain, Seattle (1984).
Imai, H.; Muramatsu, Y.; Niu, K.; Nozaki, M. and Fujimura, H.: Inhibitory effect of TN-762 (suprofen) on the platelet aggregation. Folia Pharmacologica Japonica 80: 61-68 (1982).
Ishibashi, K.; Asada, K.; Hashimoto, F.; Nakagawa, Y.; Doi, Y.; Ohtsubo, K. and Tanaka, T.: A double-blind study of a new non-steroidal anti-inflammatory analgesic agent, suprofen, after tooth extraction. Oral Therapeutics and Pharmacology 1: 53-64 (1982).
Lagu, A.L.; Young, R.; McGonigle, E. and Lane, P.A.: High-performance liquid chromatographic determination of suprofen in drug substance and capsules. Journal of Pharmaceutical Sciences 71: 85-88 (1982).
Littlejohns, D.W. and Vere, D.W.: The clinical assessment of analgesic drugs. British Journal of Clinical Pharmacology 11: 319-332 (1981).
Lorenzi, G.L.; Bertini, G.; Peveraro, A.; Rosso, V. and Rossi, E.: A single-dose, double-blind evaluation of suprofen and dipyrone in post-operative pain. Royal Society of Medicine International Congress and Symposium Series 90: 31-40 (1985).
Markus, A.F. and Gough, D.: A clinical trial of suprofen and aspirin in post-operative dental pain. International Journal of Oral Surgery 9: 477-479 (1980).
McGuire, J.E.; Niemegeers, C.J.E.; Shriver, D.A. and Awouters, F.: Antinociceptive properties of suprofen, a new analgesic agent. (Abstract No. 2915.) Federation Proceedings 37: 769 (1978).
Mehlisch, D.R.: Double-blind evaluation of analgesic efficacy and safety of suprofen, aspirin, aspirin plus codeine, and placebo in patients with post-operative dental pain. Royal Society of Medicine International Congress and Symposium Series 90: 41-50 (1985).
Mehlisch, D.R. and Eglsaer, M.: A double-blind evaluation of analgesic efficacy and safety of suprofen 200mg compared to Darvon Compound-65, Darvocet-N 100, aspirin 650mg and codeine 60mg, and placebo in patients with postoperative pain. (Abstract No. 362.) Presented at the II World Conference on Clinical Pharmacology and Therapeutics, Washington DC, July 31-August 5 (1983).
Mehlisch, D.R.; Friedman, N. and Van Horn, A.W.: A double-blind evaluation of suprofen, aspirin and an oxycodone combination analgesic in post-operative pain. Poster presented at the 4th World Conference on Pain, Seattle (1984).
Michos, N. and Zulliger, H.: Local and systemic tolerance of suprofen, diclofenac and placebo, and plasma levels of suprofen given intramuscularly in normal subjects for 7 days. Royal Society of Medicine International Congress and Symposium Series 90: 11-22 (1985).
Michos, N.; Zulliger, H.W. and Fenzl, C.E.: Local and systemic tolerability of suprofen. Arzneimittel-Forschung 35: 745-748 (1985a).
Michos, N.; Zulliger, H.W. and Fenzl, E.: Pharmacokinetics and tolerability of suprofen. Arzneimittel-Forschung 35: 738-745 (1985b).
Mok, M.S.; Steen, S.N. and Lippmann, M.: Suprofen in the relief of pain. IRCS Medical Science; Clinical Medicine; Clinical Pharmacology and Therapeutics 6: 511 (1978).
Mori, Y.; Kuroda, N.; Sakai, Y.; Yokoya, F.; Toyoshi, K. and Baba, S.: Species differences in the metabolism of suprofen in laboratory animals and man. Drug Metabolism and Disposition 13: 239-245 (1985).
Mori, Y.; Yokoya, F.; Sakai, Y.; Toyoshi, K.; Furuta, T. and Baba, S.: Absorption and excretion of suprofen in both sexes of rats, guinea-pigs, and rabbits. Radioisotopes 32: 416-418 (1983a).
Mori, Y.; Yokoya, F.; Sakai, Y.; Toyoshi, K. and Baba, S.: Absorption, distribution, and excretion of suprofen in mice of both sexes. Chemical and Pharmaceutical Bulletin 32: 1106-1112 (1984a).
Mori, Y.; Yokoya, F.; Sakai, Y.; Toyoshi, K. and Baba, S.: Distribution of suprofen in rats of both sexes. Radioisotopes 33: 284-290 (1984b).
Mori, Y.; Yokoya, F.; Toyoshi, K.; Baba, S. and Sakai, Y.: Absorption and excretion of suprofen in rats. Drug Metabolism and Disposition 11: 387-391 (1983b).
Müller, H.; Zulliger, H.W.; Dörig, B.A. and Egli, R.A.: Quantitative determination of suprofen in human plasma and urine by fully automated high-performance liquid chromatography. Arzneimittel-Forschung 32: 257-260 (1982).
Nevelsteen, A.; De Clerck, F.; Loots, W. and De Gryse, A.: Restoration of post-thrombotic peripheral collateral circulation in the cat by ketanserin, a selective 5-HT_2-receptor antagonist. Archives Internationales de Pharmacodynamie et de Therapie 270: 268-279 (1984).
Niemegeers, C.J.E. and Janssen, P.A.J.: Suprofen, a potent antagonist of sodium urate crystal-induced arthritis in dogs. Arzneimittel-Forschung 25: 1512-1515 (1975).
Niemegeers, C.J.E.; Awouters, F.; Lenaerts, F.M. and Janssen, P.A.J.: The activity of suprofen on nystatin-induced paw oedema in rats. Arznemittel-Forschung 25: 1516-1519 (1975a).
Niemegeers, C.J.E.; Lenaerts, F.M. and Janssen, P.A.J.: The antipyretic effect of suprofen in rats with yeast-induced fever. Arzneimittel-Forschung 25: 1519-1524 (1975b).
Niemegeers, C.J.E.; Lenaerts, F.M.; Awouters, F. and Janssen, P.A.J.: Gastrointestinal effects and acute toxicity of suprofen. Arzneimittel-Forschung 25: 1537-1542 (1975c).
Niemegeers, C.J.E.; Van Bruggen, W.; Awouters, F. and Janssen, P.A.J.: The effects of suprofen in rats with implanted cotton pellets. Arzneimittel-Forschung 25: 1524-1526 (1975d).
Niemegeers, C.J.E.; Van Bruggen, J.A.A. and Janssen, P.A.J.: Suprofen, a potent antagonist of acetic acid-induced writhing in rats. Arzneimittel-Forschung 25: 1505-1509 (1975e).
Olson, N.; Sunshine, A.; Roure, C.; Colon, A.; Laska, E. et al.: Analgesic efficacy of suprofen, codeine and placebo. Poster presented at the 4th World Conference on Pain, Seattle (1984).
Porzio, F.: A double-blind evaluation of suprofen and diclofenac in acute exacerbations of osteoarthritic pain. Royal Society of Medicine International Congress and Symposium Series 90: 51-60 (1985).
Pujalte, J.; Valdez, E. and de la Paz, R.: Clinical comparison of the analgesic efficacy of suprofen and mefenamic acid in the treatment of musculoskeletal pain. Current Therapeutic Research 36: 245-252 (1984).
Rainsford, K.D.: The comparative gastric ulcerogenic activities of non-steroid anti-inflammatory drugs. Agents and Actions 7: 573-577 (1977).
Rainsford, K.D.: The effects of aspirin and other non-steroid anti-

inflammatory/analgesic drugs on gastro-intestinal mucus glycoprotein biosynthesis *in vivo* relationship to ulcerogenic actions. Biochemical Pharmacology 27: 877-885 (1978).

Rizzo, S.C.; Sarchi, C.; Pacchiarini, L. and Ricevuti, G.: Studio comparativo sull'attività antipyretica del suprofen. Bollettino Chimico Farmaceutico 122: 28S-36S (1983).

Rosenthale, M.E.; McGuire, J.L. and Capetola, R.J.: Pharmacological properties of a new peripheral analgesic, suprofen. European Journal of Rheumatology 4: 469-480 (1981).

Salzman, R.T. and Brobyn, R.D.: Long-term comparison of suprofen and propoxyphene in patients with osteoarthritis. Pharmacology 27 (Suppl. 1): 55-64 (1983).

Schuermans, Y.: Comparison of suprofen and ibuprofen in the treatment of pain secondary to osteoarthritis. Pharmacology 27 (Suppl. 1): 41-47 (1983).

Schichikawa, K.; Orihara, M.; Kimura, M.; Komatsubara, Y.; Maeda, A. et al.: The clinical evaluation of suprofen on low back pain – multi-center double-blind study in comparison with indomethacin. Japanese Pharmacology and Therapeutics 11: 225-242 (1983).

Silberman, H.M.: Multiple-dose comparison of suprofen, aspirin and placebo in the treatment of musculoskeletal pain. Pharmacology 27 (Suppl. 1): 65-73 (1983).

Singh, P.P.; Junnarkar, A.Y.; Rao, C.S.; Varma, R.K. and Shridhar, D.R.: Acetic acid and phenylquinone writhing test: a critical study in mice. Methods and Findings in Experimental and Clinical Pharmacology 5: 601-606 (1983).

Smith, R.J.: Nonsteroid anti-inflammatory agents: Regulators of the phagocytic secretion of lysosomal enzymes from guineapig neutrophils. Journal of Pharmacology and Experimental Therapeutics 207: 618-629 (1978).

Stark, W.J.; Maumeree, A.E.; Fagadau, W.; Datiles, M.M.; Baker, C.C. et al.: Cystoid macular edema in pseudophakia. Survey of Ophthalmology 28 (Suppl.): 442-451 (1984).

Sunshine, A.; Marrero, I.; Olson, N.Z.; Laska, E.M. and McCormick, N.: Oral analgesic efficacy of suprofen compared to aspirin, aspirin plus codeine, and placebo in patients with postoperative dental pain. Pharmacology 27 (Suppl. 1): 31-40 (1983).

SuSace, A.; Previtera, A.M.; Sarchi, C. and Pietrogrande, V.: Sull'impiego di un nuovo antiflogistico in ortopedia. Ortopedia e Traumatologia Oggi 2: 407-411 (1982).

Tolman, E.L.; McGuire, J.L. and Rosenthale, M.E.: Pharmacology of nonsteroidal anti-inflammatory drugs and their use in dysmenorrhea; in Dawood et al. (Eds) Premenstrual Syndrome and Dysmenorrhea, pp. 159-175 (Urban and Schwarzenberg, Baltimore 1985).

Tolman, E.L.; Rosenthale, M.E.; Capetola, R.J. and McGuire, J.L.: Suprofen: The pharmacology and clinical efficacy of a new nonnarcotic peripheral analgesic. Clinics in Rheumatic Diseases 10: 353-368 (1984).

Tong, E.Y.; Leibowitz, H.M. and Kupferman, A.: Suppression of prostaglandin release from the inflamed cornea. (Abstract No. 3916.) Federation Proceedings 43: 954 (1984).

Tosato, F.; Fossaluzza, V. et al.: Acute haemolytic anaemia induced by suprofen. (Abstract.) British Medical Journal 290: 1042 (1985).

Tsurumi, K. and Fujimura, H.: Effect of anti-inflammatory drugs on endotoxin-induced diarrhea in mice. Japanese Journal of Pharmacology 33: 165-173 (1983).

Van Daele, P.G.H.; Boey, J.M.; Sipido, V.K.; De Bruyn, M.F.L. and Janssen, P.A.J.: Synthesis of α-methyl-4-(2-thienylcarbonyl) benzeneacetic acid, suprofen, and derivatives. Arzneimittel-Forschung 25: 1495-1501 (1975).

Van Nueten, J.M.; Hoebeke, J.; De Clerck, F.; Awouters, F. and Janssen, P.A.J.: Inhibition by suprofen and other non-narcotic analgesic drugs of the effects of prostaglandin precursors on isolated tissues and platelets. Archives Internationales de Pharmacodynamie et de Therapie 220: 297-310 (1976).

Vane, J.R.: Mode of action of aspirin and similar compounds; in Robinson and Vane (Eds) Prostaglandin Synthetase Inhibitors, pp. 155-163 (Raven Press, New York 1974).

Vargha von Szeged, A. and Michos, N.: Erfahrungen mit Suprofen bei akuten und chronische Schmerzen in der neurologischen Praxis. Arzneimittel-Forschung 33: 1334-1338 (1983).

Vericat Cadesas, F.; Igual, A. and Giralt, J.: Estudio comparativo de la actividad de LC-R 505 frente a otros antiinflamatorios. Archivos de Farmacologia y Toxicologia 5: 259-261 (1979).

Wagenberg, B.; Eskow, R.; Zissu, J. and Cooper, S.A.: Relative analgesic efficacy of suprofen 200mg, d-propoxyphene 65mg, codeine 60mg, and placebo. (Abstract No. C36.) Clinical Pharmacology and Therapeutics 33: 199 (1983).

Weintraub, H.S.: Human acute pharmacokinetics and comparative bioavailability of suprofen from various dosage forms. (Abstract.) Clinical Research 26: 595A (1978).

Weippl, G.: Effect of suprofen on fever and pains in young children with infection of the upper respiratory tract and otitis media. (Abstract No. 91.) Pain (Suppl. 2): S63 (1984).

Weippl, G.: Treatment of fever in children: clinical comparison of seven different doses of suprofen. Royal Society of Medicine International Congress and Symposium Series 90: 23-30 (1985).

Willkens, R.F.: Long-term clinical evaluation of suprofen and aspirin in patients with osteoarthritis. Pharmacology 27 (Suppl. 1): 48-54 (1983).

Wong, S. and Gardocki, J.F.: Anti-inflammatory and antiarthritic evaluation of acetaminophen and its potentiation of tolmetin. Journal of Pharmacology and Experimental Therapeutics 226: 625-632 (1983).

Yeadon, A.; Gardner, M.C.; Milak, D.M. and Smith, K.E.: Suprofen: an overview of long-term safety. Pharmacology 27 (Suppl. 1): 87-94 (1983).

Yokoya, F.; Mori, Y.; Toyoshi, K.; Sakai, Y.; Baba, S. and Horie, M.: Disposition of suprofen in rats following intravenous injection. Radioisotopes 33: 137-141 (1984a).

Yokoya, F.; Nakayama, T.; Sakamoto, K.; Ohhira, K.; Ohshika, Y. et al.: Effect of (±)-2-[p-(2-thenoyl)phenyl] propionic acid (suprofen) on experimental allergic reactions. Japanese Journal of Pharmacology 34: 23-31 (1984b).

Zulliger, H.: Comparison of local and systemic tolerability of suprofen I.M. 200 mg/ml versus diclofenac I.M. 25 mg/ml and placebo I.M. 1 ml: Determination of 'steady state' plasmakinetics of suprofen in 15 volunteers each. Poster presented at the 4th World Congress on Pain, Seattle (1984).

Zulliger, H.W. and Fassolt, A.: Suprofen kinetics in healthy male volunteers after intramuscular injection of increasing dosages. Arzneimittel-Forschung 33: 1322-1326 (1983).

Zulliger, H.W. and Fassolt, A.: Pharmacokinetics and bioavailability of suprofen injection solution after intravenous application *versus* capsules on six healthy male volunteers. Arzneimittel-Forschung 35: 976-980 (1985).

Zulliger, H.W.; Michos, N. and Fenzl, E.: Local and systemic tolerability of suprofen. Arznemittel-Forschung 35: 748-755 (1985).

Zusman, R.M. and Keiser, H.R.: Prostaglandin biosynthesis by rabbit renomedullary interstitial cells in tissue culture: Stimulation by angiotensin II, bradykinin and arginine vasopressin. Journal of Clinical Investigation 60: 215-223 (1977).

Authors' address: *P.A. Todd*, ADIS Drug Information Services, Private Bag, Mairangi Bay, Auckland 10 (New Zealand).

Review Article

Drugs 30: 539-551 (1985)
0012-6667/85/0012-0539/$06.50/0

Newer Methods of Delivery of Opiates for Relief of Pain

P.J. Slattery and *R.A. Boas*

Department of Pharmacology and Clinical Pharmacology, University of Auckland School of Medicine, Auckland

Summary

Successful pain management using opiates requires both an analgesic with sufficient intrinsic activity and an effective administration system. Most instances of unsatisfactory pain control, however, are due to failure to achieve and maintain adequate blood concentrations of the chosen drug. Newer techniques of administration aim to overcome this problem.

Oral opiate therapy with conventional or sustained-release formulations of morphine provide good control of terminal cancer pain provided that a regular dosing pattern is established and reviewed according to the patient's needs. This represents a significant departure from the traditional 'as required' prescription of this type of drug. In the management of acute severe pain, sublingual and intravenous opiates – self-administered as needed, or given by mandatory dosing schedules – have also been shown to overcome the limitations of intermittent intramuscular injections. A further novel development, stemming from basic neuroscience research, is the selective application of opiates to the spinal cord via the epidural or intrathecal route. This controversial technique has led to major improvements in treatment of some types of acute and chronic pain.

Recent advances in the neurophysiology and neurochemistry of pain have come at a time when medical and nursing staff are increasingly aware that pain is an important component of many disease states, and deserves better management than previously. The result has been an expansion of interest in, and increased clinical investigation of, pain – exemplified by the establishment of an international association for the study of pain and the emergence of pain clinics as separate entities in most hospitals.

It has become apparent that careful choice of both drug and delivery system is important for successful treatment of pain. Although important advances have been made in the synthesis of new classes and examples of opiates, morphine remains the standard for the majority of applications and the development of more effective administration systems has been of greater clinical significance than development of new drugs. An important study by Marks and Sachar (1973) noted failure in pain control in over 70% of patients treated, and identified inappropriate use of the available narcotic analgesics as the immediate cause. Many other workers (Keeri-Szanto and Heaman, 1972; Stapleton et al., 1978) have also drawn attention to inadequate administration regimens as the prime cause for failure in pain management.

This review is not exhaustive, but covers the more important new administration techniques as well as some traditional techniques which have undergone reappraisal and significant improvement in recent years.

1. Oral Administration

1.1 Orally Administered Opiates: Conventional Formulations

The effectiveness of orally administered opiates such as morphine and diamorphine (heroin) is modified by their extensive and variable presystemic elimination in the gut and liver (Iwatomo and Klaassen, 1977). The renewed importance of this route of administration as a cornerstone of modern management of moderate and severe chronic cancer pain has been amply stressed by Twycross (1978). Recent studies also review the effectiveness of different opiates and their use in combination with stimulants, antiemetics and tranquillisers (e.g. Melzac et al., 1979; Twycross, 1977; Walsh, 1984).

The use of orally administered opiates to treat severe pain provides a good example of the dual importance of efficacy and practicality as determinants of the clinical usefulness of any new treatment regimen. The high patient acceptance of palatable orally administered drugs together with an increasing readiness on the part of medical and nursing staff to recognise the wide variation in dose requirements between patients, has meant that this simple way of using opiates now has a prime role in treatment of chronic cancer pain.

1.1.1 Pharmacokinetic Considerations

Single-dose studies on morphine kinetics in cancer patients after oral administration (Sawe et al., 1981) show pronounced differences between individuals in volume of distribution (0.95 to 3.75 L/kg), serum clearance (5 to 16 ml/min/kg), elimination half-life (58 to 467 min) and oral bioavailability (15 to 64%). Subsequent studies of steady-state kinetics in similar groups of patients (Neumann et al., 1982; Sawe et al., 1983) show no accumulation of morphine after regular oral dosing (20 to 40mg 4- or 6-hourly), but variable average steady-state concentrations of morphine which were linearly related to dose. The clinical implication of these studies is that dosing needs must be established individually and that predetermined limits of drug dose are totally inappropriate without prior trial in each patient.

The effects of liver disease on metabolism and bioavailability of oral pethidine (meperidine) were studied by Pond et al. (1981). Cirrhotic patients had a lower systemic clearance, greater bioavailability (85%) and a longer half-life of pethidine than normal subjects; these findings are also likely to hold for other high clearance opiates. Pond also noted that a fixed proportion of pethidine was metabolised to norpethidine irrespective of the route of administration, which suggests that it is unsuited to oral administration since high dosage is likely to be associated with high norpethidine blood concentrations with a potential for adverse side effects (Austin et al., 1981; Mather and Glynn, 1982).

1.1.2 Clinical Experience

Extensive hospice experience with orally administered opiates shows the efficacy of this technique when a policy of mandatory dosing at fixed intervals is followed. Individual dose requirements vary widely (2.5 to 180mg morphine 4-hourly; Twycross, 1983). Requirements tend to increase for the first few weeks of treatment only. Tolerance is not a problem in practice, nor is physical dependance in this setting. Clinically important respiratory depression is also rarely a problem when opiates are used in individually determined doses to treat chronic pain (Twycross, 1983).

Diamorphine has been traditionally recommended for use in terminal cancer care, but studies do not substantiate any advantage over morphine, either with parenteral or oral administration. The potency ratio of oral diamorphine : morphine is 1.5 : 1 (Twycross, 1977). Diamorphine is available in few countries outside the UK and in any case is rapidly deacylated *in vivo* first to monoacetyl morphine and then to active morphine (Way et al., 1965).

Whilst many patients with chronic pain will require multiple medications, the use of cocktails, such as the Brompton mixture, is not recommended. Melzack et al. (1979) compared morphine solution with Brompton mixture and found no difference in degree of pain relief (good with both) or incidence of side effects such as drowsiness, confusion or nausea (all low).

1.2 Orally Administered Opiates: Controlled Release Formulations

The use of oral opiates in conventional formulation necessitates that they be given regularly and frequently (commonly every 4 hours). A short interval between dosing may be inconvenient or prove too difficult in some settings, so controlled release tablets of morphine sulphate 10, 30, 60 and 100mg have been introduced into clinical studies with the aim of overcoming this.

1.2.1 Pharmacokinetic Considerations

In studies involving healthy volunteers, comparisons of the plasma morphine concentration-time profiles resulting from oral ingestion of conventional encapsulated morphine sulphate 10mg and controlled release morphine 10 and 20mg ('MST Continus'; Leslie et al., 1980) show a similar bimodal pattern. In the case of the controlled release formulation, however, the initial rise in plasma morphine concentrations is slower and more prolonged, whilst the secondary rise (thought to be due to a substantial enterohepatic circulation) is more pronounced (fig. 1a,b). These effects in combination are thought to provide the basis for the prolonged clinical effects of this preparation.

1.2.2 Clinical Experience

Orally administered medications have been traditionally eschewed in the early postoperative period because of occasional prolonged drowsiness and the relatively frequent occurrence of vomiting and ileus. Modern anaesthetic practice has shortened recovery times and usually includes an antiemetic and analgesic. Thus, reassessment of the role of slow-onset oral analgesic therapy for postoperative pain is appropriate.

There have been conflicting reports of the efficacy of sustained release morphine tablets in the management of acute pain. Used as a sole analgesic after surgical dental extractions by Hanks et al. (1981), both a sustained release tablet 20mg and conventional morphine sulphate solution 20mg produced poor pain relief. In a comparison with intramuscular morphine as analgesic after intra-abdominal surgery, however, both treatments produced satisfactory pain control and the same incidence of side effects (Fell et al., 1982). A significant difference between this and the previous study was the use of an intravenous loading dose of the drug during surgery. This would seem to be a consistent requirement for the success of any relatively slow onset drug in relieving postoperative or other acute pain (see section 2.1).

Controlled release morphine preparations are now also used in management of chronic cancer pain, and preliminary reports are generally favourable, although no controlled comparisons with conventional morphine formulations are yet available.

2. Sublingual Administration

The sublingual route of administration holds many advantages for self-administered opiate medication since it combines the convenience and cost advantages of the oral route with a relatively high and, more importantly, a relatively predictable bioavailability. This is due to the extremely good blood supply to the oral mucosa and the fact that venous drainage is into the systemic rather than portal circulation, so the potential for presystemic clearance is limited. The sublingual use of phenazocine was described by Brown in 1966, but buprenorphine is currently the only opiate marketed in a sublingual preparation.

2.1 Sublingual Buprenorphine

Buprenorphine is ideally suited for sublingual self-administration for several reasons:

1. It is a highly lipophilic substance and well absorbed across biological membranes

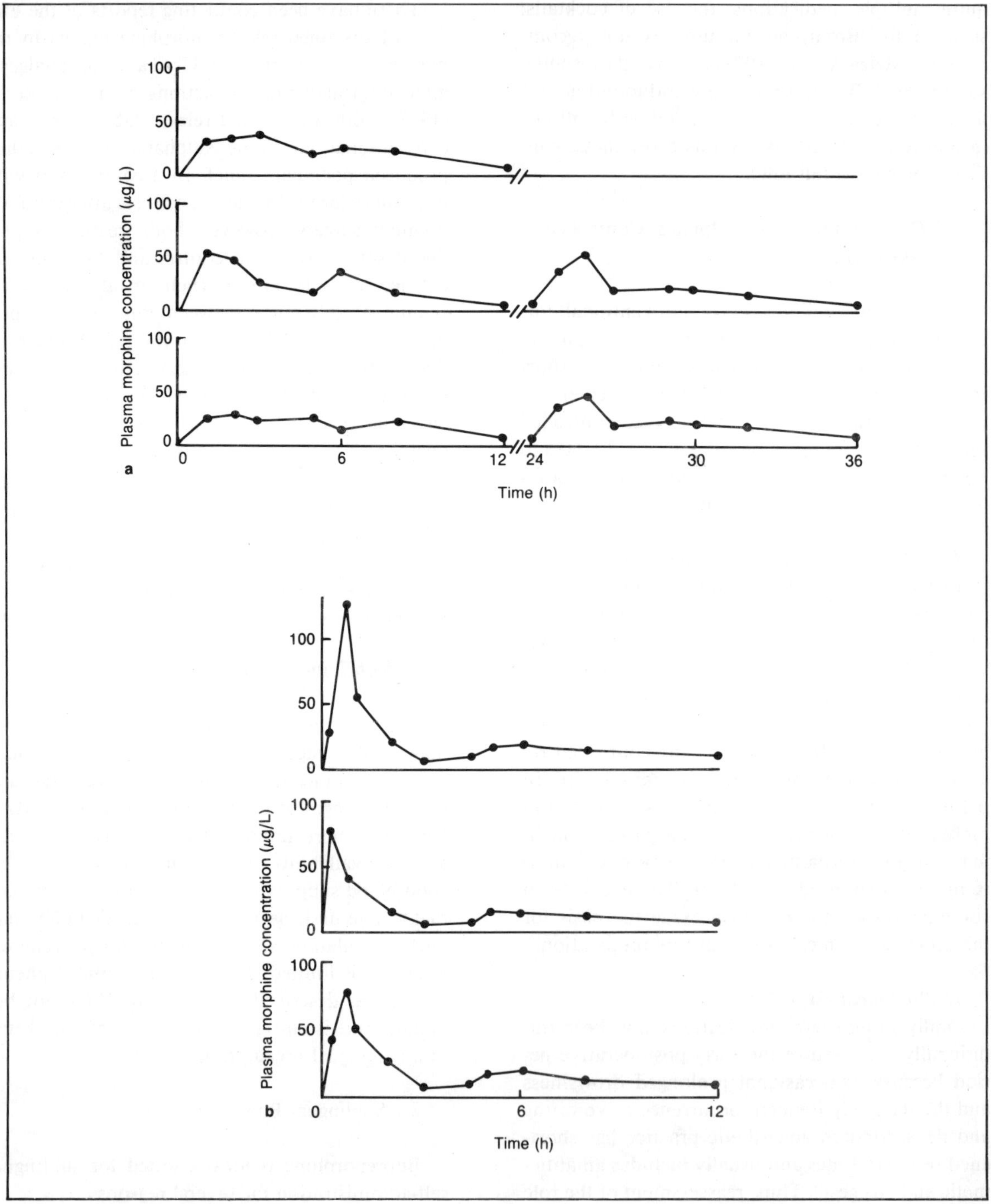

Fig. 1. a: Plasma morphine concentrations in 3 subjects after 10mg controlled release morphine sulphate; **b:** Plasma morphine concentrations in 3 subjects after 10mg encapsulated morphine sulphate (reproduced with permission from Leslie et al. 1980).

2. It has a high hepatic clearance – thus, tablets accidentally swallowed are effectively eliminated and do not contribute significantly to the drug effect
3. It is a partial agonist with long duration of action and low addiction potential (Cowan et al., 1977).

Sublingual buprenorphine is established as an effective analgesic for the treatment of postoperative and chronic pain, although it has a slower onset of action than intramuscular morphine (Edge et al., 1979; Heel et al., 1979). As with oral medication in the treatment of acute severe pain, sublingual buprenorphine may need to be preceded by a parenterally administered opiate. It has proved to be a convenient and effective therapy for both acute and chronic pain, but two problems have arisen with its use. In ambulant patients buprenorphine produces a relatively high incidence of nausea (this association is recognised with other opiates and buprenorphine appears to be no exception), and despite having a low addiction potential its limited euphoriant effects and initial widespread prescription have resulted in occasional instances of abuse.

2.1.1 Pharmacokinetic Considerations

Absorption after sublingual administration is slow, with peak plasma buprenorphine concentrations occurring on average about 200 minutes after administration, and bioavailabity reaching about 55% of the dose (Bullingham et al., 1982). Early studies on the kinetics of buprenorphine after intravenous administration (McQuay et al., 1980) demonstrated that there was a disparity between plasma concentration-time profile and analgesic effect, with analgesia persisting despite a rapid decline in plasma concentration. The unusual nature of the buprenorphine-opiate receptor interaction [high affinity but slow association and even slower dissociation (Boas and Villiger, 1985; Hambrook and Rance, 1976)] is a likely explanation for these effects. These considerations, together with the high lipid solubility of buprenorphine, also help to explain why the drug is so effective by the sublingual route despite slow absorption and relatively low (but sustained) plasma concentrations.

2.1.2 Clinical Experience

Double-blind comparisons of sublingual buprenorphine with intramuscular morphine (Edge et al., 1979) and papaveretum (Fry, 1979) show a relatively slow onset and prolonged duration of action of buprenorphine, the quality of pain relief and incidence of side effects being the same as with the parenteral opiate. The slow onset and long duration of action suggest that sublingual buprenorphine might be most appropriately used pre-emptively in the management of postoperative pain – giving the drug on a predetermined fixed dose and interval regimen rather than on the more usual 'as required' basis. Indeed, Ellis et al. (1982) produced good results using regular administration; they found a higher incidence of nausea and sedation than with conventional intramuscular or intravenous on-demand analgesia, but did not consider these effects clinically important and commented instead on the relative ease of administration of the sublingual drug. Bullingham et al. (1984) studied the efficacy of mandatory sublingual buprenorphine over a 3-day period in patients after total hip replacement. The quality of analgesia, which was always good, improved as the study progressed, while the incidence of nausea and vomiting decreased. The authors suggested that the higher incidence of side effects noted in the early postoperative period might be due principally to the operation and anaesthetic, rather than the analgesic.

3. Intravenous Administration

3.1 Continuous Intravenous Infusions

Continuous intravenous infusion represents an important advance in administration of drugs for relief of postoperative pain – it can reliably provide total relief of pain at rest, though it may not provide full cover with coughing or other activity. So long as realistic expectations are observed in terms of pain relief, this system seems to have a more than adequate safety margin. It does not require expensive or complex equipment, preoperative preparation of the patient, or any unusual skills of the nursing and medical staff. It is in theory less able to cater for individual differences in analgesic requirement than some form of on-demand apparatus (see section 3.2), but in practice the low initial cost and the ready availability of apparatus mean that this system is most suitable for routine use in the management of severe postoperative pain.

3.1.1 Pharmacokinetic Considerations

The development of better assays for opiates has enabled investigation of the relationship between the pain-relieving effects of these drugs and their blood concentrations. The concept that for any patient there is a minimum effective analgesic concentration has proved useful in promoting and rationalising the use of opiates by constant infusion. Thus, Shih et al. (1976) investigated serum pethidine concentrations following oral and intramuscular administration, and reported the existence of a minimum effective concentration. Stapleton et al. (1978) used pharmacokinetic modelling to construct a 3-step pethidine infusion regimen which would rapidly attain and maintain plateau levels for extended periods. In this study a steep transition to a median pain score of zero (no pain) was noted in 10 patients after lower abdominal surgery when the blood pethidine concentration exceeded 0.46 mg/L. This estimate was supported by Austin et al. (1980), who studied concentrations resulting from multiple intramuscular injections of pethidine. Austin also noted a steep blood concentration-effect curve, with transition from no analgesia to complete analgesia between 0.35 and 0.45 mg/L on the first postoperative day, and between 0.4 and 0.5 mg/L on the second day.

Basic pharmacokinetic data are available for all commonly used opiates, but these data are usually derived from healthy volunteers or from single-dose studies in patients immediately after operation. There remains considerable uncertainty about the effects of disease and surgery on these kinetic parameters. Commonly used opiates have high hepatic clearance, and would be susceptable to alterations in hepatic blood flow. The plasma clearance of pethidine in healthy subjects ranges from 36 to 54 L/h, but in cirrhosis the total systemic clearance is significantly (50%) reduced (Pond et al., 1981). Anaesthesia and surgery produce significant changes in cardiac output and patterns of hepatic and other regional blood flows. Studies on the pharmacokinetics of pethidine under these circumstances (Mather et al., 1975; Tamsen et al., 1982a) suggest a 25% reduction in systemic clearance, which persists into the immediate postoperative period.

3.1.2 Clinical Experience

Continuous intravenous infusions of opiates are commonly employed in intensive care units and for the management of postoperative pain. Early reports (Church, 1979) described the infusion of dilute analgesic solutions on an hourly basis, but wider availability of portable infusion pumps has favoured continuous infusion of more concentrated solutions. Most opiates have been administered in this way and been found to be highly effective if there is provision for variation in the infusion rate to cater for individual patient requirements. Church (1979) and Fry (1979) noted that the amount of analgesic given intravenously was in excess of that administered to similar patients via the intramuscular route. Catling et al. (1980) compared the analgesic and respiratory effects of continuous intravenous and intermittent intramuscular administration of papaveretum, and again noted the relatively larger amounts of analgesic given by infusion. They found the higher dose produced superior analgesia, but more respiratory depression together with a higher incidence of what were described as potentially life-threatening apnoeic episodes. Comparable results in terms of analgesia were reported from a contemporary controlled trial conducted by Rutter et al. (1980), although no estimates of respiratory depression were made in this study.

In clinical practice there is rarely any opportunity to tailor loading and maintenance infusion rates on the basis of known kinetic parameters for the individual, so a more empirical approach is taken. An intravenous loading dose is invariably used, based either on the amount of drug required to produce initial analgesia or on averaged data for the steady-state volume of distribution and minimum effective blood concentration. Maintenance infusion rates are then adjusted by monitoring response to pain and the occurrence of respiratory rate depression (below 8 breaths per minute). A typical prescription for a postoperative morphine infusion in an adult is 8 to 10mg over 30 minutes, then 2 to 2.5 mg/hour.

3.2 Patient-Controlled Intravenous Infusions

This is a slight misnomer since the prescribing physician retains overall control of the type and total dose of the drug administered, as well as the minimum interval between increments and the rate at which each increment is administered. Within these constraints, however, the awake and responding patient is able to modify analgesic intake to match their individual requirement. Described by Sechzer in 1968 as a component of a pain evaluation system, this concept is being widely studied and purpose-built equipment has been described by Evans et al. (1976), Tamsen et al. (1979) and Hull et al. (1981).

The basis of this technique is as follows: the patient perceiving pain triggers an infusion of analgesic drug which reduces or abolishes the pain thus 'closing the loop' (fig. 2). When the analgesic effect wanes this sequence is repeated, the patient thus maintaining a mainly pain-free state. The simpler commercially available apparatus such as the 'Cardiff Palliator' closely follow this principle, but more complex microprocessor controlled infusion pumps (Hull and Sibbald, 1981) provide, in addition, a background continuous infusion which is updated automatically according to the patient's demand pattern. In this way the pain episodes (which trigger the infusion) are kept at a minimum consistent with the on-demand principle.

Although a fascinating research tool, and by definition the best way to control drug therapy for the symptomatic relief of pain, patient-controlled analgesic infusions have several limitations at the clinical level. The equipment is expensive, the patient requires previous instruction in its use, and it requires that the patient be awake and responding to maintain drug delivery. Periods of sleep may thus result in inadequate plasma concentrations of analgesic, and pain recurrence.

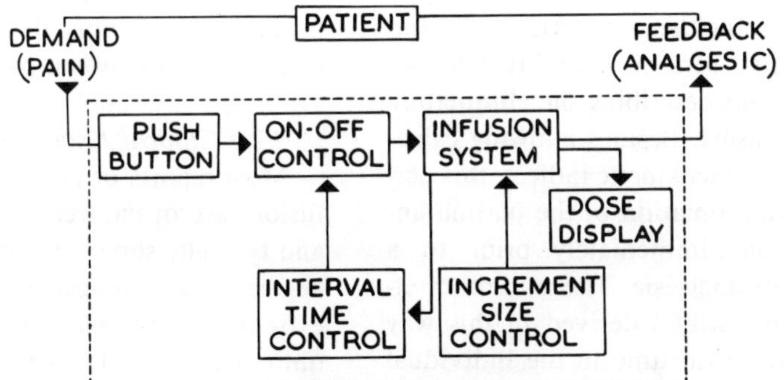

Fig. 2. Diagrammatic representation of control system for a simple patient controlled-analgesia system. Patient input is usually by means of a hand-held button.

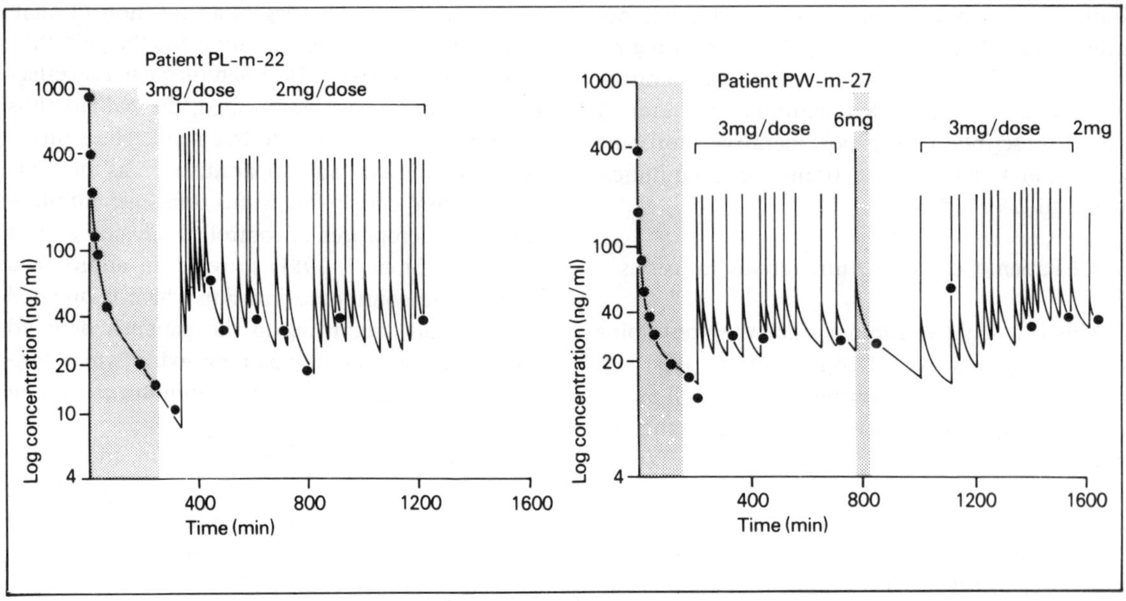

Fig. 3. Computer-calculated plasma concentration of morphine base during surgery under general anaesthesia ▩ and postoperative patient-controlled analgesic therapy in 2 patients; ● = measured plasma concentrations (Dahlström et al. 1982).

3.2.1 Pharmacokinetic Considerations

Tamsen et al. (1982a,b,c) and Dahlstrom (1982) used patient-controlled analgesia to study the multiple-dose pharmacokinetics of pethidine, ketobemidone and morphine. Plasma concentration data accumulated during the peroperative and immediate postoperative periods were fitted to polyexponential functions describing the elimination of drug from the plasma. Besides allowing calculation of various pharmacokinetic indices, this permitted retrospective estimation of the plasma analgesic concentrations immediately prior to a patient's demand for analgesia. The minimum effective concentration (MEC) derived in this way changed only slightly with time in the individual patient, and the patients self-administered analgesic to maintain a pseudo-steady state (figs 3 and 4). The mean plasma MECs of pethidine in these studies were in agreement with the analgesic concentration suggested by Stapleton et al. (1979) and Austin (1980), but individual MEC means varied 7-fold within the group of 20 patients. Individual analgesic requirements correlated with individual MEC, but not with any anthropomorphic or pharmacokinetic variables (total plasma clearance, elimination half-life, etc.). This suggests that pharmacodynamic factors (variation in individual MECs) are more important than pharmacokinetic factors in explaining the large variation in analgesic demand between patients.

3.2.2 Clinical Experience

Most reports of patient-controlled analgesic infusions are in the treatment of postoperative pain and typically show very good relief of pain, a high degree of patient acceptance and, incidentally, an extreme between-patient variation in analgesic requirement (e.g. Harmer et al., 1983; Sprigge and Otton, 1983). A further obvious application is in making comparisons between drugs. Slattery et al. (1981) compared pethidine and meptazinol after upper abdominal surgery and found both drugs were able to produce good relief of pain, although meptazinol produced significantly more nausea at the dose level required. The amount of drug consumed in this type of double-blind study is a relatively unbiased estimate of true requirement and sometimes grossly at variance with results from single-dose observer-scored studies of dose and effect.

4. Spinal Administration

The pioneering animal studies conducted by Yaksh and Rudy (1976), which showed a spinal site of action of intrathecally injected opiates, ushered in a new and exciting era in clinical pain therapy. Extension of this concept to intrathecal and epidural injection in man (Behar et al., 1979; Wang et al., 1979) was subsequently followed by many clinical reports and scientific studies examining the specific actions, dose-response relationships, pharmacokinetics and long term responses of spinal opiate injections.

4.1 Intrathecal Administration

Opioid receptors (including sub-types 'μ' and 'k') are present at several sites in the outer laminae of the dorsal horn of the spinal cord. It is not known which of these receptors subserve nociception in man nor is the mechanism of analgesic action known, though excitation (or disinhibition) of inhibitory interneurons or direct post-synaptic inhibition of transmitter cells is proposed. Generation of direct analgesic action at a spinal level requires an exogenously administered agent to first penetrate the superficial neurons of the cord before gaining access to deeper opioid receptor sites. Even with direct intrathecal injections, this leads to a delay of 30 minutes before the full effect is developed (Baraka et al., 1981).

Studies on intrathecal opiates provide an important insight into the contribution of spinally mediated analgesia to the total analgesic effect. An intrathecal injection of morphine 0.5mg is a massive dose by comparison with that which enters the CNS after a single administration by any other route. Paalzow (1982) calculated that only 0.1% of the amount given distributes to the entire CNS – i.e. 10μg for a normal 10mg dose. Despite this, the resultant analgesic effect is not as profound as might

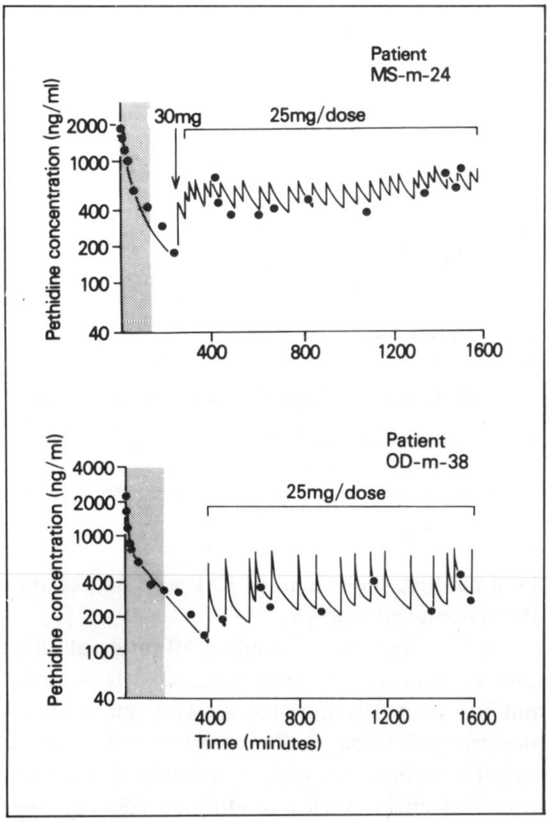

Fig. 4. Computer-calculated plasma concentrations of pethidine base during surgery and general anaesthesia ▨ and postoperative patient-controlled analgesic therapy in 2 patients; ● = measured plasma concentrations (Tamsen et al. 1982b).

be expected, for two reasons. Firstly, much of the analgesic action of opiates is derived from higher levels in the CNS at the periaqueductal grey neurons in the midbrain, nucleus raphe magnus and rostral ventral medulla, and drug concentration at these sites may be relatively low. Secondly, the spinal actions appear to be more specific for some forms of pain than for others. Deep and duller forms of somatic pain are better relieved than sharp pains of acute injury or the pain of primary neurological disease.

4.1.1 Drug Disposition

After entry into the cerebrospinal fluid (CSF), drug disposition will be determined by factors of

Table I. *In vitro* receptor binding affinities

Opioid	K_D (nmol/L)
Lofentanil[a]	0.06
Sufentanil[a]	0.13
Fentanyl[b]	0.5
Buprenorphine[b]	1.13
Naloxone[a]	5.2
Morphine	10 (approx.)
Pethidine	10,000 (approx.)

a Data from Leysen et al. (1983).
b Data from Boas and Villiger (1985).

local binding, movement of CSF and uptake into the systemic circulation.

The *in vitro* specific binding affinities of clinically available opiates range from K_D 10,000 to 0.5 nmol/L, with pethidine the weakest and fentanyl the strongest (table I). This feature will to some extent determine the dose required and the time-course of effect: weaker binding necessitates high doses whilst strong binding gives extended duration and smaller dosage requirements.

Circulation patterns within the dural sac are of importance since the cephalad flow of CSF as it traverses the cisterns to be absorbed at the arachnoid villae will transport intrathecally administered opiate to the brain stem. Reports both of extension of analgesia (Bromage et al., 1982) and delayed respiratory depression (Gustaffson et al., 1982) have drawn attention to the clinical relevance of this drug movement.

The rate of uptake into the systemic circulation is primarily determined by the lipid solubility of the opiate. Intrathecal injection of buprenorphine (a highly lipid-soluble drug) is followed by rapid systemic uptake so that the plasma concentrations are almost the same as those following intramuscular injections of similar doses (unpublished data, Boas and Villiger). Morphine is retained within the dural sac to a far greater extent and – with very little systemic uptake – has a more marked regional specificity of action.

4.1.2 Drug Choice

It is likely that there will prove to be a close correlation between duration and intensity of spinally mediated analgesic action and the risk of undesired side effects such as respiratory depression, itch and urinary retention. Morphine is currently the 'standard' since it produces the longest duration of analgesia (12 to 24 hours in patients who have not previously received opiates), although it also has the greatest incidence of side effects. Prolonged duration of action is desirable since intrathecal injection is a 'once only' technique (unlike epidural injections where a 16 or 18 guage nylon cannula can be left *in situ* for repeated injections). Spinal injections of other more lipid-soluble opiates would not appear to confer any great therapeutic advantage over conventional routes of administration because of their rapid transfer out of the CSF.

There is no strong evidence to support the use of preservative-free opiate solutions. Preliminary data suggest that ordinary commercial preparations for parenteral use are free of irritant effects (Boas et al., 1982).

4.1.3 Clinical Experience

Current use of intrathecal opiates is limited to concurrent administration with local anaesthetics in spinal anaesthesia (Cunningham et al., 1983), and to occasional use in the treatment of cancer pain. In obstetrics, intrathecal morphine provided adequate analgesia for the first stage of labour but required supplementation with local anaesthetic drugs for the second stage (Baraka et al., 1981; Scott et al., 1980). The development of itch, nausea and vomiting, urinary retention and respiratory depression in particular (Davies et al., 1980) have restricted use of all intrathecal opiates, so that this technique is no longer advocated for routine use in obstetric or postoperative pain relief. As mentioned above, small doses of morphine in conjunction with spinal anaesthesia give postoperative extension of analgesia, although the risk of severe respiratory depression of approximately 1 case per 600, occurring as late as 6 to 12 hours post-injection (Gustaffson et al., 1982) is sufficient to make this a high risk procedure for an unsupervised patient.

4.2 Epidural Administration

The epidural route provides a major advantage in that, as with local anaesthetic drugs, the use of epidural cannulae allow for repeat injections to sustain analgesia. Duration of effect is not then so critical a factor in the choice of opiate, although the analgesia is potentially associated with the same side effects and depressant actions as direct intrathecal injection.

The true role of epidural opiates in routine pain management is not yet known. The choice of drugs other than morphine, for reasons of safety, inevitably means that any differences between epidural and conventionally administered parenteral opiates become harder to discern. Whether the benefits available in terms of pain control outweigh the side effects and the added expenses of close patient supervision, remains to be seen.

4.2.1 Disposition

The critical distinction between the epidural and intrathecal routes is the extent to which drug in the epidural space is transferred to the intrathecal as opposed to the systemic circulation. *In vitro* studies on dural transfer by Moore et al. (1982) suggest molecular weight rather than lipid solubility as the most important factor. However, transfer into the CNS is by a number of other routes apart from dural transfer (via spinal cord blood supply, and diffusion along axons), so there are multiple factors to consider. These studies also predict a far higher *in vitro* degree of transdural transfer of morphine than buprenorphine (20% *vs* 0.17%) and indeed in clinical practice morphine seems to be readily transferred since doses of about 6mg produce analgesia for 8 to 12 hours. The systemic levels attained with this dose barely reach analgesic concentrations in the arterial blood, and then only for the first hour.

As with intrathecal administration, opiate is not restricted solely to the level of injection within the spinal cord. Irrespective of the particular drug, the volume used or the segmental level of the epidural injection, once within the CSF drug is carried towards the brain stem. However, clinical evidence of this spread is not readily observed with drugs other than morphine, again probably because their higher lipid solubility allows for greater systemic uptake from the dural sac as the drug is transported.

4.2.2 Drug Choice

Within the range of commercially available agents, drug choice is determined to some extent by the clinical objective. The most profound and extended analgesic action is obtained with morphine in doses of about 5 to 7mg, with 1 : 200,000 adrenaline (epinephrine) added to provide a faster onset and further prolongation of analgesia. Other drugs studied include pethidine, fentanyl, methadone and the partial agonists buprenorphine and nalbuphine. Analgesia tends to be less profound, less regionally specific and of lesser duration with all these agents than with morphine. Systemic blood concentrations reach analgesic concentrations because higher doses need to be given more frequently (every 4 to 6 hours) to sustain good analgesia, and some of the selectivity of action is inevitably lost.

On a theoretical basis, agonist agents with high affinity for spinal receptors and with high lipid solubility might be expected to give enhanced regional specificity. A small dose given intrathecally or epidurally could then bind firmly with the receptor site so that subsequent kinetic shifts would not diminish analgesic intensity or duration, and rostral intrathecal spread could be readily absorbed. Newer opiates such as lofentanyl and sufentanyl exhibit some of these pharmacological features, and clinical studies on their use are awaited with interest.

4.2.3 Clinical Experience

In comparative studies morphine has generally proved to be the most effective agent for epidural analgesia but risk-to-benefit considerations have confined its use to those patients at greatest risk from pain-induced complications, such as those with coronary ischaemia and chest disease. The management of crushed chest injury has been quite dramatically improved allowing patients with major chest wall injury to be managed with epidural morphine rather than assisted ventilation. Some centres routinely use epidural pethidine or fentanyl to provide postoperative analgesia following epidural local anaesthetic block for lower abdominal surgery, especially caesarean section. Accepting a relatively shorter duration of effect than with morphine, the epidural is 'topped up' with more opiate as necessary. A typical initial dose would be pethidine 50mg in 10ml.

5. Conclusions

Important advances in methods of administering opiates for analgesia have occurred in recent years. Oral administration of regular or sustained-release preparations at fixed intervals, the availability of buprenorphine for sublingual administration, continuous intravenous infusions, patient-controlled intravenous administration, and intrathecal or epidural administration of opiates all offer potential advantages over traditional 'as needed' parenteral administration in certain clinical settings.

References

Austin KL, Stapleton JV and Mather LE. Multiple intramuscular injections: a major source of variability in analgesic response to meperidine. Pain 8: 47-62, 1980

Austin KL, Stapleton JV and Mather LE. Rate of formation of norpethidine from pethidine. British Journal of Anaesthesia 53: 255-258, 1981

Baraka A, Noueihid R and Hajj S. Intrathecal injection of morphine for obstetric analgesia. Anesthesiology 54: 136-140, 1981

Behar M, Magora F, Olshwang D and Davidson JT. Epidural morphine in treatment of pain. Lancet 1: 527-529, 1979

Boas RA, Taylor KM, Villiger JW, Cahill V and Synek B. Epidural opiate analgesia. New Zealand Medical Journal 95: 84, 1982

Boas RA and Villiger JW. Clinical actions of fentanyl and buprenorphine. British Journal of Anaesthesia 57: 192-196, 1985

Bromage PR, Camporesi EM, Duvant PA and Neilson, CH. Rostral spread of epidural morphine. Anesthesiology 56: 431-436, 1982

Brown AS. Absorption of analgesics from the buccal mucous membrane. Practitioner 196: 125-126, 1966

Bullingham RES, McQuay HJ, Porter EJB, Allen MC and Moore RA. Sublingual buprenorphine used postoperatively: ten hour plasma drug concentration analysis. British Journal of Clinical Pharmacology 13: 665-673, 1982

Bullingham RES, O'Sullivan G, McQuay HJ, Poppleton P, Rolfe M, et al. Mandatory sublingual buprenorphine for postoperative pain. Anaesthesia 39: 329-334, 1984

Catling JA, Pinto DM, Jordan C and Jones RG. Respiratory effects of analgesia after cholecystectomy: comparison of continuous and intermittent papaveretum. British Medical Journal 280: 12-13, 1980

Church JJ. Continuous narcotic infusions for relief of postoperative pain. British Medical Journal 1: 977-979, 1979

Cowan A, Lewis JW and Macfarlane IR. Agonist and antagonist properties of buprenorphine, a new antinociceptive agent. British Journal of Pharmacology 60: 537-545, 1977

Cunningham AJ, McKenna JA and Skene DS. Single injection spinal anaesthesia with amethocaine and morphine for transurethral prostatectomy. British Journal of Anaesthesia 55: 423-427, 1983

Dahlstrom B, Tamsen A, Paalzow L and Hartvig P. Patient controlled analgesic therapy, Part IV: Pharmacokinetics and analgesic plasma concentrations of morphine. Clinical Pharmacokinetics 7: 266-279, 1982

Davies GK, Tolhurst-Cleaver CL and James TL. Respiratory depression after intrathecal narcotics. Anaesthesia 35: 1080-1083, 1980

Edge WG, Cooper GM and Morgan M. Analgesic effects of sublingual buprenorphine. Anaesthesia 34: 463-467, 1979

Ellis R, Haines D, Shah R, Cotton B and Smith, G. Pain relief after abdominal surgery – a comparison of I.M. morphine, sublingual buprenorphine and self-administered I.V. pethidine. British Journal of Anaesthesia 54: 421-427, 1982

Evans JM, Rosen M, MacCarthy J and Hogg MIJ. Apparatus for patient controlled administration of intravenous narcotics during labour. Lancet 1: 17-18, 1976

Fell D, Chmielewski A and Smith G. Postoperative analgesia with controlled-release morphine sulphate: Comparison with intramuscular morphine. British Medical Journal 285: 92-94, 1982

Fry ENS. Relief of pain after surgery – a comparison of sublingual buprenorphine and intramuscular papaveretum, Anaesthesia 34: 549-551, 1979

Gustafsson LL, Schildt B and Jacobsen K. Adverse effects of extradural and intrathecal opiates: report of a nationwide survey in Sweden. British Journal of Anaesthesia 54: 479-486, 1982

Hambrook JM and Rance MJ. The interaction of buprenorphine and the opiate receptor: lipophilicty as a determining factor in drug receptor kinetics. In Kosterlitz (Ed.) Opiates and endogenous opioid peptides, p. 295, Elsevier, Amsterdam, Biomedical Press, North Holland, 1976

Hanks GW, Rose NM, Aherne GW and Piall EM. Controlled release morphine tablets – a double blind trial in dental patients. British Journal of Anaesthesia 53: 1259-1263, 1981

Harmer M, Slattery PJ, Rosen M and Vickers MD. Comparison between buprenorphine and pentazocine given i.v. on demand in the control of postoperative pain. British Journal of Anaesthesia 55: 21-25, 1983

Heel RC, Brogden RN, Speight TM and Avery GS. Buprenorphine: a review of its pharmacological properties and therapeutic efficacy. Drugs 17: 81-110, 1979

Hull C and Sibbald A. Control of postoperative pain by interactive demand analgesia. British Journal of Anaesthesia 53: 385-391 1981

Iwamoto K and Klaassen, CD. First-pass effect of morphine in rats. Journal of Pharmacology and Experimental Therapeutics 200: 236-243, 1977

Keeri-Szanto M and Heaman S. Postoperative on-demand analgesia. Surgery, Gynaecology and Obstetrics 134: 647-651, 1972

Leslie ST, Rhodes A and Black FM. Controlled release morphine

sulphate tablets – a study in normal volunteers. British Journal of Clinical Pharmacology 9: 531-534, 1980
Leysen JE, Gommeren W and Niemegeers CJE. [^{3}H] Sufantanil, a spurerior lingand for opiate receptors binding properties and regional distribution in rat brain and spinal cord. European Journal of Pharmacology 87: 209-225, 1983
Marks RM and Sachar EJ. Undertreatment of medical inpatients with narcotic analgesics. Annals of Internal Medicine 78: 173-181, 1973
Mather LE, Tucker GT, Phlug AE, Lindop MJ and Wilderson C. Meperidine kinetics in man. Clinical Pharmacology and Therapeutics 17: 21-30, 1975
Mather LE and Glynn CJ. The minimum effective analgetic blood concentration of pethidine in patients with intractable painBritish Journal of Clinical Pharmacology 14: 385-390, 1982
McQuay HJ, Bullingham RES, Paterson GMC and Moore RA. The clinical effects of buprenorphine during and after operation. British Journal of Anaesthesia 52: 1013-1019, 1980
Melzack R, Mount BM and Gordon JM. The Brompton mixture versus morphine solution given orally: effects on pain. Canadian Medical Association Journal 120: 435-438, 1979
Moore RA, Bullingham RES, McQuay HJ, Hand CW, Aspel JB et al. Dural permeability to narcotics: in vitro determination and application to extradural administration. British Journal of Anaesthesia 54: 1117-1128, 1982
Neumann PB, Henrickson H, Grosman N and Christensen CB. Plasma morphine concentrations during chronic oral administration in patients with cancer pain. Pain 13: 247-252, 1982
Nordberg G, Hedner T, Mellstrand T and Dahlstrom B. Pharmacokinetic aspects of intrathecal morphine analgesia. Anesthesiology 60: 448-454, 1984
Nordberg G, Hedner T, Mellstrandt T and Borg, L. Pharmacokinetics of epidural morphine in man. European Journal of Clinical Pharmacology 26: 233-237, 1984
Paalzow LK. Pharmacokinetic aspects of optimal pain treatment. Acta Anaesthesiologica Scandanavica 74 (Suppl.): 37-43, 1982
Pond SM, Tong T, Benowitz NL, Jacob P and Rigod J. Presystemic metabolism of meperidine to normeperidine in normal and cirrhotic subjects. Clinical Pharmacology and Therapeutics 30: 183-188, 1981
Rutter PR, Murphy F and Dudley HAF. Morphine: controlled trial of different methods of administration for postoperative pain relief. British Medical Journal 280: 12-13, 1980
Sawe J, Dahlstrom B, Paalzow L and Rane A. Morphine kinetics in cancer patients. Clinical Pharmacology and Therapeutics 30: 629-635, 1981
Sawe J, Dahlstrom B and Rane A. Steadystate kinetics and analgesic effect of oral morphine in cancer patients. European Journal of Clinical Pharmacology 24: 537-542, 1983
Scott PV, Bowen FE, Cartwright P, Mohan Rao BC, Deeley D, et al. Intrathecal morphine as sole analgesic during labour. British Medical Journal 281: 351-353, 1980
Sechzer PH. Objective measurement of pain. Anesthesiology 1: 209-210, 1968
Shih APL, Robinson K and Au WYW. Determination of therapeutic serum concentration of oral and parenteral meperidine by gas liquid chromatography. European Journal of Clinical Pharmacology 9: 451-456, 1976
Slattery PJ, Harmer M, Rosen M and Vickers MD. Comparison of meptazinol and pethidine given I.V. on demand in the management of postoperative pain. British Journal of Anaesthesia 53: 927-931, 1981
Sprigge JS and Otton PE. Nalbuphine versus meperidine for postoperative analgesia: a double-blind comparison using the patient controlled analgesic technique. Canadian Anaesthetists Society Journal 30: 517-521, 1983
Stapleton JV, Austin KL and Mather LE. Postoperative pain. British Medical Journal 2: 1499, 1978
Stapleton JV, Austin KL and Mather LE. A pharmacokinetic approach to postoperative pain: continuous infusion of pethidine. Anaesthesia and Intensive Care 7: 25-32, 1979
Tamsen A, Hartvig P, Dahlstrom B, Lindstrom B and Holmdahl MH. Patient controlled analgesic therapy in the early postoperative period. Acta Anaesthesiologica Scandinavica 23: 462-470, 1979
Tamsen A, Hartvig P, Fagerlund C and Dahlstrom B. Patient controlled analgesic therapy I: Pharmacokinetics of pethidine in the perioperative and postoperative period. Clinical Pharmacokinetics 7: 149-163, 1982a
Tamsen A, Hartvig P, Fagerlund C and Dahlstrom B. Patient-controlled analgesic therapy, part II: Individual analgesic demand and analgesic plasma concentrations of pethidine in postoperative pain. Clinical Pharmacokinetics 7: 164-175, 1982b
Tamsen A, Bondesson U, Dahlstrom B and Hartvig P. Patient-controlled analgesic therapy, part III. Pharmacokinetics and plasma concentrations of ketobemidone. Clinical Pharmacokinetics 7: 252-265, 1982c
Twycross RG. Choice of strong analgesic in terminal cancer: diamorphine or morphine? Pain 3: 93-104, 1977
Twycross RG. Relief of pain. In Saunders (Ed.) The management of terminal disease, pp. 65-92, Arnold, London, 1978
Twycross RG. Narcotic analgesics in clinical practice. In Bonica et al., (Eds) Advances in pain research and therapy, Vol. 5, pp. 435-459, Raven Press, New York, 1983
Walsh TD. Oral morphine in chronic cancer pain. Pain 18: 1-11, 1984
Wang JK, Nauss LA and Thomas JE. Pain relief by intrathecally applied morphine in man. Anesthesiology 50: 149-151, 1979
Way EL, Young JM and Kemp JW. Metabolism of heroin and its pharmacological implications. Bulletin on Narcotics 17: 25, 1965
Yaksh TL and Rudy TA. Analgesia mediated by a direct spinal action of narcotics. Science 192: 1357-1358, 1976

Address for correspondence and reprints: Dr *P.J. Slattery*, Department of Pharmacology and Clinical Pharmacology, University of Auckland School of Medicine, Private Bag, Auckland (New Zealand).

Drugs 30: 552-560 (1985)
0012-6667/85/0012-0552/$04.50/0

The Urticarias
Current Concepts in Pathogenesis and Treatment

Kenneth P. Mathews

Division of Allergy, Department of Internal Medicine, University of Michigan Medical School, Ann Arbor

Summary

Urticaria is a very common disease which is often associated with angioedema. Release of histamine and perhaps other mediators from the cutaneous mast cells is believed to be the likeliest cause for the development of these wheals in most instances, but there may be both non-immunological as well as immunological inputs into this final common pathway. The former include trauma, cholinergic mechanisms and non-immunological histamine release by drugs. Immune mechanisms most commonly are of the IgE-mediated type, but occasionally the activation of complement or other mediators of hypersensitivity may be involved.

Drug and food allergy are among the most common causes of acute urticaria, but there are numerous other possibilities which mandate a thorough general medical history and physical examination (including ruling out infection, connective tissue disease and neoplasms). In cases of chronic *urticaria, when the lesions have persisted for longer than about 2 months, no cause for the disease is discernable in most instances. However, in these cases, as well as in acute urticaria, symptomatic treatment generally can provide substantial symptom relief, with emphasis on the astute use of various types of antihistamines.*

It has been estimated that in North America about 20% of the populace experiences at least 1 episode of urticaria during their lifetime (Mathews, 1983). It occurs in all age groups, but chronic urticaria (where lesions occur frequently or continuously for longer than about 6 weeks) is more common in middle age, especially in women. As discussed below, certain types of urticaria appear to occur more often in atopic persons, but the majority of afflicted individuals are not atopic. About half of adult urticaria patients also experience angioedema (Warin and Champion, 1974).

1. Pathophysiology

Historically, efforts to delineate the pathogenesis of urticaria initially focused on a possible role for histamine, since intracutaneous injections of histamine in humans reproduce the pruritic wheal-and-flare reaction typical for urticaria. More recently it has been shown that cutaneous mast cell and histamine content are increased in chronic urticaria patients (Natbony et al., 1983; Phanuphak et al., 1980). Although the capacity of antihistaminic drugs to inhibit urtication in many instances is suggestive, it does not firmly prove a role for histamine, since most of these drugs have additional pharmacological effects. Some of the most impressive evidence in support of a role for histamine in urticaria comes from the study of urticarias arising from a physical stimulus. Several investigators have found that if one places the distal extremity of a patient with cold urticaria in cold water, there is a transient elevation of histamine levels in venous plasma from the chilled extremity as it i3rewarmed. Transient elevations in plasma histamine have also been found after challenging some patients with solar urticaria, dermographism, cholinergic urticaria, and aquagenic urticaria. However, it should be noted that these observations do not prove that histamine actually is causing the skin lesions, since other mast cell products can also be found in these venous effluents, including a high-molecular-weight neutrophil chemotactic factor and 3 types of eosinophil chemotactic factors (Wasserman et al., 1982).

Sir Thomas Lewis (1927) in particular called attention to the possible role of histamine in the pathogenesis of urticaria during the 1920s in an era when the concept had also evolved that allergic symptoms were due to histamine. Accordingly, the conclusion was reached that urticaria must be due to allergy, a concept that completely dominated thinking about urticaria for decades. Although the concept is valid for many cases of *acute* urticaria, it gradually became apparent that no IgE-mediated allergy could be discovered in the large majority of cases of *chronic* urticaria. One possibility is that histamine release may occur as a result of non-immunological mechanisms or by immune processes not involving IgE. An example of the former is cholinergic urticaria. Patients afflicted with this disorder have hives featuring tiny wheals surrounded by large areas of erythema; these lesions are brought on by exertion, heat, or emotional stress (Grant et al., 1936). Trauma is another mechanism for non-immunological histamine release: examples include welts resulting from a whip lash or the urtication that develops when one rubs cutaneous lesions of urticaria pigmentosa, which are benign mast cell tumours. In addition, pharmacologists have known for decades that there are a large number of compounds which produce histamine release the first time that animal tissues are perfused with them (Paton, 1957). These include many drugs used clinically, including morphine, codeine, pethidine (meperidine), d-tubocurarine, polymyxin antibiotics, and thiamine. Indeed, it is a common practice to use codeine as a positive control in performing ordinary allergy skin testing, since almost all normal humans give a wheal-and-erythema response to this agent. Thus, one may conceptualise a final pathway leading to urticaria from mast cell mediator release into which there may be both non-immunological and immunological inputs (fig. 1).

The possible role of complement has been assessed in an attempt to account for urticaria not explicable on an IgE-mediated allergic basis. Since the C5a, C3a, and C4a anaphylatoxins are known to be very potent histamine releasers from mast cells, their generation would provide a means whereby complement activation could result in urticaria (Schwartz et al., 1982). This might explain some cases of urticaria associated with cryoglobulinaemia, connective tissue disease (e.g. systemic lupus erythematosus), leucocytoclastic vasculitis, localised heat urticaria (sometimes), idiopathic urticaria or angioedema (rarely), and on rare occasions some drugs such as lignocaine (lidocaine) and procarbazine.

In addition to histamine and complement, other biologically active substances such as kinins, arachidonic acid metabolites, plasmin, or serotonin (5-hydroxytryptamine) could play a pathogenetic role in some cases of urticaria and/or angioedema. Kinin generation could occur secondarily as a result of either the secretion of basophil kallikrein or the cleavage of kininogen after its escape into connective tissue consequent to increased vascular permeability produced by histamine or other mediators. The possible involvement of arachidonic acid metabolites is suggested by the clinical observation that aspirin and other cyclo-oxygenase inhibitors often exacerbate chronic urticaria, suggesting a possible role for lipoxygenase metabolites. There also is evidence that substance P, a neuropeptide, is a histamine liberator and may be responsible for the 'flare' surrounding urticarial wheals. Another plausible approach is to postulate a deficiency of an inhibitor of some urticariogenic substance. The documented role of complement Cl inhibitor deficiency in hereditary angioedema lends credence to this possibility. However, my studies of a large number of sera from patients with chronic idiopathic urticaria and angioedema have shown very infrequent subnormal values of the major serum protease inhibitors. We have reported a single family afflicted with serum carboxypeptidase N (anaphylatoxin inactivator) deficiency (Mathews et al., 1980).

It is presumed that impaired breakdown of the anaphylatoxins or bradykinin predisposed the propositus of this family to the frequent attacks of angioedema and urticaria which he has had for the past 19 years.

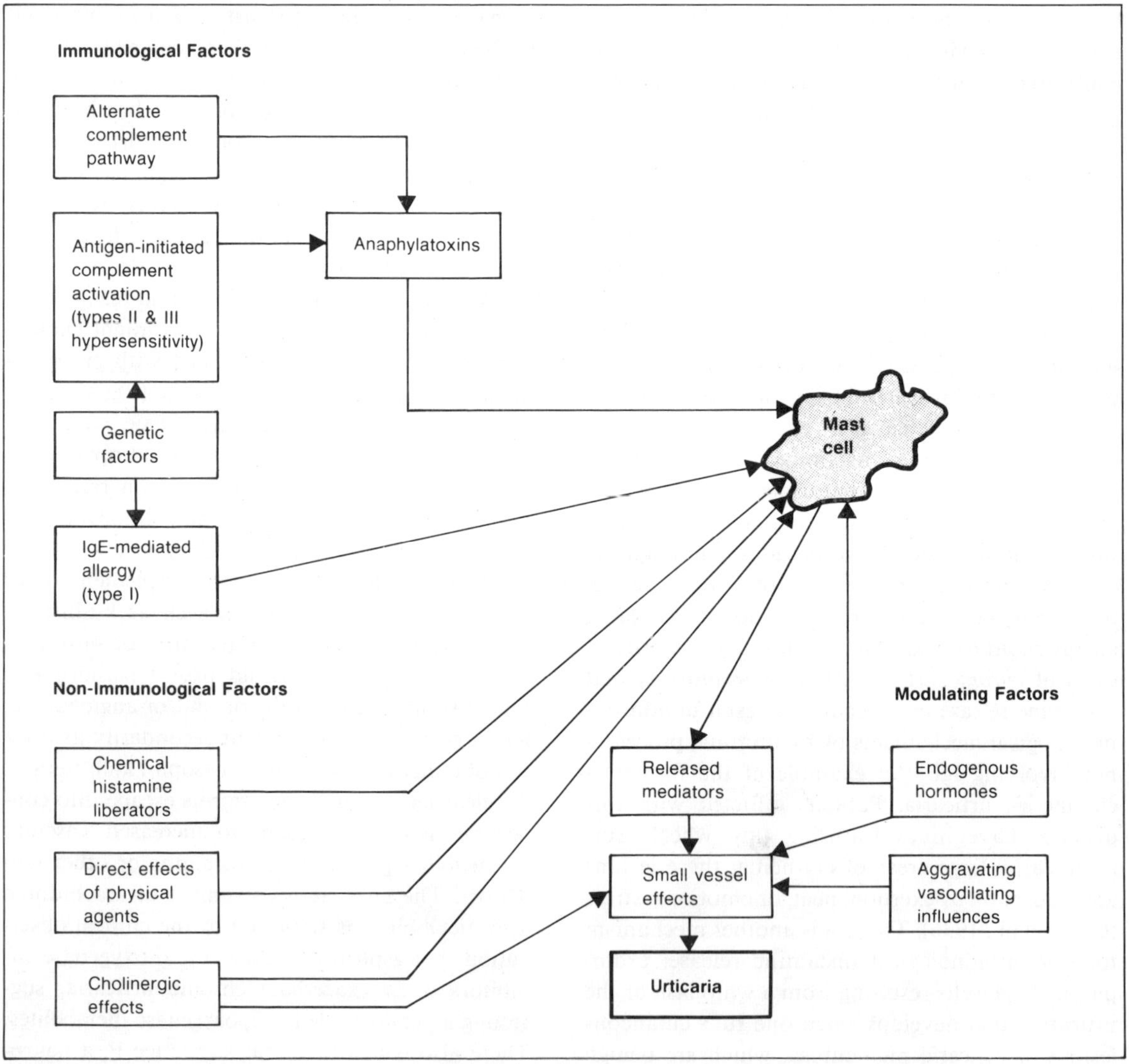

Fig. 1. Schematic representation of factors involved in producing urticaria (from Mathews, 1974).

As well as these factors that might play an underlying role in urticaria and angioedema, there are also a number of modulating factors which often are rather conspicuous clinically. These include factors and agents that produce cutaneous vasodilation, such as heat, exertion, alcoholic drinks, fever, emotional upsets, and hyperthyroidism. Other endocrine factors also may play a modulating role either by regulating mediator secretion or by direct effects on blood vessels. Also, some women have striking premenstrual exacerbations of their chronic urticaria, and in a few cases lesions appear only at such times. Finally, as discussed below, genetic factors are also involved in the pathogenesis of some types of urticaria.

2. *Clinical Assessment*

In a few instances the appearance of the lesions gives a clue to pathogenesis: cholinergic urticaria has been described above; linear wheals suggest dermographism; lesions limited to exposed areas suggest possible solar or cold urticaria; hives mainly on the lower extremities suggest urticarial vasculitis or papular urticaria; small perifollicular hives occur in aquagenic urticaria; and in urticaria pigmentosa there are persistent, pigmented, macular, papular or nodular lesions which urticate when rubbed. Unfortunately, however, in the vast majority of cases the appearance of the lesions gives no indication of the cause of urticaria or angioedema.

The search for possible clues about pathogenesis is appropriately initiated by the types of questions used to assess patients with other types of potentially allergic disease. When and where does the patient have symptoms? What agents has the patient suspected to cause difficulty? Especially vigorous 'detective work' is more likely to be productive in acute or intermittent cases, although at the outset one cannot differentiate acute urticaria from the beginning of chronic, idiopathic disease. Even in chronic cases the patient merits a reasonable effort at trying to identify a specific aetiology, but the low yield of success in such instances argues against an exhaustive and expensive assessment that is most likely to yield only frustration. Possibilities which should be considered are: drugs and foreign sera; foods and food additives; infection; psychic factors; inhalants; bites and stings; contact urticaria; connective tissue diseases; neoplasms; physical agents; genetic types; and miscellaneous factors.

Drugs and foreign sera are two of the most commonly identifiable causes of urticaria. Often IgE antibodies to a drug metabolite are presumed to cause the reaction, but, as discussed above, some drugs are pharmacological histamine liberators. The penicillins are the most common offenders, but numerous other medications have also been implicated. A careful history of *all* drugs taken by all possible routes of administration remains the cornerstone for diagnosing drug allergy.

In addition to drugs actually causing the difficulty, it is noteworthy that aspirin is said to cause exacerbations in up to 40% of cases of chronic urticaria, even though these patients continue to have difficulty when aspirin is assiduously avoided. Accordingly, it is common to advise patients with chronic urticaria that they should avoid this drug. Other drugs that inhibit cyclo-oxygenase, such as indomethacin, phenylbutazone, and other nonsteroidal anti-inflammatory agents, also have the potential for flaring urticaria. Paracetamol (acetaminophen) is a preferable analgesic for these patients.

In the community at large, many cases of *acute* urticaria or angioedema are caused by food allergy. Fish, seafood, nuts, peanuts, and egg are among the most common offenders, although numerous other foods are also culprits at times. This type of urticaria or angioedema appears to be more frequent in atopic than in non-atopic individuals, presumably because it is IgE mediated. As a cause for *chronic* urticaria or angioedema, however, food allergy only rarely can be implicated. A retrospective food diary is of value in making the diagnosis in acute, sporadic cases, whereas elimination diets are employed when symptoms are frequent or continuous.

In addition to the food antigens themselves, there has been much interest in the possibility that

Table I. Physical agents producing urticaria (from Mathews, 1980)

1. **Mechanical Urticarias**
   Dermatographism
   Primary: idiopathic; allergic
   Secondary: cutaneous mastocytosis
   Transient forms
   Delayed-pressure urticaria
   Immediate-pressure urticaria
2. **Thermal Urticarias**
   Cold
   Acquired: idiopathic; associated with cryoglobulinaemia, cryofibrinogenaemia, or cold haemolysins; transient forms associated with other factors
   Delayed cold-induced urticaria
   Familial cold urticaria
   Heat
   Cholinergic
   Localised heat urticaria
   Familial localised heat urticaria of delayed type
3. **Solar Urticarias**
   Probably allergic types
   Associated with abnormal protoporphyrin metabolism
   Idiopathic types

food additives may cause urticaria or angioedema. An example is the use of sodium or potassium sulphite or metabisulphite as antioxidants in such foods as lettuce, shrimp, or wines. Vegetable gums such as acacia, gum arabic, tragacanth, quince, carob seed, or carregeenan also have been known as occasional allergens for many years. Tartrazine yellow dye also is added to a large variety of foodstuffs — particularly coloured soft drinks. However, I doubt that this dye is a major and common cause of urticaria, partly since the amount required to provoke a response often substantially exceeds the amount likely to be encountered in an ordinary diet. It is also noteworthy that some elimination diets commonly used to rule out food allergy are essentially tartrazine free, thus indicating that the usual failure to improve speaks against tartrazine reactivity as well as to food allergy. Similar concerns apply to the question of whether other azodyes, benzoic acid, 4-hydroxybenzoic acid, and salicylates in foods are as important as claimed by some investigators.

Without reviewing in detail the other potential causes of urticaria noted above, it again should be emphasised that a thorough general medical assessment is needed to rule out such conditions as infection, connective tissue disease, or underlying neoplasms. With regard to the former, viral infection (especially in children) and occasionally parasitic infestation must be kept in mind, while previously emphasised chronic focal bacterial infection is of dubious importance. Physical agents producing urticaria are outlined in table I. Types which have been passively transferred by IgE include immediate type dermographism, idiopathic cold urticaria, and some types of solar urticaria. Genetic types are listed in table II. Miscellaneous forms include aquagenic urticaria and hives due to implanted materials, such as 'Vitallium' cups or retained myelographic contrast media.

2.1 Diagnostic Procedures

Needless to say, if the history or physical examination gives any clues about the cause(s) of the patient's urticaria, this should be pursued by the appropriate tests; these might include dietary intervention, tests for systemic lupus erythematosus, exercise test for cholinergic urticaria, the ice cube test, and delayed-pressure test. Skin tests with atopic allergens are likely to be helpful only in exceptional patients with suspected inhalant allergy or in some cases of suspected food allergy where the history is not diagnostic. In the many cases of chronic urti-

Table II. Hereditary forms of urticaria[a]

Urticaria, deafness and amyloidosis (Muckle-Wells syndrome)
Familial cold urticaria
Delayed cold-induced urticaria
Erythropoietic protoporphyria with solar urticaria
C3 inhibitor deficiency

a Hereditary and vibratory angioedema are not listed here since they are not associated with urticaria.

Table III. Diagnostic procedures to be considered in cases of apparently idiopathic, chronic urticaria

Detailed history
Test for dermographism
CBC, urinalysis, sedimentation rate, ANA and test panel
Food and food additive evaluation
?T3, T4, antithyroid microsomal antibodies
?Fresh stools for ova and parasites
?Chest roentgenogram
Complement tests (CH_{50}, C3, C4, Cl_q)[a]
?Skin biopsy[a]
Hepatitis B antigens and antibodies
?Cryoglobulins[a]
?Other tests for immune complexes[a]
?'Create history' by trying environmental changes

a Consider primarily in cases of suspected vasculitis, as suggested by high sedimentation rate, arthralgias, abnormal urine or other systemic symptoms or signs.

caria and angioedema where the history provides no clues about aetiology, it is reasonable to supplement the complete physical examination (which should include testing for dermographism) with a complete blood count, urinalysis, test panel, sedimentation rate, and antinuclear antigen test. In sporadic cases it is simple enough to have patients retroactively keep a diary of food ingested within 6 to 12 hours of their attacks. Beyond this point, the physician faces a difficult dilemma: there are many additional tests that may be helpful in a few patients, but the cost-effectiveness of these procedures is very poor when applied routinely to patients with chronic urticaria or angioedema (Jacobson et al., 1980). At some point the judicious physician must call a halt to diagnostic testing, accepting that these conditions often have no known cause, given our present state of knowledge. Endless testing not only is wasteful but also leads to increasing frustration on the part of both the patient and physician. Indeed, in cases of *chronic* urticaria, it generally is advisable to tell the patient at the outset that no specific cause is likely to be found (though an effort will be made) but that usually the disease can be controlled symptomatically until a spontaneous remission occurs. Some other diagnostic procedures which can be considered on a selective basis are listed in table III.

3. Treatment of Urticaria (Table IV)

3.1 Non-Drug Treatment

Obviously the preferred form of treatment for urticaria is *avoidance* of the causative agent(s) when this can be identified and when avoidance is feasible. This generally is the case when allergy to drugs, foods, inhalants, insects, and contactants is involved. In cases of papular urticaria due to insect bites, the family pets also may require therapy. An explanation of the disease process and its triggers should be helpful for patients with cholinergic urticaria, dermatographism, and perhaps delayed-pressure urticaria. Patients with cold allergy should be forewarned about the dangers of swimming in

Table IV. Therapeutic procedures: summary of the treatment of urticaria

Avoid identifiable cause(s) when possible	
Acute urticaria	
0.3ml 1:1000 adrenaline SC for adults; 0.1 ml/kg for children	
50mg diphenhydramine IM or IV when adrenaline is contraindicated	
Possibly teach self-administration of adrenaline	
Long term treatment	
None – if very mild	
H_1-antihistamines: gradually increase dose to big doses if needed and not excessively sedating (e.g. hydroxyzine, cyproheptadine, doxepin)	
New generation H_1-antihistamine (less sedative; e.g. astemizole, mequitazine, terfenadine)	
H_1-antihistamine plus ephedrine or terbutaline	
H_1- plus H_2-antihistamine	
Corticosteroid 'burst'	For disabling disease
Low-dose alternate day corticosteroid	For disabling disease
Treat underlying disease	

cool water and should never swim alone. Such common-sense measures as wearing warm socks and gloves help to protect against cold air, but in extreme cases wrapping most of the face in a scarf or wearing a ski face mask may be necessary. In cases of mild solar urticaria, simple precautionary measures such as wearing broad-brimmed hats and long sleeves may suffice. In more severe cases sun screens containing paraminobenzoic acid help to protect against light in the 285 to 320nm wavelengths may be required, and chloroquine has been reported to be helpful in some instances. Of course, if an underlying disease has been identified, therapy should be focused on this. Genetic counselling should be offered to families with the hereditary forms of these diseases. In addition to avoidance of possible causative factors, patients with chronic urticaria or angioedema are appropriately advised to avoid, to the extent feasible, previously mentioned potentiating factors such as alcoholic drinks, heat, exertion and aspirin.

Reassurance is another important aspect of therapy, since the cutaneous lesions often are more frightening in appearance than the generally favourable prognosis warrants. In reassuring patients, however, the physician should observe two caveats. One is the threat of laryngealoedema, particularly in patients who already have experienced swelling in the throat. The other caveat concerns the possible presence of a significant underlying disorder, such as a connective tissue disease, which is not apparent when the patient is first seen. Accordingly, periodic follow-up is important even though the skin lesions may be under control with suitable medications.

Desensitisation or immunotherapy has little to offer in the management of patients with urticaria and angioedema. The main exception would be patients with hymenoptera sensitivity together with occasional cases of prophylactic desensitisation to penicillin, insulin, or equine antisera. There also may be rare indications for immunotherapy with inhalants when urticaria accompanies respiratory allergy. Procedures to desensitise to cold and light are cumbersome and generally not very successful, although good results with psoralen-ultraviolet A (PUVA) treatment have been reported recently.

In actual practice, symptomatic treatment plays a prominent role in providing temporary relief of acute symptoms, in controlling the problem while investigations about possible pathogenesis are in progress, and in providing the main source of treatment in the majority of cases of chronic urticaria when no aetiological agent can be identified or eliminated.

3.2 Drug Treatment

At the outset it should be recalled that drugs themselves, taken perhaps for another purpose, are a common cause of urticaria, and thus stopping previously used drugs, when possible, is an important aspect of assessing these patients.

3.2.1 Adrenaline

Subcutaneously administered adrenaline (epinephrine) usually is the drug of choice for severe acute urticaria. Generally 0.3 ml of 1 : 1000 aqueous adrenaline is the dose for older children and adults, small children being given 0.01 ml/kg. If necessary, such doses could be repeated once or twice at intervals of 15 minutes or longer. Of course, another drug usually should be substituted in cases when adrenaline is contraindicated, such as in the older patient with a history of myocardial infarction or cardiac arrhythmias. A parenteral antihistamine, such as diphenhydramine 50mg intramuscularly or intravenously, could be tried in such cases. If the patient has had laryngeal oedema, the possible serious consequences of upper airway obstruction should be explained, and at the very least such an individual should be urged to seek medical assistance (which should include an injection of adrenaline) at the first symptoms suggesting a recurrence of laryngeal oedema. If this has been a recurrent problem, teaching such individuals to administer adrenaline to themselves should be considered. This involves having the patients practice self-injection (in the thigh with saline). However, ordinary solutions of adrenaline deteriorate rather rapidly unless kept refrigerated and in the dark. Accordingly, if available, it is desirable to have the patient carry a syringe preloaded with adrenaline solution containing a preservative which conserves its potency for more than a year even without refrigeration. An alternative device which injects adrenaline without resorting to a visible syringe or needle is also available in some countries. However, only in rare cases of unusually severe, acute urticaria is it necessary to have adrenaline immediately available for injection. Even in these instances it is important not to generate undue anxiety about laryngeal oedema. The only actual deaths from this cause which I am aware of followed hymenoptera stings or were associated with the hereditary form of angioedema.

3.2.2 Antihistamines

Antihistamines are the drugs of first choice in the more usual patients afflicted with mild or moderately severe recurrent or chronic urticaria. Most antihistamines of the H_1-blocking type provide some degree of benefit for most patients – especially in relieving pruritus. Sometimes larger-than-usual doses are required. The main problem is the frequently associated side effects, especially sedation; these tend to decrease in severity after a few days but may be persistently annoying. It is especially important when patients' work might result in injury if alertness is impaired. Sometimes giving these drugs only in the evening for the first few days may be helpful. Hydroxyzine is a potent antihistamine, but since drowsiness frequently occurs with its use, one may elect to start with a low dose, such as a 10mg tablet 4 times daily, and then increase the number of tablets taken at each dose (e.g. up to 50mg) until relief is obtained or the patient becomes excessively drowsy. Cyproheptadine is another commonly used H_1-type antihistamine and is generally considered to be the drug of choice in cold urticaria. Its side effects also include increased appetite and possible effects on pituitary function.

Although most commonly used as an antidepressant, doxepin is also a potent antihistamine, and is often effective in urticaria, but drowsiness again is a common side effect.

A new generation of very potent H_1-antihistamines is becoming available which do not cross the blood-brain barrier and thus do not produce drowsiness or other central nervous system effects includes astemizole, terfenadine and mequitazine. They are well worth a trial in patients in whom drowsiness with traditional antihistamines is a problem.

If a trial of several antihistamines fails to provide benefit, consideration can be given to supplementing these with an adrenergic agent, such as ephedrine or terbutaline. Indeed, ephedrine was the most commonly used drug for treating urticaria before the advent of the antihistamines. However, it infrequently has a potent effect in severe urticaria, but its side effects may tend to counteract drowsiness induced by antihistamines. Another option is to supplement H_1-antihistamines with an H_2-antagonist, such as cimetidine 300mg 4 times daily, or ranitidine. Although not regularly efficacious, controlled trials have shown benefit in some cases (Monroe et al., 1981). It is important not to give H_2-blockers alone, since urticaria may actually become worse – perhaps by blocking a negative feedback through H_2-receptors or by inhibiting histamine N-methyl transferase.

3.2.3 Corticosteroids

There are a few patients with severe urticaria/angioedema who do not respond to any of these measures but are benefited by corticosteroid therapy. In very refractory cases of disabling disease, it is therefore of interest to see whether the patient is benefited by a short 'burst' of prednisone or a similar drug. Of course, recurrence in a few days is the rule, but if the response to corticosteroids is dramatic, one may wish to reinstitute such treatment periodically during exacerbations. Rarely one may need to maintain the patient for a more prolonged period on a low dose preferably given every other day if possible. Prolonged treatment with large daily doses of corticosteroids is not acceptable, however, since the potential side effects of such treatment pose more of a threat to the patient's general health than the disease being treated.

3.2.4 Miscellaneous

Over the years innumerable other forms of

treatment for urticaria/angioedema have been tried but abandoned. In general, angioedema is less responsive than urticarial lesions. Patients with delayed pressure urticaria are especially refractory to treatment; they may respond to corticosteroids, and in a few cases indomethacin has provided relief (Sussman et al., 1982). Other recently used drugs have included doxantrazole and dapsone for urticaria associated with systemic lupus erythematosus. Of course, if urticaria is associated with some underlying disease process, such as an infection, connective disease or a neoplasm, appropriate treatment of the latter is imperative. No specific treatment is available for the rarer hereditary forms of urticaria listed above. Hereditary angioedema is a treatable disease which is beyond the scope of this discussion (Mathews, 1983).

References

Grant, R.T.; Pearson, R.S.B. and Comeau, W.J.: Observations on urticaria provoked by emotion, by exercise and by warming the body. Clinical Science 2: 253 (1936).

Jacobson, K.W.; Branch, L.B. and Nelson, H.S.: Laboratory tests in chronic urticaria. Journal of the American Medical Association 243: 1644 (1980).

Lewis, T.: The Blood Vessels of the Human and Their Responses (Shawn and Sons, London 1927).

Mathews, K.P.: A current view of urticaria. Medical Clinics of North America 58: 185 (1974).

Mathews, K.P.: Management of urticaria and angioedema. Journal of Allergy and Clinical Immunology 6: 347 (1980).

Mathews, K.P.: Urticaria and angioedema. Journal of Allergy and Clinical Immunology 72: 1 (1983).

Mathews, K.P.; Pan, P.M.; Gardner, N.J. and Hugli, T.E.: Familial carboxypeptidase N deficiency. Annals of Internal Medicine 99: 443 (1980).

Monroe, E.W.; Cohen, S.H.; Kalbfleisch, J. and Schulz, C.I.: Combined H_1 and H antihistamine therapy in chronic urticaria. Archives of Dermatology 117: 404 (1981).

Natbony, S.F.; Phillips, M.E.; Elias, J.M.; Godfrey, H.P. and Kaplan, A.P.: Histologic studies of chronic idiopathic urticaria. Journal of Allergy and Clinical Immunology 71: 177 (1983).

Phanuphak, P.; Schocket, A.C.; Arroyave, L.M. and Kohler, P.F.: Skin histamine in chronic urticaria. Journal of Allergy and Clinical Immunology 65: 371 (1980).

Paton, W.D.M.: Histamine release by compounds of simple chemical structure. Pharmacological Review 9: 269 (1957).

Schwartz, H.R.; McDuffie, F.C.; Black, L.F., Schroeter, A.L. and Conn, D.L.: Hypocomplementemic urticarial vasculitis. Mayo Clinic Proceedings 57: 231 (1982).

Sussman, E.L.; Harvey, R.P. and Schocket, A.L.: Delayed pressure urticaria. Journal of Allergy and Clinical Immunology 70: 337 (1982).

Warin, R.P. and Champion, R.H.: Urticaria. (W.B. Saunders, Philadelphia 1974).

Wasserman, S.I.; Austen, K.F. and Soter, N.A.: The functional and physicochemical characterization of three eosinophilotactic activities released into the circulation by cold challenge of patients with cold urticaria. Clinical and Experimental Immunology 47: 570 (1982).

Address for correspondence and reprints: Dr *K.P. Mathews*, P.O. Box 027, D3259 SACB, University of Michigan Medical Center, Ann Arbor, MI 48109 (USA).

A New Angiotensin-Converting Enzyme Inhibitor: Treatment of Hypertension and Congestive Heart Failure

Proceedings of an international symposium on enalapril, sponsored by Merck Sharp & Dohme International, held in São Paulo, Brazil, on November 10, 1984

Guest Editor
M.G. Nicholls

Technical Editor
M. Chaffman

Drugs

Contents Vol. 30, Suppl. 1, 1985

Section 1: Genesis and Development of Angiotensin-Converting Enzyme Inhibitors: Focus on Enalapril
Moderator: *J.A.F. Ramires*

1-5 *S.H. Ferreira*
History of the Development of Inhibitors of Angiotensin I Conversion

6-12 *A.B. Ribeiro, O. Kohlmann Jr, M.A.S. Saragoça, O. Marson* and *O.L. Ramos*
The Renin-Angiotensin System in the Control of Systemic Arterial Pressure

13-24 *H.J. Gomez, V.J. Cirillo* and *J.D. Irvin*
Enalapril: A Review of Human Pharmacology

25-34 *F.H. Messerli* and *H.O. Ventura*
Cardiovascular Pathophysiology of Essential Hypertension: A Clue to Therapy

35-46 *J. Herrera-Acosta, H. Pérez-Grovas, M. Fernández* and *J. Arriaga*
Enalapril in Essential Hypertension

47-48 General Discussion

Section 2: Enalapril: Pharmacodynamic Findings and Therapeutic Efficacy in Hypertension and Heart Failure
Moderator: *M.G. Nicholls*

49-58 *R.A. Sánchez, E. Marcó, H.B. Gilbert, P. Raffaele, M. Brito, M. Giménez* and *L.I. Moledo*
Natriuretic Effect and Changes in Renal Haemodynamics Induced by Enalapril in Essential Hypertension

59-69 *G.P. Reams* and *J.H. Bauer*
Enalapril versus Triple-Drug Therapy in the Treatment of Renovascular Hypertension

70-73 *C.R. Ayers, K.M. Baker, B.A. Weaver* and *M.R. Lehman*
Enalapril Maleate versus Captopril. A Comparison of the Hormonal and Antihypertensive Effects

74-81 *M.W.I. Webster, M.A. Fitzpatrick, E.J. Hamilton, M.G. Nicholls, H. Ikram, E.A. Espiner* and *J.E. Wells*
Effects of Enalapril on Clinical Status, Biochemistry, Exercise Performance and Haemodynamics in Heart Failure

82-89 *F. Moncloa, J.A. Sromovsky, J.F. Walker* and *R.O. Davies*
Enalapril in Hypertension and Congestive Heart Failure. Overall Review of Efficacy and Safety

90-93 General Discussion

94-96 Summary

Contributors

Symposium Chairman

E. Sabbaga
Av. Brig. Luiz Antonio, 3333 3 Andar, São Paulo (Brazil)

Section Moderators

M.G. Nicholls
Department of Endocrinology, The Princess Margaret Hospital, Christchurch (New Zealand)

J.A.F. Ramires
University São Paulo, Hospital Clinic, Faculty of Medicine, Institute Coraçao, São Paulo (Brazil)

Contributors

J. Arriaga
Department of Nephrology, Instituto Naciónal de la Nutrición Salvador Zubirán, Mexico City (Mexico)

C.R. Ayers
Department of Internal Medicine, Division of Cardiology, University of Virginia Medical Center, Charlottesville, Virginia (USA)

K.M. Baker
Geisinger Medical Center, Danville, Pennsylvania (USA)

J.H. Bauer
Harry S. Truman Memorial Veterans Hospital, Medical Service, Columbia, Missouri (USA)

M. Brito
Hospital Instituto de Cardiología, Academia Nacional de Medicina, Buenos Aires (Argentina)

V.J. Cirillo
Department of Cardiovascular Clinical Research, Merck Sharp & Dohme Research Laboratories, Rahway, New Jersey (USA)

R.O. Davies
Merck Sharp & Dohme Research Laboratories, Rahway, New Jersey (USA)

E.A. Espiner
Department of Endocrinology, The Princess Margaret Hospital, Christchurch (New Zealand)

M. Fernández
Department of Nephrology, Instituto Nacional de la Nutrición Salvador Zubirán, Mexico City (Mexico)

S.H. Ferreira
Department of Pharmacology, Faculty of Medicine of Ribeirão Preto, São Paulo (Brazil)

M.A. Fitzpatrick
Department of Cardiology, The Princess Margaret Hospital, Christchurch (New Zealand)

H.B. Gilbert
Hospital Instituto de Cardiología, Academia Nacional de Medicina, Buenos Aires (Argentina)

M. Giménez
Hospital de Niños Ricardo. Gutierrez, Buenos Aires (Argentina)

H.J. Gomez
Department of Cardiovascular Clinical Research, Merck Sharp & Dohme Research Laboratories, Rahway, New Jersey (USA)

E.J. Hamilton
The Princess Margaret Hospital, Christchurch (New Zealand)

J. Herrera-Acosta
Department of Nephrology, Instituto Nacional de Cardiología Ignacio Chávez, Mexico City (Mexico)

H. Ikram
Department of Cardiology, The Princess Margaret Hospital, Christchurch (New Zealand)

J.D. Irvin
Merck Sharp & Dohme Research Laboratories, West Point, Pennsylvania (USA)

O. Kohlmann, Jr
Nephrology-Hypertension Division, Escola Paulista de Medicina, São Paulo (Brazil)

M.R. Lehman
Hypertension/Atherosclerosis Unit, University of Virginia, School of Medicine, Charlottesville, Virginia (USA)

E. Marcó
Hospital Instituto de Cardiología, Academia Nacional de Medicina, Buenos Aires (Argentina)

O. Marson
Nephrology-Hypertension Division, Escola Paulista de Medicina, São Paulo (Brazil)

F.H. Messerli
Department of Internal Medicine (Section on Hypertension), Ochsner Clinic and Alton Ochsner Medical Foundation, New Orleans, Louisiana (USA)

L.I. Moledo
Hospital Instituto de Cardiología, Academia Nacional de Medicina, Buenos Aires (Argentina)

F. Moncloa
Merck Sharp & Dohme Research Laboratories, Rahway, New Jersey (USA)

M.G. Nicholls
Department of Endocrinology, The Princess Margaret Hospital, Christchurch (New Zealand)

H. Pérez-Grovas
Department of Nephrology, Instituto Nacional de Cardiología Ignacio Chávez, Mexico City (Mexico)

P. Raffaele
Hospital Instituto de Cardiología, Academia Nacional de Medicina, Buenos Aires (Argentina)

O.L. Ramos
Nephrology-Hypertension Division, Escola Paulista de Medicina, São Paulo (Brazil)

G.P. Reams
University of Missouri School of Medicine, Columbia (USA)

A.B. Ribeiro
Nephrology-Hypertension Division, Escola Paulista de Medicina, São Paulo (Brazil)

R.A. Sánchez
Hospital Instituto de Cardiología, Academia Nacional de Medicina, Buenos Aires (Argentina)

M.A.S. Saragoça
Nephrology-Hypertension Division, Escola Paulista de Medicina, São Paulo (Brazil)

J.A. Sromovsky
Merck Sharp & Dohme Research Laboratories, Rahway, New Jersey (USA)

H.O. Ventura
Department of Internal Medicine (Section on Hypertension), Ochsner Clinic and Alton Ochsner Medical Foundation, New Orleans, Louisiana (USA)

J.F. Walker
Merck Sharp & Dohme Research Laboratories, Rahway, New Jersey (USA)

B.A. Weaver
Hypertension/Atherosclerosis Unit, University of Virginia, School of Medicine, Charlottesville, Virginia (USA)

M.W.I. Webster
The Princess Margaret Hospital, Christchurch (New Zealand)

J.E. Wells
The Princess Margaret Hospital, Christchurch (New Zealand)

Section 1:
Genesis and Development of Angiotensin-Converting Enzyme Inhibitors: Focus on Enalapril

Drugs 30 (Suppl. 1): 1-5 (1985)
0012-6667/85/0100-0001/$2.50/0

History of the Development of Inhibitors of Angiotensin I Conversion

S.H. Ferreira

Department of Pharmacology, Faculty of Medicine of Ribeirão Preto, São Paulo

Summary *The major steps in the initial development of angiotensin I conversion inhibitors are described, from the discovery of the* Bothrops *peptides (bradykinin potentiating factor) to the demonstration of the therapeutic potential. It is a history where chance, serendipity and clear scientific reasoning weaved together the work of several scientists. It is also a classical example of drug development for which the initial basic research was made at the university, but the useful product was achieved by industry.*

The history of the development of the angiotensin converting enzyme (ACE) inhibitors reflects the summation of the efforts of basic and drug-orientated research, a classical example of the relationship between university and industry research.

The major pre-clinical discoveries were made in universities or research institutes, while the practical development of useful compounds was accomplished by industry. Research in the university is rarely task-orientated and the initial stepping-stones in the discovery of this new class of antihypertensive drugs clearly illustrate this point.

In 1961, I started work in the laboratory of Professor M. Rocha e Silva in Ribeirão Preto, searching for substances capable of blocking the enzymatic inactivation of bradykinin. Following the observation of Erdös and Sloane (1962) suggesting that the major inactivating enzyme in plasma had the characteristics of a carboxypeptidase, and that pancreatic carboxypeptidase B was a metal-enzyme (Vallee, 1961), we demonstrated that several metal chelating agents (in particular dimercaptopropanol) inhibited bradykinin inactivation by plasma, and potentiated its pharmacology and actions *in vitro* and *in vivo* (Ferreira and Rocha e Silva, 1962, 1963; Ferreira et al., 1962; Rocha e Silva, 1963). The cardiovascular action of these compounds was confirmed by Erdös and Wöhler (1963). Following this line of research I intended to investigate the ability of dimercaptopropanol to potentiate the contractions of isolated guinea-pig ileum induced by the venom of a Brazilian snake, *Bothrops jararaca.* I found that the venom itself had a strong bradykinin potentiating activity. The biological activity of this new group of substances was associated with a family of peptides present in the venom. The crude preparation was named bradykinin potentiating factor or BPF (Ferreira, 1965). Bradykinin potentiating factor inhibited plasma kininase activity, and potentiated the spasmogenic activity of bradykinin upon isolated smooth muscle preparations as well as increasing its vasodilation and permeability effects. Bradykinin potentiating factor had no potentiating effect upon the pharmacological effects of histamine, acetylcholine, angiotensin II or eledoisin (Amorim et al., 1967a,b; Capek et al., 1966; Ferreira, 1965, 1966; Ferreira and Rocha e Silva, 1965; Graeff et al., 1965). Bradykinin potentiating factor was the most powerful bradykinin potentiating substance described at that time. It was present in the venom of *Bothrops* but not in the Crotalus family (Ferreira, 1966).

I continued this line of research, on the metabolism of bradykinin, in the Department of Pharmacology at the Royal College of Surgeons of England, working with Professor J.R. Vane. We discovered that the major site of inactivation of circulating bradykinin *in vivo* was in the pulmonary vascular bed (Ferreira and Vane, 1967a). Bradykinin potentiating factor increased the half-life of bradykinin in the circulation (Ferreira and Vane, 1967b). At that time synthetic angiotensin I became available and Ng and Vane (1968) found that during its passage through the pulmonary vascular beds it was converted to angiotensin II. This conversion appeared to be similar to bradykinin inactivation since the carboxyterminal amino acids of both peptides were hydrolysed. They found that bradykinin potentiating factor had a very strong inhibitory action upon angiotensin I conversion by the lung vascular bed (Ng and Vane, 1970). However, it was Dr Bakhle, in the same Department, who first demonstrated the inhibitory action of bradykinin potentiating factor on the *in vitro* enzymatic conversion of angiotensin I (Bakhle, 1968; Bakhle et al., 1969). Thus, bradykinin potentiating factor provided the first demonstration of the association of the conversion of angiotensin I with kininase activity. This was later confirmed by Yang et al. (1971) with purified kininase II.

In 1968, I started a very effective partnership with Dr L.T. Greene of Brookhaven National Laboratory which resulted in the isolation and characterisation of 9 low molecular weight, pharmacologically active peptides (Ferreira et al., 1970a; Greene et al., 1970). A general parallelism between kininase inhibition (indicated by potentiation of bradykinin contractile activity upon guinea-pig ileum) and inhibition of enzymatic angiotensin I conversion was demonstrated for the peptides (Ferreira et al., 1970b). The sequence of the pentapeptide bradykinin potentiating factor$_{5a}$ (PCA-Lys-Tryp-Ala-Pro) was reported in 1970 (Ferreira et al., 1970b). These peptides were named bradykinin potentiating peptides (BPP) and the pentapeptide was named as BPP_{5a}. The knowledge of the structure of BPP_{5a} allowed us, together with Dr J.M. Stewart, to synthetise the peptide and demonstrate its activity for bradykinin potentiation and inhibition of angiotensin I conversion *in vivo* (Stewart et al., 1971).

Our studies were concluded when, together with Dr Krieger in Brazil, we used BPP_{5a} to provide the first demonstration that an inhibitor of converting enzyme lowers the blood pressure in models possessing an overactive renin system. It was also shown that angiotensin I- (but not angiotensin II-) induced hypertension was blocked by BPP_{5a} (Krieger et al., 1971). Because BPP_{5a} was short-lived, we suggested it could be used as a test to select patients with renin-dependent hypertension.

Our work clearly demonstrated that among the *Bothrops* peptides the nonapeptide (BPP_{9a}) was the most potent (Ferreira et al., 1970a,b). Its structure (SQ 20,881), however, was established by Ondetti et al. (1971). SQ 20,881 was instrumental in demonstrating the possibility of the therapeutic use of an ACE inhibitor either as a diagnostic tool (Rosenthal et al., 1979) or in the control of hypertensive patients (Gavras et al., 1974). However, the main hindrance to the therapeutic use of BPP_{9a} was its lack of oral activity. The discovery of orally active compounds certainly was the last major step in the development of the ACE inhibitors, which established a new class of antihypertensive drugs.

Knowledge of the structure of the *Bothrops* peptides, and in particular of the site of cleavage of BPP_{5a} by the angiotensin converting enzyme (kininase II), allowed Cushman et al. (1977) in the USA, to devise an elegantly rational approach in the search for synthetic ACE inhibitors. It was assumed that the active site of ACE was analogous to that of carboxypeptidase A. It was known that the carboxy-terminal amino acid of a carboxypeptidase A substrate would interact with the active site of the enzyme, and that the carbonyl of the peptide bond interacted with a zinc ion tightly bound to the enzyme. Based upon this model, inhibitors of carboxypeptidase A, such as D-2 benzylsuccinic acid, were designed (Byers and Wolfenden, 1972). Considering that the converting enzyme was a dipeptidase (it splits the Ala-Pro carboxyl-terminal of BPP_{5a}), it was assumed that the distance between the carboxyl-binding group and the zinc ion was greater than that in carboxypeptidase A. Thus, to the last amino acid of BPP_{5a} (proline) a succinyl radical was added (Cushman et al., 1977). The resulting molecule was a weak ACE inhibitor, but its oral activity and specificity opened the way to the synthesis of analogous substances, leading to the invention of the presently available, potent orally-active inhibitors, such as captopril and enalapril.

It is frequently stated that the development of the ACE inhibitors has been, since pre-clinical animal studies, very rational. This idea implies a rather successful task-orientated research, in both university and industry. This view is incorrect. Bradykinin potentiating factor was discovered in Rocha e Silva's laboratory, which was totally devoted to the study of bradykinin. At that time we believed in developing a specific probe to evaluate the participation of bradykinin in physiological or pathological situations, as eserine was used for acetylcholine during early studies on parasympathetic transmission.

Serendipity played a definite role in this story. The initial test of bradykinin potentiating factor upon angiotensin I conversion occurred in the same laboratory. While I was studying the inactivation of bradykinin by the lungs in one room, the pulmonary conversion of angiotensin I was being discovered in another room. It was sheer luck that later I met Dr Lewis Greene who was an expert on peptide purification and sequencing, and was invited to Brazil by Professor Rocha e Silva to study the effect of proteinase inhibitors on bradykinin liberation. Little do people realise that the idea of developing ACE inhibitor drugs from bradykinin potentiating factor was not born in an industrial laboratory devoted to the search for antihypertensive drugs. In fact, the subject was introduced by Professor J.R. Vane, as consultant to a very learned peptide group which was about to be disbanded due to industrial reorganisation (personal communication). At that time there was no clear evidence that ACE inhibitors could be useful for controlling hypertension. This evidence was later supplied by our experiments with the synthetic pentapeptide, BPP_{5a}. I believe that from that moment the research could be classified as drug-orientated. It is only when a physiopathologically meaningful screening test can be established, based upon experimental evidence, that drug-orientated research can really start.

Awareness that the pathway for the development of new therapeutic agents may start in universities or research institutes (Conroe and Dripps, 1976) is of fundamental importance for the survival of university non-orientated research, especially in the third world. On the other hand, the present history also tells us that an invention never comes to fruition without the existence of competent industrial development. In this context it must be pointed out that the initial discovery of bradykinin potentiating factor did not occur solely because of the wisdom of a young scientist, but could only take place at a laboratory like that of Professor Rocha e Silva where, in addition to his obvious expertise with bradykinin, there was a solid knowledge of peptides and snake venoms.

During the overall developmental period of the ACE inhibitors, we thought that their antihypertensive action depended upon a reduction of circulating angiotensin II. However, evidence has accumulated that its antihypertensive mechanism is not solely due to this effect. It appears that local tissue conversion of angiotensin I plays an important role. The inhibition of the formation of angiotensin in the vessel walls seems to abolish the facilitatory action of angiotensin II on neurogenic vasoconstriction. Furthermore, blockade of the formation of angiotensin II in the brain seems to be responsible for the reduction of sympathetic tone (Unger et al., 1983). Thus, in addition to its therapeutic antihypertensive actions, this new class of drugs, the ACE inhibitors, are presently helping us understand the interplay between the renin-angiotensin system and the sympathetic system in the control of blood pressure.

In this paper I have described what I believe to

be the most relevant contributions in the initial development of the ACE inhibitors. In 1970, I realised that as a basic pharmacologist, my contribution to the field was completed, since I was neither an expert in hypertension, nor a clinical pharmacologist, nor an inspired chemist able to transform those expensive peptides into useful drugs. At that time there were less than 20 papers in the relevant literature and the majority of these were associated with our work (Greene et al., 1972). With the availability of the synthetic nonapeptide (SQ 20,881), and the first orally-active ACE inhibitor, the growth in this field was explosive, as attested by the comprehensive review of Cushman and Ondetti (1980), where more than 300 papers are cited. By now, the number of publications has multiplied greatly.

The marketing of another ACE inhibitor is a clear indication that the use of this class of drugs is now consolidating. I am happy that this meeting took place here in São Paulo, the State where bradykinin potentiating factor was discovered.

Last but not least I would like to draw attention to the central role of the bioassay in the development of this area. The discovery of angiotensin, bradykinin and bradykinin potentiating factor, and the demonstration of the conversion of angiotensin I by lungs or tissue homogenates and its inhibition by bradykinin potentiating factor, illustrates this point. It is important for medical students and young scientists alike to understand that it is not only with the use of sophisticated methodology that relevant discoveries can be made. Indeed, contractions of a guinea-pig ileum led to the discovery of a new class of antihypertensive drugs.

References

Amorim, D.S.; Manço, J.C.; Ferreira, S.H.; Sader, A.A. and Cardoso, S.S.: Cardiovascular responses in the anesthetized dog to the central venous infusion of bradykinin and eledoisin; in Rocha e Silva and Rothschild (Eds) International Symposium on Vaso-Active Polypeptides: Bradykinin and Related Kinins pp. 53-63 (1967a).

Amorim, D.S.; Ferreira, S.H.; Manço, J.C.; Tanaka, A.; Sader, A.A. and Cardoso, S.: Potentiation of circulatory effects of bradykinin by a factor contained in the *Bothrops jararaca* venom. Cardiologia 50: 23-32 (1967b).

Bakhle, Y.S.: Conversion of angiotensin I to angiotensin II by cell-free extracts of dog lung. Nature (London) 220: 919-921 (1968).

Bakhle, Y.S.; Reynard, A.M. and Vane, J.R.: Metabolism of the angiotensins in isolated perfused tissues. Nature (London) 222: 956 (1969).

Byers, L.D. and Wolfenden, R.: A potent reversible inhibitor of carboxypeptidase A. Journal of Biological Chemistry 247: 606-608 (1972).

Capek, R.; Corrado, A.P.; Ferreira, S.H. and Rocha e Silva, M.: The effect of bradykinin on the electroencephalogram. Activitas Nervosa 8 (Suppl.): 419-420 (1966).

Conroe, J.H. and Dripps, R.R.: Scientific basis for the support of biomedical science. Science 192: 105-111 (1976).

Cushman, D.W.; Cheung, H.S.; Sabo, E.F. and Ondetti, M.A.: Design of potent competitive inhibitors of angiotensin-converting enzyme carboxyalkanoyl and mercaptoalkanoyl amino acids. Biochemistry 16: 5484-5491 (1977).

Cushman, D.W. and Ondetti, M.A.: Inhibitors of angiotensin-converting enzyme; in Ellis and West (Eds) Progress in Medicinal Chemistry, Volume 17, pp. 41-104 (Elsevier/North Holland Biomedical Press, Amsterdam 1980).

Erdös, E.G. and Sloane, E.M.: An enzyme in human blood plasma that inactivates bradykinin and kallidin. Biochemistry and Pharmacology 11: 585-592 (1962).

Erdös, E.G. and Wöhler, J.R.: Inhibition 'in vivo' of the enzymatic inactivation of bradykinin and kallidin. Biochemistry and Pharmacology 12: 1193-1199 (1963).

Ferreira, S.H.: A bradykinin-potentiating factor (BPF) present in the venom of *Bothrops jararaca.* British Journal of Pharmacology 24: 163-169 (1965).

Ferreira, S.H.: Bradykinin-potentiating factor; in Erdös and Sicuteri (Eds) Hypotensive Peptides, pp.356-367 (Springer-Verlag, New York 1966).

Ferreira, S.H.; Corrado, A.P. and Rocha e Silva, M.: Potenciação do efeito hopotensor da bradicinina por inibição da enzima bradicininolítica plasmática. Ciências e Cultura 14: 238 (1962).

Ferreira, S.H. and Rocha e Silva, M.: Potentiation of bradykinin by dimercaptopropanol (BAL) and other inhibitors of its destroying enzyme in plasma. Biochemical Pharmacology 11: 1123-1128 (1962).

Ferreira, S.H. and Rocha e Silva, M.: Potenciação de polipeptideos por um fator presente no veneno de *Bothrops jararaca.* Ciências e Cultura 15: 276 (1963).

Ferreira, S.H. and Rocha e Silva, M.: Potentiation of bradykinin and eledoisin by BPF (Bradykinin Potentiating Factor) from *Bothrops jararaca* venom. Experientia 21: 347-349 (1965).

Ferreira, S.H. and Vane, J.R.: The disappearance of bradykinin and eledoisin in the circulation and vascular beds of the cat. British Journal of Pharmacology and Chemotherapy 30: 417-424 (1967a).

Ferreira, S.H. and Vane, J.R.: The detection and estimation of bradykinin in the circulating blood. British Journal of Pharmacology and Chemotherapy 29: 367-377 (1967b).

Ferreira, S.H.; Bartelt, D.C. and Greene, L.J.: Isolation of bradykinin-potentiating peptides from *Bothrops jararaca* venom. Biochemistry 9: 2583-2593 (1970a).

Ferreira, S.H.; Greene, L.J.; Alabaster, V.A.; Bakhle, Y.S. and Vane, J.R.: Activity of various fractions of bradykinin potentiating factor against angiotensin I converting enzyme. Nature 225: 379-380 (1970b).

Gavras, H.; Brunner, H.R.; Laragh, J.; Sealey, J.E.; Gavras, I. and Vukovich, R.A.: An angiotensin converting-enzyme inhibitor to identify and treat vasoconstrictor and volume factors in hypertensive patients. New England Journal of Medicine 291: 817-821 (1974).

Graeff, F.G.; Ferreira, S.H.; Corrado, A.P. and Rocha e Silva, M.: Potentiation of the cerebral vascular action of bradykinin by

the 'Bradykinin Potentiating Factor' (BPF) in the dog. Experientia 21: 607-608 (1965).
Greene, L.J.; Stewart, J.M. and Ferreira, S.H.: Bradykinin-potentiating peptides from the venom of *Bothrops jararaca;* in Sicuteri, Rocha e Silva and Back (Eds) Bradykinin and Related Kinins: Cardiovascular, Biochemical and Neural Actions, Volume 8, pp.81-87 (Plenum Press, New York 1970).
Greene, L.J.; Camargo, A.C.M.; Krieger, E.M.; Stewart, J.M. and Ferreira, S.H.: Inhibition of the conversion of angiotensin I to II and potentiation of bradykinin by small peptides present in *Bothrops jararaca* venom. Circulation Research 30 (Suppl. 2): 62-71 (1972).
Krieger, E.M.; Salgado, H.C.; Assan, C.J.; Greene, L.J. and Ferreira, S.H.: Potential screening test for detection of overactivity of renin-angiotensin system. Lancet 1: 269-271 (1971).
Ng, K.K.F. and Vane, J.R.: Fate of angiotensin I in the circulation. Nature (London) 218: 144-150 (1968).
Ng, K.K.F. and Vane, J.R.: Some properties of angiotensin converting enzyme in the lung, in vivo. Nature (London) 225: 1142-1144 (1970).
Ondetti, M.A.; Williams, N.J.; Sabo, E.F.; Plušcěc, J.; Weaver, E.R. and Kocy, O.: Angiotensin-converting enzyme inhibitors from the venom of *Bothrops jararaca.* Isolation, elucidation of structure and synthesis. Biochemistry 10: 4033-4039 (1971).
Rocha e Silva, M.: The physiological significance of bradykinin. Annals of the New York Academy of Sciences 104: 190-211 (1963).
Rosenthal, T.; Kissin, E.; Jacob, E.T.; Stern, N.; Levi, J. and Adar, R.: Angiotensin-converting enzyme inhibitor (SQ 20881) in the diagnosis of renovascular hypertension. Angiology 30: 123-128 (1979).
Stewart, J.M.; Ferreira, S.H. and Greene, L.J.: Bradykinin potentiating peptide PCA-Lys-TRP-Ala-Pro. An inhibitor of the pulmonary inactivation of bradykinin and conversion of angiotensin I to II. Biochemical Pharmacology 20: 1557-1567 (1971).
Unger, T.; Ganten, D. and Leng, E.R.: Converting enzyme inhibitors: antihypertensive drugs with unexpected mechanisms. TIPS 4: 514-519 (1983).
Vallee, B.L.: The 'active catalytic site' an approach through metaloenzymes. Federation Proceedings 20 (Suppl. 10): 71-80 (1961).
Yang, H.Y.T.; Erdös, E.G. and Lewin, Y.: Characterisation of a dipeptide hydrolase (Kininase II: Angiotensin I converting enzyme) Journal of Pharmacology and Experimental Therapeutics 177: 291-300 (1971).

Address for correspondence and reprints: Dr *S.H. Ferreira,* Department of Pharmacology, Faculty of Medicine of Ribeirão Preto, 14100 – Ribeirão Preto-SP (Brazil).

Drugs 30 (Suppl. 1): 6-12 (1985)
0012-6667/85/0100-0006/$3.50/0

The Renin-Angiotensin System in the Control of Systemic Arterial Pressure

Artur B. Ribeiro, Osvaldo Kohlmann Jr, Manoel A.S. Saragoça, Odair Marson and *Oswaldo L. Ramos*
Nephrology-Hypertension Division, Escola Paulista de Medicina, São Paulo

Summary *The renin-angiotensin system through its active octapeptide, angiotensin II, has an important role in systemic arterial pressure control. Angiotensin II is a potent direct vasoconstrictor and is also the main regulator of aldosterone secretion. The complete analysis of the role of angiotensin II has to take into account the prevailing sodium balance for a given level of angiotensin II and also its indirect action upon the sympathetic nervous system as well as other hormonal systems. A number of studies have provided evidence for an important role for the renin-angiotensin system in renovascular hypertension, malignant and severe hypertension, as well as in mild to moderate forms of essential hypertension.*

The role of the renin-angiotensin system in both normotensive and hypertensive states has been widely studied. A major step in our understanding of the role of the renin-angiotensin system in blood pressure control has been the development of specific peptide inhibitors such as saralasin, and more recently angiotensin-converting enzyme (ACE) inhibitors such as captopril and enalapril. It has become clear that, in considering the participation of the renin-angiotensin system in the control of systemic arterial pressure, one has to consider not only the levels of circulating angiotensin II, but also the prevailing sodium balance, as well as the multiple interactions of angiotensin II with the sympathetic nervous system. To draw a clear picture of the role of the renin-angiotensin system in normotension and hypertension, one must consider not only the direct vasoconstrictor action of angiotensin II upon vascular smooth muscle, but also its indirect actions via aldosterone secretion and the central and peripheral sympathetic nervous system. Renin-angiotensin system participation in cardiac failure is beyond the scope of this paper.

1. Angiotensin II as a Direct Vasoconstrictor

The octapeptide angiotensin II, the active end product of the renin-angiotensin system, is a potent direct vasoconstrictor. With the availability of renin-angiotensin system blocking agents, the role of angiotensin II-mediated vasoconstriction has been evaluated. In some patients with essential hypertension (Case et al., 1976), coarctation of the aorta (Ribeiro and Krakoff, 1976), and those with malignant (Saragoça et al., 1983) and renovascular hypertension (Krakoff et al., 1980), an angiotensin II-mediated vasoconstrictor component has been identified. In these patients it is clear that angiotensin II participates in the maintenance of the elevation in arterial blood pressure in spite of a normal dietary salt intake.

Table I. Blood pressure responses in normal volunteers studied after sodium depletion and sodium repletion. Data from Brunner et al. (1976)

Patient	Mean arterial pressure (mm Hg)					
	Na depletion			Na repletion		
	control	angiotensin inhibition		control	angiotensin inhibition	
	supine	supine	upright	supine	supine	upright
1	80	73	(52)	73	77	93
2	87	70	(37)	73	83	83
3	92	95	(57)	89	89	95
4	79	73	(20)	78	84	90
5	97	(40)	—	79	81	78

Numbers in parentheses represent lowest blood pressure.

2. *Aldosterone Regulation*

Angiotensin II is the most important stimulus for aldosterone secretion by the adrenal gland. Aldosterone is an important contributor to extracellular volume regulation and has, accordingly, a pivotal role in circulatory homeostasis.

3. *Angiotensin II-Sodium Interactions*

In some circumstances, the role of angiotensin II-mediated vasoconstriction may not be apparent unless the state of sodium balance is considered. In a healthy man eating a diet containing normal amounts of sodium, plasma renin activity is relatively low. Under these conditions, acute blockade of the direct pressor action of angiotensin II, through the infusion of saralasin, causes no significant fall in arterial pressure. If these individuals are now submitted to sodium depletion, a significant fall in arterial pressure will occur in some of them during saralasin infusion. This fall in arterial pressure will be even more dramatic with upright body posture (table I). From this observation it is clear that the renin-angiotensin system is of pivotal importance for control of normal systemic arterial pressure during sodium depletion. More recent reports have also documented decreases in blood pressure following administration of captopril and enalapril in normotensive subjects studied while on normal sodium intake (MacGregor et al., 1981a, b). These data were interpreted as implicating the renin-angiotensin system in blood pressure control even in the presence of a normal sodium intake. However, the possibility that these agents may also diminish blood pressure through other mechanisms than blockade of the renin-angiotensin system should also be considered (Marks et al., 1980; Mimram et al., 1980; Moore et al., 1981). Regardless of the explanation, it is clear that a direct angiotensin II-dependent vasoconstrictor component in normotensive man is more readily apparent during sodium restriction.

In patients with essential hypertension, manipulations of dietary salt may reveal a pattern similar to that observed in normotensive controls. In these patients, manipulations of the sodium balance may alter the degree of renin dependency of the hypertensive state. As shown in table II, the mean arterial pressure of patients with high renin essential hypertension exhibited significant reductions during saralasin infusion following sodium depletion. Repeat saralasin infusion following sodium repletion caused only minor variations in mean arterial

Table II. Mean arterial pressure (MAP) responses to saralasin infusion in patients with high renin essential hypertension studied after sodium depletion and sodium repletion. Data from Gavras et al. (1976)

	MAP before	MAP during saralasin infusion	
		supine	erect
Sodium depletion	119±6	90±4	70±2
Sodium repletion	116±7	123±8	133±21

MAP (mm Hg), mean ± SEM.

pressure. The same type of results have been observed in patients with normal or low renin essential hypertension (Gavras et al., 1976). Thus, secondary activation of the renin-angiotensin system may explain therapeutic failure in patients with hypertension treated with dietary sodium restriction and by the use of diuretics.

4. Participation of the Renin-Angiotensin System as a Function of the Phase of the Hypertensive State

Well-documented observations have shown that the degree of participation of the renin-angiotensin system may vary with the duration of the hypertensive state. In one-clip, two kidney hypertension in the rat, activation of the renin-angiotensin system is well-documented during the early, but not in the late phases of the hypertensive state (Gavras et al., 1975). A possibility is that this change in the mechanism maintaining the hypertension may reflect alterations in sodium handling capacity by the unclipped kidney exposed to the high blood pressure. Similar observations were made in methylprednisolone hypertension in the rat. Administration of methylprednisolone in a wide dose range was accompanied by a clear elevation of blood pressure (fig. 1). Four weeks after administration of methylprednisolone the renin-angiotensin system was clearly activated, and both saralasin and captopril administration caused a fall in arterial pressure (fig. 2). The same animals studied after 8 weeks of methylprednisolone administration showed no significant degree of renin dependency (fig. 2).

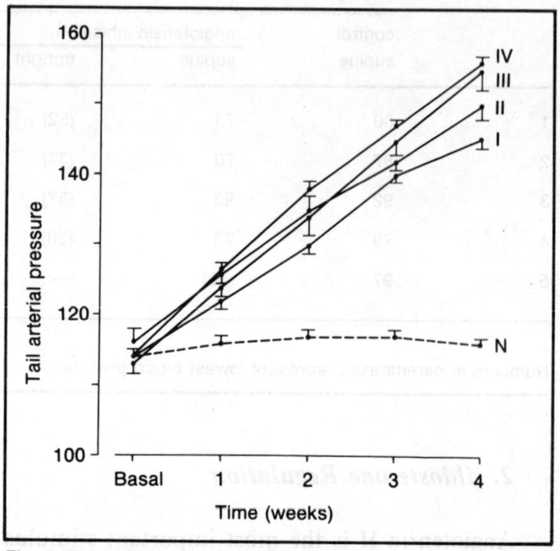

Fig. 1. Tail arterial pressure values in Wistar rats treated with four different doses of methylprednisolone groups (I = 2.5mg; II = 5mg; III = 10mg; IV = 20mg) and in control (group N). Data from Ribeiro et al. (1981).

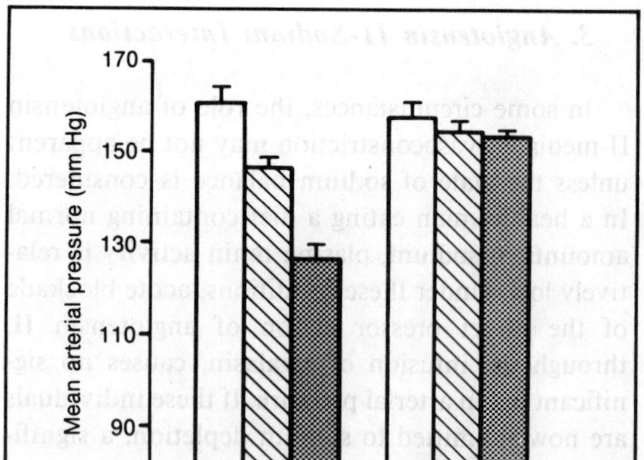

Fig. 2. Mean arterial pressure values before and during acute administration of captopril (▩) or saralasin (▧) in rats treated with methylprednisolone (20 mg/kg/week) for 4 and 8 weeks. Control (□). Data from Ribeiro et al. (1981).

Furthermore, concomitant administration of methylprednisolone and captopril did not prevent this hypertensive state pointing to the fact that mechanisms other than renin-angiotensin system activation must be involved (Ribeiro et al., 1981). It is tempting to speculate that this change in the degree of participation of the renin-angiotensin system in the maintenance of the hypertension, so well-documented in animal models, is also at work in human hypertension.

5. Central Actions of Angiotensin II

When evaluating participation of the renin-angiotensin system in hypertension, the central actions of renin-angiotensin II should be considered (table III). It is well-known that angiotensin II has a central hypertensive effect which is mediated by an increase in sympathetic outflow (Bickerton and Buckley, 1961). Angiotensin II also increases water intake when administered centrally (Epstein et al., 1970).

In the rat, the main site of action of centrally-administered angiotensin II is the AV3V area (Buggy et al., 1975; Hoffman and Phillips, 1976). As shown in table IV, angiotensin II (20ng) injected directly into the third ventricle of a normotensive rat caused a 32.6 ± 1.9mm Hg increase in systemic mean arterial pressure and a 9.0 ± 0.4ml angiotensin II-induced water intake. The same type of study repeated 56 days after the AV3V lesion, showed that following angiotensin II, mean arterial pressure elevation and water intake were dramatically diminished to about 20% of those values observed before the AV3V lesion. It is clear, therefore, that pressor and dipsogenic actions of angiotensin II depend on the integrity of the AV3V area in the rat. Destruction of the AV3V may alter the development and maintenance of the hypertensive state in several experimental models (Buggy et al., 1977a,b; 1978; Fink et al., 1977; Haywood et al., 1978; Marson et al., 1981a) pointing to a central role for angiotensin II in these models of experimental hypertension.

As can be seen in figs 3 and 4 from work by our group (Marson et al., 1983) the AV3V lesions partially prevented the hypertension associated with the one-clip, two kidney rat model. Furthermore, once the hypertensive state is stabilised (fig. 4), the AV3V lesions cause a dramatic fall in blood pressure. Interestingly enough, in this study we showed that the mild hypertensive state obtained after the AV3V lesion is not accompanied by activation of the renin-angiotensin system as evaluated by the lack of a depressor response to saralasin and captopril. These observations confirm that the AV3V area plays a pivotal role in some hypertensive states in the rat.

The area postrema is the main central site of angiotensin II action in other species (Gildenberg et al., 1973; Marson et al., 1984).

The existence of an independent brain renin-angiotensin system is now well established (Ganten et al., 1978). However, angiotensin II generated in the blood may also act centrally because a functional blood-brain barrier is lacking in the circum-

Table III. Central actions of angiotensin II

Increase in sympathetic efferent nerve activity
Increase in water intake
Secretion of vasopressin
Secretion of adrenocorticotrophic hormone
Modulation of baroreflex activity
Reduction in vagal activity

Table IV. Effect of AV3V lesion upon central actions of angiotensin II n = 5. All values mean ± SEM. Data from Marson et al. (1981b)

	MAP (mm Hg)	Water intake (ml)
Control[a]	32.6 ± 1.9	9.0 ± 0.4
AV3V lesion[b]	7.2 ± 0.4	1.4 ± 0.2

a Control indicates injection of angiotensin II (20ng) into the 3rd ventricle.

b AV3V lesion indicates injection of angiotensin II 56 days after the AV3V lesion.

ventricular organs (Broadwell and Brightman, 1976). The problem of the local versus systemic origin of angiotensin II acting in the central nervous sytem is not settled at the present time. In addition to the central actions noted above, angiotensin II may also increase vasopressin and ACTH secretion (Scholkens et al., 1982; Severs and Daniels-Severs, 1973) which can directly or indirectly increase arterial pressure. Angiotensin II also causes a resetting of the baroreflex curve (Hatton et al., 1981) and a reduction in vagal efferent activity (Lee et al., 1980). Taken together, these central actions are important for systemic arterial pressure control and must be considered when evaluating the participation of the renin-angiotensin system in hypertensive states.

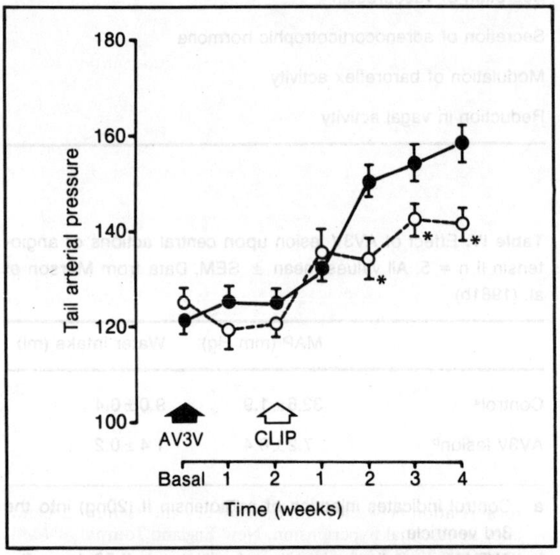

Fig. 3. Increases in tail arterial pressure after clipping of the left renal artery in rats (two kidney, one-clip model) with lesions (○) or sham lesions (●) of AV3V area. *$p < 0.001$. Data from Marson et al. (1983).

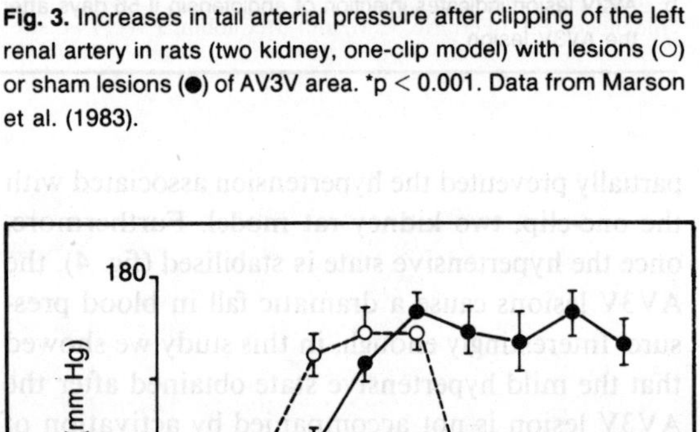

Fig. 4. Changes in tail arterial pressure with lesion (○) or sham lesion (●) of AV3V area in rats during the phase of established hypertension by clipping of the left renal artery (two kidney, one-clip model). * $p < 0.001$. Data from Marson et al. (1983).

6. Angiotensin II and Peripheral Sympathetic Nervous System Interactions

Angiotensin II has a series of interactions with the peripheral nervous systems which may influence systemic arterial pressure (table V). Accordingly, angiotensin II can facilitate the vasoconstrictor response to both sympathetic nerve stimulation and to exogenously administered noradrenaline (Khairallah, 1972; Zimmerman, 1978). Furthermore, angiotensin II increases the release of noradrenaline from the sympathetic nerve terminals (Zimmerman, 1978), facilitates transmission at sympathetic ganglia (Reit, 1972), inhibits reuptake of noradrenaline (Khairallah, 1972), facilitates biosyntheses of noradrenaline (Roth, 1972), and releases catecholamines from the adrenal medulla (Reit, 1972).

Some of these actions, which are well documented *in vitro,* and have been demonstrated (Antonaccio and Kerwin, 1981; Atkinson et al., 1980; Kohlmann et al., 1984) and denied (Nicholls et al., 1981) *in vivo,* may help to explain some of the antihypertensive aspects of ACE inhibitors.

In clinical practice the importance of the renin-angiotensin system has become more apparent to physicians with the availability of ACE inhibitors. These agents, which may also lower blood pressure through mechanisms other than blockade of the renin-angiotensin system, have been most helpful in diagnosing and treating renovascular hypertension and severe and malignant hypertension, all

Table V. Peripheral sympathetic nervous system actions of angiotensin II

Potentiates release of noradrenaline at sympathetic nerve terminals
Facilitates transmission in sympathetic ganglia
Inhibits re-uptake of noradrenaline
Increases biosynthesis of noradrenaline
Releases catecholamines from adrenal medulla
Potentiates post-junctional actions of noradrenaline

conditions known to involve activation of the renin-angiotensin system. Furthermore, blockade of the renin-angiotensin system has also become a practical approach for treating mild and moderate essential hypertension.

In conclusion, the renin-angiotensin system plays an important role in circulatory homeostasis. Complete assessment of renin-angiotensin system participation must include the direct vasoconstrictor action of angiotensin II, as well as its interaction with sodium metabolism and the sympathetic nervous system.

References

Antonaccio, M.J. and Kerwin, L.: Pre- and post-junctional inhibition of vascular sympathetic function by captopril in SHR. Hypertension 3 (Suppl. I): I54-I62 (1981).

Atkinson, A.B.; Brown, J.J.; Frazer, R.; Lever, A.F.; Morton, J.J.; Reigger, A.J.G. and Robertson, J.I.S.: Angiotensin II and renal hypertension in dog, rat and man: Effect of converting enzyme inhibition. Clinical and Experimental Hypertension 2: 499-524 (1980).

Bickerton, R.K. and Buckley, J.P.: Evidence for a central mechanism in angiotensin induced hypertension. Proceedings of the Society for Experimental Biology and Medicine 106: 834-836 (1961).

Broadwell, R.D. and Brightman, N.W.: Entry of peroxidase into neurons of the central and peripheral nervous system from extracerebral and cerebral blood. Journal of Comparative Neurology 166: 257-283 (1976).

Brunner, H.R.; Gavras, H.; Ribeiro, A.B. and Postenak, L.: Angiotensin II blockade in normal man and patients with essential hypertension. Progress in Biochemical Pharmacology 12: 145-162 (1976).

Buggy, J.; Fisher, A.E.; Hoffman, W.E.; Johnson, A.K. and Phillips, M.I.: Ventricular obstruction: Effect on drinking induced by intracranial injection of angiotensin. Science 190: 72-74 (1975).

Buggy, J.; Fink, G.D.; Brody, M.J. and Johnson, A.K.: Interruption of the course of renal hypertension by anteroventral third ventricle (AV3V) lesions. Federation Proceedings 36: 547 (1977a).

Buggy, J.; Fink, G.D.; Johnson, A.K. and Brody, M.J.: Prevention of the development of renal hypertension by anteroventral third ventricular tissue lesions. Circulation Research 40 (Suppl. 1): S110-S117 (1977b).

Buggy, J.; Fink, G.D.; Haywood, J.R.; Johnson, A.K. and Brody, M.J.: Interruption of the maintenance phase of established hypertension by ablation of the anteroventral third ventricle (AV3V) in rats. Clinical and Experimental Hypertension 1: 337-353 (1978).

Case, D.B.; Wallace, J.M.; Kein, H.J.; Sealy, J.E. and Laragh, J.H.: Usefulness and limitations of saralasin, a partial competitive agonist of angiotensin II for evaluating the renin and sodium factor in hypertensive patients. American Journal of Medicine 60: 825-836 (1976).

Epstein, A.N.; Fitzsimons, J.T. and Rolls, B.J.: Drinking induced by injection of angiotensin into the brain of rat. Journal of Physiology 210: 457-474 (1970).

Fink, G.D.; Buggy, J.; Johnson, A.K. and Brody, M.J.: Prevention of steroid-salt hypertension in the rat by anterior forebrain lesions. Circulation 56 (Suppl. 3): III 242 (1977).

Ganten, D.; Fuxe, K.; Phillips, M.I.; Mann, J.F.E. and Ganten, U.: The brain isorenin-angiotensin system: Biochemistry localisation and possible role in drinking and blood pressure regulation. Frontiers in Neuroendocrinology 5: 61-99 (1978).

Gavras, H.; Brunner, H.R.; Thurston, H. and Laragh, J.H.: Reciprocation of renin dependency with sodium volume dependency in renal hypertension. Science 188: 1316-1317 (1975).

Gavras, H.; Ribeiro, A.B.; Gavras, I. and Brunner, R.H.: Reciprocal relation between renin dependency and sodium dependency in essential hypertension. New England Journal of Medicine 295: 1278-1283 (1976).

Gildenberg, P.L.; Ferrario, C.M. and McCubbin, J.W.: Two sites of cardiovascular action of angiotensin II in the brain of the dog. Clinical Science 44: 417-420 (1973).

Hatton, R.; Clough, D.P.; Faulkner, K.L. and Conway, J.: Angiotensin converting enzyme interferes with baroreceptor reflex in conscious dogs. Hypertension 3: 676-681 (1981).

Haywood, J.R.; Fink, G.D.; Buggy, J.; Boutelle, S. and Brody, M.J.: Prevention and reversal of 2 kidney – 1 clip Goldblatt hypertension by the ablation of anteroventral third ventricular tissues. Federation Proceedings 37: 804 (1978).

Hoffman, W.E. and Phillips, M.I.: Regional study of cerebroventricle sensitivity sites to angiotensin II. Brain Research 110: 313-317 (1976).

Khairallah, P.A.: Action of angiotensin in adrenergic nerve endings: Inhibition of norepinephrine uptake. Federation Proceedings 31: 1351-1357 (1972).

Krakoff, L.R.; Ribeiro, A.B.; Gorkin, J.V. and Felton, K.F.: Saralasin infusion in screening patients for renovascular hypertension. American Journal of Cardiology 45: 609-613 (1980).

Kohlmann, J.R.O.; Bresnahan, M. and Gavras, H.: Central and peripheral indices of sympathetic activity after blood pressure lowering with enalapril (MK 421) or hydralazine in normotensive rats. Hypertension 6 (Suppl. I): I1-I6 (1984).

Lee, W.B.; Ismay, M.J. and Lumbers, E.P.: Mechanism by which angiotensin II affects the heart rate of the conscious sheep. Circulation Research 47: 286-292 (1980).

MacGregor, G.A.; Markanou, N.D.; Bayliss, J.; Roulston, J.E.; Squire, M. and Morton, J.J.: Non sulfhydryl-containing angiotensin converting enzyme inhibitor (MK-421): Evidence for role of renin system in normotensive subjects. British Medical Journal 283: 401-403 (1981a).

MacGregor, G.A.; Markanou, N.D.; Roulston, J.E.; Jones, J.C. and Morton, J.J.: Maintenance of blood pressure by the renin angiotensin system in normal man. Nature 291: 329-331 (1981b).

Marks, E.S.; Bing, R.F.; Thurston, H. and Swales, J.D.: Vasodepressor property of the converting enzyme inhibitor captopril (SQ 14225): The role of factors other than renin-angiotensin blockade in the rat. Clinical Science 58: 1-6 (1980).
Marson, O.; Ribeiro, A.B.; Tufik, S.F.; Fo, G.A.; Saragoçca, M.A. and Ramos, O.L.: Role of the anteroventral third ventricle region and the renin-angiotensin system in methylprednisolene hypertension. Hypertension 3 (Suppl. II: II142-II146 (1981a).
Marson, O.; Ribeiro, A.B.; Tufik, S.; Kohlmann Jr, O. and Ramos, O.L.: Inhibition of central angiotensin I conversion by oral captopril. Brazilian Journal of Medical Biological Research 14: 73-76 (1981b).
Marson, O.; Saragoça, M.A.; Ribeiro, A.B.; Bossolan, D.; Tufik, S. and Ramos, O.L.: Anteroventral third ventricle and renin-angiotensin system interaction in the two kidney-one clip hypertensive rat. Hypertension 5 (Suppl. V): V90-V93 (1983).
Marson, O.; Chernicky, C.L.; Slugg, R.C.; Barnes, K.L. and Ferrario, C.M.: The AV3V region does not participate in the pathophysiology of renal hypertension in the dog. (Abstract.) Annual Fall Conference and Scientific Sessions. Council for High Blood Pressure Research, Cleveland, Ohio USA (1984).
Mimram, A.; Targhetta, R. and Laroche, B.: The antihypertensive effect of captopril. Evidence for an influence of kinins. Hypertension 2: 732-737 (1980).
Moore, T.J.; Grantz, F.R.; Hollenberg, N.K.; Kolestsky, R.J.; Leboff, M.S.; Swartz, S.L.; Levine, L.; Podolsky, S.; Dluhy, R.G. and Williams, G.H.: Contribution of prostaglandins to the antihypertensive action of captopril in essential hypertension. Hypertension 3: 168-173 (1981).
Nicholls, M.G.; Espiner, E.A.; Mils, K.B.; Swifler, A.J. and Julius, S.: Evidence against an interaction of angiotensin II with the sympathetic nervous system in man. Clinical Endocrinology 15: 423-430 (1981).
Reit, E.: Actions of angiotensin on the adrenal medulla and autonomic ganglia. Federation Proceedings 31: 1338-1343 (1972).
Ribeiro, A.B. and Krakoff, L.R.: Angiotensin blockade in coarctation of the aorta. New England Journal of Medicine 295: 148-150 (1976).
Ribeiro, A.B.; Franco, R.J.S.; Kohlmann Jr, O.; Marson, O. and Ramos, O.L.: Etiopathogenesis of excess methylprednisolone arterial hypertension in the rat. Clinical and Experimental Hypertension 3 (6): 1219-1237 (1981).
Roth, R.H.: Action of angiotensin on adrenergic nerve endings: Enhancement of norepinephrine biosynthesis. Federation Proceedings 31: 1358-1364 (1972).
Saragoça, M.A.S.; Homsi, E.; Ribeiro, A.B.; Ferreira, Filho, S.R. and Ramos, O.L.: Hemodynamic mechanism of blood pressure response to captopril in human malignant hypertension. Hypertension 5 (Suppl. I): I53-I58 (1983).
Scholkens, B.A.; Jung, W.; Rascher, W.; Dietz, R. and Ganten, D.: Intracerebroventricular angiotensin II increases arterial blood pressure in rhesus monkeys by stimulation of pituitary hormones and the sympathetic nervous system. Experientia 38: 469-470 (1982).
Severs, W.B. and Daniels-Severs, A.E.: Effects of angiotensin on the central nervous system. Pharmacology Review 25: 415-449 (1973).
Zimmerman, B.G.: Actions of angiotensin on adrenergic nerve endings. Federation Proceedings 37: 199-202 (1978).

Address for correspondence and reprints: Dr *A.B. Ribeiro*, Associate Professor of Medicine, Escola Paulista de Medicina, Division of Nephrology, Rua Botucatu 740, 04023 São Paulo, SP (Brasil).

Drugs 30 (Suppl. 1): 13-24 (1985)
0012-6667/85/0100-0013/$6.00/0

Enalapril: A Review of Human Pharmacology

Hector J. Gomez, Vincent J. Cirillo and *John D. Irvin*

Department of Cardiovascular Clinical Research, Merck Sharp & Dohme Research Laboratories, Rahway, and West Point

Summary *Enalapril, an orally-active, long-acting, nonsulphydryl angiotensin-converting enzyme (ACE) inhibitor, is extensively hydrolysed* in vivo *to enalaprilat, its bioactive form. Bioactivation probably occurs in the liver. Metabolism beyond activation to enalaprilat is not observed in man. Administration with food does not affect the bioavailability of enalapril; excretion of enalapril and enalaprilat is primarily renal. Peak serum enalaprilat concentrations are reached 4 hours post-dose, and the profile is polyphasic with a prolonged terminal half-life (> 30 hours) due to the binding of enalaprilat to ACE. Steady-state is achieved by the fourth daily dose, with no evidence of accumulation. The effective accumulation half-life following multiple dosing is 11 hours. Higher serum concentrations and delayed urinary excretion occur in patients with severe renal insufficiency.*

Enalapril reduces blood pressure in hypertensive patients by decreasing systemic vascular resistance. The blood pressure reduction is not accompanied by an increase in heart rate. Furthermore, cardiac output is slightly increased and cardiovascular reflexes are not impaired. Once- and twice-daily dosage regimens reduce blood pressure to a similar extent. Enalapril increases renal blood flow and decreases renal vascular resistance. Enalapril also augments the glomerular filtration rate in patients with a glomerular filtration rate less than 80 ml/min. Enalapril reduces left ventricular mass, and does not affect cardiac function or myocardial perfusion during exercise. There is no rebound hypertension after enalapril therapy is stopped.

Enalapril does not produce hypokalaemia, hyperglycaemia, hyperuricaemia or hypercholesterolaemia. When combined with hydrochlorothiazide, enalapril attenuates the undesirable diuretic-induced metabolic changes. Therapeutic doses of enalapril do not affect serum prolactin and plasma cortisol in healthy volunteers or T_3, rT_3, T_4 and TSH in hypertensive patients. Enalapril has natriuretic and uricosuric properties.

The antihypertensive effect of enalapril is potentiated by hydrochlorothiazide, timolol and methyldopa, but unaffected by indomethacin and sulindac. No interactions occur between enalapril and frusemide, hydrochlorothiazide, digoxin and warfarin. The bioavailability of enalapril is slightly reduced when propranolol is coadministered, but this does not appear to be of any clinical significance.

Enalapril increases cardiac output and stroke volume and decreases pulmonary capillary wedge pressure in patients with congestive heart failure refractory to conventional treatment with digitalis and diuretics. Exercise capacity improves during chronic treatment. Human experience to date (6000 patients/subjects) indicates that enalapril is safe and well tolerated.

There is ample evidence that angiotensin-converting enzyme (ACE) inhibitors are effective therapeutic agents for the treatment of hypertension and congestive heart failure (Gomez and Cirillo, 1983). Ten years ago a basic research programme began at the Merck Sharp & Dohme Research Laboratories, which had as its purpose the development of a nonsulphydryl, orally-active ACE inhibitor. Enalapril[1], N-[(S)-1-(ethoxycarbonyl)-3-phenylpropyl]-L-alanyl-L-proline, was selected as a drug development candidate from more than 200 compounds synthesised (Patchett et al., 1980).

1. Pharmacokinetic Studies

Enalapril, as the maleate salt, is well absorbed following oral administration and extensively hydrolysed to enalaprilat[2], its bioactive form (fig. 1). Human plasma is devoid of enalapril esterolytic activity. Since human liver homogenates do possess appropriate activity (Jackson et al., 1984b; Tocco et al., 1982), bioactivation is thought to occur in the liver. Metabolism beyond activation to enalaprilat has not been observed in man.

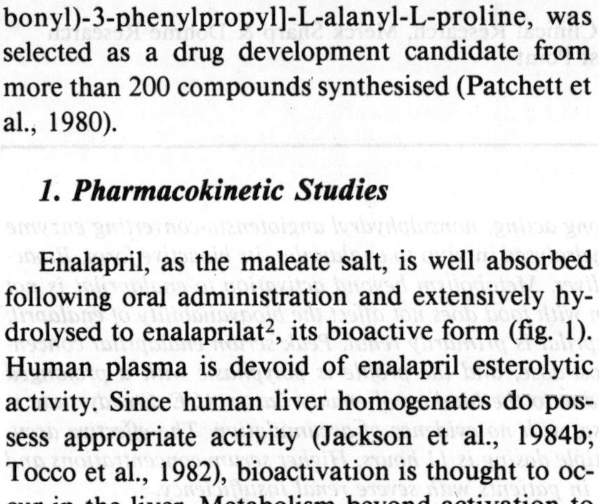

Fig. 1. Chemical structures of enalapril and enalaprilat.

1 Identified during its early development as MK-421.
2 Identified during its early development as MK-422 and enalaprilic acid.

Enalapril is absorbed intact, achieving peak serum concentrations by 1 hour and disappearing from the blood by approximately 4 hours after dosing (fig. 2). Its bioavailability is not significantly affected by the presence of food in the gastrointestinal tract (Ferguson et al., 1983). The extent of absorption and hydrolysis of enalapril are similar for various doses over the proposed therapeutic dose range (fig. 3) [Kukovetz, W.R.; unpublished data]. Peak serum concentrations of enalaprilat occur 4 hours post-dose (fig. 2) and its serum concentration profile is polyphasic, with a prolonged terminal phase. Enalaprilat is still detectable in serum 96 hours post-dose, the terminal half-life being approximately 35 hours (Ulm et al., 1982). This protracted terminal phase may be a function of the binding of enalaprilat to converting enzyme (Till et al., 1982), though it is not highly bound to protein (< 60%). Excretion of enalapril and enalaprilat is primarily renal (Ulm et al., 1982).

Steady-state serum concentrations of enalaprilat are achieved by the fourth daily dose of enalapril, with no evidence of accumulation thereafter. The effective accumulation half-life following multiple dosing is 11 hours (Till et al., 1984). Increased and delayed peak concentrations of enalaprilat are observed in patients with severe renal impairment (Saris et al., 1984). Glomerular filtration rates less than 20 to 30 ml/min were associated with markedly increased enalaprilat levels and accumulation (Kelly et al., 1984).

2. Pharmacodynamic Studies

The principal known action of enalapril in man is the inhibition of ACE activity. Maximum inhibition is observed 2 to 4 hours after drug administration, and inhibition persists for more than 24 hours (fig. 4) [Brunner et al., 1981]. The biological consequence of ACE inhibition is a reduction in plasma angiotensin II and aldosterone with a simultaneous increase in plasma renin activity. Enalapril produces a dose-related increase in plasma renin activity and decrease in plasma levels of angiotensin II and aldosterone (Shoback et al., 1983).

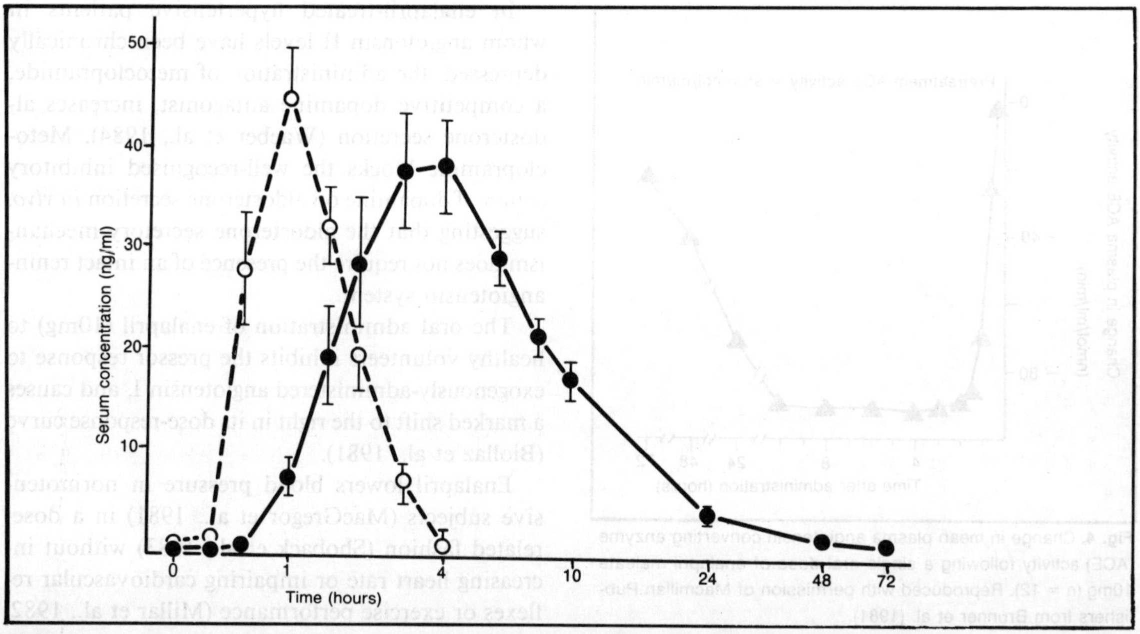

Fig. 2. Serum concentrations of enalapril (○---○) and its bioactive metabolite, enalaprilat (●---●), after a single oral dose of enalapril maleate 10mg (n = 12). Reproduced with permission of Blackwell Scientific Publications from Biollaz et al. (1982b). All values mean ± SEM.

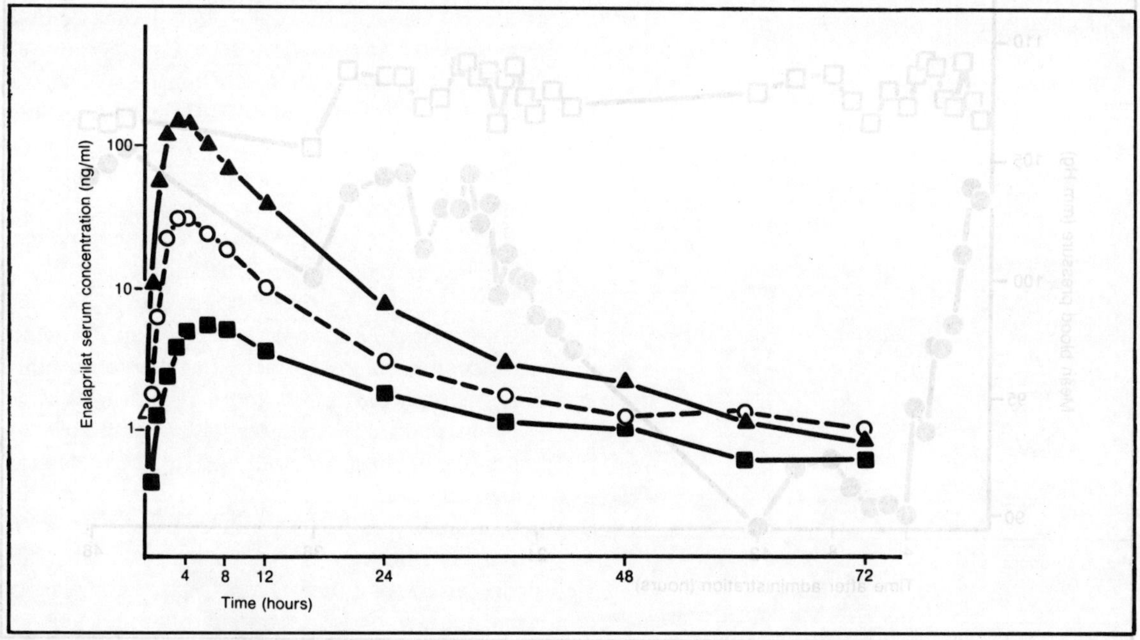

Fig. 3. Mean serum concentrations of enalaprilat after single oral doses of enalapril maleate, 2.5mg (■—■), 10mg (○—○) and 40mg (▲—▲) (n = 12). Reproduced with permission of Gower Medical Publishing from Gomez et al. (1983a).

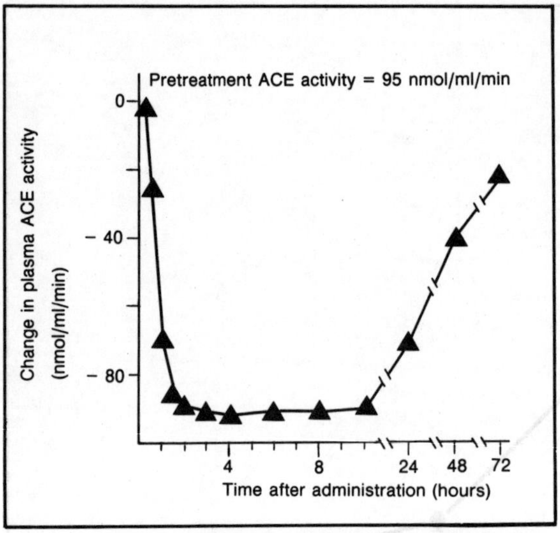

Fig. 4. Change in mean plasma angiotensin converting enzyme (ACE) activity following a single oral dose of enalapril maleate 10mg (n = 12). Reproduced with permission of Macmillan Publishers from Brunner et al. (1981).

In enalapril-treated hypertensive patients in whom angiotensin II levels have been chronically depressed, the administration of metoclopramide, a competitive dopamine antagonist, increases aldosterone secretion (Waeber et al., 1984). Metoclopramide blocks the well-recognised inhibitory action of dopamine on aldosterone secretion *in vivo*, suggesting that the aldosterone secretory mechanism does not require the presence of an intact renin-angiotensin system.

The oral administration of enalapril (10mg) to healthy volunteers inhibits the pressor response to exogenously-administered angiotensin I, and causes a marked shift to the right in its dose-response curve (Biollaz et al., 1981).

Enalapril lowers blood pressure in normotensive subjects (MacGregor et al., 1981) in a dose-related fashion (Shoback et al., 1983) without increasing heart rate or impairing cardiovascular reflexes or exercise performance (Millar et al., 1982;

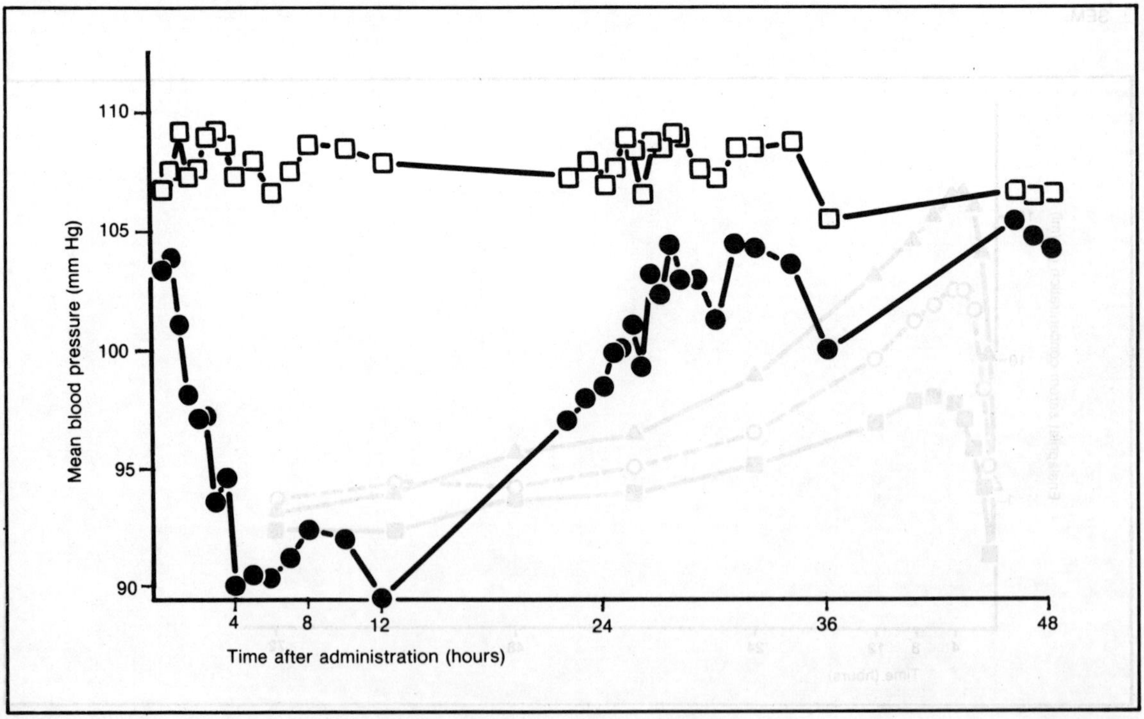

Fig. 5. Mean supine diastolic blood pressure in hospitalised patients after placebo (□—□) and optimal doses of enalapril maleate (●—●) [2.5 to 20 mg/day] (n = 33). Reproduced with permission of Blackwell Scientific Publications from Gomez et al. (1983a).

Shoback et al., 1983). Blood pressure reductions are greater in sodium-restricted subjects (Jackson et al., 1984a; Shoback et al., 1983).

3. Therapeutic Studies

3.1 Essential Hypertension

Single oral doses of enalapril (2.5 to 40mg) significantly reduce blood pressure in hospitalised patients with mild to severe hypertension. The onset of antihypertensive activity occurs 1 hour post-administration, with a peak effect at 3.5 to 8 hours which corresponds with peak serum concentrations of the bioactive moiety. Approximately 50% of the maximal antihypertensive effect is still present 24 hours after taking the drug (fig. 5) [Gomez et al., 1983a].

Since enalaprilat has a long serum half-life, it was of interest to determine if once-daily administration of enalapril would control hypertension. Studies were conducted using 20 and 40 mg/day. The data from the 20 mg/day study (table I) indicate that enalapril administered as 20mg once-daily or 10mg twice-daily reduces blood pressure to a similar extent (Bergstrand et al., 1982; Gomez et al., 1983b). Results from the 40 mg/day study (Saris et al., 1983) support the conclusion that once-daily dosing is as effective as half the dose administered twice-daily.

At least 60% of patients with mild to moderate hypertension are controlled (supine diastolic blood pressure ≤ 90mm Hg) by treatment with enalapril alone in doses up to 40 mg/day (Biollaz et al., 1982a). An even greater proportion (90%) can be controlled by the addition of a diuretic (Biollaz et al., 1982a; Ferguson et al., 1982; Gomez et al., 1984b; Nelson et al., 1983b).

Enalapril does not produce hypokalaemia, hyperglycaemia, hyperuricaemia or hypercholesterolaemia. When combined with hydrochlorothiazide, enalapril attenuates the undesirable diuretic-induced metabolic side effects (Gomez et al., 1984b; Nelson et al., 1983a). Also, it has been shown that enalapril reverses the hypokalaemia associated with primary and secondary hyperaldosteronism (Griffing and Melby, 1983).

Table I. The antihypertensive effect of enalapril 20mg daily, administered either as a single or divided daily dose in 53 patients with mild to moderate essential hypertension. Data from Gomez et al. (1983b).

Regimen	Blood pressure (mm Hg)		Change[a]
	initial	at 4 weeks	
Supine			
20mg qd	162/104	146/92	−17/−11
10mg bid	161/102	145/92	−16/−11
Erect			
20mg qd	162/106	142/94	−20/−12
10mg bid	159/105	139/93	−20/−12

a All within-treatment changes $p < 0.001$.

Long term treatment with a fixed daily dose of enalapril causes a progressive reduction in blood pressure which does not reach a maximum before 3 weeks of therapy. Although significant blood pressure reduction can be obtained with doses of enalapril 2.5 to 80 mg/day, the recommended dose is 10 to 40 mg/day, administered as a once- or twice-daily regimen. The usual starting dose of enalapril is 10mg/day (Bergstrand et al., in press 1985).

The antihypertensive effect of enalapril is characterised haemodynamically by a reduction in systemic vascular resistance and a moderate increase in cardiac output with no change in heart rate (Velasco et al., 1983). The change in cardiac output is due to an increase in stroke volume, since heart rate does not change. Cardiac output and oxygen consumption are unchanged during exercise (Morioka and Moriyama, 1983). A decrease in limb vascular resistance has been observed in hypertensive patients, and is representative of the change in systemic vascular resistance. The total peripheral resistance index decreased 16% during maximal bicycle exercise in patients with moderately severe essential hypertension treated for 6 to 8 months with enalapril. There were no significant changes in their cardiac output, heart rate or stroke volume (Lund-Johansen and Omvik, 1984). Haemodynamic changes appear to persist during long term treatment with enalapril, without significant expansion in total blood volume (Fouad et al., 1983). A reversal of left ventricular hypertrophy without reducing left ventricular performance has been observed in hypertensive patients treated with enalapril (Dunn et al., 1984; Nakashima et al., 1983). Enalapril does not affect myocardial perfusion during exercise (Rosendorff et al., 1984).

Enalapril antagonises the vasoconstrictor effects of angiotensin II on cat coronary arteries, probably by a direct antagonism of angiotensin receptors (Lefer and Lefer, 1984). This angiotensin II antagonism may explain the anecdotal reports of beneficial effects of enalapril in instances of human myocardial ischaemia. Cardioprotective effects of enalapril in experimental myocardial ischaemia have been reported recently (Lefer and Peck, 1984). Controlled clinical trials in this area are being carried out.

Enalapril produces profound changes in thc forearm arterial system: brachial artery diameter, blood velocity and blood flow increased significantly, while forearm vascular resistance decreased (Simon et al., 1984). Enalapril thus dilates both the large artery and arterioles involved in the forearm circulation. It has no effect, however, on veins. Enalapril produces a greater systolic blood pressure effect than other antihypertensive agents, viz., metoprolol (O'Connor et al., 1984) and propranolol (Beevers et al., 1984). This suggests that enalapril could be useful in the treatment of systolic hypertension.

Biochemical changes in hypertensive patients treated with single doses of enalapril are similar to those observed in healthy subjects: reductions in plasma angiotensin II and aldosterone with a simultaneous increase in plasma renin activity. Chronic enalapril therapy results in increased angiotensin I and plasma renin activity, and depressed renin substrate (Boer and Geyskes, 1984) without affecting inactive renin (Golub et al., 1984). The increase in plasma renin activity is probably due to an increase in active renin concentration. Increases in active renin concentration have been reported to be greater in responders to enalapril than in nonresponders, suggesting that unresponsiveness to enalapril may be associated with an abnormality in the feedback mechanism which regulates renin release (Gomez et al., 1984a). Similar results have recently been reported for captopril in patients with congestive heart failure, wherein responders were distinguished from nonresponders by their reactive hyperreninaemia (Packer et al., 1984).

In patients treated for up to 10 months, the blood pressure remains controlled even though plasma angiotensin II and aldosterone return to baseline levels 12 to 16 hours after drug administration, while ACE remains inhibited and plasma renin activity elevated (Biollaz et al., 1982a). However, 6 hours after each subsequent daily dose of enalapril, angiotensin II, aldosterone and ACE activity are further reduced in patients chronically treated with enalapril (Brunner et al., 1983). These results suggest that tachyphylaxis to the blockade of angiotensin II generation does not occur with prolonged enalapril administration. Although assays for angiotensin II have been criticised because of the crossreactivity with angiotensin I, especially in samples treated with converting enzyme inhibitors, the radioimmunoassay for angiotensin II has been greatly improved by using new methods of peptide extraction and a more selective antiserum (Nussberger et al., 1984).

Sympathetically mediated cardiovascular reflexes are not impaired in hypertensive patients chronically treated with enalapril (Fouad et al., 1984). Enalapril attenuates the rise of plasma noradrenaline during exercise (Morioka and Moriyama, 1983).

Renal plasma flow increases significantly in patients with mild essential hypertension after acute and chronic enalapril therapy (Bauer, 1984; Simon et al., 1983). Bauer (1984) reported no changes in glomerular filtration rate in hypertensive patients with a normal glomerular filtration rate, but significant increases in those with a glomerular filtration rate less than 80 ml/min. The renal effects of enalapril have been reviewed recently (Davies et al., 1984). Enalapril increases urinary urate and sodium excretion in healthy volunteers on a normal dietary sodium intake (Lant et al., 1984), and produces natriuresis in hypertensive patients (Johnston et al., 1984) on a normal sodium diet, but not in those with a low sodium intake.

In a study where patients with mild to moderately severe hypertension were treated for 1 month with enalapril 5 to 80 mg/day, no rebound hypertension was observed after abrupt withdrawal of the drug (Guthrie et al., 1982).

3.2 Renovascular Hypertension

Experience to date indicates that long term treatment with enalapril (10 to 40 mg/day) produces good blood pressure control (Hodsman et al., 1982; Karlberg et al., 1984). Blood pressure control improves with time (several months), such that the dose of enalapril may be reduced. Most of these patients do not need the addition of a diuretic (Hodsman et al., 1983). Patients chronically treated with single daily doses of enalapril have reduced levels of circulating angiotensin II and aldosterone throughout the day (Hodsman et al., 1983).

3.3 Congestive Heart Failure

Enalapril has been administered to patients with congestive heart failure refractory to conventional treatment with digitalis and diuretics. Significant increases are observed in cardiac output and stroke

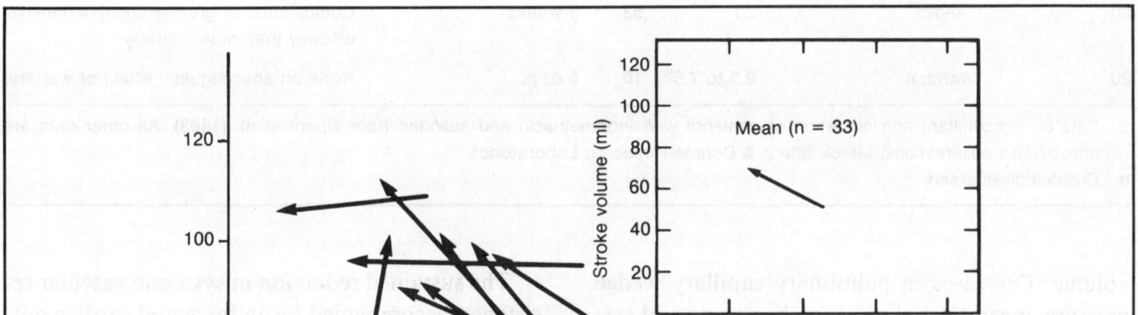

Fig. 6. Left ventricular function curve after 1 to 4 months of enalapril therapy. Each arrow represents the response of a single patient and points from baseline to follow-up. The insert arrow represents the mean response (n = 33), PCWP = pulmonary capillary wedge pressure. (Unpublished data, Merck Sharp & Dohme).

Table II. Summary of pharmacokinetic and pharmacodynamic studies of enalapril in combination with various drugs[a]

Drug and daily dose (mg) enalapril	other agent		n	Duration of concomitant treatment	Pharmacokinetic and/or pharmacodynamic effect
10	Digoxin	0.25	12	single dose	None on bioavailability of enalapril
10	Frusemide	80	12	single dose	None on bioavailability of either drug
20	Hydrochlorothiazide	50	12	1 week	As above
10		50	11	2 weeks	Combination of greater antihypertensive efficacy than monotherapy
40	Indomethacin	100	33	4 weeks	None on hypotensive effect of enalapril
20	Methyldopa	500	23	single dose	Combination of greater antihypertensive efficacy than monotherapy
10	Propranolol	10	12	single dose	Increase in propranolol bioavailability Decrease in enalapril bioavailability
40	Sulindac	400	33	4 weeks	None on hypotensive effect of enalapril
20	Timolol	20	53	3 weeks	Combination of greater antihypertensive efficacy than monotherapy
20	Warfarin	2.5 to 7.5[b]	10	5 days	None on anticoagulant effect of warfarin

a Data on concomitant administration of enalapril with indomethacin and sulindac from Oparil et al. (1983). All other data are unpublished observations, Merck Sharp & Dohme Research Laboratories.
b Doses individualised.

volume. Decreases in pulmonary capillary wedge pressure, mean arterial pressure, heart rate and systemic vascular resistance occur in patients treated for up to 4 months with enalapril (10 to 20 mg/day) [Gomez et al., in preparation].

Chronic therapy results in a sustained favourable change in the haemodynamic indices. The left ventricular function curve shifts upward and to the left (fig. 6). Significant improvements in patients' NYHA functional classification, ejection fraction and exercise tolerance are also observed. Furthermore, in most cases the dose of diuretic needed can be decreased after enalapril treatment has been instituted (Fitzpatrick et al., 1983a). Recently, it was reported that enalapril reduces the ventricular ectopic rate in patients with severe congestive heart failure who are receiving digitalis and diuretics. This important effect may be a consequence of improved cardiac function and an increase in serum potassium and magnesium concentrations (Cleland et al., 1985).

The sustained reduction in systemic vascular resistance, accompanied by an increased cardiac output and a decrease in pulmonary capillary wedge pressure all indicate that enalapril is a vasodilator with balanced effects on preload and afterload. These changes are accompanied by a gradual, smooth reduction in blood pressure without increased heart rate. There is no first-dose effect as described for captopril (Ader et al., 1980; Dzau et al., 1980; Sharpe et al., 1980). The gradual, smooth reduction in blood pressure, observed during the first 8 hours post-drug is an important pharmacological characteristic of enalapril which is rarely associated with symptomatic hypotension (Fitzpatrick et al., 1983b). However, severe hypotension may occur in hyponatraemic and/or hypovolaemic patients with high plasma renin activity.

It has been reported that there is no reduction in the formation of enalaprilat from enalapril in patients with liver dysfunction associated with severe heart failure, suggesting that the esterolytic capacity is adequate and that dosage modification may not be necessary in such cases (Jackson et al., 1984b).

4. Drug Interactions

Studies were performed to determine if enalapril has clinically meaningful interactions with antihypertensive drugs, cardiac glycosides, anticoagulants and nonsteroidal anti-inflammatory agents. The results are summarised in table II.

The antihypertensive effect of enalapril is potentiated by hydrochlorothiazide, propranolol, timolol and methyldopa (unpublished observations, Merck Sharp & Dohme), but unaffected by indomethacin and sulindac (Oparil et al., 1983). No pharmacokinetic interactions occur between enalapril and frusemide, hydrochlorothiazide and digoxin. The bioavailability of enalapril is slightly reduced when propranolol is coadministered, but this does not appear to be of any clinical significance. Enalapril does not affect the anticoagulant action of warfarin.

5. Side Effects

It is advantageous to treat hypertension with ACE inhibitors, because they do not induce reflex tachycardia, orthostatic hypotension or central nervous system and autonomic side effects, and they may improve renal blood flow and glomerular filtration.

Impotence and loss of libido have not been reported following treatment with enalapril. Enalapril does not affect serum T_3, rT_3, T_4 and TSH in hypertensive patients (Wilhelmsson, C.E. and Berglund, G.; unpublished data), serum prolactin in healthy volunteers (McNabb et al., 1983), plasma cortisol in either normal subjects (Hodsman et al., 1984) or patients with congestive heart failure (Fitzpatrick et al., 1983a).

To date, approximately 6000 people have received treatment with enalapril (2.5 to 80 mg/day), over 1000 for more than 1 year, approximately 600 for more than 2 years and over 100 for more than 3 years. Dysgeusia (0.5%), proteinuria (> 1 g/24 hour; 0.51%), skin rash (1.2%) and leucopenia (< 3000/mm^3; 0.5%) have been reported. There was one instance of leucopenia < 1000/mm^3 (Studer and Vetter, 1982). If one uses the criteria established for captopril by Frohlich et al. (1984), then neither leucopenia nor proteinuria are observed with enalapril. A single case of glycosuria and azotaemia has been reported following the administration of enalapril together with high doses (100 mg/day) of hydrochlorothiazide (Cressman et al., 1982). A man taking enalapril reported a burning sensation in his mouth comparable with having been scalded; however, his taste perception was normal (Vlasses et al., 1982).

Four hypertensive patients with previously documented adverse reactions to captopril (including maculopapular rash, pruritus and fever) have been treated for several months with enalapril without the reoccurrence of the side effects (Gavras and Gavras, 1983). Another hypertensive patient with a history of skin rash to methimazole developed a similar cutaneous reaction to a low dose of captopril. When enalapril was substituted for captopril, the rash gradually disappeared without the loss of blood pressure control (Rotmensch et al., 1983).

Adverse effects with most drugs are dose-related; i.e., higher doses are associated with an increased incidence and severity. No such dose response is seen for enalapril within its therapeutic dose range of 10 to 40 mg/day (Smith et al., 1984).

6. Conclusions

Enalapril is a potent, orally-active, long-acting, nonsulphydryl ACE inhibitor which effectively lowers blood pressure in patients with essential and renovascular hypertension and improves the signs and symptoms of congestive heart failure. Human experience to date (6000 patients/subjects) indicates that enalapril in most patients is safe and well tolerated.

References

Ader, R.; Chatterjee, K.; Ports, T.; Brundage, B.; Hiramatsu, B. and Parmley, W.: Immediate and sustained hemodynamic and clinical improvement in chronic heart failure by an oral angiotensin converting enzyme inhibitor. Circulation 61: 931-937 (1980).

Bauer, J.H.: Role of angiotensin converting enzyme inhibitors in essential and renal hypertension. Effects of captopril and enalapril on renin-angiotensin-aldosterone, renal function and hemodynamics, salt and water excretion and body fluid composition. American Journal of Medicine 77 (2A): 43-51 (1984).

Beevers, D.G.; Weissberg, P.L.; Thurston, H.; Bing, R.F.; Breckenridge, A.; L'Orme, M.; Grimmer, S.F.M.; Goodwin, F.J.; Barnes, J.N.; Drew, P.J.; Skeehan, J.D.; Davies, J.R.; Kapila, H.; Currie, W.J.C.; Vandenburg, M.J.; Cooper, W.D.; Arr, S. and Wollard, M.: Enalapril in essential hypertension: A comparative study with propranolol. British Journal of Clinical Pharmacology 18: 51-56 (1984).

Bergstrand, R.; Herlitz, H.; Johansson, S.; Berglund, G.; Vedin, A.; Wilhelmsson, C.; Gomez, H.J.; Cirillo, V.J. and Bolognese, J.A.: Effective dose range of enalapril in mild to moderate essential hypertension. British Journal of Clinical Pharmacology, in press (1985).

Bergstrand, R.; Johansson, S.; Vedin, A. and Wilhelmsson, C.: Comparison of once-a-day and twice-a-day dosage regimens of enalapril (MK-421) in patients with mild hypertension. British Journal of Clinical Pharmacology 14: 136P (1982).

Biollaz, J.; Brunier, M.; Turini, G.A.; Brunner, D.B.; Porchet, M.; Gomez, H.J.; Jones, K.H.; Ferber, F.; Abrams, W.B.; Gavras, H. and Brunner, H.R.: Three new long-acting converting enzyme inhibitors: relationship between plasma converting enzyme activity and response to angiotensin I. Clinical Pharmacology and Therapeutics 29: 665-670 (1981).

Biollaz, J.; Brunner, H.R.; Gavras, I.; Waeber, B. and Gavras, H.: Antihypertensive therapy with MK-421: angiotensin II-renin relationships to evaluate efficacy of converting enzyme blockade. Journal of Cardiovascular Pharmacology 4: 966-972 (1982a).

Biollaz, J.; Schelling, J.L.; Jacot des Combes, B.; Brunner, D.B.; Desponds, G.; Brunner, H.R.; Ulm, E.H.; Hichens, M. and Gomez, H. J.: Enalapril maleate and a lysine analogue (MK-521) in normal volunteers: Relationship between plasma drug levels and the renin-angiotensin system. British Journal of Clinical Pharmacology 14: 363-368 (1982b).

Boer, P. and Geyskes, G.G.: Plasma renin substrate concentration during chronic enalapril and propranolol therapy. Hypertension 6 (1): 132-133 (1984).

Brunner, D.B.; Desponds, G.; Biollaz, J.; Keller, I.; Ferber, F.; Gavras, H.; Brunner, H.R. and Schelling, J.L.: Effect of a new angiotensin converting enzyme inhibitor MK-421 and its lysine analogue on the components of the renin system in healthy subjects. British Journal of Clinical Pharmacology 11: 461-467 (1981).

Brunner, H.R.; Waeber, B.; Nussberger, J.; Schaller, M.D. and Gomez, H.J.: Long-term clinical experience with enalapril in essential hypertension. Journal of Hypertension 1 (Suppl. 1): 103-107 (1983).

Cleland, J.G.F.; Dargie, H.J.; Gillen, G.; Hodsman, G.P.; Ball, J.G. and Robertson, J.I.S.: Effects of enalapril on clinical state and serum electrolytes in congestive heart failure. British Journal of Clinical Pharmacology, in press (1985).

Cressman, M.D.; Vidt, D.G. and Acker, C.: Renal glycosuria and azotemia after enalapril maleate (MK-421). Lancet 2: 440 (1982).

Davies, R.O.; Gomez, H.J.; Irvin, J.D. and Walker, J.F.: An overview of the clinical pharmacology of enalapril. British Journal of Clinical Pharmacology 18: 215S-229S (1984).

Dunn, F.G.; Oigman, W.; Ventura, H.O.; Messerli, F.H.; Kobrin, I. and Frohlich, E.D.: Systemic and renal effects of enalapril and its effects on cardiac mass. Journal of Hypertension 2 (Suppl. 2): 57-61 (1984).

Dzau, V.J.; Colucci, W.S.; Williams, G.H.; Curfman, G. and Meggs, L.: Sustained effectiveness of converting enzyme inhibition in patients with severe congestive heart failure. New England Journal of Medicine 302: 1373-1379 (1980).

Ferguson, R.K.; Vlasses, P.H.; Swanson, B.N.; Mojaverian, P.; Hichens, M.; Irvin, J. and Huber, P.: Effects of enalapril, a new converting enzyme inhibitor, in hypertension. Clinical Pharmacology and Therapeutics 32: 48-53 (1982).

Ferguson, R.K.; Irvin, J.D.; Swanson, B.N.; Vlasses, P.H.; Bergquist, P.A.; Till, A.E. and Feinberg, J.A.: Food does not alter the absorption of enalapril maleate (MK-421) as measured by the disposition of its active metabolite (MK-422). Clinical Pharmacology and Therapeutics 33: 254 (1983).

Fitzpatrick, D.; Nicholls, M.G.; Ikram, H. and Espiner, E.A.: Hemodynamic, hormonal and electrolyte effects of enalapril in heart failure. British Heart Journal 50: 163-169 (1983a).

Fitzpatrick, D.; Nicholls, M.G.; Ikram, H. and Espiner, E.A.: Acute hemodynamic, hormonal and electrolyte effects and short term clinical response to enalapril in heart failure. Journal of Hypertension 1 (Suppl. 1): 147-153 (1983b).

Fouad, F.M.; Tarazi, R.C. and Bravo, E.L.: Cardiac and haemodynamic effects of enalapril. Journal of Hypertension 1 (Suppl. 1): 135-142 (1983).

Fouad, F.M.; Tarazi, R.C.; Bravo, E.L. and Textor, S.C.: Hemodynamic and antihypertensive effects of the new oral angiotensin-converting enzyme inhibitor MK-421 (enalapril). Hypertension 6: 167-174 (1984).

Frohlich, E.D.; Cooper, R.A. and Lewis, E.J.: Review of the overall experience of captopril in hypertension. Archives of Internal Medicine 144: 1441-1444 (1984).

Gavras, I. and Gavras, H.: Captopril and enalapril. Annals of Internal Medicine 98: 566-567 (1983).

Golub, M.; Eggena, P.; Barrett, J. and Sambhi, M.P.: Renin-angiotensin, hemodynamic and renal responses to enalapril with and without hydrochlorothiazide in essential hypertension. Clinical Research 32 (2): 242A (1984).

Gomez, H.J. and Cirillo, V.J.: Angiotensin converting enzyme inhibitors: The clinical pharmacology of captopril and enalapril maleate. In Velasco (Ed.) Clinical Pharmacology and Therapeutics (International Congress Series No. 604), pp. 52-57 (Excerpta Medica, Amsterdam 1983).

Gomez, H.J.; Cirillo, V.J. and Jones, K.H.: The clinical pharmacology of enalapril. Journal of Hypertension 1 (Suppl. 1) 65-70 (1983a).

Gomez, H.J.; Velasco, M.; Bolognese, J.A. and Cirillo, V.J.: Enalapril: Comparison of once-a-day and twice-a-day dosage regimens in essential hypertension. Proceedings of the IInd World Conference on Clinical Pharmacology and Therapeutics, Abstract 577 (1983b).

Gomez, H.J.; Lutterbeck, P.M.; Cirillo, V.J.; Bolognese, J.A.; Wilhelmsson, C. and Berglund, G.: Diminished renin compensatory increase in nonresponders to enalapril. Clinical Pharmacology and Therapeutics 35: 244 (1984a).

Gomez, H.J.; Walker, J.F.; Moncloa, F.; Cirillo, V.J.; Sromovsky, J.A. and Gabriel, M.: Enalapril attenuates hydrochlorothiazide-induced hypokalemia, hyperglycemia, hyperuricemia and hypercholesterolemia; in Puschett and Greenberg (Eds) Diuretics. Chemistry, Pharmacology and Clinical Applications, pp. 263-265 (Elsevier, New York 1984b).

Griffing, G.T. and Melby, J.C.: The therapeutic use of a new potassium-sparing diuretic, amiloride, and a converting enzyme inhibitor, MK-421, in preventing hypokalemia associated with primary and secondary hyperaldosteronism. Clinical and Experimental Hypertension. Theory and Practice A5 (6): 779-801 (1983).

Guthrie, G.P.; Hammond, J. and Kotchen, T.A.: Abrupt cessation of enalapril (MK-421) in essential hypertension. Clinical Research 30: 733A (1982).

Hodsman, G.P.; Brown, J.J.; Davies, D.L.; Fraser, R.; Lever, A.F.; Morton, J.J.; Murray, G.D. and Robertson, J.I.S.: Converting enzyme inhibitor enalapril (MK-421) in treatment of hypertension with renal artery stenosis. British Medical Journal 285: 1697-1699 (1982).

Hodsman, G.P.; Brown, J.J.; Cumming, A.M.M.; Davies, D.L.; East, B.W.; Lever, A.F.; Morton, J.J.; Murray, G.D. and Robertson, J.I.S.: Enalapril (MK-421) in the treatment of hypertension with renal artery stenosis. Journal of Hypertension 1 (Suppl. 1): 109-117 (1983).

Hodsman, G.P.; Zabludowski, J.R.; Zoccali, C.; Fraser, R.; Morton, J.J; Murray, G.D. and Robertson, J.I.S.: Enalapril (MK-421) and its lysine analogue (MK-521): A comparison of acute and chronic effects on blood pressure, renin-angiotensin system and sodium excretion in normal man. British Journal of Clinical Pharmacology 17: 233-241 (1984).

Jackson, B.; Cubela, R. and Johnston, C.I.: Effect of dietary sodium on angiotensin-converting enzyme (ACE) inhibition and the acute hypotensive effect of enalapril (MK-421) in essential hypertension. Journal of Hypertension 2: 371-377 (1984a).

Jackson, B.; Larmour, I.; McGrath, B. and Johnston, C.: Bioactivation of enalapril to enalaprilic acid in man: In vitro and in vivo studies. 10th Scientific Meeting of the International Society of Hypertension, Abstract 471 (1984b).

Johnston, C.I.; Jackson, B.; Cubela, R. and Arnolda, L.: Mechanism for hypotensive action of angiotensin converting enzyme inhibitors. Clinical and Experimental Hypertension, Theory and Practice A6(1-2): 551-561 (1984).

Karlberg, B.E.; Fyhrquist, F.; Gronhagen-Riska, C.; Tikkanen, I. and Ohman, K.P.: Enalapril and lisinopril in renovascular hypertension. Antihypertensive and hormonal effects of two new angiotensin-converting enzyme (ACE) inhibitors. Scandinavian Journal of Urology and Nephrology (Suppl. 79): 103-106 (1984).

Kelly, J.; Doyle, G.; Donohoe, J.; Laher, M.; Vandenburg, M.J.; Currie, W.J.C. and Cooper, W.D.: The pharmacokinetic profile of enalaprilat in normal subjects and patients with renal impairment. British Journal of Clinical Pharmacology 18: 274P (1984).

Lant, A.F.; McNabb, R.W. and Noormohamed, F.H.: Kinetic and metabolic aspects of enalapril action. Journal of Hypertension 2 (Suppl. 2): 37-42 (1984).

Lefer, D.J. and Lefer, A.M.: Coronary vascular actions of the converting enzyme inhibitor, enalapril. Proceedings of the Society for Experimental Biology and Medicine 175: 211-214 (1984).

Lefer, A.M. and Peck, R.C.: Cardioprotective effects of enalapril in acute myocardial ischemia. Pharmacology 29: 61-69 (1984).

Lund-Johansen, P. and Omvik, P.: Long-term hemodynamic effects of enalapril (alone and in combination with hydrochlorothiazide) at rest and during exercise. Journal of Hypertension 2 (Suppl. 2): 49-56 (1984).

MacGregor, G.A.; Markandu, N.D.; Bayliss, J.; Roulston, J.E.; Squires, M. and Morton, J.J.: Non-sulfhydryl-containing angiotensin converting enzyme inhibitor (MK-421): evidence for role of renin system in normotensive subjects. British Medical Journal 283: 401-403 (1981).

McNabb, W.R.; Brooks, B.A.; Noormohamed, F.; Lant, A.F.; Gomez, H. J.; Cirillo, V.J.; Hichens, M. and Bolognese, J.A.: The effect of enalapril on serum prolactin. British Journal of Clinical Pharmacology 15: 752-754 (1983).

Millar, J.A.; Derkx, F.H.M.; McLean, K. and Reid, J.L.: Pharmacodynamics of converting enzyme inhibition: The cardiovascular, endocrine and autonomic effects of MK-421 (enalapril) and MK-521. British Journal of Clinical Pharmacology 14: 347-355 (1982).

Morioka, S. and Moriyama, K.: Cardiac and hormonal effects of enalapril (MK-421) therapy in hypertension. Japanese Journal of Medicine 22 (4): 333 (1983).

Nakashima, Y.; Fouad, F.M.; Tarazi, R.C. and Bravo, E.L.: Left ventricular function with reversal of left ventricular hypertrophy in hypertensive patients. Journal of the American College of Cardiology 1 (2): 599 (1983).

Nelson, E.B.; Pool, J.L.; Taylor, A.A.; Mitchell, J.R. and Irvin, J.D.: Metabolic effects of hydrochlorothiazide + enalapril in hypertensive patients. Clinical Research 31 (5): 834A (1983a).

Nelson, E.B.; Pool, J.L.; Taylor, A.A. and Mitchell, J.R.: Long-term efficacy of enalapril plus hydrochlorothiazide in the treatment of essential hypertension. Clinical Pharmacology and Therapeutics 33: 230 (1983b).

Nussberger, J.; Re, R.; Matsueda, G.R. and Haber, E.: A simplified radioimmunoassay for physiologically active angiotensin peptide [(1-8) Octa- and (2-8) Heptapeptides]. Hormone Metabolism Research 16: 596-600 (1984).

O'Connor, D.T.; Mosley, C.A.; Cervenka, J. and Bernstein, K.N.: Contrasting renal haemodynamic responses to the angiotensin converting enzyme inhibitor enalapril and the beta-adrenergic antagonist metoprolol in essential hypertension. Journal of Hypertension 2 (Suppl. 2): 89-92 (1984).

Oparil, S.; Horton, R.; Wilkins, L.H.; Irvin, J.; Hammett, D.K. and Dustan, H.P.: Antihypertensive effects of enalapril (MK-421) in low renin essential hypertension: Role of vasodilator prostaglandins. Clinical Research 31 (2): 538A (1983).

Packer, M.; Medina, N. and Yushak, M.: Efficacy of captopril in low-renin congestive heart failure: Importance of sustained reactive hyperreninemia in distinguishing responders from nonresponders. American Journal of Cardiology 54: 771-777 (1984).

Patchett, A.A.; Harris, E.; Tristram, E.W.; Wyvratt, M.J.; Wu, M.T.; Taub, D.; Petersen, E.R.; Ikeler, T.J.; tenBroeke, J.; Payne, L.G.; Ondeyka, D.L.; Thorsett, E.D.; Greenlee, W.J.; Lohr, N.S.; Hoffsommer, R.D.; Joshua, H.; Ruyle, W.V.; Rothrock, J.W.; Aster, S.D.; Maycock, A.L.; Robinson, F.M.; Hirschmann, R.; Sweet, C.S.; Ulm, E.H.; Gross, D.M.; Vassil, T.C. and Stone, C.A.: A new class of angiotensin converting enzyme inhibitors. Nature 288: 280-283 (1980).

Rosendorff, C.; Goodman, C. and Coull, A.: Effect of antihypertensive therapy on left ventricular function and myocardial perfusion at rest and during exercise. Journal of Hypertension 2 (Suppl. 2): 63-68 (1984).

Rotmensch, H.H.; Vlasses, P.H. and Ferguson, R.K.: Resolution of captopril-induced rash after substitution of enalapril. Pharmacotherapy 3: 131-133 (1983).

Saris, S.; Affrime, M.B.; Lowenthal, D.T.; Irvin, J.; Viau, J.; Dickerman, D. and Onesti, G.: Similar antihypertensive effect of once- and twice-daily enalapril. Clinical Research 31 (2): 334A (1983).

Saris, S.; Lowenthal, D.; Klein, L.; Irvin, J.D.; Merrill, D.; Till, A.E.; Hichens, M. and Harris, K.E.: Enalapril maleate in renal failure. Clinical Pharmacology and Therapeutics 35: 272 (1984).

Sharpe, D.N.; Coxon, R.J.; Douglas, J.E. and Long, B.: Low dose captopril in chronic heart failure. Acute hemodynamic effects and long-term treatment. Lancet 2: 1154-1157 (1980).

Shoback, D.M.; Williams, G.H.; Swartz, S.L.; Davies, R.O. and Hollenberg, N.K.: Time course and effect of sodium intake on vascular and hormonal responses to enalapril (MK-421) in normal subjects. Journal of Cardiovascular Pharmacology 5 (6): 1010-1018 (1983).

Simon, A.C.; Levenson, J.A.; Bouthier, J.D.; Benetos, A.; Achimastos, A.; Fouchard, M.; Maarek, B.C. and Safar, M.E.: Comparison of oral MK-421 and propranolol in mild to moderate essential hypertension and their effects on arterial and venous vessels of the forearm. American Journal of Cardiology 53: 781-785 (1984).

Simon, G.; Morioka, S.; Synder, D.K. and Cohn, J.N.: Increased renal plasma flow in long term enalapril treatment of hypertension. Clinical Pharmacology and Therapeutics 34: 459-465 (1983).

Smith, W.M.; Kulaga, S.F.; Moncloa, F.; Pingeon, R. and Walker, J.F.: Overall tolerance and safety of enalapril. Journal of Hypertension 2 (Suppl. 2): 113-117 (1984).

Studer, A. and Vetter, W.: Reversible leucopenia associated with angiotensin converting enzyme inhibitor MK-421. Lancet 1: 458 (1982).

Till, A.E.; Irvin, J.D.; Hichens, M.; Lee, R.B.; Davies, R.O.; Swanson, B. and Vlasses, P.H.: Pharmacodynamics and disposition of intravenous MK-422, the diacid metabolite of enalapril maleate. Clinical Pharmacology and Therapeutics 31: 275 (1982).

Till, A.E.; Gomez, H.J.; Hichens, M.; Bolognese, J.A.; McNabb, W.R.; Brooks, B.A.; Noormohamed, F. and Lant, A.F.: Pharmacokinetics of repeated single oral doses of enalapril maleate (MK-421) in normal volunteers. Biopharmaceutics and Drug Disposition 5: 273-280 (1984).

Tocco, D.L.; deLuna, F.A.; Duncan, A.E.W.; Vassil, T.C. and Ulm, E.H.: The physiological disposition and metabolism of enalapril maleate (MK-421) in laboratory animals. Drug Metabolism and Disposition 10: 15-19 (1982).

Ulm, E.H.; Hichens, M.; Gomez, H.J.; Till, A.E.; Hand, E.; Vassil, T.C.; Biollaz, J.; Brunner, H.R. and Schelling. J.L.: Enalapril maleate and a lysine analogue (MK-521): Disposition in man. British Journal of Clinical Pharmacology 14: 357-362 (1982).

Velasco, M.; Murillo, J.; Urbina, A.; Hernandez-Pieretti, O.; Cirillo, V.J. and Gomez, H.J.: Hemodynamic effects of enalapril maleate in patients with essential hypertension. Proceedings of IInd World Conference on Clinical Pharmacology and Therapeutics, Abstract 578 (1983).

Vlasses, P.H.; Rotmensch, H.H. and Ferguson, R.K.: 'Scalded mouth' caused by angiotensin converting enzyme inhibitors. British Medical Journal 284: 1672-1673 (1982).

Waeber, B.; Nussberger, J.; Schaller, M.D.; Gomez, H.J. and Brunner, H.R.: Dopaminergic control of aldosterone secretion in hypertensive patients chronically treated with an angiotensin converting enzyme inhibitor. Hormone Metabolism Research, in press (1984).

Address for correspondence and reprints: Dr *H.J. Gomez,* Department of Cardiovascular Clinical Research, Merck Sharp & Dohme Research Laboratories, Rahway, NJ 07065-0914 (USA).

Drugs 30 (Suppl. 1): 25-34 (1985)
0012-6667/85/0100-0025/$5.00/0

Cardiovascular Pathophysiology of Essential Hypertension: A Clue to Therapy

Franz H. Messerli and *Hector O. Ventura*

Department of Internal Medicine (Section on Hypertension), Ochsner Clinic and Alton Ochsner Medical Foundation, New Orleans

Summary

Arterial hypertension is by definition a haemodynamic disorder. At least 3 different subsets of cardiovascular pathophysiological features can be identified in so-called essential hypertension:

1. The young lean patient characterised by an elevated cardiac output and renal blood flow, elevated plasma renin activity and circulating catecholamine levels, as well as symptoms and signs of hyperadrenergic hypertension.

2. The elderly patient characterised by a low cardiac output often with left ventricular hypertrophy, elevated total peripheral resistance, nephrosclerosis, and symptoms and signs of target organ disease.

3. The obese patient (and to a lesser degree the black patient) characterised by expanded fluid volume state, elevated cardiac output, a normal to low total peripheral resistance, and symptoms and signs of volume overload.

To initiate antihypertensive therapy, the drug of choice in the young patient is a β-adrenergic receptor blocker; in the elderly it is a haemodynamic vasodilator (anti-adrenergic drug, slow channel calcium blocker, or converting enzyme (ACE) inhibitor), and in black or obese patients it remains a thiazide diuretic. Enalapril, a new ACE inhibitor is indicated as a first-step agent in the great majority of hypertensive patients in whom the elevated arterial pressure should be reduced by a decrease in total peripheral resistance, without compromising systemic or regional blood flow. In contrast to other antihypertensive agents, enalapril will lower preload and afterload to the left ventricle while improving systemic and regional flow in elderly patients with latent or manifest congestive heart failure.

Arterial hypertension, by definition, has to be considered a haemodynamic disorder. The classic haemodynamic picture of the patient with established essential hypertension is characterised by an elevated arterial pressure due to an increase in total peripheral resistance and a normal cardiac output. However, investigations over the past few years have indicated that haemodynamic, endocrine and fluid volume findings are not homogeneous in essential hypertension and that at least 3 distinctly different pathophysiological profiles can be identified. The following review describes these different pathophysiological findings in patients with essential hypertension and their effect on cardiac adaptation, and also stresses possible consequences for the selection of specific antihypertensive agents.

1. *Borderline and Early Established Hypertension*

1.1 Haemodynamic Findings

Numerous studies worldwide have indicated that young patients with borderline hypertension (defined as an arterial pressure around 140/90mm Hg) are characterised haemodynamically by an elevated cardiac output and renal blood flow (Esler et al., 1977; Frohlich et al., 1970; Hollenberg and Merrill, 1970; Julius et al., 1971; Kioschos et al., 1967; Messerli et al., 1978; Tuck et al., 1973; Widimsky et al., 1957). Since arterial pressure is only mildly elevated, total peripheral resistance remains numerically normal. However, total peripheral resistance has to be considered still inappropriately high with regard to the elevated cardiac output, since in a normotensive person, total peripheral resistance would be expected to be lower in the presence of a similar (elevated) cardiac output. Indices of activity of the adrenergic nervous system such as resting heart rate, plasma renin activity, and circulating plasma noradrenaline levels tend to be elevated (Esler et al., 1977; Tuck et al., 1973). Intravascular volume may be slightly contracted. Freis (1960) used the illustrative term 'cardiogenic hypertension' to describe such patients haemodynamically. Although that term may no longer be entirely correct, it still describes the primary haemodynamic abnormality associated with borderline hypertension, i.e., an elevated cardiac output.

1.2 Cardiac Adaptation

Several groups of investigators have independently identified cardiac changes that occur very early in the development of primary hypertension (Culpepper et al., 1983; Goldring et al., 1979; Laird et al., 1981; Schieken et al., 1981; Zahka et al., 1981). Echocardiographic evidence of left ventricular hypertrophy has been found to be present in 10 to 15% of adolescents whose blood pressure was above the 90th percentile. Not unexpectedly, the relationship between left ventricular mass and random measurements of arterial pressure was not very close in these teenagers since arterial pressure is often very labile (Culpepper et al., 1983; Goldring et al., 1979; Laird et al., 1981; Schieken et al., 1981; Zahka et al., 1981). Although factors other than arterial pressure also influence the development of left ventricular hypertrophy, these findings indicate that the left ventricle responds to a persisting pressure load, however small, with an increase in contractile elements. Whether or not these adaptive changes ultimately fulfil arbitrarily defined criteria of left ventricular hypertrophy (such as a posterior wall thickness of more than 1.1cm on the echocardiogram or a Sokoloff index of 35cm on the electrocardiogram) becomes irrelevant.

2. *Hypertension in the Elderly*

2.1 Haemodynamic Findings

In contrast to juvenile patients with borderline hypertension, elderly hypertensive patients are characterised by a low cardiac output and, as a consequence, by a very high total peripheral resistance (fig. 1). Resting cardiac output has recently been reported to be well preserved in normotensive subjects throughout the seventh and even the

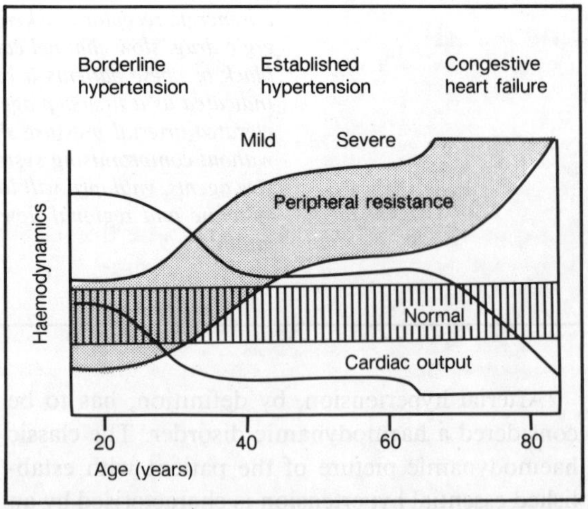

Fig. 1. Change of haemodynamic profile as hypertension progresses from a borderline stage to established hypertension, followed by hypertension with congestive heart failure in the elderly patient. High cardiac output hypertension evolves into high peripheral resistance low cardiac output hypertension.

eighth decade (Rodeheffer et al., 1984), although in previous studies a decline in cardiac output with age was found (Brandfonbrener et al., 1955; Cournand et al., 1945; Standell, 1964). However, in patients with essential hypertension, the left ventricle is burdened with a high afterload which accelerates the age-induced decline of left ventricular performance. The more severe the arterial hypertension, the faster left ventricular function declines and the earlier the stage of congestive heart failure will be reached. However, even those elderly hypertensive patients who are not in overt congestive heart failure, still present with a distinctly lower cardiac output than younger patients with the same arterial pressure (Messerli et al., 1983a). At the same time, renal blood flow often falls even faster than systemic flow because of progressive nephrosclerosis (Hollenberg and Adams, 1976; Meade et al., 1983). In parallel with the increase in total peripheral resistance, intravascular volume becomes more and more contracted (Hollenberg and Merrill, 1970). This volume contraction makes elderly hypertensive patients particularly susceptible to volume depletion (such as induced by diuretic medication). Circulating noradrenaline levels are usually elevated, whereas plasma renin activity has been shown to be low and less responsive in elderly hypertensive patients, unless congestive heart failure is present (Meade et al., 1983).

2.2 Cardiac Changes

More than 50% of elderly patients with essential hypertension have left ventricular hypertrophy by echocardiographic criteria (Report of the Hypertension Task Force, 1979). An increase in posterior wall thickness with age has been documented in a population that was free of cardiovascular disease – in particular, free of arterial hypertension (Gardin et al., 1979; Gerstenblith et al., 1977). Not surprisingly, the increased afterload in arterial hypertension accelerates both the decline in cardiac output as well as the increase in left ventricular mass (fig. 2). Although the classic response to an increased afterload is concentric hypertrophy, congestive heart failure may ultimately ensue, and the left ventricle will become progressively dilated (eccentric hypertrophy).

3. Consequences of Left Ventricular Hypertrophy

3.1 Ventricular Ectopy

We recently documented that patients with left ventricular hypertrophy by electrocardiographic criteria averaged between 40 and 50 times more ventricular (but not atrial) premature contractions than those with essential hypertension without left ventricular hypertrophy or normotensive subjects (Messerli et al., 1984a). Higher grade ventricular ectopy, such as coupled and multifocal premature ventricular contractions, was present in 5 of 16 patients with left ventricular hypertrophy (table I). These data on increased ventricular ectopy provide an electrophysiological correlate of the findings of the Framingham cohort, indicating that left ventricular hypertrophy was a pressure-independent risk factor for sudden death and other cardiovascular morbidity and mortality (Kannel, 1983). Clearly, the appearance of premature ventricular contractions in asymptomatic patients with left ventricular hypertrophy is an ominous electrocardiographical sign that requires aggressive and specific therapeutic intervention.

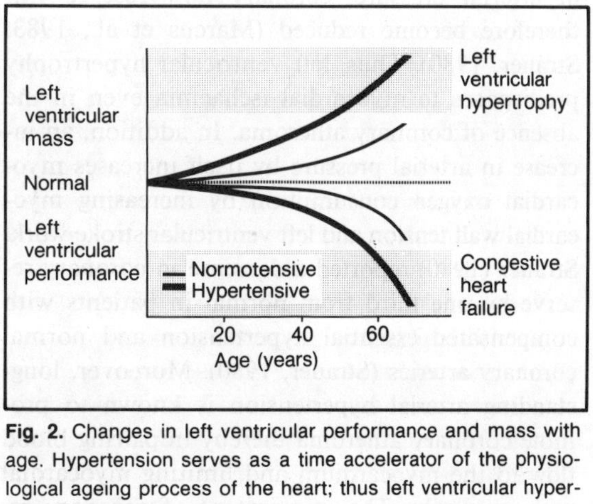

Fig. 2. Changes in left ventricular performance and mass with age. Hypertension serves as a time accelerator of the physiological ageing process of the heart; thus left ventricular hypertrophy and congestive heart failure may develop earlier in life in the patient with hypertension.

Table I. Prevalence and severity of ectopic ventricular activity in patients with left ventricular hypertrophy (LVH) and control groups

Maximal Lown class	Normotensive	Hypertensive	
		without LVH	with LVH[a]
0	10	6	3
I	4	4	6
II	0	0	4
III	0	0	1
IV	0	0	2

a $p < 0.004$ versus both other groups.

3.2 Myocardial Ischaemia and Coronary Artery Disease

Left ventricular hypertrophy occurring beyond infancy does not sufficiently increase the cross-sectional area of the coronary vascular bed but enhances total myocardial oxygen consumption in proportion to muscle mass (Hoffman et al., 1983; Marcus et al., 1983; Strauer, 1980). To supply the increased demand, resting ventricular blood flow must be increased and resting coronary arteries must dilate more than normal. For any given level of arterial pressure, coronary flow reserve will therefore become reduced (Marcus et al., 1983; Strauer, 1980). Thus, left ventricular hypertrophy predisposes to myocardial ischaemia even in the absence of coronary atheroma. In addition, an increase in arterial pressure by itself increases myocardial oxygen consumption by increasing myocardial wall tension and left ventricular stroke work. Strauer (1980) reported a decrease in coronary reserve by one third from normal in patients with compensated essential hypertension and normal coronary arteries (Strauer, 1980). Moreover, longstanding arterial hypertension is known to promote coronary atheroma thereby impairing blood flow to the myocardium and limiting myocardial oxygen supply. The impairment of coronary reserve in left ventricular hypertrophy corroborates clinical experience that patients with accelerated hypertension often exhibit symptoms of angina pectoris despite the absence of overt coronary artery disease.

4. Hypertension in the Obese

4.1 Haemodynamic Findings

Obesity can be defined as an increase in body mass caused by an excessive amount of adipose tissue. An increase in body mass requires an increase in cardiac output and intravascular volume to fulfil metabolic requirements. This increase, however, exceeds by far the amount needed to perfuse excessive adipose and supportive tissue (Messerli et al., 1983b). Thus, obesity is characterised by a relative volume expansion in the presence of a restricted vascular capacitance. Moreover, total peripheral resistance will be lower in obese patients than in lean patients having a similar arterial pressure (Coleman et al., 1971; Messerli et al., 1983b). These haemodynamic changes in obesity (elevated cardiac output, expanding total blood volume, and decreased total peripheral resistance) are very similar to those observed in the experimental situation with salt-loading in a partially nephrectomised dog in which, invariably, arterial hypertension will develop.

4.2 Cardiac Adaptations

Since heart rate remains unchanged, the increased cardiac output in obesity results in an expanded stroke volume (Kaltman and Goldring, 1976; Messerli et al., 1983c). Thus, left ventricular filling pressure and filling volume (preload) become elevated. When this burden persists, the left ventricle responds to it with eccentric left ventricular hypertrophy (Messerli et al., 1983c) [fig. 3]. Indeed, left ventricular mass has been shown to correlate with bodyweight in a heterogeneous population of 171 patients (Messerli et al., 1984b) [fig. 4]. In contrast, arterial hypertension alone stimulates the left ventricle to undergo concentric hypertrophy. A combination of the two evils (obesity and hypertension) will create a double burden for the heart; hence, both preload and afterload will become elevated. Not surprisingly, such an evil combination will lead to early left ventricular dysfunction (Alexander and Pettigrove, 1967; Divitis et al., 1981) [fig. 3]. Indeed, premature congestive heart failure has been found to be a common consequence of longstanding obesity and hypertension (Gordon and Kannel, 1976; Hubert et al., 1983; US Department of Health, Education and Welfare, 1964).

5. *Hypertension and Race*

Hypertension is more prevalent in blacks than whites, and systemic vascular and target organ disease such as hypertensive heart disease, stroke and nephrosclerosis is more rapid and severe (Cruickshank and Beevers, 1982; Entwisle et al., 1977;

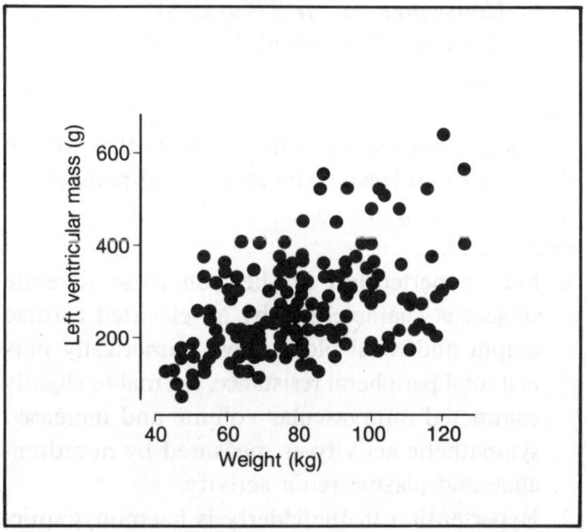

Fig. 4. Correlation of left ventricular mass (as determined by M-mode echocardiography) and bodyweight in 171 patients of a heterogeneous population.

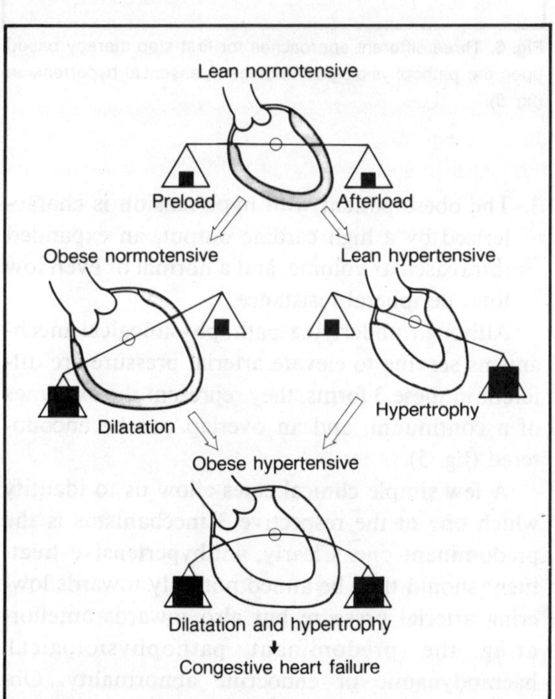

Fig. 3. Obesity increases the left ventricular preload thereby producing dilatation and eccentric left ventricular hypertrophy. On the other hand hypertension increases the afterload, and left ventricular adaptation consists of an increase of relative wall thickness, i.e. concentric left ventricular hypertrophy.

Freis, 1973; Gillum, 1979; HDFP Cooperative Group, 1978; Levy et al., 1978; McDonough et al., 1964; Stamler et al., 1975). However, when comparing systemic haemodynamics and intravascular volume among black and white patients with essential hypertension, we did not find a significant difference in cardiac output, total peripheral resistance or intravascular volume (Messerli et al., 1979). Only resting heart rate and its response to upright tilt were somewhat slower in black patients. When we subsequently studied the renal and hepatic circulation, we found that although hepatic blood flow was similar in black and white patients, renal blood flow was lower and renal vascular resistance was higher at any level of renal arterial pressure in blacks (Frohlich et al., 1984). Also, black patients had increased left ventricular mass when compared with white patients that were matched with regard to mean arterial pressure (Messerli et al., 1983d). These pathophysiological findings clearly lend credence to those epidemiological reports suggesting that for any given level of arterial pressure, hypertensive target organ disease in the kidneys and in the heart can be expected to be more severe in black than in white patients.

6. Consequences for Treatment

6.1 Matching Pathophysiology with Pharmacology

The previous sections demonstrate that we are dealing with at least 3 different sets of pathophysiological findings in so-called 'essential' hypertension (fig. 5).

1. Mild hypertension in the non-obese juvenile subject is characterised by an elevated cardiac output and renal blood flow, numerically normal total peripheral resistance, normal to slightly contracted intravascular volume and increased sympathetic activity as measured by noradrenaline and plasma renin activity.
2. Hypertension in the elderly is haemodynamically characterised by a low cardiac output, very often with left ventricular hypertrophy, elevated total peripheral resistance, contracted intravascular volume and low plasma renin activity as well as elevated circulating catecholamine levels.

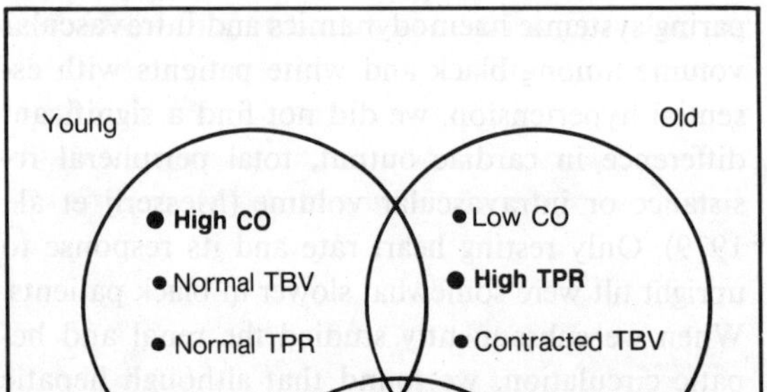

Fig. 5. Three different sets of pathophysiological findings in essential hypertension which may overlap to some extent. CO = cardiac output; TBV = total blood volume; TPR = total peripheral resistance.

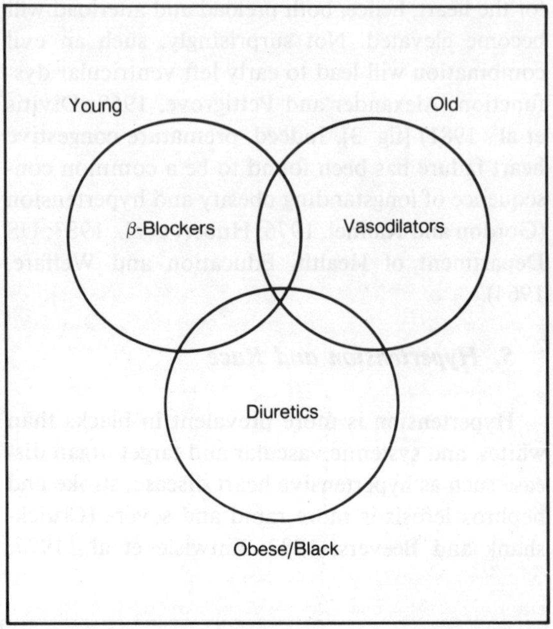

Fig. 6. Three different approaches for first-step therapy based upon the pathophysiological findings in essential hypertension (fig. 5).

3. The obese patient with hypertension is characterised by a high cardiac output, an expanded intravascular volume, and a normal or even low total peripheral resistance.

Although underlying pathophysiological mechanisms serving to elevate arterial pressure are different in these 3 forms, they represent the extremes of a continuum, and an overlap can be encountered (fig. 5).

A few simple clinical clues allow us to identify which one of the respective 3 mechanisms is the predominant one. Clearly, antihypertensive treatment should then be aimed not only towards lowering arterial pressure but also towards ameliorating the predominant pathophysiological, haemodynamic or endocrine abnormality. Obviously a β-adrenoceptor blocker is the first-step drug to be used in juvenile patients with hyperadrenergic 'cardiogenic' hypertension (fig. 6). β-Adrenoceptor blockade will bring cardiac output and heart rate back to normal and also decrease plasma renin activity and shield the β-receptors against surges in circulating catecholamine levels.

In contrast, in the elderly hypertensive patient, a vasodilating agent should be used in an attempt to unburden the heart that has to put up with a high afterload (fig. 6). Vasodilator agents include antiadrenergic drugs, slow channel calcium blockers and ACE inhibitors. All of these agents lower total peripheral resistance and, to a variable degree, decrease preload to the left ventricle, thereby maintaining or even increasing systemic, as well as renal, blood flow.

In the obese patient with expanded intravascular volume and also in most black subjects, the first step antihypertensive agent remains a thiazide diuretic (fig. 6). Black patients have been shown to be more sensitive to diuretic treatment than to β-adrenoceptor blockade, whereas the obese subject is characterised by volume expansion and, frequently, a high sodium intake.

6.2 Angiotensin Converting Enzyme (ACE) Inhibition and Enalapril

Laragh (1984) stated that 'maintenance or improvement of tissue flow will prove a more relevant goal of antihypertensive therapy than lowering of blood pressure *per se*, especially when the latter is achieved at the expense of blood supply.' Although the importance of maintaining or improving regional blood flow when lowering blood pressure was recognised many years ago by Page et al. (1961), it only recently evolved as a major principle of antihypertensive therapy. Evidence is growing that lowering of arterial pressure at the expense of systemic or organ blood flow may often do more harm than good. Thus, the ideal antihypertensive agent should not only lower arterial pressure but should also improve or at least preserve blood flow to the target organs (i.e. the heart, the brain and the kidneys) that are commonly damaged by longstanding arterial hypertension. Target organ damage clinically presents as left ventricular hypertrophy, hypertensive heart disease, nephrosclerosis, renal failure and cerebrovascular damage.

6.2.1 Effects on Haemodynamics

How do ACE inhibitors fit into this concept? We recently evaluated the antihypertensive effect of enalapril by measuring systemic and renal haemodynamics, biochemical and cardiac adaptive changes in 8 patients with essential hypertension before and after 12 weeks of therapy (Dunn et al., 1984). Enalapril was given in an average dose of 20 mg/day. Mean arterial pressure decreased from 110 to 90mm Hg corresponding to a fall of 18% from the baseline. This decrease was mediated through a fall in total peripheral resistance without a significant change in cardiac output or heart rate (fig. 7). At the same time, renal blood flow increased by 16% above pretreatment values, and renal vascular resistance fell by almost 40% (fig. 8). Our data confirm previous studies with enalapril (Fouad et al., 1984; Simon et al., 1983) and captopril (Schalekamp et al., 1982; Tarazi et al., 1980; Ventura et al., 1984) and also indicate that the haemodynamic effects of ACE inhibition fulfil the above postulated requirements: it maintains systemic blood flow, opens up constricted vascular beds and improves blood supply to the kidneys. An increase in renal blood flow occurring 12 weeks after treatment is begun does not necessarily indicate reversal of nephrosclerosis. However, Bauer (1984) and Reams and Bauer (1985) have reported an increase in effective renal plasma flow of up to 100%

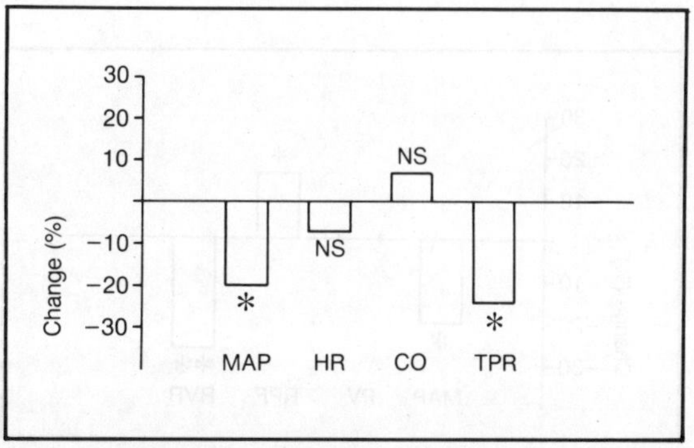

Fig. 7. Enalapril lowers arterial pressure by a decrease in total peripheral resistance without affecting cardiac output. Data from Dunn et al. (1984). MAP = mean arterial pressure; HR = heart rate; CO = cardiac output; TPR = total peripheral resistance; NS = not significant; * $p < 0.05$.

in single patients after 2 years of continuous enalapril treatment. These findings clearly imply structural changes in the renal vasculature.

6.2.2 Cardiac Effects

In our study, enalapril also produced a regression in left ventricular mass as determined by M-mode echocardiography and a decrease in voltage precordial ECG leads (Dunn et al., 1984). Logically, a reduction in left ventricular mass should also lower the risk of sudden death and acute myocardial infarction, both of which have been shown to be increased in patients who have left ventricular hypertrophy.

6.2.3 Effects on Intravascular Volume

Plasma volume as well as total blood volume did not change with enalapril (fig. 8), arguing against sodium and fluid retention – a problem that is occasionally encountered with antiadrenergic drugs. Thus, pseudoresistance (mitigation or abolition of the antihypertensive effect by fluid and salt retention) does not seem to occur with enalapril.The absence of pseudoresistance is hardly surprising in view of the fact that ACE inhibition diminishes aldosterone release from the adrenal cortex. Despite the fall in arterial pressure (which by itself would predispose to sodium and fluid retention), a mild natriuretic effect is commonly seen when enalapril is given.

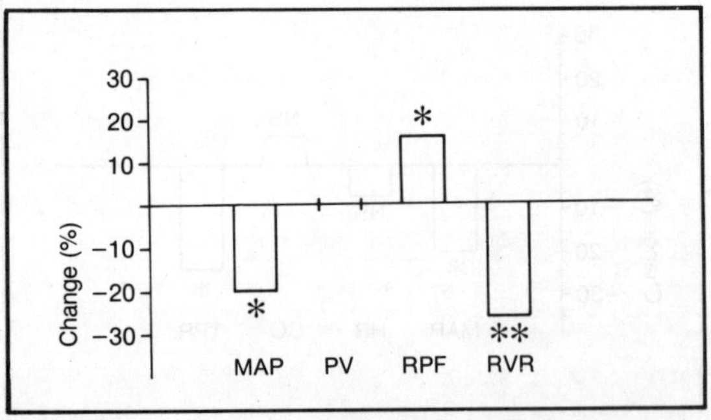

Fig. 8. Renal blood flow increases with enalapril, while renal vascular resistance falls and plasma volume remains unchanged. Data from Dunn et al. (1984). MAP = mean arterial pressure; PV = plasma volume; RPF = renal plasma flow; RVR = renal vascular resistance; * p = 0.05; ** p = 0.01.

Where do these properties place enalapril in the armamentarium of antihypertensive agents? Its final place will not be determined solely by its effect on the cardiovascular pathophysiological profile of established hypertension, but also by patient and physician acceptance, cost, safety, adverse effects, etc. All antihypertensive drugs lower arterial pressure, by definition. However, the trade-off of a lower pressure is often a reduced blood flow to target organs that have been damaged by longstanding arterial hypertension. The patient experiences this relative ischaemia as reduced vigour, hypothermia, fatigue, decreased exercise capacity, or orthostatic hypotension. In sharp contrast, ACE inhibition may lower arterial pressure by improving blood flow to the regional vascular beds in the heart, the kidneys and the brain. This improved blood flow may result in a feeling of well-being which is quite different from the adverse effects seen with other antihypertensive drugs.

Present data with regard to safety and convenience indicate that enalapril could become a first-step agent in the treatment of essential hypertension. Its antihypertensive potency seems quite independent of pretreatment plasma renin activity (Wilkins et al., 1983). From a haemodynamic point of view, enalapril is clearly the agent of choice for first-step treatment of established essential hypertension in the great majority of patients, in whom an elevated total peripheral resistance is the haemodynamic hallmark. However, in contrast to other antihypertensive agents, ACE inhibition will lower preload and afterload to the left ventricle without impairing systemic or regional flow in elderly patients with low cardiac output, and particularly in those with congestive heart failure. Enalapril has no effect on cardiac output in patients whose cardiac output is normal (such as in essential hypertension). In contrast, enalapril increases cardiac output in patients whose cardiac output is low because of manifest or latent congestive heart failure. These unique properties of enalapril will redefine the place of ACE inhibitors in antihypertensive therapy. According to its cardiovascular effects, enalapril shows promise of becoming the first-step agent in all patients with established essential hypertension, perhaps excepting young subjects with hyperadrenergic symptoms or those few patients with hypertension characterised by extracellular fluid volume excess.

Acknowledgement

Part of the material in this article was previously submitted in 'Hemodynamic and Cardiac Adaptation in Essential Hypertension: Consequences for Therapy' by F.H. Messerli for publication in the Journal of Clinical Hypertension, submitted 1984.

References

Alexander, J.K. and Pettigrove, J.R.: Obesity and congestive heart failure. Geriatrics 22: 101-108 (1967).

Bauer, J.H.: Role of angiotensin converting enzyme inhibitors in essential and renal hypertension. Effects of captopril and enalapril on renin-angiotensin-aldosterone, renal function and hemodynamics, salt and water excretion, and body fluid composition. American Journal of Medicine 77: 43 (1984).

Brandfonbrener, M.; Landowne, M. and Shock, N.W.: Changes in cardiac output with age. Circulation 12: 557-566 (1955).

Coleman, T.G.; Granger, H.J. and Guyton, A.C.: Whole-body circulatory autoregulation and hypertension. Circulatory Research 28 and 29: 76-87 (1971).

Cournand, A.R.; Riley, L.; Breed, E.S.; Baldwin, W.F. and Richards, D.W. Jr: Measurements of cardiac output in man using the technique of catheterization of the right auricle or ventricle. Journal of Clinical Investigation 24: 106-116 (1945).

Cruickshank, J.K. and Beevers, D.G.: Epidemiology of hypertension: Blood pressure in blacks and whites. Clinical Science 62: 1-6 (1982).

Culpepper, W.S.; Sodt, P.C.; Messerli, F.H.; Ruschhaupt, D.G. and Arcilla, R.A.: Cardiac status in juvenile borderline hypertension. Annals of Internal Medicine 98: 1-7 (1983).

Divitis, O.; Fazio, S.; Pettito, M.; Maddalena, G.; Contaldo, F. and Mancini, M.: Obesity and cardiac function. Circulation 64: 477-482 (1981).

Dunn, F.G.; Oigman, W.; Ventura, H.O.; Messerli, F.H.; Kobrin, I. and Frohlich, E.D.: Enalapril improves systemic and renal hemodynamics and allows regression of left ventricular mass in essential hypertension. American Journal of Medicine 53: 105-108 (1984).

Entwisle, G.; Apostolides, A.Y.; Hebel, J.R. and Henderson, M.M.: Target organ damage in black hypertensives. Circulation 55: 792-796 (1977).

Esler, M.; Julius, S.; Zweifler, A.; Randall, O.; Harburg, E.; Gardiner, H. and DeQuattro, V.: Mild high-renin essential hypertension. Neurogenic human hypertension? New England Journal of Medicine 296: 405-411 (1977).

Fouad, F.M.; Tarazi, R.C.; Bravo, E.L. and Textor, S.C.: Hemodynamic and antihypertensive effects of the new oral angiotensin-converting-enzyme inhibitor MK-421 (enalapril). Hypertension 6: 167-174 (1984).

Freis, E.D.: Hemodynamics of hypertension. Physiological Reviews 40: 27-54 (1960).

Freis, E.D.: Age, race, sex, and other indices of risk in hypertension. American Journal of Medicine 55: 275-280 (1973).

Frohlich, E.D.; Kozul, V.J.; Tarazi, R.C. and Dustan, H.P.: Physiological comparison of labile and essential hypertension. Circulatory Research 27: 55-69 (1970).

Frohlich, E.D.; Messerli, F.H.; Dunn, F.G.; Oigman, W.; Ventura, H.O. and Sundgaard-Riise, K.: Greater renal vascular involvement in the black patient with essential hypertension: A comparison of systemic and renal hemodynamics in black and white patients. Mineral and Electrolyte Metabolism 10: 173-177 (1984).

Gardin, J.M.; Henry, W.L.; Savage, D.D.; Ware, J.H.; Burn, C. and Borer, J.S.: Echocardiographic measurements in normal subjects: Evaluation of an adult population without clinically apparent heart disease. Journal of Clinical Ultrasound 7: 439-447 (1979).

Gerstenblith, G.; Frederiksen, J.; Yin, F.C.; Fortuin, N.J.; Lakatta, E.G. and Weisfeldt, M.L.: Echocardiographic assessment of normal adult aging population. Circulation 56: 273-278 (1977).

Gillum, R.F.: Pathophysiology of hypertension in blacks and whites. A review of the basis of racial blood pressure differences. Hypertension 1: 468-475 (1979).

Goldring, D.; Hernandez, A.; Choi, S.; Lee, J.Y.; Londe, S.; Lundgren, F.T. and Burton, R.M.: Blood pressure in a high school population. II. Clinical profile of the juvenile hypertensive. Journal of Pediatrics 95: 298-304 (1979).

Gordon, T. and Kannel, W.B.: Obesity and cardiovascular disease: The Framingham study. Clinics in Endocrinology and Metabolism 5: 367-374 (1976).

HDFP Cooperative Group: Sex and race differences in end organ damage among 10,940 hypertensives. (Abstract.) American Journal of Cardiology 41: 402 (1978).

Hoffmann, J.I.E.; Grattan, M.T.; Hanley, F.L. and Messina, L.M.: Total and transmural perfusion of the hypertrophied heart; in Ter, Keurs and Schipperheyn (Eds) Cardiac Left Ventricular Hypertrophy, pp. 130-151 (Martinus Nijhoff Publishers, Boston 1983).

Hollenberg, N.K. and Merrill, J.P.: Intrarenal perfusion in the young 'essential' hypertensive: A subpopulation resistant to sodium restriction. Transactions of the Association of American Physicians 83: 93-101 (1970).

Hollenberg, N.K. and Adams, D.F.: The renal circulation in hypertensive disease. American Journal of Medicine 60: 773-784 (1976).

Hubert, H.B.; Feinleib, M.; McNamara, P.M. and Castelli, W.P.: Obesity as an independent risk factor for cardiovascular disease: A 26-year follow-up of participants in the Framingham Heart Study. Circulation 67: 968-977 (1983).

Julius, S.; Pascual, A.V.; Sannerstedt, R. and Mitchell, C.: Relationship between cardiac output and peripheral resistance in borderline hypertension. Circulation 43: 382-390 (1971).

Kaltman, A.J. and Goldring, R.M.: Role of circulatory congestion in the cardiorespiratory failure of obesity. American Journal of Medicine 60: 645-653 (1976).

Kannel, W.B.: Prevalence and natural history of electrocardiographic left ventricular hypertrophy. American Journal of Medicine 75 (Suppl. 3A): 4-11 (1983).

Kioschos, J.M.; Kirkendall, W.M.; Valenca, M.R. and Fitz, A.E.: Unilateral renal hemodynamics and characteristics of dye dilution curves in patients with essential hypertension and renal disease. Circulation 35: 229-249 (1967).

Laird, W.P. and Fixler, D.E.: Left ventricular hypertrophy in adolescents with elevated blood pressure: Assessment by chest roentgenography, electrocardiography, and echocardiography. Pediatrics 67: 255-259 (1981).

Laragh, J.H.: Concept of anti-renin system therapy: Historic perspective. American Journal of Medicine 77: 1-6 (1984).

Levy, S.B.; Talner, L.B.; Coel, M.N.; Holle, R. and Stone, R.A.: Renal vasculature in essential hypertension: Racial differences. Annals of Internal Medicine 88: 12-16 (1978).

Marcus, M.L.; Koyanagi, S.; Harrison, D.G.; Doty, D.B.; Hiratzka, L.F. and Eastham, C.L.: Abnormalities in the coronary

circulation that occur as a consequence of cardiac hypertrophy. American Journal of Medicine 75: 62-66 (1983).
McDonough, J.R.; Garrison, G.E. and Hames, C.G.: Blood pressure and hypertensive disease among negroes and whites. Annals of Internal Medicine 61: 208-228 (1964).
Meade, T.W.; Imerson, J.D.; Gordon, D. and Peart, W.S.: The epidemiology of plasma renin. Clinical Science 64: 273-280 (1983).
Messerli, F.H.; DeCarvalho, J.G.; Christie, B. and Frohlich, E.D.: Systemic and regional hemodynamics in low, normal and high cardiac output borderline hypertension. Circulation 58: 441-448 (1978).
Messerli, F.H.; DeCarvalho, J.G.R.; Christie, B. and Frohlich, E.D.: Essential hypertension in balck and white subjects: Hemodynamic findings and fluid volume state. American Journal of Medicine 67: 27-31 (1979).
Messerli, F.H.; Ventura, H.O.; Glade, L.B.; Sundgaard-Riise, K.; Dunn, F.G. and Frohlich, E.D.: Essential Hypertension in the elderly: Haemodynamics, intravascular volume, plasma renin activity, and circulating catecholamine levels. Lancet 2: 983-986 (1983a).
Messerli, F.H.; Sundgaard-Riise, K.; Reisin, E.; Dreslinski, G.; Dunn, F.G. and Frohlich, E.: Disparate cardiovascular effects of obesity and arterial hypertension. American Journal of Medicine 74: 808-812 (1983b).
Messerli, F.H.; Sundgaard-Riise, K.; Reisin, E.D.; Dreslinski, G.R.; Ventura, H.O.; Oigman, W.; Frohlich, E.D. and Dunn, F.G.: Dimorphic cardiac adaptation to obesity and arterial hypertension. Annals of Internal Medicine 99: 757-761 (1983c).
Messerli, F.H.; Sundgaard-Riise, K.; Ventura, H.O.; Dunn, F.G. and Frohlich, E.D.: Cardiovascular adaptation in elderly hypertensive patients. (Abstract.) Journal of the American College of Cardiology 3: 518 (1983d).
Messerli, F.H.; Ventura, H.O.; Elizardi, D.J.; Dunn, F.G. and Frohlich, E.D.: Hypertension and sudden death: Increased ventricular ectopic activity in left ventricular hypertrophy. American Journal of Medicine 77: 18-22 (1984a).
Messerli, F.H.; Sundgaard-Riise, K.; Ventura, H.O.; Dunn, F.G.; Oigman, W. and Frohlich, E.D.: Clinical and hemodynamic determinants of left ventricular dimensions. Archives of Internal Medicine 144: 477-481 (1984b).
Page, I.H.; Hurley, R.E. and Dustan, H.P.: The prolonged treatment of hypertension with guanethidine. Journal of the American Medical Association 175: 543 (1961).
Reams, G.P. and Bauer, J.H.: Enalapril versus triple-drug therapy in the treatment of renovascular hypertension. Drugs 30 (Suppl. 1): 59-69 (1985).
Report of the Hypertension Task Force: Vol. 9, DHEW Publication No. 79-1631 [NIH] (1979).
Rodeheffer, R.J.; Gerstenblith, G.; Becker, L.C.; Fleg, J.L.; Weisfeldt, M.L. and Lakatta, E.G.: Exercise cardiac output is maintained with advancing age in healthy human subjects: Cardiac dilatation and increased stroke volume compensate for a diminished heart rate. Circulation 69: 203-213 (1984).
Schalekamp, M.A.D.H.; Wenting, G.J.; DeBruyn, J.H.B.; Man-in'T Veld, A.J. and Derkx, F.H.M.: Hemodynamic effects of captopril in essential and renovascular hypertension: Correlations with plasma renin activity. Cardiovascular Review Report 3: 651-685 (1982).
Schieken, R.M.; Clarke, W.R. and Lauer, R.M.: Left ventricular hypertrophy in children with blood pressures in the upper quintile of the distribution (The Muscatine Study). Hypertension 3: 669-675 (1981).
Simon, G.; Morioka, S.; Snyder, D.K. and Cohn, J.N.: Increased renal plasma flow in long-term enalapril treatment of hypertension. Clinical Pharmacology and Therapeutics 34: 459-465 (1983).
Stamler, J.; Rhomberg, P.; Schoenberger, J.A.; Shekelle, R.B.; Dyer, A.; Shekelle, S.; Stamler, R. and Wannamaker, J.: Multivariate analysis of the relationship of seven variables to blood pressure: Findings of the Chicago Heart Association Detection Project in Industry, 1967-1972. Journal of Chronic Diseases 28: 527-548 (1975).
Standell, T.J.: Circulatory studies on healthy old men. Acta Medica Scandinavica 175: 1-44 (1964).
Strauer, B.E.: Hypertensive Heart Disease. (Springer, New York 1980).
Tarazi, R.C.; Bravo, E.L.; Fouad, F.M.; Omvik, P. and Cody, R.J.: Hemodynamic and volume changes associated with captopril. Hypertension 2: 576-585 (1980).
Tuck, M.L.; Sullivan, J.M.; Hollenberg, N.K.; Dluhy, R.G. and Williams, G.H.: Hemodynamic and endocrine response patterns in young patients with normal renin essential hypertension. Clinical Research 21: 505 (1973).
U.S. Department of Health, Education, and Welfare: National Health Survey, National Center for Health Statistics Series 11: No. 5 (1964).
Ventura, H.O.; Frohlich, E.D.; Messerli, F.H.; Kobrin, I. and Kardon, K.B.: Immediate regional blood flow distribution following angiotensin converting enzyme inhibition in patients with essential hypertension. American Journal of Medicine 76: 58-61 (1984).
Widimsky, J.; Fejfarova, M.D. and Ferfar, Z.: Changes in cardiac output in hypertensive disease. Cardiologia 31: 381 (1957).
Wilkins, L.H.; Dustan, H.P.; Walker, J.F. and Oparil, S.: Enalapril in low-renin essential hypertension. Clinical Pharmacology and Therapeutics 34: 297-302 (1983).
Zahka, K.G.; Neill, C.A.; Kidd, L.; Cutiletta, M.A. and Cutiletta, A.F.: Cardiac involvement in adolescent hypertension. Hypertension 3: 664-668 (1981).

Address for correspondence and reprints: Dr *F.H. Messerli*, Ochsner Clinic, 1516 Jefferson Highway, New Orleans, Louisiana 70121 (USA).

Drugs 30 (Suppl. 1): 35-46 (1985)
0012-6667-85-0100-0035/$6.00/0

Enalapril in Essential Hypertension

Jaime Herrera-Acosta, Héctor Pérez-Grovas,* Margarita Fernández†* and *Jaime Arriaga†*

* Department of Nephrology, Instituto Nacional de Cardiología Ignacio Chávez and † Department of Nephrology, Instituto Nacional de la Nutrición Salvador Zubirán, Mexico City

Summary *It is now well recognised that the renin-angiotensin system plays a key role in the control of blood pressure not only through circulating angiotensin II but through its interaction with the autonomic and central nervous systems. Angiotensin-converting enzyme (ACE) inhibitors have proved to be effective in lowering blood pressure in different types of hypertension. This study evaluates the antihypertensive effects of enalapril, a new, potent, long acting ACE inhibitor.*

50 patients with uncomplicated essential hypertension were included in 4 groups. Group I was used to compare the effects of enalapril and propranolol on blood pressure, renal function, plasma renin activity, aldosterone excretion and plasma lipids in 24 patients after 23 weeks. Group II was used to evaluate long term effects (48 weeks) of these drugs in 13 patients. Group III included 32 patients that received enalapril as monotherapy for 6 to 12 weeks. Group IV was studied to estimate the antihypertensive effect of low doses of hydrochlorothiazide in 18 patients receiving enalapril.

The effect on mean blood pressure was similar with enalapril and propranolol (enalapril 117 versus 103mm Hg and propranolol 115 versus 104mm Hg); however, the glomerular filtration rate decreased with propranolol (105 versus 87 ml/min; $p < 0.05$) and was unaltered with enalapril (102 versus 98 ml/min). Triglycerides rose with propranolol (179 versus 231 mg/dl; $p < 0.05$) and did not change with enalapril (157 versus 121 mg/dl). In the long term, antihypertensive effects were similar and no significant side effects were observed. In 14/32 patients blood pressure became normal with enalapril alone. Low doses of hydrochlorothiazide (12.5 to 25mg) decreased mean blood pressure by 10mm Hg when added to enalapril.

The antihypertensive effect of enalapril was similar to that of propranolol; however, the lowering effect on glomerular filtration rate of propranolol did not occur with enalapril. A slight rise in triglycerides occurred only with propranolol. No significant side effects were observed with either propranolol or enalapril. Used as monotherapy, enalapril normalised blood pressure in 44% of cases. Addition of low doses of hydrochlorothiazide significantly increased the antihypertensive effect of enalapril.

It is well established that the renin-angiotensin system plays a key role in the control of blood pressure, not only through circulating angiotensin II but through other mechanisms as well (Peart, 1983). Angiotensin converting enzyme (ACE) inhibitors have proved to be effective antihypertensive agents (Biollaz et al., 1982; Chrysant et al., 1983; Fernández et al., 1984; Groel et al., 1983). Their mechanism of action, however, is still a matter of some controversy. It is generally accepted that suppression of circulating angiotensin II is the principal mechanism of the blood pressure lowering effect when hypertension is associated with increased renin secretion (Brunner et al., 1979). However, since ACE inhibitors are active when there is no concomitant activation of the renin-angiotensin system, some workers have postulated additional non-renin-mediated antihypertensive effects (Ito et al., 1981; Thurston and Swales, 1978; Zusman 1984). Another possibility is that ACE inhibitors attenuate the normal facilitatory effects of angiotensin II on the autonomic and central nervous systems (Antonaccio and Kerwin, 1981; Unger et al., 1983).

Captopril, the first orally active ACE inhibitor, has been used with good results in a vast number of patients with hypertension (Captopril Collaborative Study Group, 1982; Veteran's Administration Cooperative Study Group, 1982, 1983). More recently, enalapril maleate has been developed. It has a longer antihypertensive effect and its molecule lacks the sulphydryl moiety to which some of the adverse effects of captopril have been attributed (Gavras et al., 1981; Gross et al., 1981).

To evaluate the efficacy of this new ACE inhibitor in the treatment of hypertension, we compared it with other antihypertensive drugs with different mechanisms of action. The present studies were designed to compare hormonal, renal haemodynamic, and antihypertensive effects of enalapril with propranolol, to assess the adverse effects of both drugs, and to evaluate the efficacy of enalapril alone and in association with small doses of hydrochlorothiazide. Some of these studies were part of a multicentre study (Merck Sharp & Dohme, 1983).

1. Methods

50 patients with mild to moderate essential hypertension were randomly selected from the hypertension clinic. Age varied between 33 and 68 years with a mean of 52 ± 6.2 years, and the known duration of hypertension varied from 7 to 280 months (mean of 100 ± 20.1 months). Retinal examination findings were normal in 13 patients, grade I (KW) in 31 and grade II in 6. 60% of patients had some degree of left ventricular hypertrophy as assessed by electrocardiographical criteria. Patients with the following conditions were excluded from the studies: secondary forms of hypertension, malignant hypertension, pregnancy, congestive heart failure, myocardial infarct, angina pectoris, valvular heart disease, A-V conduction defects, strokes, diabetes mellitus, asthma, collagen disease, neoplastic disease, significant renal or hepatic disease, and haemolytic anaemia. Patients treated with other ACE inhibitors, or having a history of skin rash, allergies or abnormal antinuclear antibody titre, were also excluded.

All blood pressure measurements were recorded after 10 minutes' rest in the supine position. The average of 2 or 3 consecutive readings was recorded. The 1st and 5th Korotkoff sounds were used to determine systolic and diastolic blood pressures, respectively. Four different studies were conducted.

1.1 Study I: Enalapril and Propranolol Compared

24 patients were included in this study comparing enalapril with propranolol. After the withdrawal of previous antihypertensive treatment, patients received 2 placebo tablets daily for 4 weeks. At the end of this period the patients were randomly assigned to receive either enalapril (10 to 40 mg/day) or propranolol (80 to 240 mg/day) for 12 weeks.

During placebo and active treatment periods, patients attended the clinic every 2 weeks. In addition to measurements of blood pressure, pulse rate and weight, the patients underwent a complete physical examination (including fundoscopy), audiometry, chest x-rays, ECG, blood chemistry and urine analysis.

Hormonal and renal haemodynamic studies were performed every 4 weeks. Hormone measurements included plasma renin activity while supine and after 4 hours of upright posture (Haber et al., 1969), and 24-hour urinary excretion of aldosterone, adrenaline, noradrenaline and vanillyl mandellic acid.

Renal haemodynamic studies included measurements of glomerular filtration rate and renal plasma flow by a constant intravenous infusion of ^{131}I-iothalamate (for glomerular filtration rate) and ^{125}I-hippuran (for renal plasma flow). After 60 min of equilibration, four 30-min clearances were obtained.

1.2 Study II

13 patients of the previous group continued active treatment for a total of 48 weeks; 7 were on enalapril (40 mg/day) and 6 on propranolol (240 mg/day). Hydrochlorothiazide in doses of 25 to 50 mg/day was added to their treatment after 4 weeks if diastolic blood pressure readings remained greater than 90mm Hg. Patients attended the clinic every 2 weeks up to 30 weeks and every 4 weeks thereafter for blood pressure measurements, physical examination and routine laboratory measurements.

1.3 Study III

24 additional patients received enalapril 20 mg/day for 6 weeks after a placebo period of 2 weeks. Blood pressure, heart rate and weight were recorded before and after placebo, and on weeks 3 and 6 of active treatment. In addition, patients underwent a physical examination, ECG and blood chemistry measurements.

1.4 Study IV

18 patients whose diastolic blood pressure remained higher than 90mm Hg after receiving enalapril in a single dose of 20mg for 6 weeks were randomly assigned to one of the following treatments for an additional 4 weeks: (a) enalapril (20 mg/day) plus placebo; (b) enalapril (20mg) plus hydrochlorothiazide (12.5 mg/day); (c) enalapril (20mg) plus hydrochlorothiazide (25 mg/day). Patients attended the clinic for blood pressure measurements, physical examination and laboratory determinations before and once every 2 weeks during the combined treatment period.

1.5 Data Analysis

Blood pressure is given as mean blood pressure [diastolic + 1/3 (systolic−diastolic)]. All data are shown as mean ($\bar{X} \pm$ SEM) values. Statistical analyses made use of the paired or unpaired t-test. A p value of less than 0.05 was considered significant.

2. Results

2.1 Study I

2.1.1 Hormone Determinations

The effects of treatment with enalapril and propranolol on plasma renin activity are shown in table I. Basal values of plasma renin activity were higher in the propranolol group due to the fact that two hyperreninaemic patients were randomly assigned to this group.

Plasma renin activity rose with enalapril both for supine and upright-posture although the increments were significant only after 8 weeks of treatment. In contrast, propranolol suppressed plasma renin activity, the changes being significant by the fourth week. At the end of the treatment period, striking differences in plasma renin activity were apparent between the two groups both in the supine position ($p < 0.05$) and the upright position ($p < 0.05$).

Aldosterone excretion was studied in 8 patients receiving enalapril and 9 receiving propranolol (table II). Basal values were very similar in the two groups. During active treatment, there was a slight decrease with the two drugs, however, the change was significant only with enalapril after 12 weeks of treatment.

The results of catecholamine excretion are shown in table III. A small increment in adrenaline excretion was observed during treatment but the changes did not reach statistical significance with either drug. Noradrenaline excretion decreased slightly with enalapril from 35.7 ± 5.1 to 25.2 ± 4.2 μg/24 hours after 12 weeks of treatment, but

Table I. Plasma renin activity (PRA) during treatment with enalapril and propranolol. All values mean ± SEM

Time (weeks)		0	4	8	12
Propranolol	Supine	1.94 ± 0.43	0.58 ± 0.11[a]	0.56 ± 0.12[a]	0.62 ± 0.11[a]
(PRA ng/ml/hour)	Upright[c]	4.72 ± 1.47	1.18 ± 0.25[a]	1.84 ± 0.37	1.59 ± 0.49[a]
Enalapril	Supine	0.7 ± 0.14[b]	1.27 ± 0.33 ns	1.94 ± 0.50[a,b]	2.33 ± 0.59[a,b]
(PRA ng/ml/hour)	Upright	1.87 ± 0.34	3.33 ± 1.10 ns	5.39 ± 1.80[a]	6.53 ± 2.16[a,b]

a $p < 0.05$ versus week 0.
b $p < 0.05$ propranolol versus enalapril.
c After 4 hours of upright body posture.
ns = not significant.

Table II. Aldosterone excretion during treatment with enalapril and propranolol. All values mean ± SEM

Time (weeks)		0	4	8	12
Urine aldosterone excretion	Enalapril (n = 8)	10.0 ± 2.3	9.1 ± 2.4	8.1 ± 2.4	6.9 ± 1.8[a]
(μg/24 hours)	Propranolol (n = 9)	9.5 ± 1.8	7.8 ± 1.3	8.0 ± 2.0	8.0 ± 1.5

a $p < 0.05$ compared to week 0.

Table III. Catecholamine excretion during treatment with enalapril (E) and propranolol (P). All values mean ± SEM

Time (weeks)		0	4	8	12
Adrenaline	E	2.1 ± 0.61	1.73 ± 0.49	2.63 ± 0.58	3.56 ± 0.76
(μg/24 hour)	P	2.6 ± 0.6	1.87 ± 0.48	2.65 ± 0.85	4.11 ± 0.97
Noradrenaline	E	35.7 ± 5.1	26.5 ± 2.3	32.4 ± 4.9	25.2 ± 4.2
(μg/24 hour)	P	31.3 ± 2.0	26.1 ± 1.5	28.0 ± 3.2	33.7 ± 4.4
Vanillyl mandellic acid	E	6.1 ± 0.64	5.30 ± 0.65	6.80 ± 1.1	3.79 ± 0.3[a]
(μg/24 hour)	P	5.97 ± 0.42	5.13 ± 0.42	3.4 ± 0.66	3.98 ± 0.62[a]

a $p < 0.05$ versus week 0.

did not change with propranolol; vanillyl-mandellic acid decreased significantly with both drugs at week 12 (table III).

2.1.2 Renal Haemodynamics

The effects of enalapril and propranolol on renal haemodynamics are shown in table IV. Glomerular filtration rates measured by ^{131}I-iothalamate clearances were within the normal range, and were very similar in the two groups during the placebo period (table IV). During treatment there was a slight but significant fall with both drugs (≥ 10%) which was already apparent by the 4th week of treatment. In the group that received enalapril, the glomerular filtration rate remained low at week 8 but recovered to control values at the end of the treatment period. In contrast, for patients who received propranolol, the fall in glomerular filtration rate persisted throughout the entire treatment period.

Table IV. Renal haemodynamics during treatment with enalapril and propranolol. All values mean ± SEM

Week	0	4	8	12
Glomerular filtration rate (^{131}I-iothalamate clearance, ml/min/m^2)				
Enalapril	102 ± 6.7	89 ± 6.1[a]	88 ± 7.3[a]	98 ± 8.9
Propranolol	105 ± 7.2	90 ± 4.2[a]	84 ± 6.3[a]	87 ± 5.0[a]
Renal plasma flow (^{125}I-hippuran clearance, ml/min/m^2)				
Enalapril	358 ± 26	350 ± 23	388 ± 18	378 ± 33
Propranolol	368 ± 38	358 ± 30	334 ± 35	365 ± 44

a $p < 0.05$ versus week 0.

The changes in glomerular filtration rate were not due to decreased renal perfusion since renal plasma flow did not change with either drug. Mean values were very similar for the two groups during placebo administration and remained steady throughout the study (table IV).

The fall in glomerular filtration rate in the presence of a constant renal plasma flow indicates a fall in filtration fraction. In fact, filtration fraction decreased in both groups. With enalapril, it fell from 0.29 ± 0.02 to 0.23 ± 0.02 after 8 weeks, but returned to control values (0.28 ± 0.04) by the end of treatment. With propranolol it fell to the same extent (from 0.30 ± 0.01 to 0.26 ± 0.01) but remained low at the end of treatment.

2.1.3 Antihypertensive Effect of Enalapril and Propranolol

The effects on blood pressure were very similar with both drugs. Figure 1 shows average values of mean blood pressure at each visit. After placebo, the mean blood pressure was 117 ± 2mm Hg for the enalapril group and 115 ± 2mm Hg for the propranolol group. At week 4 of active treatment, a significant decrease in mean blood pressure was apparent with the two drugs. Average mean blood pressure values continued to decline gradually after 12 weeks to 108 ± 1mm Hg ($p < 0.05$) with enalapril and to 104 ± 2mm Hg ($p < 0.05$) with propranolol. Differences between the final values were not significant. Changes in systolic and diastolic blood pressures were also very similar with both drugs. With enalapril it decreased from 148 ± 5.5/98 ± 1.8 to 139 ± 3.1/89 ± 2.1mm Hg ($p < 0.025$) and with propranolol it decreased from 149 ± 3.8/102 ± 2.1 to 137 ± 2.7/88 ± 1.4mm Hg ($p < 0.025$).

10 of 12 patients responded to enalapril and 8 of them became normotensive: those who responded received a dose of 20 mg/day or less. With propranolol, all patients responded but only 10 became normotensive: 4 patients required 240 mg/day and only 3 responded to 80 mg/day.

Heart rate did not change with either drug. With enalapril it was 69 ± 3 beats/minute during the placebo period and 73 ± 3 beats/minute after treatment. With propranolol, it was 68 ± 2 beats/minute during the placebo phase and 65 ± 1 beats/minute after treatment.

2.1.4 Routine Laboratory Measurements and Side Effects

No significant changes occurred in any of the routine laboratory tests including haemoglobin, blood chemistry, plasma electrolytes and antinuclear antibodies. A slight but significant increase in plasma triglycerides was observed with propranolol from 179 ± 23 mg/dl during placebo to 231 ± 40.5 mg/dl ($p < 0.05$) after 12 weeks of active treatment. In contrast, a slight but significant decrease was observed with enalapril from 157 ± 15.2 to 121 ± 5.3 mg/dl ($p < 0.05$). The final values were also significantly different when comparing propranolol with enalapril groups ($p < 0.05$). Total cholesterol did not change in either group. With propranolol it fell from 214 ± 13.9 to 206.9 ±

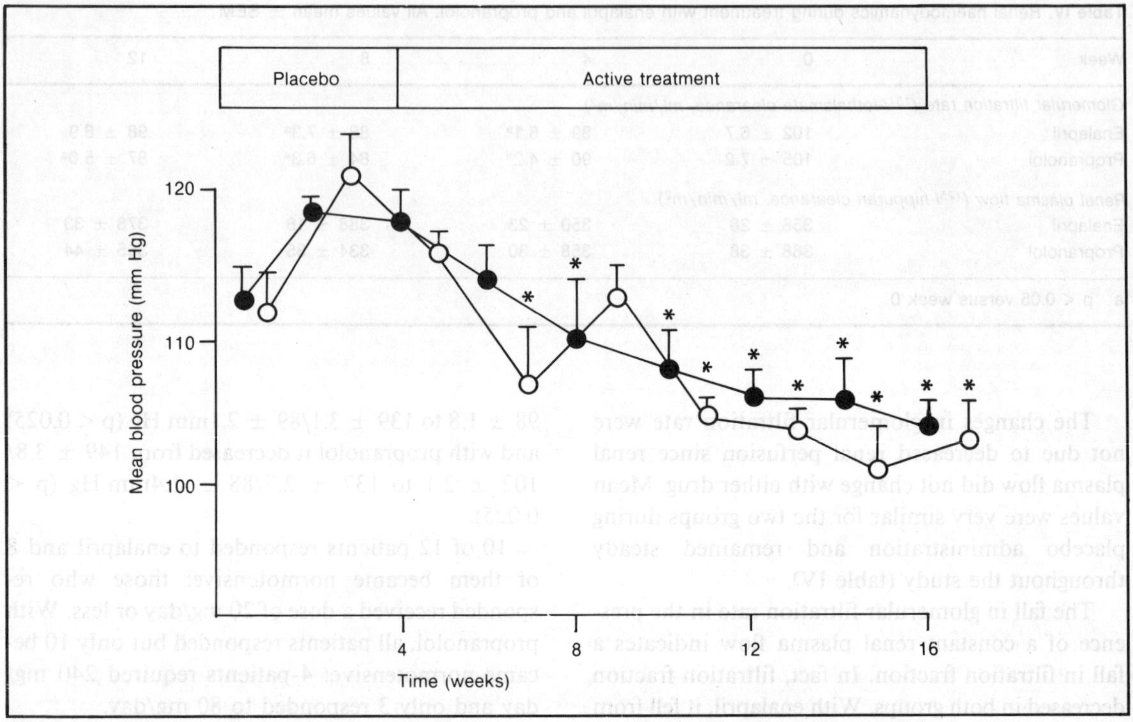

Fig. 1. Mean blood pressure values during placebo and during active treatment with enalapril (●—●) and propranolol (○—○). A significant decrease in mean blood pressure occurred with both drugs after 4 weeks of active treatment and continued to decrease gradually for 12 weeks. Mean blood pressure values between drugs were not statistically different. * $p < 0.05$ versus week 0.

11.9 mg/dl and from 233.4 ± 15.8 to 216.7 ± 14.9 mg/dl with enalapril.

Two patients developed slight transient proteinuria with enalapril, 1 of whom had a urinary tract infection before proteinuria developed. Four patients receiving propranolol and 1 with enalapril had slight transient dizziness. One patient on propranolol complained of headache.

2.2 Study II

13 patients from group I continued on active treatment for 48 weeks; 7 were on enalapril and 6 on propranolol. The drugs were given in increasing doses, and if the supine diastolic blood pressure remained above 90mm Hg, hydrochlorothiazide 25mg daily was added. Four patients on enalapril and one on propranolol received hydrochlorothiazide. The effects on blood pressure are shown in fig. 2. At the end of the placebo period, the blood pressure was 150 ± 6.6/97 ± 1.5mm Hg for the enalapril group, decreasing after 48 weeks of treatment to 132 ± 5.4/83 ± 3mm Hg ($p < 0.05/ < 0.005$). In the propranolol group, it decreased from 150 ± 7.6/99 ± 2.5 to 140 ± 8.5/84 ± 3.2mm Hg; only the fall in diastolic pressure was significant ($p < 0.0025$).

Heart rate tended to decrease with propranolol (73.2 ± 2 versus 69 ± 2 beats/minute, $p < 0.05$) whereas it did not change with enalapril (77 ± 2 versus 77 ± 2 beats/minute). No significant changes in routine laboratory tests nor significant side effects were observed in either group of patients.

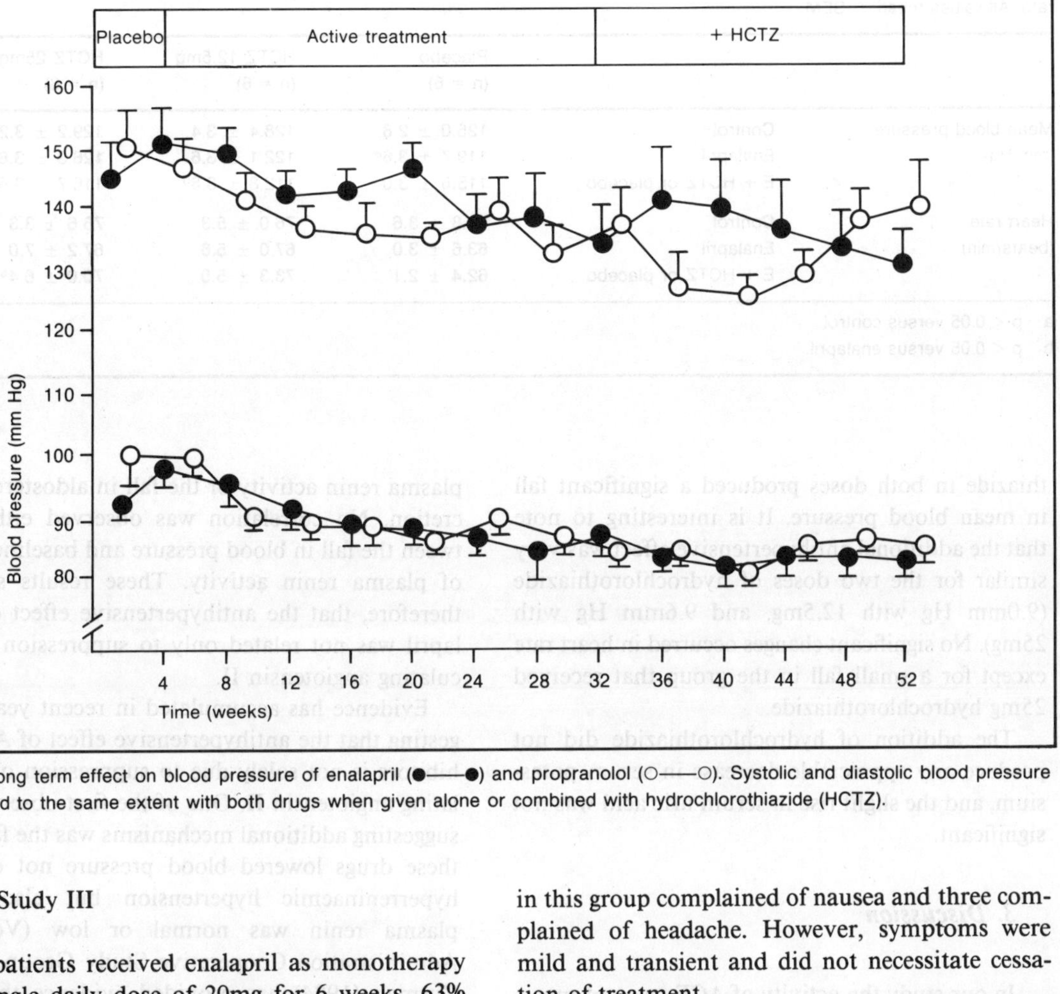

Fig. 2. Long term effect on blood pressure of enalapril (●—●) and propranolol (○—○). Systolic and diastolic blood pressure decreased to the same extent with both drugs when given alone or combined with hydrochlorothiazide (HCTZ).

2.3 Study III

24 patients received enalapril as monotherapy in a single daily dose of 20mg for 6 weeks. 63% (15/24) responded to the drug with a fall in mean blood pressure greater than 7mm Hg; in 11 patients the fall was greater than 10mm Hg; and in 25% (6/24) the blood pressure became normal (mean blood pressure < 107mm Hg). The average values at the end of the placebo period were 169.5 ± 4.2/106.8 ± 1.7mm Hg decreasing to 161.2 ± 5.03/99.5 ± 5mm Hg after treatment. However, only the fall in diastolic blood pressure was significant ($p < 0.05$). The heart rate did not change during treatment (74.6 ± 7.4 versus 70 ± 6.8 beats/minute, $p < 0.05$). No significant change was observed in any of the routine laboratory parameters. Two patients in this group complained of nausea and three complained of headache. However, symptoms were mild and transient and did not necessitate cessation of treatment.

2.4 Study IV

This group consisted of 18 patients in whom the diastolic blood pressure remained above 90mm Hg after 6 weeks of treatment with enalapril 20 mg/day. In addition to enalapril, 6 patients were given 25mg hydrochlorothiazide, 6 received 12.5mg hydrochlorothiazide, and 6 received a placebo.

The effects on mean blood pressure are shown in table V. Addition of placebo to enalapril decreased mean blood pressure slightly, but the change was not significant. In contrast, hydrochloro-

Table V. Effect of enalapril (E) in combination with hydrochlorothiazide (HCTZ) 12.5 or 25mg on mean blood pressure and heart rate. All values mean ± SEM

		Placebo (n = 6)	HCTZ 12.5mg (n = 6)	HCTZ 25mg (n = 6)
Mean blood pressure (mm Hg)	Control	125.0 ± 2.8	128.4 ± 3.4	129.2 ± 3.2
	Enalapril	119.7 ± 3.6[a]	122.1 ± 3.6	126.3 ± 3.6
	E + HCTZ or placebo	115.6 ± 3.0	112.8 ± 3.8[b]	116.7 ± 3.6[b]
Heart rate (beats/min)	Control	64.8 ± 3.6	76.0 ± 5.3	76.6 ± 3.3
	Enalapril	63.6 ± 3.0	67.0 ± 5.6	67.2 ± 7.0
	E + HCTZ or placebo	62.4 ± 2.1	73.3 ± 5.0	70.0 ± 6.4[b]

a $p < 0.05$ versus control.
b $p < 0.05$ versus enalapril.

thiazide in both doses produced a significant fall in mean blood pressure. It is interesting to note that the additional antihypertensive effect was very similar for the two doses of hydrochlorothiazide (9.0mm Hg with 12.5mg, and 9.6mm Hg with 25mg). No significant changes occurred in heart rate except for a small fall in the group that received 25mg hydrochlorothiazide.

The addition of hydrochlorothiazide did not produce any appreciable decrease in serum potassium, and the slight rise in serum uric acid was not significant.

3. Discussion

In our study the activity of ACE was not measured. However, we can assume that enalapril inhibited the enzyme, since there was a significant rise in plasma renin activity, as expected when circulating angiotensin II falls, thereby releasing its normal inhibitory effect on renin secretion (Hofbauer et al., 1983). The opposite occurred with propranolol which suppresses β-adrenergic stimulation of renin secretion (Bühler et al., 1972). Further indirect evidence of ACE inhibition and angiotensin II suppression was the observed decrease in aldosterone secretion (Brunner et al., 1981). No correlation was observed, however, between the antihypertensive effect of enalapril and the rise in plasma renin activity or the fall in aldosterone excretion. No correlation was observed either between the fall in blood pressure and baseline levels of plasma renin activity. These results suggest, therefore, that the antihypertensive effect of enalapril was not related only to suppression of circulating angiotensin II.

Evidence has accumulated in recent years suggesting that the antihypertensive effect of ACE inhibitors is not solely due to suppression of circulating angiotensin II. One of the first observations suggesting additional mechanisms was the fact that these drugs lowered blood pressure not only in hyperreninaemic hypertension but also when plasma renin was normal or low (Veteran's Administration Cooperative Study Group, 1983). Zusman (1984) has provided evidence that captopril increases prostaglandin synthesis, in part by the stimulatory effect of kinins, and most importantly by direct stimulation of phospholipase A_2 which releases arachidonic acid, the precursor of prostaglandins.

Another possible explanation for the lack of correlation between the antihypertensive effect and circulating angiotensin II is the facilitatory effect of angiotensin II on the autonomic and central nervous systems. Normally, angiotensin II increases the release of noradrenaline from sympathetic nerve endings and inhibits its reuptake. These effects enhance the vasoconstricting action of the adrenergic nervous system (Zimmerman et al., 1972). Accordingly, inhibition of angiotensin II formation may lower blood pressure in part by decreasing adrenergic-mediated vasoconstriction (Antonnacio and Kerwin, 1981).

In the present study, enalapril (and propranolol) produced a slight decrease in noradrenaline excretion and a more significant decrease in vanillyl mandellic acid. This effect probably relates to withdrawal of the facilitatory effect of angiotensin II on catecholamine release.

Finally, the presence of all elements of the renin-angiotensin system in the arterial wall as well as in other tissues (Thurston et al., 1979), makes it possible that angiotensin II can be generated locally. ACE inhibition could, therefore, lower blood pressure by suppressing local angiotensin II, independently of circulating levels.

During chronic hypertension, renal function adapts to a high level of arterial pressure. There is a shift to the right of the pressure-natriuresis curve (Guyton et al., 1972). This adaptation appears to be due, at least in part, to an increase in afferent arteriolar resistance, which tends to prevent excessive increases in intraglomerular pressure and filtration. Another mechanism of adaptation however, is a decrease in the permeability coefficient of glomerular capillaries. This would prevent an increase in filtration in spite of a high glomerular pressure (Herrera-Acosta et al., 1983).

Recent studies from our laboratory involving untreated patients with essential hypertension showed that acute protein intake did not produce any rise in filtration rate, which suggests that the kidney is filtering at almost maximum capacity. This could be interpreted as meaning that intraglomerular pressure is elevated and maintains a high filtration rate in the remaining nephrons (Herrera-Acosta et al., 1984). A drug-induced fall in blood pressure would be expected to decrease glomerular filtration rate by lowering perfusion pressure. A number of studies have shown that renal function decreases with antihypertensive treatment (Epstein and Oster, 1982). In our study, both enalapril and propranolol initially decreased glomerular filtration rate. After 12 weeks, however, it returned to normal in patients receiving enalapril, but remained low in those taking propranolol. This difference in the response to the two drugs has been described before (Weber and Drayer, 1980). Several studies have reported a persistent fall in glomerular filtration rate and renal plasma flow with propranolol for periods as long as 1 year (Epstein and Oster, 1982; Weber and Drayer, 1980). In contrast, recent reports indicate that both captopril and enalapril maintain glomerular filtration rate or even increase it in spite of the fall in blood pressure (Bauer and Gaddy, 1984). However, in experimental animals with volume depletion, ACE inhibition with captopril decreases renal vascular resistance and increases the permeability coefficient of the glomerular capillaries (Navar and Rosivall, 1984). It is conceivable, therefore, that these functional changes could contribute to the maintenance of renal function in patients receiving ACE inhibitors for prolonged periods. In contrast, patients receiving propranolol, in whom cardiac output is low, have increased renal vascular resistance and decreased glomerular filtration rate as a result of alpha-adrenergically mediated reflex vasoconstriction (Hansson et al., 1974; Tarazi and Dustan, 1972; Warren et al., 1981).

To evaluate the efficacy of a new drug in the treatment of hypertension, it is useful to compare it with other current antihypertensive drugs with different mechanisms of action. Propranolol has been the most widely used β-adrenergic blocking agent for the last 20 years, and has proved to be an effective antihypertensive agent. In this study, the antihypertensive effect of enalapril was very similar to that of propranolol in both the short and long term. When used as monotherapy for 12 weeks, blood pressure decreased by 9mm Hg with enalapril and by 11mm Hg with propranolol in a comparable group of patients with mild to moderate essential hypertension. In a larger group of patients (enalapril, 242 patients; propranolol, 243 patients) that were treated following the same protocol as part of a multicentre study, diastolic blood pressure decreased by 16.5mm Hg with enalapril and by 13.4mm Hg with propranolol ($p < 0.05$) (Merck Sharp & Dohme, 1983). In our study, the number of patients who became normotensive, and requirements for additional therapy to lower blood pressure, were similar for both drugs. On long term follow up (48 weeks), both drugs alone, or in combination with small doses of hydrochlorothiazide lowered blood pressure to normal in all patients in our study. In the multicentre study, 97 patients taking enalapril and 99 on propranolol required the addition of hydrochlorothiazide because diastolic readings were higher than 90mm Hg. Of these patients, 85% on enalapril and 72% on propranolol became normotensive.

In summary, these results clearly demonstrate that the antihypertensive effect of enalapril is similar or slightly greater than that of propranolol in patients with mild to moderate essential hypertension.

At the present time, a great deal of controversy exists regarding the medication of first choice in treating patients with essential hypertension. Traditionally, diuretics or β-blockers have been used in this role (Gifford, 1983). Diuretics have a lower cost and can be as effective as other drugs. They are well tolerated, and given in a single daily dose they can control approximately 50% of patients with mild to moderate hypertension. β-blockers sometimes require several doses per day. In a study of 81 patients taking propranolol as monotherapy, 52% became normotensive, but 34 patients required high doses (Berlung and Anderson, 1981). In our study, propranolol alone controlled blood pressure in 10 of 12 patients. Of all patients included in the multicentre study, however, only 95 out of 184 (52%) became normotensive with doses lower than 240 mg/day.

Captopril has been used recently as monotherapy with good results in patients with mild to moderate essential hypertension. Because of its short duration of action, however, the drug has to be given twice or three times daily. Enalapril has a longer duration of action and can be administered in a single daily dose. In this study, 36 patients received enalapril as monotherapy, 24 in a single dose of 20 mg/day for 6 weeks, and 12 in increasing doses administered twice-daily. When given as a single daily dose, 63% of patients responded, but only 25% (6/24) became normotensive. With increasing doses (up to 40 mg/day), 10 out of 12 responded and 8 became normotensive. For all patients included in the multicentre study, 98 out of 182 (54%) became normotensive. These findings demonstrate that enalapril as monotherapy, given once or twice-daily can be at least as effective as other drugs currently used as initial therapy. Combined use of ACE inhibition and diuretics produces a substantially greater pressure lowering effect than either drug alone. This has been demonstrated in several studies using captopril (Stumpe et al., 1982; Veteran's Administration Cooperative Study Group, 1982; Vlasses et al., 1982). In this study, the effect of adding small doses of hydrochlorothiazide was studied in a group of patients in whom the diastolic blood pressure remained above 90mm Hg after 6 weeks on enalapril monotherapy. In these patients, adding 12.5 or 25mg hydrochlorothiazide induced a drop in blood pressure greater than that produced by enalapril alone. Similarly, in long term studies (Study II) in which hydrochlorothiazide was added to enalapril, 7 of 7 patients became normotensive and 85% of the 182 patients of the multicentre study achieved normotension with this combination (Merck Sharp & Dohme, 1983). These data confirm that diuretics potentiate the antihypertensive effect of the ACE inhibitors.

In this study, very few side effects were associated with enalapril or propranolol. Proteinuria occurred in two cases on enalapril, but it was a transient phenomenon and possibly a consequence of urinary tract infection rather than drug-related. Other complaints reported by patients were of minor importance. The small number of patients included in this study makes it difficult to draw conclusions regarding the true frequency of side effects. A more realistic assessment can be obtained from the multicentre study (Merck Sharp & Dohme, 1983). In this series, 485 patients of both sexes entered the study and the most significant adverse experiences were dizziness (4.5%) and headache (2.1%) with enalapril, and bradycardia (3.3%), dizziness (2.9%), headache (2.1%) and paraesthesiae (2.9%) with propranolol. A larger series of patients was recently reviewed by Stumpe et al. (1984). 2203 patients receiving enalapril were compared with 4849 receiving captopril. The most common side effects with enalapril were dizziness (6.3%), headache (5.6%), and hypotension (2.4%). Rash and taste disturbance were more frequent in patients on captopril (6.0 versus 1.5% and 3.1 versus 0.5%), but no difference was found in the frequency of proteinuria.

Routine laboratory measurements did not show significant alteration except for a rise in the plasma levels of triglycerides with propranolol which was not observed with enalapril. No changes occurred in total cholesterol with either drug. Although disturbances in lipid metabolism have been described with the use of β-blockers, the significance of hypertriglyceridaemia in our patients is difficult to evaluate since it was not apparent when analysing all the patients included in the multicentre study (Merck Sharp & Dohme, 1983). It is possible that our finding was due to the random inclusion of two hyperlipidaemic patients in the propranolol group.

Finally, it is worth mentioning that no significant change occurred in serum potassium or serum uric acid in patients receiving the combination of enalapril and hydrochlorothiazide. Amelioration of the metabolic effects of thiazides by captopril has been described (Veteran's Administration Cooperative Study Group, 1983). Although the mechanism for this is not completely understood, it represents a considerable advantage in the use of ACE inhibitors.

References

Antonaccio, M.J. and Kerwin, L.: Pre- and postjunctional inhibition of vascular sympathetic function by captopril in SHR. Hypertension 3 (Suppl. 1): 54-62 (1981).

Bauer, J. and Gaddy, P.: Long-term enalapril/hydrochlorothiazide therapy markedly improves impaired renal function in patients with essential hypertension. Abstracts of the IXth International Congress of Nephrology, Los Angeles, California, USA pp.201A (1984).

Berglünd, G. and Anderson, O.: Beta-blockers or diuretics in hypertension? A six year follow-up of blood pressure and metabolic side effects. Lancet 1: 744-747 (1981).

Biollaz, J.; Brunner, H.R.; Waeber, B. and Gavras, H.: Antihypertensive therapy with MK-421: Angiotensin II renin relationship to evaluate efficacy of converting enzyme blockade. Journal of Cardiovascular Pharmacology 4: 966-972 (1982).

Brunner, D.B.; Desponds, G.; Biollaz, J.; Keller, I.; Ferber, F.; Gavras, H.; Brunner, H.R. and Schelling, H.L.: Effect of a new angiotensin converting enzyme inhibitor MK-421 and its lysine analogue on the components of the renin system in healthy subjects. British Journal of Clinical Pharmacology 11: 461-467 (1981).

Brunner, H.R.; Gavras, H.; Waeber, B.; Kershaw, G.R.; Turini, G.A.; Vukovich, R.A.; Mckinstry, D.N. and Gavras, I.: Oral angiotensin converting enzyme inhibitor in long term treatment of hypertensive patients. Annals of Internal Medicine 90: 19-23 (1979).

Bühler, F.R.; Laragh, J.H.; Baer, L.; Vaughan, E.D. and Brunner, H.R.: Propranolol inhibition of renin secretion. A specific approach to diagnosis and treatment of renin-dependent hypertensive disease. New England Journal of Medicine 287: 1209-1214 (1972).

Captopril Collaborative Study Group: Does captopril cause renal damage in hypertensive patients? Lancet 2: 988-990 (1982).

Chrysant, S.G.; Brown, R.D.; Kem, D.C. and Brown, J.L.: Antihypertensive and metabolic effects of a new converting enzyme inhibitor, enalapril. Clinical Pharmacology and Therapeutics 33: 741-746 (1983).

Epstein, M. and Oster, J.R.: Beta-blockers and the kidney. Mineral and Electrolyte Metabolism 8: 237-254 (1982).

Fernández, P.G.; Kim, B.K. and Galway, A.B.: An appraisal of antihypertensive efficacy and adverse reactions with two drugs regimes: Enalapril maleate as a part of triple therapy compared to conventional therapy in moderate to severe hypertension. Pharmacotherapeutica 3: 505-514 (1984).

Gavras, H.; Biollaz, J.; Waeber, B.; Brunner, H.R.; Gavras, I. and Davies, R.O.: Antihypertensive effect of the new oral angiotensin converting enzyme inhibitor MK-421. Lancet 2: 543-547 (1981).

Gifford, R.W.: Management and treatment of essential hypertension including malignant hypertension and emergencies; in Genest; Kuchel; Hamet and Cantin (Eds) Hypertension, pp. 1127-1170 (McGraw Hill, New York 1983).

Groel, J.T.; Tadros, S.S.; Dreslinski, G.R. and Jenkins, A.C.: Long-term antihypertensive therapy with captopril. Hypertension 5 (Suppl. 3): 145-151 (1983).

Gross, D.M.; Sweet, C.S.; Ulm, E.H.; Backlund, E.P.; Morris, A.A.; Weitz, D.; Bohn, D.L.; Wenger, H.C.; Vassill, T.C. and Stone, C.A.: Antihypertensive effect of N-S[-1-carboxy-3 phenyl propyl]-L-Ala-Pro and its ethyl ester (MK-421) on angiotensin converting enzyme in vitro and angiotensin I pressor responses in vivo. Journal of Pharmacology and Experimental Therapeutics 216: 552-557 (1981).

Guyton, A.C.; Coleman, T.G.; Cowley, A.W.; Scheel, K.W.; Manning, R.D. and Normal, R.A.: Arterial pressure regulation. American Journal of Medicine 52: 584-594 (1972).

Haber, E.; Koerner, T.; Page, L.B.; Kliman, B. and Puronde A.: Application of a radioimmunoassay for angiotensin I to the physiologic measurements of plasma renin activity in normal human subjects. Journal of Clinical Endocrinology and Metabolism 29: 1349-1355 (1969).

Hansson, L.; Zweifler, A.J.; Julius, S. and Hungor, S.N.: Hemodynamic effects of acute and prolonged beta-adrenergic blockade in essential hypertension. Acta Medica Scandinavica 196: 27-34 (1974).

Herrera-Acosta, J.; Gabbai, F.; Franco, M.; Tapia, E.; Linfa, G.; Díaz, L. and Campos, J.: Glomerular hemodynamics in persistent renovascular hypertension in the rat. Hypertension 5 (Suppl. 5): 110-114 (1983).

Herrera-Acosta, J.; Fernández, M.; Gabbai, F.; Moscoso, J.; López, G.; Romero, E. and Peña, J.C.: Renal hemodynamic response to protein loading in essential hypertension. Abstracts of the IXth International Congress of Nephrology, Los Angeles, California USA pp.210A (1984).

Hofbauer, K.G.; Hulthen, L.V. and Bühler, F.R.: Antagonist inhibitors of the renin angiotensin system for the treatment of hypertension; in Genest, Kuchel, Hamet and Cantin (Eds) Hypertension, pp.1225-1238 (McGraw-Hill, New York 1983).

Ito, K., Koike, H.; Miyumoto, M.; Ozaki, H.; Kishimoto, T. and Urakawa, N.: Long term effects of captopril on cellular sodium content and mechanical properties of aortic smooth muscle from spontaneously hypertensive rats. Journal of Pharmacology and Experimental Therapeutics 219: 520-525 (1981).

Merck Sharp & Dohme Research Laboratories. Multicenter Study for evaluation of the antihypertensive effect of enalapril maleate compared with propranolol as single entities and/or hydrochlorothiazide (25 and 50mg) in patients with mild or moderate essential hypertension. Data on File (1983).

Navar, L.G. and Rosivall, L.: Contribution of the renin-angiotensin system to the control of intrarenal hemodynamics. Kidney International 25: 857-868 (1984).

Peart, W.S.: General review of hypertension; in Genest, Kuchel, Hamet and Cantin (Eds) Hypertension, pp.3-14 (McGraw Hill, New York 1983).

Stumpe, K.O.; Overlack, A.; Kolloch, R. and Schreyer, S.: Long term efficacy of angiotensin converting enzyme inhibition with captopril in mild to moderate essential hypertension. British Journal of Clinical Pharmacology 14 (Suppl. 2): S121-S126 (1982).

Stumpe, K.O.; Kolloch, R. and Overlack, A.: Captopril and enalapril: evaluation of therapeutic efficacy and safety. Practical Cardiology 10, No. 7 (1984).

Tarazi, R.C. and Dustan, H.P.: Beta-adrenergic blockade in hypertension. Practical and theoretical implications of long-term hemodynamic variations. American Journal of Cardiology 29: 633-640 (1972).

Thurston, H. and Swales, J.D.: Converting enzyme inhibitor and saralasin infusion in rats. Evidence for an additional vasodepressor property of converting enzyme inhibitor. Circulation Research 42: 588-592 (1978).

Thurston, H.; Swales, J.D.; Bing, R.F.; Hurst, B.C. and Marck, E.S.: Vascular renin-like activity and blood pressure maintenance in the rat. Hypertension 1: 643-649 (1979).

Unger, T.; Ganten, D. and Lang, R.E.: Pharmacology of converting enzyme inhibitors: New aspects. Clinical and Experimental Hypertension A5: 1333-1354 (1983).

Veteran's Administration Cooperative Study Group on Antihypertensive Agents: Captopril: Evaluation of low doses, twice-daily doses and the addition of diuretic for the treatment of mild to moderate hypertension. Clinical Science 63 (Suppl. 8): S443-S445 (1982).

Veteran's Administration Cooperative Study Group on Antihypertensive Agents: Low dose captopril for the treatment of mild to moderate hypertension. Hypertension 5 (Suppl. 3): 131-144 (1983).

Vlasses, P.H.; Rotmensch, H.H.; Swanson, B.N.; Mojaverian, P. and Ferguson, R.K.: Low dose captopril. Its uses in mild to moderate hypertension unresponsive to diuretic treatment. Archives of Internal Medicine 142: 1098-1101 (1982).

Warren, S.E.; O'Connors, D.T.; Cohen, I.M. and Mitas, J.A.: Renal hemodynamic changes during long-term antihypertensive therapy. Clinical Pharmacology and Therapeutics 29: 310-317 (1981).

Weber, M.A. and Drayer, J.I.M.: Renal effects of beta-adrenoreceptor blockade. Kidney International 18: 686-699 (1980).

Zimmerman, B.G.; Gomer, S.F. and Liao, J.C.: Action of angiotensin on vascular adrenergic nerve endings: Facilitation of norepinephrine release. Federation Proceedings 31: 1344-1350 (1972).

Zusman, R.M.: Renin and non-renin-mediated antihypertensive actions of converting enzyme inhibitors. Kidney International 25: 969-983 (1984).

Address for correspondence and reprints: Dr *J. Herrera-Acosta*, Instituto Nacional de Cardiología, Ignacio Chávez, Juan Badiano 1, Del. Tlalpan, 14080 Mexico DF (Mexico).

Drugs 30 (Suppl. 1): 47-48 (1985)
0012-6667/85/0100-0047/$1.00/0

General Discussion

Moderator: *J.A.F. Ramires*

1. Genesis and Development of Angiotensin-Converting Enzyme Inhibitors: Focus on Enalapril

Dr *Ramires:* I understood that angiotensin III has some physiological functions. What is its place in the secretion of aldosterone? Secondly, do you have any comments on the role of atrionatrin (atrial natriuretic factor) in the control of fluid balance?

Dr *Ribeiro:* It has been said that angiotensin III is equivalent to angiotensin II in terms of aldosterone control, and it was postulated that at the adrenal level angiotensin II can release aldosterone only after being converted to angiotensin III. The latter point is no longer considered valid, but there is no doubt that angiotensin III can be measured in the plasma in normal individuals. Further, when injected into experimental animals or normal man it stimulates aldosterone secretion and has a weak action to raise blood pressure.

In relation to atrionatrin, I do not know if there is an interaction between this peptide of cardiac origin and the renin-angiotensin system. What is interesting is that if we administer the peptide to experimental animals with an activated renin-angiotensin system, there is a marked fall in arterial blood pressure, and in some preparations it is able to inhibit practically all known vasoconstrictive stimuli. This includes angiotensin II.

Anon: Have there been studies on the relationship between liver function and the conversion of enalapril to enalaprilat?

Dr *Gomez:* Studies are being carried out at the present time. Looking at available data we see no limitation of hydrolysis for the conversion of enalapril to enalaprilat, but we do not yet have the final answer.

Anon: Have there been studies of enalapril in dialysis patients?

Dr *Gomez:* Enalaprilat is dialysable. It can be removed completely by haemodialysis.

Dr *H. Calvo:* I would like to ask if it is known if any effects from high levels of renin occur during treatment with ACE inhibitors?

Dr *Gomez:* Experience with ACE inhibitors includes some years with captopril and, in our case, with enalapril in approximately 6000 patients, some of whom have been treated for up to 4 years. As far as we know, there is no problem attributed to hyperreninaemia.

Dr *Calvo:* Why does arterial pressure fall during ACE inhibition, and how do you explain the continuing decline in pressure seen with enalapril? My second question is: the paper by Gomez and colleagues showed a decrease in converting enzyme activity with enalapril, and I would like to know if there are any results of measurements of converting enzyme concentrations?

Dr *Gomez:* The first question is complicated. We know very well that the main pharmacological mechanism of action of ACE inhibition is the consequent reduction of blood angiotensin II levels. We can only measure angiotensin II in the plasma and not in the tissues, where it is possibly more important. Although I have no data to support it, I dare say that apart from this mechanism there must be a mechanism *not* related to the renin-angiotensin system, but at present I am speculating completely. With regard to the second question, the most important effect is inhibition of converting enzyme activity. We know that in chronic therapy, and this has been demonstrated in animals, the total concentration of converting enzyme increases, apparently due to enzyme induction.

Dr *F. Fardel:* I do not entirely agree with some points made within the report by Drs Messerli and Ventura. Peripheral vascular resistance has different connotations in young and elderly hypertensive subjects. There are anatomical differences between the young and the elderly that lead to this inappropriately high peripheral vascular resistance. Secondly, one area that cannot be ignored is coronary insufficiency, which is clearly much more common in the elderly than in the young. Thirdly, I do not agree with the statement that hypertrophy is so prejudicial. In reality, hypertrophy is a normal reaction of the heart to the inappropriate stimulus of hypertension, and in an attempt to reduce the peak systolic 'stress', the heart reacts with hypertrophy and in the final analysis this is to reduce myocardial oxygen consumption.

Dr *Messerli:* Let me answer your last question first. With regard to left ventricular hypertrophy we are used to thinking that this was just a physiological process that serves to overcome or to compensate for the high afterload. However, it was initially shown by the Framingham study that the so-called physiological process is not so physiological since these patients are indeed at high risk of sudden death, they are at higher risk of acute myocardial infarction, and they are also at higher risk from developing congestive heart failure. From these epidemiological studies I think it becomes clear that what we have been thinking is not correct anymore.

Your second point is well taken. It is quite clear that when left ventricular hypertrophy is produced, there is at the same time a factor that produces a relative reduction in coronary blood flow. Thus, these patients are more prone to develop ischaemia and therefore they have a higher ventricular irritability. Regarding your first point, I am not implying that the pathological substrate is different in the young or in the old. What we did was to measure haemodynamics in the old and in the young, and I think it is well established that in young patients we are dealing with a high cardiac output hypertension, and with increasing age the cardiac output falls and resistance goes up. You may be perfectly right that this is secondary to arteriosclerosis, but we did not address this question.

Dr *Herrera-Acosta:* Is it correct that only 2 of the patients of Drs Messerli and Ventura had increased ventricular mass, and these are the patients in whom ventricular mass decreased during treatment?

Dr *Messerli:* This is correct. But I think the point is that left ventricular hypertrophy is not a 'yes' or 'no' diagnosis. As pressure goes up slowly, posterior wall thickness will go from 0.9 to 1 cm, then 1.1 cm then 1.2 cm, and once it is greater than 1.2 cm we say this is left ventricular hypertrophy. This is an arbitrary criterion, so the fact that we had only 2 patients with left ventricular hypertrophy does not really mean anything because what we did in some patients was to reduce posterior wall thickness from 1.1 to 0.8 cm, and I find that we still did something good for these patients.

Anon: What diet were the patients of Dr Herrera-Acosta and colleagues allowed? What was the salt intake?

What was the maximum dose of propranolol used?

Dr *Herrera-Acosta:* The patients took their normal diet. We did not attempt to modify salt intake. We increased the propranolol dose up to 240 mg/day and achieved normotension in 10 of the 12 patients.

Dr *R. Sánchez:* Regarding the reduction of glomerular filtration rate in the study by Herrera-Acosta et al., could this account for variability in the method used?

Dr *Herrera-Acosta:* Any non-systematic error in the method ought to eliminate any change in one direction or another. The fact that the values decreased would speak against a variation in the method. In addition, this method has been validated by us over the years and we have obtained an excellent correlation with results from other laboratories.

Section 2:
Enalapril: Pharmacodynamic Findings and Therapeutic Efficacy in Hypertension and Heart Failure

Drugs 30 (Suppl. 1): 49-58 (1985)
0012-6667/85/0100-0049/$5.00/0

Natriuretic Effect and Changes in Renal Haemodynamics Induced by Enalapril in Essential Hypertension

R.A. Sánchez, E. Marcó, H.B. Gilbert, P. Raffaele, M. Brito, M. Giménez and *L.I. Moledo*

Hospital Instituto de Cardiologia, Academia Nacional de Medicina and Hospital de Niños Ricardo Gutierrez, Buenos Aires

Summary *The purpose of this study was to evaluate the natriuretic effect and renal haemodynamic changes induced by enalapril in patients with essential hypertension. In a group of 11 patients with mild to moderate hypertension with normal renal function, and on a controlled sodium intake (80 mmol/day), a decrease in systolic and diastolic blood pressure was observed ($p < 0.001$) after 16 weeks of enalapril treatment (20 mg/day), without a change in heart rate. An increase in plasma renin activity ($p < 0.05$) without changes in serum aldosterone, and a decrease in exchangeable sodium ($p < 0.001$) were present at the end of the treatment period.*

In 10 hypertensive patients also taking a dietary sodium of 80 mmol/day, the renal haemodynamics, humoral changes, and urinary sodium excretion were measured during 4 days of enalapril treatment (20 mg/day). There was an increase in urinary sodium excretion on the 3rd and 4th days of treatment ($p < 0.01$). The effective renal plasma flow and fractional sodium excretion increased 72 hours after the beginning of treatment ($p < 0.01$); the glomerular filtration rate did not change, and filtration fraction decreased at 72 hours. Mean blood pressure fell 2 hours after the first dose ($p < 0.01$), and the maximum drop in intrarenal vascular resistance occurred after 72 hours of treatment ($p < 0.01$). Plasma renin activity increased ($p < 0.05$) and serum aldosterone decreased ($p < 0.01$) 2 hours after the first dose. Thereafter, serum aldosterone increased progressively until it reached values similar to those with placebo at 48 and 72 hours of treatment. Urinary kallikrein fell during the 2nd and 3rd day of treatment ($p < 0.01$). It was concluded that the decrease in exchangeable sodium was due to a natriuretic effect of enalapril. This effect presumably results from renal haemodynamic changes due to the reduction of angiotensin II. Other mechanisms, such as the reduction of aldosterone and accumulation of kinins, could be contributory factors.

The angiotensin-converting enzyme (ACE) inhibitors have proved effective in the treatment of hypertension and congestive heart failure (Brunner et al., 1980; Johnston et al., 1982; Ondetti et al., 1977; Wenting et al., 1983). Captopril, the first orally-active inhibitor, has been extensively used in both situations (Atkinson and Robertson, 1979; Atkinson et al., 1980; Romankiewicz et al., 1983; Wenting et al., 1983). Enalapril, a new ACE inhibitor whose molecule does not have the sulphydryl group, has also shown its effectiveness in the treatment of hypertension (Brunner et al., 1983; Gavras et al., 1981; Hodsman et al., 1983) and congestive heart failure (Fitzpatrick et al., 1983; Kjekshus et al., 1983). Aside from their therapeutic effects, the availability of ACE inhibitors has resulted in a better knowledge of the function of the renin-angiotensin system in several physiological and pathological conditions (Brunner et al., 1981; Cody et al., 1983; Hollenberg and Williams, 1983; MacGregor et al., 1981; Shoback et al., 1983).

The kidney plays an essential role in the control of angiotensin production. This organ is the principal source of renin, and several observations have indicated that angiotensin II has important regulatory functions within the kidney. In this respect, the extreme sensitivity of the kidney vascular bed to the constrictor action of angiotensin II is well known (Levens et al., 1981).

It is important that we document the hormonal and renal haemodynamic changes induced by ACE inhibitors, since the kidney is considered to play a central role in the pathogenesis of essential hypertension.

The purpose of this paper was to evaluate the natriuretic effect and renal haemodynamic and humoral changes induced by enalapril in patients with mild to moderate essential hypertension. In one group of patients, changes in exchangeable sodium ($E_{Na}+$), plasma renin activity and serum aldosterone were studied before and after 16 weeks of enalapril treatment. In the second group, changes in renal haemodynamics, urinary sodium ($U_{Na}+$) excretion, plasma renin activity, serum aldosterone and urinary kallikrein excretion induced by short term enalapril treatment, were evaluated.

1. Methods

21 patients with mild to moderate essential hypertension were selected. Renal function was normal in all cases (creatinine clearance was between 98 and 136 ml/min/1.73m^2), and none had proteinuria. They were divided into two groups. The first group consisted of 11 patients (7 men and 4 women, aged 35 to 61 years). Antihypertensive treatment was discontinued 4 weeks before beginning the study. Two weeks prior to the study, they received a placebo tablet daily, and took a diet of 80 mmol/day sodium and 100 mmol/day potassium. This diet was continued throughout the study. Systolic and diastolic blood pressures were measured weekly during the placebo period using a Dinamap 845 machine. The average of 3 consecutive readings at 1-minute intervals, in the supine position, was recorded. For the purpose of this study, the baseline (placebo) blood pressure was recorded on the first day of treatment, before the first dose of enalapril was administered.

At the end of the placebo period, plasma renin activity and serum aldosterone were determined in peripheral blood by previously described radioimmunoassay methods (Sánchez et al., 1979; Underwood and Williams, 1972) and $E_{Na}+$, expressed in mmol/kg, with $^{22}Na^+$, as previously reported (Sánchez et al., 1981). During the 16-week treatment phase, the patients received 20mg enalapril daily as a single dose in the morning. Blood pressure was measured, once weekly in the morning before taking the daily dose of enalapril (24 hours after the last dose). The final blood pressure reading (after 16 weeks on enalapril) was recorded. At that time, $E_{Na}+$, plasma renin activity and serum aldosterone determinations were again made. Blood samples for plasma renin activity and serum aldosterone measurements were taken 24 hours after the last dose of enalapril.

The second group consisted of 10 patients (7 men and 3 women, aged 15 to 60 years). Antihypertensive medications were discontinued 4 weeks before beginning the study. Each patient received a placebo tablet daily for 2 weeks before initiation of enalapril treatment. During the placebo and treatment periods, the patients followed the diet mentioned earlier. For the treatment period of 4 days, the patients were given 20mg enalapril daily in a single dose at 10am. The mean blood pressure was recorded with the Dinamap 845 apparatus before the first dose of enalapril (placebo value), 2 hours after the first dose and, on the next 3 days, 24 hours after the previous dose of enalapril.

Table I. Group 1. Systolic blood pressure, diastolic blood pressure, heart rate, plasma renin activity, serum aldosterone and exchangeable sodium ($E_{Na}+$) values corresponding to the placebo period and after 16 weeks of treatment (mean ± SEM)

Parameters	Placebo period	16 Weeks	p value
Systolic blood pressure (mm Hg)	170.5 ± 1	138.4 ± 4	< 0.001
Diastolic blood pressure (mm Hg)	112.4 ± 1	87.6 ± 3	< 0.001
Heart rate (beats/min)	74.8 ± 4	76.7 ± 2	NS
Plasma renin activity (ng/ml/h)	2.2 ± 0.3	11.3 ± 2	< 0.05
Aldosterone (pg/ml)	138.9 ± 11	133.0 ± 14	NS
$E_{Na}+$ (mmol/kg)	39.8 ± 0.6	35.6 ± 0.6	< 0.001

Also, 24-hour urine collections were made on the final 3 placebo days and the 4 days of enalapril treatment for the measurement of $U_{Na}+$ excretion by flame photometry. Before the first dose of enalapril and 2, 24, 48 and 72 hours thereafter, effective renal plasma flow, glomerular filtration rate and filtration fraction (glomerular filtration rate/effective renal plasma flow) were determined by the simultaneous clearances of para-amino-hippuric acid and inulin (Schnurr et al., 1980; Smith et al., 1938). An index of intrarenal vascular resistance (mean blood pressure/effective renal plasma flow), expressed in mm Hg/ml minute, was calculated. Sodium concentrations in blood and urine were also determined and the fractional excretion of sodium [$FE_{Na}+ = C_{Na}+$/glomerular filtration rate × 100 (% glomerular filtration rate)] was calculated as follows:

$$FE_{Na}+ = U_{Na}+ \cdot P_{In}/P_{Na} \cdot U_{In} \times 100$$
(% glomerular filtration rate),

where $U_{Na}+$ is the sodium concentration in urine, P_{In} the concentration of inulin in plasma, $P_{Na}+$ the Na^+ concentration in plasma, and U_{In} the urine concentration of inulin. Plasma renin activity and serum aldosterone were measured before the first dose of enalapril (baseline or placebo value), and 2, 24, 48 and 72 hours thereafter. Three final blood samples were taken 24 hours after the final dose of enalapril. Urinary kallikrein excretion, expressed in units of kallikrein/24 hours, was determined on the final placebo day and also on the second and third days of enalapril treatment (Claeson et al., 1978; Giménez et al., 1982). Data from the first group of patients were analysed statistically using the Student's t-test for paired samples. Values were expressed as means and standard errors of the mean (SEM), and statistical significance was taken as $p < 0.05$. For the second group, one-way analysis of variance (ANOVA) was used, with the Tuckey criterion for the limit of significance between mean values.

2. *Results*

Data from group 1 are shown in table I and fig. 1. Systolic and diastolic blood pressures decreased after 16 weeks of treatment with enalapril (table I, $p < 0.001$). There was no change in heart rate. Plasma renin activity increased significantly ($p < 0.05$), but there was no change in serum aldosterone. After 16 weeks of treatment, $E_{Na}+$ showed a significant decrease ($p < 0.001$; table I, fig. 1).

Results from the second study are shown in table II and figs 2 to 4. There was a significant decrease in mean blood pressure 2 hours after the first dose of enalapril ($p < 0.01$), and a further fall had occurred by 24 hours. Little further change was seen at 48 and 72 hours (table II, fig. 2). Effective renal plasma flow was increased significantly, compared with the placebo value, 72 hours after the begin-

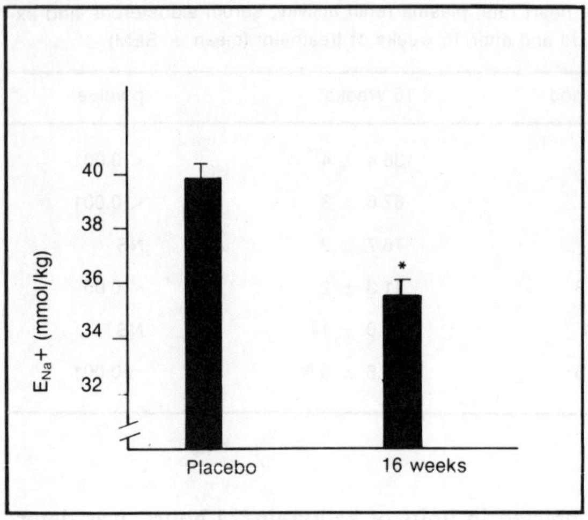

Fig. 1. Group 1. Exchangeable sodium (E_{Na}+) expressed as mmol/kg on placebo and after 16 weeks of enalapril therapy (mean ± SEM; * $p < 0.001$).

ning of treatment ($p < 0.01$). Glomerular filtration rate did not change. As a result, a significant fall in filtration fraction occurred 72 hours after the initiation of enalapril treatment ($p < 0.01$). Compared with the placebo value, the intrarenal vascular resistance dropped rapidly, reaching statistical significance after 24 hours ($p < 0.05$). Plasma renin activity increased 2 hours after the first dose ($p < 0.05$), and remained elevated thereafter (table II). Serum aldosterone decreased significantly 2 hours after the first dose of enalapril, then returned toward baseline levels (table II, fig. 3). Urinary kallikrein excretion fell to low levels during enalapril treatment (fig. 3).

Figure 4 shows the sodium balance in group 2. There was an increase in sodium excretion on the third and fourth days of treatment with enalapril compared with that during the placebo period and

Table II. Group 2. Mean blood pressure, effective renal plasma flow, glomerular filtration rate, filtration fraction, fractional sodium excretion (FE_{Na}+), intrarenal vascular resistance, plasma renin activity, serum aldosterone and urinary kallikrein in the placebo period and 2, 24, 48 and 72 hours after beginning enalapril[a]

Parameters measured	Placebo period	2 hours	24 hours	48 hours	72 hours
MBP (mm Hg)	120.6 ± 3.5	110.4 ± 3.0[b]	104.4 ± 3.0[b]	102.6 ± 2.0[b]	100.5 ± 1.0[b]
ERPF (ml/min/1.73m^2)	486.8 ± 9.0	496.0 ± 9.0	502.2 ± 7.0	513.5 ± 10.0	587.5 ± 11.0[b,c]
GFR (ml/min/1.73m^2)	113.9 ± 5.0	109.9 ± 4.0	108.7 ± 4.0	112.4 ± 3.0	108.7 ± 3.0
FF (GFR/ERPF)	0.23 ± 0.01	0.22 ± 0.01	0.22 ± 0.01	0.22 ± 0.01	0.18 ± 0.01[b,c]
FE_{Na}^+[C_{Na}^+/GFR × 100 (% GFR)]	0.31 ± 0.01	0.30 ± 0.01	0.30 ± 0.01	0.30 ± 0.01	0.58 ± 0.02[b,c]
IVR (mm Hg/ml min)	0.25 ± 0.01	0.23 ± 0.01	0.21 ± 0.01[b]	0.20 ± 0.01[b]	0.17 ± 0.01[b,d]
PRA (ng/ml/h angiotensin I)	0.68 ± 0.6	10.0 ± 1.7[e]	9.33 ± 1.6[e]	9.67 ± 1.7[e]	10.5 ± 1.9[e]
Aldosterone (pg/ml)	141.9 ± 8.2	77.4 ± 2.5[b]	94.7 ± 5.0[e]	106.7 ± 6.0	118.5 ± 7.2
Urinary kallikrein (UK/24h)	10.8 ± 1.0	–	–	2.9 ± 0.6[b]	2.2 ± 0.4[b]

a Mean ± SEM.
b $p < 0.01$ significant with respect to placebo.
c $p < 0.01$ significant with respect to previous values.
d $p < 0.05$ significant with respect to previous values.
e $p < 0.05$ significant with respect to placebo.

Abbreviations: MBP = intrarenal vascular resistance; ERPF = mean blood pressure; GFR = filtration fraction; FF = glomerular filtration rate; FE_{Na}+ = effective renal plasma flow; IVR = fractional sodium excretion; PRA = plasma renin activity.

on the first 2 days of treatment ($p < 0.01$). Coincidentally, a significant increase in the $FE_{Na}+$ compared with previous levels ($p < 0.01$) was noted at 72 hours (table II, fig. 2).

3. Discussion

This study confirms the effectiveness of enalapril in the treatment of essential hypertension (Biollaz et al., 1982; Brunner et al., 1983; de Leeuw et al., 1983). Enalapril induced a persistent increase in plasma renin activity, presumably a result of the decrease in angiotensin II and the fall in blood pressure. This effect is well documented (Biollaz et al., 1982; de Zeeuw et al., 1983) and is similar to that seen with captopril (Case et al., 1978).

Of interest in the current study is the decrease of $E_{Na}+$ after 16 weeks of treatment. A similar observation was made by Hodsman et al. (1983) in hypertension associated with renal artery stenosis during treatment with enalapril. ACE inhibitors would be the only antihypertensive drugs, apart from the diuretics, to lower the body sodium content.

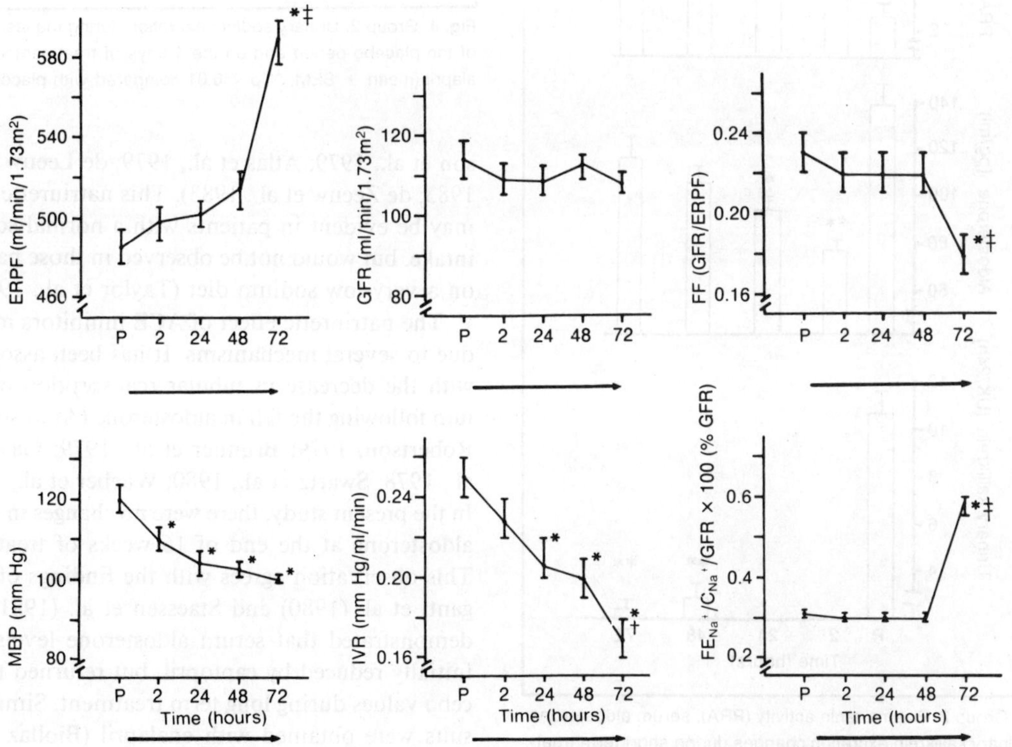

Fig. 2. Group 2. Effective renal plasma flow (ERPF), glomerular filtration rate (GFR), filtration fraction (FF), mean blood pressure (MBP), intrarenal vascular resistance (IVR) and fractional sodium excretion ($FE_{Na}+$) changes induced by enalapril treatment. Measurements were made on placebo (P), 2 hours after the first dose of enalapril and 24, 48 and 72 hours after the onset of treatment (mean ± SEM; * $p < 0.01$ compared with placebo; † $p < 0.05$ compared with the previous value; ‡ $p < 0.01$ compared with the previous value).

The results from group 2 confirm that the decrease in $E_{Na}+$ found in group 1 was due to a natriuretic effect of the drug, which in this study was apparent in the third day of treatment and occurred in spite of the fall in blood pressure. This finding agrees with previous observations (Atkinson et al., 1979; Atlas et al., 1979; de Leeuw et al., 1983; de Zeeuw et al., 1983). This natriuretic effect may be evident in patients with a normal sodium intake, but would not be observed in those patients on a very low sodium diet (Taylor et al., 1984).

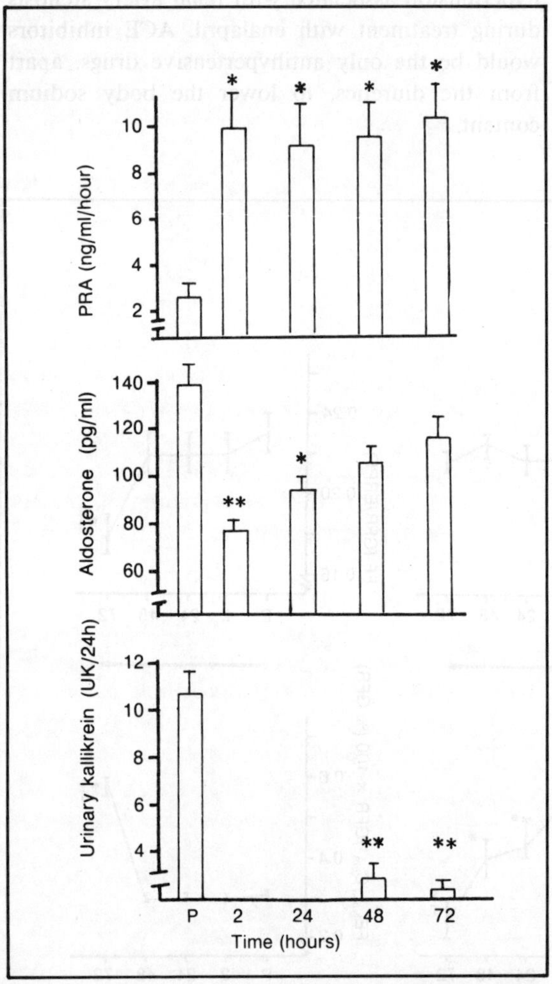

Fig. 3. Group 2. Plasma renin activity (PRA), serum aldosterone and urinary kallikrein excretion changes during short term treatment with enalapril. Plasma renin activity and aldosterone determinations were made on placebo (P), 2 hours after the first dose of enalapril, and 24, 48 and 72 hours after the onset of treatment. Urinary kallikrein measurements were made on placebo and on the second and third days of enalapril treatment (mean ± SEM; * $p < 0.05$ compared with placebo; ** $p < 0.01$ compared with placebo).

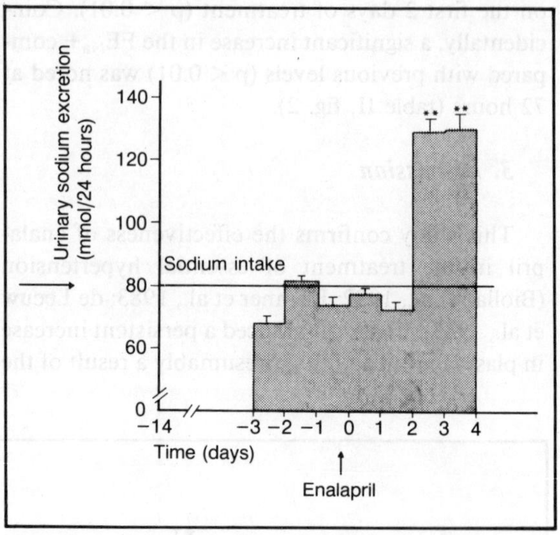

Fig. 4. Group 2. Urinary sodium excretion during the last 3 days of the placebo period and on the 4 days of treatment with enalapril (mean ± SEM; ** $p < 0.01$ compared with placebo).

The natriuretic effect of ACE inhibitors may be due to several mechanisms. It has been associated with the decrease in tubular reabsorption of sodium following the fall in aldosterone (Atkinson and Robertson, 1979; Brunner et al., 1979; Gavras et al., 1978; Swartz et al., 1980; Waeber et al., 1980). In the present study, there were no changes in serum aldosterone at the end of 16 weeks of treatment. This observation agrees with the findings of Morganti et al. (1980) and Staessen et al. (1981) who demonstrated that serum aldosterone levels were initially reduced by captopril, but returned to placebo values during long term treatment. Similar results were obtained with enalapril (Biollaz et al., 1982; Hodsman et al., 1983). Biollaz et al. (1982), during a 6-month study, showed that serum aldosterone, and to a lesser extent angiotensin II, tended to return to baseline levels 12 to 16 hours after enalapril administration, while the ACE inhibition, the increase in plasma renin activity, and the antihypertensive effect were maintained. In the present study we observed in the short term that serum aldosterone was clearly lowered after 2 hours, was still significantly low after 24 hours, but it had risen in the 48- and 72-hour blood samples obtained 24 hours after the previous dose of enalapril. These observations confirm the complexity of aldosterone's regulation, since adrenocorticotrophic hormone (ACTH), potassium and plasma sodium concentrations affect its secretion (Brown et al., 1979; Davies et al., 1979; Fraser et al., 1979), although the presence of at least some angiotensin II seems obligatory. Our findings do not enable us to discard *a priori* the reduction of aldosterone as a natriuretic mechanism. Brunner et al. (1983) demonstrated that, in spite of the restoration of aldosterone levels 24 hours after the last dose of enalapril, administration of a further dose again reduced the levels to those observed at the beginning of treatment.

However, the reduction of aldosterone was probably a minor contributory factor in the loss of body sodium. In our study, there was no increase in FE_{Na^+} 2 hours after drug administration, nor was there an increase in sodium excretion during the first day of treatment in spite of the fall in serum aldosterone. Besides, it was recently demonstrated that enalapril increased sodium excretion in adrenalectomised dogs in a similar fashion to that found in sodium-replete intact dogs (Sweet et al., 1983). The patients in group 2 of our study showed changes in renal haemodynamics which were most evident after 72 hours of treatment. The sustained increase in effective renal plasma flow due to a pronounced fall of vascular resistance during enalapril therapy has also been shown by other investigators (de Zeeuw et al., 1983; Simon et al., 1982), and similar findings have been reported with captopril (Hollenberg et al., 1981; Meggs and Hollenberg, 1980). In the present study, there were no changes in glomerular filtration rate, which was in agreement with previous observations (de Leeuw et al., 1983; Zimmerman and Wong, 1981). It must be pointed out, however, that glomerular filtration rate responses can differ according to the pathophysiological conditions. Thus, in the case of marked hypovolaemia or bilateral renal artery stenosis, the reduction in glomerular filtration rate can be critical (Hricik et al., 1983). On the other hand, there can be increases in the glomerular filtration rate in patients who initially are azotaemic (Hollenberg et al., 1979). The reduction in filtration fraction, as reported also by others (de Zeeuw et al., 1983; Levens et al., 1981), indicates predominant vasodilatation of the efferent arteriole. This fits with the concept that angiotensin II has a greater vasoconstrictor action on the efferent arteriole (Edwards, 1982). Zimmerman and Wong (1981) stated that the renal vasodilatory effect of the ACE inhibitors is primarily due to the reduction in circulating angiotensin II. Nevertheless, it is possible that the increase in renal blood flow could result from either inhibition of circulating angiotensin II or local angiotensin II formation (de Zeeuw et al., 1983).

In the present study, the concurrent increase in sodium excretion and renal haemodynamic changes raises the possibility of a causal relationship between the two. On the other hand, the increase in FE_{Na^+} 72 hours after the beginning of enalapril treatment in group 2, indicates that the natriuretic effect was due to a reduction of the tubular reabsorption of sodium. It is likely that the fall in filtration fraction would induce a reduction of oncotic pressure in peritubular blood, with a subsequent reduction in the proximal reabsorption of sodium. A relative decrease in reabsorption in more distal segments would be necessary to account for the natriuretic effect. Only the effective cortical plasma flow was measured, which does not provide confirmation as to whether or not there was an increase of flow in juxtamedullary nephrons and in the medulla which might lead to a reduction in sodium reabsorption in the long loops of Henle (Osgood et al., 1977; Stein et al., 1976). A further mechanism by which the ACE inhibitors could promote an increase in sodium excretion would be by blocking the stimulant effect of angiotensin II on the distal sodium reabsorption (Hall et al., 1977, 1979).

Another mechanism that could contribute to the decrease of intrarenal vascular resistance, to the increase in renal blood flow, to the increase in sodium excretion, and even to the antihypertensive effect, is the reduction in kinin degradation and a subsequent increase in prostaglandin synthesis. In the present study, a significant fall in urinary kallikrein excretion on the second and third days of treatment was observed, similar to observations in essential hypertensive patients treated with captopril (Karlberg et al., 1980). This effect may result from an increase in kinins induced by ACE inhibitors (Karlberg et al., 1980; McCaa et al., 1978), but a contribution from the reduction in aldosterone levels is possible. Studies in man aimed at clarifying these uncertainties have given differing results, in part because of assay difficulties (Anderson et al., 1980; Johnston et al., 1979). Finally, it should be pointed out that the kinins and prostaglandins are hormones found predominantly in tissues, and that changes in synthesis, biological activity and degradation are not necessarily reflected by changes in their plasma concentrations.

4. Conclusions

The effective treatment of essential hypertension with enalapril is accompanied by a decrease in body sodium content due to an increase in urine sodium excretion. The natriuretic effect is due to a decrease in tubular reabsorption of sodium. It is related to renal haemodynamic changes characterised by a decrease of intrarenal vascular resistance, an increase of effective renal plasma flow, and a decrease of filtration fraction, which are basically the result of the reduction in plasma angiotensin II and blockade of its local action within the kidney. The fall in aldosterone and the accumulation of kinins are probably minor contributory factors. Whatever the underlying mechanisms, the renal haemodynamic changes and the natriuretic effect of ACE inhibitors are probably central to their antihypertensive action.

References

Anderson, G.H.; Springer, J.; Tivnan, E.; Kearney, H. and Streeten, D.H.P.: Hypotensive mechanism of captopril. Clinical Research 28: 328A (1980).

Atkinson, A.B.; Brown, J.J.; Fraser, R.; Leckie, B.; Lever, A.F.; Morton, J.J. and Robertson, J.I.S.: Captopril, angiotensin II and sodium in blood pressure regulation. Lancet 1: 1140 (1979).

Atkinson, A.B. and Robertson, J.I.S.: Captopril in the treatment of clinical hypertension and cardiac failure. Lancet 2: 836-839 (1979).

Atkinson, A.B.; Morton, J.J.; Brown, J.J.; Davies, D.L.; Kelly, P.; Leckie, B.; Lever, A.F. and Robertson, J.I.S.: Captopril in clinical hypertension. Changes in components of the renin-angiotensin system and in body composition in relation to fall in blood pressure with a note on measurement of angiotensin II during converting enzyme inhibition. British Heart Journal 44: 290-296 (1980).

Atlas, S.A.; Case, D.B.; Sealey, J.E.; Laragh, J.H. and McKinstry, D.N.: Interruption of the renin-angiotensin system in hypertensive patients by captopril induces sustained reduction in aldosterone secretion, potassium retention and natriuresis. Hypertension 1: 274-280 (1979).

Biollaz, J.; Brunner, H.R.; Gavras, I.; Waeber, B. and Gavras, H.: Antihypertensive therapy with MK 421: Angiotensin II-renin relationships to evaluate efficacy of converting enzyme blockade. Journal of Cardiovascular Pharmacology 4: 966-972 (1982).

Brown, J.J.; Casals-Stenzel, J.; Cumming, A.M.M.; Davies, D.L.; Fraser, R.; Lever, A.F.; Morton, J.J.; Semple, P.F.; Tree, M. and Robertson, J.I.S.: Angiotensin II, aldosterone and arterial pressure: A quantitative approach. Hypertension 1: 159-179 (1979).

Brunner, D.B.; Desponds, G.; Biollaz, J.; Keller, I.; Ferber, F.; Gavras, H.; Brunner, H.R. and Schelling, J.L.: Effect of a new angiotensin converting enzyme inhibitor MK-421 and its lysine analogue on the components of the renin system in healthy subjects. Journal of Cardiovascular Pharmacology 11: 461-467 (1981).

Brunner, H.R.; Gavras, H.; Waeber, B.; Korshow, G.R.; Turini, G.A.; Vukovich, R.A.; McKinstry, D.N. and Gavras, I.: Oral angiotensin converting inhibitor in long-term treatment of hypertensive patients. Annals of Internal Medicine 90: 19-23 (1979).

Brunner, H.R.; Gavras, H.; Waeber, B.; Textor, S.G.; Turini, G.A. and Wanters, J.P.: Clinical use of an orally acting converting enzyme inhibitor: Captopril. Hypertension 2: 558-564 (1980).

Brunner, H.R.; Waeber, B.; Nussberg, J.; Schaller, M.D. and Gomez, H.J.: Long-term clinical experience with enalapril in essential hypertension. Journal of Hypertension 1 (Suppl. 1): 103-107 (1983).

Case, D.B.; Atlas, S.A.; Laragh, J.H.; Sealey, J.E.; Sullivan, P.A. and McKinstry, D.M.: Clinical experience with blockade of the renin-angiotensin-aldosterone system by an oral converting enzyme inhibitor (S.Q. 14224, captopril) in hypertensive patients. Progress in Cardiovascular Diseases 21: 195-206 (1978).

Claeson, G.; Friberger, E.; Knos, O. and Eriksson, E.: Methods for determinations of prekallikrein in plasma, glandular kallikrein and urokinase. Haemostasis 7: 76-78 (1978).

Cody, R.J.; Laragh, J.H.; Atlas, S.A. and Case, D.B.: Converting enzyme inhibition to identify and treat renin-mediated or sodium volume related forms of increased peripheral resistance in hypertension and in congestive heart failure. Journal of Hypertension 1 (Suppl. 1): 77-84 (1983).

Davies, D.L.; Beevers, D.G.; Brown, J.J.; Cumming, A.M.M.; Fraser, R.; Lever, A.F.; Mason, P.A.; Morton, J.J.; Robertson, J.I.S.; Titterington, M. and Tree, M.: Aldosterone and its stimuli in normal and hypertensive man: Are essential hypertension and primary hyperaldosteronism without tumour the same condition? Journal of Endocrinology 81: 79P-91P (1979).

de Leeuw, P.W.; Hoogma, R.P.L.M.; van Soest, G.A.W.; van Es, P.N. and Birkenhäger, W.H.: Physiological effects of short-term treatment with enalapril in hypertensive patients. Journal of Hypertension 1 (Suppl. 1): 87-91 (1983).

de Zeeuw, D.; Navis, G.J.; Donker, A.J.M. and deJong, P.E.: The angiotensin converting enzyme inhibitor enalapril and its effects on renal function. Journal of Hypertension 1 (Suppl. 1): 93-97 (1983).

Edwards, R.M.: Response of isolated renal microvessels to intraluminal pressure, norepinephrine and angiotensin II. Abstracts of the 15th Annual Meeting of the American Society of Nephrology, Chicago p.150 (1982).

Fitzpatrick, D.; Nicholls, M.G.; Ikram, H. and Espiner, E.A.: Acute haemodynamic, hormonal and electrolyte effects and short-term clinical response to enalapril in heart failure. Journal of Hypertension 1 (Suppl. 1): 147-153 (1983).

Fraser, R.; Brown, J.J.; Lever, A.F.; Mason, P.A. and Robertson, J.I.S.: Control of aldosterone secretion. Clinical Science 56: 389-392 (1979).

Gavras, H.; Gavras, I.; Textor, S.; Volices, L.; Brunner, H.R. and Rolieska, E.J.: Effect of angiotensin converting enzyme inhibition on blood pressure, plasma renin activity and plasma aldosterone in essential hypertension. Journal of Clinical Endocrinology and Metabolism 46: 220-226 (1978).

Gavras, H.; Biollaz, J.; Waeber, B.; Brunner, H.R.; Gavras, I. and Davies, R.D.: Antihypertensive effect of the new oral angiotensin converting enzyme inhibitor 'MK-421'. Lancet 2: 543-547 (1981).

Giménez, M.; Grunfeld, B.; Simsolo, R.; Mendilharzu, F.; Barontini, M. and Becú, L.: Kalicreína urinaria en distintas formas de hipertensión en pediatría. Medicina (Buenos Aires) 42: 736-737 (1982).

Hall, J.E.; Guyton, A.C.; Trippodo, N.C.; Lohmeier, T.E.; McCaa, R.E. and Cowley, A.W.: Intrarenal control of electrolyte excretion by angiotensin II. American Journal of Physiology 233: F538-F544 (1977).

Hall, J.E.; Coleman, T.G.; Guyton, A.C.; Balfe, J.W. and Salgado, H.C.: Intrarenal role of angiotensin II and (des-Asp[1]) angiotensin II. American Journal of Physiology 236: F252-F259 (1979).

Hodsman, G.P.; Brown, J.J.; Cumming, A.M.M.; Davies, D.L.; East, B.W.; Lever, A.F.; Morton, J.J.; Murray, G.D. and Robertson, J.I.S.: Enalapril (MK-421) in the treatment of hypertension with renal artery stenosis. Journal of Hypertension 1 (Suppl. 1): 109-117 (1983).

Hollenberg, N.K.; Swartz, J.L.; Passan, D.R. and Williams, G.H.: Increased glomerular filtration rate after converting enzyme inhibition. New England Journal of Medicine 301: 9-12 (1979).

Hollenberg, N.K.; Meggs, L.G.; Williams, G.H.; Katz, J.; Garnic, J.D. and Harrington, D.P.: Sodium intake and renal responses to captopril in normal man and in essential hypertension. Kidney International 20: 240-245 (1981).

Hollenberg, N.K. and Williams, G.H.: Volume control and altered renal and adrenal responsiveness to angiotensin in essential hypertension: Implications for treatment with converting enzyme inhibition. Journal of Hypertension 1 (Suppl. 1): 119-128 (1983).

Hricik, D.E.; Browning, P.J.; Kopeleman, R.; Goormo, W.E.; Madias, N.E. and Dzau, V.J.: Captopril induced functional renal insufficiency in patients with bilateral renal artery stenosis or renal artery stenosis in a solitary kidney. New England Journal of Medicine 308: 373-376 (1983).

Johnston, C.I.; McGrath, B.P.; Millar, J.A. and Matthews, P.G.: Long-term effects of captopril (SQ 14225) on blood pressure and hormone levels in essential hypertension. Lancet 2: 493-495 (1979).

Johnston, C.I.; McGrath, B.P.; Matthews, P.G. and Jackson, B.: Treatment of hypertension with angiotensin converting enzyme inhibitors. Clinical and Experimental Pharmacology and Physiology 7 (Suppl.): 135-144 (1982).

Karlberg, B.E.; Ohman, K.P.; Nilsson, O.R. and Wettre, S.: Captopril lowers urinary kallikrein in hypertensive patients. Lancet 1: 150-151 (1980).

Kjekshus, J.K.; Søyland, E.; Dickstein, K.; Abrahamsen, A.M. and Gundersen, T.: Sustained haemodynamic effects of enalapril in left ventricular failure. Journal of Hypertension 1 (Suppl. 1): 143-145 (1983).

Levens, N.R.; Peach, M.J. and Casey, R.M.: Role of the intrarenal renin-angiotensin system in the control of renal function. Circulation Research 48: 157-167 (1981).

MacGregor, G.A.; Markandu, N.D.; Bayliss, J.; Roulston, J.E.; Squires, M. and Morton, J.J.: Non sulphydryl containing angiotensin converting enzyme inhibitor (MK-421); evidence for a role of renin system in normotensive subjects. British Medical Journal 23: 401-403 (1981).

McCaa, R.E.; Hall, J.E. and McCaa, C.S.: The effects of angiotensin I converting enzyme inhibitors on arterial blood pressure and urinary sodium excretion. Role of renal renin-angiotensin and kallikrein-kinin systems. Circulation Research 43 (Suppl. 1): 32-39 (1978).

Meggs, L.G. and Hollenberg, N.K.: Converting enzyme inhibition and the kidney. Hypertension 2: 551-557 (1980).

Morganti, A.; Pickering, T.G.; López Ovejero, J.A. and Laragh, J.H.: Endocrine and cardiovascular influences of converting enzyme inhibition with SQ 14225 in hypertensive patients in the supine position and during head-up tilt before and after sodium depletion. Journal of Clinical Endocrinology and Metabolism 50: 748-754 (1980).

Ondetti, M.A.; Rubin, B. and Cushman, D.W.: Design of specific inhibitors of angiotensin converting enzyme. Science 196: 441-444 (1977).

Osgood, R.W.; Reineck, H.J. and Stein, J.H.: Effect of volume expansion on sodium transport in the proximal tubule of juxtamedullary nephrons. Clinical Research 25: 444A-450A (1977).

Romankiewicz, J.A.; Brogden, R.N.; Heel, R.C.; Speight, T.M. and Avery, G.S.: Captopril: An update review of its pharmacological properties and therapeutic efficacy in congestive heart failure. Drugs 25: 6-40 (1983).

Sánchez, R.A.; Cavarra, O.; Brea, S.A.; Marcó, E.J.; Ravera, M. and Moledo, L.I.: Actividad renínica plasmática en la hipertensión esencial. Medicina (Buenos Aires) 39: 171-177 (1979).

Sánchez, R.A.; Marcó, E.J.; Brea, S.A.; Bourgés, M.M.; Gilbert, B.H. and Moledo, L.I.: Sodio total intercambiable en la hipertensión esencial e hipertensión con insuficiencia renal crónica. Medicina (Buenos Aires) 41: 153-156 (1981).

Schnurr, E.; Lahme, W. and Kuppers, H.: Measurement of renal clearance of inulin and PAH in the steady state without urine collection. Clinical Nephrology 13: 26-29 (1980).

Shoback, D.M.; Williams, G.H.; Swartz, S.L.; Davies, R.O. and Hollenberg, N.K.: Time course and effect of sodium intake on vascular and hormonal responses to enalapril (MK-421) in normal subjects. Journal of Cardiovascular Pharmacology 5: 1010-1018 (1983).

Simon, G.; Morioka, S.; Snyder, D.K. and Cohn, J.N.: Increased renal plasma flow during long-term treatment of essential hypertension with MK-421. (Abstract 660.) Circulation 66: 166 (1982).

Smith, H.W.; Goldring, W. and Chasis, H.: The measurement of the tubular excretory mass, effective blood flow and filtration rate in the normal human kidney. Journal of Clinical Investigation 17: 263-278 (1938).

Staessen, J.; Lijnen, P.; Fagard, R.; Verschueren, L.J. and Amery, A.: Rise of plasma aldosterone during long-term captopril treatment. New England Journal of Medicine 304: 1110 (1981).

Stein, J.H.; Osgood, R.W. and Kunau, R.T.: Direct measurement of papillary collecting duct sodium transport in the rat: Evidence for heterogeneity of nephron function during Ringer's loading. Journal of Clinical Investigation 58: 767-773 (1976).

Swartz, S.L.; Williams, G.H.; Hollenberg, N.F.; Grantz, F.R.; Moore, T.J.; Levine, L.; Sadahra, A.A. and Dluhy, R.G.: Endocrine profile in the long-term phase of converting enzyme inhibition. Clin. Pharmacol. and Ther. 28: 499-504 (1980).

Sweet, C.S.; Gaul, S.L.; Reitz, P.M.; Blaine, E.H. and Ribeiro, L.T.: Mechanism of action of enalapril in experimental hypertension and acute left ventricular failure. Journal of Hypertension 1 (Suppl. 1): 53-63 (1983).

Taylor, T.; Moore, T.J.; Hollenberg, N.K. and Williams, G.H.: Converting-enzyme inhibition corrects the altered adrenal response to angiotensin II in essential hypertension. Hypertension 6: 92-99 (1984).

Underwood, R.H. and Williams, G.H.: The simultaneous measurement of aldosterone cortisol and corticosterone in human peripheral plasma by displacement analysis. Journal of Laboratory and Clinical Medicine 79: 848-862 (1972).

Waeber, B.; Brunner, H.R.; Brunner, D.B.; Curtet, A.; Turini, G.A. and Gavras, H.: Discrepancy between antihypertensive effect and angiotensin converting enzyme inhibition by captopril. Hypertension 2: 236-242 (1980).

Wenting, G.J.; Man Int'Veld, A.J.; Woitteuz, A.J.; Boomsma, F.; Laird-Meeter, K.; Simoons, M.L.; Hugenholtz, P.G. and Schalekamp, M.A.D.: Effects of captopril in acute and chronic heart failure. Correlations with plasma levels of noradrenaline, renin and aldosterone. British Heart Journal 49: 65-73 (1983).

Zimmerman, B.G. and Wong, P.C.: Alterations in renal function produced by angiotensin converting enzyme inhibitors; in Horovitz (Ed.) Angiotensin Converting Enzyme Inhibitors, pp. 239-253 (Urban and Schwarzenberg, Baltimore 1981).

Address for correspondence and reprints: Dr *Luis I. Moledo,* Hospital Instituto de Cardiologia, Coronel Diaz 2423, 1425 Buenos Aires (Argentina).

Drugs 30 (Suppl. 1): 59-69 (1985)
0012-6667/85/0100-0059/$5.50/0

Enalapril versus Triple-Drug Therapy in the Treatment of Renovascular Hypertension

Garry P. Reams and *John H. Bauer*

The Harry S. Truman Memorial Veterans Hospital and University of Missouri School of Medicine, Columbia

Summary *18 renovascular hypertensive patients were entered into a randomised, double-blind protocol to assess the safety and efficacy of enalapril (5 to 20mg twice-daily) and hydrochlorothiazide (50 to 100 mg/day), versus triple-drug therapy employing hydrochlorothiazide (50 to 100 mg/day), timolol (10 to 30mg twice-daily) and hydralazine (50 to 150mg twice-daily). Specifically monitored were the effects of each drug regimen on blood pressure, plasma renin activity and angiotensin II, glomerular filtration rate by inulin clearance, and effective renal plasma flow by para-aminohippurate clearance. Results indicate that enalapril/hydrochlorothiazide was more effective than triple-drug therapy in lowering blood pressure. All patients on enalapril/hydrochlorothiazide had excellent control of blood pressure, and there were no adverse effects. In contrast, 50% of the patients on triple-drug therapy had either uncontrolled blood pressure or significant drug-related side effects. Patients who were uncontrolled or intolerant of triple-drug therapy were well controlled on enalapril/hydrochlorothiazide. Patients on enalapril/hydrochlorothiazide demonstrated stimulation of plasma renin activity with inhibition of plasma angiotensin II, indicating adherence with therapy. Therapy for both unilateral and bilateral renovascular hypertension with enalapril/hydrochlorothiazide did not result in reductions in either glomerular filtration rate or effective renal plasma flow, except in 1 patient with a functional solitary stenotic kidney. In contrast, triple-drug therapy was generally associated with modest reductions in glomerular filtration rate and effective renal plasma flow, with a severe reduction in glomerular filtration rate and effective renal plasma flow occurring in 1 patient with bilateral symmetrical renovascular disease. We conclude that the combination of enalapril and hydrochlorothiazide is a safer and more effective regimen, compared with triple-drug therapy, for the treatment of renovascular hypertension.*

Enalapril is an angiotensin II converting enzyme (ACE) inhibitor which has been shown to be effective in reducing blood pressure in patients with renovascular hypertension. However, it has been reported that the use of ACE inhibitors may precipitate a serious deterioration in glomerular filtration rate and renal blood flow. Such findings have been described in patients with bilateral renal artery stenosis (Aldigier et al., 1982; Bender et al., 1984; Chrysant et al., 1983; Fotino and Sporn, 1983; Grossman et al., 1980; Hricik et al., 1983; Textor et al., 1984), renal artery stenosis in the solitary kidney (Hricik et al., 1983; Kawamura et al., 1982) and in renal artery stenosis in the transplant kidney (Collste et al., 1979; Curtis et al., 1983; Farrow and Wilkinson, 1979; Mason and Hilton, 1983). Deterioration in renal function is thought to be related to the blockade of angiotensin II formation in the presence of reduced renal perfusion pressure, with a resultant disturbance in the autoregulation of glomerular filtration and renal blood flow (Blythe, 1983; Edwards, 1982; Hall et al., 1977; Helmchen et al., 1982).

Treatment with triple-drug therapy employing a diuretic, β-blocker and vasodilator has also been shown to be effective in reducing blood pressure in patients with renovascular hypertension (Alpert and Bauer, 1982; Brooks and Bauer, 1979; Felts and Charler, 1980; Larochelle et al., 1980). Triple-drug therapy has not been reported to produce adverse renal effects. However, no prospective, double-blind studies have been reported assessing the renal effects and efficacy of triple-drug therapy versus ACE inhibitor therapy in the treatment of renovascular hypertension.

The purpose of this study was to investigate the antihypertensive effects (safety and efficacy) of enalapril/hydrochlorothiazide versus triple-drug therapy in the treatment of renovascular hypertension. Most importantly, it was the intent of this study to define and compare in a randomised, double-blind, prospective manner, the effects of these treatments on renal haemodynamics and renal function.

1. Methods

1.1 Subjects

18 hypertensive patients were selected for the study. Each patient had renovascular hypertension (see Results section), and a mean 5-minute recumbent diastolic (fifth phase) blood pressure > 95mm Hg while on hydrochlorothiazide therapy (50mg). Patient adherence to therapy was monitored by count of returned tablets. Informed consent was obtained according to the principles of the Declaration of Helsinki. All studies were approved by the Harry S. Truman Memorial Veterans Hospital and the University of Missouri Health Sciences Center joint Institutional Review Board (committee for research involving human subjects).

1.2 Patient Protocol

The patients were randomly assigned to either the enalapril and placebo, or the timolol and hydralazine arm of the protocol. The hydrochlorothiazide dosage remained fixed at 50 mg/day. An optional increase of hydrochlorothiazide to 100mg was allowed in patients with a creatinine clearance between 40 and 60 ml/min/1.73m^2. Patients were titrated either to achieve blood pressure control (supine diastolic blood pressure < 90mm Hg) or to maximum dosages allowed by the protocol. Titration of enalapril progressed from 5mg twice-daily to 10 and 20mg twice-daily. The number of placebo tablets were titrated similarly. Titration of hydralazine progressed from 50mg twice-daily to 100 and 150mg twice-daily in combination with timolol from 10mg twice-daily to 20 and 30mg twice-daily. Titration periods ranged from 2 to 5 days, depending on the severity of the hypertension. Criteria for titrating drugs to the next dosage was a supine diastolic blood pressure > 90mm Hg. At the end of the titration period, controlled patients were maintained on blind drug therapy for an additional period of 6 weeks. In uncontrolled patients (supine diastolic pressure > 90mm Hg) the treatment code was broken and they were given the option of switching to the alternate therapy. Following 6 weeks of maintenance therapy, the treatment code was broken in all patients. Patients on enalapril/hydrochlorothiazide were permitted to continue their antihypertensive (open label) therapy for an additional 6-month period. Patients on triple-drug therapy were maintained on individualised triple-drug therapy and discontinued from further protocol assessment.

1.3 Procedures

Blood pressure was monitored using a standard mercury sphygmomanometer. Three blood pressures were recorded after the patient had been supine for 5 min. The 3 pressures were averaged to give a mean representation of the patient's blood pressure. Mean arterial pressure was calculated as diastolic blood pressure plus 1/3 of the pulse pressure. The mean heart rate was recorded from the average of 3 supine determinations, obtained prior to each blood pressure measurement.

Clearances of inulin, para-aminohippurate and 24-hour urinary protein excretions were determined as previously described (Bauer and Jones, 1984) prior to randomisation, 2 weeks following titration of effective antihypertensive therapy (maintenance period 1), at the completion of 6 weeks of therapy (maintenance period 2), and following 6 months of open label therapy (maintenance period 3). Blood was drawn for determination of plasma renin activity and plasma angiotensin II as previously described (Bauer and Jones, 1984) prior to randomisation, and at completion of maintenance periods 1, 2 and 3.

Data were analysed by non-parametric methods; the Wilcoxon signed rank test was used to make comparisons between matched groups, and the Wilcoxon rank sum test (Mann-Whitney test) was used to make comparisons between independent groups. A difference was considered statistically significant when $p < 0.05$.

2. Results

2.1 Patient Characteristics, Blood Pressure and Subdivisions of Renovascular Hypertensive Disease

18 patients (4 female, 14 male: mean age 53 years) were prospectively selected for the protocol. The diagnosis of renovascular hypertension was made on the basis of an abnormal renal arteriogram and lateralised (ratio > 1.5) or bilaterally elevated split renal vein renin determinations. All patients met the above criteria within 1 year of entrance into the protocol. Nine patients were initially randomised to the enalapril/hydrochlorothiazide arm, and 9 to the triple-drug therapy arm of the protocol. Of the 9 patients who entered the enalapril/hydrochlorothiazide group, all successfully completed the titration and maintenance periods. No side effects were reported. Both systolic and diastolic blood pressures were well controlled (fig. 1). Of the 9 patients who entered the triple-drug therapy group, 5 patients successfully completed the titration and 6-week maintenance phase of the protocol (fig. 2). Four patients were discontinued; 2 developed disabling hydralazine headaches and 2 had uncontrolled hypertension. Three of the 4 patients who were discontinued from the protocol elected to switch to the alternative enalapril therapy with subsequent control of both systolic and diastolic blood pressures. In addition, 1 patient on triple-drug therapy developed elevated supine diastolic pressure (> 90mm Hg) 2 months after completion of the 6-week maintenance period. This patient was switched to the alternative enalapril/

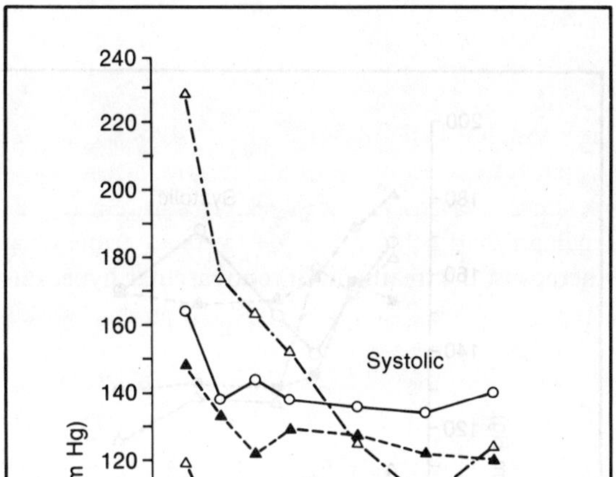

Fig. 1. Mean systolic and diastolic blood pressure response to enalapril/hydrochlorothiazide therapy in patients with: unilateral renovascular hypertension (○——○) n = 8, n = 6 at 6 months; asymmetrical bilateral renovascular hypertension (▲---▲) n = 4, n = 2 at 6 months; renovascular hypertension plus contralateral parenchymal (small kidney) disease (△—·—△) n = 1.

hydrochlorothiazide therapy with subsequent control of both systolic and diastolic blood pressures.

Because of the heterogeneous nature of renovascular hypertension, patients were subdivided into 4 categories based on angiographic and humoral determinations:

2.1.1 Unilateral Renovascular Hypertension

This is defined as (a) angiographic evidence of unilateral involvement, and (b) having ipsilateral renal vein renin lateralisation with a ratio > 1.5.

2.1.2 Asymmetrical Bilateral Renovascular Hypertension

This is defined as (a) angiographic evidence of bilateral involvement with 1 side being more severely involved, and (b) having a lateralisation ratio > 1.5 of the split renal vein renins to the more involved side.

2.1.3 Unilateral Renovascular Disease plus Contralateral Renal Parenchymal (Small Kidney) Disease

This is defined as (a) angiographic involvement on only 1 side with a small contralateral kidney, secondary to renal parenchymal disease, and (b) having non-lateralising high split renal vein renins.

2.1.4 Symmetrical Bilateral Renovascular Disease

This is defined as (a) angiographic involvement of both sides, and (b) having non-lateralising, high split renal vein renins.

Applying the above definitions to the group successfully treated with enalapril/hydrochlorothiazide therapy, there were 8 patients with unilateral renovascular hypertension, 4 patients with asymmetrical bilateral renovascular hypertension, and 1 patient with unilateral renal artery stenosis plus contralateral renal parenchymal (small kidney) disease. In the group successfully treated with triple-drug therapy, there was 1 patient with unilateral renovascular hypertension, 2 patients with asymmetrical bilateral renovascular hypertension, 1 patient with unilateral renal artery stenosis plus contralateral renal parenchymal (small kidney) disease, and 1 patient with symmetrical bilateral renal artery stenosis and non-lateralising, high renal vein renins. Patient characteristics are presented in tables I and II. Medication doses and duration of treatment for each subgroup treated with enalapril/hydrochlorothiazide therapy or triple-drug therapy are given in tables III and IV. There were no significant changes in weight throughout the therapy periods in either group of patients.

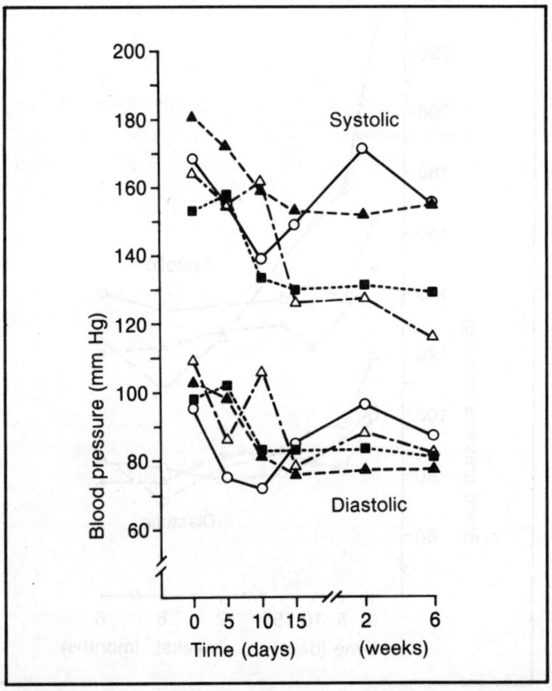

Fig. 2. Mean systolic and diastolic blood pressure response to triple-drug therapy in patients with: unilateral renovascular hypertension (○——○) n = 1; asymmetrical bilateral renovascular hypertension (▲-----▲) n = 2; unilateral renovascular hypertension plus contralateral parenchymal (small kidney) disease (△—·—△) n = 1; symmetrical bilateral renovascular hypertension (■-----■) n = 1.

2.2 Humoral Response to Therapy

Enalapril/hydrochlorothiazide therapy was associated with mean increases in plasma renin activity and mean decreases in plasma angiotensin II in maintenance periods 1 and 2 in subjects with unilateral renovascular hypertension and asymmetrical bilateral renovascular hypertension (fig. 3). However, by maintenance period 3, plasma angiotensin II inhibition was attenuated in subjects with asymmetrical bilateral renovascular hypertension. The patient with unilateral renovascular disease plus contralateral renal parenchymal (small kidney) disease receiving enalapril/hydrochlorothiazide exhibited a slight decrease in plasma renin activity, but a marked decrease in plasma angiotensin II at maintenance period 2 compared to baseline. The inhibition of plasma angiotensin II was maintained in maintenance period 3 (fig. 3).

The patient with unilateral renovascular hypertension receiving triple-drug therapy had mean decreases in plasma renin activity and plasma angiotensin II following maintenance period 2 compared to baseline (fig. 4). The 2 patients with asymmetrical bilateral renovascular hypertension receiving triple-drug therapy had mean decreases in plasma renin activity and plasma angiotensin II in maintenance period 2 compared to baseline (fig. 4). The patient with unilateral renovascular disease plus contralateral renal parenchymal (small kidney) disease receiving triple-drug therapy had a decrease in plasma renin activity, but an increase in plasma

Table I. Patient characteristics: enalapril

	Unilateral renovascular	Asymmetrical bilateral renovascular	Unilateral renovascular contralateral small kidney
Number	8	4	1
Female/male	1/7	1/3	1/0
Diagnosis	1 fibromuscular 7 atherosclerotic	1 fibromuscular 3 atherosclerotic	1 fibromuscular
Mean age (years)	55	49	39
Mean duration of hypertension (years)	6.6	6.7	8.0
Baseline blood pressure (mm Hg)	164/99	148/102	231/119
Ipsilateral renin vein ratio (range)	1.5-2.6	1.6-3.1	1.4

Table II. Patient characteristics: triple-drug therapy

	Unilateral renovascular	Asymmetrical bilateral renovascular	Unilateral renovascular contralateral small kidney	Symmetrical bilateral renovascular
Number	3	3	2	1
Female/male	1/2	1/2	2/0	0/1
Diagnosis	1 fibromuscular 2 atherosclerotic	3 atherosclerotic	2 fibromuscular	1 atherosclerotic
Mean age (years)	48	58	43	52
Mean duration of hypertension (years)	3.2	10.5	7	12
Baseline blood pressure (mm Hg)	144/98	171/102	198/114	153/98
Ipsilateral renin vein ratio (range)	1.7-2.6	1.7-2.8	1.1-1.4	1.2

Table III. Maintenance doses and duration of treatment: enalapril

	Unilateral renovascular	Asymmetrical bilateral renovascular	Unilateral renovascular contralateral small kidney
Maintenance–1			
Number	8	4	1
Mean duration (days)	26	27	36
Mean dose (mg)			
Hydrochlorothiazide	56	50	50
Enalapril	22.5	10	40
Maintenance–2			
Number	8	4	1
Mean duration (days)	53	57	64
Mean dose (mg)			
Hydrochlorothiazide	56	50	50
Enalapril	20	27.5	20
Maintenance–3			
Number	6	2	1
Mean duration (months)	7.2	6.2	8.1
Mean dose (mg)			
Hydrochlorothiazide	37.5	37.5	50
Enalapril	21.6	12.5	20

Table IV. Maintenance doses and duration of treatment: triple-drug therapy

	Unilateral renovascular	Asymmetrical bilateral renovascular	Unilateral renovascular contralateral small kidney	Symmetrical bilateral renovascular
Maintenance–1				
Number	1	2	1	1
Mean duration (days)	36	29	31	23
Mean dose (mg)				
Hydrochlorothiazide	50	50	50	50
Timolol	20	20	60	40
Hydralazine	100	100	300	200
Maintenance–2				
Number	1	2	1	1
Mean duration (days)	62	61	60	51
Mean dose (mg)				
Hydrochlorothiazide	50	50	50	50
Timolol	60	20	60	40
Hydralazine	300	100	300	200

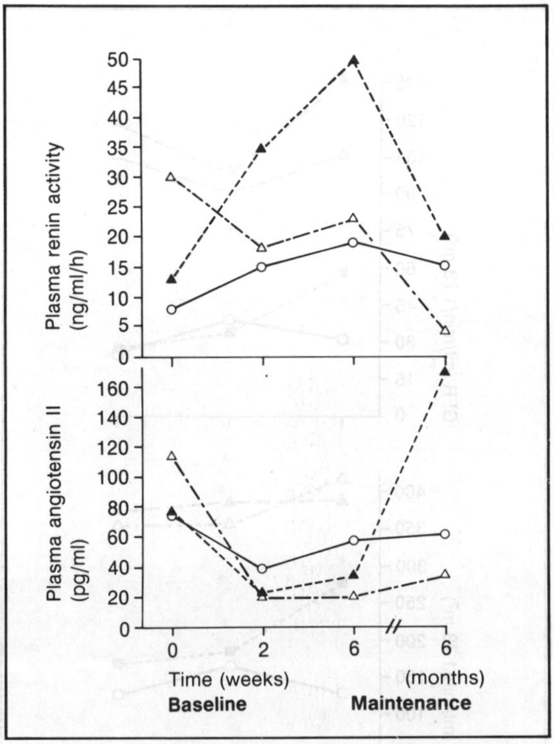

Fig. 3. Plasma renin activity and plasma angiotensin II response to enalapril/hydrochlorothiazide therapy in patients with: unilateral renovascular hypertension (○——○) n = 8, n = 6 at 6 months; asymmetrical bilateral renovascular hypertension (▲----▲) n = 4, n = 2 at 6 months; unilateral renovascular hypertension plus contralateral parenchymal (small kidney) disease (△—·—△) n = 1.

angiotensin II (fig. 4). The patient with symmetrical bilateral renovascular disease and non-lateralising, high renal vein renins receiving triple-drug therapy had an increase in plasma renin activity and plasma angiotensin II at maintenance period 2 compared to baseline (fig. 4).

2.3 Renal Function and Renal Haemodynamic Responses to Therapy

There were no significant changes in mean inulin or para-aminohippurate clearances with enalapril/hydrochlorothiazide therapy during maintenance periods 1, 2 or 3 in patients with either unilateral renovascular hypertension or asymmetrical bilateral renovascular hypertension (fig. 5). The patient with unilateral renovascular disease plus contralateral renal parenchymal (small kidney) disease receiving enalapril/hydrochlorothiazide had a 50% reduction in inulin clearance and a 30% reduction in para-aminohippurate clearance at the end of maintenance period 1 (fig. 5). This deterioration in renal function was sustained at maintenance periods 2 and 3.

The patient with unilateral renovascular hypertension receiving triple-drug therapy had a mild decrease in inulin clearance and essentially no change in para-aminohippurate clearance at main-

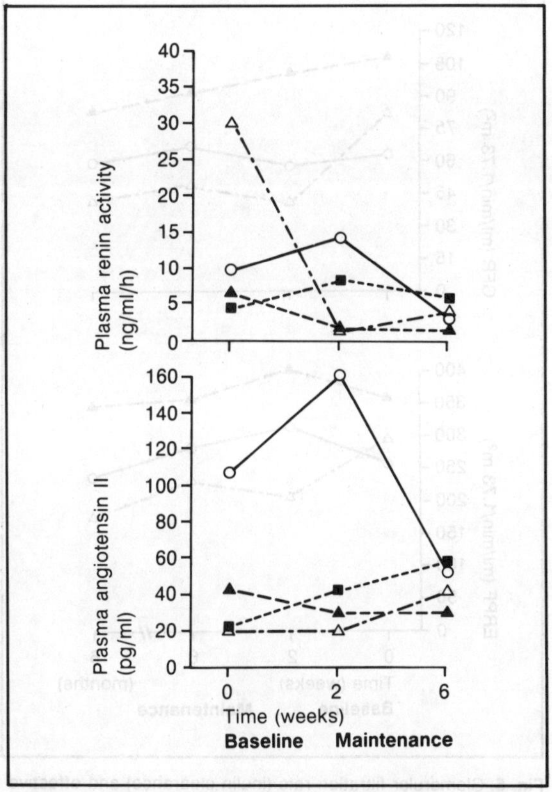

Fig. 4. Plasma renin activity and plasma angiotensin II response to triple-drug therapy in patients with: unilateral renovascular hypertension (○——○) n = 1; asymmetrical bilateral renovascular hypertension (▲----▲) n = 2; unilateral renovascular hypertension plus contralateral parenchymal (small kidney) disease (△—·—△) n = 1; symmetrical bilateral renovascular hypertension (■----■) n = 1.

tenance period 2 compared to baseline (fig. 6). The 2 patients with asymmetrical bilateral renovascular hypertension receiving triple-drug therapy had either a decrease or no change in both inulin clearance and para-aminohippurate clearance at maintenance period 2 compared to baseline (fig. 6). The patient with unilateral renovascular disease plus contralateral renal parenchymal (small kidney) disease receiving triple-drug therapy had no change in inulin clearance and a decrease in the para-aminohippurate clearance at maintenance period 2 compared to baseline (fig. 6). The patient with symmetrical bilateral renovascular disease and nonlateralising, elevated renal vein renin receiving triple-drug therapy, had marked decreases in inulin and para-aminohippurate clearances at maintenance period 2 compared to baseline (fig. 6).

Neither enalapril/hydrochlorothiazide combination therapy nor triple-drug therapy altered the 24-hour urine protein excretion in any subgroup (tables V and VI).

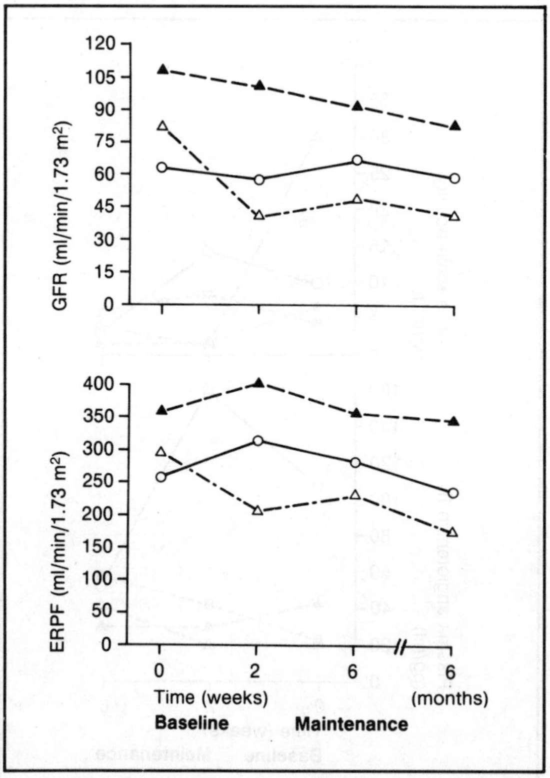

Fig. 5. Glomerular filtration rate (inulin clearance) and effective renal plasma flow (para-aminohippurate clearance) response to enalapril/hydrochlorothiazide therapy in patients with: unilateral renovascular hypertension (○——○) n = 8; n = 6 at 6 months; asymmetrical bilateral renovascular hypertension (▲-----▲) n = 4, n = 2 at 6 months; unilateral renovascular hypertension plus contralateral parenchymal (small kidney) disease (△—·—△) n = 1.

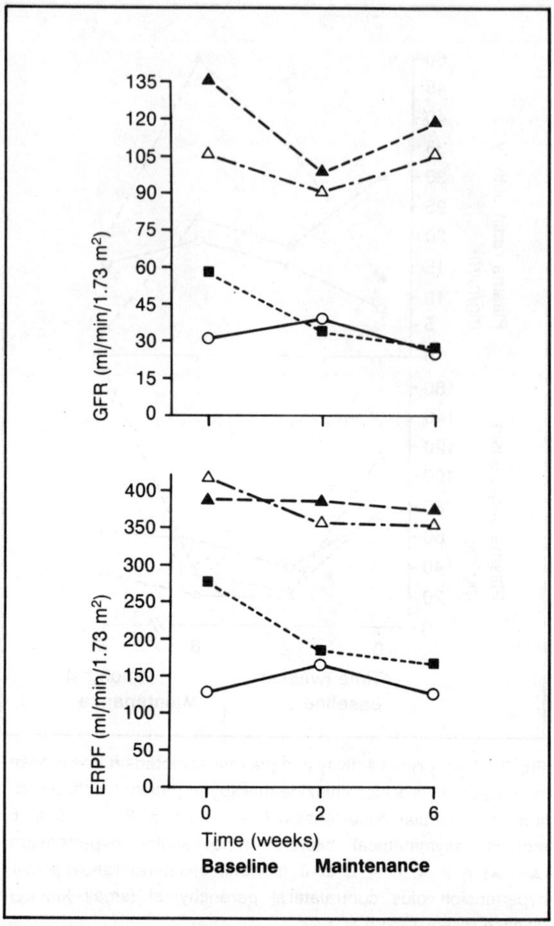

Fig. 6. Glomerular filtration rate (inulin clearance) and effective renal plasma flow (para-aminohippurate clearance) response to triple-drug therapy in patients with: unilateral renovascular hypertension (○——○) n = 1; asymmetrical bilateral renovascular hypertension (▲-----▲) n = 2; unilateral renovascular hypertension plus contralateral parenchymal (small kidney) disease (△—·—△) n = 1; symmetrical bilateral renovascular hypertension (■----■) n = 1.

Table V. Effects of enalapril on 24-hour urinary protein excretion*

	n	Baseline	Maintenance–1	Maintenance–2	Maintenance–3
Unilateral renovascular	8	0.22	0.13	0.12	0.13 (n = 6)
Asymmetrical bilateral renovascular	4	0.10	0.12	0.05	0.31 (n = 2)
Unilateral renovascular contralateral small kidney	1	0.20	0.63	0.08	0.04

* Mean (g protein/g creatinine).

Table VI. Effects of triple-drug therapy on 24-hour urinary protein excretion*

	n	Baseline	Maintenance–1	Maintenance–2
Unilateral renovascular	1	0.03	0.03	0.17
Asymmetrical bilateral renovascular	2	0.03	0.07	0.00
Unilateral renovascular contralateral small kidney	1	0.04	0.05	0.00
Symmetrical bilateral renovascular	1	0.14	0.15	0.08

* Mean (g protein/g creatinine).

3. Discussion

Our results demonstrate that the combined therapy of enalapril (dosages ranging from 10 to 40mg) and hydrochlorothiazide (50mg) was an effective antihypertensive regimen for the treatment of renovascular hypertension. Indeed, all patients randomised to enalapril/hydrochlorothiazide therapy had good blood pressure control (supine diastolic blood pressure < 90mm Hg) throughout 6 months of therapy. Triple-drug therapy (hydrochlorothiazide, timolol and hydralazine) was less effective in controlling blood pressure; only 5 of the 9 patients originally randomised to triple-drug therapy had reductions in supine diastolic blood pressure to < 90mm Hg at weeks 2 and 6 of maintenance therapy. The remaining 4 patients did not complete the treatment protocol due either to the development of significant side effects (2 patients), or the lack of blood pressure control (2 patients). One of the 5 patients who achieved blood pressure control on triple-drug therapy developed uncontrolled blood pressure (supine diastolic blood pressure > 95mm Hg) 2 months following completion of maintenance period 2. Four of the above 5 patients were subsequently crossed over from triple-drug therapy to enalapril/hydrochlorothiazide therapy and achieved good blood pressure control without side effects; the fifth patient declined further investigational study.

Enalapril/hydrochlorothiazide therapy was associated with increases in plasma renin activity and decreases in plasma angiotensin II, indicating drug adherence. Triple-drug therapy resulted in variable responses of plasma renin activity and plasma angiotensin II, probably reflecting the combination of renin-inhibiting β-adrenergic blockade and the renin stimulating effects of diuretic-induced volume contraction and hydralazine-induced vasodilatation.

Enalapril/hydrochlorothiazide therapy was not associated with reductions in inulin clearance (a sensitive marker of glomerular filtration rate), or para-aminohippurate clearance (a sensitive marker of effective renal plasma flow), in renovascular hypertensive patients with unilateral or bilateral (but asymmetrical) disease. Reduction in renal function has been reported in patients with bilateral renovascular hypertension following ACE inhibitor therapy (Aldigier et al., 1982; Bender et al., 1984; Chrysant et al., 1983; Fotino and Sporn, 1983; Grossman et al., 1980; Hricik et al., 1983; Textor et al., 1984). However, those patients, unlike our group of asymmetrical bilateral renovascular hypertensive patients, had either severely decreased renal function prior to treatment, or extensive renovascular involvement with occluded renal arteries or functional dependence on a unilateral stenotic kidney. Our group of bilateral renovascular hypertensive patients had relatively preserved renal function, and their disease was asymmetrical, with one side more severely involved, as demonstrated by both angiography and lateralisation of the renal vein renin activity. Renal function in these patients was not dependent on blood flow to the most severely involved kidney. In contrast, the patient receiving enalapril/hydrochlorothiazide therapy and who had unilateral renovascular disease plus a small contracted contralateral kidney (hence, a functional solitary stenotic kidney) demonstrated a marked reduction in inulin clearance and para-aminohippurate clearance. In this patient the deterioration in renal function may have been related to angiotensin II inhibition with loss of autoregulatory control of renal perfusion (Bender et al., 1984; Blythe, 1983) and may be a predictable complication of this generic class of antihypertensive drugs in patients with functionally solitary stenotic kidneys.

Four of the 5 patients completing 6 weeks of triple-drug therapy had a mean decrease in inulin clearance and either no change (2 patients) or a decrease (3 patients) in para-aminohippurate clearance. Conventional therapy for renovascular hypertension, employing a diuretic, β-blocker and vasodilator is not without apparent risk to glomerular filtration rate and renal blood flow. Changes in renal function following triple-drug therapy cannot be attributed to inhibition of angiotensin II, and its consequent effect on renal haemodynamics; most likely, the decrease is related to reduced renal perfusion pressure.

Renovascular hypertension is clearly a heterogeneous disease, having a varying effect on the extent of renovascular involvement (in degree of stenosis and number of renal arteries involved) and on the extent of renal ischaemia. Only when there is pre-existing, severe compromise in renal function and where the primary functional dependence resides within the stenotic kidney, is the patient's overall renal function at risk from ACE inhibitor therapy.

It can be concluded that enalapril/hydrochlorothiazide therapy is an effective antihypertensive regimen in renovascular hypertension. None of the patients studied experienced intolerance to this combination. Renal function deteriorated only in the patient with a functional unilateral stenotic kidney. Although triple-drug therapy employing hydrochlorothiazide, timolol and hydralazine was an effective antihypertensive regimen for some patients, there was a high incidence of treatment withdrawal due to either poorly controlled blood pressure or intolerable side effects. Triple-drug therapy was not without risk; 4 out of 5 patients treated had a decrease in glomerular filtration rate after 6 weeks of therapy. If the long term safety of enalapril is confirmed, it may become an important mode of therapy for the treatment of renovascular hypertension.

Acknowledgements

We wish to thank Rebecca DeCourley, Denise Redding and Judy Todd for their assistance in preparation of this manuscript. We would also like to thank Pat Gaddy, Alisa Lau, Karla Wilson and Ann Hamory for their nursing support.

References

Aldigier, J.; Plorin, P.; Guyene, T.; Thibonnier, M.; Corvol, P. and Ménard, J.: Comparison of the hormonal and renal effects of captopril in severe essential and renovascular hypertension. American Journal of Cardiology 49: 1447-1452 (1982).

Alpert, M.A. and Bauer, J.H.: Rapid control of severe hypertension with minoxidil. Archives of Internal Medicine 142: 2099-2014 (1982).

Bauer, J.H. and Jones, L.B.: Comparative studies: Enalapril versus hydrochlorothiazide as first-step therapy for the treatment of primary hypertension. American Journal of Kidney Diseases 4: 55-62 (1984).

Bender, W.; LaFrance, N. and Walker, W.G.: Mechanism of deterioration in renal function in patients with renovascular hypertension treated with enalapril. Hypertension 6 (Suppl. 1): I193-I197 (1984).

Blythe, W.B.: Captopril and renal autoregulation. New England Journal of Medicine 308: 390-391 (1983).

Brooks, C.S. and Bauer, J.H.: Treatment of refractory hypertension with minoxidil. Cardiac Medicine (4) 6: 683-690 (1979).

Chrysant, S.G.; Dunn, M.; Marples, D. and DeMasters, K.: Severe reversible azotemia from captopril therapy. Archives of Internal Medicine 143: 437-441 (1983).

Collste, P.; Haglund, K.; Lundgren, G.; Magnusson, G. and Ostman, J.: Reversible renal failure during treatment with captopril. British Medical Journal 2: 612-613 (1979).

Curtis, J.J.; Luke, R.G.; Whelchel, J.D.; Diethelm, A.G.; Jones, P. and Dustan, H.P.: Inhibition of angiotensin-converting enzyme in renal-transplant recipients with hypertension. New England Journal of Medicine 308: 377-381 (1983).

Edwards, R.M.: Response of isolated renal microvessels to intraluminal pressure, norepinephrine and angiotensin II. (Abstract.) American Society of Nephrology 150A (1982).

Farrow, P.R. and Wilkinson, R.: Reversible renal failure during treatment with captopril. British Medical Journal 1: 1680 (1979).

Felts, J.H. and Charler, J.: Minoxidil in refractory hypertension. Journal of Cardiovascular Pharmacology 2 (Suppl. 2): S114-S122 (1980).

Fotino, S. and Sporn, P.: Nonoliguric acute renal failure after captopril therapy. Archives of Internal Medicine 143: 1252-1253 (1983).

Grossman, A.; Eckland, D.; Price, P. and Edwards, C.R.W.: Captopril: Reversible renal failure with severe hyperkalaemia. Lancet 1: 712 (1980).

Hall, J.E.; Guyton, A.C.; Jackson, T.E.; Coleman, T.G.; Lohmeier, T.E. and Trippodo, N.C.: Control of glomerular filtration rate by renin-angiotensin system. American Journal of Physiology 233: F366-F372 (1977).

Helmchen, U.; Gröne, H.J.; Kirchertz, E.J.; Bader, H.; Bohle, R.M.; Kneissler, U. and Khosla, M.C.: Contrasting renal effects of different antihypertensive agents in hypertensive rats with bilaterally constricted renal arteries. Kidney International 22 (Suppl. 12): S198-S205 (1982).

Hricik, D.E.; Browning, P.J.; Kopelman, R.; Goorno, W.E.; Madias, N.E. and Dzau, V.J.: Captopril-induced functional renal insufficiency in patients with bilateral renal-artery stenoses or renal-artery stenosis in a solitary kidney. New England Journal of Medicine 308: 373-376 (1983).

Kawamura, J.; Okada, Y.; Nishibuchi, S. and Yoshida, O.: Transient anuria following administration of angiotensin II converting enzyme inhibitor (SQ14225) in a patient with renal artery stenosis of the solitary kidney successfully treated with renal auto-transplantation. Journal of Urology 127 (1): 111-113 (1982).

Larochelle, P.; Beronrade, V.; Hamet, P. and Kuchel, O.: Treatment of refractory hypertension with minoxidil. Journal of Cardiovascular Pharmacology 2 (Suppl. 2): S107-S113 (1980).

Mason, J.C. and Hilton, P.J.: Repeated renal failure with use of captopril in a stenotic renal allograft recipient. British Medical Journal 286: 145-146 (1983).

Textor, S.C.; Tarazi, R.C.; Novick, A.C.; Bravo, E.L. and Fouad, F.M.: Regulation of renal hemodynamics and glomerular filtration in patients with renovascular hypertension during converting enzyme inhibition with captopril. American Journal of Medicine 76: 29-37 (1984).

Address for correspondence and reprints: Dr *Garry P. Reams*, Department of Medicine, Division of Nephrology (Rm. M-472), University of Missouri School of Medicine, Columbia, Missouri 65212 (USA).

Drugs 30 (Suppl. 1): 70-73 (1985)
0012-6667/85/0100-0070/$2.00/0

Enalapril Maleate *versus* Captopril
A Comparison of the Hormonal and Antihypertensive Effects

Carlos R. Ayers, Kenneth M. Baker, Barbara A. Weaver and *Marcia R. Lehman*

University of Virginia Medical Center, Charlottesville, and Geisinger Medical Center, Danville

Summary *24 hypertensive patients were randomised into 2 groups to compare the antihypertensive effects of enalapril and captopril over a 10-week period. In the hydrochlorothiazide run-in period, blood pressure was reduced from 171 ± 4/109 ± 1mm Hg to 160 ± 4/103 ± 1mm Hg (p < 0.05). Angiotensin-converting enzyme (ACE) inhibition decreased blood pressure to 132 ± 3/87 ± 2mm Hg. Captopril decreased diastolic blood pressure significantly more after 3 hours than enalapril (−24 versus −17mm Hg, p < 0.05). After 10 weeks of therapy, this antihypertensive response was maintained at 134 ± 3/83 ± 1mm Hg. There was no difference between the captopril and enalapril treated groups. Acute and chronic responses of plasma renin activity, plasma aldosterone and ACE were determined. There was an acute positive correlation between the rise in plasma renin activity and the fall in blood pressures with captopril but not with enalapril. With chronic treatment there was no difference in the ability of either of the 2 drugs to reduce blood pressure, inhibit ACE, reduce aldosterone or stimulate plasma renin activity.*

In 1973 it was shown that teprotide, a parenteral angiotensin-converting enzyme (ACE) inhibitor, was effective in lowering blood pressure (Gavras et al., 1974). Since then, 2 oral ACE inhibitors have been developed – enalapril maleate and captopril. Both these drugs have been found to be effective in reducing blood pressure in several animal species (Bengis et al., 1978; Harris et al., 1978; Muirhead et al., 1978; Murthy et al., 1977, 1978; Vollmer and Boccagno, 1977) as well as in man (Bravo and Tarazi, 1979; Brunner et al., 1979; Case et al., 1978; Gavras et al., 1978; Johns et al., 1980). Captopril has been associated with several side effects such as rash, taste disturbance, leucopenia and proteinuria. These side effects are thought to be due to the presence of the sulphydryl group in the compound. Many efforts have been made to develop an orally effective ACE inhibitor without the sulphydryl group. Enalapril maleate is such a drug, and is the major focus of this report.

The study was carried out on 24 patients who were randomised and assigned to receive either enalapril or captopril. The antihypertensive effects of both drugs were compared, together with their ability to increase plasma renin activity, to decrease plasma aldosterone and to decrease ACE.

1. Methods

1.1 Patients

24 patients with essential hypertension were randomised to receive either enalapril or captopril therapy. There were 18 men and 6 women, aged 35-62 years. Average duration of hypertension was 10.6 years (1.2-25 years) and mean arterial pressure was 114-145mm Hg.

1.2 Experimental Design

All patients signed a consent form approved by the Institutional Review Board prior to entry into the study. All antihypertensive medications were withdrawn, and sympatholytic drugs were appropriately tapered over 3 weeks prior to randomisation and treatment. Patients continued on their customary diet unless the sodium content was judged to be unusually high. A 24-hour urine collection was obtained to measure sodium and potassium excretion rates. Blood samples were obtained in the upright position to determine plasma renin activity, plasma aldosterone concentration and ACE activity. The samples were stored at −20°C until assayed, except for ACE which was stored under liquid nitrogen.

The subjects were then started on 50 mg/day hydrochlorothiazide. After 4 weeks, 24-hour urine and 3-hour upright plasma samples were collected for measurement of sodium and potassium excretion rates and plasma renin activity, plasma aldosterone concentration and ACE activity. Double-blind randomisation was then carried out. A single dose of captopril (25mg) or enalapril (5mg) was then given, and blood samples for plasma renin activity, plasma aldosterone concentration and ACE activity were obtained after 3 hours in the upright position. Patients were treated for 10 weeks on hydrochlorothiazide (50mg) plus either captopril or enalapril. The maximum dose of captopril was 100mg thrice-daily and for enalapril 20mg twice-daily. After 10 weeks of ACE inhibition, blood pressure, sodium and potassium excretions, plasma renin activity, plasma aldosterone concentration and ACE activity were re-evaluated.

Plasma renin activity was determined by measuring angiotensin I generated at 37°C and pH 5.7 according to the method of Sealey et al. (1972). Plasma aldosterone concentration was measured using the radioimmunoassay of Kubasik et al. (1979). ACE activity was determined by the radioassay of Rohatgi and Ryan (1980). Urine sodium and potassium were determined by flame photometry.

2. Statistical Analysis

Student's paired and unpaired t-test, or a one-way analysis of variance was used, and a p value of less than 0.05 was considered statistically significant. Data are expressed as the mean ± 1 standard error of the mean.

3. Results

3.1 Blood Pressure

13 patients were randomised to receive captopril and 11 to receive enalapril therapy.

There was a significant ($p < 0.05$) decrease in diastolic blood pressure in both groups 4 weeks after hydrochlorothiazide therapy. Three hours after acute administration of the ACE inhibitors, there was a significantly greater decrease in diastolic blood pressure with captopril when compared with enalapril (−24 versus −17mm Hg, $p < 0.05$). After 10 weeks of ACE inhibition, the decrease in diastolic blood pressure was the same with the 2 drugs (−26 and −25mm Hg, respectively).

Plasma renin activity increased from a control level of 3.0 ± 0.8 to 10.1 ± 3.0ng angiotensin I/ml/hour ($p < 0.05$) after 4 weeks of hydrochlorothiazide therapy. After 3 hours of captopril and enalapril therapy, plasma renin activity increased to 33 ± 3.8 ($p < 0.05$) and 37 ± 3.9ng angiotensin I/ml/hour ($p < 0.05$), respectively. There was a further increase in plasma renin activity after 10 weeks of ACE inhibition – 53 ± 11ng angiotensin I/ml/hour for captopril and 72 ± 15ng angiotensin I/ml/hour for enalapril. The increase from their 3-hour level was significant for both drugs ($p < 0.05$).

ACE activity was normal (96 ± 4 units) and

did not change with 4 weeks of hydrochlorothiazide treatment. The ACE activity decreased to 0 units at 3 hours with both ACE inhibitors and the inhibition was maintained during the 10 weeks of treatment.

Control aldosterone level was 26 ± 5.4 ng/dl in the captopril group and was 29 ± 5.1 ng/dl (not significant) after 4 weeks of hydrochlorothiazide treatment. The enalapril control aldosterone level was 17 ± 5.1 ng/dl and increased to 29 ± 5.1 ng/dl ($p < 0.05$) after 4 weeks of hydrochlorothiazide treatment. After 3 hours of ACE inhibition, aldosterone concentration decreased to 10 ± 2 ng/dl in both groups ($p < 0.05$). After 10 weeks of treatment, plasma aldosterone concentration was 15 ± 6.8 and 17 ± 2 ng/dl for the captopril and enalapril groups. This was not significantly different from the 3-hour plasma aldosterone concentration, but was less ($p < 0.05$) than the plasma aldosterone concentration prior to ACE inhibition.

4. Discussion

Teprotide (SQ 20881) was the first ACE inhibitor that was demonstrated to be antihypertensive. In 1977 the first oral ACE inhibitor, captopril, was synthesised. Captopril was shown to be efficacious in treating renovascular, essential and renal hypertension, as well as hypertension due to scleroderma. In addition, it reduced afterload in congestive heart failure.

Captopril has been shown to have a low incidence of toxicity when used in low effective doses in hypertensive patients (Veterans Administration Cooperative Study Group, 1982). There are groups of patients known to be at a higher risk from captopril side effects. These are patients with renal dysfunction, collagen vascular disorders and patients with immunological diseases. The side effects that have been described are rash, proteinuria, leucopenia, taste disturbance and mouth ulcers. Enalapril is a member of a new class of ACE inhibitors which do not contain a sulphydryl group.

The 2 drugs compared in this study, captopril and enalapril, are equally effective in the long term control of blood pressure, in inhibiting ACE, in decreasing plasma aldosterone levels and in stimulating renin release. The initial (3 hour) decrease in blood pressure with captopril compared to enalapril is probably explained by the delay in converting enalapril in the body to its active diacid form.

References

Bengis, R.G.; Coleman, T.G.; Young, D.B. and McCaa, R.E.: Long-term blockade of angiotensin formation in various normotensive and hypertensive rat models using converting enzyme inhibitor (SQ 14,225). Circulation Research 43 (Suppl. 1): I45-I53 (1978).

Bravo, E.L. and Tarazi, R.C.: Converting enzyme inhibition with an orally active compound in hypertensive man. Hypertension 1: 39-46 (1979).

Brunner, H.R.; Gavras, H.; Baeber, B.; Kershaw, G.R.; Turini, G.A.; Vukovich, R.A.; McKinstry, D.N. and Gavras, I.: Oral angiotensin-converting enzyme inhibitor in long-term treatment of hypertensive patients. Annals of Internal Medicine 90: 19-23 (1979).

Case, D.B.; Atlas, S.A.; Laragh, J.H.; Sealey, J.E.; Sullivan, P.A. and McKinstry, D.N.: Clinical experience with blockadc of the renin-angiotensin-aldosterone system by an oral converting enzyme inhibitor (SQ 14,225, captopril) in hypertensive patients. Progress in Cardiovascular Diseases 21: 195-206 (1978).

Gavras, H.; Brunner, H.R.; Laragh, J.H.; Sealey, J.E.; Gavras, I. and Vukovich, R.A.: An angiotensin converting enzyme inhibitor to identify and treat vasoconstriction and volume factors in hypertensive patients. New England Journal of Medicine 291: 817-821 (1974).

Gavras, H.; Brunner, H.R.; Turini, G.A.; Kershaw, G.R.; Tefft, C.P.; Cuttelod, S.; Gavras, I.; Vukovich, R.A. and McKinstry, D.N.: Antihypertensive effect of the oral angiotensin converting enzyme inhibitor SQ 14,225 in man. New England Journal of Medicine 298: 991-995 (1978).

Harris, D.N.; Heran, C.L.; Goldenberg, H.J.; High, J.P.; Laffow, R.J.; Rubin, B.; Antonaccio, M.J. and Goldberg, M.E.: Effects of SQ 14,225, an orally active inhibitor of angiotensin-converting enzyme on blood pressure, heart rate and plasma renin activity of conscious normotensive dogs. European Journal of Pharmacology 51: 345-349 (1978).

Johns, D.W.; Baker, K.M.; Ayers, C.R.; Vaughan, E.D. Jr; Carey, R.M.; Peach, M.J.; Yancey, M.R.; Ortt, E.M. and Williams, S.C.: Acute and chronic effect of captopril in hypertensive patients. Hypertension 2: 567-575 (1980).

Kubasik, N.P.; Warren, K. and Sine, H.E.: Evaluation of a new commercial radioassay kit for aldosterone using an iodinated tracer. Clinical Biochemistry 12: 59-61 (1979).

Muirhead, E.E.; Prewitt, R.L.; Brooks, B. and Brosius, W.L. Jr: Antihypertensive action of the orally active converting enzyme inhibitor (SQ 14,225) in spontaneously hypertensive rats. Circulation Research 43 (Suppl. 1): I53-I59 (1978).

Murthy, V.S.; Waldron, T.L.; Goldberg, M.E. and Vollmer, R.R.: Inhibition of angiotensin converting enzyme by SQ 14,225 in conscious rabbits. European Journal of Pharmacology 46: 207-212 (1977).

Murthy, V.S.; Waldron, T.L. and Goldberg, M.E.: The mechanism of bradykinin potentiation after inhibition of angiotensin-converting enzyme by SQ 14,225 in conscious rabbits. Circulation Research 43 (Suppl. 1): I40-I45 (1978).

Rohatgi, P.K. and Ryan, J.W.: Simple radioassay for measuring serum activity of angiotensin-converting enzyme in sarcoidosis. Chest 78: 69-76 (1980).
Sealey, J.E.; Gerten-Banes, J. and Laragh, J.H.: The renin system: Variations in man measured by radioimmunoassay or bioassay. Kidney International 1: 240-253 (1972).
Veterans Administration Cooperative Study Group on Antihypertensive Agents: Captopril: Evaluation of low doses, twice-daily doses and the addition of diuretic for the treatment of mild to moderate hypertension. Clinical Science 63: 443S-445S (1982).
Vollmer, R.R. and Boccagno, J.A.: Central cardiovascular effects of SQ 14,225, an angiotensin-converting enzyme inhibitor in chloralose-anesthetized cats. European Journal of Pharmacology 45: 117-125 (1977).

Address for correspondence and reprints: Dr *Carlos R. Ayers,* Box 146, University of Virginia Medical Center, Charlottesville, VA 22908 (USA).

Drugs 30 (Suppl. 1): 74-81 (1985)
0012-6667/85/0100-0074/$4.00/0

Effects of Enalapril on Clinical Status, Biochemistry, Exercise Performance and Haemodynamics in Heart Failure

M.W.I. Webster, M.A. Fitzpatrick, E.J. Hamilton, M.G. Nicholls, H. Ikram, E.A. Espiner and *J.E. Wells*

Departments of Cardiology and Endocrinology, The Princess Margaret Hospital and Department of Community Health, Christchurch Hospital, Christchurch

Summary

The effects of enalapril on clinical well-being, treadmill exercise performance, haemodynamic measurements, hormone levels, and plasma biochemistry in patients with moderate heart failure, were assessed in a 12-week placebo-controlled, double-blind study. Maintenance frusemide and digoxin treatment was continued throughout the study. Compared with placebo, enalapril treatment improved clinical status and increased exercise capacity. The most obvious haemodynamic change was a fall in pulmonary artery wedge pressure and pulmonary artery pressure. Enalapril-induced increases in left-ventricular ejection fraction and cardiac index, and falls in systemic arterial pressure, were small. Of the hormone indices measured, plasma renin activity rose 4-fold, angiotensin II and aldosterone fell slightly, and plasma catecholamines were unaltered by enalapril. Plasma potassium increased on average by 0.3 mmol/L during enalapril therapy. No adverse clinical or biochemical effects were observed. Enalapril has a sustained beneficial action in patients with moderate heart failure.

Cardiac failure is a common disorder in western society (Gibson et al., 1966; McKee et al., 1971). Its prevalence is likely to rise as longevity increases in the population at large and with the decline in mortality from ischaemic heart disease (Stern, 1979). The angiotensin-converting enzyme (ACE) inhibitors are now established in the treatment of severe cardiac failure. They have predictable effects on plasma hormone levels (Dzau et al., 1980; Maslowski et al., 1981) which translate into beneficial haemodynamic changes in the short term (Fitzpatrick et al., 1983; Maslowski et al., 1981; Wenting et al., 1983). More important, careful studies have demonstrated sustained clinical improvement during long term treatment with captopril (Captopril Multicenter Research Group 1983; Cowley et al., 1982; Kramer et al., 1983). Many questions, however, remain to be answered. For example, do ACE inhibitors other than captopril provide sustained beneficial effects? Is well-being, measured objectively, improved by these drugs? There are conflicting reports on plasma catecholamine responses to short term therapy with ACE inhibitors, and long term changes are unclear. These and other questions are addressed in the current 12-week study of enalapril in cardiac failure. A preliminary report of some aspects from this study was presented by Nicholls et al. (1984).

1. Methods

We studied 20 patients aged 37 to 74 years, 17 males and 3 females, with chronic congestive heart failure (NYHA functional class II or III). All were stable clinically, free of peripheral oedema, and taking frusemide (80 to 750 mg/day) and digoxin (0.125 to 0.375 mg/day), apart from 1 patient who was not on digoxin. 14 patients had myocardial ischaemia and 6 had idiopathic cardiomyopathy as the basis for heart failure. The study protocol was approved by the Hospital's Ethical Committee, and informed consent was obtained from each patient.

At the time of randomisation the patients were admitted to hospital for biochemical and invasive haemodynamic measurements. Venous blood was drawn at approximately 9a.m. for the measurement of routine biochemical indices (SMAC II autoanalyser). At 8a.m. the next day they underwent catheterisation of a brachial artery for pressure recording, and the pulmonary artery (triple lumen Swan-Ganz catheter) for pressure and cardiac output measurements. Digoxin and frusemide were withheld until completion of the haemodynamic recordings. Two hours after catheter insertion, baseline haemodynamic measurements were taken at rest, and again after 3 min of supine bicycle exercise (at 70% of their previously-determined maximum workload). The first dose of placebo or enalapril (5mg) was then taken, and repeat haemodynamic recordings were made 2 hours (resting) and 5 hours later (resting, and after 3 min of supine bicycle exercise). Pressure measurements used transducers maintained at the level of the mid-axillary line and a Mennen Response 10 monitor with Yokogawa E.W. Photorecorder. Upon completion of these baseline recordings the patients continued their maintenance treatment of frusemide and digoxin and either enalapril 5mg twice-daily, or a matching placebo in a double-blind fashion, for 12 weeks.

They were then seen at regular intervals as outpatients. At 12 weeks, the biochemistry and invasive haemodynamic recordings were repeated, as described above.

Before randomisation and again after 4 and 12 weeks of placebo or enalapril treatment, the patients underwent measurement of resting left ventricular ejection fraction using technetium-99_m-labelled red cells and a Nuclear Stethoscope (Bios Inc.) [Wagner et al., 1976]. Also on these 3 occasions they undertook a symptom-limited treadmill exercise test (Patterson et al., 1972). Blood samples were drawn from an indwelling venous cannula (inserted at least 30 min before the treadmill test) just before exercise with the patient sitting, after 6 min of treadmill exercise, immediately upon completion of exercise, and finally 15 and 60 min after exercise while resting, again in the sitting position. The blood was placed in containers on ice, centrifuged at +4°C, and the plasma stored at −20 or −80°C, for measurements of plasma renin activity (Dunn and Espiner, 1976), angiotensin II (Nicholls and Espiner, 1976), aldosterone (Lun et al., 1983), noradrenaline and adrenaline (Peuler and Johnson, 1977), and cortisol (by means of radioimmunoassay using kits from Diagnostic Products, Los Angeles). All samples from each patient were run in the same assay. Interassay variability (coefficient of variation) was between 7% (for cortisol) and 17% (for angiotensin II). An assessment of clinical status with particular reference to dyspnoea, fatigue and chest pain was made at the beginning and end of the trial using an objective scoring system based on that of Feinstein and Wells (1975).

Statistical tests used were the Wilcoxon matched-pairs signed-rank test, a t-test for within-group comparisons, and the Mann-Whitney U-test for assessing between-group changes. Results are expressed as mean ± SEM.

2. Results

One patient receiving placebo was withdrawn from the trial after 3 weeks because of worsening cardiac failure. Two others, 1 on placebo and 1 on enalapril, died suddenly between the 4- and 12-week recording times. The dose of digoxin was stable throughout but frusemide was increased because of worsening heart failure in 2 patients on placebo and in 1 patient on enalapril.

2.1 Bodyweight

Bodyweight in placebo patients was initially 84.4 ± 6.7kg, and was unchanged after 4 weeks (84.0 ± 6.6kg) and 12 weeks (84.3 ± 6.9kg). In contrast, bodyweight fell in enalapril patients from a baseline of 66.5 ± 3.5kg to 64.2 ± 3.5kg after 12 weeks of treatment ($p < 0.05$).

2.2 Routine Biochemistry

Mean plasma potassium concentration increased by 0.3 mmol/L over 12 weeks in enalapril-treated patients ($p < 0.05$, table I). Changes in plasma sodium, urea, creatinine, glucose, γGT, bilirubin, uric acid and cholesterol concentrations were minor in both groups (table I) and generally failed to reach levels of statistical significance.

2.3 Clinical Status

No pattern of change was observed in placebo patients whereas every subject taking enalapril recorded clinical improvement over 12 weeks as scored on the 'Yale Scale' ($p < 0.05$, fig. 1).

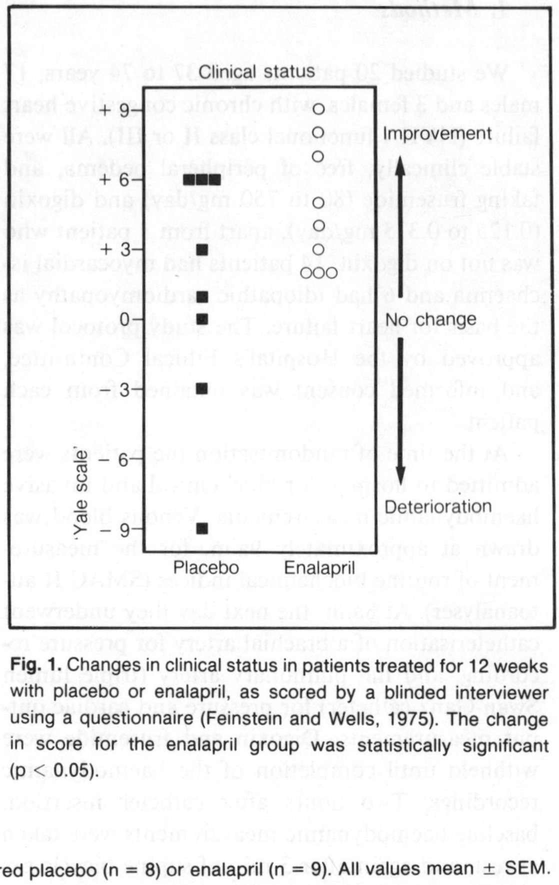

Fig. 1. Changes in clinical status in patients treated for 12 weeks with placebo or enalapril, as scored by a blinded interviewer using a questionnaire (Feinstein and Wells, 1975). The change in score for the enalapril group was statistically significant ($p < 0.05$).

Table I. Plasma biochemistry in patients with heart failure administered placebo (n = 8) or enalapril (n = 9). All values mean ± SEM. * = $p < 0.05$, compared to week 0

	Normal range in plasma	Placebo			Enalapril		
		week 0	week 4	week 12	week 0	week 4	week 12
Sodium	(136-146 mmol/L)	138.0 ± 0.9	139.9 ± 0.5*	137.6 ± 0.6	138.0 ± 0.7	137.9 ± 0.5	137.6 ± 0.6
Potassium	(3.5-5 mmol/L)	4.00 ± 0.13	3.80 ± 0.12	3.81 ± 0.10	3.58 ± 0.10	3.70 ± 0.09	3.94 ± 0.10*
Urea	(2.7-7.8 mmol/L)	7.8 ± 0.6	8.4 ± 0.6	7.8 ± 0.4	7.2 ± 0.5	7.9 ± 0.7	8.0 ± 0.9
Creatinine	(0.05-0.11 mmol/L)	0.101 ± 0.005	0.105 ± 0.004	0.103 ± 0.006	0.112 ± 0.008	0.116 ± 0.018	0.127 ± 0.016
Glucose	(3.5-8 mmol/L)	5.9 ± 0.3	5.4 ± 0.3	5.9 ± 0.3	6.1 ± 0.4	6.9 ± 0.7	6.6 ± 0.9
γGT	(<50 iu/L)	60 ± 13	47 ± 12	53 ± 10	44 ± 9	45 ± 13	56 ± 16
Bilirubin	(3-21 μmol/L)	14.1 ± 1.3	12.1 ± 1.6	14.0 ± 2.6	12.7 ± 2.4	9.4 ± 2.2	11.2 ± 2.6
Uric acid	0.15-0.48 mmol/L)	0.60 ± 0.04	0.62 ± 0.04	0.59 ± 0.04	0.50 ± 0.03	0.52 ± 0.05	0.50 ± 0.04
Cholesterol	(age dependent, mmol/L)	5.4 ± 0.6	—	5.5 ± 0.4	6.3 ± 0.6	—	6.8 ± 0.6

Left ventricular ejection fractions, measured by the Nuclear Stethoscope while the patients rested, showed little change in the placebo group (23.4 ± 4.7% at baseline; 26.0 ± 3.9% at 12 weeks). Those taking enalapril increased their ejection fraction from 22.1 ± 3.9% to 25.9 ± 3.3% at 4 weeks (not significant) and 29.5 ± 3.4% at 12 weeks ($p < 0.05$).

2.4 Treadmill Exercise Testing

Placebo patients showed variable changes in maximum exercise tolerance over 12 weeks, whereas those taking enalapril exhibited little change, or an improvement ($p < 0.05$, fig. 2). Venous hormone levels were drawn before, during and after treadmill testing. Plasma renin activity, aldosterone, and especially catecholamine levels increased during the initial treadmill exercise test in both groups (fig. 3). Peak levels were achieved at the time of maximum exercise for the catecholamines but occurred later for plasma aldosterone (fig. 3). Placebo patients exhibited almost identical hormone responses at 4 weeks (not shown) and 12 weeks to those observed in the baseline test (fig. 3). The enalapril group showed a 4-fold increase in resting plasma renin activity at 4 weeks, and this was maintained at 12 weeks. Further, the rise in plasma renin activity with exercise was both accentuated and prolonged (fig. 3). In contrast, there was a minor fall in resting plasma aldosterone (487 ± 93 pmol/L at baseline, 348 ± 75 pmol/L at 12 weeks, not significant) and little change in the aldosterone response to exercise (fig. 3). Resting plasma angiotensin II concentrations (data not shown) were not high before randomisation in either the placebo patients (16 ± 3 pg/ml) or the enalapril group (22 ± 3 pg/ml). As with plasma renin activity and aldosterone, there were minor increments with exercise. At 12 weeks, angiotensin II levels were slightly lower in patients taking enalapril than those receiving placebo both at rest and with exercise, the mean difference between the groups being 7 pg/ml (not significant). Baseline catecholamines were slightly lower in enalapril patients both at rest and with exercise (fig. 3). This was generally so also after 12 weeks of treatment.

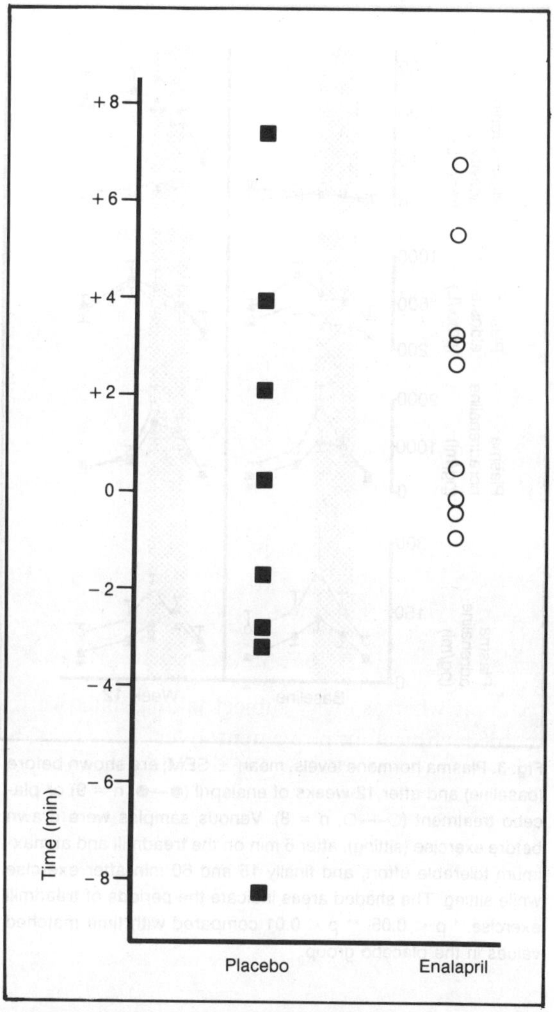

Fig. 2. Change in treadmill exercise duration over 12 weeks of treatment with enalapril (n = 9) or placebo (n = 8). The change in exercise time for enalapril patients was statistically significant ($p < 0.05$).

Although between-group differences reached statistical significance on 3 occasions (fig. 3), treatment for 12 weeks did not alter plasma catecholamine levels in either the enalapril or the placebo group. Plasma cortisol levels were much the same in the 2 groups at the start of the study (resting levels 494 ± 31 nmol/L placebo group; 450 ± 41 nmol/L enalapril group), and were not altered by 12 weeks

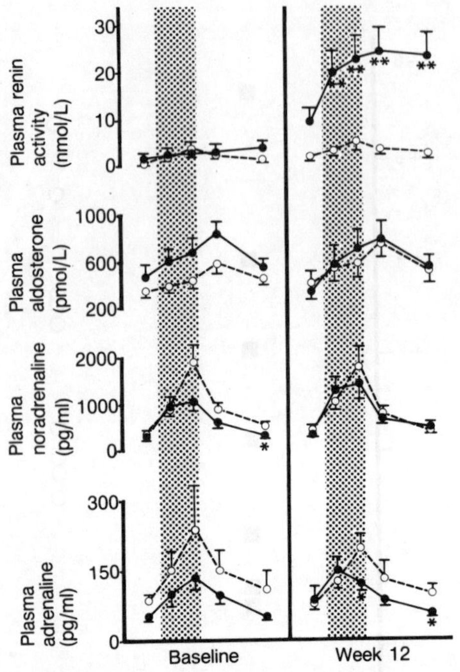

Fig. 3. Plasma hormone levels, mean ± SEM, are shown before (baseline) and after 12 weeks of enalapril (●—●, n = 9) or placebo treatment (○---○, n = 8). Venous samples were drawn before exercise (sitting), after 6 min on the treadmill and at maximum tolerable effort, and finally 15 and 60 min after exercise while sitting. The shaded areas indicate the periods of treadmill exercise. * $p < 0.05$, ** $p < 0.01$ compared with time matched values in the placebo group.

of enalapril or placebo treatment. Exercise induced minor increases in plasma cortisol in both groups.

2.5 Haemodynamics

Haemodynamic results are given in table II. Recordings made 2 hours after insertion of catheter, at rest and with exercise, are shown in fig. 4. Before the first dose of placebo or enalapril, measurements were similar in the 2 groups. After the first dose of enalapril, mean arterial pressure fell from 90.9 ± 7mm Hg to 79.1 ± 5mm Hg at 2 hours ($p < 0.05$) and 86.2 ± 5.1mm Hg at 5 hours (not significant). There was little acute change in cardiac index or right-heart pressures, either at rest or with exercise (table II). Pulmonary artery wedge pressure, pulmonary artery pressure, and right atrial pressures were lower after 12 weeks of enalapril treatment than before therapy, whereas no change was seen in placebo-treated patients (table II, fig. 4). Arterial pressure and cardiac index were altered little in the long term by enalapril (table II), although the exercise-induced rise in cardiac index increased after 12 weeks of enalapril therapy whereas no alteration occurred in placebo patients (fig. 4).

2.6 Adverse Effects

There were no side effects reported by patients taking enalapril. None developed proteinuria or change in the white cell count, platelets or haemoglobin.

3. Discussion

The ACE inhibitors offer a new approach to the treatment of heart failure. They are often successful in combination with a diuretic and digoxin where other vasodilators have failed (Dzau et al., 1980; Fitzpatrick et al., 1983; Maslowski et al., 1981; Wenting et al., 1983). Controlled studies have shown that captopril induces a sustained improvement in exercise tolerance, haemodynamic indices and clinical status (Captopril Multicenter Research Group, 1983; Cowley et al., 1982; Kramer et al., 1983). In the present study we determined the effects of the second ACE inhibitor, enalapril, on clinical status, exercise tolerance, hormones, biochemistry and haemodynamics, in patients with heart failure of moderate severity.

Clinical status, as assessed by a questionnaire, improved in those taking enalapril but not in placebo patients. Likewise, enalapril induced a significant increase in treadmill exercise capacity although individual responses were variable. These changes are similar to those reported in a 3-month placebo-controlled, double-blind study of enalapril in cardiac failure (Sharpe et al., 1984).

Hormone levels were stable throughout the study

Table II. Haemodynamic measurements[a] in patients with heart failure administered placebo (n = 8) or enalapril (n = 9). All values mean ± SEM

	Time (hours)	Placebo				Enalapril			
		week 0		week 12		week 0		week 12	
		rest	exercise	rest	exercise	rest	exercise	rest	exercise
Cardiac index ($L/min/m^2$)	0	2.3 ± 0.2	3.2 ± 0.3	2.4 ± 0.2	3.5 ± 0.3	2.4 ± 0.2	3.2 ± 0.3	2.6 ± 0.2	3.6 ± 0.3
	5	2.6 ± 0.2	3.5 ± 0.3	2.5 ± 0.3	3.7 ± 0.3	2.5 ± 0.2	3.3 ± 0.4	2.7 ± 0.2	3.5 ± 0.3
Mean arterial pressure (mm Hg)	0	88.8 ± 5.3	106.4 ± 10.2	87.6 ± 3.5	101.4 ± 6.0	90.9 ± 7.0	100.4 ± 6.9	87.8 ± 5.7	96.1 ± 6.2
	5	97.7 ± 6.8	110.4 ± 8.9	91.2 ± 5.5^{c}	108.4 ± 5.8	86.2 ± 5.1	97.3 ± 5.3	83.3 ± 4.8	94.9 ± 4.8
Pulmonary artery wedge pressure (mm Hg)	0	26.9 ± 2.0	37.1 ± 2.2	24.5 ± 3.8	31.8 ± 2.2^{c}	22.9 ± 3.2	32.2 ± 3.1	15.2 ± 2.5^{c}	23.1 ± 2.5^{bd}
	5	26.9 ± 2.5	37.1 ± 1.5	25.9 ± 3.3	32.0 ± 3.7	22.4 ± 3.4	34.1 ± 3.4	15.9 ± 3.0^{c}	23.9 ± 3.6^{c}
Mean pulmonary artery pressure (mm Hg)	0	36.6 ± 1.7	51.0 ± 1.9	37.5 ± 4.4	50.5 ± 3.1	33.1 ± 3.8	46.2 ± 4.4	23.2 ± 1.9^{bc}	39.9 ± 3.2^{b}
	5	36.6 ± 2.8	53.4 ± 2.0	35.9 ± 3.4	51.2 ± 5.3	34.1 ± 4.4	51.2 ± 4.9	26.7 ± 3.2	42.8 ± 3.0
Mean right atrial pressure (mm Hg)	0	8.0 ± 1.0	15.9 ± 0.7	10.6 ± 1.7	16.8 ± 1.7	9.9 ± 1.8	15.1 ± 2.5	7.1 ± 1.4^{c}	15.2 ± 4.0
	5	9.4 ± 0.9	16.1 ± 1.1	10.3 ± 1.2	20.1 ± 1.7^{c}	10.6 ± 2.4	16.7 ± 3.4	9.2 ± 1.9	15.9 ± 2.8

a Rest and exercise recordings were made at time 0 (2 hours after catheter insertion) and repeated 5 hours after placebo or enalapril administration. Exercise readings were taken after 3 min of supine bicycle exercise at 70% maximum load.

b $p < 0.05$ comparing time-matched results from placebo versus enalapril patients.

c $p < 0.05$ comparing within-group data between week 0 and week 12.

d $p < 0.01$ comparing within-group data between week 0 and week 12.

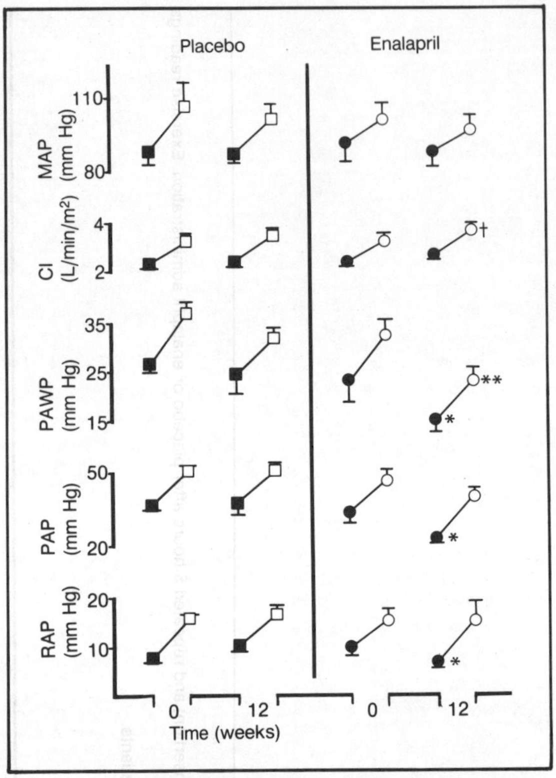

Fig. 4. Haemodynamic recordings (mean ± SEM) taken approximately 2 hours after insertion of arterial and right-heart cannulae before randomisation, and again 12 weeks after treatment with placebo (□, ■) or enalapril (○, ●). Readings were made with the patients supine at rest (●, ■) and after 3 min of supine bicycle exercise at 70% of maximum load (○, □). * $p < 0.05$, ** $p < 0.01$ change within the enalapril group over 12 weeks. † $p < 0.05$ a significant increase in cardiac index over 12 weeks in those on enalapril compared to the placebo group. MAP = mean arterial pressure; CI = cardiac index; PAWP = mean pulmonary artery wedge pressure; PAP = mean pulmonary artery pressure; RAP = mean right atrial pressure.

in the placebo group. Those taking enalapril showed the expected clearcut rise in plasma renin activity at 4 and 12 weeks. They also had slightly lower circulating levels of immunoreactive angiotensin II than placebo subjects. That enalapril might not have blocked angiotensin II formation completely was suggested by the measurable levels of immunoreactive angiotensin II, and the fact that plasma aldosterone concentrations showed a very small decline. Under different circumstances, in patients with hypertension due to renal artery stenosis, Hodsman et al. (1982) noted incomplete inhibition of angiotensin II formation with 1.25 to 5mg enalapril compared to larger doses of the drug. The possibility exists, then, that higher doses of enalapril than used here will block converting enzyme more completely in cardiac failure. Whether this would enhance clinical efficacy is not known.

In our patients taking enalapril, there was no clear fall in circulating noradrenaline levels over 12 weeks, either at rest or with exercise. We (Fitzpatrick et al., 1983) and others (Creager et al., 1981; Dicarlo et al., 1983; Silberbauer et al., 1983; Wenting et al., 1983) have noted a decline in plasma noradrenaline during treatment with ACE inhibitors, but most of these were short term studies in severely ill patients and without a parallel group of untreated subjects. The patients in the present study did not have particularly high baseline levels of catecholamines, and a major fall with enalapril might not necessarily be expected, especially as the decline in plasma angiotensin II was small. We await further studies to clarify the role of the renin-angiotensin system in modulating activity of the sympathetic nervous system in heart failure.

Haemodynamic indices in placebo patients remained stable over 12 weeks. The first dose of enalapril reduced arterial pressure significantly and right-heart pressures declined, but cardiac output was not altered. Invasive recordings at 12 weeks demonstrated a sustained reduction of right-heart pressures with enalapril administration, a small increase in cardiac index, and little change in arterial pressure. A minor but significant rise in left ventricular ejection fraction was observed. These haemodynamic changes are similar to those observed by others in 3-month studies of enalapril in patients with heart failure of similar or greater severity (Kjekshus et al., 1983; Sharpe et al., 1984).

Routine plasma biochemistry testing failed to show definite changes in plasma concentrations of sodium, urea, creatinine, glucose, uric acid or cholesterol in either the placebo or enalapril groups, and liver function tests were stable. Plasma potassium increased slightly but significantly, as has been reported previously with both captopril (Maslowski et al., 1981) and enalapril (Fitzpatrick et al., 1983) in shorter studies. Our study does not clarify the mechanisms behind the rise in potassium, but a contribution from the decline in plasma aldosterone, though minor and not statistically significant, seems possible. The improved clinical well-being may have resulted in an increase in appetite and thence in dietary potassium intake. Whatever the mechanisms, an increase in plasma potassium toward the middle of the normal range is likely to be beneficial for patients such as ours, on digoxin.

No patient developed subjective side effects during 12 weeks of treatment with enalapril.

In summary, we found that enalapril, when added to maintenance frusemide and digoxin therapy, induced improvements in exercise performance, and in clinical and haemodynamic status. There were no adverse clinical or biochemical events and the drug had sustained beneficial effects in moderate heart failure.

Acknowledgements

We are grateful for the assistance of the Dietary and Biochemistry Department, Steroid Laboratory, Special Test Sisters, Endocrine and Cardiology Department technicians and Mrs Natalie Purdue. Financial assistance was from the New Zealand Medical Research Council.

References

Captopril Multicenter Research Group: A placebo-controlled trial of captopril in refractory chronic congestive heart failure. Journal of the American College of Cardiology 2: 755-763 (1983).

Cowley, A.J.; Rowley, J.M.; Stainer, K.L. and Hampton, J.R.: Captopril therapy for heart failure: A placebo controlled study. Lancet 2: 730-732 (1982).

Creager, M.A.; Halperin, J.L.; Bernard, D.B.; Faxon, D.P.; Melidossian, C.D.; Gavras, H. and Ryan, T.J.: Acute regional circulatory and renal hemodynamic effects of converting-enzyme inhibition in patients with congestive heart failure. Circulation 64: 483-489 (1981).

Dicarlo, L.; Chatterjee, K.; Parmley, W.W.; Swedberg, K.; Atherton, B.; Curran, D. and Cucci, M.: Enalapril: A new angiotensin-converting enzyme inhibitor in chronic heart failure; acute and chronic hemodynamic evaluations. Journal of the American College of Cardiology 2: 865-871 (1983).

Dunn, P.J. and Espiner, E.A.: Outpatient screening tests for primary aldosteronism. Australian and New Zealand Journal of Medicine 6: 131-135 (1976).

Dzau, V.J.; Colucci, W.S.; Williams, G.H.; Curfman, G.; Meggs, L. and Hollenberg, N.K.: Sustained effectiveness of converting-enzyme inhibition in patients with severe congestive heart failure. New England Journal of Medicine 302: 1373-1379 (1980).

Feinstein, A.R. and Wells, C.K.: Two new indexes for assessing clinical improvement in angina pectoris. Transactions of the Association of the American Physician 88: 161-167 (1975).

Fitzpatrick, D.; Nicholls, M.G.; Ikram, H. and Espiner, E.A.: Haemodynamic, hormonal, and electrolyte effects of enalapril in heart failure. British Heart Journal 50: 163-169 (1983).

Gibson, T.C.; White, K.L. and Klainer, L.M.: The prevalence of congestive heart failure in two rural communities. Journal of Chronic Diseases 19: 141-152 (1966).

Hodsman, G.P.; Brown, J.J.; Davies, D.L.; Fraser, R.; Lever, A.F.; Morton, J.J.; Murray, G.D. and Robertson, J.I.S.: Converting-enzyme inhibitor enalapril (MK421) in treatment of hypertension with renal artery stenosis. British Medical Journal 285: 1697-1699 (1982).

Kjekshus, J.K.; Soyland, E.; Dickstein, K.; Abrahamsen, A.M. and Gundersen, T.: Sustained haemodynamic effects of enalapril in left ventricular failure. Journal of Hypertension 1 (Suppl. 1): 143-145 (1983).

Kramer, B.L.; Massie, B.M. and Topic, N.: Controlled trial of captopril in chronic heart failure: A rest and exercise hemodynamic study. Circulation 67: 807-816 (1983).

Lun, S.; Espiner, E.A.; Nicholls, M.G. and Yandle, T.G.: A direct radioimmunoassay for aldosterone in plasma. Clinical Chemistry 29: 268-271 (1983).

Maslowski, A.H.; Ikram, H.; Nicholls, M.G. and Espiner, E.A.: Haemodynamic, hormonal, and electrolyte responses to captopril in resistant heart failure. Lancet 1: 71-74 (1981).

McKee, P.A.; Castelli, W.P.; McNamara, P.M. and Kannel, W.B.: The natural history of congestive heart failure: The Framingham Study. New England Journal of Medicine 285: 1441-1446 (1971).

Nicholls, M.G. and Espiner, E.A.: A sensitive, rapid radioimmunoassay for angiotensin II. New Zealand Medical Journal 83: 399-403 (1976).

Nicholls, M.G.; Ikram, H.; Espiner, E.A.; Webster, M.W.I. and Fitzpatrick, M.A.: Enalapril in heart failure. British Journal of Clinical Pharmacology 18: 163S-167S (1984).

Patterson, J.A.; Naughton, J.; Pietras, R.J. and Gunnar, R.M.: Treadmill exercise in assessment of the functional capacity of patients with cardiac disease. American Journal of Cardiology 30: 757-762 (1972).

Peuler, J.D. and Johnson, G.A.: Simultaneous single isotope radioenzymatic assays of plasma norepinephrine, epinephrine and dopamine. Life Sciences 21: 625-636 (1977).

Sharpe, D.N.; Murphy, J.; Coxon, R. and Hannan, S.F.: Enalapril in patients with chronic heart failure: A placebo-controlled, randomized, double-blind study. Circulation 70: 271-278 (1984).

Silberbauer, K.; Punzengruber, C. and Sinzinger, H.: Endogenous prostaglandin E_2 metabolic levels, renin-angiotensin system and catecholamines versus acute hemodynamic response to captopril in chronic congestive heart failure. Cardiology 70: 297-307 (1983).

Stern, M.P.: The recent decline in ischemic heart disease mortality. Annals of Internal Medicine 91: 630-640 (1979).

Wagner, H.N.; Wake, R.; Nickoloff, E. and Natarajan, T.K.: The nuclear stethoscope: A simple device for generation of left ventricular volume curves. American Journal of Cardiology 38: 747-750 (1976).

Wenting, G.J.; Man in't veld, A.J.; Woittiez, A.J.; Boomsma, F.; Laird-Meeter, K.; Simoons, M.L.; Hugenholtz, P.G. and Schalekamp, M.A.D.H.: Effects of captopril in acute and chronic heart failure: Correlations with plasma levels of noradrenaline, renin, and aldosterone. British Heart Journal 49: 65-76 (1983).

Address for correspondence and reprints: Dr *M.G. Nicholls,* Department of Endocrinology, The Princess Margaret Hospital, Christchurch (New Zealand).

Drugs 30 (Suppl. 1): 82-89 (1985)
0012-6667/85/0100-0082/$4.00/0

Enalapril in Hypertension and Congestive Heart Failure

Overall Review of Efficacy and Safety

F. Moncloa, J.A. Sromovsky, J.F. Walker and *R.O. Davies*

Merck Sharp & Dohme Research Laboratories, Rahway

Summary *Multiclinic controlled studies have shown that enalapril alone 10 to 40 mg/day orally is effective in lowering blood pressure in patients with essential hypertension. Enalapril has been compared with thiazides and β-blockers (propranolol, metoprolol and atenolol). The effect on systolic blood pressure has been greater with enalapril than with β-blockers. The proportion of patients who respond to enalapril alone with a decrease in diastolic blood pressure (≥ 10mm Hg) is around 70%. When a thiazide is added to the treatment, the proportion is above 90%.*

Enalapril improves the signs and symptoms associated with congestive heart failure. Patients increased their exercise tolerance by an average of 148 sec and improved in their NYHA cardiac status and prognosis classification.

The overall incidence of side effects is similar to that seen in the placebo control groups. Side effects such as agranulocytosis, taste loss, rash, proteinuria were not characteristic of enalapril. This supports the hypothesis that the improved safety profile of enalapril is the result of being a nonsulphydryl angiotensin-converting enzyme (ACE) inhibitor. The most common side effects reported were dizziness, headache and asthenia. Abnormalities in electrolytes, uric acid, glucose or in lipids have generally not been associated with enalapril.

Enalapril maleate is an angiotensin-converting enzyme (ACE) inhibitor developed by Merck Sharp & Dohme Research Laboratory (Gross et al., 1981; Patchett et al., 1980) that is well absorbed after oral administration. Food has no influence on its absorption. Enalapril is hydrolysed to the active molecule, enalaprilat, predominantly by the liver. There is no further metabolism of the compound, and elimination is primarily by the kidney. Enalapril has a long duration of action with an effective serum half-life of 11 hours (Gomez et al., 1983). The maximum inhibition of the plasma-converting enzyme occurs 2 to 4 hours after administration and substantial inhibition persists for over 24 hours (Given et al., 1984). The consequences of ACE inhibition are a decrease in the serum concentrations of angiotensin II and aldosterone and a simultaneous increase in plasma renin activity (Gavras et al., 1982).

The results of the overall clinical experience with enalapril in the treatment of hypertension and congestive heart failure in relation to efficacy and safety are presented in this review. Studies from a number of clinics have been reported elsewhere (Brunner et al., 1984; Cody et al., 1983; Davies et al., 1984; Enalapril in Hypertension Study Group, 1984; Sharpe et al., 1984; Smith, 1984; Winer and Carter, 1983).

Table I. Antihypertensive effects of enalapril (once- or twice-daily) and placebo in patients with mild hypertension. Blood pressures expressed as mean supine systolic/diastolic (mm Hg)

Treatment week	Daily dose[a]	Enalapril once-daily			Enalapril twice-daily			Placebo		
		no. of patients	baseline	treatment	no. of patients	baseline	treatment	no. of patients	baseline	treatment
4[b]	10	54	142/95	137/89	50	148/95	139/88	50	148/95	150/94
8[b]	20	54	142/95	135/88	50	148/95	139/87	44	148/95	150/93
12[b]	40	52	142/96	135/87	46	147/95	137/87	40	146/95	150/95

a Either mg/24h of enalapril or matching placebo.
b Significant difference ($p < 0.05$) between both enalapril groups (once- and twice-daily) and placebo with regard to mean reductions from baseline.

Table II. Antihypertensive effects of enalapril and hydrochlorothiazide and their combination in patients with essential hypertension. Blood pressures expressed as mean supine systolic/diastolic (mm Hg)

Treatment week	Enalapril (10-40 mg/day)			Hydrochlorothiazide (50-100 mg/day)			Enalapril + hydrochlorothiazide (10-40mg/ 50-100 mg/day)		
	no. of patients	baseline	treatment	no. of patients	baseline	treatment	no. of patients	baseline	treatment
8	176	162/105	146/94	189	160/105	142/94	90	159/104	128/84[a]

a Significant difference ($p < 0.01$) between the combination and each of its components, with regard to mean reductions from baseline. All decreases from baseline were significant ($p < 0.01$).

1. Essential Hypertension

Enalapril treatment has been tested as first-line therapy in several multiclinic controlled studies. The antihypertensive effect of the drug is related to a decrease in peripheral resistance without having important effects on cardiac output, and without reflex tachycardia. Table I shows the antihypertensive effect of enalapril compared to placebo. Its efficacy is similar given once- or twice-daily. The comparison versus hydrochlorothiazide (table II) showed similar efficacy of the 2 drugs, and a complementary effect when they were administered together. Figure 1 summarises the results of 3 multiclinic studies comparing enalapril to propranolol, atenolol and metoprolol. The degree of efficacy was similar to that of β-blockers in terms of diastolic blood pressure; however, enalapril had a consistently greater effect on systolic blood pressure. A possible explanation is that enalapril, in contrast to β-blockers, dilates both large arteries and arterioles (Simon et al., 1984), thereby improving arterial compliance. This may result in a greater effect on systolic blood pressure, which correlates well with arterial compliance (Randall, 1982). Figure 2 combines the results of several multiclinic studies and stratifies the patients according to the severity of hypertension. As would be expected, the patients with more severe hypertension showed a larger decrease in blood pressure than those with milder disease.

The decrease obtained with a 10mg dose is sufficient in most patients with mild hypertension to achieve diastolic blood pressures of ≤ 90mm Hg.

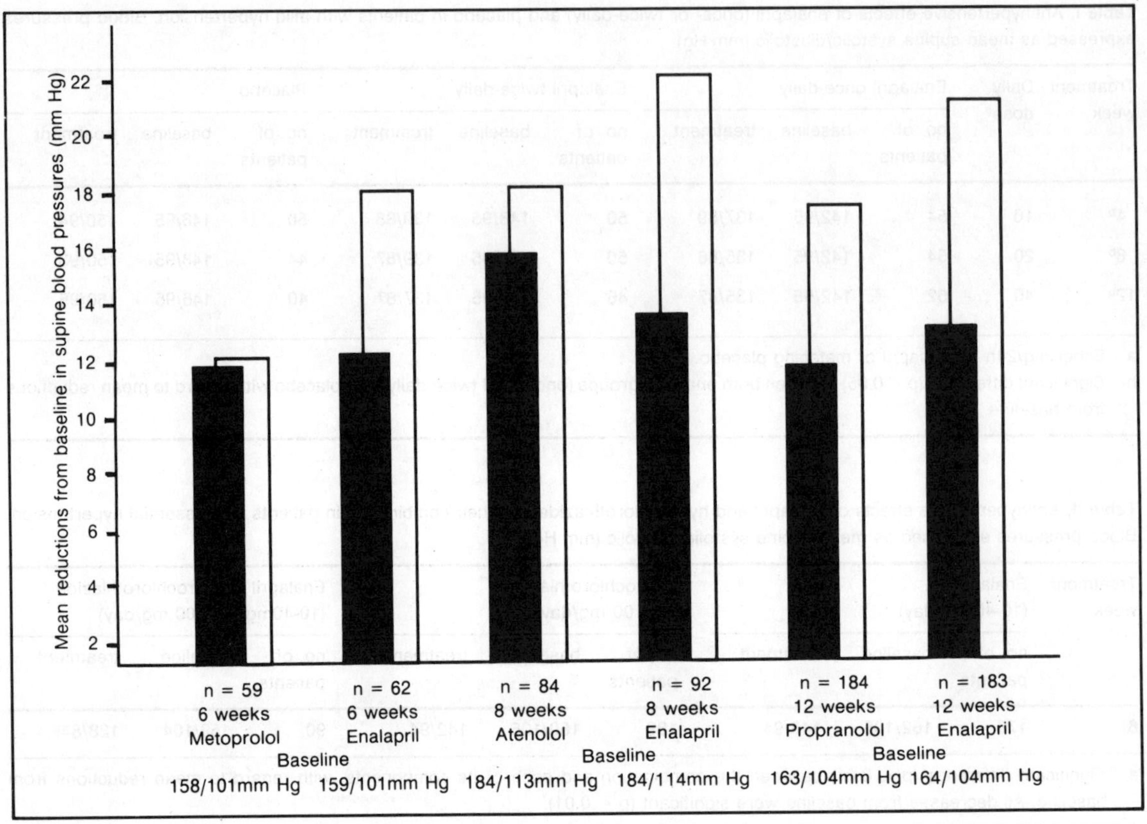

Fig. 1. Enalapril versus β-adrenergic blockade in patients with essential hypertension: Results of three multiclinic studies. ■ = diastolic blood pressure, □ = systolic blood pressure.

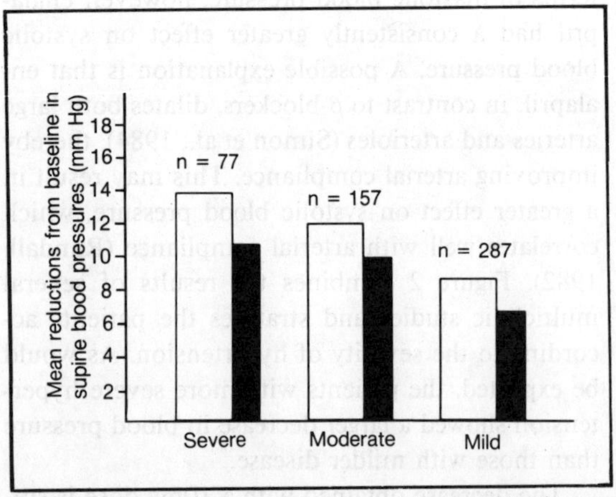

Fig. 2. Decreases in supine systolic and diastolic blood pressures after 2 weeks' treatment with enalapril 10 mg/day. ■ = diastolic blood pressure, □ = systolic blood pressure.

However, in moderate and severe cases, the addition of hydrochlorothiazide is often required (table III).

Approximately 70% of the patients studied experienced a decrease of 10mm Hg or more in diastolic blood pressure. This increased to above 90% of patients with mild to moderate hypertension when hydrochlorothiazide was added. About 20% of the more severe cases required the addition of a third agent to obtain adequate antihypertensive results.

There was no apparent age-related difference in the magnitude of the antihypertensive response to enalapril comparing those older or younger than 65 years (table IV). This contrasts with reports for captopril (Lijnen et al., 1983).

Table III. Proportion of hypertensive patients achieving normotension[a] with enalapril alone or in combination with hydrochlorothiazide

Baseline diastolic blood pressure (mm Hg)	No. of patients	Percentage of patients achieving normotension (%)					
		enalapril (mg/day)			total on enalapril alone[b]	additional effect of hydrochlorothiazide up to 50mg[c]	total
		10	20	40			
90-104	104	38	7	0	45	–	–
95-115	180	20	18	16	54	31	85
110-130	117	5	10	13	28	42	70

a Normotension: in the 90-104mm Hg group the criterion was ⩽ 85mm Hg. In the other groups, the criteria were diastolic ⩽ 90mm Hg and a decrease in diastolic ⩾ 10mm Hg.
b Duration of treatment 12 weeks.
c Duration of treatment 16 to 26 weeks.

Table IV. Antihypertensive effect of enalapril by age category. A 'responder' is defined as a patient with a normal diastolic blood pressure (⩽ 90mm Hg)

Treatment week	Age ⩾ 65 years				Age < 65 years			
	no. of patients	mean supine systolic/diastolic blood pressure (mm Hg)		responders (%)	no. of patients	mean supine systolic/diastolic blood pressure (mm Hg)		responders (%)
		baseline	treatment			baseline	treatment	
4	37	174/106	151/91	57	1197	163/105	146/94	43
12	38	172/106	146/87	68	1041	163/105	136/88	69

2. *Congestive Heart Failure*

Enalapril has been tested in 3 multiclinic studies in patients with congestive heart failure (NYHA class II to IV).

The first study was an open label, invasive haemodynamic study in which patients were treated for 1 to 4 months. The second and third studies were double-blind, placebo-controlled studies. Patients were maintained on their standard treatments of digitalis and diuretics. In addition, these patients received either enalapril or placebo for a 12-week period.

The effects on exercise tolerance and NYHA classifications are presented in tables V and VI. There was a significant improvement in the groups treated with enalapril compared to baseline, as well as compared to the control (placebo) group. There was no difference in the response of older patients (⩾ 65 years) compared to those aged less than 65 years. The most commonly used initial dose was 10 mg/day and the maintenance dose was in the range of 10-40 mg/day.

These results show that enalapril is effective in the treatment of congestive heart failure. Invasive studies indicated that enalapril is a balanced vasodilator acting on both preload and afterload (Gomez et al., 1983). Aldosterone secretion is also reduced, and this presumably contributes to the therapeutic effect. The possible benefits of protecting the heart from the effects of angiotensin II are speculative at present.

Table V. Mean duration of exercise (seconds) in patients with heart failure treated with enalapril or placebo

	Enalapril								Placebo							
	age < 65 years				age ⩾ 65 years				age < 65 years				age ⩾ 65 years			
	no.	pre	post	change	no.	pre	post	change	no.	pre	post	change	no.	pre	post	cha
Double-blind studies																
12 weeks																
Bicycle	20	546	715	169^{b,e}	6	549	657	108	18	638	667	29	5	446	454	8
Treadmill	57	606	703	97^{e}	11	677^{a}	917	239^{b,c,e}	51	590	671	81^{e}	14	519	509	−10
Combined	77	590	706	116^{a,e}	17	632^{a}	825	193^{b,e}	69	602	670	68^{e}	19	500^{c}	494	−6
Open study																
4-16 weeks																
Bicycle	14	393	525	132^{e}	5	236	470	234								
Treadmill	13	641	739	98	4	288	523	235								
Combined	27	512	628	116^{e}	9	259	494	234^{d}								

a Significant difference between treatments within the same age group, $p < 0.05$.
b Significant difference between treatments within the same age group, $p < 0.01$.
c Significant difference between age groups within the same treatment, $p < 0.05$.
d Significant within group change, $p < 0.05$.
e Significant within group change, $p < 0.01$.

Table VI. Change in functional class NYHA status and prognosis in patients with heart failure treated with enalapril or placebo

Variable	Week	Enalapril				Placebo			
		age < 65 years		age ⩾ 65 years		age < 65 years		age ⩾ 65 years	
		no. of patients	improved (%)^{a}	no. of patients	improved (%)^{a}	no. of patients	improved (%)^{a}	no. of patients	impro (%)^{a}
Prognosis (double-blind studies)	12	82	26^{d}	18	28	68	13	21	10
Status (double-blind studies)	12	82	45^{c,e}	18	50^{b,d}	68	18	21	14
Status (open study)	4-16	22	68^{c}	10	70^{b}				

a Improved means by at least one category.
b Significant improvement within the indicated group, $p < 0.05$.
c Significant improvement within the indicated group, $p < 0.01$.
d Significant difference between treatments within the same age group, $p < 0.05$.
e Significant difference between treatments within the same age group, $p < 0.01$.

Table VII. Adverse experiences with enalapril, placebo, and other treatments in controlled studies. Incidence expressed as percentage of patients evaluated

Category of patients	Enalapril				Placebo				Other treatments			
	no.	incidence	discontinued	serious	no.	incidence	discontinued	serious	no.	incidence	discontinued	serious
Mild hypertension	113	38.9	1.8	0	56	46.4	3.6	0				
Mild to moderate hypertension	751	33.0	5.3	4.4					430	29.3	5.1	1.9
Moderate to severe hypertension	272	37.8	3.7	0.7					271	39.1	8.1	4.8
Renovascular hypertension	14	14.3	0	0					15	20.0	0	0
Congestive heart failure	243	31.7	2.5	8.2	178	36.5	9.6	11.8				

3. Safety

The overall incidence of adverse reactions is presented in table VII. It should be noted that this table includes all adverse reactions reported, whether considered to be drug-related or not by the investigator. It also shows the proportion of patients who had to discontinue treatment because of side effects.

Special consideration was given to the analysis of rash, taste disturbances, proteinuria, leucopenia and changes in serum creatinine. In terms of clinical side effects we may consider the following categories: those related to the antihypertensive effect; those related to ACE inhibition; and toxic effects of the compound unrelated to its mechanism of action.

Enalapril had pharmacological side effects related to its antihypertensive action. Dizziness was reported by 6% of the patients with hypertension. Hypotension and/or orthostatic hypotension was seen in about 2%. A hypotensive effect from the first dose of captopril seems to be relatively frequent (Hodsman et al., 1983a; Whiteworth et al., 1982); however, first dose hypotension seems to be less common with enalapril (Davies et al., 1984) probably because of its slower onset of action. Enalapril is also effective in patients with renovascular hypertension (Hodsman et al., 1983b). However, precautions should be taken in these patients, especially in those with bilateral renal artery stenosis, since there is the possibility of an acute deterioration of renal function in that subgroup which has a so-called 'angiotensin II dependent' kidney.

Side effects such as rash, ageusia, proteinuria and severe leucopenia/neutropenia, which theoretically could be due either to ACE inhibition or to the chemical structure, have not been characteristic of enalapril, a non-sulphydryl ACE inhibitor. Differences in the reported incidence of rash and taste alteration are 4- to 8-fold more with captopril, even with low doses. In relation to proteinuria, severe leucopenia and neutropenia, Stumpe et al. (1984) have claimed that low doses of captopril are as safe as enalapril. However, a more careful review shows this not to be the case. The definitions of proteinuria and leucopenia in the reports on captopril have required that abnormal values be seen on more than

Table VIII. Incidence of rash, taste disturbance, severe leucopenia and proteinuria[a] in patients administered captopril (Frohlich et al., 1984) or enalapril

	Captopril (%) [no. evaluated]	Enalapril (%) [no. evaluated]
Rash	(5-10) [C5000]	(1.2) [2249]
Taste disturbance	(4-7) [C5000]	(0.5) [2249]
Neutropenia		
Normal renal function	(0.2) [4544]	(Nil) [C6000]
Previous renal impairment	(0.5) [997]	(Nil) [143]
Concomitant collagen disease	(4.7) [172]	(Nil) [30]
Proteinuria		
No prior renal disease (hypertensive patients)	(0.2-1.0) [3573]	(Nil) [2164]
Prior renal impairment	(1.0-3.5) [2196]	(Nil) [143]

a The definitions of leucopenia and proteinuria are those of Frohlich et al. (1984). The percentage range indicates low and high doses of captopril.

one occasion before the observation is considered to be valid (Frohlich et al., 1984). If the same criteria are applied to our data on patients with hypertension, neither proteinuria nor leucopenia has been seen with enalapril (table VIII).

At present, precautions should be taken in the presence of renovascular hypertension and renal insufficiency. To date, there are no studies available on the effects of enalapril in pregnant women, nursing mothers or children.

A number of increases in creatinine and/or BUN have been reported which may require an adjustment of dosage either of enalapril or of the concomitant diuretic. In terms of biochemical side effects, enalapril is usually not associated with disturbances in water balance or alterations of serum electrolytes, glucose, lipids or uric acid. On the contrary, enalapril has been reported to minimise the biochemical side effects of thiazides, especially hypokalaemia and hyperuricaemia (Gomez et al., 1984).

4. Implications for the Clinical Use of Enalapril

Enalapril is indicated in essential hypertension with a dosage range of 10 to 40 mg/day. There is no apparent age-related difference in the response to enalapril.

Enalapril demonstrates a consistently greater effect on systolic blood pressure than β-blockers. It appears that enalapril improves arterial compliance by dilation of the large arteries and arterioles.

Enalapril is effective in the treatment of congestive heart failure in a dosage range of 10 to 40 mg/day. There was significant improvement in exercise tolerance in the group treated with enalapril compared to baseline as well as the placebo group.

The overall incidence of side effects with enalapril is similar to that experienced in placebo control groups. The side effects are related primarily to its antihypertensive effect. Precaution is recommended in patients with renal impairment. There have been no studies to date in pregnant women, children or in nursing mothers.

Side effects reported for ACE inhibitors with the sulphydryl radical such as rash, ageusia, proteinuria and severe leucopenia, have not been characteristic of enalapril. Enalapril has been reported to minimise the biochemical side effects of thiazide therapy, especially hypokalaemia and hyperuricaemia.

References

Brunner, H.R.; Biollaz, J.; Waeber, B.; Nussberger, J. and Turini, G.A.: Experience with enalapril in normotensive volunteers and in patients with hypertension and congestive heart failure; in Doyle and Bearn (Eds) Hypertension and the Angiotensin System: Therapeutic Approaches, pp. 193-207 (Raven Press, New York 1984).

Cody, R.J.; Covit, A.S.; Schaer, G.L. and Laragh, J.H.: Evaluation of a long-acting converting enzyme inhibitor (enalapril) for the treatment of chronic congestive heart failure. Journal of the American College of Cardiology 1: 1154-1159 (1983).

Davies, R.O.; Irvin, J.D.; Kramsch, D.K.; Walker, J.F. and Moncloa, F.: Enalapril worldwide experience. American Journal of Medicine 77 (No. 2A): 23-25 (1984).

Enalapril in Hypertension Study Group (UK): Enalapril in essential hypertension: A comparative study with propranolol. British Journal of Clinical Pharmacology 18: 51-56 (1984).

Frohlich, E.D.; Cooper, R.A. and Lewis, E.J.: Review of the overall experience of captopril in hypertension. Archives of Internal Medicine 144: 1441-1444 (1984).

Gavras, H.; Biollaz, J.; Walker, B.; Brunner, H.R.; Gavras, I. and Davies, R.O.: Effects of the new oral angiotensin converting enzyme inhibitor MK-421 in human hypertension. Clinical and Experimental Hypertension – Theory and Practice A4: 303-314 (1982).

Given, B.D.; Taylor, T.; Hollenberg, N.K. and Williams, G.: Duration of action and short-term hormonal responses to enalapril (MK-421) in normal subjects. Journal of Cardiovascular Pharmacology 6: 436-441 (1984).

Gomez, H.J.; Cirillo, V.J. and Jones, K.H.: The clinical pharmacology of enalapril. Journal of Hypertension 1 (Suppl. 1): 65-70 (1983).

Gomez, H.J.; Walker, J.F.; Moncloa, F.; Cirillo, V.J.; Sromovsky, J.A. and Gabriel, M.: Enalapril attenuates hydrochlorothiazide-induced hypokalemia, hyperglycemia, hyperuricemia and hypercholesterolemia; in Puschett (Ed.) Diuretics. Chemistry, Pharmacology and Clinical Applications. Proceedings of the First International Conference on Diuretics, pp.263-265 (Elsevier Scientific Publishing Company, Amsterdam 1984).

Gross, D.M.; Sweet, C.S.; Ulm, E.H.; Backlund, E.P.; Morris, A.A.; Weitz, D.; Bohn, D.L.; Wenger, H.C.; Vassil, T.C. and Stone, C.A.: Effect of N-[(s)-1-carboxy-3-phenylpropyl]-L-Ala-L-Pro and its ethyl-ester (MK-421) on angiotensin I pressor responses in vivo. Journal of Pharmacology and Experimental Therapeutics 216: 552-557 (1981).

Hodsman, G.P.; Isles, C.G.; Murray, G.D.; Usherwood, T.P.; Webb, D.J. and Robertson, J.I.S.: Factors related to first dose hypotensive effect of captopril: Prediction and treatment. British Medical Journal 286: 832-834 (1983a).

Hodsman, G.P.; Brown, J.J.; Cumming, A.M.M.; Davies, D.L.; East, B.W.; Lever, A.F.; Morton, J.J.; Murray, G.D. and Robertson, J.I.S.: Enalapril (MK-421) in the treatment of hypertension with renal artery stenosis. Journal of Hypertension 1 (Suppl. 1): 109-117 (1983b).

Lijnen, P.; Fagard, R.; Groeseneken, D.; M'Buyamba, J.R.; Staessen, J. and Amery, A.: The hypotensive effect of captopril in hypertensive patients is age-related. Methods and Findings in Experimental and Clinical Pharmacology 5: 655-660 (1983).

Patchett, A.; Harris, E.; Tristram, E.; Wyvratt, M.; Wu, M.T.; Taub, D.; Peterson, E.; Ikeler, T.; Ten Broeke, J.; Payne, L.; Ondeyka, D.; Thorsett, E.; Greenlee, W.; Lohr, N.; Hoffsommer, R.; Joshua, H.; Ruyle, W.; Rothrock, J.; Aster, S.; Robinson, R.M.; Sweet, C.S.; Ulm, E.H.; Gross, D.M.; Vassil, T.C. and Stone, C.A.: A new class of angiotensin converting enzyme inhibitors. Nature (London) 288: 280-283 (1980).

Randall, O.S.: Effect of arterial compliance on systolic blood pressure and cardiac function. Clinical and Experimental Hypertension - Theory and Practice A4: 1045-1057 (1982).

Sharpe, D.N.; Murphy, J.; Coxon, R. and Hannan, S.F.: Enalapril in patients with chronic heart failure: A placebo-controlled, randomized, double-blind study. Circulation 70: 271-278 (1984).

Simon, A. Ch.; Levenson, J.A.; Bouthier, J.D.; Benetos, A.; Achimastos, A.; Fouchard, M.; Maarek, B.G. and Safar, M.E.: Comparison of oral MK-421 and propranolol in mild to moderate essential hypertension and their effects on arterial and venous vessels of the forearm. American Journal of Cardiology 53: 781-785 (1984).

Smith, W. McF.: Long-term clinical experience with enalapril; in Doyle and Bearn (Eds) Hypertension and the Angiotensin System: Therapeutic Approaches, pp.261-279 (Raven Press, New York 1984).

Stumpe, K.O.; Kolloch, R. and Overlack, A.: Captopril and enalapril: Evaluation of therapeutic efficacy and safety. Practical Cardiology 10: No. 7, pp.111-124 (1984).

Whiteworth, J.A.; Walter, N.M.A.; Kincaid-Smith, P.: First dose effect of captopril. Australian and New Zealand Journal of Medicine 12: 325-326 (1982).

Winer, N. and Carter, C.H.: Effect of enalapril (MK-421) and metoprolol (MTP) on blood pressure, converting enzyme, renin, and catecholamines. Clinical Pharmacology and Therapeutics 33: 232 (1983).

Address for correspondence and reprints: Dr *F. Moncloa,* Merck & Co. Inc., P.O. Box 2000, Rahway, NJ 07065-0914 (USA).

Drugs 30 (Suppl. 1): 90-93 (1985)
0012-6667/85/0100-0090/$2.00/0

General Discussion

Moderator: *M.G. Nicholls*

1. Enalapril: Pharmacodynamic Findings and Therapeutic Efficacy in Hypertension and Heart Failure

Dr *C. Piovano:* Dr Moledo, did you measure potassium levels and potassium balance in your study of patients with essential hypertension?

Dr *L.I. Moledo:* There was a minor nonsignificant rise in plasma potassium. We did not undertake potassium balance studies.

Anon: To my knowledge there are no data that support a sustained natriuretic effect with ACE inhibitors. Secondly, results have been published showing that enalapril enhances free water clearance, and it is believed that this mechanism is mediated perhaps through the fall in angiotensin II.

Dr *Moledo:* With respect to the natriuretic effect of the ACE inhibitors, it would be impossible to have a continuing negative sodium balance. With diuretics, after 5 days or so of treatment, the negative balance ceases. We encountered a marked decrease in exchangeable sodium after 16 weeks of enalapril therapy, and we believe that this was governed by a natriuretic effect that lasted for no more than 5 or 6 days.

Dr *Sánchez:* I am interested to know the age of the patients in the study conducted by Drs Reams and Bauer. Secondly, one way of evaluating the participation of the renin-angiotensin system in renovascular hypertension is by measuring the blood pressure response to surgical correction or balloon dilatation. Did Drs Reams and Bauer have such information in their patients with renovascular hypertension?

Dr *Bauer:* With respect to age, our patients were between 40 and about 65 years, with a mean age of about 50 years. Most of our patients had atherosclerotic disease. Secondly, I agree that there is a place for surgical revascularisation and percutaneous transluminal angioplasty. We frequently perform these procedures in our hospital. However, it was the intent of this study to determine the renal haemodynamic effect of these drugs. Some of these patients did undergo angioplasty after completion of the protocol. Some, because they were totally free from side effects on the enalapril-hydrochlorothiazide regime, chose not to undergo the uncertainty of revascularisation surgery. Finally, there was a category of patient who had diffuse vascular disease that placed them at high risk for surgery, or who had a proximal stenotic lesion which makes transluminal angioplasty less likely to be successful. In these patients we felt that stabilised renal function, an asymptomatic state, and excellent control of blood pressure warranted continuation of medical therapy.

Dr *Ayers:* The response of renal function obtained in renovascular hypertension is dependent upon the state of sodium balance. The relationship between angiotensin II, blood pressure, and sodium seems to have been forgotten in recent literature, but is very important. I would like to ask, what was the state of sodium balance in the patients studied by Drs Reams and Bauer? Finally, I am not sure if I have ever seen exactly balanced renal artery stenosis, and I am curious if these investigators have noted this abnormality with any frequency?

Dr *Bauer:* Our patients were all studied on an outpatient basis and were advised to follow a no-added-salt diet. Time constraints prevent me from showing results on sodium. The bottom line is that these patients were consuming somewhere between 4 and 6g sodium daily as monitored by 24-hour urinary sodium excretion, and that their urinary sodium excretion did not vary statistically throughout the study. I firmly agree with you that if we had severely salt-restricted these people, or alternatively salt-expanded them, we might have got very different results.

Regarding balanced renal artery stenosis, we find that bilateral severe renovascular disease, as depicted in that last radiograph I showed, is very unusual. It does occur, and I think in those patients there may be an adverse response to ACE inhibitors, whether captopril or enalapril. I think that we need to respect the ACE inhibitors, but not fear their appropriate application in renovascular disease and hypertension.

Dr *Gomez:* Dr Bauer, I understand that you also have experience with enalapril in essential hypertension. We would be interested in knowing what happens in patients with essential hypertension who have low glomerular filtration rates.

Dr *Bauer:* We have published the results of patients that have low glomerular filtration rates (inulin clearances below 80), and it has been shown that on average, in patients on enalapril monotherapy, the glomerular filtration rate increases from a mean of about 60 to a mean of about 90 ml/min. Comparable changes are seen in PAH clearance.

Anon: I would like to hear your comments on the very high incidence of side effects in the multicentre efficacy study in patients with heart failure, both in the placebo group and in the group treated with enalapril.

Dr *Nicholls:* Many patients were quite unwell, some being in NYHA Functional Class IV. I think it is inherent in a study such as this that one is going to see problems perceived by such unwell patients. In addition, the patients were encouraged to report all adverse experiences, whether or not they might relate to drug therapy.

Dr *E. Daysi:* Is there any work on enalapril in children?

Dr *Nicholls:* I am not aware of any studies whatsoever. There have been anecdotal reports of captopril in congestive heart failure in children, with good results, but I am not aware of anything as yet with enalapril.

Dr *Messerli:* Dr Nicholls, I find the data of your group on ventricular irritability in patients with heart failure very provocative. There is no doubt that you improve the haemodynamic situation, but could it be that enalapril has a direct electrophysiological stabilising effect on the myocardium, or what is your own feeling?

Dr *Nicholls:* I really would be guessing. Even though we found no statistical relationship between potassium change and ectopic frequency, I still have the feeling that potassium may be important, perhaps in combination with magnesium and other electrolytes.

Dr *A. Guimpel:* In the study of patients with hypertension or congestive heart failure were impotence or other sexual disorders encountered during treatment with enalapril?

Dr *Moncloa:* We have not undertaken any studies with specific attention to impotence, but sexual problems have not been reported.

Dr *A. Souza:* Dr Moncloa, are any studies being undertaken on measurements of magnesium levels? Might enalapril be magnesium-sparing and therefore reduce ventricular irritability?

Dr *Moncloa:* I do not believe that there have been studies of magnesium.

Dr *E.S. Navarro:* Have any studies have been undertaken on the administration of enalapril to pregnant women?

Dr *Moncloa:* We know of only 2 pregnant women who received enalapril. In the first case, the doctor substituted captopril for enalapril, and a normal baby was delivered. In the second case, enalapril therapy was withdrawn during the pregnancy, and the outcome is awaited. In animals, enalapril has not induced genetic damage, but it is fetotoxic if given in the second half of pregnancy in the rabbit. Because of this, our position is that enalapril should not be used in pregnant women, unless the possible benefits should outweigh the risks.

Dr *E. Paolasso:* Dr Moncloa, in patients with advanced heart failure, hyponatraemia is quite common. It was recently reported that captopril combined with frusemide corrected the hyponatraemia. Have you any experience with enalapril in this respect and, if so, what would be the mechanisms involved?

Dr *Moncloa:* No. Dr Nicholls, do you have such results?

Dr *Nicholls:* We have not set out to study this problem, but it is well reported that the hyponatraemic patient given an ACE inhibitor will often normalise the plasma sodium concentration. This might be due to a fall in circulating antidiuretic hormone, a lessening of thirst, and withdrawal of water-retaining actions of angiotensin II on the kidneys. These effects would result in a decreased water intake, and water excretion slightly in excess of sodium excretion.

Dr *R. Shubber:* Are there drug interactions which complicate treatment with enalapril?

Dr *Gomez:* We have studied kinetic interactions with diuretics of the frusemide type and of the hydrochlorothiazide type. The results are completely negative. Digoxin has been studied, also with negative results. With analgesics, antipyretics and anti-inflammatory drugs, the results have been negative, as with anticoagulants. In summary, the sole positive kinetic interaction has been found with propranolol. When enalapril and propranolol are administered concomitantly, serum enalapril concentrations are slightly reduced. However, this reduction appears to have no clinical relevance.

Dr *A. Agnus:* The Framingham study highlighted the problem of systolic hypertension as a risk factor, yet there seems no successful treatment for systolic hypertension. I have heard it said here that enalapril modifies arterial compliance. Has any study been carried out in a large number of patients with enalapril in systolic hypertension?

Dr *Moncloa:* In pure systolic hypertension with normal diastolic values, the answer is no.

Dr *Messerli:* Dr Moncloa, since ACE inhibitors have the potential to raise serum potassium, especially in patients with impaired kidney function, it would seem to me that the concomitant use of potassium-sparing agents should be avoided. Do you have any comment?

Dr *Moncloa:* There is rarely a need to combine enalapril with a potassium-sparing diuretic. For patients with normal renal function, the combination seems to cause no problem. In those with renal impairment, however, the combination is best avoided.

Anon: Is it necessary to alter the dose of enalapril in the presence of liver failure?

Dr *Moncloa:* A study in patients with liver failure has recently been started. What we can anticipate is that the dose of enalapril will probably have to be adjusted. In patients with heart failure many of whom have compromised liver function, the hydrolysis of enalapril to enalaprilat is somewhat diminished during the first few days, but with the passage of time, the conversion is identical to that in patients with normal liver function. In studies undertaken in Australia by Professor C.I. Johnston when livers from cadavers of patients who had liver failure in life were incubated, the hydrolysis to enalaprilat was, as expected, reduced.

Dr *S. Luguini:* Does enalapril alter the frequency of angina pectoris?

Dr *Moncloa:* In the multicentre heart failure study, the frequency of chest pain decreased in the enalapril group compared with the placebo group, but without statistical significance. To extrapolate from this, however, that there is a specific antianginal effect, is debatable. Studies in angina are now in progress.

Dr *R.A. Pinto:* Is there any advantage in combining spironolactone with enalapril in patients with refractory heart failure?

Dr *Moncloa:* As I see it, the use of any potassium-sparing agent would only be justified if the patient had a low potassium level. Dr Nicholls, would you like to comment?

Dr *Nicholls:* We have added spironolactone when the combination of frusemide and an ACE inhibitor (with or without digoxin) has failed to mobilise oedema fluid in cardiac failure. Such a combination can induce a diuresis in our experience, but azotaemia and hyperkalaemia tends to occur when the diuretic response is past its peak. Such patients often have impaired renal function to begin with, and they represent the most resistant form of heart failure. We have not used triamterene or amiloride.

Dr *Gomez:* I would like to comment on the use of spironolactone and enalapril. We have 8 patients with hypertension, and some with congestive heart failure, who were hypokalaemic despite treatment with enalapril. Spironolactone was added and the hypokalaemia was corrected. There have been no problems on follow-up.

Dr *Ayers:* One has to use potassium-sparing diuretics carefully, but they can be used with ACE inhibitors in hypertensive patients who are also receiving a conventional thiazide or loop diuretic, but the patients do need to be monitored carefully.

Dr *J.A. Salvador:* I understand that the vasodilatation obtained with captopril is very variable depending on the area being considered. A marked reduction of hepatic flow has been reported with captopril. I would like to know if there are any data of this type for enalapril, and whether such an effect might contraindicate the use of the drug in patients with liver failure?

Dr *Moncloa:* For patients with liver failure we are at present unable to give a specific recommendation on the use of enalapril. With regard to the effect on hepatic blood flow, we have no information.

Drugs 30 (Suppl. 1): 94-96 (1985)
0012-6667/85/0100-0094/$1.50/0

Summary

M.G. Nicholls

Endocrinology and Cardiology Departments, The Princess Margaret Hospital, Christchurch

Angiotensin-converting enzyme (ACE) inhibitors have clarified the role of the renin-angiotensin system in some physiological circumstances and in a number of clinical disorders. More important, they are a major advance in the treatment of hypertension and heart failure.

This conference directed its attention to the renin-angiotensin system, to the hormonal, haemodynamic, renal and electrolyte effects of blocking this system, and to the use of ACE inhibitors in patients with hypertension and cardiac failure. The emphasis was on the second oral ACE inhibitor, enalapril. Papers were presented by authors from different countries, and data from multicentre studies were shown. The resulting articles, published here, require little discussion from me. Rather, I will give a personal perspective on the ACE inhibitors, and especially on their place in clinical medicine.

Regarding the mechanisms of action of ACE inhibitors, most workers accept that the decline in angiotensin II in plasma (and perhaps in some tissues and organs) is central to the changes in arterial pressure, myocardial and renal function, and regional blood flow in patients with heart failure or hypertension. The decline in circulating aldosterone, which is secondary to withdrawal of angiotensin II, probably contributes to the tendency for loss of body sodium and retention of body potassium. Less clear is the role played by other factors such as bradykinin, vasoactive prostaglandins and the sympathetic nervous system. This uncertainty reflects, to a large extent, limitations of measurement technique. For example, the level of sympathetic stimulation to an organ before and after blockade of angiotensin II formation can be recorded in experimental animals, but in man we tend to rely on changes in plasma catecholamines which give, at best, a crude estimate of 'global' sympathetic tone.

As emphasised for enalapril in this conference, ACE inhibitors given alone for essential hypertension have a useful hypotensive effect which seems slightly greater than that with β-blockers, especially for systolic readings. Because of its sustained inhibition of ACE, enalapril can be taken as a single daily dose. Its antihypertensive action is maintained during long term treatment, and there is no sudden rebound hypertension if the drug is stopped. The tendency towards a minor loss of body sodium and retention of potassium should be advantageous. In combination with thiazide diuretics, the antihypertensive effect of ACE inhibitors is amplified. Further, ACE inhibitors lessen diuretic-induced hypokalaemia and hyperuricaemia.

In severe grades of heart failure, ACE inhibitors reduce symptoms, and improve haemodynamic functioning and exercise performance. Body potassium content, which is usually low in cardiac failure, increases during treatment with ACE inhibitors. It is possible that the fall in frequency of cardiac arrhythmias, observed during ACE inhibitor therapy by at least 2 groups (Cleland et al., 1984; Webster et al., submitted for publication), relates to this positive cumulative balance of potassium, although other potential explanations exist. A natriuresis is sometimes observed when an ACE inhibitor is started, and a reduction in the maintenance dose of diuretic becomes possible for some patients. On the other hand, clinical and haemodynamic improvement can occur while body sodium content increases in response to the introduction of an ACE inhibitor. What is clear in this complex issue, is that beneficial effects from ACE inhibitors may be seen whether body sodium content is, in the short term, increasing or decreasing.

The ACE inhibitors are a major advance in the treatment of moderate-to-severe heart failure. Although not yet demonstrated, it is likely that they will increase longevity in this common disorder.

Not mentioned in the conference because of time constraints, are the effects of ACE inhibitors on blood flow to the brain and the myocardium. It was shown in experimental animals that captopril administration induced a downward shift in the range of cerebral autoregulation (Barry et al., 1984). A similar phenomenon probably occurs during treatment with ACE inhibitors in severe heart failure, where cerebral blood flow is well-maintained even when the arterial pressure reaches levels below the expected range of autoregulation (Paulson et al., 1984; Rajagopalan et al., 1984). Although few studies have been reported, and we lack information on changes in regional flow within the myocardium, it seems that the ACE inhibitors induce little change or a fall in coronary blood flow, which is appropriate to the decline in myocardial oxygen demand (Chatterjee et al., 1982; Faxon et al., 1984; Halperin et al., 1982). These data fit with the clinical impression that symptomatic cerebral and myocardial ischaemia are uncommon in hypertensives and in patients with heart failure, even when the fall in arterial pressure is vigorous.

What of the side effects from treatment with enalapril? An update from experience throughout the world is given in the paper by Dr Moncloa and colleagues. The infrequency of serious adverse effects is pleasing. There are some circumstances, however, where particular caution should be exercised in the use of ACE inhibitors. First, patients with extreme activation of the renin-angiotensin system can develop dangerous hypotension with the first dose of an ACE inhibitor. Patients at risk are those with severe grades of heart failure or hypertension (particularly if diuretic doses are high and if hyponatraemia is present), and patients with renal artery stenosis. Where possible, these particular subjects should be admitted to hospital, the diuretic dose reduced or stopped, the initial dose of ACE inhibitor should be small (captopril 6.25mg or less, enalapril 5mg or less), arterial pressure must be measured regularly after the first dose, and intravenous saline and angiotensin II should be available if severe hypotension occurs. Secondly, until more information is available, the combination of an ACE inhibitor and a potassium-sparing diuretic (spironolactone, amiloride or triamterene) should be reserved for the rare hypertensive patient with persistent hypokalaemia, or patients in heart failure whose oedema is resistant to the usual diuretics-ACE inhibitor regimen. When the drug combination is contemplated it is mandatory to watch for hyperkalaemia and azotaemia. Thirdly, experience with ACE inhibitors during pregnancy is limited. They should, therefore, be avoided until efficacy and safety have been demonstrated. A final note of caution is based on the fact that converting enzyme is present in most organs of the body, yet the role of the renin-angiotensin system, if any, is uncertain. Likewise, we do not know the consequences, if any, of blocking this system in various organs. To date, no worrying, unexpected adverse effects have occurred with enalapril. The same comment, however, was frequently made until very recently, about thiazide-like diuretics, yet there is now a degree of concern regarding their routine use in mild hypertension. All clinicians prescribing ACE inhibitors must be alert to the possibility of unexpected side effects.

What does the future hold for ACE inhibitors? When given in the early phases of experimental heart failure, they prevent or limit the development of severe haemodynamic deterioration (Riegger et al., 1984). There is every reason to determine, with carefully planned studies, whether the same applies to man. If so, the current sequence of prescribing drugs for heart failure (a diuretic or digoxin initially, then an ACE inhibitor) may be reversed. In hypertension, there must be some hope that the ACE inhibitors, through their antihypertensive action, their favourable effect on body potassium and sodium, and possibly through a decline in sympathetic activity and circulating angiotensin II, may prove superior to other medications in preventing the complications of a high blood pressure. Again, careful, long term comparative studies are needed.

References

Barry, D.I.; Paulson, O.B.; Jarden, J.O.; Juhler, M.; Graham, D.I. and Strandgaard, S.: Effects of captopril on cerebral blood flow in normotensive and hypertensive rats. American Journal of Medicine 76 (5B): 79-85 (1984).

Chatterjee, K.; Rouleau, J.-L. and Parmley, W.W.: Haemodynamic and myocardial metabolic effects of captopril in chronic heart failure. British Heart Journal 47: 233-238 (1982).

Cleland, J.G.F.; Dargie, H.J.; Robertson, J.I.S.; Ball, S.G. and Hodsman, G.P.: The use of captopril in the management of cardiac failure. Scottish Medical Journal 29: 129-130 (1984).

Faxon, D.P.; Creager, M.A.; Halperin, J.L.; Bernard, D.B. and Ryan, T.J.: Redistribution of regional blood flow following angiotensin-converting enzyme inhibition. American Journal of Medicine 76 (5B): 104-110 (1984).

Halperin, J.L.; Faxon, D.P.; Creager, M.A.; Bass, T.A.; Melidossian, C.D.; Gavras, H. and Ryan, T.J.: Coronary hemodynamic effects of angiotensin inhibition by captopril and teprotide in patients with congestive heart failure. American Journal of Cardiology 50: 967-972 (1982).

Paulson, O.B.; Jarden, J.O.; Godtfredsen, J. and Vorstrup, S.: Cerebral blood flow in patients with congestive heart failure treated with captopril. American Journal of Medicine 76 (5B): 91-95 (1984).

Rajagopalan, B.; Raine, A.E.G.; Cooper, R. and Ledingham, J.G.G.: Changes in cerebral blood flow in patients with severe congestive cardiac failure before and after captopril treatment. American Journal of Medicine 76 (5B): 86-90 (1984).

Riegger, G.A.J.; Liebau, G.; Holzschuh, M.; Witkowski, D.; Steilner, H. and Kochsiek, K.: Role of the renin-angiotensin system in the development of congestive heart failure in the dog as assessed by chronic converting-enzyme blockade. American Journal of Cardiology 53: 614-618 (1984).

Address for correspondence and reprints: Dr *M.G. Nicholls*, Department of Endocrinology, The Princess Margaret Hospital, Christchurch (New Zealand).